On Moral Medicine

Theological Perspectives in Medical Ethics

Edited by
STEPHEN E. LAMMERS
ALLEN VERHEY

Grand Rapids, Michigan
William B. Eerdmans Publishing Company

255 Jefferson Ave. S.E., Grand Rapids, Mich. 49503

Printed in the United States of America

Reprinted, March 1989

Library of Congress Cataloging-in-Publication Data

On moral medicine.

Includes bibliographies.
1. Medical ethics. 2. Medicine — Religious aspects.
I. Lammers, Stephen. II. Verhey, Allen. [DNLM:
1. Ethics, Medical. 2. Religion and Medicine.
W 50 058]
R724.058 1986 174'.2 86-19656

ISBN 0-8028-3629-1

Contents

Preface

A little over two decades ago Kenneth Boulding first suggested that the twentieth century would witness a "biological revolution" with consequences as dramatic and profound as those of the industrial revolution of the eighteenth century.[1] The years since Boulding made his prophetic remark have seen advances in medical science and technology which have made his words seem almost reserved. Not all of the advances have been as dramatic as "cracking" the genetic code or the birth of a "test-tube baby"; not every advance has been as striking as the implantation of an artificial heart into a human patient or the electrical stimulation of the brain; but each of the advances has contributed to a rapidly expanding human control over the human and natural processes of giving birth and dying, over human genetic potential, and over behavioral performance. With the help of biological and behavioral sciences, human beings are seizing control over human nature and human destiny. That is what makes the biological revolution "revolutionary": the nature now under human dominion is *human* nature. We are the stakes as well as the players.[2]

The new powers have raised new moral questions, and the public discussion of the complex issues raised by developments in medicine has been vigorous (and sometimes rancorous). Although the questions are raised by the developments in science and technology, they are not fundamentally scientific and technological questions. They are inevitably moral and political. Science can tell us a lot of things, but it cannot tell us what ends we ought to seek with the tools it gives us or how to use those tools without morally violating the human material on which they work. Answers to the novel questions posed by new developments in medicine always assume or contain some judgments both about the good to be sought and done and about the justice of certain ways of seeking it.

Thus among reflective people the novel questions posed by developments in medicine lead quickly to some of the oldest questions of all. The new powers have raised new moral problems, but any attempt to deal with them soon confronts fundamental questions about the meaning of life, death, health, freedom, and the person, and about the goals worth striving for and the limits to be imposed on the means to reach them. And these questions inevitably raise the most ancient question of all: What are human beings meant to be and to become? It could hardly be any different, for the nature now under human dominion is human nature.

Public discussion of the novel questions raised by these new powers has seldom candidly raised the ancient and fundamental questions about human nature and human flourishing, however. The public debate has tended to focus instead on two issues: freedom or autonomy and the weighing of risks versus benefits. This is not accidental. Many contemporary moral philosophers have identified the moral point of view with the so-called impartial perspective and have defended either a right to equal freedom or the principle of the greatest good for the greatest number as required by that perspective. Since the Enlightenment the project of philosophical morality has been to identify and justify some impartial and rational principle—some principle which we can and must hold on the basis of reason alone, quite apart from our loyalties and identities, quite apart from our particular histories and communities with their putatively partial visions of human flourishing.[3] The development of bioethics as a discipline, as a branch of applied philosophy, in the last two decades has led many to the task of applying that impartial perspective with its purely rational principles to the concrete and complex quandaries posed by the new developments in medical science and technology. The literature has become increasingly governed by (and limited to) utilitarian and formalist accounts of morality. There remains considerable practical discussion about which impartial principle is the *right* impartial principle, whether respect for autonomy or the greatest good for the greatest number, but the assumption still seems to be that public discourse must be limited and governed by an impartial rational principle. That assumption has affected the anthologies in medical ethics, too.

This anthology starts from different assumptions. It is our conviction that theological reflection on the issues raised by advances in medical research and technology is critically important. It is important, first, of course, for communities of faith with visions of what it means for human beings to flourish, for they want to live in faith, and to live with integrity to the identity they have been given and to which they are called. But it is also important for the broader community, for a genuinely pluralistic society requires the candid expression of different perspectives. Candid attention to the religious dimensions of morality, including medical morality, could prevent the reduction of morality to a set of minimal expectations necessary for pluralism and could remind all participants in the public discourse of broader and more profound questions about what human beings are meant to be and to become.

Classes and programs in medical ethics have sprung up all over the country in response to the new developments in medicine and the public controversy concerning them. Many of the courses are in religious studies departments; many more are in institutions which preserve and nurture a lively sense of the

Christian tradition. It is primarily for such courses that we produced this anthology, but we hope it will be useful as well to a broader audience as a demonstration of the possibility and promise of candidly theological reflection about these issues.

The criteria for selection of articles for inclusion in this anthology have been these: First, the article should articulate a theological perspective; short of that, it must at least be of significant theological interest. Second, the article should be readable and interesting. Third, the articles should be representative of the diversity of theological opinion and approaches. And fourth, the articles should be either recent pieces or "classic" pieces. It was still difficult to decide what to include and what to leave out, and many of the articles listed in the suggestions for further reading in each chapter are worthy of inclusion. Nevertheless, we think we have assembled a collection which can be used in reading and in teaching to become acquainted with and appreciative of the contributions of theological reflection to medical ethics.

To produce an anthology is to be reminded of one's indebtedness to others, not only to the authors of the essays included in the anthology but also to those who have assisted us in preparing it.

We are especially grateful to Robert Burt and Richard Mouw for permission to print previously unpublished essays.

Jon Pott of William B. Eerdmans Publishing Company has been consistently patient with us and ready with his encouragement and help. Many other friends and colleagues have encouraged us in the project and advised us concerning it: Jim Childress, Rich Mouw, Stan Hauerwas, Lisa Cahill, David Cook. A special debt of gratitude is due David H. Smith, the director of the National Endowment for the Humanities seminar in medical ethics at which we met and began to collaborate on this project and a good friend and valued colleague ever since.

Our institutions have been helpful to us not only by providing leaves and sabbaticals and faculty grants, but also by supplying colleagues and support personnel and students. To mention any names means that many more whose help and support deserve acknowledgment are slighted, but we must risk at least mentioning our secretaries, Karen Michmerhuizen at Hope College and Jacqueline Wogotz at Lafayette College. And all teachers know they are indebted to their students for the simple possibility of owning the identity of teacher—and for a good deal more besides. So, thanks are due the students in IDS 454, Medicine and Morals, at Hope College, and in Religion 302, Medical Ethics, at Lafayette, on whom we have tried some of our ideas and some of these articles.

Stephen E. Lammers
Allen Verhey

Notes

1. Kenneth Boulding, *The Meaning of the Twentieth Century* (New York: Harper and Row, 1964), p. 7.
2. Pierre Teilhard de Chardin, *The Phenomenon of Man* (New York: Harper and Row, 1959), p. 229: "We have become aware that, in the great game that is being played, we are the players as well as being the cards and the stakes."
3. Alasdair MacIntyre, *After Virtue* (Notre Dame: University of Notre Dame Press, 1981).

Part I
PERSPECTIVES ON RELIGION AND MEDICINE

Chapter One
RELIGION AND MEDICINE

Introduction

The author of the little piece, "Honor the Physician," which is included in the selections below, was a Jew living in a Hellenistic culture. He faced the problem of solving the discrepancy between how a model of divine activity and a medical model explain and deal with sickness. The Old Testament tradition of the Lord's "healing monopoly"[1] is accepted by the author but modified to acknowledge the place of the physician. Because God is the creator of the world and of the physician, magical remedies have no place, but a person's vision is freed for a natural view of the world, and the empirical medicine of Hellenistic physicians was made available to the community of faith in the diaspora.

That solution, unusual and innovative then, became commonplace. People began, as Walter Rauschenbusch did much closer to our own day, to give thanks to God for medicine and its practitioners and petition God for blessing upon "the white light of science" (see below). Such prayers seem to have been answered, but the white light of science has given an aura to medicine that has prompted the question about the relation between religion and scientific medicine to be raised anew. What do religion and scientific medicine have to do with one another? That question opens up a number of other questions: Should they be kept independent? Should one be subordinated to the other? What contributions does or can one make to the other? The selections here provide some perspective on these questions and ways of answering them.

Roy Branson reminds us in this chapter that the scientific form of medicine has been used to advance the power and the authority of the physician. This has led to the promotion of a religious aura around the doctor. The physician is the one who holds the rational and objective knowledge that may save our lives. Given this understanding of their practice, it is not surprising that some physicians arrogated to themselves the power of life and death. Nor is it surprising that in response others with significant religious commitments have sought to secularize American medicine. Why is this so?

Persons committed to the claim that God alone is the source of life and death are suspicious of any profession that claims the power over life and death. Thus, as Donald Shriver reminds us, we must critique on religious grounds the pretensions of medicine.

But the connections between religion and medicine in the West do not end only in critique of one by the other. For the medical practitioner who has the power of modern medicine at her disposal must still confront questions concerning the point and purpose of our lives and of medical practice as a service to them. All that medical power cannot prevent the eventual death of patients. Further, that power may be used either appropriately or inappropriately. And finally, even with the best of efforts, the practitioner may err. How is the practitioner to understand all of this?

Donald Shriver argues that Western religion makes a contribution to medicine precisely at these points. Medical practitioners are reminded that they are fallible and sinful—especially so when they are pretentious. At the same time, human life is worth caring for, even when it proceeds under the shadow of death. This feature of human life means that physicians must explore with patients the meaning of their life and must care for more than the body. It is the *person* who is the object of care.

But Shriver's claims themselves raise further questions about the caregiver. It seems obvious that the caregiver must be technically competent. But what other characteristics must they possess so that they will continue to care for us when we are very ill, in pain, and unpleasant to be with; in short, what characteristics do they need so that they will not abandon those who need their care?

What is an appropriate vision of life to sustain this person? Are physicians to understand what they do as a ministry, as Rauschenbusch's prayer suggests? Paul Tournier would say yes and emphasize that medicine is not only a ministry to individuals. It is also a ministry to the entire society. Thus physicians and health care personnel fail in their responsibility if they do not raise questions about injustices in the health care system.

Most of us are not and will not be health care givers. But we are all persons who will be patients. The critique of the pretensions of medicine is for us as well. We are the persons who expect miracles of medical science and who blame the physician when the miracle does not occur. Along with the physician we must ask what kind of medicine we want and must learn to critique our unrealistic expectations of medicine. In our era, one response to the priestly aura surrounding the doctor has been an emphasis upon responsibility for one's own health. Thus one ought not turn to the physician for miracles after a lifetime of bad habits.

Even this kind of emphasis has its dangers according to Karl Barth, who questions the cult of the body. As long as we seek to maintain our health as part of our responsibility to fully exercise our potentialities as human beings, care for the body is sensible, according to Barth; but when this care becomes an end in itself, it becomes another form of idolatry. Barth also joins Tournier in making the concern for health more than a concern for an individual's wellbeing. Health is a social issue as well.

All of these problems lead us to a consideration of a further question: "What are the proper limits of medicine?" Do we limit medicine to the organic and chemical, as Barth would have us do? Are we to broaden the scope, and thus the power of medicine, to care for the "whole patient" as Shriver suggests? This issue is an important one in resolving our understanding of healing. Some would limit the physician's healing to the body and thus argue that only scientific knowledge is appropriate or necessary. Others argue that physicians heal *persons* and claim with Roy Branson that more than scientific knowledge is involved.

In summary, there are a number of important questions that we face today that involve the relationship of religion and medicine. Perhaps the question we might ask ourselves is, "What kind of medicine do we want?" This is not a question either for religious people only or for nonreligious people only but a question which has implications for all of us. If we seek a medicine that will work "miracles," then it might not be surprising to find that we have created a medicine that claims for itself the power of life and death.

Note

1. Klaus Seybold and Ulrich B. Mueller, *Sickness and Healing,* trans. Douglas Stott (Nashville: Abingdon, 1981).

Suggestions for Further Reading

Belgum, David, ed. *Religion and Medicine: Essays on Meaning, Values, and Health.* Ames, Iowa: Iowa State University Press, 1967.

Edmunds, Vincent, and Charles G. Scorer, eds. *Ideals in Medicine: A Christian Approach to Medical Practice.* London: Tyndale, 1958.

Fox, Renee C., and Judith W. Swazey. "Medical Morality is not Bioethics—Medical Ethics in China and the United States." *Perspectives in Biology and Medicine* 27 (Spring 1984).

Hauerwas, Stanley. "Salvation and Health: Why Medicine Needs the Church." In *Theology and Bioethics: Exploring the Foundations and Frontiers,* edited by Earl E. Shelp. Dordrecht: D. Reidel, 1985.

Heineken, Martin J. "Medicine and Theology." In *Man, Medicine and Theology.* New York: Board of Social Ministries, Lutheran Church in America, 1967.

Kelly, David F. *The Emergence of Roman Catholic Medical Ethics in North America: An Historical-Methodological-Bibliographical Study.* New York: Edwin Mellen, 1979.

Marty, Martin E., and Kenneth L. Vaux, eds. *Health/Medicine and the Faith Traditions: An Inquiry into Religion and Medicine.* Philadelphia: Fortress, 1982.

Sheils, W. J., ed. *The Church and Healing.* Oxford: Basil Blackwell, 1982.

Shriver, Donald W., Jr., ed. *Medicine and Religion: Strategies of Care.* Pittsburgh: University of Pittsburgh Press, 1980.

White, Dale, ed. *Dialogue in Medicine and Theology.* Nashville: Abingdon, 1968.

1.
For Doctors and Nurses

WALTER RAUSCHENBUSCH

We praise thee, O God, for our friends, the doctors and nurses, who seek the healing of our bodies. We bless thee for their gentleness and patience, for their knowledge and skill. We remember the hours of our suffering when they brought relief, and the days of our fear and anguish at the bedside of our dear ones when they came as ministers of God to save the life thou hadst given. May we reward their fidelity and devotion by our loving gratitude, and do thou uphold them by the satisfaction of work well done.

We rejoice in the tireless daring with which some are now tracking the great slayers of mankind by the white light of science. Grant that under their teaching we may grapple with the sins which have ever dealt death to the race, and that we may so order the life of our communities that none may be doomed to an untimely death for lack of the simple gifts which thou hast given in abundance. Make thou our doctors the prophets and soldiers of thy kingdom, which is the reign of cleanliness and self-restraint and the dominion of health and joyous life.

Strengthen in their whole profession the consciousness that their calling is holy and that they, too, are disciples of the saving Christ. May they never through the pressure of need or ambition surrender the sense of a divine mission and become hirelings who serve only for money. Make them doubly faithful in the service of the poor who need their help most sorely, and may the children of the workingman be as precious to them as the child of the rich. Though they deal with the frail body of man, may they have an abiding sense of the eternal value of the life residing in it, that by the call of faith and hope they may summon to their aid the mysterious spirit of man and the powers of thy all-pervading life.

From Walter Rauschenbusch, *Prayers of the Social Awakening* (New York: The Pilgrim Press, 1909), pp. 77–78. Used by permission.

2.
Honor the Physician

SIRACH 38:1–15

Honor the physician with the honor due him, according to your need of him,
for the Lord created him;
for healing comes from the Most High,
and he will receive a gift from the king.
The skill of the physician lifts up his head,
and in the presence of great men he is admired.
The Lord created medicines from the earth,
and a sensible man will not despise them.
Was not water made sweet with a tree
in order that his power might be known?
And he gave skill to men
that he might be glorified in his marvelous works.
By them he heals and takes away pain;
the pharmacist makes of them a compound.
His works will never be finished;
and from him health is upon the face of the earth.

My son, when you are sick do not be negligent,
but pray to the Lord, and he will heal you.
Give up your faults and direct your hands aright,
and cleanse your heart from all sin.
Offer a sweet-smelling sacrifice, and a memorial portion of fine flour,
and pour oil on your offering, as much as you can afford.
And give the physician his place, for the Lord created him;
let him not leave you, for there is need of him.
There is a time when success lies in the hands of physicians,
for they too will pray to the Lord
that he should grant them success in diagnosis
and in healing, for the sake of preserving life.
He who sins before his Maker,
may he fall into the care of a physician.

3. The Will to Be Healthy

KARL BARTH

Let us now raise the question of respect for life in the human sphere. In its form as the will to live, it will also include the will to be healthy. The satisfaction of the needs of the impulses corresponding to man's vegetative and animal nature is one thing, but health, although connected with it, is quite another. Health means capability, vigour and freedom. It is strength for human life. It is the integration of the organs for the exercise of psycho-physical functions. . . .

If man may and should will to live, then obviously he may and should also will to be healthy and therefore to be in possession of this strength too. But the concept of this volition is problematical for many reasons and requires elucidation. For somehow it seems to be part of the nature of health that he who possesses it is not conscious of it nor preoccupied with it, but hardly ever thinks about it and cannot therefore be in any position to will it. . . .

If this is so, we must ask whether a special will for health is not a symptom of deficient health which can only magnify the deficiency by confirming it. And a further question which might be raised with reference to this will is whether we can reasonably affirm and seek health independently, or otherwise than in connexion with specific material aims and purposes. . . .

Yet included in the will to live there is a will to be healthy which is not affected by these legitimate questions but which, like the will to live, is demanded by God and is to be seriously achieved in obedience to this demand. By health we are not to think merely of a particular physical or psychical something of great value that can be considered and possessed by itself and therefore can and must be the object of special attention, search and effort. Health is the strength to be as man. It serves human existence in the form of the capacity, vitality and freedom to exercise the psychical and physical functions, just as these themselves are only functions of human existence. We can and should will it as this strength when we will not merely to be healthy in body and soul but to be man at all: man and not animal or plant, man and not wood or stone, man and not a thing or the exponent of an idea, man in the satisfaction of his instinctive needs, man in the use of his reason, in loyalty to his individuality, in the knowledge of its limitations, man in his determination for work and knowledge, and above all in his relation to God and his fellow-men in the proffered act of freedom. We can and should will this, and therefore we can and should will to be healthy. For how can we will, understand or desire the strength for all this unless in willing it we put it into operation in the smaller or greater measure in which we have it? And in willing to be man, how can we put it into operation unless we also will and seek and desire it? We gain it as we practise it. We should therefore will to practise it. This is what is demanded of man in this respect.

Though we cannot deny the antithesis between health and sickness when we view the problem in this way, we must understand it in its relativity. Sickness is obviously negative in relation to health. It is partial impotence to exercise those functions. It hinders man in his exercise of them by burdening, hindering, troubling and threatening him, and causing him pain. But sickness as such is not necessarily impotence to be as man. The strength to be this, so long as one is still alive, can also be the strength and therefore the health of the sick person. And if health is the strength for human existence, even those who are seriously ill can will to be healthy without any optimism or illusions regarding their condition. They, too, are commanded, and it is not too much to ask, that so long as they are alive they should will this, i.e., exercise the power which remains to them, in spite of every obstacle. Hence it seems to be a fundamental demand of the ethics of the sick bed that the sick person should not cease to let himself be addressed, and to address himself, in terms of health and the will which it requires rather than sickness, and above all to see to it that he is in an environment of health. From the same standpoint we cannot count on conditions of absolute and total health, and therefore on the existence of men who are already healthy and do not need the command to will to be so. Even healthy people have great need of the will for health, though perhaps not of the doctor. Conditions of relative and subjectively total ease in relation to the psycho-physical functions of life may well exist. But whether the man who can enjoy such ease is healthy, i.e., a man who lives in the power to be as man, is quite another question which we need only ask, and we must immediately answer that in reality he may be severely handicapped in the exercise of this power, and therefore sick, long before this makes itself felt in the deterioration of his organs or their functional disturbance, so that he perhaps stands in greater need of the summons that he should

From Karl Barth, *Church Dogmatics,* III/4, trans. A. T. Mackay et al. (Edinburgh: T&T Clark, 1961), pp. 357-63. Used by permission.

be healthy than someone who already suffers from such deterioration and disturbance and is therefore regarded as sick in soul or body or perhaps both. And who of us has not constantly to win and possess this strength? A fundamental demand of ethics, even for the man who seems to be and to a large extent really is "healthy in body and soul," is thus that he should not try to evade the summons to be healthy in the true sense of the term.

On the same presupposition it will also be understood that in the question of health we must differentiate between soul and body but not on any account separate the two. The healthy man, and also the sick, is both. He is the soul of his body, the rational soul of his vegetative and animal body, the ruling soul of his serving body. But he is one and the same man in both, and not two. Health and sickness in the two do not constitute two divided realms, but are always a single whole. It is always a matter of the man himself, of his greater or lesser strength, and the more or less serious threat and even increasing impotence. It is he who has been predominantly ill and he who may be predominantly well. Or it is he who must perhaps go the opposite way from predominant health to predominant sickness. It is he who is on the way from the one or the other. Hence he does not have a specific healthy or sick life of the soul with particular dominating or subjugated, unresolved or resolved inclinations, complexes, ties, prohibitions and impulses, and then quite apart from this, in health or sickness, in the antithesis, conflict and balance of the two, an organic vegetative and animal life of the body. On the contrary, he lives the healthy or sick life of his soul in his body and with the life of his body, so that in both, and in their mutual relationship, it is a matter of his life's history, his own history. Again, he does not have a specific physical life in the sound or disordered functions of his somatic organs, his nervous system, his blood circulation, digestion, urination and so on, and then in an upper storey a separate life of the soul. But he lives the healthy or sick life of his body together with that of his soul, and again in both cases, and in their mutual relationship, it is a matter of his life's history, his own history, and therefore himself. And the will for health as the strength to be as man is obviously quite simply, and without duplication in a psychical and physical sphere, the will to continue this history in its unity and totality. A man can, of course, orientate himself seriously, but only secondarily, on this or that psychical or physical element of health in contrast to sickness. But primarily he will always orientate himself in this contrast on his own being as man, on his assertion, preservation and renewal (and all this in the form of activity) as a subject. In all his particular decisions and measures, if they are to be meaningful, he must have a primary concern to confirm his power to be as man and to deny the lack of power to be this. In all stages of that history the question to be answered is: "Wilt thou be made whole?" (Jn. 5:6), and not: "Wilt thou have healthy limbs or be free of their sickness?" The command which we must always obey is the command to stand upright and not to fall.

From exactly the same standpoint again there can be no indifference to the concrete problems of getting and remaining well. If in the question of health we were concerned with a specific psychical or physical quantity, we might be interested at a distance in the one or the other, and seek health and satisfaction first in psychology and then in a somatic form of healing, only to tire no less arbitrarily of one or the other or perhaps both, and to let things take their course. But if on both sides it is a matter of the strength to be as man, on both sides we are free from the anxious or fanatical expectation that real decisions can and must be made, but also free to give to the psychical and physical spheres the attention due to them in this respect because they are the field on which the true decisions of the will for health must be worked out. It is precisely in the continuation of his life of soul and body that the history of man must continue in the strength to be as man. What he *can* do for the continuation and therefore against every restriction of his life of soul and body, he ought to *will* to do if he is to be healthy, if he is to live in this strength, and if his history is to proceed in the strength of his being as man. In order that this strength may not degenerate into a process in which he is only driven as an object and is therefore no longer man, in order that he may remain its subject and therefore man, he must be on the watch and active for the continuation and against the constriction of his psychical and physical life. The fact that he wills to rise up and stand in this power, and not to fall into weakness, is not in the least decided by the various measures which he might adopt to maintain and protect his psychical and physical powers. He could adopt a thousand measures of this kind with full zeal and skill, and yet not possess the will to maintain this strength, thus lacking the will for health and falling in spite of all his efforts. But if he possesses the will to win and maintain this strength, it is natural that he should be incidentally concerned to take the necessary precautions to preserve and protect his psychical and physical powers, and this in a responsible and energetic way in which the smallest thing is not too small for him nor the greatest too great.

At this point, therefore, we may legitimately ask,

and must do so in all seriousness, what is good, or not good, or more or less good, for the soul and body. There is a general and above all a particular hygiene of the psychical and physical life concerning the possibilities and limitations of which we must all seek individual clarity by investigation and experience and also by instruction from a third party, and to which we must all keep in questions of what we may or may not do. In such a hygiene God's gifts of sun, air and water will be applied as the most important factors, effective positively in the psychical no less than the physical sphere. Hygiene is the foundation of every prophylactic against possible illness, as it is also the main basis of therapy where illness has already commenced. We have to realise, however, that in all the negative or positive measures which may be taken it is a matter of maintaining, protecting and restoring not merely a strength which is necessary and may be enjoyed in isolation, but the strength even to be at all as man. It is because so much is at stake, because being as man is a history enacted in space and developing in, with and by the exercise of the psychical and physical functions of life, that attention is demanded at this point and definite measures must be incidentally taken by all of us. Sport may also be mentioned in this connexion. But sport has, legitimately, other dimensions, namely, those of play, of the development of physical strength and of competition, so that it may even constitute a threat to health in the true sense of the term as it now concerns us. We shall thus content ourselves with the statement that sport may form a part of hygiene, and therefore ought to do so in specific instances.

The question has often been raised, and will never find a wholly satisfactory answer, whether the measures to be adopted in this whole sphere really demand the consultation of a doctor. The doctor is a man who is distinguished from others by his general knowledge of psychical or physical health or sickness on the basis of tradition, investigation and daily renewed and corrected experience. He is thus in a position to pass an objective verdict on the psychical or physical health or sickness of others. He is capable of assisting them in their necessary efforts to maintain or regain health by his advice or orders or even, if necessary, direct intervention. What objections can there be to consulting a doctor? If we acknowledge the basic fact that we are required to will the strength to be as man, that we are thus required to will psycho-physical forces, and that we are thus commanded to take all possible measures to maintain or preserve this basic power, there seems to be no reason why consultation of a doctor should not find a place among these measures. This is the wise and prudent verdict of Ecclesiasticus in a famous passage (*c.* 38): "For of the Most High cometh healing . . . the Lord has created medicines out of the earth, and he that is wise will not abhor them. . . . And he has given men skill that he might be honoured in his marvellous works. With such doth the physician heal men, and taketh away their pains. Of such doth the apothecary make a confection; and of his works there is no end, and from him is peace over all the earth" (vv. 2 ff.). Therefore, "give place to the physician, for the Lord has created him; let him not go from thee, for thou hast need of him. There is a time when in their hands there is good success. For they shall also pray unto the Lord, that he would prosper that which they give for ease and remedy to prolong life" (vv. 12 ff.).

What do we have against the medical man? Apart from a general and illegitimate passivity in matters of health and sickness, the main point seems to be that there are reasons to suspect the objectivity of the knowledge, diagnosis and therapy of a stranger to whom we are required to give place and confidence at the very heart of our own history, handing over to him far-reaching powers of authority and instruction. The more a man understands the question of health and sickness correctly, i.e., the question of his own strength to be as man and therefore of the continuation of his own life history, the more he will entertain this kind of suspicion in relation to the doctor, not in spite of but just because of his science as general knowledge, and the objectiveness of his verdict, orders and interventions. Is not health or sickness, particularly when it is understood as strength or weakness to be as man, the most subjective thing that there is? What can the stranger with his general science know of this strength or weakness of mine? How can he really help me? How can I surrender myself into his hands?

Yet this form of argument, and the suspicion based upon it, is quite mistaken, and Ecclesiasticus is in the right against it. For it rests on a misunderstanding in which the doctor himself may share through a presumptuous conception of his position, but which may well exist only on the part of the suspicious patient. Health in the true sense of the term as strength to be as man is not to be expected from any of the measures which can be adopted in the sphere of psychical and physical functions as a defence against sickness or for the preservation or restoration of health. There exists, more perhaps in the imagination of others than on the part of experts, or at any rate of genuine and serious experts, a medical and especially in our own day a psychological totalitarianism and imperialism which would have it that the doctor is the one who really heals. In this form, he must truly be warded off as an unpleasant stranger. There is, in fact, an ancient and in itself interesting connexion between medical and priestly craft. But both doctors and others are urgently asked not to think of the medical man as occupying the position and role of a priest. In all these or similar presumptuous forms, he will probably not be able to help even in the sphere and sense in which he might actually do so. It was probably in some such form that he confronted the woman of whom it is written in Mk. 5^{26}: "She had suffered many things of many physicians, and had spent all that she had, and was nothing bettered, but rather grew worse." But in his true form, why should not the doctor be the man who is really able to assist others in his own sphere? And why should he not be looked upon in this way even when he perhaps appears in that perverted form?

In what way can he help? Can he promote the strength to be as man? No, this is something which each can only will, desire and strive for, but not procure nor attain of himself. This is something which even the best doctor can only desire for him. And he will be a better doctor the more consciously he realises his limitations in this respect. For in this way he can draw the attention of others to the fact that the main thing in getting well is something in which neither he nor any human measure can help. If he is a Christian doctor, in certain cases he will explicitly draw attention to this fact. He will then be free to help where he can and should do so, namely, in the sphere of the psychical and physical functions. In relation to these, to their organic, chemical and mechanical presuppositions, to their normal progress and its laws, to their difficulties and degeneracies, to their immediate causes, and to that which can be done in certain circumstances to promote their normal progress and prevent their disturbance, in short, to human life and its health and sickness, there exists more than individual knowledge and opinion. Within the limits of all human knowledge and ability, there are general insights the knowledge of which is based on a history, rich in errors but also in genuine discoveries, of innumerable observations, experiences and experiments, and there are also the general rules to apply this history in the diagnosis and therapy of the individual case. For in this sphere every man, irrespective of his uniqueness before God and among men, is also a specimen, a case among many cases to be classified in the categories of this science, an object to which its rules may be applied. To be sure, each is a new and individual case in which the science and its rules take on a new and specific form. It is the task and business of the doctor to find and apply the new and specific form of the science and its application to the individual case. Hence he is not for any of us an absolute stranger in this sphere. He is a relative newcomer to the extent that each case is necessarily new. But from the standpoint of his science and its practice he is a competent newcomer, and as such he deserves trust rather than suspicion, not an absolute confidence, but a solid relative confidence that in this matter he has better general information than we have, and that for the present we can hopefully submit to his judgment, advice, direction and even intervention in our own particular case. Those who cannot show this confidence ought not to trouble the doctor, nor to be troubled by him. But why should we not show this modest confidence when dealing with a modest doctor?

Ecclesiasticus is quite right to say: "The Lord has created him too." Medical art and science rest like others on a legitimate use of the possibilities given to man. If the history of medicine has been as little free from error, negligence, one-sidedness and exaggeration as any other science, in its main development it has been and still is, to lay eyes at least, as impressive, honourable and promising as, for instance, theology. There is no real reason to ignore its existence or refuse its offer. How can the doctor help? Obviously by giving free play, and removing the obstacles, to the will for real health, i.e., the will to exist forcefully as man, which he cannot give to any of us but to which he may supremely exhort us. Psychical and physical illness is naturally a hindrance to this will. It restricts its development. It constitutes an external damaging of it. The doctor's task is to investigate the particular type and form of illness in any given case, to trace its causes in the heredity, constitution, life history and mode of life of the patient, and to study its secondary conditions and consequences, its course thus far, its present position and threatened progress. If humanly speaking everything depends on that will, is it not a great help to be able to learn with some degree of reliability what is really wrong, or more positively what possibilities of movement and action still remain in spite of the present injury, and within what limits one may still will to be healthy? And these limits might, of course, be extended. The doctor goes on to treat the patient with a view to arresting at least the damage, to weakening its power and effect, perhaps even to tackling its causes and thus removing it altogether, so that the patient is well again at least in the medical sphere. And even if the doctor cannot extend the limits of life available, he can at least make the restrictive ailment tolerable, or at worst, if there is no remedy and the limits become progressively narrower, he can do everything possible to make them relatively bearable. All this may be done by the doctor within the limits of his subjective mastery of his medical science and skill. He cannot do more, but at least he cannot do less. And in this way he can assist the will to live in its form as the will to be healthy. In this respect he can encourage man in the strongest sense of the word, and by removing, arresting or palliating the hampering illness he can give him both the incentive to do what he may still do, i.e., to will to be healthy, and also joy and pleasure in doing it. Having done this to the best of his ability, he should withdraw. He has no power in the crucial issue of the strength or weakness of the patient to be as man. He has no control over the will of the patient in this antithesis. Indeed, he has only a very limited power even over the health or sickness of his organs, of the psychical and physical functions in which that strength and the will for it must express themselves in conflict against the weakness. But if he does his best where he can, we must be grateful to him.

Finally, we have to remember that, when seriously posed, the whole question of measures to be adapted for the protection or recovery of the freedom of vital functions necessarily goes beyond the answers given by each of us individually. The basic question of the power to be as man, and therefore of the will for this power and therefore for real health, and the associated question of its expression and exercise, are questions which are not merely to be raised and answered individually but in concert. They are social questions. Hygiene, sport and medicine arrive too late, and cannot be more than rather feeble palliatives, if such general conditions as wages, standards of living, working hours, necessary breaks, and above all housing are so ordered, or rather disordered, that instead of counteracting they promote and perhaps even cause illness, and therefore the external impairing of the will for life and health. Respect for life in the form in which we now particularly envisage it necessarily includes responsibility for the standard of living conditions generally, and particularly so for those to whom they do not constitute a personal problem because they personally need not suffer or fear any threat from this angle, being able to enjoy at least the possibility of health, and to take measures for its protection or recovery, in view of their income, food, working hours, rest and wider interests. The principle *mens sana in corpore sano* can be a highly short-sighted and brutal one if it is only understood individually and not in the wider sense of *in societate sana.* And this extension cannot only mean that we must see to it that the benefits of hygiene, sport and medicine are made available for all, or at least as many as possible. It must mean that the general living conditions of all, or at least of as many as possible, are to be shaped in such a way that they make not just a negative but a positive preventative contribution to their health, as is the case already in varying degrees with the privileged. The will for health of the individual must therefore take also the form of the will to improve, raise and perhaps radically transform the general living conditions of all men. If there is no other way, it must assume the form of the will for a new and quite different order of society, guaranteeing better living conditions for all. Where some are necessarily ill the others cannot with good conscience will to be well. Nor can they really do it at all if they are not concerned about neighbours who are inevitably sick because of their social position. For sooner or later the fact of this illness will in some way threaten them in spite of the measures which they take to isolate themselves and which may be temporarily and partially successful. When one person is ill, the whole of society is really ill in all its members. In the battle against sickness the final human word cannot be isolation but only fellowship. In this present context the bald assertion must suffice.

4.
The Interrelationships of Religion and Medicine

DONALD W. SHRIVER, JR.

As a start on the validation of the hypothesis that the study of religion does indeed hold promise of making tangible contributions to medical care, let us consider some substantive attempts at such a contribution, at least on the level of history and theory. Our attempt to do so will be divided into two sections, representing two broad concerns of the medical members of our dialogue group: concern for better care of individual patients and concern for the just distribution of health care in our society as a whole. How religion may enter into the understanding and the practices of the medical profession on either of these counts has thus far been barely suggested. The aim of the next few pages is to make good on the claim that, in both an individual and a social context, religious studies have a contribution to make to the improvement of medical practice.

How Might Religious Studies Contribute to Patient Care?

The Critique of Idolatry

Religious studies might contribute to a humane critique of the pretensions and idolatries of both religion and medicine. The theme of illicit pretense to power and the idolizing of something human as rival to something divine is old in the history of religion. Many patients come into doctors' offices speaking some version of a line from W. H. Auden: "We who must die demand a miracle."[1] Doctors shoulder an inhuman burden if they pretend to work miracles. They need deliverance from the pretension of patients who cast them in that role. Speaking from within the Hebrew-Christian tradition, one may say that a lot of anger against doctors in today's medical public—anger about the continuing realities of suffering and death—needs to be transferred, Job-like, to a more proper object, God the Creator. Among other things, deliverance from the status of powerful miracle-maker will involve the medical person in a self-conscious affiliation with the patient in the category of fellow sufferer.

More broadly, the classic religious problem of idolatry needs to be understood and attacked in the medical profession (and in all professions) in its institutional, social guises. All professions want to regulate themselves. As self-regulators, they tend toward self-insulation and thence to autocracy. The medical profession in modern times seems to command the total loyalty and total energy of its members in ways analogous to the historic demands of the monastic order. So we get the complaint of a young M.D. about the consuming pressures of being a house physician in the early days of his postgraduate clinical practice: "The virtual enslavement of house officers to a hospital for years of training and the idea that only one who eats, sleeps, and breathes medicine can become a competent and caring physician, are traditions that cannot withstand the scrutiny of reasonable persons. Osler was a fine and humane physician, but he was not God; and his way of approaching medicine does not represent the only right way."[2]

Protest against *any* human way of doing things as "the only right way" has been called by some theologians the "Protestant principle," the anti-idol principle inherent in all high religions. The worship of the human as unchallengeably divine degrades the human; Hebrew scripture circles back again and again to that claim. The scientific method circles back to it, too. But, ironically enough, scientific authority in modern medicine may become institutionalized in ways that oppress physicians and patients alike. It is no casual hope that a genuine religious consciousness, on both sides of the doctor-patient relation, will guard that relation against degradations of idolatry in either personal or institutional terms. At stake is the right of all parties in the clinical situation to be human.

The Meaning of Suffering

Another classic religious question is, *Why* do I suffer? Empirical and speculative answers to this question, in all times and places, are bound to be complex. Our suffering has many causes, but the mind of the modern physician has been trained to ferret out those immediate causes which, acted upon, can alleviate suffering. Preoccupation with the quick fix of near causes, however, has often led doctors and patients to concentrate on manipulation at the expense of meaning. At its worst this has yielded the great tranquilizer culture of Americans who want to avoid pain on all levels including the mental. It has produced an expectation that fundamental experiences in human life such as childbirth and death must be abandoned to unconsciousness. And, most seriously from a reli-

---

This work originally appeared as "The Interrelationships of Religion and Medicine," in *Medicine and Religion: Strategies of Care,* Donald W. Shriver, Jr., editor. Published in 1980 by the University of Pittsburgh Press. Used by permission.

gious perspective, it has cut short the exploration of a certain grandeur that sometimes hides beneath the surface of human misery. Hardly a religion in the world rests content with the proposal that the securing of pleasure and the avoidance of pain are the chief purposes of a human life.

Some suffering is meaningless, but not all suffering is so. Good medical care might be defined in part as that which enables the patient and the physician to explore all possible dimensions of pain and its alleviation. Here one has to raise the philosophical question of what the word *meaning* means. Someone has said, "Explanation is where the mind is at rest." Since the human mind can rest in any number of places, none of us can say with certainty where the resting place has to be. An explanation of liver ailment that ends with "You drink too much" may be the end of patient and physician curiosity; but the deeper question, "Why do you drink too much?" camps just below the surface. How broadly should the philosophical exploration of such questions be allowed to range in the medical situation? Merely by following the rule to "let the patient decide," the exploration might range deep and far indeed. Should the doctor resist such exploration? Should any of the patient's associates resist it? Religion and religious ethics reply with a firm no, qualified only by those considerations of time and place which suggest a tactical delay to asking certain questions. Job's "comforters," for example, hastened to offer theological reasons for his suffering, when plain empathy would have probably been the most religious initial comfort. But the theological meaning of his suffering is for Job an unavoidable question as it is for religious persons generally.

Some meanings of suffering, of course, are quite beyond either the expert understanding or the manipulations of the medical profession. It may do a victim of byssinosis little good to be told that his or her lifelong inhalation of cotton dust could have been prevented by technical precautions known twenty years ago. It may do even less immediate good to glimpse the faults in the American economic system that led to this sort of suffering; but, given five predictable years of continued life, it may do this patient *great* good to be invited into a social movement aimed at the deliverance of a new generation of textile workers from the scourge of byssinosis. Might not such ranges of meaning be far more important for the full medical treatment of this person than any treatment confined to the biological framework of congested lung tissue? To be sure, the answer "We live in an unjust society" to the question "Why do I suffer?" is ethical more than strictly religious. But the ethical and the religious are often inseparable in most Western religions, and the physician or patient who has been freed of captivity to biologism may be experiencing a taste of life in its wholeness which some consider *religio sui generis.* The modest, minimal claim here is that the exploration of the meaning of human suffering is likely to be a long pilgrimage for every human person, physician and patient alike. The attempt to limit that search to the mechanisms of the body can easily be the anxious avoidance of other dimensions of life that are the very sources of the human experience of triumph and tragedy.

The Understanding of Death

The medical profession is rightly preoccupied with the fact of death. Death is the enemy that physician and patient are most solidly allied against; yet it is the enemy that will ultimately win. Striving against a reality which ultimately will defeat you is the classic theme of tragedy. What to believe and what to do about this tragedy is a classic theme of religion. There are other important themes in the engagement of medicine and religion, but the two can hardly focus on those other themes unless they first wrestle together over the meaning of death in human life. It is the test case of their ability to strike up a partnership.

Death is a very important test for the practice of medicine, as many doctors can testify. When a patient dies, the caring physician may suffer a great loss. He or she may suffer that loss personally—we like people whom we come to know well—as well as professionally, because one great meaning of the profession is its ability to delay death. But what is the meaning of the death that every human one of us *must* suffer?

The various religions have their various ways of clothing death with significance. Each tries to exorcize death of its demonic power, to subject it to some benevolence, and thus to deliver the death-expecting human from the tragedy that all humans feel in the presence of death. Not to join one's personhood and one's profession in the search for some such deliverance would seem to be a mark of profoundest inhumanity in the medical practitioner. Sheer agnosticism about death and its meaning is one of the philosophic-religious options that anyone might adopt, of course. Sheer combativeness in the face of tragedy is another. But either of these options is difficult to implement beside any deathbed without the felt implication of cruelty. In the roster of professional medical virtues, what is more imperative than kindness? In the New Testament Paul says, "The sting of death is sin" (1 Cor. 15.56). Not wholly removed from that opinion is the fear of some dying people that the sting of their death will be abandonment.

The corollary here is the help that medical experience, in turn, can give to religious professionals in this same matter—a theme on which we expand below. Partly under the influence of a medicalized culture, religious intellectuals in the twentieth century have sometimes practiced their own brand of agnosticism about dying. Some Christians, for example, have written off as excessive the preoccupations of a previous generation with heaven and hell, only to draw a blank when asked what death means in the perspective of a New Testament believer. The experience of medical professionals, we have reason to think, might help a lot of clergypeople, first, to recover their interest in the "art of holy living—and dying," and second, to recover their faith, old in the traditions of many religions, that makes death a part of life continuous in meaning with the other parts. New Testament Christian faith, for example, calls for the acceptance of the creature's status before a Creator, the acceptance of judgment against the pathogenic events in human life that are subject to human repentance, and even the acceptance of a benevolent, divine intention that new life should be ours beyond this old one.

The Value of Human Life

At some level of "final analysis," the values of life must be assumed. They cannot be further proved. But the study of philosophy, religion, and ethics suggests that values can be divided between final and instrumental, between ultimate and secondary, between higher and lesser orders. The medical profession has a number of values which it seeks to institutionalize but which, thoughtfully analyzed, may not qualify as ultimate. The focus of much American medicine upon a system of fee for service, for example, presupposes an important but not ultimate value. The Hippocratic oath suggests that service to any person in need is more important than payment for the service; this is a professional presupposition that links medicine at once with those traditions in religion that sanction unselfish love as the highest motive of human relationships. Again, the insistence of modern medical practitioners that they be free to serve others, as they see fit, accounts for some of the profession's resistance to various sorts of legal or governmental control. "We must be free to serve a higher obligation than the laws that politicians are apt to make." In turn, politicians may claim that they, too, have a right to stress the value of service—public service, for example—and to invoke that value in the medical profession.

The point here is that arguments over values quickly become assertions about priority among values and the subordination of some to others. The logic of religion may play an important role at this point, if only at the intellectual level. Religion by definition involves assertions about what in human life must be accounted worthy of one's highest allegiance. Or, to reverse direction, religion concerns the deepest roots of our deepest sense of worth, purpose, and meaning. The values in which the rest of life is "rooted" could, by one definition, comprise the most religious dimension of life.

Religion might be especially important to medical practice by offering answers to a question which doctors seldom take time to answer: What is the value of human life itself? Yet some answer seems implied in the very existence of a medical profession. In a recent lecture, Ronald Berman laid down the axiom, *"In order to fight sickness there has to be a real and demonstrable connection between the fight and what is saved."* He goes on to say that in one Western religious tradition—English Puritanism—death is "an act of recognition and not of civility," for "the dignity of death resided in its meaning. And meaning depended upon two assumptions, one governing the special value of life, and another concerning its place in the universe."[3] Together these two assumptions are integral to the content of most religions. They relate to philosophical propositions on which the medical profession itself seems to rest.

A patient's uncertainty that doctors believe in the value of a human life may strike the doctor as odd. Isn't the whole apparatus of medical practice geared to the preservation of life? Ironically, as many patients will testify, the apparatus itself sometimes seems to deny the value. New medical technologies make many patients feel that they are being constantly shoved around. Reduced to feeling like things, patients want some human voice to say, by word and other gesture, "We are caring for you; and what's more, you are worth caring for." The presence of one's family at times of serious illness may chiefly be related to this kind of reassurance; perhaps only a family can fill out the care offered by a physician. The custom in Africa and Asia that families accompany patients to the hospital may thus be an example of very good medicine.

The final worth of human life, its status in the world, is inescapably a religious issue. Members of a "caring" profession have abundant reason to think about their most fundamental reasons for saying yes to the question, Are humans worth caring for? Such thought might be considered part of the groundwork that prepares a physician to *be* a physician, "in spirit and in truth," as a New Testament passage would put it. One member of our dialogue group remembers the conversation he had as a college student with a surgeon acquaintance. In a philosophical moment the surgeon explained that "the struggle of the bugs in the grass to compete with the birds for survival is the same struggle that goes on among human beings." A long time afterward, no thanks to the surgeon's philosophy but with the help of the writings of Loren Eiseley, he was able to understand the doctrine of evolution in a way that made sense of human care as itself a clue to the meaning of evolution. "My surgeon friend would have been puzzled, I feel sure, if I had been astute enough to ask him, 'How on the grounds of that philosophy of life do you justify your own profession as a surgeon?'"

Definition of the moral and religious grounds for affirming the value of a human being remains a very practical question for the medical profession. As suicide and anorexia nervosa would suggest, among many other examples of the human capacity to will self-destruction, we cannot assume automatic commitments to life in ourselves or our neighbors. Many a patient is lost to a physician because the mysterious will to live is somehow absent. A cultural suspicion about the worth of human existence has infected some segments of the ecological movement ("humanity is one of nature's mistakes"); and many Western young people, obsessed with pessimism over possible nuclear annihilation of the race, reflect gloomily that the race does not deserve to survive. Some religious views of human history are allies to this very pessimism—views, for example, that proclaim antiworldly dualism, the evil of the material world, and the purity of life beyond death.

The medical profession has a stake in religions that sustain the belief that humans are worth caring for. It has a similar stake in resisting those interpretations of the human drama which reduce its significance to that of a trash pile or otherwise weaken the significance of the actors' commitment to taking part in that drama. At stake here is not only the quantitative question of whether human life is worth prolonging, but also the qualitative question of what kind of life is worth prolonging.

Of course the traditional religions may not offer convincing grounds-of-value to many a modern mind. New religions are always possible, as are new choices between old religions—options that religious studies may help to pose. But in this array of possibilities the medical profession can hardly be value free or neutral. In the long or short run, care for people that presupposes the valuelessness of people undermines itself. Medical professionals may need the help of religious studies in the search for the substrata of their own and their patients' sense of worth. The rock or the quicksand "in the depths" is heavy with promise and threat for the ground where we stand.

The Professional Decision

Religious studies might help the medical profession to detect and to endure the ambiguity, the limit, and the power of "the professional decision." Fortified intellectually by the prestige of science, sustained by the professional loyalty of colleagues, and trusted to the point of pathos by many a patient, the modern doctor has an impressive array of defenses against the thought which Roman generals at their triumphs had whispered in their ears: "Remember, thou art mortal." On the other hand, members of our dialogue group can testify that most medical professionals are only too aware of their mortality and wish only too sincerely that modern society's infatuation with "the miracles of modern medicine" were cut down to reality. The issue here is companion to that of idolatry above: Once you know that you are indeed a mortal among mortals, how do you interpret that awareness in professional and personal terms? The mounting anxiety of doctors over the cost of medical insurance and the mounting rage of the public over occasional mistakes, carelessness, and incompetence in the profession are all part of this picture. How shall the public learn to accept the limits of medical knowledge and skill? How shall patients make peace with uncertainty and ambiguity in the most competent medical decision?

The study of religion might come to the assistance of doctor, patient, and public here. It might help all parties to the medical decision to breathe a sigh of acceptance of their common humanity. Indeed, as an academic study, religion's claim to classification as one of the humanities seems especially strong, because of its insistence that we are all human beings first, and only secondly are we professionals or members of a social class or specialists of various sorts. The statement does not hold true for all religions. Some of them have helped legitimate vast caste systems, as in Hinduism. Some have promoted a spiritual aristocracy, as in Buddhism. And some have given divine sanction to slavery, as in some expressions of Christianity. Yet the broad, nonspecialist concern for the human as such seems endemic to religion. One of its services, even at the level of intellectual inquiry, is to invite the student to step aside inwardly from the specifics of social role, special knowledge, and individual experience to consider the universally human. "What is man that thou are mindful of him?" asks the author of Psalm 8, as he looks up at the "moon and the stars which Thou hast ordained." Another psalmist (139) wonders at the mystery of his own birth when the Creator "knit me together in my mother's womb." Such a reflection has little to do with biological explanations of the process by which a human being comes to birth. The psalmist is wondering at what a sophisticated Western philosopher would call the "contingency" of his existence. There was a time when he was not. There will be a time when he will not be. Yet before his beginning and after his end, there is God—or so the viewpoint of his faith compels him to believe.

Ambiguity and limit camp about every human existence. No one who fails to acknowledge this can be fully human. The powers of scientific medicine remain afflicted by ambiguity and limit: What medical procedure is truly "foolproof"? And in cases where the foolishness of the medical professional or the medical institution wreaks havoc on the life of some patient, what can be done? The wrong drug is prescribed, the therapy too late and a grief-stricken new widow asks the doctor, "Why?" The medical profession, like other professions that make mistakes, has its own characteristic ways of "covering up." The ability to admit limitations, mistakes, and genuine foolishness remains rare in most of the professions, including the clergy. But some religious points of view have their own therapy for these things: life and death endured in the presence of a larger intelligence than our own; unwitting and willful mistakes given over to forgiveness; and the pain of inadequacy in this instance given some meaning as an occasion for reformation and repentance in the next. It is hard to describe this "context of creaturehood" for the medical decision without seeming to commend a particular religion to the decision maker. But some point of view has to be adopted for making answer to the widow. What truly humane professional will answer out of his or her own scientific jargon, "You lost your husband to the law of averages"? At the last the more human and more acceptable answer may well be, "We didn't know enough, we made some mistakes, but we tried." The study of religion might help empower one to make that sort of answer. Above all, it might empower everyone around a sickbed to say a word that is due in all seasons of a human life: "We care for you."

How Might Religious Studies Contribute to a More Just Distribution of Health Care in Our Society?

Like religion itself, medical practice involves some irreducible personal dimensions. One philosopher, Alfred North Whitehead, has even defined religion as "what one does with solitude." That definition fits nicely the bias of some mystical and some Protestant traditions which claim that religious faith is an exclusively personal matter.

In the book *Medicine and Religion* some members of the dialogue group summarized a religious argument for medical concern for public health as well as for the individual health of patients in offices and hospitals. It will seem mysterious to some readers that such a concern should enter at all into a discussion of religious studies and medicine. Granted that religion may rightly be concerned with the dignity of the sick, the meaning of death, and the like; but what does religion have to do with the politics and economics of national health policy?

Behind this rhetorical question may lie the honest belief that religion really is a personal affair; that politics and religion do not and should not mix; that the attempt to derive guidance from religion for complex social questions is an insult to both religion and society. Theologians and historians know this as a very old debate in the history of religion itself. In quest of "spiritual" purity, some radically religious persons (such as the medieval monks) cast themselves loose from "secular" society, living in their own separate social enclaves. Equally radical mystics have reduced their religious quest to a personal life of prayer. Culturally nearer at hand is the individualistic American Protestant, ready to claim that "my religion is my business." Ever and again in history, however, the prophets of many great religions have reminded their adherents that piety without ethics is empty, just as ethics without piety is rootless. Neither religion nor ethics is what one does with one's solitude but what one does in relationship to other human beings. In the Hebrew, Christian, and other great world religions, religion always bears ethical fruit, just as ethics always has spiritual roots. Moreover, in many of these traditions, the distinction between personal and social ethics hardly exists. Such a distinction may arise in a liberal democratic society like the United States where many people have the freedom to segregate their personal lives drastically from their social involvements. Most human beings in history have had no such luxury. All early religions were social in almost every aspect. Anthropologists have demonstrated that so-called primitive religion is difficult to distinguish from the structure of entire social orders. And most of the so-called great world religions (Judaism, Christianity, Islam) developed society-wide prescriptions for human behavior. The idea of a purely individual religion would have appeared absurd to most of the religiously inclined people who have ever lived. Especially in the case of the great world religions, their proponents have inclined toward universal claims which are intended to apply to human beings and all their relationships.

More particularly, the question of better distribution of health care arose for many members of our dialogue group out of their specific commitments to their own religious tradition, which happened to be Judeo-Christian. This tradition makes much of "the justice of God," a notion embedded in the Old Testament account of the exodus of the Hebrew people from their political captivity in Egypt. According to this account, the God of Israel displays justice by actively saving the weak and exploited people of society. This is the emphasis of the prophetic strain in the Old and New Testaments. The deity of this faith has a characteristic "bias toward the weak," and justice is not less universal but more so because of this bias. The prophets knew that societies often build institutions to provide benefits to some members while excluding others. Even the most inclusive society has its marginal members. The God of the Bible seems to specialize in care for those members in particular and thereby remedies the deficiencies of justice in human history by looking out for neglected people—through the words of the prophets, for example. H. Richard Niebuhr was alluding to this feature of biblical religion when he compared religion at its best to science at its best: "Like pure religion pure science seems to care for 'widows and orphans'—for bereaved and abandoned facts, for processes and experiences that have lost meaning because they did not fit into an accepted framework of interpretation."[4]

An illustration of an inadequate framework of interpretation would be one that permitted the interpreter of personal religious experience to ignore certain social sources of that experience. The "free individual" is something of an abstraction, realistically considered, as abstract as the existence of a child considered apart from his or her parentage and social setting. The same abstraction may be present in a physician's preoccupation with the one-to-one relationship of bedside medicine. Dozens, even hundreds or thousands, of other people have some relation to a sick person and to the physician. One thinks of a single sick baby being treated in a Harlem hospital. Does the attending physician "see" only *a* sick baby or one of a crowd of babies who die in Harlem every year from causes associated with poverty (including inadequate prenatal and postnatal care)? Harlem's infant mortality statistics should hang heavy in the minds of the medical profession in New York City. To be born and to live in Harlem is to have more chance of dying before the age of one, and indeed at almost any age of life, than in many other neighborhoods in New York. The personal health of infants and socioeconomic conditions of life are glaringly intertwined.

Do religious studies have anything to contribute to the enhancement of just and caring delivery of health services to all the people of society? Most members of our dialogue group answered yes from several lines of reasoning.

Institutional Systems

Contemporary concern for "good medical care" is understood by some students of religion as analogous to religious concern for the total welfare of human beings; religious studies might help medical professionals to reexamine the social institutional structures and cultural norms that tend to frustrate the delivery of good care to large segments of the human community.

Medical advocates of individual patient care in this country often display an intense commitment to human welfare that matches closely the call of this book for meaningful, as opposed to manipulatory, care. Sometimes this commitment has a profoundly religious quality to it. A doctor committed to the well-being of a single acutely ill patient may stay up all night watching that bedside—as faithfully as any priest carrying the sacrament to a parishioner on the verge of death. Such religiously committed care deserves much honor. But religious imagination and prophetic passion call for an intensification, a universalization of such commitment until it includes all the people whom Jesus called "the least of these my brethren" (Matt. 25:40). From this point of view, medical care, in any society, cannot be judged truly "good" until it extends to all members of that society. The work of achieving that goal in practice will inevitably involve the criticism of institutions, and such criticism may derive from deep religious and ethical conviction. To become such critics, medical practitioners may have to distinguish sharply between (1) those values acclaimed by the profession which are yet to be adequately institutionalized, and (2) those values of the profession that are subject to criticism in the light of yet higher values. The first form of criticism is the least difficult; but as many medical reformers can testify, it is difficult enough. Some years ago a doctor in a small South Carolina town discovered cases of severe malnutrition among children and adults living in the county. His attempts to call this condition to the attention of his local colleagues met with rejection and even reprisal. Eventually he moved away. Yet he was merely calling attention to people in distress who would be legitimately the object, one would suppose, of the Hippocratic oath or any of the higher canons of medical care. The second form of criticism is inescapably prophetic. No profession takes kindly to the attempt of any of its members to subject it to "outside" standards. The pluralism of religious attitudes in the modern medical profession keeps most of its members from calling for change in the name of standards like those of the

Bible suggested above. But when Steven Levenson, quoted above, attributes the exploitation of house officers to a kind of idolatry, he invokes a standard of human behavior from the realm of religion. He appeals to horizons of meaning not particular to the medical profession. Such invocations of a religiously rooted ethic can threaten vested interests, not merely in medical institutions but in all institutions whatsoever.

Nothing is more common in organized society than a confusion of means and ends. Vested interest usually implies the danger of such a confusion. Sometimes the stated ends of an institution must be invoked over against its means. Sometimes the ends themselves deserve criticism in the light of larger ends. The courage to move along this spectrum may be one of the gifts of religious faith and religious community to the inhabitants of all institutions, including religious institutions.

Social Commitments

Religious studies might provide context and encouragement for the ethical reflection and political commitment of health professionals who seek more justice in medical care systems. In the current controversy over national health insurance in the United States, nonmedical critics often assume that membership in the American Medical Association is synonymous with opposition to "socialized medicine." Such critics tend to ignore the real diversities of political and economic opinion among the 438,000 physicians of this country. Not even on so controversial a matter as government-sponsored health programs would doctors cast unanimous votes. Furthermore, the rigor of medical training and practice does not tend to equip medical professionals with great interest or competence in political and economic policy questions. Yet further, even if medical leaders had the unanimity and the competence to recommend health policy for legislatures and bureaucrats, they would often not have the power to get their recommendations accepted. Public policy regarding health care is precisely that: the policy of a public, by a public, and for a public. Of that public, the medical community composes only a part. Controversy over the social dimensions of health, in short, will surely occur inside and outside the medical profession.

In this controversy, as in many others, churches, synagogues, university departments of religion, and other institutions may have little specialized knowledge to contribute. Religious concern often commits a person to certain ends (e.g., better health for the poor and oppressed) without any illumination of the proper means to those ends. Here the religiously concerned medical leader may be in quite the same boat with others outside the profession. Together what they both may need is not wisdom from on high on the best design of a national health policy, but free space in which to explore their mutual concerns outside the immediate constraints of professional tradition, economic interests, and political ideology. The religious institution can be such a free space. A congregation can be the place where some members envision a society in which "the least of these my brethren" have justice done to their needs. It may also be the place where those members search together for mutual illumination of difficult questions of great moment to society. In more academic ways, seminaries and departments of religion can offer the same freedom of exploration to many parties to public controversy. Our society has few institutions that can stand between other institutions, inviting their constituents into open dialogue on important public questions. Religion and its institutions can be sponsors of just such dialogue. Religion does not have all the answers, but it can offer the rationale and the organization for the human search for better answers than single-function institutions are likely to cultivate.

In recent years religious organizations have sponsored programs that have opened conversation between health professionals and others around these issues. One example is our dialogue group, as well as the Society for Health and Human Values itself. Another example is the Christian Medical Commission of the World Council of Churches, a body in which Dr. John Bryant has been a leading member. In 1973 Bryant developed a paper for the commission in which he follows John Rawls—and the prophets of the Old Testament—in adopting a principle of justice that favors the needs of the "worst off" people of society: "Whatever health services are available should be equally available to all. Departures from equality of distribution are permissible only if those worst off are made better off." Bryant goes on to specify this principle of distributive justice in four secondary principles: (1) "There should be a floor or minimum of health service for all. . . . (2) Resources above the floor should be distributed according to need. . . . (3) In those instances where health care resources are nondivisible or necessarily uneven, their distribution should be of advantage to the least favored. . . . (4) The population actually or potentially receiving health care should participate in decisions on the distribution of those resources."[5]

A leading Christian ethicist, Paul Ramsey, has said that the task of religion in modern society is to "nurture the moral and political ethos" but not to prescribe or to make specific social policy.[6] The church, says Ramsey, should be "a community of unlimited discussion and discourse." The nourishing of this kind of thought may constitute an indispensable service of a religious institution to the improvement of health in our society through the improvement of citizens' ability to deliberate together.

Giving Voice to the Neglected

Religious studies might help health professionals understand the historic concern of some religions and their institutions to give voice to the voiceless, ailing people of the world. Continuous with the potential of religion as a support to people inside the medical profession concerned with social justice is its potential support for neglected people themselves. Among the various communities into which the human race is divided, perhaps none are so varied sociologically, politically, and geographically as the communities of the world's great religions. Christianity is only one example of the social diversity of a single religious community, but it is a notable example. It is no coincidence that the World Council of Churches is concerned about medical care for poor people: the Bible enjoins special care for the poor. Moreover, many of the Council's member churches work in countries inhabited primarily by the poor.

History tells us that religion has great power for creating vicious human divisions; but the contrary side of religious communal life is equally striking. Certainly most religious communities provide their members with an experience of social diversity greater than that available in the typical professional association. Again, as illustrated by the World Council of Churches, social diversity provides an opportunity for the breakdown of the specialism and the professionalism that afflict modern society. In a church or a synagogue, a professional may hear opinions quite contrary to the opinions of colleagues on the job. The same diversity and contradiction will reign, of course, in the public arena of politics. One of the services of religion to public politics is the equipment of diverse, specialized persons with the ability to listen to each other. And the particular duty of the religious community, in the prophetic tradition, is to enable the powerful to hear the powerless. At its best, the religious institution in this tradition becomes an irritant to the complacency of the body politic in regard to the good of the weakest of its members. In this sense, the politics of better health care belong to the central role of religion in modern society.

How Might Medicine Contribute to Religion and Religious Studies?

By now readers may suspect religious imperialism. So far we have concentrated on the possible contributions of religious studies to medicine. That has been, and will continue to be, our chief assignment. But for the long dialogue between these disciplines that lies ahead, such one-sidedness would be unjust indeed. What are the contributions of medicine to religion and the study of religion? Though the burden of our own dialogue was on the complement of this question, we were aware of both questions. Our most systematic answers we reserved for the first, but here are our suggestions for an answer to the second.

Despiritualization

Medicine might help to despiritualize and deplatitudinize the advocacy and the study of religion. By returning again and again to the problems of the real people who suffer daily on sickbeds, medical members of our group sometimes provided us the best examples of "true humanism." Human problems, they said, are more serious, complex, and difficult to resolve than any theories, faiths, formulas, or preachments can cope with. However necessary the symbols and philosophical grounds of religion may be, they do not substitute for that relief of pain, restoration of health, and acceptance of loss which are the ordinary human needs of the medical situation. One of our medical members remembered an incident from his own time in medical school:

> I was on rounds with a senior physician as an intern. We were about to enter the patient's room, and almost instinctively I put one hand on the door knob and the other on my stethoscope around my neck. My instructor looked at me and said quietly, "Why not leave your technical equipment hanging on the door?" Somewhat abashed, I did so and went into the room to see a patient as a fellow human being like myself, minus "technical equipment." The same requirement I would recommend to the students and practitioners of religion in their relation to medical professionals and to their patients. We are not intolerant of technical academic equipment, but mostly we want to be useful to people. We hope that religion can be useful to people, too.

The Historical Influence

Medicine might remind students of religion how much influence religion has exercised in human history for better or for worse. This contribution has two sides. On the one, the history of Western medicine over the past two or three centuries has frequently involved conflict with religious leaders, customs, and doctrines. Thus medical people cannot be blamed for their suspicion of religion, which around the world still accounts for resistance to medical measures as diverse as inoculation, birth control, fluoridation, and even sanitation. On the other, the modern practitioner and student of a religious faith may need reminding of religion's power to mold human behavior for good and for evil. The easy secularism of many Westerners tempts them to forget that mere beliefs can introduce vast changes in human society. The nightmare of Nazism should have demonstrated that to all inhabitants of the twentieth century. Too readily do some religious people, including academics, accept the secularity of the age and assume that "the great days of religious influence are past." Neither of these theories stands the test of history and experience—the clinical test. Religion may have been bad for some people in the past, but it was nonetheless powerful. Religion may need reforming if it is to benefit the present; but the reformation can come only from people who take its influence very seriously. Ironically enough, the great religious skeptic may not be the religious amateur who happens to be a doctor, but the religious professional who happens to be a theologian! The medical profession would be ill served by members who do not appreciate the real powers of medicine. So also with the field of religion. "Be not eager for self-negation," medical people may need to say to students and practitioners of religion.

Language

Medicine might enrich the language, the images, and the basic theories of religion. The language of religion may become more eloquent and communicative in our time when rightly enriched by the language of biology, medicine, and science. Theologians like Teilhard de Chardin have taken this suggestion with utmost seriousness in their intellectual formulations, for example, in Teilhard's evocation of the "turning points" in human evolution. The Clinical Pastoral Education movement has already led the way, in church circles, toward treatment-oriented collaboration between the medical and clerical professions; and from this collaboration have emerged many contributions to the language and symbols of religion. Words like *sin, alienation, bondage,* and *redemption* acquire new significance when used in knowledgeable connection with the plight of people suffering from depression, ulcers, and suicidal resistance to therapy. Some contemporary Western theologians have said that the classical doctrine that most needs redefinition is theological anthropology—theology's answer to the question, What is human? In helping theology to answer this question, the sciences, including the medical sciences, may not be authoritative, but their help may be indispensable.

The Cost of Caring

Medicine might help teach the leaders of religious thought and religious practice the cost of caring. Like other academics, scholars, teachers, and preachers in the field of religion put high value on "the right word." Words are the tools of their trade. Facility in the use of those tools may lure them, on occasion, into what one famous theologian called "cheap grace." At their best, teachers know that splendid lectures may not be enough for the real teaching of students; and at their best, clergy know that good sermons may not be enough to demonstrate the meaning of the statement, "God loves you." To the verbal costs of caring must be added the emotional, economic, organizational, and political costs of caring. One member of our dialogue group has spent some years helping the government of Thailand to improve the country's medical systems. What medical care can be provided an entire population when the budget available amounts to less than one dollar per capita annually? Even in the rich United States, popular demands for expensive health care may outrun all the available budgets. Religious people's call for personal attention to certain neglected groups (e.g., the dying, the poor) may require more expenditures of time, money, and other resources than taxpayers want spent. On a more personal level, the minister who wants a doctor to pay more individual attention to a dying cancer patient should know, through his own experience, the emotional costliness of such care. Doctors can teach this, along with the skill to achieve the combination of personal empathy and professional distance necessary in all the helping arts.

The Public Role of Religion

Medicine might help religious institutions to recognize their public role in remedying the deficiencies of medical care in our society. Complaining about each other over their respective institutional walls constitutes a low level of dialogue between any two professional groups. Often the upshot of such complaint is, "Improve your own shop, please." But in a society as complex as ours, improvements in one shop often depend heavily on improvements elsewhere. The example just given about the cost of caring is suggestive. If the voters refuse to authorize taxes to support the human services in municipal and state budgets, the case loads of social workers will go up, the public hospital will lack enough professional help to pay attention to even routine patient needs, and the vulnerability of the central city slums to disease will mount. Where, if not in the religious organizations of a community, can public outcry about immoral economizing be raised? The medical profession—the doctors and nurses who worship in churches and synagogues regularly—has its own teaching to do in such organizations outside their profession. The levers for change may lie there, even the levers for change of the medical institution itself. One benefit of such teaching to the leaders of religious institutions will be greater accuracy of information about the problems of the medical system. Often, in our dialogue group, the sternest critics of both medicine and religion were their respective practitioners. Insiders often know best the inadequacies of their systems. They may need the help of outsiders in the search for remedies. To get that help, they must engage in their own version of missionary work.

A Common Pilgrimage

Medicine might join religion in a common pilgrimage through unexplored human territory. One image of the religious life, prominent in the Bible, is the pilgrimage. Such an image conflicts somewhat with images of professionalism. The professional, who has acquired training, skills, colleagues, knowledge, and experience, presumably knows what to do about certain human problems. But, unfortunately for a sense of professional security, many human problems yield very little to professional powers. Death is only one perennial illustration. The problem of building a modern medical system in Thailand is another, and convincing a nation to spend more money on medicine and less on armaments may be yet another. Ordinarily professions work on that range of human problems whose solution is already known; but this may confine the professional, like the man in the famous story, to looking for a lost key inside the patch of light under the streetlamp. Some of the most sensitive physicians in our dialogue group have insisted that both religion and medicine need to relate to one another more in a research mode than in an interprofessional or mutual teaching mode. As in pioneering scientific research, the moment of a breakthrough may be the moment of the disturbing question to which there are literally no answers. "I have occasionally had to confess," said one physician, "to a mismatch between my professional preparation and the questions which get directed at me by people in great need. Sometimes these questions are basic religious questions, such as, What is human life for? I know a theologian who has helped me bear that question in the human situation where I work, and he was wise enough to confess that he had no pat answers to the question. He was also faithful enough to walk with me in my search for an answer. We human beings need more often simply to accompany one another on a 'walk through the wilderness.' To be human sometimes means to encounter *aphoria,* waylessness. Such waylessness is not random, but it is mysterious. And it is endurable only with the help of comrades for the journey."

Auden imagined the future as "the Land of Unlikeness," where humans "will see rare beasts, and have unique adventures."[7] Such adventures seem to multiply in the experience of twentieth-century humans. Medical and religious professionals may need each other's comradeship as seldom before in history.

Notes

1. "For the Time Being: A Christmas Oratorio," in *Religious Drama I,* ed. Marvin Halverson (New York: Meridian Books, 1957), p. 17.
2. Steven Levenson, "The Self-Contradictions of a 'Humane' Profession," in *Humanizing the Process of Medical Education: Winning Essays of the Medical Student and Housestaff Essay Contest* (Philadelphia: Society for Health and Human Values, 1976), p. 12.
3. Ronald Berman, "The Favour of the Gods," annual oration of the Society for Health and Human Values (Philadelphia: Society for Health and Human Values, 1977), pp. 15-16. Italics in original.
4. H. Richard Niebuhr, *Radical Monotheism and Western Culture* (New York: Harper and Brothers, 1960), p. 87.
5. "Principles of Justice as a Basis for Conceptualizing a Health Care System," mimeo, 1973.
6. Paul Ramsey, *Who Speaks for the Church?* (Nashville: Abingdon Press, 1967), pp. 152, 155.
7. Auden, "For the Time Being," p. 68.

5.
The Meaning of Medicine

PAUL TOURNIER

We have seen that healing is an effect and a sign of God's mercy, extending the term of our life. And so, as Professor Courvoisier writes, the vocation of medicine is 'a service to which those are called who through their studies and the natural gifts with which the Creator has endowed them . . . are specially fitted to tend the sick and to heal them. Whether or not they are aware of it, whether or not they are believers, this is from the Christian point of view fundamental, that doctors are, by their profession, fellow workers with God. . . . because their activity is itself a sign of God's patience. It is not His will that men should be lost, but that they should all come to the knowledge of His Son and of His salvation.'

This is the meaning of medicine for us. From this it derives its greatness and its beauty. And it is also this that lays upon us such a heavy load of responsibility. 'Sickness and healing are acts of grace', writes Dr. Pouyanne.[1] 'The doctor is an instrument of God's patience', writes Pastor Alain Perrot.[2] 'Medicine is a dispensation of the grace of God, who in His goodness takes pity on men and provides remedies for the evil consequences of their sin', writes Dr. Schlemmer.[3] Calvin described medicine as a gift from God.[4]

Thus every doctor, Christian or not, is a collaborator with God, as Ambroise Paré said, in these well-known words: 'I tended him. God healed him.' Some of my colleagues may be thinking that, in repeating the affirmations of these theologians and doctors, I am breaking down doors that are already open. I do not think so. It is important to have a solid conviction as the basis of action, and to be sure that it is in accordance with God's purpose. I have mentioned elsewhere that there are Christians who condemn medicine in the name of their faith; and others who hesitate to have recourse to it, as if one had to choose between God's help and that of the doctor. I should like to give another charming quotation from Ambroise Paré, in which he well expresses this marriage of intellect and faith, technology and prayer: 'The Marquis d'Auret had a bullet wound in the joint of his knee and seemed at death's door. . . . Howbeit, to give him courage and a good hope, I told him that I should soon set him on his feet. . . . When I had seen him I went for a walk in a garden, where I prayed God that He would grant me this grace, that the Marquis be healed, and that He would bless our hands, and the physics that were needed to fight so many complicated maladies. . . . I discoursed in my mind on the means I must adopt to do this.'

To know ourselves to be called by God is to believe in our vocation with as much conviction as St. Paul when he declares himself to be 'separated unto the gospel of God' (Rom. 1.1). And it is St. Paul who speaks of the 'diversities of ministrations' (I Cor. 12.5). Our profession is a priestly ministry. I should like to see the Church consecrating doctors just as it ordains its ministers. This would be in conformity with the gospel. It is this conviction which makes us give ourselves with our hearts and minds and souls to our vocation—with our 'spiritual hearts', as Dr. Stocker says,[5] quoting Pascal.

Even when the doctor believes he is obeying only his own feelings, his compassion for human suffering, he is at that moment the instrument of the divine compassion: Jesus 'saw a great multitude, and he had compassion on them, and healed their sick' (Matt. 14.14). Even the prophets who speak of God's wrath tell us that He repents of His anger: 'For I will not contend for ever, neither will I be always wroth. . . . For the iniquity of his covetousness was I wroth and smote him, I hid my face and was wroth: and he went on frowardly in the way of his heart. I have seen his ways, and will heal him: I will lead him also, and restore comforts unto him and to his mourners. . . . I will heal him' (Isa. 57.16-19).

And so the command rings out in our ears also: 'Heal the sick' (Matt. 10.8). We all know the parable of the Last Judgement (Matt. 25.31-46), in which Jesus takes as His criterion not this or that sin, but the charity or the hardness of the heart. And he adds: 'Inasmuch as ye did it unto one of these my brethren, even these least, ye did it unto me' (Matt. 25.40). Similarly, the prophet Ezekiel castigates the shepherds of Israel: 'Ye feed not the sheep. The diseased have ye not strengthened, neither have ye healed that which was sick, neither have ye bound up that which was broken, neither have ye brought again that which was driven away, neither have ye sought that which was lost' (Ezek. 34.3-4).

We have here the whole task of medicine, which is not only to heal, but also to protect the weak: 'Ye shall not respect persons in judgement; ye shall hear the small and the great alike; ye shall not be afraid of the face of man' (Deut. 1.17). Again, medicine is to bring back to obedience those who are neglecting the

---

From Paul Tournier, *A Doctor's Casebook in the Light of the Bible,* trans. Edwin Hudson (London: SCM Press, 1954; New York: Harper & Row, 1960), pp. 215-21. Used by permission.

laws of life: 'Thou, O son of man, I have set thee a watchman . . . therefore thou shalt hear the word at my mouth, and warn them from me. . . . If thou dost not speak to warn the wicked man from his way, that wicked man shall die in his iniquity; but his blood will I require at thine hand' (Ezek. 33.7-8, A.V.).

The Bible makes no distinction between spiritual and temporal action, between supernatural and natural healing. The Bible, of course, preceded scientific medicine and so could make no allusion to it; but it is not silent on the art of healing. See, for example, the passage in Ecclesiasticus (38.1), which speaks of the physician as created by the Lord. Isaiah uses a cake of figs to cure King Hezekiah (II Kings 20.7); our Lord applies clay to the eyes of a blind man (John 9.6); music was used to calm King Saul when he was suffering from mental disease (I Sam. 16.16). Mention is made in the Bible of plants that are used for healing (Ezek. 47.12), of the oil that is poured on sores (Isa. 1.6), of the balm that is applied to wounds (Jer. 8.22), of wine used as a disinfectant (Luke 10.34), of appliances for containing fractures (Ezek. 30.21), of therapeutic baths (John 5.2), and of the calling in of physicians (Jer. 8.22). St. Paul concerned himself with Timothy's diet (I Tim. 5.23), and invited his companions to recruit their strength by taking some food on board their ship buffeted by the storm, adding: 'This is for your safety' (Acts 27.34). There are also many instructions regarding rest (Ex. 20.8), fasting (Acts 27.9), and on feeding (Deut. 14), many of which have a medical basis, as, for example, abstention from alcohol during pregnancy (Judg. 13.4).

Thus the doctor collaborates with God through his remedies, his techniques, and the skill of his hands, as well as through his intercession for his patients (Jas. 5.14), by his personal asceticism (Matt. 17.21, R.V. marg.), by the laying on of hands (Luke 4.40), and the unction of oil (Mark 6.13). 'And I find occasion here', writes Ambroise Paré, 'to praise God for that it hath pleased Him to call me to the work of medicine, which is commonly called surgery, the which may not be bought with gold or silver, but rather only by virtue and by long experience. Nevertheless it is stable in all countries, for the cause that the sacred laws of medicine are not subject to those of Kings and Princes, nor to the changing ordinance of time, as having their origin from God, 'whom I beseech that it please Him to bless this mine undertaking, that it be to His eternal glory.'

I should like further to call attention to the words of St. Paul—words which the doctor may make his own—on dedication, even to death, to the service of others: 'So then death worketh in us, but life in you' (II Cor. 4.12). But however great his knowledge and his dedication, the doctor does not always succeed in snatching his patient from death. I have already spoken several times of the 'death complex' in doctors. Those who have no other conscious source of vocation than their zeal for the relief of suffering find the death of their patients very hard to bear. They feel it to be a personal failure.

It is appropriate here to recall what I have said about death also being considered, in the Bible, as a blessing and as one of the elements in God's purpose. The doctor who in tending the sick is conscious of being God's instrument will be fired with an equal zeal, but will also accept more easily the death of a patient. Professor Courvoisier speaks of this at the close of his study. He writes: 'It is the same God who is there . . . whether the patient lives or dies. That is why success and failure are . . . elements of one and the same truth.'

We are shown David fasting and spending the night lying on the ground when his son is sick, then rising and eating when the child is dead (II Sam. 12.15-23). It is in this sense also, I think, that we are to understand the words of our Lord: 'Leave the dead to bury their own dead' (Matt. 8.22). The dead no longer belong to us. They are in God's peace. Let us turn towards the living. I should like to stress the psychological importance of the Biblical view on this point. We often see families in which a member who has passed on still holds a place that ought to be taken by the living. There are parents, for example, who have lost a child, and who make him the centre of all their thoughts. It can become a sort of religious cult, having serious consequences for the remaining children.

But it is clear that to accept death we must believe in resurrection. I am very sorry for those of my colleagues who do not. Their vocation must be a singularly disappointing one, always striving to prolong lives which will inevitably finish in an endless night of death.

There is no need to emphasize that on this subject the Bible is categorical. It assures us of God's final victory over death: 'He hath swallowed up death for ever' (Isa. 25.8); 'Death shall be no more' (Rev. 21.4); 'I will redeem them from death: O death, where are thy plagues? O grave, where is thy destruction?' (Hos. 13.14). The Bible promises us the resurrection of our whole person: 'He that raised up Christ Jesus from the dead shall quicken also your mortal bodies' (Rom. 8.11).

But the Bible does more than promise. It shows us the bodily Resurrection of Jesus Christ as the proof of its affirmations: 'Reach hither thy finger, and see my hands; and reach hither thy hand, and put it into my side: and be not faithless, but believing. Thomas answered and said unto him, My Lord and my God' (John 20.27-8).

St. Paul in his discussion with the Corinthians lays great stress on this proof of our resurrection by that of Christ: 'If there is no resurrection of the dead, neither hath Christ been raised. . . . If in this life only we have hoped in Christ, we are of all men most pitiable. But now hath Christ been raised from the dead, the first-fruits of them that are asleep' (I Cor. 15.13, 19-20). To Timothy he writes: 'Christ Jesus . . . abolished death, and brought life and incorruption to light' (II Tim. 1.10).

There are many more texts that I could quote, but I will desist, not wishing to desert the sphere of medicine for that of theology. It is, however, impossible to over-emphasize the concrete practical importance of this certainty to the doctor at the bedside of a dying man. When science has done all it can do, when the doctor is, as we said before, accompanying his patient to the gates of death, this inner conviction of the certainty of resurrection is the only true consolation that remains. Whether, at God's instance, he voices it, or whether he communicates it only by his own silent confidence, he is the messenger of hope: 'Neither death, nor life, nor angels, nor principalities, nor things present, nor things to come, nor powers, nor height, nor depth, nor any other creature, shall be able to separate us from the love of God, which is in Christ Jesus our Lord' (Rom. 8.38-9).

Reassurance and consolation. It has been said of medicine that its duty is sometimes to heal, often to afford relief, and always to bring consolation. This is exactly what the Bible tells us that God does for suffering humanity. Sometimes God heals, but not always. But He gives relief, He protects and sustains us in times of affliction; and His consolation is unending. Here too we may say that the doctor in his vocation works hand in hand with God. . . .

As for God's protection when we are in affliction and even when we are in rebellion, there is an interesting Biblical reference. When Cain had murdered Abel (Gen. 4.3-15), God said to him: 'What hast thou done? the voice of thy brother's blood crieth unto me from the ground. And now cursed art thou . . . ; a fugitive and a wanderer shalt thou be in the earth.' And yet when the terrified Cain says to Him: 'Whosoever findeth me shall slay me,' the Lord replies: 'Whosoever slayeth Cain, vengeance shall be taken on him sevenfold. And the Lord appointed a sign for Cain, lest any finding him should smite him.'

Thus, in the Biblical perspective, although affliction and disease are bound up with sin, and although they are occasionally represented as the expression of the wrath of God, man still remains under His protection; even when man is cursed, he is never completely abandoned. A particular illustration of this truth is furnished by the forty years spent by the Israelites wandering in the desert. Rebellious as they were, and always earning God's maledictions, they nevertheless also enjoyed His succour in their afflictions: 'The Lord thy God . . . humbled thee, and suffered thee to hunger, and fed thee with manna' (Deut. 8.2-3). God tried them, but they remained His people and lived under His protection.

This is the experience of every believer. This is the meaning of God's answer to St. Paul when the Apostle asked for healing and was not granted it: 'My grace is sufficient for thee' (II Cor. 12.9). We find it in the mouth of the Psalmist: 'Yea, though I walk through the valley of the shadow of death, I will fear no evil; for thou art with me' (Ps. 23.4). This certainty of divine protection whatever happens fills the whole Bible: 'Fear not, for I have redeemed thee; I have called thee by thy name, thou art mine. When thou passest through the waters, I will be with thee; and through the rivers, they shall not overflow thee: when thou walkest through the fire, thou shalt not be burned; neither shall the flame kindle upon thee' (Isa. 43.1-2).

Notes

1. See Pouyanne, "Le Médicin et la vie chrétienne," in *Les Deux Cités,* No. 4, Cahiers des Associations professionelles protestantes, 5 rue Cermeschi, Paris.

2. *Notes sur la signification que la Révélation biblique donne à la mort,* unpublished.

3. André Schlemmer 'Médecine', in *La foi chrétienne et l'Université,* 'Foi et Vie' Books, 139 Bd. Montparnasse, Paris.

4. Jean Calvin, *Contre la secte phantastique et furieuse des libertins qui se nomment spirituels,* Op. VIII, p. 246, 1545.

5. A. Stocker, *Amour et sensualité,* Œuvre de Saint-Augustin, St. Moritz, 1951.

6. The Secularization of American Medicine

ROY BRANSON

Physicians have reason to be frightened. The American Medical Association opposes national health insurance because it knows voting of such a proposal by Congress will mark the end of medicine's privileged status among professions in America. It will memorialize the transferring of power from the professional in medicine to the layman. Under the pressure of increasingly powerful outside forces, America's most cloistered profession has already begun conforming to the values, norms and practices of the society around it. Physicians know that with comprehensive health insurance Congress will be celebrating nothing less than the secularization of American medicine.

Enough has been written by sociologists and historians to demonstrate that health and disease are not purely physiological, but conditions defined by the whole matrix of human expectations, beliefs and habits. Medicine has always been practiced within the context of what a society conceived as normative in thought and action. The enormous prestige of medicine in the recent history of America derives, to a large extent, from its adherence to values and norms that have been central to American society. The problem for medicine today is that these values sometimes stand in opposition to other values, equally fundamental to American society.

Medicine continues to have faith in the inherent value of reason to discover order in empirical facts, continues to believe scientific and technological knowledge testify to a rational order.[1] It is an unquestioned good that man should know this order. Medicine believes man should not only discern order intellectually, but he should also act according to rationally ordered patterns. Because it adheres to the value of order in both thought and action, medicine acts according to the criterion of effectiveness. Medicine could not help but flourish in an America loyal to scientific rationality and bureaucratic efficiency.

But now values as basic to America as rationality and order are being powerfully articulated. There are increasing demands that the self-evident truths of freedom and equality of all men be extended throughout American society. It is being argued that no group has the right, because of its knowledge and effectiveness—no matter how impressive—to dictate the terms of life and death to the rest of society. Every group of experts, including medical doctors, must recognize the basic equality of all men to set the conditions of their existence. Doctors are faced with the norm they so treasure—effectiveness—losing precedence to free participation of equals as the criterion society follows in deciding problems of medical care.

This fundamental shift in emphasis from order and technical knowledge to equality and freedom, from efficiency of the expert to participation of the citizen, will affect the roles of doctor and patient. As much as loss of revenue, this is what frightens the physician. Patients will not as easily allow themselves to be treated as deviants from the doctor's marvelously rational world. They will not revere the physician as the mediator of special knowledge. Patients will quite likely regard themselves as fellow-citizens demanding technical information. Certainly any sense that medical care is a privilege that the physician mediates to those he chooses will give way to the community asserting, indeed enforcing, its right to medical care.

The Religion of Medicine

Alterations in medical care have been analyzed from the perspectives of economics and political theory. But if the controversy and deep emotion accompanying basic alterations in medical practice are to be understood, it must be realized that medicine in America has not been merely one more occupation in our economic system or an effective power bloc in American polity. Medicine's roots go deeper. If we are to understand why the conflicts over federal health care legislation have been so passionate, we must realize that medicine has acted in America as a kind of religious system, with its own symbols, values, institutions and rituals.

Robert Bellah defines religion "as a set of symbolic forms and acts which relate man to the ultimate conditions of his existence."[2] Thomas O'Dea concurs: "Religion is a response to the ultimate which becomes institutionalized in thought, practice and organization."[3] Agreement with his fellow sociologists on a functional definition of religion allows J. Milton Yinger to describe science as an attempt to deal with ultimate questions, to characterize science as a religious enterprise.

> Few men can avoid the problem of struggling with questions of salvation (how can man be

From the *Hastings Center Studies* 1, no. 2 (1973): 17-28. Used by permission of the publisher and the author.

> saved from his most difficult problems?), of the nature of reality, of evil (why do men suffer?), and the like. Science as a way of life is an effort to deal with these questions.[4]

Science affirms that there is an ideal natural order, a set of laws or patterns, and that, as Stephen Toulmin puts it, "these ideals of natural order have something absolute about them."[5] Science has believed that ultimate questions could be answered by knowing the order it affirms. The scientist has seemed to say to his fellow men that "if we know or are aware of everything, if we understand all relevant causes and factors, we can control everything." The scientist, quintessential modern man, has genuinely believed and committed his life to what Langdon Gilkey calls "faith in the healing power of knowledge."[6]

Medicine, of course, is the healing knowledge par excellence. Medicine assumes that disorders can be treated by relying on the order science proclaims. "The science of medicine depends on the faith that it is not chance which operates, but cause."[7]

Talcott Parsons argues that while the cosmos proclaimed by traditional religion no longer dominates modern culture, society depends for its very existence on some sense of order. He suggests that the pattern of beliefs and values integrating contemporary culture is maintained by the "intellectual disciplines," among which science is pre-eminent.[8] If Parsons is right that science has replaced religion (narrowly defined) as the unifying focus of modern culture, then medicine is part of the central faith of our times.

Because medicine has identified itself so closely with science it has gained great authority as a profession. One of America's foremost sociologists of medicine, Eliot Freidson, is convinced that

> medicine is not merely one of the major professions of our time. Among the traditional professions established in the European universities of the Middle Ages, it alone has developed a systematic connection with science and technology. . . . Medicine has displaced the law and the ministry from their once dominant positions.[9]

Much of the credit physicians receive for knowing the true order of things, for being experts, comes from medicine's widely proclaimed commitment to the scientific ideals of knowledge and order.

Medicine, of course, is not a purely scholarly profession. It would not be supported by the public for simply possessing knowledge. Medicine is expected to transmute science into therapy, knowledge into action. As they move from theory to practice, physicians adhere strictly to their scientific faith, trying not only to think but act in orderly fashion. Physicians who believe in a reality that is coherent regulate their actions by strict patterns of behavior. Medical doctors are committed to following procedures that have the least waste motion, that cure in the shortest amount of time. Physicians believe they should move as directly as possible from symptom to cause, from cause to treatment. The profession of medicine combines the values of scientific faith—knowledge and order—with concrete norms for regulating medical practice—effectiveness and efficiency. Medicine, then, not only conforms to what has been the fundamental perspective of modern, scientific culture, but energetically follows some of the guiding principles of pragmatic, American society. It is no wonder medicine has enjoyed enormous prestige in America.

So great has been the respect accorded medicine by American society that some commentators have come to describe it as more than an ordinary profession. Freidson believes "medicine's position today is akin to that of the state religions yesterday—it has an officially approved monopoly of the right to define health and illness and to treat illness."[10]

It is understandable that medicine would achieve such an exalted status in American society; that it would be trusted not only to control but define deviancy. What would be more appropriate than a group so obviously dedicated to order and effectiveness deciding what constitutes deviance from these values and standards?

Talcott Parsons, who has done as much as anyone to show disease to be not simply a physical condition but a social role, goes so far as to call disease the primary type of deviance in American society.[11] He does so because a person in a diseased condition cannot be effective, cannot achieve.[12] Of course, the diseased person not only violates norms regulating behavior in society. He is at fundamental odds with the natural order. Parsons follows the logic of his reasoning. He explicitly correlates illness with original sin.[13]

Freidson agrees that the stigma of having been a deviant stays with the diseased person, even after he has recovered; that someone who has received grace remains in some sense a sinner, or at least an ex-sinner. But Freidson insists that there are still important variations in society's abhorrence of disease. He suggests that two independent criteria, personal responsibility and seriousness of condition, are used to distinguish, for example, among a careless youngster sniffling from a cold, a drunk bleeding from a brawl, a bachelor suffering from venereal disease, and a gunman critically wounded in an attempted homicide.[14] Freidson's clarifications do not contradict Parsons' basic point. Indeed both men assume the same premise. "Quite unlike neutral scientific concepts like that of 'virus' or 'molecule,' the concept of illness is inherently evaluational. Medicine is a moral enterprise."[15]

Indeed, in a scientific age, where illness becomes the most ubiquitous label for deviance, medicine emerges as a crucial agent in the application of the scientific creed to a variety of problems. Consider the importance of medical testimony in courts and the influence of medical opinion in defining alcoholism and drug addiction as not strictly ecclesiastical or legal issues but as health problems. Imperceptibly, physicians, as loyal defenders of rationality, order and effectiveness, become the group that defines normality, that arbitrates orthodoxy in modern culture.[16]

Of course, physicians are not content to identify sin. They have the ability to combat it. Their knowledge of science and their extended training in applying that knowledge in a rational, disciplined manner give them confidence that evil can be purified. Men who are not in harmony with the basic order of existence can be restored. Those who have capitulated, who believe they cannot perform according to acceptable standards, can be rehabilitated. Medicine has the means.[17]

For those means to be effective the agents of order and rationality must be trusted. The sick and those responsible for them must realize that they cannot find restoration by their own efforts. They must rely on those who are competent in these matters; those who possess the proper knowledge. Furthermore, it is impossible for each practitioner to be asked to prove and re-prove his merit every time he heals. Patients must come to trust physicians as such; not the admittedly fluctuating worth of individual doctors, but the office of physician.[18] It will not do for patients to take their own medical records from one waiting room to another demanding evidence of a doctor's competence. The sick must put themselves in the hands of the professional. Patients must believe in physicians. "Their therapy depends upon faith. And we may be wise to recognize that there is a faithful quality to medical practice."[19]

The most obvious way for the diseased to show their trust in the representatives of science and their desire to return to a life of rationality and order is for patients to follow the procedures outlined for them by their physicians. It is "the patient's obligation faithfully to accept the implications of the fact that he is 'Dr. X's patient' and so long as he remains in that status he must 'do his part' in the common enterprise."[20] The patient is out of harmony with the basic order of existence. He suffers from the power of disruptive forces distorting his life. Through the course of action outlined by the physician, the patient can experience the power of rationality in his own life. By means of carefully planned actions the physician mediates the mysteries of scientific research for the benefit of ordinary, diseased patients. In the process, medicine creates a ritual system, and the doctor becomes a priest.

As is the case in all religious systems, medicine's symbols are effective because they arise from generally accepted truths. The impact of these symbols is familiar. With the separation of the priest from the layman, the mystery enshrouding the priest expands and his authority increases.

A desire to avoid contamination may be the basis for the physicians' dress, but their spotless white apparel instantly conveys an aura that divides the diseased from the holy. Even when their attire cannot contribute to asepsis, physicians cling to their peculiar vestments.[21] Traditional clerics and theologians have begun to refer to their new colleagues and rivals as "the men in the white coats."[22] Technical language may be precise and convenient, but it also allows conversations among physicians which the laymen are not ready to hear. If the laymen did understand, their questions would impede the efficiency of efforts to rescue them from their grave condition.[23]

Asking a deviant for the location of records of his past actions, requiring him to give a recital of his previous deeds and present attitudes, demanding that he disrobe for a careful examination of the visible signs of his polluted state, all have good, scientific justification. They also comprise an interrogation as old as Egyptian medical rites and as intimidating as any confession taken in the Inquisition.[24] After this ritual there is no question as to where authority in the doctor-patient relationship lies.

If any doubt lingers, it is soon expelled. The fully-robed, impressively self-contained examiner pronounces a verdict on the condition of the diseased. He may grant complete absolution, saying that the problem is imaginary, or he may absolve the diseased of any guilt for his present condition; none of his past actions have led to his present deplorable state. Quite likely the inquisitor points out where there have been some past transgressions contributing to the present turmoil, and prescribes a series of penitential acts by which purity may be regained.[25] The discipline may include the purchase of objects with special powers to assist in achieving full release.[26] If the condition is serious a sentence of separation from the healthy may be pronounced. Those untouched by the corruption deserve protection, and the diseased must be encouraged to seek a new life.[27]

The authority of the physician reaches its heights

when men face the ultimate threat of death. The terror is greatest because the secrecy is absolute. Nothing is more mysterious or tremendous than death, nothing more daunting. Before this final specter men become desperate for the reliable knowledge of science. They gladly deliver themselves into the hands of its representative, pleading for him to effectively impose rational order on lives being drawn into chaos. As Parsons observes,

> It is striking that the medical is one of the few occupational groups which in our society have regular, expected contact with death in the course of their occupational roles.... It is presumed that this association with death is a very important factor in the emotional toning of the role of the physician.[28]

He goes on to say that while he believes the physician is not identical to a clergyman, he "has very important associations with the sacred."[29] Certainly the patient, desperate to achieve salvation from death, regards a physician offering him medicine with the same awe as he does a priest extending the wafer. The physician is providing a visible means by which man may receive salvation.

Parsons' own illustrations of the sacred within clinical training and practice point less in the direction of internal medicine and more towards surgery.

> Dissection is not only an instrumental means to the learning of anatomy, but is a symbolic act, highly charged with affective significance. It is in a sense the initiatory rite of the physician-to-be into his intimate association with death and the dead.[30]

If dissection of an already dead cadaver is an initiatory rite, how is cutting into a living body to be regarded? Clearly, at the present time, the medical profession itself looks on this act with the greatest awe. Medical students list surgery as a desirable specialty because it is "one which offers a wide variety of experience and in which responsibility is symbolized by the possibility of killing or disabling patients in the course of making a mistake."[31] Training to become a surgeon is the longest in medicine, and the profession has agreed that performing an operation should bring the highest financial reward of any single act in medical practice.

As for the sick, nothing in medicine frightens them more than surgery.[32] They know that the potential benefits are great. Patients feel that an operation, if survived, promises the fastest and most efficient recovery from a major illness.[33] But the sick also know that for a major operation, they must knowingly relinquish to the doctor complete control over their destiny. On previous occasions the patient has been dependent on the physician, but at no other time is the act of submission into the hands of a doctor so carefully considered, so self-conscious.

Once the decision is made, a prescribed, carefully planned sequence of actions is set in motion. The force of these lengthy preparations comes from the knowledge that they are required by the rational, orderly faith of science. Deviations will bring evil consequences, severe complications.

Days before the operation the patient enters a rigid discipline. His actions are restricted. His diet becomes even more controlled than before. The day of the operation he receives special, cleansing ministrations.

Few know exactly what transpires within the secluded area where surgery is performed. Ordinary functionaries are not allowed entrance; only those with special training. Even these enter only after purifying themselves. The surgeon himself must unvaryingly observe necessary ablutions before approaching the body. Reports indicate that drugs administered to the patient bring a deep sleep. Special ointments applied to the body complete the rituals anticipating the climactic act. Then, according to the requirements of science, the knife falls.

Of course, some are lost though their death often advances the cause of science. But sacrifice is not the culminating rite of this religion. Many recover from surgery. When they do, the religion of medicine has been able to do nothing less than ritualize the miracle of miracles. Through the surgeon's knowledge of the fundamental order of reality and his performance in the most efficient manner possible, a body has been laid to rest, and risen again.[34]

Not surprisingly, no believer testifies more zealously to his faith than the newly-recovered surgical patient. In his previous, broken condition he felt himself the least knowledgeable, least effective member of the medical community. Within the medical hierarchy it seemed appropriate that he occupy the lowest position. Grateful for his astonishing recovery, the patient regards the surgeon as high priest.

Profanation of the Religion

Except for the years from the Renaissance to the nineteenth century in the West, the physician has always been regarded as a priest. Only during the relatively brief period when faith in miraculous healing through incantation and prayer was being lost and trust in a substitute authority had not yet emerged, did the physician lose his aura of possessing sacred powers. In primitive tribes, in the high cultures of

Mesopotamia, Egypt, China, India, Greece and Rome, right into the Christian Middle Ages, the physician was a religious functionary.[35]

Universally, disease was considered an evidence of sin. Not only in primitive tribes, but in Mesopotamia, Egypt, India, Mexico and Christian countries, confession necessarily preceded cure.[36] Potions with mysterious powers and rituals with guaranteed purgative effect have been prescribed by all civilizations. In Egypt, India and Greece, incubation was a central part of medical treatment.[37] The building to which the patient traveled for his healing sleep (when he was visited by the gods) were temples, presided over by physicians who were priests.[38] Especially charismatic physicians evolved from mediators of the sacred into its incarnation; for example, Akhnaten in Egypt and Aesculapius in Greece.[39]

As late as the seventeenth century the clergy were the principal healers in America.[40] Even today in America, there are hospitals with religious sponsorship, operated by ecclesiastical orders.

However, it is undeniable that from the Renaissance into the nineteenth century, medicine, in the West, suffered a crisis of confidence. No potion, no priesthood, no prayers, could stay the ravages of the Plague. As many people died under medical care as survived. Increasingly, the masses were unwilling to dismiss this record as the all-wise will of God. Hospitals, far from being temples, were shunned as repositories of those already enduring the final agonies of death.[41]

The recovery of medicine's influence and authority followed the rise of a new confidence in science. Though it came late, long after basic scientific discoveries, medicine finally discovered vaccines for immunizing mass populations and developed aseptic and anesthetic procedures, allowing the performance of extensive surgery.[42] Medicine had found the effective means to mediate the new, scientific world view.

The buildings where the new scientific wonders were discovered or performed ceased to be shunned as charnel houses. The population, as they had not since perhaps the days of Egypt and Greece, were awed by the new mysterious power active in these edifices. They flocked to them, seeking release from their grievous condition. Once again, in the twentieth century, the physician found amidst the marvels of scientific technology, the appropriate setting for his traditional role of wonder-worker. Never has he been more revered.

But medicine faces a crisis as challenging to its authority as the Renaissance and Enlightenment's diminished faith in the efficacy of prayer and miracle. Just as men's reliance on their own ability to think and act during that time undercut the influence of priestly physicians so today's demand for self-determination in every sector of society threatens medicine's independence of action. The process by which the laity in some parts of the West seized control of the church in the sixteenth century, the state in the eighteenth and nineteenth centuries and the economy in the twentieth, is now threatening the autonomy of science and technology. Medicine, so proudly identified as a bastion of scientific orthodoxy, must brace itself for this latest wave of reformation.[43]

Talcott Parsons identifies the present stage of reformation as an "education revolution" that insists that all institutions, groups and professions must operate in accordance with wider cultural values. Groups can find their own special areas of concern, but they must conform to the culture's general values. If they do not, if a group insists on remaining isolated, acting according to its own idiosyncratic principles, it is falling into a fundamentalism. Examples could include the American Amish, the Roman Catholic Curia, as well as such twentieth-century political movements as Fascism and Stalinism.[44] If the scientific community rejects the basic values of a culture, it too is fundamentalist.

Reformers of contemporary culture, concerned about segments of society resisting universal values, understandably concentrate their attention on the professions. From Emile Durkheim on, social philosophers have regarded the professions as pivotal elements in modern society. With the disappearance of the tribe and the weakening of the family and church, the professions have become crucial as moral orders, drawing men not only into common tasks, but common interpretations of life.[45] Parsons goes so far as to say that

> the professional complex, though obviously still incomplete in its development, has already become the most important single component in the structure of modern societies . . . the massive emergence of the professional complex, not the special status of capitalistic or socialistic modes of organization is the crucial development in twentieth-century society.[46]

As we have already noted, with the waning of faith, the clergy has differentiated into distinct professions. These newer orders of service within society have gained recognition because of their technical knowledge, their mastery of a particular set of facts and skills, but the professions have also become influential because they have been relied upon to continue the traditional function of the clergy: inculcating within individuals the overarching values of a culture.

Max Weber quite consciously called the scientific professions a "calling," with the clear religious overtones that word carries, to underline the central role of these particular professions in mediating the values of the modern, scientific age.[47] If our previous analysis is correct, medicine is the profession within the scientific callings that has most clearly assumed the function of the clergy.[48]

Protestants against this new priesthood do not dispute the technical expertise of physicians, but they do object to medical doctors thinking that mastery of scientific data qualifies them to act as moral arbiters. Influence and leadership within a society, they say, should result from adherence to universally acknowledged moral principles.

Of course physicians, and others in the scientific callings, have thought that they already lived according to the basic beliefs of the age. Certainly science has kept faith with rationality and order. It is startling to hear contemporary reformers inveighing against science as a new orthodoxy blind to more inclusive concerns. Today's reformers declare that knowledge is not sacrosanct. They demand that science recognize the priority of equality and freedom.

Appeals to equality and freedom may initially seem harmless enough. But when the reformers begin to draw out the implications of these values physicians become aware that a full-dress challenge is under way to their profession and its hallowed status. Equality means extension of power beyond the privileged few. Today's laity, like their predecessors in previous centuries, claim that equality gives them the right to participate in making decisions affecting their own lives and destiny.

Participation in medicine means invading the heart of its authority: defining the nature of disease.[49] Physicians can list a set of symptoms, but it is up to the general population to decide whether or not the condition described by the physician is normal or abnormal, acceptable or unacceptable. Definition of sin cannot be the exclusive preserve of those ordained by the community to wage war against evil.[50]

If equality means the laity involves itself to the point of defining illness, it certainly means laymen can set priorities as to which diseases are especially abhorrent, and which will receive less attention. Allocation of medical resources is the prerogative of the donors, not the functionaries receiving funds to perform designated services. Equality, for many reformers, even means that laymen retain the right to decide whether or not the method by which a physician treats a deviant conforms to generally accepted standards of behavior and practice.[51] Regional medical programs, comprehensive health planning, public review boards, and even the courts, are all ways in which laymen are already beginning to exercise authority over professionals in medicine.[52]

As this process of secularization continues, the roles of the patient and doctor will be affected. The patient will approach the physician, not as a suppliant, but as a fellow-citizen. He will not request expiation of his condition, but affirm his right, as a member of the community, to medical care. The physician can continue to have authority, but in a much more limited sphere. The function of the physician will be much more specific. He will provide information concerning the etiology and rehabilitation of various physical disorders.

Secularization seems always to affect ritual last. As long as death, or the possibility of death, continues to strike fear in human beings, actions that are able to ward it off, or at least postpone its advent, will elicit confidence. No doubt the rite of surgery will continue to create a response of dread and awe. Certainly individual acts of healing will result in grateful patients according respect to their own physician.

But as medicine enters a new era, the rituals of cure are less impressive than the cooperative efforts of a community trying to improve its general health. The citizenry is becoming less inclined to measure the adequacy of medicine by miraculous deeds in the temple, and more interested in finding a way of life that makes spectacular cures unnecessary. Participation is moving beyond citizens asserting their control over the processes of cure to their assuming responsibility for bettering the conditions for health. The goal is not simply reforming the ministrations of physicians, but improving the health of the community to the point where their mediation is almost unnecessary.[53]

Of course, the majority of American physicians stress the dangers of this secularization of medicine. As the goal of medicine moves from cure to health, they warn that medicine's task will become much more diffuse and ill-defined. It will be less easy to integrate into a coherent pattern the knowledge needed for this expanded enterprise. It will be impossible to rely on a stable body of information to achieve specific ends. Furthermore, as the task broadens, individuals from increasingly diverse disciplines will be needed. The process of coordinating these increasingly differentiated roles will make medicine less precise. As the widened goal of health is pursued, previous standards of effectiveness in cure will be impossible to maintain. When these developments coincide with common citizens insisting on exercising their influence in medical matters, barbarism will have engulfed the orderly, scientific practice of medicine in America.[54]

The American medical community may be correct that the efficacy of their expertise is threatened by present trends. If our analysis is correct, the changes coming in American medicine are so thoroughgoing, affecting, as they do, its values, norms, roles and practices, that no one can guarantee that the future will improve on the past. However, for better or worse, one thing is certain about American medicine: it must either narrow its understanding of itself or broaden its vision.

Medicine can become one occupation among many dealing with the improvement of a community's health; that occupation responsible for the technical question of finding the physical causes and cures of disease. It can remain committed exclusively to rationality, order and effectiveness. Physicians can become ever more efficient in performing their unending round of therapeutic rituals. There is no doubt that a culture needs these tasks performed.

Or, medicine can accept the vast challenge of improving America's health. It can embrace the values of equality and freedom, and recognize the right of the whole population to involve itself in determining the nature of disease and the priorities of medical care. Medicine can redefine its task as not exclusively ceremonial, but increasingly educational. To a population with rising expectations of participation it can respond with full disclosure concerning the facts of health and cure. If physicians want to continue to enjoy the enormous respect and influence they have heretofore received in American society, they must consider assuming the crucial job of dramatizing, for the public, conditions preventing a general improvement in health.

The days when the mysteries of science could be relied upon to awe the credulous are fading quickly. Faith in the power of technical reason to save man is dead. Physicians cannot survive as mediators of the holy. With the secularization of medicine, doctors will most likely endure as civil-service technicians.

The only alternative is for physicians to launch themselves into a life where scientific knowledge gives no automatic advantage, where worth depends on sensitivity to principles known to all. Among the most highly respected individuals in American society today are those who point out to the community those places where its disregard for basic values maims and kills; those who arouse the citizenry to correct injustices and thereby improve and save the lives of thousands.[55]

Recognition that science can no longer be a religion will lead physicians to realize that they can no longer be priests performing mysterious healing rites. Instead, physicians adopting the role of pointing out the relevance of universal values and norms to particular evils will have found a new way of life. They will be demonstrating a loyalty to the freedom, dignity and worth of man. They will have put their trust in the enduring validity of morality. They will have become prophets. The secularization of medicine may prove to be its salvation.

Notes

1. Paul Tillich, *Systematic Theology,* I (Chicago: University of Chicago Press, 1951), pp. 53-54, 72-74. Reason here refers to what Tillich called *technical reason.* "By the technical concept of reason, reason is reduced to the capacity for reasoning. Only the cognitive side of reason remains and within the cognitive realm only those cognitive acts which deal with the discovery of means for ends" (pp. 72, 73). Tillich contrasts technical reason with ontological reason. "According to the classical philosophical tradition reason is the structure of the mind which enables the mind to grasp and to transform reality. It is effective in the cognitive, aesthetic, practical and technical functions of the mind" (p. 72). Elsewhere, he identifies ontological reason with ecstatic and existential reason. "Ecstatic reason is reason grasped by an ultimate concern" (p. 53). What Tillich calls ontological reason, could not be opposed to a sense of equality and freedom; but rationality, narrowly defined as technical reason, can be. Cf. Langdon Gilkey, *Religion and the Scientific Future* (New York: Harper & Row, 1970), p. 96. "Knowing for Greek philosophy, was not *techne,* knowing how to do something; it was rather *wisdom,* knowledge of the self. . . . Modern knowing is science, on the other hand; it represents objective knowledge of external structure unrelated to the self, or to the mystery of its freedom."

2. Robert Bellah, "Religious Evolution," *American Sociological Review* 29 (June, 1964), p. 359.

3. Thomas O'Dea, *The Sociology of Religion* (Englewood Cliffs, N.J.: Prentice-Hall, Inc., 1966), p. 27; cf. Milton J. Yinger, *The Scientific Study of Religion* (New York, N.Y.: Macmillan Co., 1970), p. 7. "Religion, then, can be defined as a system of beliefs and practices by means of which a group of people struggle with these ultimate problems of human life."

4. Yinger, *The Scientific Study of Religion,* p. 12.

5. Stephen Toulmin, *Foresight and Understanding* (New York: Harper & Row, 1961), p. 57.

6. Gilkey, *Religion and the Future,* p. 52. "Use of knowledge for control over physical nature has until the present raised few moral problems, and so the model taken from engineering and medicine has seemed to validate over and over this hope for a better scientific technology" (p. 85). Cf. pp. 79, 85-89, 95, 96.

7. Lester S. King, *The Growth of Medical Thought* (Chicago: University of Chicago Press, 1963), p. 36.

8. Talcott Parsons, *The System of Modern Societies* (Englewood Cliffs, N.J.: Prentice-Hall, Inc., 1971), p. 99.

9. Eliot Freidson, *Profession of Medicine* (New York: Dodd, Mead & Co., 1970), p. xviii; cf. Talcott Parsons, "A Sociologist Looks at the Legal Profession," in *Essays in Sociological Theory* (New York: Free Press, 1949), p. 376.

"Established scientific knowledge *does* constitute a highly stable point of reference. Hence the 'authority' of the relevant professional groups for interpretations can always be referred to such established knowledge."

10. Freidson, *Profession of Medicine,* p. 5.

11. Talcott Parsons, "Definitions of Health and Illness in the Light of American Values and Social Structure," in *Patients, Physicians and Illness,* ed. by E. Gartley Jaco (New York: Free Press, 1958), p. 186.

12. Ibid., p. 185; cf. Talcott Parsons, *The Social System* (New York: Free Press, 1951), pp. 437-439.

13. Parsons, "Definitions of Health and Illness," p. 175; cf. Freidson, *Profession of Medicine,* p. 231.

14. The specific examples are mine, not Freidson's.

15. Freidson, *Profession of Medicine,* pp. 208, 233, 236, 252; cf. pp. 339-340. "Furthermore, an essential component of what is said to be knowledge is the designation of illness, which, I have insisted, is in and of itself, evaluative and moral rather than technical in character."

16. Ibid., pp. 244, 248-249; cf. Parsons, *The Social System,* p. 445.

17. Parsons, "Definitions of Health and Illness," p. 178.

18. Parsons, *The Social System,* p. 439.

19. Yinger, *Study of Religion,* p. 77; cf. Eliot Freidson, *Professional Dominance: The Social Structure of Medical Care* (New York: Atherton Press, 1972), pp. 119, 143.

20. Parsons, *The Social System,* p. 465.

21. Julius A. Roth, "Ritual and Magic in the Control of Contagion," *American Sociological Review* 20 (June, 1957), pp. 310-314; cf. Freidson, *Profession of Medicine,* p. 9.

22. Gilkey, *Religion and the Future,* p. 79.

23. Raymond S. Duff and August B. Hollingshead, *Sickness and Society* (New York: Harper & Row, 1968), pp. 132, 327.

24. Erwin H. Ackerknecht, *A Short History of Medicine* (New York: Ronald Press, 1968), p. 16; cf. Henry E. Sigerist, *A History of Medicine* (New York: Oxford University Press, 1951), pp. 188, 196.

25. Freidson, *Profession of Medicine,* p. 228.

26. Yinger, *Study of Religion,* p. 77.

27. Freidson, *Profession of Medicine,* pp. 228, 313-314; cf. Talcott Parsons and Renée Fox, "Illness, Therapy and the Modern Urban American Family," *Patients, Physicians and Illness,* pp. 241, 244.

28. Parsons, *The Social System,* pp. 444-445.

29. Ibid., p. 445.

30. Ibid.

31. Eliot Freidson, "Medical Personnel," *International Encyclopedia of the Social Sciences,* 2nd edition, 10, p. 107; based on data from Howard S. Becker, et al., *Boys in White; Student Culture in Medical School* (Chicago: University of Chicago Press, 1961).

32. Duff and Hollingshead, *Sickness and Society,* p. 273.

33. Ibid., p. 294.

34. For a concurring analysis of surgery (though the two analyses were developed independently of each other) see Robert N. Wilson, "Teamwork in the Operating Room," *Human Organization* 12 (Winter, 1954), pp. 9-14.

35. In addition to the works of Ackerknecht and Sigerist already cited, I am especially indebted for the historical background given by the following authors: Lester S. King, *The Growth of Medical Thought* and George Rosen, "The Hospital: Historical Sociology of a Community Institution," in *The Hospital in Modern Society,* ed. by Eliot Freidson (Glencoe, Ill.: Free Press, 1963).

36. Ackerknecht, *History of Medicine,* pp. 27-28, 31, 38; Sigerist, *History of Medicine,* pp. 188, 196.

37. Ackerknecht, *History of Medicine,* pp. 21, 41, 50.

38. Rosen, *Hospital in Society,* pp. 26, 29.

39. Ackerknecht, *History of Medicine,* pp. 21, 50.

40. Ibid., pp. 219, 220.

41. Rosen, *Hospital in Society,* pp. 26-29.

42. Ackerknecht, *History of Medicine,* p. 171; King, *Growth of Medical Thought,* p. 221; Freidson, *Profession of Medicine,* p. 16.

43. Parsons, *System of Modern Societies,* p. 99. Although Parsons does not interpret changes within medicine as a process of secularization, he does note that significant developments within the field are taking place. He analyzes the changes in medicine in terms that he elsewhere uses to describe developments in religious structures; developments which he calls secularization. See in particular, Parsons, "Some Theoretical Considerations Bearing on the Field of Medical Sociology," *Social Structure and Personality* (New York: Free Press, 1964), p. 257. "A further highly significant feature of the general process of change which has been going on is the generalization of the value complex involving health problems. This is a relatively intangible matter to which little explicit research attention has been devoted." Ibid., p. 355. Freidson does put changes within medicine in a historical continuity with secularization of institutional religion. See *Profession of Medicine,* pp. xviii, 250.

44. Parsons, *System of Modern Societies,* p. 100.

45. Emile Durkheim, *On the Division of Labor in Society,* trans. by George Simpson (New York: 1893); Cornelia Brookfield, *Professional Ethics and Civic Morals* (London: 1898-1900). Theodore M. Steeman, "Durkheim's Professional Ethics," *Journal for the Scientific Study of Religion* 2 (April, 1963), pp. 163-181. C. P. Wold, "The Durkheim Thesis: Occupational Groups and Moral Integration," *Journal for the Scientific Study of Religion* 2 (Spring, 1970), pp. 17-32.

46. "Professions," the *International Encyclopedia of the Social Sciences,* 2nd edition, 12, p. 545.

47. *From Max Weber,* ed. and trans. by H. H. Gerth and C. Wright Mills (New York: Oxford University Press, 1936), pp. 129-156; Robert M. Veatch, "Medical Ethics; Professional or Universal?" Working Paper for the Institute of Society, Ethics and the Life Sciences. Hastings-on-Hudson, New York, p. 2. A comparison of professional to universal ethics in medicine.

48. Freidson, *Profession of Medicine,* pp. 335, 348.

49. Ibid., p. 206.

50. Ibid., pp. 252, 342-343, 345.

51. Ibid., pp. 345, 374; Veatch, "Medical Ethics," pp. 16-18.

52. See Barbara Ehrenreich, *American Health Empire* (New York: Random House, 1970) for criticisms of these

programs and arguments for more radical proposals for community control of health care.

53. See Bellah's article "Religious Evolution" for helpful periodization of religious change. Within Bellah's stages of primitive, archaic, historic, early modern and modern, medicine might be described as in transition from historic to early modern. There is a shift from an emphasis on sacrifice to morality, from dependence on the rituals of the temple to a kind of "inner-worldly" maintenance of health. As medicine moves on from its present point of maturation there will likely be increased emphasis on each person maintaining his own health through measures that heretofore have not been considered "medical." Living a well-rounded life, with its appropriate measure of recreation, reflection and aesthetic endeavors will all be seen as part of the good, healthy life, with each person free to combine the various elements according to what is best for him. At that point, medicine will have reached Bellah's modern stage of religion, where each man echoes Jefferson's statement that "I am a sect myself." Cf. Parsons, *Social Structure and Personality,* p. 355.

54. Freidson, *Profession of Medicine,* pp. 352–353.

55. Robert F. Buckhorn, *Nader: The People's Lawyer* (Englewood Cliffs, N.J.: Prentice-Hall, Inc., 1972), p. 276. "Pollster Louis Harris ran a survey of 1,620 families in March, 1971, asking a nationwide cross-section this question: 'Do you feel that in his attacks on American industry, consumer-advocate, Ralph Nader, has done more good than harm, or more harm than good?' The result: a lopsided 53 percent to 9 percent agreed that Nader was doing more good than harm. . . . Louis Harris said the survey showed that, basically, the efforts of Nader 'have been extremely well received by the American public.' A poll by George Gallup taken in the same month showed that out of 1,571 persons sampled, Nader was known to 50 percent of American men and 37 percent of the women. That would be a recognition factor at the time higher than most of the announced presidential candidates."

Chapter Two
THEOLOGY AND MEDICAL ETHICS

Introduction

In the article which heads this section James Gustafson observes that a good deal of the literature on medical ethics, even when written by people trained as theologians, makes no explicit reference to theological affirmations or to religious convictions. He acknowledges that there are sometimes good reasons for bracketing one's religious convictions but laments nevertheless the paucity of material which candidly attends to the relevance of religious traditions and theological reflection to issues in medical ethics. The first question set before the readers of this chapter, then, is whether it makes sense to share Gustafson's lament. Does theology have a contribution to make to medical ethics? Should people with religious convictions set them aside in order to engage in public discussion about issues in medical ethics? Can medical ethics be theological? Should it be? In what contexts is it appropriate to engage in theological reflection about medical ethics, and why?

If one shares Gustafson's lament, then a second set of questions becomes inescapable: What is the contribution of theology to medical ethics? How should theological reflection about these issues be conducted? The remaining essays in this chapter provide proposals for theological reflection about medical ethics. Taken together they raise some significant methodological questions.

One question is the appropriate mode of moral analysis. Richard McCormick would have us attend to certain values or goods to be sought and realized, but never repudiated. Richard Mouw, on the other hand, directs our attention to biblical commands. Paul Ramsey proposes that we attend to "canons of loyalty" or "relationally objective norms," as he calls them in another place. And Karen Labacqz finally recommends that questions of character, integrity, and virtue should be given first and central consideration.

To some extent, these alternative proposals simply rehearse the old debate in philosophical morality between theories which analyze and test conduct in terms of its relation to some good end (teleological theories), theories which analyze and test conduct in terms of its conformity to some right rule (deontological theories), and theories which analyze and test conduct in terms of its integrity and virtuous character. But in a theological account of morality the appropriate mode of moral analysis will have to be coherent with the way God is judged to be related to human moral agents, and that judgment will have to be coherent with the sources acknowledged as authoritative in and for the community. One might note and discuss, for example, Ramsey's emphasis on covenant, McCormick's attention not only to the creative and providential design of God but also to his redemptive intention in Jesus Christ, Mouw's emphasis on God as commander and lawgiver, and Lebacqz's attention to God as an agent in the narratives that Christian communities read and live.

A second set of methodologically significant questions has to do with the relation of a religious morality to the "natural" morality or, to state the issue differently, the relation of a theological perspective to an impartial perspective on the moral questions raised by advances in medical research and technology. Two interesting responses to Gustafson's lament raised this question. Stanley Hauerwas shares that lament but urges that Christian ethics "pay closer attention to its particularistic claims."[1] In other writings he has called attention to the fundamental irrelevance of the "natural morality" or impartial, universal, and purely rational morality. Over against its claims, he urges attention to an explicitly theological ethic. Richard McCormick, on the other hand, while applauding Gustafson's concern for theological reflection concerning medical morality, insists that the integrity of natural morality be recognized.[2]

Between the positions of Hauerwas and McCormick are those who would acknowledge "natural morality" or the moral truth which can be seen from an impartial perspective and nevertheless demand its transformation and a radical reorientation of perspective. The Christian tradition for example illumines and supports natural morality; it does not disown it. The options may be styled after H. Richard Niebuhr's famous typology in *Christ and Culture:*[3] theological ethics *of* natural morality, theological ethics *over against* natural morality, theological ethics *above* natural morality, theological ethics and natural morality *in creative tension,* or theological ethics *transforming* natural morality.

The backing for any methodological proposal will include theological affirmations about the relation of God to the world and correlative claims about human persons in relation to God. Specifically, if God's creative and redemptive relation to persons is emphasized but the significance of his relation to persons as judge (and the correlative recognition of persons as sinners) is ignored or disavowed, then natural morality will have a strong theological backing. If, on the other hand, God as judge and man as sinner—as fallen, even noetically—is emphasized, then the theologian will have considerably less confidence in natural morality. The theological affirmations need not be the only backing for such methodological proposals, of course. Philosophical judgments, social scientific judgments, and human experience are all relevant and provide tests for the adequacy of such methodological proposals. Even so, some coherence between theological judgments and the methodological proposal is not only a desideratum but a requirement.

A third methodological question is one of style. Mouw distinguishes a "priestly" and a "prophetic" style of reflection and calls for more prophetic critique. Gustafson's essay honors the "radically prophetic stance" but challenges its holders to the much more priestly exercise of helping people with the choices open to them in their social and historical circumstances.

Prophetic criticism is at risk of being tiresome and irrelevant without the mediation of the priest; yet priestly concern, assuming for the most part the legitimacy (or at least the inevitability) of current practices and institutions and attempting to be loving and fair within them, is at risk of being coopted by the establishment without the prophet. Perhaps a purely "priestly" contribution to bioethics would also be lamentable, as lamentable as any "prophetic" criticism that stands proud and aloof from the real world where people suffer within historical contexts and not just from them.

Finally, there is the matter of sources for a theological account of medical morality. To be sure methodological proposals here are related to the previous questions. If, for example, one defended theologically a position which honored the integrity of natural morality, then the moral philosophy which articulates that position will be a source as well as a conversation partner for a theological account of medical morality. Similarly, the priestly style might have an initial sympathy for and readiness to use the conventional or customary standards of medical practice as a source. But what of other sources: the sciences; the history of technology; legal and political traditions; the medical tradition; the Christian tradition, including ecclesiastical statements and the canonical part of that tradition, Scripture; and, finally, the experience of human beings, especially of those human beings who are Christian? How are these sources related to each other? Is any one authoritative compared to the others? Richard Mouw is quite candid about the authority of Scripture, for example, and that conviction is shared by many Christians. But how is this source to be used? What does it provide? If one granted the authority of Scripture as a source, one would still have to articulate its authority for particular uses in moral claims about medicine. Although Ramsey may share Mouw's affirmation about the authority of Scripture, for example, he seems content to extract "the Biblical norm of *fidelity to covenant*" and to fill in the meaning of that norm from the social and biological order. And Lebacqz is as candid as Mouw when she identifies the experience of the oppressed as a "primary source," presumably even for the interpretation of Scripture.

These are hard and complex questions. And there are more besides. But they are worth pondering and discussing if one is at all sympathetic with Gustafson's lament.

Notes

1. Stanley Hauerwas, "Can Ethics be Theological?" *Hastings Center Report* 8 (October, 1978): 47-49.
2. Richard A. McCormick, "Notes on Moral Theology," *Theological Studies* 40 (1979): 98-99.
3. H. Richard Niebuhr, *Christ and Culture* (New York: Harper and Row, 1951)

Suggestions for Further Reading

Ashley, Benedict M., O. P., and Kevin D. O'Rourke, O. P. *Health Care Ethics: A Theological Analysis.* 2d ed. St. Louis: Catholic Hospital Association of the United States, 1982.

Carney, F. S. "Theological Ethics." In *Encyclopedia of Bioethics.* New York: Macmillan, 1978. 1:429-37.

Dyck, Arthur. *On Human Care.* Nashville: Abingdon, 1977.

Gustafson, James M. *The Contributions of Theology to Medical Ethics.* Milwaukee: Marquette University Press, 1975.

Gustafson, James M., and Stanley M. Hauerwas, eds. *Theology and Medical Ethics.* Issue of *The Journal of Medicine and Philosophy* 4 (December 1979).

MacIntyre, Alasdair. "Can Medicine Dispense with a Theological Perspective on Human Nature?" In *The Roots of Ethics,* edited by Daniel Callahan and H. Tristam Englehardt. New York: Plenum Press, 1981.

Moltmann, Jürgen. "Hope and the Biomedical Future of Man." In *Hope and the Future of Man,* edited by Evert H. Cousins. Philadelphia: Fortress, 1972.

Shelp, Earl E., ed. *Theology and Bioethics: Exploring the*

Foundations and Frontiers. Philosophy and Medicine, vol. 20. Dordrecht: D. Reidel, 1985.
Simmons, Paul D. *Birth and Death: Bioethical Decision-Making.* Biblical Perspectives on Current Issues. Philadelphia: Westminster, 1983.

7. Theology Confronts Technology and the Life Sciences

JAMES M. GUSTAFSON

That persons with theological training are writing a great deal about technology and the life sciences is clear to those who read *The Hastings Center Report, Theological Studies* and many other journals. Whether *theology* is thereby in interaction with these areas, however, is less clear. For some writers the theological authorization for the ethical principles and procedures they use is explicit; this is clearly the case for the most prolific and polemical of the Protestants, Paul Ramsey. For others, writing as "ethicists," the relation of their moral discourse to any specific theological principles, or even to a definable religious outlook is opaque. Indeed, in response to a query from a friend (who is a distinguished philosopher) about how the term "ethicist" has come about, I responded in a pejorative way, "An ethicist is a former theologian who does not have the professional credentials of a moral philosopher."

Much of the writing in the field is by persons who desire to be known as "religious ethicists" if only to distinguish themselves for practical reasons from those holding cards in the philosophers' union. Exactly what the adjective "religious" refers to, however, is far from obvious. If it refers to something as specific as "Christian" or "Jewish," or even "Protestant" or "Catholic," presumably writers would be willing to use the proper term. Again Ramsey is to be commended; one can ask for nothing more forthright than his 1974 declaration, "I always write as the ethicist I am, namely a Christian ethicist, and not as some hypothetical common denominator." If "religious ethicists" would even say what the "religious dimensions" of the problems were, we could place the adjective in some frame of reference: Tillichian, Deweyan, Luckmannian, Geertzian or what have you.

The difficulties in formulating a theological (and not merely moral) confrontation with technology and the life sciences are real, and not just apparent, as any of us who have written in this area knows. Unless the intended readership is one internal to the theological

---

From *Commonweal* 105 (June 16, 1978): 386-92. Used by permission.

community, communication problems are exacerbated beyond the ordinary. Much of the writing is done for persons who are making policy or choices in the areas of technology, biological experimentation and clinical medicine. While there is a self-consciously Catholic constituency among these professional persons (for example, the members of the National Federation of Catholic Physicians' Guilds who sponsor *The Linacre Quarterly*), and while there may well be constituencies from the evangelical wing of Protestantism, most of the professional persons the writers seek to influence are judged not to be interested in the theological grounds from which the moral analysis and prescription grows. (I recall attending a party after a day of meetings with biologists and physicians at which a biologist, made friendlier by the ample libations provided, said to me, "Say something theological, Gustafson." I had the presence of mind to utter a guttural and elongated "Gawd.")

Not only is the audience frequently uninterested in the theological principles that might inform moral critique, but also the problems that are addressed are defined by the non-theologians, and usually are problems that emerge within a very confined set of circumstances. Should one cut the power source to a respirator for patient *y* whose circumstances are *a, b,* and *c?* Although the stakes are much higher, this is not utterly dissimilar to asking whether $8.20 an hour or $8.55 an hour ought to be paid to carpenter's helpers in Kansas City. Even a clear and well developed principle of distributive justice would not easily answer the latter question. To ask what "theology" might say to that question is patently more difficult. Obviously it is not easy to give a clearly theological answer to a question that is formulated so that there are no theological aspects to it. To make the practical moral question susceptible to any recognizably theological answer requires nursing, massaging, altering, and maybe even transforming processes. When these processes are completed one might discover that a different set of issues are under discussion from those that originated the interaction.

To respond to specific questions requires more acumen in moral reasoning than it requires theological learning and acumen. I am sure that the writers of the manuals in medical moral theology were well schooled in the tractates on the Trinity; the bearing of these texts on their medical moral discussions, however, is at best remote. It is quite understandable, then, that theology (either as doctrine from an historic tradition, or ideas about the "religious dimensions" of life) tends to be displaced in the attention of the writer by ethical theory and by procedures of practical moral reasoning.

In the Catholic tradition with its continued development of natural law as a basis for ethics an intellectual legitimation for the autonomy of moral theology developed; the natural moral order was itself created by God so the natural order was God's order. Ethical analysis and prescription were theological in principle; moralists were theologians by being moralists. Enough said about theology. Unfortunately, in this tradition the resources and dimensions of theological reflection became confined to a basic theological authorization for ethics, and almost nothing more. And the ethical questions were stirred by particular acts about which judgments of moral rightness or wrongness could be made. It did not occur to these moralists, for example, to wonder if the prophets' critiques of the worship of Baal might not provide, by an act of imagination if not by well developed analogy, some basis for a theological criticism of the excessive scrupulosity that the moral enterprise itself might promote.

A brute fact, and a source of some embarrassment in discourse with the professionals in technology and the life sciences, is the lack of consensus among theologians on some rather simple matters. What is it that theologians think about and write about? What is the subject matter of theology? The high degree of *anomie* among practicing theologians, and the uncertainty among some as to what defines their work as theological, is hardly an asset to any interaction between "theology" and technology and the life sciences. A tired old story from the years of the banquet circuit of the National Conference of Christians and Jews comes to mind. A priest, a Protestant minister and a rabbi were asked to respond to the same question. The priest began, "The Church teaches that . . . " The rabbi began, "The tradition teaches that . . . " The minister began, "Now I think that . . . " There are very good historical and intellectual explanations for the extension of a kind of Protestant *anomie* to the theological enterprise as a whole, but explanations of why it is hard to answer the simple question "what is the subject matter of theology?" do little to identify a melody in a collective cacophonous response. I can readily cite coherent passages from Tillich on technology, Barth on clinical medical moral problems, Rahner on the uses of genetic knowledge, and Ramsey on why Richard McCormick's Jesuit probabilism requires a rigorist response, but I see no way in which I can find from among them a basis for a generalization about how theology confronts technology and the life sciences.

We know what many of the *moral* issues are in technology and the life sciences; we are not sure what the "religious" or *theological* issues are. While debate continues about what moral principles ought to be decisive in determining courses of action in the life sciences and technology, at least the principles under debate can be formulated with some conceptual precision. Much of the literature deals with such matters as the rights of individuals, the preservation of individual self-determination, the conditions under which others might exercise their own self-determination, and the consideration of what benefits and whose good might justify overriding the rights of individuals. Certain principles are invoked constantly: informed consent, risk-benefit ratios, distributive justice, and so forth. There are procedures for justifying particular judgments; there are complex prescriptions like double-effect.

Nothing of comparable detail and precision exists in the more strictly theological realm of discourse; and for various theological reasons the sorts of questions a previous generation asked—such as "What is God doing in these circumstances?" or "What is God saying to us through these crises?"—appear to be very odd and unanswerable. Ethics provides a basis for a new casuistry that is indispensable as long as the issues are framed by the professional persons who have to make particular choices, and as long as the terms of discussion are those on which there can be some consensus, namely ethical terms. No doubt there can be a theological justification for the casuistry, but then there can also be a lot of other, non-theological justification for it. The ethical questions have become fairly clear, and to an ethical question one gives an ethical answer, whether one is a physician, engineer, philosopher or theologian. The theological questions are not clear, and as a result frequently even those writers trained in theology neither attempt to make them clear, nor attempt to answer those that can be asked.

Matters of Belief

I have long believed, and often said, that many of the debates that are passionately conducted within the framework of ethics are misplaced, and that the issues that divide persons are matters of beliefs (whether theological in function or in fact, or whether moral or something else we need not decide here) and loyalties which determine our value choices. Paul Ramsey's Beecher Lectures at Yale, from which came the widely read *The Patient As Person,* provoked a discussion between an internist and surgeon both of whom worked in the renal program. The internist was much taken by Ramsey's argument, and vehemently supported the Uniform Anatomical Gifts Act, an act stipulating in precise detail the consent procedures for using an organ from a corpse. The surgeon strongly expressed the opinion that hospitals and their staffs ought legally to be authorized to "salvage" from corpses any usable organs that might benefit the health and prolong the life of patients. There certainly are ways to deal with the controversy between these two that might lead to some agreement—that might determine whether to pay the carpenter's helpers $8.20 or $8.55 an hour. The precision of the debates at the level of casuistry is not to be demeaned. But the difference between these two physicians really stemmed from more general beliefs and valuations, and these divergences will not be settled, or even addressed, by the latest refinement of the principle of double-effect and its application to cases in the operating room.

Who ought to address these differences? What is the agenda for exploring them? What are the grounds for convictions about the "limit questions," to use Stephen Toulmin's phrase? In a most technical sense, perhaps, these are not yet "theological" questions; but surely they demand a response that is more "theological" than casuistic. And surely there are resources in the religious traditions, in speculative natural theologies, and in the discussions of "religious dimensions" that can be used at least to frame the questions and explore answers to them.

A different example reveals the need for another kind of discourse which at least approaches "theology" if it is not theology. How one understands the relation of self and society, how this relationship is interpreted and conceptualized has profound effects upon the outcome of very specific answers to specific questions. I shall illustrate this too simply by suggesting that the competing metaphors used to depict this relationship are the mechanistic and the organic. The first understands society basically in contractual terms; society is a structure that individuals voluntarily agree to institute and develop. The second understands society, obviously, in organic terms; society is a network of interrelatedness and interdependence in which the relations of the parts are "internal" (I do not intend to invoke a whole Hegelian view by using this term), and in which the development of the well-being of the whole must be considered, if not supreme, at least on par with the well-being of its individual members. The population geneticist tends to take the latter view; when he or she speaks of "benefits," the reference is to the human species. When the ecologist speaks of benefits, the reference is to the well-being of life on the planet. Physicians and most persons writing about ethical issues in medicine and the life sciences have consciously or implicitly adopted the more mechanistic metaphor, and not without some good reasons. Those who use the organic metaphor are more ready to justify overriding an individual "right." If there is any plausibility to my observations, it is fair to ask who is responsible to think about such matters of basic perception, in this case of the relations of individuals to society. What data and warrants support alternative views, and which view in the end appears more adequate?

Another example refers more specifically to Christians and their doctrinal differences. I have argued elsewhere that Karl Rahner's apparent openness to certain kinds of experimentation on humans is a reasonable conclusion from his philosophical and theological anthropology, and from his understanding of the relations of grace and nature. This openness so alarmed Paul Ramsey that he described it as "remarkably like a priestly blessing over everything, doing duty for ethics" and yet Rahner's attitude rests firmly on theological and philosophical grounds.

If one does not like Rahner's openness (which is really very guarded and has several severely restraining principles) one has to argue with his theological and philosophical anthropology and with his views of the relations of grace and nature. If one is persuaded that Rahner's theology is the best available for the Catholic Church today (and the number of dissertations sympathetically exploring his thought suggests that quite a few people are so persuaded), then one ought to come out in moral theology somewhere within the range of his conclusions. If one is concerned that Rahner's openness is morally dangerous in its potential consequences, perhaps one ought to examine one's own theological anthropology, and one's own views of grace and nature. The proper argument is not to be confined to the consequences of relatively closed or open positions but must pursue the question further, to the adequacy of doctrines of God and different anthropologies. A *real* theological discussion then becomes unavoidable.

In the course of such an argument an apparently astounding matter might be seen, namely that one's theological convictions and their articulation in principles about the character of ultimate reality and about human life have a fundamental bearing on one's attitude toward the life sciences and technology. This bearing, in fact, might be more significant in determining one's particular moral preferences than the specific principles chosen to justify a particular decision. It might turn out that passionate ethical debates about technology and the life sciences are missing the crucial point where the real differences lie, and (my goodness!) "ethicists" might have to become theologians! They might find an agenda that would give them something distinctive to do!

To be trained in theology should alert one to aspects of discussions that are otherwise hidden. Several years ago a number of us participated in an intensive conference with research and clinical geneticists. One of the papers was rather more utopian in outlook than the others; its author limned out a vision of the vast benefits to the human race that would accrue from vigorous pursuit of genetic research. I call such scientists "hawks." The paper generated a very passionate discussion, mostly by other scientists and clinicians. Among them were the "doves." Indeed, the rhetoric in the discussion was what those of us alert to religious language could only call apocalyptic. One could interpret the whole discussion as a contest between competing eschatologies: prospects for a universal salvation pitted against prospects for eternal annihilation. The arguments were finally not about matters of hard science; there were some discussions about whose extrapolations from the known to the unknown were most reliable, and about the time frame in which certain possibilities (such as cloning of humans) might occur. But what really divided the disputants were questions that traditionally have been judged to be religious in character.

Most apparent was the question "For what can we hope?" And that could not be answered without asking, in effect, "In whom can we trust?" and "In what can we trust?" Also in dispute were answers to the question "What is desirable?"—which to my mind, incorrigibly saturated with Biblical and theological language, becomes "What are the proper objects of our love?" I feel I do not unduly alter what went on there if I say we were in the midst of a discussion of hope, faith and love. We were also in a discussion of the proper objects of hope, faith and love. No one proposed the Pauline answer, "Your hope is in God." Or the more general Christian answer, "Trust in God." Or the Augustinian answer, "God is the proper object of desire." But the discussion was about whether one should trust chance, or the evolutionary process with minimal intervention, or scientists and statesmen who have power to intervene. The house could readily have been divided between the Augustinians and Pelagians on other questions: the extent of "free will" and the depths of human corruption. It cannot be said that my intervention, in which I pointed out these themes, turned the conversation to one about theology, and certainly about Christian theology, as a subject in itself. I do believe, however, that something dawned in the consciousness of some participants: theology might not provide answers you like to accept, but it can force questions you ought to be aware of. To paraphrase the title of an article by H. Richard Niebuhr, in these circumstances theology is not queen, but servant.

This article ought to have made clear my criticisms of the interchange between theology and technology and the life sciences as long as that interchange is confined merely to the "ethical." With equal severity I would criticize those who confine the theological discussion to *Zeitgeist,* ethos and other comparably general terms. To be honored in such theologians is their radically prophetic stance. They know golden calves when they see them, and they see them sooner than persons preoccupied with how to get from one oasis to the next in the Sinai of contemporary culture and society. I have been accused, in my preoccupation with some matters of a casuistic sort, of "rearranging the deck chairs on the *Titanic.*" Valid charge. My equally nasty retort to those critics is that they think the only proper response is to jump in the North Atlantic and push the icebergs away.

Whether or not one uses the religious language of idolatry, the attack on ethos and *Zeitgeist* implies a call to radical repentance, to a turning away from the Baals of technology whose reliability is bound to fail, and to whom cultural devotion can only lead to desolation for the coming generations. What the culture is to turn from is clear; that it is to return to Yahweh is not necessarily proclaimed. That persons and society are in bondage to the powers of technology, that they are looking for a "salvation" in medical therapy that therapy cannot give them, these are poignantly indicated by the contemporary prophets. That the need is for liberation from bondage, and that some fundamental conversion of individuals and of ethos is required, these points are well made. The sickness is "global" and the antidote must be sufficient for the poison. The creative and exasperating French Protestant Jacques Ellul is one such prophet; he works out of a highly biblical and confessional theology. Not only technology and science, but programs of social revolution and churches feel the sting of his prophetic rhetoric. For him and others like him, technology tends to become reified as a demonic power which only the power of the crucifixion can overcome.

Myopic casuists need strong enough lenses to see the point of the radical theological critics. On the other hand, the perspectives of the radical prophets make conversation with persons who specialize in technology and the life sciences very difficult. If they cannot address the specific and concrete manifestation of the ethos (if it can be said to exist independently) in the particularities of cases and policy choices, if they cannot show how their theologies address the issues as they arise out of specific activities, conversation never gets down to the ground. Many theologians who are critics of culture write for other theologians and for a half-converted religious readership even when they are writing as theologians of culture—technological culture, "modern" culture, or what have you. Indeed, often when they write about the *need* for theology to be engaged in criticism of technological and scientic culture, they are addressing a like-minded group. Why not *test* the need and the practice on an endocrinologist who researches testosterone levels?

Sometimes it turns out that those who are famous as prophetic critics of culture have nothing very specific to say about any particular event in technology and the use of the life sciences. We are told, for example, that a theology of hope addresses social and cultural issues. It turns out that the principal point of the address is that present institutions and cultural values are ephemeral and relative, and we ought not to absolutize them. Thanks a lot! Any student of the history of science and technology knows that. That does not assist the committees on experimentation on human subjects on which I sit to decide whether protocol #6172 is acceptable from a moral perspective. That particular *Titanic* has not yet sunk, and there is merit in arranging things so that it can stay afloat for some time in the future, or at least in organizing things so the lifeboats can be used effectively. Theology cannot push the icebergs away. It might at least help to develop the radar technology that aids in avoiding them.

The moralists find a vocabulary enabling them to interact with the professionals from technology and the life sciences; this tends to limit the theological questions. The prophetic theologians find a vocabulary that is somewhat "theological" in some sense which enables them to interact with other theologians and with other prophetic critics of the ethos; this tends to limit their capacities to relate to the specific occasions in which critical choices have to be made.

Since this is my occasion for broadsides, yet another group of writers can be noted. They are those concerned about the relations between "religion" and "science." Frequently both terms are abstractions: these writers are not concerned about the relations of Judaism to human genetics. They frequently publish in that very interesting journal called *Zygon.* Their intention is to humanize technology and science with some sense of the sacred, and to scientize theology with arguments that presumably support "religion." While it is the case that all modern theology continues to reel from the impact of the Enlightenment, and that theologians continue to find philosophical bases on which to justify the existence of religion (or "the religious" as some like to call it), on the whole this synthetic enterprise is not in the best of repute philosophically, scientifically, or theologically and for some substantial reasons.

"Sciences are a fundamental resource for theology," writes Ralph Wendell Burhoe, a person seldom cited by professional theologians but more widely known than Van Harvey or Gordon Kaufman or David Tracy by groups of scientists interested in the relations of science and religion. Burhoe is confident. He writes, "I suggest that before this century is out we shall see all over the world an increasing integration of information from the sciences into the heart of the belief systems of traditional religions. I prophesy human salvation through a reformation and rehabilitation of religion at a level superior to any reformation in earlier histories, a level high above that of Jasper's axial age as that was above the primitive religions of 10,000 B.C. . . . The new religious and theological language will be as high above that of five centuries ago as contemporary cosmology is above the Ptolemaic, as contemporary medicine, agriculture, communications and transportation concepts are above those of the fifteenth century." Burhoe's program is in sharpest contrast with those theologians that Kai Nielsen has called "Wittgensteinian fideists" who separate religious consciousness and language from scientific consciousness and language in such a way that the former is virtually rendered immune from any criticism by the latter.

In effect the writers of whom Burhoe is fairly typical aspire to develop both theology and ethics on the basis of science, and the life sciences seem to have a privileged place in these proposals. The enterprise is not novel, and different proposals come forward from it about the biological bases for ethics, for knowledge of ultimate reality, and for other matters. Now, no less than in previous decades, it is fraught with difficulties that have frequently been indicated by philosophers of science, philosophers of religion, and moral philosophers. Inferences from scientific data and theories to theological and ethical conclusions are often weakly warranted. The enterprise has the merit of a challenge, however. Can we think theologically and ethically on the basis of what we know about biology? If we find an affirmative answer to the question unacceptable, at least we have to give our reasons for that, and we are left with the chore of figuring out just how knowledge of biology relates to ethics and theology. That is a philosophical and theological problem as important for one aspect of culture as the relation of Marxist theory to ethics and theology for another.

What can be anticipated about theology's "confrontation" with technology and the life sciences? I have amply distributed my criticisms so that few, if any, theologically trained writers in this field are exempt, including myself. I have not described the social, historical and institutional contexts in which the discussions increasingly occur. As far as the ethical responses are concerned, what was a lively, interdisciplinary enterprise even a decade ago has increasingly become a separate profession, if only because the volume of literature has exponentially increased so that it takes a fulltime effort to be in control of it. Theologically trained writers had a prominence a decade ago that is receding and will continue to do so. Their prominence was in part the effect of the concern that religious communities had for practical moral questions, a concern that moral philosophers, until very recently, looked upon with haughty disdain. Now philosophers, physicians and many other professions are contributing a larger portion of the literature than was the case. Separate institutes, national commissions, advisory committes and other organizations have come into being. Theologically trained persons have not been excluded from participation in these, and indeed continue to be significant contributors, but insofar as the contribution of the "theologians" has been and continues to be "practical moral philosophy," the basis of their being attended to is shared by practitioners who are at least as skillful as they are. Competence in argumentation is the criterion by which their contributions will be judged, and a number of them will continue to be highly respected.

Usage and Interpretation

But what if "theologians" choose to be clearer about what the theological issues, or the "religious dimensions," are in the life sciences and technology? I grant that some anxieties will arise. There is not a wide world waiting to hear about these ideas, since they do not immediately assist in determining what constitutes a just distribution of health care resources. There may, however, be more people out there who are interested than we presently recognize. Traditional theological language, and perhaps also the efforts to decontaminate its historical particularities with the language of natural theology or of religious dimensions, will require some skillful usage and significant interpretation. Timidity might be as much a restraining factor as are the objectively real problems in undertaking such discourse. Theologians and other religious thinkers seem highly self-conscious of their own cultural relativity; they often forget that other areas of thought share the same plight. It will have to be accepted that not everyone in that highly esteemed secular technological culture will be interested in the contributions of theologians, but that some persons (even some with social power) might.

In the meantime there are still a large number of people who attend churches, and who seem not fully alienated from traditional religious language and practice. They fall sick, have unexpected pregnancies, vote for legislators who in turn vote on health insurance plans and funding of research. Catholic moral theologians are more conscious of that constituency than are Protestants. Perhaps there is quite a bit to be done to help these persons understand technology in the light of their religious faith and convictions!

In the matters I have been discussing as in so many others, my impression is that much theological or "religious" writing is directed to the justification of an enterprise in the eyes of persons who are not really interested enough to care whether the justification is adequate or not. (I worked for years on a book *Can Ethics Be Christian?* with the nagging sense that most persons who answer in an unambiguous affirmative would not be interested in my supporting argument, that a few fellow professional persons might be interested enough to look at it, and that for those who believe the answer is negative the question itself is not sufficiently important to bother about.) While theologians ought to continue to participate competently in the public debates about matters of technology and the life sciences, they would also do well to attend to the home folks who *might* care more about what they have to say. I am not suggesting that theologians are the best retail communicators, but that the historically identifiable religious communities are fairly obvious loci to be taken into account in writing theology and theological ethics in relation to technology and the life sciences.

It is the "religious ethicists" who have most to be anxious about, in my judgment. They will have either to become moral philosophers with a special interest in "religious" texts and arguments, or become theologians: Christian theologians, or natural theologians, or "religious dimensions" theologians. Only indifference to what they are writing, or exceeding patience with inexcusable ambiguity, can account for the tolerance they have enjoyed.

8.
Preface to *The Patient as Person*

PAUL RAMSEY

The problems of medical ethics that are especially urgent in the present day are by no means technical problems on which only the expert (in this case, the physician) can have an opinion. They are rather the problems of human beings in situations in which medical care is needed. Birth and death, illness and injury are not simply events the doctor attends. They are moments in every human life. The doctor makes decisions as an expert but also as a man among men; and his patient is a human being coming to his birth or to his death, or being rescued from illness or injury in between.

Therefore, the doctor who attends *the case* has reason to be attentive to the patient as person. Resonating throughout his professional actions, and crucial in some of them, will be a view of man, an understanding of the meaning of the life at whose first or second exodus he is present, a care for the life he attends in its afflictions. In this respect the doctor is quite like the rest of us, who must yet depend wholly on him to diagnose the options, perhaps the narrow range of options, and to conduct us through the one that is taken.

To take up for scrutiny some of the problems of medical ethics is, therefore, to bring under examination at once a number of crucial human moral problems. These are not narrowly defined issues of medical ethics alone. Thus this volume has—if I may say so—the widest possible audience. It is addressed to patients as persons, to physicians of patients who are persons—in short, to everyone who has had or will have to do with disease or death. The question, What ought the doctor to do? is only a particular form of the question, What should be done?

This, then, is a book *about ethics,* written by a Christian ethicist. I hold that medical ethics is consonant with the ethics of a wider human community. The former is (however special) only a particular case of the latter. The moral requirements governing the relations of physician to patients and researcher to subjects are only a special case of the moral requirements governing any relations between man and man.

From Paul Ramsey, *The Patient as Person* (New Haven: Yale University Press, 1970), pp. xi-xviii. Used by permission.

Canons of loyalty to patients or to joint adventurers in medical research are simply particular manifestations of canons of loyalty of person to person generally. Therefore, in the following chapters I undertake to explore a number of medical covenants among men. These are the covenant between physician and patient, the covenant between researcher and "subject" in experiments with human beings, the covenant between men and a child in need of care, the covenant between the living and the dying, the covenant between the well and the ill or with those in need of some extraordinary therapy.

We are born within covenants of life with life. By nature, choice, or need we live with our fellowmen in roles or relations. Therefore we must ask, What is the meaning of the *faithfulness* of one human being to another in every one of these relations? This is the ethical question.

At crucial points in the analysis of medical ethics, I shall not be embarrassed to use as an interpretative principle the Biblical norm of *fidelity to covenant,* with the meaning it gives to *righteousness* between man and man. This is not a very prominent feature in the pages that follow, since it is also necessary for an ethicist to go as far as possible into the technical and other particular aspects of the problems he ventures to take up. Also, in the midst of any of these urgent human problems, an ethicist finds that he has been joined—whether in agreement or with some disagreement—by men of various persuasions, often quite different ones. There is in actuality a community of moral discourse concerning the claims of persons. This is the main appeal in the pages that follow.

Still we should be clear about the moral and religious premises here at the outset. I hold with Karl Barth that covenant-fidelity is the inner meaning and purpose of our creation as human beings, while the whole of creation is the external basis and condition of the possibility of covenant. This means that the conscious acceptance of covenant responsibilities is the inner meaning of even the "natural" or systemic relations into which we are born and of the institutional relations or roles we enter by choice, while this fabric provides the external framework for human fulfillment in explicit covenants among men. The practice of medicine is one such covenant. *Justice, fairness, righteousness, faithfulness, canons of loyalty,* the *sanctity* of life, *hesed, agapé* or *charity* are some of the names given to the moral quality of attitude and of action owed to all men by any man who steps into a covenant with another man—by any man who, so far as he is a religious man, explicitly acknowledges that we are a covenant people on a common pilgrimage.

The chief aim of the chapters to follow is, then, simply to explore the meaning of *care,* to find the actions and abstentions that come from adherence to *covenant,* to ask the meaning of the *sanctity* of life, to articulate the requirements of steadfast *faithfulness* to a fellow man. We shall ask, What are the moral claims upon us in crucial medical situations and human relations in which some decision must be made about how to show respect for, protect, preserve, and honor the life of fellow man?

Just as man is a *sacredness in the social and political order,* so he is a *sacredness in the natural, biological order.* He is a sacredness in bodily life. He is a person who within the ambience of the flesh claims our care. He is an embodied soul or ensouled body. He is therefore a sacredness in illness and in his dying. He is a sacredness in the fruits of the generative processes. (From some point he is this if he has any sanctity, since it is undeniably the case that men are never more than, from generation to generation, the products of human generation.) The sanctity of human life prevents ultimate trespass upon him even for the sake of treating his bodily life, or for the sake of others who are also only a sacredness in their bodily lives. Only a being who is a sacredness in the social order can withstand complete dominion by "society" for the sake of engineering civilizational goals—withstand, in the sense that the engineering of civilizational goals cannot be accomplished without denying the sacredness of the human being. So also in the use of medical or scientific technics.

It is of first importance that this be understood, since we live in an age in which *hesed* (steadfast love) has become *maybe* and the "sanctity" of human life has been reduced to the ever more reducible notion of the "dignity" of human life. The latter is a sliver of a shield in comparison with the awesome respect required of men in all their dealings with men if man has a touch of sanctity in this his fetal, mortal, bodily, living and dying life.

Today someone is likely to say: "Another 'semanticism' which is somewhat of an argument-stopper has to do with the sacredness or inviolability of the individual."[1] If such a principle is asserted in gatherings of physicians, it is likely to be met with another argument-stopper: It is immoral not to do research (or this experiment must be done despite its necessary deception of human beings). This is then a standoff of contrary moral judgments or intuitions or commitments.

The next step may be for someone to say that medical advancement is hampered because our "society" makes an absolute of the inviolability of the individual. This raises the spectre of a medical and scientific community freed from the shackles of that cultural norm, and proceeding upon the basis of an ethos all its own. Alternatively, the next move may be for someone to say: Our major task is to reconcile the welfare of the individual with the welfare of mankind; both must be served. This, indeed, is the principal task of medical ethics. However, there is no "unseen hand" guaranteeing that, for example, *good* experimental designs will always be morally *justifiable.* It is better not to begin with the laissez-faire assumption that the rights of men and the needs of future progress are always reconcilable. Indeed, the contrary assumption may be more salutary.

Several statements of this viewpoint may well stand as mottos over all that follows in this volume. "In the end we may have to accept the fact that some limits do exist to the search for knowledge."[2] "The end does not always justify the means, and the good things a man does can be made complete only by the things he refuses to do."[3] "There may be valuable scientific knowledge which it is morally impossible to obtain. There may be truths which would be of great and lasting benefit to mankind if they could be discovered, but which cannot be discovered without systematic and sustained violation of legitimate moral imperatives. It may be necessary to choose between knowledge and morality, in opposition to our long-standing prejudice that the two must go together."[4] "To justify whatever practice we think is technically demanded by showing that we are doing it for a good end . . . is both the best defense and the last refuge of a scoundrel."[5] "A[n experimental] study is ethical or not in its inception; it does not become ethical or not because it turned up valuable data."[6] These are salutary warnings precisely because by them we are driven to make the most searching inquiry concerning more basic ethical principles governing medical practice.

Because physicians deal with life and death, health and maiming, they cannot avoid being conscious or deliberate in their ethics to some degree. However, it is important to call attention to the fact that medical ethics cannot remain at the level of surface intuitions or in an impasse of conversation-stoppers. At this point there can be no other resort than to ethical theory—as that elder statesman of medical ethics, Dr. Chauncey D. Leake, Professor of Pharmacology at the University of California Medical Center, San Francisco, so often reminds us. At this point physicians must in greater measure become moral philosophers, asking themselves some quite profound questions about the nature of proper moral reasoning, and how moral dilemmas are rightly to be resolved. If they do not, the existing medical ethics will be eroded more and more by what it is alleged *must* be done and technically *can* be done.

In the medical literature there are many articles on ethics which are greatly to be admired. Yet I know that these are not part of the daily fare of medical students, or of members of the profession when they gather together as professionals or even for purposes of conviviality. I do not believe that either the codes of medical ethics or the physicians who have undertaken to comment on them and to give fresh analysis of the physician's moral decisions will suffice to withstand the omnivorous appetite of scientific research or of a therapeutic technology that has a momentum and a life of its own.

The Nuremberg Code, The Declaration of Helsinki, various "guidelines" of the American Medical Association, and other "codes" governing medical practice constitute a sort of "catechism" in the ethics of the medical profession. These codes exhibit a professional ethics which ministers and theologians and members of other professions can only profoundly respect and admire. Still, a catechism never sufficed. Unless these principles are constantly pondered and enlivened in their application they become dead letters. There is also need that these principles be deepened and sensitized and opened to further humane revision in face of all the ordinary and the newly emerging situations which a doctor confronts—as do we all—in the present day. In this task none of the sources of moral insight, no understanding of the humanity of man or for answering questions of life and death, can rightfully be neglected.

There is, in any case, no way to avoid the moral pluralism of our society. There is no avoiding the fact that today no one can do medical ethics until someone first does so. Due to the uncertainties in Roman Catholic moral theology since Vatican Council II, even the traditional medical ethics courses in schools under Catholic auspices are undergoing vast changes, abandonment, or severe crisis. The medical profession now finds itself without one of the ancient landmarks—or without one opponent. Research and therapies and actionable schemes for the self-creation of our species mount exponentially, while Nuremberg recedes.

The last state of the patient (medical ethics) may be worse than the first. Still there is evidence that this can be a moment of great opportunity. An increasing number of moralists—Catholic, Protestant, Jewish and unlabeled men—are manifesting interest, devoting their trained powers of ethical reasoning to questions of medical practice and technology. This same galloping technology gives all mankind reason to ask how much longer we can go on assuming that what can be done has to be done or should be, without uncovering the ethical principles we mean to abide by. These questions are now completely in the public forum, no longer the province of scientific experts alone.

The day is past when one could write a manual on medical ethics. Such books by Roman Catholic moralists are not to be criticized for being deductive. They were not; rather they were commendable attempts to deal with concrete cases. These manuals were written with the conviction that moral reasoning can encompass hard cases, that ethical deliberation need not remain highfalutin but can "subsume" concrete situations under the illuminating power of human moral reason. However, the manuals can be criticized for seeking finally to "resolve" innumerable cases and to give the once and for all "solution" to them. This attempt left the impression that a rule book could be written for medical practice. In a sense, this impression was the consequence of a chief virtue of the authors, i.e., that they were resolved to think through a problem, if possible, *to the end* and precisely with relevance and applicability in concrete cases. Past medical moralists can still be profitably read by anyone who wishes to face the challenge of how he would go about prolonging ethical reflection into action.

Medical ethics today must, indeed, be "casuistry"; it must deal as competently and exhaustively as possible with the concrete features of actual moral decisions of life and death and medical care. But we can no longer be so confident that "resolution" or "solution" will be forthcoming.

While no one can do ethics in the medical and technological context until someone first does so, anyone can engage in the undertaking. Anyone can do this who is trained in one field of medicine and willing to specialize for a few years in ethical reasoning about these questions. Anyone can who is trained in ethics and willing to learn enough about the technical problems to locate the decisional issues. This is not a personal plea. It is rather a plea that in order to become an ethicist or a moral theologian doctors have only to quit resisting being one. An ethicist is only an ordinary man and a moral theologian is only a religious man endeavoring to push out as far as he can the frontier meaning of the practice of a rational or a charitable justice, endeavoring to draw forth all the actions and abstentions that this justice requires of him in his vocation. I am sure that by now there are a number of physicians who have felt rather frustrated as they patiently tried to explain to me some technical medical circumstance I asked about. At the same time, I can also testify to some degree of frustration as I have at times patiently tried to explain some of the things that need to be asked of the science and methods of ethics. Physicians and moralists must go beyond these positions if we are to find the proper moral warrants and learn how to think through moral dilemmas and resolve disagreements in moral judgment concerning medical care.

To this level of inquiry we are driven today. The ordinary citizen in his daily rounds is bound to have an opinion on medical ethical questions, and physicians are bound to look after the good moral reasons for the decisions they make and lead society to agree to. This, then, is a plea for fundamental dialogue about the urgent moral issues arising in medical practice.

No one can alter the fact that not since Socrates posed the question have we learned how to teach virtue. The quandaries of medical ethics are not unlike that question. Still, we can no longer rely upon the ethical assumptions in our culture to be powerful enough or clear enough to instruct the profession in virtue; therefore the medical profession should no longer believe that the personal integrity of physicians alone is enough; neither can anyone count on values being transmitted without thought.

To take up the questions of medical ethics for probing, to try to enter into the heart of these problems with reasonable and compassionate moral reflection, is to engage in the greatest of joint ventures: the moral becoming of man. This is to see in the prism of medical cases the claims of any man to be honored and respected. So might we enter thoughtfully and actively into the moral history of mankind's fidelity to covenants. In this everyone is engaged.

Notes

1. Wolf Wolfensberger, "Ethical Issues in Research with Human Subjects," *Science* 155 (January 6, 1967): 48.
2. Paul A. Freund, "Is the Law Ready for Human Experimentation?" *Trial* 2 (October-November, 1966): 49; "Ethical Problems in Human Experimentation," *New England Journal of Medicine* 273, No. 10 (September 10, 1965): 692.
3. Dunlop (1965), quoted in Douglass Hubble, "Medical Science, Society and Human Values," *British Medical Journal* 5485 (February 19, 1966): 476.
4. James P. Scanlan, "The Morality of Deception in Experiments," *Bucknell Review* 13, No. 1 (March, 1965): 26.
5. John E. Smith, "Panel Discussion: Moral Issues in Clinical Research," *Yale Journal of Biology and Medicine* 36 (June, 1964): 463.
6. Henry K. Beecher, *Research and the Individual: Human Studies* (Boston: Little, Brown, 1970), p. 25.

9.
Bioethics and Method: Where Do We Start?

RICHARD A. McCORMICK

We live at a time when nearly every morning's newspaper brings us another biomedical breakthrough—and problem. Some of the recent ones would include the following: surgery on the fetus *in utero* to correct bladder pathology; laparoscopic introduction of relief valves into the fetal cranium to prevent hydrocephalus and the subsequent retardation associated with neural tube defects; the transitional use of the totally artificial heart; *in vitro* fertilization procedures to overcome tubal occlusion. In the next few years we will witness the production of hybridomas (man-made hybrid cells that can be introduced into the body to produce swarms of disease-fighting antibodies). We will see the production of interferon from DNA technology as well as the development of nuclear magnetic resonance body imaging—to do what x-rays do now.[1] And on and on it goes.

With scientific and technological breakthroughs come the usual set of questions and concerns. Will this procedure promote or undermine the *humanum?* Is it overstepping the line of human stewardship? On what criteria do we decide? And who decides? Is public regulation called for? These questions are, of course, ethical questions. Their answers are not only important in themselves. They are also a paradigm. How we go about them will tell us how we will be acting twenty years from now. For the type of moral reasoning employed, its premises, its sensitivity, its precision, its combination of finality of commitment with appropriate tentativeness of formulation will reappear wherever bioethical issues reappear.

The dangers that confront us in facing the bioethical problems cast up by advancing technology are quite well known, but easily overlooked in practice. The dangers are that such problems will be "solved" by one-eyed approaches such as power, fiat, prestige, economics or even tradition in its narrow and, I think, untenable sense (the application of old and presumably invariable injunctions to new data). That is why it is important to ask: "Where do we start?" Our beginnings are like the first chapter of a novel: they foreshadow and sometimes even determine what is to come.

From *Theology Digest* 29 (Winter 1981): 303-18. Used by permission.

There are many aspects about method that are important. I am sure that any listing that claims to be exhaustive or *the* list will turn out to be idiosyncratic and transparent of its author's major and present concerns. My listing will make no such claim. It has the much more modest aim of stating areas that cannot be neglected if the moral discourse that undergirds our common search for values in our time is to be serious and to be of help to those who have both the responsibility for and the power to influence societal policy in these matters.

Two preliminary warnings are called for here. First, in developing the considerations that follow, I will take or imply certain positions. That fact will, I hope, not function as a distraction; for what is important is not primarily the position taken or implied. What is crucial is that we appreciate the need for serious moral discourse around these points.

Second, within a sharply limited time, one can only *outline* certain areas of concern. One cannot treat them elaborately, or even at times with sufficient depth and detail to avoid oversimplification. These two warnings are not intended to exempt me from objection. They are offered rather in an effort to put objections within a broader context, and to guide attention to this context.

1. The Origin of Our Basic Moral Commitments

I mean this title to be synonymous with the phrase "the origin of moral obligation." It is an attempt to respond to the question: How do our value commitments arise?

Negatively, I think most philosophers and theologians would admit that such commitments do not *originate* with rational arguments and analyses. Let slavery be an example. We find this demeaning and immoral not because of rational (discursive) argument—which is not to say that rational arguments will not support the conclusion. Rather, over time our sensitivities are sharpened to the meaning and dignity of human persons. We then experience the out-of-jointness, inequality and injustice of slavery. We then judge it to be morally wrong. Then we develop analyses to criticize, modify and communicate that judgment. Discursive reasoning does not discover the right (and wrong) but only *analyzes* it. Perhaps this is why Malcolm Muggeridge is fond of saying that clowns, artists and poets are nearer the truth than theologians and philosophers.

Let me attempt to put this in more positive terms. How do we arrive at definite moral obligations—prescriptions and proscriptions? How does the general thrust of our persons toward good and away from evil become concrete? In attempting to answer this question, I shall follow closely the school of J. de Finance, G. de Broglie, G. Grisez, John Finnis and others. It is a school of thought with obvious roots in the Thomistic *inclinationes naturales.*

We can proceed by asking: What are the goods or values persons can seek, the values that define their human opportunity, their flourishing? We can answer this by examining our basic tendencies; for it is impossible to act without having an interest in the object, and it is impossible to be attracted by, to have an interest in something without some inclination already present. What then are the basic inclinations?

With no pretense at being exhaustive, we could list some of the following as basic inclinations of the human person: the tendency to preserve life; the tendency to mate and raise children; the tendency to explore and question; the tendency to seek out other persons and seek their approval (friendship); the tendency to use intelligence in guiding action; the tendency to establish good relations with unknown higher powers (religion); the tendency to develop skills and exercise them in play and the fine arts.

In these inclinations our intelligence spontaneously and without reflection grasps the possibilities to which they point, and prescribes them. Thus we form naturally and without reflection (Thomas' *naturaliter nota*) the basic principles of practical moral reasoning. As Finnis once put it:

> What is spontaneously understood when one turns from contemplation to action is not a set of Kantian or neoscholastic "moral principles" identifying this as right and that as wrong, but a set of values which can be expressed in the form of principles such as "life is a good-to-be-pursued-and-realized and what threatens it is to be avoided."[2]

We have not yet arrived at a determination of what concrete actions are morally right and wrong; but we have laid the basis. Since these basic values are equally underivative and irreducibly attractive, the morality of our conduct is determined by the adequacy of our openness to these values, for each of these values has its self-evident appeal as a participation in the unconditioned Good we call God. The realization of these values in intersubjective life is the only adequate way to love and attain God.

Further reflection by practical reason tells us what it means to remain open and to pursue these basic human values. First, we must take them into account in our conduct. Simple disregard of one or other shows we have set our mind against this good. Second, when we can do so as easily as not, we should avoid acting in ways that inhibit these values, and prefer ways that realize them. Third, we must make an effort in their behalf when their realization in another is in extreme peril. If we fail to do so, we show that the value in question is not the object of our efficacious love and concern. Finally, we must never repudiate or turn against a basic good. What is to count as rejecting or "turning against a basic good" is, of course, the crucial moral question in some concrete and controversial ethical discussions in which I find myself in disagreement with Grisez, Finnis and others.

For instance, there are a few theologians who attempt to explain the intrinsic wrongness of sterilization (and individual contraceptive acts, for that matter) by asserting that it involves us in repudiating the basic good of procreation.

I prefer the structure of reasoning proposed by Pius XII. That pontiff made two moves. First he proposed a general duty to procreate, on the basis that the individual, society, and the Church depend on fertile marriage for their existence. He concluded: "Consequently, to embrace the state of matrimony, to use continually the faculty proper to it, and in it alone, and on the other hand to withdraw always and deliberately, without a grave motive, from its primary duty, would be to sin against the very meaning of conjugal life." But Pius XII immediately continued: "Serious motives, such as those which are frequently present in the so-called 'indications'—medical, eugenic, economic and social—can exempt from this positive, obligatory office (*prestazione*) for a long time, even for the entire duration of the marriage."[3]

Several things are notable here. First, "to sin against the very meaning of conjugal life" is a fair rendering of "turn against a basic good." This failure is attributed to failure to fulfil a duty. Secondly, the Holy Father acknowledges that one does not contravene this duty when the serious indications he mentions are present. In other words, whether one "sins against the very meaning of conjugal life" is determined by the presence or absence of these indications—which he later described as "in truth very wide." This is a straightforward form of teleology. As Ford and Kelly wrote: "As for the expressions 'grave motive,' 'serious reasons,' etc. we believe that a careful analysis of all these phrases in the context would justify the interpretation that they are the equivalent of the expression 'proportionate reasons.' "[4] What this means, then, is that in the context of periodic continence Pius XII associated "turning against a basic good" with a pattern of actions, and the presence or absence of a proportionate reason. This is, I believe, as it should be. But why should it be otherwise when dealing with sterilization?

Put negatively, it is simply incomprehensible to many theologians (and others) that a couple who have seven or eight children, then encounter serious medical (economic, eugenic, social) problems that make any further procreation irresponsible, and choose sterilization as the means, must be said to be "turning against a basic good." One would think that such a "turning against" must be understood here just as it was by Pius XII when dealing with periodic continence, by looking at the couple's overall performance.

This is the point of view taken by philosopher John Langan, S.J. In an overall favorable critique of Finnis' book *Natural Law and Natural Rights,* he states:

> One thing that is not clear in Finnis' approach is the connection between a basic value in its general form and its particular exemplifications. It is hard to see a reason why one should accord overriding importance to any particular instance of sociability or aesthetic experience or play or knowledge or why one should conclude that acting against a particular instance of any of these basic values entails disrespect for the value in general. Certainly the tradition did not draw such a conclusion even with regard to the taking of a particular life.[5]

Indeed Langan regards this aspect of Finnis' theory as "hopeful to the point of being fanciful."

In summary, our more particular moral judgments are specifications (by practical reason attending to all the data relevant in particular cases and circumstances) of these more basic normative positions—positions that have their roots in spontaneous, prediscursive inclinations. My only point here is to call attention to the need of facing up to an understanding of the origin of the moral "ought." If we do not, subsequent moral analysis is likely to be based on and infected by inadequate suppositions: e.g., a concretism (act utilitarianism) that is rootless and capricious, or a revelatory fundamentalism, or a rather crude cost-benefit analysis.

2. The Threat to Our Basic Value Commitments

This is, I believe, a second step in determining where we start. Specifically, we must identify the cultural shaping of our grasp on values. Put in the language of the *inclinationes naturales,* our inclinations to values are culturally conditioned.

Let me use Philip Rieff's book *Triumph of the Therapeutic* (New York: Harper and Row, 1966) as an explanatory vehicle here. Rieff points out that a culture survives by the power of institutions to influence conduct with "reasons" that have sunk so deeply into the self that they are implicitly understood, the "unwitting part of the culture" to borrow Harry Stack Sullivan's usage. It is such "reasons" that determine the direction and drift of a culture, much more than operative structures (codes, regulations, policies, etc.). The "reasons" are our cultural ways of perceiving basic human values, the soil of our decisions and policies. Our way of perceiving the basic human values, and relating to them, is shaped by our whole way of looking at the world.

One could use any of several cultural conditionings to illustrate this point. For instance, it takes little argument to convince a reflective person that American culture is pansexualized. The cultural mandate to our youngsters is roughly this: "You have to have it. Even bad sex is better than no sex." The trivialization of sexuality has occurred through a process of objectification→autonomy→depersonalization and has arrived at the point where its cultural symbol is, as Malcolm Muggeridge has noted, a torso and a hand. The enshrinement of orgasm as the meaning and purpose of sexual intimacy has led to what Paul Ramsey occasionally refers to as "calisthenic sexuality." It is a sexuality devoid of any past or future—lived only in the present. We know with our communal memory and experience that present quality is had only when the present celebrates the past and secures the future, when sexuality is lived as a history affirming the past and promising the future. Joseph Sittler, one of my favorite authors, catches this beautifully:

> It is not a very courageous thing for two people who have found themselves mutually delectable to say, "We will shack up as long as the delectability continues." That's neither broadly human nor is it particularly commendable. It has no gallantry. It's a mutual opportunism. So that if people want to create all kinds of lovely music about what is simply one of the higher forms of self-satisfaction, I find nothing admirable about this at all. I find it completely understandable. I find it even momentarily delightful. But I don't think it has much to do with marriage. Certainly nothing to do with a promise.[6]

Sittler then refers to the "challenge to fulfill the seemingly impossible," to the risk that is a kind of madness. What he is saying is that sex and eros are fleeting, fickle and frustrative unless they exist in the atmosphere of *philia,* the covenanted friendship that has a past, present and future because solidly built on a promise. Yet we have as a culture drifted from this, and this drift will influence our reflections and judgments, because it influences our grasp on a basic value. We are knee-deep in this culture.

A good start in bioethics means identifying these cultural biases and redressing their influence on our moral judgments.

Let me take an example from the area of bioethics itself. In relating to the basic human values, several images of man are possible, as Daniel Callahan has observed.[7] First, there is a power-plasticity model. In this model, nature is alien, independent of man, possessing no inherent value. It is capable of being used, dominated, and shaped by human persons. We see ourselves as possessing an unrestricted right to manipulate in the service of our goals. Death is something to be overcome, outwitted. Johann Metz refers to this as the "anthropology of domination" and calls it "the secret regulating principle of all interpersonal relationships."[8]

Second, there is the sacral-symbiotic model. In its religious forms, nature is seen as God's creation, to be respected and heeded. We are not masters; we are stewards and nature is our trust. In secular forms, persons are seen as a part of nature. If persons are to be respected, so is nature. We should live in harmony and balance with nature. Nature is a teacher showing us how to live with it. Death is one of the rhythms of nature, to be gracefully accepted.

The model that seems to have sunk deep and shaped our moral imagination and feelings—shaped our perception of basic values—is the anthropology of domination. We are corporately *homo technologicus.* The best solution to the dilemmas created by technology is more technology. We tend to eliminate the maladapted condition (defectives, retardates) rather than adjust the environment to it. Even our language is sanitized and shades from view our relationship to basic human values. We speak of "surgical air strikes" and "terminating a pregnancy," ways of blunting the moral imagination from the shape of our conduct. We are moving, as Paul Ramsey constantly reminds us, toward "administered death." Joseph Sittler notes that technology "profoundly changes Homo operator's sense for the world." Borrowing from Tillich, he asserts that technology "injects a 'second nature' into humanity's reflective life."[9] This "second nature" shapes not only our actions, but our very perceptions.

My only point here is that certain cultural "reasons" qualify or shade our perception of and our grasp on the basic human values. These "reasons" are the cultural soil of our moral judgments. A reflexly conscious look at these cultural tintings and trappings is essential to a good start in bioethical thought.

3. The Relation of the Sources of Faith to Basic Value Commitments

I raise this question as pertinent to where we start because there are two positions on this question that represent extremes. The first is that answers to the bioethical problems we face are found in the documents of religious traditions, whether these be understood as scripture, papal teaching, the Talmud. Thus there are those who believe that the declarations of Pius XII on medical problems—rich, stimulating, and well-informed as they are—are the absolutely final word. This is a kind of ecclesiastical positivism and infallibilism that could endanger the very values that that great and learned pontiff was intent on protecting.

On the other hand there are those who think and act as if religious perspectives and commitments have no influence on bioethical problems. James Gustafson has complained about this for years in protesting the fact that in the study of the life sciences theologians have become moral philosophers. By this he means that ethical questions are getting merely ethical answers without theological input because moral theologians are no longer doing theology. This allows the question to be framed exclusively by nontheologians. He acknowledges that the problem traces partially to a lack of consensus among theologians as to what theological issues really are. Moral principles have some precision (e.g., rules on informed consent) but nothing of comparable precision exists in the theological realm of discourse.[10]

Whatever the cause of the problem, it seems clear that the differences between people are often matters of belief and loyalties. We do not settle these differences by refining ethical principles. Rather, it is, as Gustafson notes, convictions about the character of ultimate reality and life that have more bearing on answers than particular moral principles. For example, discussions on genetic research are often discussions about competing eschatologies without the discussants adverting to this.

If those two be extreme, how does a faith commitment and membership in an historical believing community influence one's analysis of bioethical problems? I am sure that there are many enriching ways of articulating this, and I claim no monopoly here. For instance, Gustafson in his Pere Marquette lecture argued that one's concept of God has immediate repercussions on our approach to this matter.[11] Thus, if God is conceived of uniquely as the creator and conserver of order, then this emphasis may all but determine certain very practical conclusions. For instance, it is possible to attach an almost mechanical significance to the *inclinationes naturales.* One sees divine providential wisdom at work in these natural purposes. *Deus (natura) nihil facit inane.* When natural ends, by appeal to God's creative wisdom, are viewed as inviolable, then certain conclusions follow rather quickly. Thus no contraception no matter what. Thus no artificial insemination by husband no matter what. These are seen as illicit tamperings with nature.[12] It is quite possible that a notion of God lies behind the conclusions just mentioned, a notion that simply identifies the creative (and conserving) will of God with the moral will of God.

If, however, God is seen as also the enabler of our possibilities (a notion strongly suggested by *STh* I-II, q. 91, a. 2: *Rationalis creatura. . . . fit providentiae particeps, sibi ipsi et aliis providens* [creatures endowed with reason participate in providence by providing for themselves and others]) then quite different perspectives dominate one's analyses. As John Macquarrie notes: the doctrines of creation and providence make possible an ultimate trust but at the cost of imposing an ultimate responsibility. We are not only creatures, but co-creators with God who "have a share in shaping an as yet fluid and plastic world—a world in which the most fluid entity is human nature itself."[13] Thus our attitude toward the world must live in paradoxical tension, combining both appreciation and manipulation.

Another way of articulating the relation of the sources of faith with bioethics is to link faith with the basic values already mentioned. In this perspective, love of and loyalty to Jesus Christ, the perfect human being, sensitizes us to the meaning of persons. The Christian tradition is anchored in faith in the meaning and decisive significance of God's covenant with persons, especially as manifested in the saving incarnation of Jesus Christ, his eschatological kingdom which is here aborning but will finally only be given. Faith in these events, love of and loyalty to their central figure, yields a decisive way of viewing and intending the world, of interpreting its meaning, of hierarchizing its values. In this sense the Christian tradition only illumines human values, supports them, provides a context for their reading at given points in history. It aids us in staying human by underlining the truly human against all cultural attempts to distort the human. By steadying our gaze on the basic human values that are the parents of more concrete norms and rules, faith influences moral judgment and decision-making.

It has been a Catholic tradition to refer to moral theological enquiry under the phrase "reason informed by faith." How does this "informing" work? I am suggesting that the stories and symbols that relate the origin of Christianity and nourish the faith of the individual affect our perspectives by intensifying and sharpening our focus on the human goods definitive of our flourishing. It is persons so informed, persons with such "Christian reasons" sunk deep in their being, who face new situations, new dilemmas and reason together as to what is right and wrong. They do not find concrete answers in their tradition, but they bring a worldview that informs their reasoning—especially by allowing the basic human goods to retain their original attractiveness and not be tainted by cultural distortions. Macquarrie notes that a distinctive tradition may help its adherents "to perceive some aspects of the general moral drive with a special clarity."[14] I am suggesting here something very close to Macquarrie's wording.

Perhaps it is something like this that Vatican II had in mind when it asserted that "faith throws a new light on everything, manifests God's design for man's total vocation, and thus directs the mind to solutions which are *fully human.*"[15] It further stated: "But only God, who created man to His own image and ransomed him from sin, provides a fully adequate answer to these questions. This He does through what He has revealed in Christ His Son, who became man. Whoever follows after Christ, the perfect man, *becomes himself more a man.*"[16] This statement has been turned around slightly by Enda McDonagh as follows: "The experience of Jesus Christ is regarded as normative because he is believed to have experienced what it is to be human in the fullest way and at the deepest level."[17] That is why Christian ethics is the objectification in Jesus Christ of what every person experiences of him/herself in his/her subjectivity.

Let me linger for a moment on Vatican II's phrase "faith throws a new light on everything." What does that mean in the area of concrete moral problems? Does it mean that faith replaces human insight and reasoning? I think not. I agree with Franz Böckle when he states that "the natural moral law must in principle be clarified by argumentation."[18] "Reason informed by faith" means neither *replaced* by faith nor *without* faith. In this matter one cannot but agree with Henrico Chiavacci that the magisterium is not a replacement for moral insight and reasoning, but an aid to it. It should function as a kind of "exemplary pedagogy" for moral "discernment."[19] But we must understand reason here in its broadest sense. Discursive moral reasoning cannot always (perhaps even ever) capture and reflect adequately the fullness of moral insight and judgment. There are factors at work in moral conviction that are reasonable but not always reducible to the clear and distinct ideas that the term "human reason" can mistakenly suggest. When all these factors are combined, they suggest that the term "moral reasoning" is quite broad and is defined most aptly by negation: "reasonable" means not ultimately mysterious.

In a more positive view, "faith throws a new light on everything" suggests that there may well be certain enlightening perspectives or themes that can be disengaged from the Christian story to form what Böckle calls "morally relevant insights." I have attempted elsewhere to develop these rather broad themes[20] and will only list them here. 1) Life as a basic but not absolute value. 2) The extension of this judgment to nascent life. 3) Human relationships as the basic quality of human physical life to be valued as the *conditio sine qua non* for other values. 4) Our essential sociality. 5) The unity of the spheres of life-giving (procreative) and love-making (unitive). 6) Heterosexual, permanent marriage as normative.

Several things ought to be noted about such themes or perspectives. First, they are by no means an exhaustive listing. One could mention, for instance, the presence of sinfulness in the world and how this impacts on our understanding of human institutions and norms.[21] One could also argue with Franz Böckle that faith forbids the absolutizing of any created good.[22] Second, these themes do not immediately yield concrete moral judgments about the rightfulness or wrongfulness of human actions.[23] Rather they direct and inform our view of the world. Third, they are not ultimately mysterious. They find resonance in broad moral experience and in this sense are not impervious to human insight. Fourth, they are capable of yielding different applications in different times and circumstances. Finally, they are themes or perspectives that stem from the Christian story in a dynamic sense: sc., as this story is continuously appropriated in a living tradition.

4. The Incorporation of Basic Values into Moral Norms

Our spontaneous knowledge of basic values must become specific and concrete in specific, concrete situations. Furthermore, it must be communicated to others, both educationally and motivationally. The need to be specific and to communicate results in the emergence of moral norms. One of the most basic and divisive areas of all of ethics and therefore of bioethics is the meaning of moral norms, how they are elaborated and interpreted. If one fails to come to grips with this problem, one's moral reasoning will very likely reflect the dominant form of popular moral discourse in bioethics, a thinly disguised act-utilitarianism with exclusive and often rather crude consideration of quantitative good and evil. This is very appealing to physicians and researchers, as Daniel Callahan notes, because "the specificity and idiosyncrasy of individual clinical cases seem a dominant feature."[24]

One can see the importance of the question raised here in the starkly different ways of doing bioethics that characterize Paul Ramsey and Joseph Fletcher. At the heart of Fletcher's ethics is "getting results" and here and now. If the greatest good of the greatest number "calls for" it, Fletcher would bioengineer parahumans and clones to undertake our dangerous or menial tasks. He would administer euthanasia on anyone (fetus, newborn, terminal patients) if this would remove "useless" suffering or eliminate "unmeaningful life." The use of the atomic bomb on Hiroshima and Nagasaki was the result of an agapeic calculus. It is consequences that count and they alone. One of my favorite Fletcher quotes is the following: "Man is a maker and a selector and a designer, and the more rationally contrived and deliberate anything is, the more human it is." Thus: "laboratory reproduction is radically human compared to conception by ordinary heterosexual intercourse. It is willed, chosen, purposed and controlled and surely these are among the traits that distinguish *Homo sapiens* from others in the animal genus . . . Coital reproduction is, therefore, less human than laboratory reproduction."[25] One need not condemn all *in vitro* fertilization to reject this sacralization of technology. One need only point out that in Fletcher's "more human" world, the fun has gone out of it. There is a wisdom—and I think it divine—that human procreation occurs amidst human love-making.

At the opposite end of the pole is Paul Ramsey. For Ramsey there are pieces of human conduct that one must never do regardless of the consequences. For instance, we may never experiment nonbeneficially (nontherapeutically) on those incapable of consent. We may never directly kill another human being. We may never licitly perform AID (artificial insemination by donor), cloning or even *in vitro* fertilization. Why these latter strictures? Because we know from the Christian story (specifically John's prologue and Ephesians 5) what human parenthood is meant to be.

> God created nothing apart from his love; and without divine love was not anything made that was made. Neither should there be among men and women, whose man-womanhood is in the image of God, any love set out of the context of responsibility for procreation or any begetting

> apart from or from beyond the sphere of their love.[26]

For Ramsey, consequences are not the prime determinant of all morality. There are covenant relations between persons and persons, and persons and God that issue in a morality of means that resists Fletcher's consequentialist calculus.

The Fletcher-Ramsey polarity in moral reasoning reflects a much broader moral-philosophical discussion—that between deontological theories and teleological theories. "A teleological theory says that the basic or ultimate criterion or standard of what is morally right, wrong, obligatory, etc., is the nonmoral value that is brought into being."[27] Deontological theories deny that the right, wrong, obligatory, etc. are wholly a "function of what is nonmorally good or of what promotes the greatest balance of good over evil for self, one's society, or the world as a whole."[28] Certain aspects of the act itself "other than the value it brings into existence" may make an act right or wrong, for instance, the fact that it "keeps a promise, is just, or is commanded by God or the state."[29]

I do not wish to rehearse here the niceties of this discussion (for instance, the distinctions between act teleology and rule teleology, act deontology and rule deontology). They are available in many reputable philosophical textbooks. But I do want to point out three things. First, the terms "teleological" and "deontological" are rather huge umbrellas. They represent a division along a *spectrum,* what Broad has referred to as "ideal limits." Most metaethical theories contain elements of both polarities of this *spectrum* and resist classification into the extreme poles of these opposing notions. I shall return to this.

Second, it is quite possible and actually frequently the case that those who call themselves either deontologists or teleologists arrive at identical practical rules and conclusions. An example would be the Childress-Beauchamp volume *Principles of Biomedical Ethics.* Beauchamp describes himself as a rule-utilitarian, Childress sees himself a rule-deontologist. Of this difference they note:

> We come to these different conclusions after testing the various theories for their consistency and coherence, their simplicity, their completeness and comprehensiveness, and their capacity to take account of and to account for our moral experience, including our ordinary judgments. Still, for each of us, the theory that we find more satisfactory is only slightly preferable, and no theory is fully satisfactory on all the tests. . . . the differences [between the two] can easily be overemphasized. In fact, we find that many forms of rule utilitarianism and rule deontology lead to identical rules and actions.[30]

My third point has to do with the identification of many recent Catholic moral theologians along the *spectrum.* I refer to theologians such as Bruno Schüller, Joseph Fuchs, Louis Janssens, Jean-Marie Aubert, Franz Böckle, Charles Curran, Peter Knauer, Franz Scholz, Helmut Weber, W. Molinski, Peter Chirico, John Dedek, Alfons Auer, Karl Rahner, Bernard Häring, Sean O'Riordan, Klaus Demmer, F. Furger, Dietmar Mieth, Daniel Maguire, Henrico Chiavacci, Marciano Vidal, Timothy O'Connell and a whole host of others. While these theologians differ from each other in significant ways, they do share a certain bottom line, so to speak: individual actions, independent of their circumstances (e.g., killing, contraception, falsehood, sterilization, masturbation), cannot be said to be intrinsically morally evil *as this term is used by the recent magisterium.* Why? Because such concepts describe an action only in terms of its *materia circa quam* (materiality) and do not take account of morally relevant circumstances. This means that such actions can at times be justified. In impoverishing summary these theologians are insisting that moral norms must take account of the conflictual character of human choices. As Janssens words it: there are times when "we cannot realize a premoral value without admitting the inseparable premoral disvalue."[31]

Where does this contention situate these theologians along the spectrum? Somewhere in the middle. Bruno Schüller has listed three possible positions on the spectrum mentioned above. (1) The moral rightness or wrongness of all actions is exclusively determined by their consequences. (2) The moral rightness or wrongness is always also but not only determined by consequences. (3) There are some actions whose moral rightness is determined in total independence of consequences.[32] The first position is called "teleological" or "utilitarian," the second and third "deontological." Unfortunately, there is no terminology that distinguishes the second and third positions.

The Catholic moral theologians mentioned above fit by and large into the second position. This second or middle position differs from a strict teleology (position one), as Charles Curran notes, because it maintains the following points: (1) moral rightness and wrongness arise from elements other than consequences; (2) the good is not separate from the right; (3) the way in which the good or evil is achieved by the agent is an important and morally relevant circumstance. Therefore, Curran rightly concludes that "as the debate progressed it became quite evident that the reforming Catholic theologians, generally speaking, do not embrace utilitarianism or what Rawls, Frankena, Williams and others have called teleology or consequentialism."[33] For this reason the middle position I have described has been called both "mixed deontology" and "mixed teleology."[34] Interestingly and autobiographically, my colleague James Childress regards my position as "mixed deontology," whereas others regard it as "consequentialist." Lisa Cahill concludes her interesting study: "The moral theory of Richard McCormick, and like-minded colleagues, is teleological. Further, the thesis is defensible that it is a non-utilitarian form of teleology, if fully understood."[35] Such is the malleability of human language, such the expanse of territory between the pure poles on the spectrum.

This matter may seem to be purely academic. But I think it is not. Any number of writers (e.g., Grisez) who resist these developments describe the position as "consequentialism" or "proportionalism." They then set forth the rather standard arguments leveled against utilitarian theories and feel that they have discredited the entire analytic development.[36] A careful reading of the literature will show that this involves the creation of some rather robust strawpersons. Specifically, in their explanations of *materia apta* (Janssens), commensurate reason (Knauer), *ratio proportionata* (Schüller), the aforementioned theologians insist very carefully and explicitly that elements other than consequences—as this term is ordinarily understood—function in their assessment of moral rightness or wrongness. For instance, they insist that promises [e.g.] have a value in themselves. They emphasize the institutional importance of some obligations. They highlight expressive actions (*Ausdruckshandlungen*) as having a meaning in themselves—the meaning of love, support, solidarity. I include myself among those who so insist. The most careful and informative discussion of these newer tendencies will appear in *Theological Studies* (December, 1981). It is by Lisa Cahill.

Whatever one's metaethical preference, it is clear that making a good start with bioethical problems means getting entangled in this discussion. For if one does not, basic presuppositions will remain unexamined and the superstructure built upon them will be vulnerable.

5. The Emergence of Public Morality

Nearly everyone has heard the term "public morality" and is vaguely conscious of the need of public morality. But what does the term mean? It suggests that the pursuit of the basic goods that define our well-being has increasingly been shifted from private one-on-one acts and has been put into the public sphere. That means that bioethics will have to have much more to say at the level of policy-making than it has. Until quite recently it has been much more concerned with the level of individual decisions. "But," as Daniel Callahan correctly notes, "on a national scale those decisions are going to be overshadowed by large structural moral and political decisions. It is these decisions that will eventually shape the individual decisions."[37]

I will begin by stating what public morality is not. First, it is not simply public participation in the directions and priorities of medical practice, research and health care. If public morality is understood in this way, it easily becomes a merely formal affair, a matter of structuring dialogue to include representative participants.

Secondly, it is not merely law or public policy. One of the prime tests of law is "its own 'possibility' " as John Courtney Murray words it,[38] or its feasibility—". . . that quality whereby a proposed course of action is not merely possible but practicable, adaptable, depending on the circumstances, cultural ways, attitudes, traditions of a people, etc."[39] Public policy must, therefore, take account of some very pragmatic considerations in a rather utilitarian way. Reducing public morality to public policy would be to undermine public morality.

A clearer grasp of the meaning of public morality becomes possible when we consider the contemporary context of health care delivery. Individual decisions will, of course, remain and will remain important. But increasingly the services of physician to patient are mediated by institutions. Such institutions have become partners in health care delivery. Thus we have group practice, third party carriers, legislative and administrative controls (FDA), etc.

Groups (whether universities, insurance companies or the government) have interests and concerns other than the immediate good of the patient. Thus the government has a legitimate interest in population control, in reducing welfare rolls, in control of illegitimacy, in the advancement of diagnostic, therapeutic, preventative medicine, in balancing the budget, in protecting life. Teaching and research hospitals have a concern for the health of future generations.

This suggests that whenever other values (than the patient's) are the legitimate concern of the mediator of health care, the good of the individual patient becomes one of several values, in competition for priority. It further suggests that the individual is in danger of being subordinated to these values.

As I understand the term, "public morality" is the pursuit of these other values without violating the needs and integrity of the individual. It is a harmonizing of public concerns with individual needs. These "other values and concerns" constitute the public dimension of biomedicine because they represent concerns other than and beyond the individual. In Callahan's words: "ways will have to be found to balance that ethic [patient-centered] off against the legitimate interests of the public . . . "[40]

Callahan has summarized this matter splendidly. He argues that the allocation of resources, the development of a just health-care delivery system, the adjudication of the rights and claims of different competing groups "are and will be the important moral problems of the future."[41] These problems will "force biomedical ethics to move into the mainstream of political and social theory, beyond the model of the individual decision maker, and into the thicket of important vested and legitimate private and group interests." Establishing the proper balance between individual patient-centered concerns and other legitimate interests is what I mean by the term "public morality."

When biomedicine is mediated by groups with other (than the individual's) concerns, the medical-research establishment is thereby deeply inserted into the value-perspectives of society at large, and begins to be shaped by these perspectives and priorities. One need not be a Cassandra to note that in the United States top cultural priorities are technology, efficiency, comfort. This means that these priorities will unavoidably penetrate the "medical-research complex" and shape its decisions. As the late Dr. Andre Hellegers used to say: "Medicine is increasingly being asked to provide heaven on earth."

Priorities of this type can very easily, if not inevitably, lead to a hierarchizing of values and priorities that is, under analysis, distorted—in the sense that the legitimate needs and claims of individuals are neglected. The ones most likely to get hurt in such policy shifts are the poor, the dependent (elderly, retarded), and the "ordinary patient" who is neglected in favor of exquisite medical virtuosities that consume undue time, energy and funds.

Contemporary reflection on bioethics must include, therefore, from the very start an awareness of and an analysis of the public character of the biomedical enterprise. This public character is always in danger of shortsuiting the individual. Public morality is the proper balance preserved, the proper hierarchizing of concerns, so that the individual is not subordinated to the collectivity, or vice versa.

In summary, to the question "Bioethics: Where Do We Start?" I have suggested a five-point answer. We begin by struggling to greater clarity on the following points:

1. The origin of our basic value commitments.
2. The threat to our basic value commitments.
3. The relation of religious belief to our basic value commitments.
4. The structure of moral reasoning making these commitments concrete and communicable.
5. The public nature of the realization of these goods and values in our time.

There are, I am sure, many other things to be said, possibly many other ways to begin where the field of bioethics is concerned. But if we neglect these five points, they will return to haunt us. Their solution is presupposed in any other beginning. For it remains true that the best beginning is the end (*finis est prima causarum*) or, better, the ends, the goods and goals that we seek, that define our well-being, and the considerations and questions that surround these goods and goals. If these are neglected in the discussion of bioethics, we will have made a start, but not a good beginning.

Notes

1. *Washington Post,* July 27, 1981.

2. John M. Finnis, "Natural Law and Unnatural Acts," *Heythrop Journal* 11 (1970) 365-87 at 373. To complete the picture "Why should one act so as to promote fundamental human goods?" Margaret Farley suggests that the "missing first principle in Aquinas' system has to be formed in his later treatment . . . of the principle, 'Love your neighbor as yourself.'" *Religious Studies Review* 7 (July, 1981) 236. Farley maintains that St. Thomas was willing to hierarchize and subordinate the various goods which are the object of our natural inclinations.

3. *AAS* 43 (1951) 835-54 at 845f.

4. John C. Ford, S.J., and Gerald Kelly, S.J., *Contemporary Moral Theology 2: Marriage Questions* (Westminster: Newman, 1963), 425.

5. John Langan, *International Philosophical Quarterly* 21 (1981) 217f. Richard Bruch warns that "one must guard against drawing too much from the [Thomistic] natural inclinations." "Intuition und Überlegung beim sittlichen Naturgesetz nach Thomas von Aquin," *Theologie und Glaube* 67 (1977) 29-54. In this connection, it may be interesting to remember that Lugo argued: *quod juste efficitur, juste intenditur* (*Just.,* d. 10, m. 149). Margaret Farley goes even further. She insists that there is nothing in St. Thomas that disallows a hierarchizing of the goods that are the objects of our spontaneous inclinations. As she words it: "There is not one of the three basic inclinations which Aquinas lists in *Summa Theologiae* I-II, 94, 3, which he is not willing at some point or other to subordinate to what may be a higher good (whether the good of the total individual being, or the common good, or the good of ultimate 'happiness'). . . . Aquinas is quite capable of building exceptions into rules or of subordinating one rule to another on

the basis of a qualifying condition. His use of the principle of double effect is extremely limited, and he does not call upon it at all when, in certain circumstances, he is willing to relativize even the value of human life (*ST* II-II, 64, 2; 124, 3; 65, 1; 66, 7)." *Loc. cit.,* 236.

6. Joseph A. Sittler, *Grace Notes and Other Fragments* (Philadelphia: Fortress Press, 1981), 17.

7. Daniel Callahan, "Living with the New Biology," *Center Magazine* 5 (1972) 4-12.

8. Johann Metz, *The Emergent Church* (New York: Crossroad, 1981), 35.

9. Joseph Sittler, cf. note 6 at 81f.

10. James M. Gustafson, "Theology Confronts Technology and the Life Sciences," *Commonweal* 105 (1978) 386-92.

11. James M. Gustafson, *The Contributions of Theology to Medical Ethics* (Milwaukee: Marquette University, 1975).

12. Cf. the very enlightening remarks of Joseph Komonchak on the "intention of nature" in *Theological Studies* 39 (1978) 254f.

13. John Macquarrie, *Christian Theology: A Case Method [Study] Approach,* ed. by Robert A. Evans and Thomas D. Parker (New York: Harper and Row, 1976), 94.

14. John Macquarrie, *Three Issues in Ethics* (New York: Harper and Row, 1970), 89.

15. *Gaudium et spes: The Documents of Vatican II* (New York: America Press, 1966), 209; italics added.

16. Ibid., 240; italics added.

17. Enda McDonagh, "Towards a Christian Theology of Morality," *Irish Theological Quarterly* 37 (1970) 187-98 at 196. Cf. also Macquarrie, note 14 at 88.

18. Franz Böckle, "Glaube und Handeln," *Concilium* 120 (1976) 641-47.

19. Enrico Chiavacci, "La fondazione della norma morale nella riflessione teologica contemporanea," *Rivista di teologia morale* 37 (1978) 9-38 at 36.

20. Richard A. McCormick, S.J., "Theology and Biomedical Ethics," *Logos* 3 (1982) 25-45.

21. Cf. Joseph Fuchs, S.J., "The 'Sin of the World' and Normative Morality," *Gregorianum* 61 (1981) 51-76.

22. Franz Böckle, cf. note 18 at 644.

23. Cf. Stanley Hauerwas, "Abortion: Why the Arguments Fail," *Hospital Progress* 61, n. 1 (1980), 38-49.

24. Daniel Callahan, "Shattuck Lecture: Contemporary Biomedical Ethics," *New England Journal of Medicine* 302 (n. 22, 1980) 1229.

25. Joseph Fletcher, "Ethical Aspects of Genetic Controls: Designed Genetic Changes in Man," *New England Journal of Medicine* 285 (1971) 776-83 at 780f.

26. Paul Ramsey, *The Vatican Council and the World of Today* (Brown University, 1966), no pagination.

27. William Frankena, *Ethics* (Englewood Cliffs: Prentice-Hall, 2nd ed., 1973), 14.

28. Ibid., 15.

29. Ibid.

30. James Childress and Tom Beauchamp, *Principles of Biomedical Ethics* (New York: Oxford University Press, 1979), 40.

31. Louis Janssens, "Norms and Priorities in a Love Ethic," *Louvain Studies* 6 (1977) 207-38.

32. Bruno Schüller, S.J., "Anmerkungen zu dem Begriffspaar 'teleologisch-deontologisch,' " *Gregorianum* 57 (1976) 315-31.

33. Charles E. Curran, "Utilitarianism and Contemporary Moral Theology: Situating the Debates," *Readings in Moral Theology No. 1: Moral Norms and Catholic Tradition* (Ramsey, NJ: Paulist Press, 1979) 341-62 at 354.

34. William May, "Ethics and Human Identity: The Challenge of the New Biology," *Horizons* 3 (1976) 17-37.

35. Lisa Cahill, "Teleology, Utilitarianism and Christian Ethics," *Theological Studies* 42 (1981).

36. This justifies Francis X. Meehan's observation: "My own fear is that the issue is beginning to be emotionally loaded with forms of code words that do not do justice to the complexities. If one wishes to react to his opponent captiously, one can then always reduce his point to absurdity." "Contemporary Theological Developments on Sexuality," in *Human Sexuality and Personhood* (St. Louis: Pope John XXIII Medico-Moral Research and Education Center, 1981), 173-90 at 190, note 31.

37. Cf. note 24 at 1232.

38. John Courtney Murray, *We Hold These Truths* (New York: Sheed and Ward, 1960), 166f.

39. Paul Micallef, "Abortion and the Principles of Legislation," *Laval théologique et philosophique* 28 (1972) 267-303.

40. Cf. note 24.

41. Ibid.

10.
Biblical Revelation and Medical Decisions

RICHARD J. MOUW

"Fear God, and keep His commandments; for this is the whole duty of man." The writer of Ecclesiastes thus summarizes a significant perspective on the nature of the good life. At the heart of this perspective is the conviction that there is a God who has offered directives to human beings, which they must acknowledge as they shape the patterns of their lives. As many Christians view things, this posture of obedience to a God who reveals his will is foundational to an adequate understanding of morality. For those who assume such a posture, it is unthinkable that we could reflect at any length on a moral issue without asking, "What does the Lord require of us?"

If divine commands have a crucial bearing on "the whole duty of man," then they must surely be taken into account when we seek to do our duty in the area of medical decision making. On such a view, Christian medical ethics cannot be pursued without careful reflection upon divine commandments as they bear on the medical dimensions of human life.

To view medical ethics in this light is to adopt a perspective whose plausibility—or even intelligibility—is not immediately obvious to all contemporary ethicists. As Peter Geach has observed: "In modern ethical treatises we find hardly any mention of God; and the idea that if there really is a God, his commandments might be morally relevant is wont to be dismissed by a short and simple argument."[1] Indeed, the assumption that divine commands are morally irrelevant even operates among contemporary Christian writers of ethical treatises.

My concern here is not so much to defend obedience to divine commands against either impious or pious critics as it is to explain one way in which divine commandments might be viewed as morally relevant and as important for shaping attitudes in the area of medical decision making. Indeed, while I will address some of my initial comments to the topic of divine commands, I am actually concerned to elucidate a somewhat broader perspective, namely, the pattern of submitting to divine revelation as it is mediated by the Bible. Divine commands, strictly speaking, constitute only part of what is involved in Biblical revelation; but I will begin by focusing on divine commandments.

My concern here is to explain a certain kind of *sola scriptura* emphasis as it applies to medical problems. This emphasis, which was a prominent feature of the Protestant Reformation and is still dear to the hearts of many conservative Protestants, differs—at least in tone and procedure—from other ways of understanding obedience to the revealed will of God. For example, some Christians understand "natural law" in such a manner that when someone makes moral decisions with reference to natural law that person is obeying divine commands. Others hold that submission to the *magisterium* of a specific ecclesiastical body counts as obedience to divine directives. Others hold that individual Christians, even those who are not members of ecclesiastical hierarchies, can receive specific and extrabiblical commands from God, such as "Quit smoking!" or "Get out of New Haven!" Still others hold that the will of God can be discerned by examining our natural inclinations or by heeding the dictates of conscience.

None of these is, strictly speaking, incompatible with a *sola scriptura* emphasis. One could hold, for example, that the Bible itself commands us to conform to natural law, or to submit to the church's teachings, or to consult our conscience. Or one could simply view these alternative sources as necessary supplements to biblical revelation. The view which I will be attempting to elucidate is not intended as a denial of the legitimacy of appeals to these other sources. Rather, I am assuming a perspective from which the Bible is viewed as a clarifier of these other modes; the Bible is viewed here as an authoritative source against which deliverances from these other sources must be tested.

Obeying Divine Commands

Before proceeding to discuss questions of medical decision making, some clarifications are in order concerning the relevance of divine commands to moral reasoning.

Christian ethicists of the past have often assumed that the Bible offers a plurality of divine commands which have continuing relevance for the moral life. That assumption seems to have been under attack in recent years by Christian ethicists who contend that there is only one divine commandment which is morally relevant, namely, the command to love God and neighbor. This seems to be Joseph Fletcher's contention when he describes himself as "rejecting all

From *The Journal of Medicine and Philosophy* 4, no. 4 (1979): 367-82. Used by permission.

'revealed' norms but the one command—to love God in the neighbor."[2]

The issue at stake here is important for a field like medical ethics. If the command to love is the only biblical command which has normative relevance for medical decision making, then much of the substance of Christian medical ethics can be established without reference to the Scriptures. But if the Bible offers other commands and considerations which bear on medical decision making, then the task will be one of finding correlations between biblical revelation and medical issues at many different points.

It is important to note, however, that when Fletcher explains the grounds for his mono-imperativism, his arguments are not so much directed against the moral relevance of other divine commands as they are against their alleged "absoluteness." To hold, however, that there is a plurality of divine commands which are morally relevant and binding is not to commit oneself to the view that each of these commands is indefeasible. It may well be that there is only one indefeasible command, the so-called "law of love"—such that in any situation in which the course of action prescribed by the law of love is one's duty, it is one's actual duty, and that only the law of love has this property. But this does not rule out the possibility—and, based on the view being assumed here, the likelihood—that there are other divine commandments which prescribe courses of action which are one's prima facie duties to perform in those situations in which the commands in question are morally relevant.

We must also insist that not all commandments which are found in the Bible are to be obeyed by contemporary Christians. For example, God commanded Abram to leave Ur of the Chaldees, and he commanded Jonah to preach in Nineveh; it would be silly to suppose that it is part of every Christian's duty to obey these commandments.

Furthermore, it would be wrong to attempt to ascertain what God commands in the Bible simply by looking at sentences which are in the imperative mood. The Bible is much more than a compendium of commandments. It contains history, prayers, sagas, songs, parables, letters, complaints, pleadings, visions, and so on. The moral relevance of the divine commandments found in the Scriptures can only be understood by viewing them in their interrelatedness with these other types of biblical writing. Divine commands, as recorded in the Bible, must be contextually understood. The history, songs, predictions, and so on of the Bible serve to sketch out the character of the biblical God; from the diversity of materials we learn what kind of God he is, what his creating and redeeming purposes are, what sorts of persons and actions he approves of, and so on. Divine commands must be evaluated and interpreted in this larger context.

But it is also the case that we will miss some of the commands which are to be "found" in the Bible if we attend only to sentences which are grammatically imperative. For example, nowhere in the New Testament is there a literal command to the followers of Jesus to stop discriminating against Samaritans. But the New Testament record has Jesus telling stories and engaging in activities which make it very clear that he is directing his followers to change their attitudes toward the Samaritans. Thus, it is accurate to say that Jesus "commanded" his disciples to love the Samaritans, even though the words (or their Greek or Aramaic equivalents) "Stop discriminating against Samaritans" never appear in the Bible.

When the writer of Ecclesiastes, then, insists that our whole duty consists in obeying God's "commandments," we must not understand him to be instructing us to attend only to divine utterances which have a specific grammatical form. He is telling us, rather, that we must conform to what God requires of us, to what he instructs us to do—whether the instruction is transmitted through parables, accounts of divine dealings with nations and individuals, or sentences which somebody commands.

Something must also be said about the relationship between obedience to divine commands and the question of moral justification. It is not within the scope of this discussion to give anything like a fully adequate account of this relationship. Instead, I will sketch out one possible way of viewing the situation.

Let us say that a person has a *direct* moral justification for a given course of action if that person directly ascertains that the course of action in question, in the light of all relevant and available factual information, satisfies what he takes to be the correct fundamental moral criteria or criterion. Furthermore, let us understand normative theories such as utilitarianism, deontology, and virtue ethics as providing different understandings of what constitutes the correct fundamental moral criterion or criteria. (This account of direct moral justification is intended as a formal one. Nothing is implied about the truth of those beliefs which are supported by direct moral justifications. A person, then, may have a direct moral justification for a course of action without being justified in pursuing that course of action.)

Thus, in one version of utilitarianism, a person who is wondering whether to keep a specific promise will ask whether the keeping of that promise will bring about a situation in which there is a greater excess of good over bad consequences than the situation which would result if the promise is not kept. Or a deontologist would ask whether, say, telling Peter that I will give him twenty-five dollars on Wednesday conforms to a rule of practice whose obligatoriness is rationally defensible (or intuitively obvious), and whether in conforming to that rule I would not be violating another rule whose obligatoriness is weightier in that situation.

When a person has gone through the proper moral operations regarding a course of action, with direct reference to fundamental moral criteria, we can say that a person has a direct moral justification for what he decides. But there are situations in which persons do not have direct moral justifications—where, for example, sufficient factual information is unavailable, or where there is no time to calculate consequences or to engage in appropriate rational reflection. Nonetheless, in such situations there may be other grounds for making justified moral judgments.

Let us say that a person has an indirect moral justification for a course of action under conditions of this sort: The course of action possesses some property distinct from the property of being supportable by fundamental moral criteria, and the person reasonably believes that the possession of this property by a course of action makes it either logically certain or inductively probable that the action has the property of satisfying the correct moral criteria.

Perhaps an analogy will be helpful. Suppose that my car engine's being fixed consists in certain adjustments having been made to the engine. But suppose I do not possess the skills to ascertain whether those adjustments have been made. But if I believe that when my mechanic, Mary, says that the engine is fixed then it is in all likelihood fixed—so that Mary's saying that it is fixed makes it highly probable that it is fixed—then knowing that Mary says so constitutes an indirect justification for the claim that it is fixed. Mary herself, in this case, has a direct justification for that claim.

The following might be a situation in which I have an indirect moral justification for some course of action: I am a utilitarian and have not calculated the consequences of some act, but I know that Jane Fonda, whom I believe to be a skilled utilitarian calculator, wants me to perform that act. Or I am a deontologist and have not engaged in the proper reflection regarding some course of action, but I know that Ralph Nader, whose intuitive powers I greatly respect, generally reacts with favor when that course of action is recommended in similar circumstances. In these cases, knowing that Jane Fonda or Ralph Nader approves of a given course of action would count as an indirect justification for my approving of that course of action.

It is important to distinguish between two questions which relate to moral decision making: What makes an action right, and how do I decide that an action is right? We can decide, of course, that an action is right by directly investigating whether it possesses what we take to be the proper right-making characteristics. But often the two questions receive very different answers. Very often people decide what to do by listening to moral authorities or by looking at moral examples. This is sometimes a dangerous basis for decision making. But not always. Sometimes, as I am suggesting, the appeal to an authority or an example can constitute an indirect justification for a specific decision. In both car repair and morality, appeals to authority or example must take into account the credentials of the person to whom reference is made.

What I mean to be arguing here is that the Christian does not have to insist that God's commanding something is what makes it morally right. It is not necessary to argue that knowing that God has commanded something constitutes a direct moral justification for that course of action; one could believe that God himself, in commanding a course of action, does so on the basis of ascertaining that that course of action satisfies certain moral criteria (which are distinct from his having commanded it). For example, God's commanding marital fidelity may not necessarily be what makes marital fidelity morally right. Indeed, in the terms which I am outlining here, the Christian believer could remain open to a number of different theoretical accounts of what constitutes a direct moral justification for a course of action. God himself might be a utilitarian, or a deontologist, or a virtue ethicist. Of course, it could be the case that God's commanding something is the correct fundamental moral criterion. But, in the view which I am suggesting, the Christian need only hold that God's commanding something is either a direct or an indirect moral justification for that course of action.

Ordinary Christian piety often leads believers to say things of this sort: "I don't know why God wants me to do that, but I am confident that he knows best." What I am suggesting here is that what goes into God's "knowing best" is subject to theoretical—even metaethical—speculation; and we do not have to answer that question in order to accept God's commands as reliable moral guidelines.

There are some who will object to this way of viewing the moral life, not so much because of any logical weakness that they perceive in it, but because of its "feel" or tone. For example, it might be thought that this perspective lacks plausibility because it is much too "heteronomous," or even "military," in its emphasis on the moral agent as a commandee, submitting to the authority of a moral commander.

Some Christian apologists seem inclined to meet this challenge head-on, claiming that if the posture of obedience to divine commands is indeed a heteronomous one, then heteronomy deserves a better reputation than it is often granted. This seems to be the thrust of Peter Geach's comments on this subject: "I shall be told by [some] philosophers that since I am saying . . . [that] it is insane to set about defying an Almighty God, my attitude is plain power-worship. So it is: but it is the worship of the Supreme Power, and as such is wholly different from, and does not carry with it, a cringing attitude towards earthly powers. An earthly potentate does not compete with God, even unsuccessfully: he may threaten all manner of afflictions, but only from God's hands can any affliction actually come upon us."[3] This is a very Hobbesian account of the relationship between God and his human creatures; we submit to God's will out of fear of his power—the appeal is not so much to a sense of the moral fittingness of that submission as it is to a prudential awareness of what is in our self-interest.

But the defense need not move along these lines. Rather, we can insist that, viewed from "inside" the Christian life, it seems quite inappropriate to describe a Christian's relationship to God as one where a human being receives commands from an "external other," although it is not difficult to see how things can be viewed in that light from other points of view (e.g., existentialism and Marxism).

In both the Old and New Testaments, there is a sense of clear movement toward an "inner-directedness" in moral decision making. The Law at Sinai may have been "handed down" from heaven on tables of stone; but it was not long before those who had received that law were talking about a word of guidance that was to be "written on the heart"—a sense of inner-directedness which culminates in the New Testament concerning the indwelling of the Holy Spirit (or receiving "the mind of Christ"). From within such a perspective, it may be difficult to identify one's posture as that of submitting to commands which are simply "handed down from above."

Similarly, a heteronomous account of Christian morality does not capture the intimacy of the relationship between commander and commandee as it is described in the Bible. The God who commands is one who has taken the human condition upon himself, who has been tempted in all of the ways in which his human creatures are tempted. The believer in turn receives his law as a gift, becoming the temple of his Spirit. The intimacy here is not, of course, one of metaphysical merger; it is an interpersonal intimacy, a unity of purpose within the context of covenant. This intimacy is such that the term "heteronomy" will seem, to those who experience it, much too formal and lifeless to account for the facts of the case.

Medical Perspectives in the Bible

How do we move from the Bible to contemporary medical decision making? How do we apply divine commandments, which were addressed to people whose cultural situations are far removed from our own, to medical questions as they arise today?

It will certainly not do to take each medically oriented divine command in the Bible and apply it directly to contemporary situations. For one thing, not all biblical directives regarding medical matters have direct application to contemporary situations. Leviticus 13 prescribes that any man who has itchy spots on the skin under his beard should present himself to the priest for examination; there follows a series of directions concerning the examination and quarantine of such persons. The elaborate steps described here are obviously developed because of a fear of various contagious diseases, grouped together under the term "leprosy." The stipulated methods and underlying concerns are clearly linked to a certain stage of disease identification and are spelled out in terms of social roles which are quite foreign to our present situation. (This is, e.g., one of the few instances in which the cultic priest is called upon to serve as both medical examiner and quarantine officer.) It would be ludicrous to view this passage as important to contemporary Christian views of skin care.

Indeed, the divine commands in the Bible which are most directly relevant to contemporary medical decision making may be commands which are not, in their biblical context, explicitly "medical" in nature. In dealing with such contemporary issues as abortion, or national health plans, or the question of a patient's consent in various situations, the most morally relevant biblical considerations may have to do with the command to love one's neighbor, or to show mercy to the oppressed, or to seek justice.

The Bible, in the view being represented here, is both a record of God's past revelation and a vehicle for his present revelation. But in some cases it takes considerable work to decide exactly what God is saying today by way of his deliverances to an ancient people. We discover what he is saying to twentieth-century Christians by attending to the record of his dealings with Semitic nomads and Palestinian fishermen, but not without considerable interpretive work.

Those who want to explore the relevance of the biblical message to contemporary medical decision making must begin by attempting to understand the Bible on its own terms. This involves at least two tasks: first, we must engage in the piecemeal descriptive task of understanding various elements of the biblical record; then, we must organize the results of that descriptive study theologically.

Let us briefly examine some elements of the first task. We have already insisted on the importance of understanding the divine commands found in the Bible in relation to their larger biblical context. This involves attempts to establish what exactly was meant by biblical directives for the people to whom they were originally addressed. The task of achieving a properly contextualized understanding of divine commands within their biblical setting must necessarily draw upon a full range of disciplines and subdisciplines which bear upon "biblical studies." With reference to medical (and I use this term in a broad sense to cover, e.g., hygienic, preventative, and curative activities) issues, this means that the Bible must be studied with the purpose of grasping the milieu within which divine commands were originally viewed as normative for medical concerns.

The descriptive task of giving an account of intrabiblical medical perspectives is an extensive one. It includes linguistic and conceptual studies focusing on biblical language regarding disease, health, bodily functions, medicinal practices, and the like. It must also involve developing something like a "historical medical sociology" of biblical cultures, which would provide accounts of the actual medical institutions, functions, and practices of, say, Israel and her neighbors.

Perspectives on the changing conceptions and practices regarding medical matters within the history covered by biblical literature are also important here. Israel experienced several major geographical and cultural shifts in her mode of social, political, and economic interaction: from slavery to nomadic life, to "landed" theocracy, to exile and diaspora, to life in Palestine under an occupying force. The New Testament also has writings which are descriptive of, and addressed to, a variety of cultural situations, with the transition from Jewish to Gentile Christianity being a dominant factor.

It should be noted that in our attempts to understand the cultural context of the biblical writings it is not always easy to distinguish or separate medical factors from other dimensions of the culture in question. This is due, in good part, to a lack of cultural differentiation in the biblical literature. The medical dimensions of life are intimately intertwined with cultic, culinary, sexual, and economic matters. What may strike us at first glance as a "medical" matter may be closely related to a cultic concern: for example, hygienic instructions may be intimately aligned to a desire for "ritual purity."

The importance of these descriptive concerns can be seen in relation to Saint Paul's reference to homosexuality in Romans 1:26-27. The apostle there describes homosexual acts as being "against nature"; and since these acts are viewed by him as being committed out of a spirit of willful rebellion against God, many Christians have understood him to be taking an unambiguous stand on the question of whether homosexuality is "sin" or "disease" or a morally neutral matter of personal preference. Some commentators have suggested, however, that what Paul is condemning here is homosexual activity as it occurred in certain specific pagan temple rituals. Others have argued that he is referring only to homosexual acts committed by persons who are "naturally" heterosexual. If either of these accounts is correct (which I personally doubt), then it would have the effect of limiting the relevance of this passage to only one subset of acts of genital contact between homosexual persons. Thus, the question of the range of acts to which Paul is referring is crucial to an understanding of the scope of his moral condemnation.

The second task which we have noted is that of organizing the results of this descriptive study theologically. This task includes elements of both "biblical theology" and "systematic theology." It might be helpful to think here in terms of a biblical-systematic theology of medicine. Such an enterprise would be rooted in a descriptive account of the variety of medical references in the Scriptures, and it would attempt to discern the overall patterns of biblical medical thought. The goal here would be that of attaining as clear an account as possible of the various nuances, and perhaps even tensions or conflicts, which emerge in considering the variety of biblical medical data.

From a conservative theological perspective, this activity would be characterized by a desire to find some coherent way of understanding the diversity of biblical data. As James Gustafson has noted, Karl Barth attempted to develop a Christian ethical perspective based on obedience to divine commands, but he did so with the insistence that those commands be viewed as fitting into the overall patterns of biblical theology. Barth recognized, as Gustafson puts it, that "while God gives specific commands on each occasion, he is not capricious; thus his commands are likely to be consistent with the Decalogue and the Sermon on the Mount."[4] The same desire for coherence should characterize (but, of course, not distort) the attempt to interpret the variety of biblical medical data.

An analogy can be drawn here to the attempt to construct a biblical understanding of poverty.[5] Some biblical references to poverty—most notably those in the Wisdom literature of the Old Testament—view economic deprivation as brought about by laziness. Proverbs 6:10-11 provides a good example of this theme: "A little sleep, a little slumber, a little folding of the hands to rest, and poverty will come upon you like a vagabond, and want like an armed man." There are many other passages, however, in which the poor are viewed as victims of injustice, as kept in bondage to poverty by the greed and hardheartedness of the rich and powerful.

A proper theological understanding of biblical references to poverty must take these differing nuances into account. One possibility, of course, is to insist that the Bible offers conflicting accounts of the causes of poverty. Or one could look (as seems quite proper) for some way of fitting these nuances into a coherent overview of poverty. One plausible way of doing so is to understand the Bible as calling human beings to engage in serious labor in order to attain their livelihood: If some refuse to do so out of sloth, they are condemned; if others are prohibited from doing so by greed of the rich and powerful, they are to be considered victims of injustice.

Similarly, a biblical theology of medicine must attempt to account for various nuances in the biblical references to disease and physical health. There is much to be explored here, since attitudes toward the role of disease in human life are closely linked to the major biblical themes of creation, sin, and redemption.

The Bible views the beginnings of creation in terms of a garden paradise in which God looked at all of the things which he had created and pronounced them to be "good." The rebellion of the first human pair against the will of the Creator shattered the original harmony of Eden. The divine curse which they brought upon themselves by their disobedience introduced experiences of physical discomfiture which they had hitherto not known: the woman would experience great pain in childbearing, while the man would eat bread "in the sweat of your face" (Gen. 3:16, 19).

Disease and serious injury are obviously viewed as incompatible with God's original creating purposes. And the hope for redemption which emerges in the life of Israel includes the expectation that human beings will be delivered from physical disease: "Bless the Lord, O my soul, and forget not all his benefits, who forgives all your iniquity, who heals all your diseases" (Ps. 103:2-3).

The New Testament consistently views Jesus as a healer. Indeed, this healing mission is viewed as one dimension of a larger confrontation with the effects of sin on human life. In the Gospel of Mark, for example, Jesus' successful efforts at healing diseases seem to be portrayed as one aspect of a ministry which has a cosmic scope: Jesus not only heals physical ailments, but he casts out demons, tames the angry sea, combats hunger and economic injustice, and even raises the dead. The elimination of disease as an element of a cosmic redemption is an important element in the eschatological expectation of a new age, in which God "will wipe every tear from their eyes, and death shall be no more, neither shall there be mourning nor crying nor pain any more, for the former things have passed away" (Rev. 21:4).

This sketchy account of the place of disease in the Bible's view of God's creating and redeeming activity points to matters which almost everyone would agree are present in the biblical perspective: intense physical suffering was not a part of the original creation; disease enters into human affairs as a result of sin and rebellion; the work of divine redemption aims at the elimination of disease from the creation.

The nuances in the biblical picture of the place of disease in human life arise primarily with regard to the significance of suffering for "this present age," that is, for the period which is no longer the original unfallen creation, but not yet the new age in which disease will be eliminated. How do we account for a specific physical affliction which enters into the life of a particular individual? How ought the contemporary Christian to deal with disease in his or her own life? The New Testament church clearly expected that Christians would be miraculously cured of physical ailments: "Is any among you sick? Let him call for the elders of the church, and let them pray over him, anointing him with oil in the name of the Lord; and the prayer of faith will save the sick man, and the Lord will raise him up" (James 5:14-15).

But even within the New Testament this encouragement to expect miraculous healing is countered by the suggestion that God sometimes desires that Christians endure physical suffering. Thus, Paul reports that he received a "thorn in the flesh," for whose removal he prayed three times, only to be convinced that God did not want to remove it, so that divine power would be manifested in Paul's weakness (2 Cor. 12:7-9).

The formulation of a clear and coherent theological account of biblical perspectives on this issue, and a variety of other topics, is necessary to provide some of the essential data for yet another task, that of wrestling with contemporary medical issues in the light of biblical teaching.

The Limitations of "Ethics"

It is not uncommon for writers of books and articles on medical ethics to give the impression that the right sort of medical decisions will be made if only we ensure that medical professional or technical expertise is wedded to an awareness of moral values. If this is to be considered an adequate portrayal of the way things ought to be, then the term "moral values" will have to carry considerable freight—which, of course, it often does—and will be a misleading label for designating that body of considerations which must supplement technical skill.

The Christian who wants to understand the full human significance of medicine will have to look to more than ethics, even to the theological and philosophical disciplines of ethics, for aid. For one thing, medical issues must be viewed from the perspectives of political, legal, and economic thought; for this reason, we can be grateful for the increased attention being given recently to "medical rights" and "the politics of health care."

But the contributions of several other philosophical and theological disciplines and subdisciplines are also important. Here is only a small sampling of issues with regard to which medicine intersects with various areas of theological and philosophical inquiry: metaphysical, epistemological, and anthropological questions concerning the genesis and cessation of human life; dualistic and monistic accounts of human composition, as they touch on basic issues concerning the significance of medical treatments in the careers of human persons; questions about the role of science in human society; issues having to do with the nature, merits, and demerits of human "technique"; analyses of the function of medical institutions in human cultural formation; theological and aesthetic criteria for deciding what counts as "deformity" and "normalcy."

We have already insisted that God's moral commands must be understood in their larger biblical context. A parallel point here is this: Christian philosophical and theological medical ethics must be understood in the context of the broader reaches of the philosophy and theology of medicine.

The upshot of all this seems to be that Christian medical decision making must take place in a context characterized by comprehensive concerns and a rather broad interdisciplinary dialogue. It will not do simply to apply biblical proof-texts to contemporary issues. Nor is "doing ethics" adequate. Admittedly, the appropriate alternative is difficult to state in terms of a precise methodology. A number of catchphrases seem, to me at least, to point in the right methodological direction: Tillich's notion of "correlating" the biblical message with contemporary problems; the call to engage in "dialogue before the Word"; the emphasis on seeking to have our contemporary struggles "disciplined" by our submission to biblical authority.

Of course, the Bible itself points in these directions. Christians are called to participate in the life of a community, in whose midst they are to "prove what is the will of God, and what is good and acceptable and perfect" (Rom. 12:2). This community is given a mandate to exercise the "gifts of the spirit," such as—to use the list of 1 Corinthians 12—"the utterance of wisdom," "the utterance of knowledge," "faith," "healing," "the working of miracles," "prophecy," "the ability to distinguish between spirits," "tongues," and the "interpretation of tongues." Perhaps it is no accident that the gift of healing is linked here to the gifts of prophecy and discernment—to say nothing of the gifts of wisdom and knowledge.

Basic Assumptions in Medicine

The Bible is a book about God and about his relationship to the creation in general and to human creatures in particular. To accept the biblical message is to grasp hold of facts—"extraordinary" facts, perhaps, but accounts nonetheless of what is the case—which, because of our sinfulness and finitude, we would not otherwise take hold of.

To believe what the Bible says about God and creation and human persons is to be thrust into a network of relationships and obligations of which we would not otherwise be aware. For example, the biblical writers describe God as a shepherd, a father (and on some occasions, a mother), a king. As James Gustafson notes, these "analogies to social roles imply certain relations, which, in turn, are sources for delineating certain moral purposes or duties."[6] The duties and purposes generated by these relationships bear on medical matters in a variety of ways.

Much attention has been given by Christian medical ethicists to questions of how biblical purposes and duties bear on medical matters as they occur within the present patterns of medical care. How is the surgeon to show agape to the patient? How can the clergy-person better coordinate his or her efforts with those of medical specialists? What does service to one's neighbor mean for the Christian social worker? How can we achieve more just and righteous patterns of health-care delivery?

My own impression is that a good many of such discussions have a rather "priestly" tone to them.

They assume, for the most part at least, the legitimacy of current standards and norms for medical practice, asking how we can be more loving or just within those patterns. The "prophetic" task of offering a critique of the fundamental patterns themselves has been left to groups who are beyond the pale of Christian medical ethics "orthodoxy." Three such prophetic groups come to mind: (1) various Marxist- and anarchist-oriented writers; (2) those who have been diagnosing the alleged "iatrogenic diseases" of Western societies; and (3) medical "fundamentalists," such as the Jehovah's Witnesses, Christian Scientists, Seventh Day Adventists, the Amish, and the "Old Reformed" Dutch Calvinists, each of whom rejects some significant item of contemporary medical orthodoxy.

If we were to take the basic concerns of these prophetic groups seriously, a result would be the development of a full-scale critique of the patterns of contemporary medicine from a point of view characterized by political, cultural, spiritual, and theological sensitivities. Attention here would be given to some of the fundamental "givens" of contemporary medical thought and practice.

This is not to say that Christian medical ethicists (or, more generally, theorists) should merely mimic the criticisms of any or all of the three groups mentioned above. In a broad-ranging dialogue on these issues, Christian thinkers will undoubtedly disagree among themselves on the merits of this or that prophetic pronouncement. The goal here is to expose contemporary medical patterns to a critical scrutiny which is disciplined by submission to biblical authority.

Take, for example, Ivan Illich's recent critique of "the medicalization of life." Illich insists that the development of medical bureaucracies leads to (among other things) conditions of this sort; "disabling dependence" on medical experts, the lowering of "levels of tolerance for discomfort or pain," the abolition of "the right to self-care," the "hospitalization" of suffering, and the labeling of "suffering, mourning, and healing outside the patient role" as "a form of deviance."[7]

Illich may be misperceiving or distorting the empirical situations, as Thomas Szasz may also be doing when he insists that "medicine now functions as a state religion."[8] But even if these writers are locating possible tendencies rather than actual states of affairs, the factors they point to are worthy of critical reflection.

Similarly, there is something to be said for the instincts, if not the hermeneutics, of the medical fundamentalists. For example, the Old Reformed refuse polio immunization, and other preventative measures, by appealing to Jesus' claim that "those who are well have no need of a physician, but those who are sick" (Matt. 9:12). Their error here is not that they think that claims made by Jesus have relevance for contemporary medical decision making, but that they misconstrue his actual intention in making this particular observation. Nonetheless, there is a kind of integrity in their insistence upon exposing medical "technique" to theological and spiritual scrutiny.

On the most favorable reading of the claims of the medical fundamentalists, what is being resisted is the absorption of the individual's struggle with suffering into the context of the patient-role. Unfortunately, many of the most vocal secular critics of the same pattern of absorption view the proper alternative in terms of the "autonomy" of the individual. Thus, the fundamental conflict is often viewed as one between medicalization and the right to self-care.

Christians (at least some Christians) will want to join the fundamentalists in viewing the basic situation in different terms. The Christian is a creature of God, "belonging" to him by virtue of God's creating and redeeming activity. All other relationships and duties and roles must be assessed in the light of this primary relationship with its attendant duties. If medical "intervention" by experts poses a threat, then, it is not to one's autonomy but rather to one's fidelity to the primary covenantal relationship with God. The danger is not so much a loss of freedom as it is a temptation to place idolatrous trust in medical technology.

Take the standard textbook case of the woman who has terminal cancer, but whose doctors think it not in her best interest to know the facts about her condition. If the patient is a Christian, then certain factors have to be taken into account in deciding what is in her best interest. For one thing, it is in the Christian's interest to be allowed to struggle with the spiritual significance of a specific affliction. Like Paul in his struggles with his "thorn in the flesh," the Christian must ask, "Why has God allowed this to happen to me, and what constitutes a faithful response to this development?" In this case, the woman must be allowed to assess the role which this experience of disease plays in her overall career as a human being. And because of what she believes by virtue of her acceptance of a Christian view of things, she will understand her own "career" as extending into the age of the Resurrection. She must go through the struggle of evaluating her own suffering and impending death in the light of the apostle's declaration: "I consider that the sufferings of this present time are not worth comparing with the glory that is to be revealed to us" (Rom. 8:18).

It is obvious simply from reading the Bible that there is an important emphasis placed there on the merits of a fully informed struggle, in the presence of

God, with the issues of personal suffering and the questions of life and death. It is an important part of the Christian experience to bargain, like King Hezekiah, for an extension of life, or to plead in agony, like Jesus himself, "Let this cup pass from me." The spiritual significance of suffering corresponds, for the Christian, to a right to know the facts about one's physical condition.

Of course, not all medical experts or ethicists will consider this view of suffering to be legitimate or plausible. But the question here is not one of asking everyone to agree with the Christian; it is a question of finding a just pattern of distributing medical information, a pattern which is built on an awareness of the existing plurality of perspectives on the issues of life and death, health and suffering.

The recent establishment of hospices and "holistic medicine clinics" may well be a positive sign in the direction of new forms of medical organization which can serve as practical alternatives for Christians who want to view health care from a self-consciously Christian perspective. These practical experiments in medical alternatives should perhaps also be viewed as a challenge and stimulus for new directions in Christian medical theorizing.

If some Christians are going to insist that their right to approach suffering in a Christian manner be respected, this has implications for broader issues having to do with medical justice. If, as the Heidelberg Catechism puts it, "I, with body and soul, both in life and death, am not my own, but belong unto my faithful Savior Jesus Christ," then questions about what other persons do to my own body will have theological—even "ideological"—significance for me. And if I claim medical rights as over against those who have differing views concerning the meaning and nature of my suffering, justice would seem to require that I be willing to generalize from my own case.

Thus, it would seem quite plausible to suggest that Christians who sense some conflict between their own medical perspectives and those of a "medicalized" society should be willing to formulate policies which grant rights to those who have even different ideologies than their own. Norman Cantor's excellent discussion of a patient's right to decline lifesaving medical treatment[9] seems to me to be an excellent starting point for a discussion that should be extended into a number of other areas which relate to issues of medical pluralism.

Medical Politics

My main concern in this discussion has been to show some of the ways in which medical questions might be approached by Christians who hold a "high" view of biblical inspiration and authority. My comments have been primarily programmatic in nature; consequently, I have skimmed over some important topics and left others untouched.

It is perhaps significant that this discussion has drifted in the direction of the sociopolitical dimensions of medical questions. The fact is that Protestant Christians who claim allegiance to a conservative or "traditional" theological perspective have not, in this century at least, demonstrated many clear sensitivities to the political dimensions of the biblical message, to say nothing of the application of that political message to medical questions.

But in very recent years many theologians—Roman Catholic, Eastern Orthodox, and Protestant (including some conservative Protestants)—have contributed to a renewed interest in the biblical address to political matters. From this ecumenical theological exploration, at least three important emphases have emerged, and each seems to have important implications for medical issues, although the connections have as yet been largely ignored.

First, and perhaps most important, has been the emphasis on the biblical call to identify with the concerns of the "poor and oppressed." Biblical passages dealing with this theme often single out specific types of persons as special objects of God's compassion and redemptive concern: the widow, the orphan, the prisoner, the sojourner, the hungry beggar (see, e.g., Ps. 146). What these types seem to have in common is that they are without rights or legal "standing" before the political, economic, and cultural structures of society.

The second emphasis is on the phenomenon of "contextualization"—a prominent notion in recent discussions carried on by Third World Christians. What is at stake here is the contention that the Christian Gospel is inevitably received in a context characterized by, among other things, the political, economic, and "class" orientation of the hearer. This emphasis has been accompanied by the insistence that Western (or "North Atlantic") Christians examine the biases which have influenced, and even distorted, their theological reflections.

A third emphasis has grown out of the work of the post-World War II "biblical theology" movement. Here there is a growing number of studies of the New Testament, especially Pauline, references to "principalities and powers," which are understood to be "invisible authorities" who influence the "minds" and structures of a society and who, as "the rulers of darkness," tempt human beings into patterns of corporate idolatry (racism, sexism, consumerism, militarism). This emphasis has led some commentators to stress the need for a discernment of the spirits as they show their influence in the systemic patterns of human interaction.

Each of these emphases—much too briefly described here—embodies a concern which deserves a special place on the agenda of contemporary Christian medical thought. No moral perspective which takes divine commands seriously can ignore the overwhelming number of occasions on which God has commanded his people to defend the cause of those who are helpless before the structures of society. Some crucial questions for medical ethics are: Who are the helpless ones in the area of medical care? Whose cries for medical attention are currently going unheeded? How best can the physically oppressed be liberated within a framework of justice?

The emphasis on contextualization indicates the need for Christian thinkers to be conscious of their own class and cultural biases in discussing medical questions—and perhaps to search for the kinds of pluralistic structures appropriate to the fact of medical contextualization. And all of this must be done out of a desire to be spiritually discerning, even if that requires us to question the basic "minds" which are often at work in medical discussions.

Notes

1. Peter Geach, *God and the Soul* (New York: Schocken Books, 1969), 117.
2. Joseph Fletcher, *Situation Ethics: The New Morality* (Philadelphia: Westminster Press, 1966), 26.
3. Geach, *God and the Soul,* 127.
4. James M. Gustafson, "The Contributions of Theology to Medical Ethics," 1975 Père Marquette Theology Lecture (Milwaukee: Marquette University, Theology Department, 1975), 84.
5. See Julio de Santa Ana, *Good News to the Poor: The Challenge of the Poor in the History of the Church* (Maryknoll, N.Y.: Orbis Books, 1979).
6. Gustafson, "The Contributions of Theology to Medical Ethics," 17.
7. Ivan Illich, *Medical Nemesis: The Expropriation of Health* (New York: Bantam Books, 1977), 33.
8. Thomas Szasz, *The Theology of Medicine: The Political-Philosophical Foundations of Medical Ethics* (New York: Harper and Row, 1977), 146.
9. Norman L. Cantor, "A Patient's Decision to Decline Lifesaving Medical Treatment: Bodily Integrity versus the Preservation of Life," *Rutgers Law Review* 26 (1973): 228-64. Reprinted in *Ethics in Medicine: Historical Perspectives and Contemporary Concerns,* ed. Stanley Joel Reiser, Arthur J. Dyck, and William J. Curran (Cambridge, Mass.: M.I.T. Press, 1977).

11.
Bio-ethics: Some Challenges from a Liberation Perspective

KAREN LEBACQZ

The Task

In Lewis Carroll's delightful story *Alice in Wonderland,* Alice has a tendency to change size, not always at will. On one such occasion, the following dialogue ensues:

"Don't squeeze so," said the Dormouse to Alice.

"I can't help it. I'm growing," she replied.

"You've no right to grow *here.*"

"Don't talk nonsense; you know you're growing, too."

"Yes, but *I* grow at a reasonable pace, and not in that ridiculous fashion."

These words describe all too accurately what many of us feel today in the face of the so-called "biological revolution": sitting next to something that appears to be growing at a ridiculous rate, we feel "squeezed" and are tempted to cry out: "You've no right to grow *here.*" Wonderland, or bad dream? Current arguments posit one or the other: proponents hold out visions of miraculous cures for human ailments and new freedoms in human living, while opponents raise the spectre of Huxley's *Brave New World.* Perhaps the only thing on which both would agree is that developments in biomedical technology threaten to change the nature of our existence.

Rather than undertake a direct discussion of ethical dilemmas raised by biomedical research and technological capacity, I wish to raise a more profound question related to our sense of being "squeezed". The great church historian Ernst Troeltsch once said: "If the present social situation is to be controlled by Christian principles, thoughts will be necessary which have not yet been thought, and which will correspond to this new situation as the older forms met the need of the social situation in earlier ages."[1]

In the conviction that advances in biomedical technology require the development of "thoughts which have not yet been thought", I shall focus on the *way* we analyse ethical issues in biomedical arenas. That

From *Faith and Science in an Unjust World.* Report of the *World Council of Churches' Conference on Faith, Science and the Future,* vol. 1: Plenary Presentations, ed. Roger L. Shinn (Geneva: World Council of Churches, 1980), pp. 272-81. Used by permission.

is, my concern will be methodological rather than substantive. In particular, I shall argue that the predominant western approach to bio-ethical issues suffers serious limitations and should be challenged in the light of some emerging ethical reflection, particularly that of feminist and liberation theology.

Bio-Ethics: The Prevailing Approach

Most contemporary writings in bio-ethics share certain characteristics. While the following list would not apply uniformly, it does suggest the predominant characteristics of the field.

1. Decision-Orientation

Like much current social ethics, both philosophical and theological, contemporary bio-ethics is largely decision-oriented. It focuses on such questions as: "Should we operate on this newborn infant with a congenital defect?", "Should we permit recombinant DNA research?" and so on. Indeed, most has been "crisis"-oriented, dealing not simply with action decisions in medical research and care, but with catastrophic events rather than routine questions about delivery of care.[2]

In short, we have focused on *doing the right thing.* This discussion of the right thing to do has resulted in increased clarity about the nature and meaning of some ethical dilemmas, some movement towards resolution of important ethical dilemmas in particular cases, and agreement about basic ethical principles applicable to certain bio-ethical dilemmas.

Nonetheless, the decision-orientation of contemporary bio-ethics has serious flaws. First, it tends to give the impression that there is *one* correct decision in every dilemma and that our only task is to find the "right" answer. It ignores the possibility that every possible action may embody some important values and that what may be at stake is not finding the "right" answer but choosing among competing values.

Second, traditional normative ethics considers at least three questions: (1) which actions are right; (2) what makes a person "good" or virtuous; and (3) what constitutes the "ideal state" or structure of human society. The decision-orientation of contemporary bio-ethics focuses on the first of these. With some exceptions, two important aspects of normative ethics have been largely ignored.

2. Individualistic Orientation

Most contemporary bio-ethics is also individualistic. It begins with the concerns of individual patients or physicians as they encounter dilemmas. Indeed, much contemporary bio-ethics takes as its starting place the "physician-patient relationship".[3]

This focus reflects the western, white culture from which such discussions originate, and is not adequate to explain the needs and experiences of most of the world. In many localities and countries, the major health questions have nothing to do with physicians and how they treat patients, but have instead to do with poor housing, inadequate sewage systems, and so on. In other localities, health care is provided through massive bureaucracies in which the primary problem may be that of getting *access* to a physician, not how one is treated once one finally sees her or him.[4] In a social structure where there is no access to physicians for major portions of the population, or in which one's "physician-patient relationship" comprises no more than 2% of one's medical and health care, a bio-ethics that takes the "physician-patient relationship" as normative is simply inapplicable. What is needed is an approach that focuses on systems and institutions and that takes seriously the entire web of relationships in the delivery of care, of which the presumed "physician-patient relationship" is only one.

3. Ahistorical Approach

Partly because of the search for norms and principles that are generally applicable, bio-ethics as currently practised tends to be ahistorical. It is assumed that once the "right" answer is found, it will be correct for all similar cases; little discussion is given to the changing historical setting within which bio-ethical decisions are made and whether this setting might affect the correctness of the decision. Resulting norms tend to be rigid.[5] While not all theorists agree with the "absolutist" position that, for example, rejects all abortion as unethical, most assume that once the proper "exceptions" are found, they hold irrespective of historical circumstance.

The "contextual" or "situational" approach to ethics, which gained popularity in the United States during the 1960's, attempted to correct this ahistorical rigidity by refusing to accept any "absolutes". However, in its own way it remains ahistorical: by failing to specify clearly *which* aspects of a situation or *which* historical changes make a difference, it also tends to focus on the immediate situation and loses any historical "bite". It leaves one with the impression that historical settings either do not matter at all, or that there is no way to sort out which do and which do not; thus, it fails to specify criteria for deciding which historical contexts are "morally relevant".

4. Scientific Evidence as Normative

Most bio-ethicists today operate out of the dominant western scientific world-view, in which science sets criteria for the acceptability of evidence. The results are, first, a minimizing of the value of individual or group experience, and second, a blurring of the value-laden nature of "facts" or data.

It is not uncommon, for example, to hear an ethicist say that the medical personnel or scientists must provide the "facts" or evidence in the case. While personal experiences are not totally ignored, they tend to be discredited: "feelings" are not an adequate basis for ethical decision-making; only logical analysis of "facts" will do. This tends to take the decision away from those most intimately involved, for they are often not in possession of all the data and are also inclined to be emotional in their responses.

Moreover, it tends to obfuscate the value-laden nature of data. Data are not value-free. We make choices about what to look for, how to measure what we find, and how to present it. Professional training determines to a large extent how we structure inquiry and how we interpret the results of that inquiry. In addition, prior value assumptions shape our interpretation and presentation of data. (E.g. is there a 50% chance of having a normal child, or a 50% chance of having a defective child? Note that the term "defective" is itself a value judgment, not a statement of fact.)

5. Grounding of Norms

Most discussions of bio-ethical issues, particularly those by Christian ethicists, either accept a wide variety of grounding sources for norms or fail to specify the grounding of particular norms; there is also little discussion of the movement from theological presuppositions to particular norms.[6] For example, in his influential book *The Patient as Person,* Ramsey introduces a number of Judeo-Christian affirmations such as *hesed* (steadfast love), covenant (faithfulness), and the like. In his discussion of concrete issues, however, he turns to norms derived from medical sources such as the Nuremberg Code with its requirement for informed consent. The link between the two sources—if, indeed, there is any—is not clear, and it is often not clear how Ramsey incorporates his Christian principles into an otherwise Kantian perspective.

It is understandable, of course, that Christian ethicists working in the field of bio-ethics would incorporate a broad base for normative statements. Many operate out of a "natural law" tradition or approach in which they affirm as a part of their Christian belief a general set of norms available to all persons and not necessarily distinctive for Christians.[7] Moreover bio-ethicists must speak to lawyers, scientists, politicians, and others who do not operate out of a specifically Christian approach. It therefore behoves the Christian ethicist not to be overly narrow.

Nonetheless, the failure to specify the grounding for norms results in confusion and disagreement as to (1) what norms there are, if any; (2) which are applicable to the situation; (3) how they are to be interpreted, e.g. does "justice" require protection of the vulnerable or simply equal treatment?; and (4) how to weigh and balance conflicting norms, e.g. does the potential social good outweigh the requirement to seek informed consent in certain types of research or genetic screening programmes? In particular, we need to know whether it makes a difference to do bio-ethics as a "Christian" and, if so, what that difference is.

Challenges and Alternatives

I shall here suggest some major alternatives to the prevailing mode of doing bio-ethics, drawing primarily on contemporary work in feminist and liberation theology.[8] I shall also indicate the sorts of questions that these alternative approaches would suggest, though it will not be possible here to answer these questions or to put them into full context.

1. Patterns of Meaning and Structural Concerns

Liberation theologians and feminists are primarily concerned not with choosing the right action, but with structures and patterns of meaning.

I believe that this is partly why there has been little attention in these writings to bio-ethical issues, important though technological advances in biomedicine may be for the lives of women and other members of oppressed and disadvantaged groups. At a recent conference on Ethical Issues in Reproductive Technology: Analysis by Women, questions about whether *in vitro* fertilization is right or wrong were transmuted into questions about who holds the power to make such decisions, what the impact of all biomedical technologies combined is on the lives of women in this society, and so on.[9] In short, questions about what is right and wrong to *do* were ignored in favour of questions about the nature of the social structures and mythologies that support these technologies.

Other liberation theologians argue that it is not merely the shape of *particular* social institutions and structures that must be analysed, but the shape of the entire *age* or epoch. For example, Roy Sano argues that Asian American liberation theologians and people turn to apocalyptic rather than prophetic literature because apocalyptic literature gives a better base from which to observe the interweavings of the various powerful institutions.[10] Dussel argues that what is at stake is recognizing the shape of evil in any and all institutions.[11] Feminist theologians analyse the myths that undergird particular institutions by defining the "masculine" and "feminine" in society.[12] Thus, it is not simply particular institutions that are to be analysed ethically, but the thought structures, myths, and loyalties that permit those institutions to exist. The very shape of the scientific world-view may be at stake.

Applied to the biomedical arena, these insights would suggest some new questions to be asked: What images of health, disease, normalcy, womanhood, sexuality, etc. undergird the present delivery of health care and development of new biomedical technologies? Who or what are our current idols? Where are our loyalties? What is the relationship between the development of new biomedical technologies and nuclear power, communications technology, and so on? The primary ethical question has to do with the shape and inter-relationship of the dominant social structures and their impact on the lives of those who are oppressed. It is in part a theological question, having to do with our loyalties and whether we give our allegiance to anything other than God—even to the scientific world-view.

2. Story and Community

As soon as one asks about patterns of meaning, one moves beyond looking at the specific decision to asking how that decision fits into the context of a life. The particular decision may either make sense or be muted in its total context within the person's life. Thus, questions of character, integrity, and virtue come to have central significance, and the telling and shaping of one's life story is crucial to the ethical task.[13]

The women's movement and feminist theology in particular have stressed the importance of life stories as the groundwork for theology. As women share their experiences, they locate patterns of meaning that emerge and give theological dimension. Theology and ethics, thus, are born of experience and its coherence in a life story.[14]

But this is partly because the interpretative framework brought to one's own life story has political significance. As women commonly put it, "the personal is political". This means that the entire context in which one interprets one's own story also matters. And so a concern for story and its patterns of meaning results in a concern for community. Indeed, it is often only when women are together in community that they make the transition from saying "I'm depressed"—an interpretative framework provided by the dominant western scientific world-view—to saying "I'm oppressed"—an interpretation possible within the context of a liberating community.

Applied to the field of bio-ethics, this concern for story and community would suggest that we ask not: "Should this woman have an abortion?" but: "What is this woman's story? What are the interpretative frameworks that give meaning to her life? Does she have a supportive community? Is she oppressed? Will the abortion be liberating for her? Will it be community-building or community destroying?"

The concern for story and community that arises from feminist and liberation perspectives is akin to Ramsey's concern for covenant, Lehmann's focus on the koinonia, and H. R. Niebuhr's concern for accountability structures, in that it focuses on one's relationship within a group. However, I believe that feminist and liberation theologians are more true to the biblical perspective when they go beyond Ramsey, Lehmann, and Niebuhr to the point of seeing one's *identity* as in some way intimately related to that group. Ramsey talks about covenants between physician and patient as though no others need be involved, whereas women and members of oppressed groups argue that those in existence today have sufficient continuity with those of the past to be able to stand in their stead and receive what was their due. This is a radically different notion of identity and I believe that it is one of the contributions that a feminist or liberation theology might make to the field of bio-ethics.

3. History (or "Herstory", as Feminists Say)

What has just been said makes it clear that feminists and liberation theologians also require a *historical* ethic—an ethic that takes seriously the oppression of people through time and asks: "Is something that was appropriate yesterday still appropriate today? Will it be appropriate tomorrow?" Yesterday's oppressions are not simply forgotten, but must be rectified today. Thus, for example, no interpretation of justice may be proffered that fails to account for retribution and compensation for past injury. Perhaps most important, this focus on history requires the rewriting of history, with a view to lifting up the role of women and other oppressed peoples—to locating the "fore-mothers" as well as the "fore-fathers" of current medical practice and technological innovation.

Applied to the arena of bio-ethics, this historical view would certainly preclude an absolute and unyielding "yes" or "no" to technological innovations. More important, however, it would require a second look at the history of development of biomedical technologies to ask how that history is perceived from the perspective of oppressed peoples, how it impacts on their lives and possibilities, and so on. One is tempted to suggest that from this perspective serious questions need to be raised about whether these technologies should be developed in the absence of basic nutritional, health, and medical care in "third world" countries.

4. Experiential Approach

To argue for the importance of history, and for the re-claiming of one's story, is also to argue for new interpretative frameworks. Thus, new criteria for evidence are emerging. Scientific data are *not* the only source of meaningful interpretation; the life histories and shared experiences of oppressed groups are the primary "facts" to be considered. Most feel that only those who have had such experiences can communicate them accurately. Thus, there is a tendency to shift from a dependence on experts to a focus on the layperson.

This new approach also suggests that there may be numerous valid value systems, not one "right" approach. At the same time, as the above analysis has shown, the primary loyalty is always to those who are oppressed, and it is their interpretations and perspectives that are given most validity.

Applied to the ethical issues posed by technological advances in medicine and science, the questions become obvious: What is the experience of women who want desperately to become pregnant and are unable to conceive? Why do they want this so desperately—i.e. what in the system creates this need? How does the development of these technologies affect the chances for life and health of the "Third World"? And, perhaps most important, are these developments really "advances" at all? Finally, a participatory decision-making model, perhaps involving community as well as individual participation, might be called for with respect to each technology and to the scientific enterprise as a whole.

5. Sources for Ethics

Since the question of norms is no longer the only question asked, the issue of grounding of norms is broadened to ask about sources of ethical insight. From the above, it is clear that a primary source for both feminists and liberation theologians is the experience of the oppressed group. Indeed, Cone goes so far as to assert that only those who are "black" can talk about God in the United States.[15]

Taking the experiences of the oppressed as central to the theological task has led some feminists to move beyond Christianity altogether, and to assert that the grounding for theological insight lies in women's bodies (e.g. menstruation and bodily cycles), dreams, and rituals.[16] Others retain a closer adherence to biblical insight, but with the proviso that the biblical message be measured and interpreted by the experiences of the oppressed.[17]

Serious questions remain for feminists and liberation theologians at this point. Is there a different norm or ethic for each group? Or is there only one ethical system, but that one discernible only by the oppressed? Is there a "natural law" or insight into ethical stances and norms provided by the natural (e.g. women's bodies)? Until such methodological questions are addressed systematically, the impact of these new approaches cannot be fully assessed. It is difficult to know thus far what the impact on bio-ethics might be of new approaches to the source of ethical insight.

Conclusions

It is not the rate of growth of biomedical technologies *per se* that makes us feel "squeezed". Rather, it is the threat they present to the meaning structures of our world. This essay is submitted in the hopes of initiating the task of creating "thoughts which have not yet been thought" and which will meet the social situation of our day. Wonderland, or nightmare? Much depends on our perspective. Will we open that perspective to the challenge of the oppressed and incorporate into the doing of bio-ethics the message of liberation theology?

Notes

1. Ernst Troeltsch: *The Social Teachings of the Christian Churches,* p. 1012. New York: Harper Torchback Edition, 1960.

2. I have criticized this "crisis" approach in an earlier essay. See Karen Lebacqz: "Peter and His Doctor". *Journal of Current Social Issues,* Fall 1975. At the same time, I wish to emphasize that I have also tended to adopt the decision-orientation in my own writings in the field of bio-ethics. Thus, the purpose of this essay is not to assign blame to those who take such an approach, but to try to be cognizant of its limits.

3. While examples are legion, one of the best known is Paul Ramsey's important volume, *The Patient as Person* (New Haven: Yale University Press, 1970).

4. I personally have not had a sustained "physician-patient relationship" with any single physician for more than 16 years; I find that my single most important problem is getting *to* the doctor—it routinely takes two hours of telephoning, two hours of waiting, and at least four contacts with clerks, receptionists, nurses, and others before I see the physician for what is generally a maximum of ten minutes. Since I am a relatively well-situated and well-educated health care consumer, I can only imagine how such problems might be multiplied for those who are less fortunate.

5. This is particularly a problem when norms are turned into governmental regulations. The norm "seek informed consent" still permits some flexibility; however, a law mandating informed consent does not permit the same flexibility.

6. Several recent volumes attempt to address this problem. See Philip Wogaman: *A Christian Method of Moral Judgment* (Philadelphia: Westminster Press, 1976).

7. For example, in his discussion of proxy consent for children, Richard McCormick argues that there are certain values that all human beings ought to uphold, and that therefore one may give consent on behalf of a child in order to foster those values. See "Proxy Consent in the Experimentation Situation". *Perspectives in Biology and Medicine,* Vol. 18, No. 1, 1974.

8. Two words of explanation are in order here. First, much "feminist" theology *is* liberation theology and can be classified under that general heading. However, some feminist theologizing does not fit neatly under the liberation approach, and I have therefore chosen to specify that I am drawing from both types of theological thought as they are emerging.

Second, feminist and liberation theologies are not the only sources of some of the alternative insights and approaches specified here. A number of male theologians and ethicists from the dominant tradition have fostered one or another of these concerns, e.g. the Niebuhr stress on community, the work of Gustafson, Stanley Hauerwas, and others on character and virtue, James McClendon's stress on biography. Nonetheless, I shall take the theology from feminists and liberation thinkers as my baseline for this analysis.

9. Held at Amherst, Massachusetts, 24–29 June 1979.

10. Roy Sano: "Ethnic Liberation Theology: Neo-Orthodoxy Reshaped or Replaced?" *Christianity and Crisis,* 10 November 1975. Others who are using apocalyptic literature and suggesting that it is the entire shape of the age that must be analysed and criticized include William Stringfellow: *An Ethic for Christians and Other Aliens in a Strange Land* (Waco, Texas: Word Books, 1973), and William Coats: *God in Public: Political Theology Beyond Niebuhr* (Grand Rapids, Michigan: William B. Eerdmans, 1974).

11. Enrique Dussel: *Ethics and the Theology of Liberation.* New York: Orbis Books, 1978.

12. See, for example, Jo Freeman (ed.): *Women: a Feminist Perspective* (Palo Alto: Mayfield, 1979); Anne Koedt *et al.*: *Radical Feminism* (New York: Quadrangle/The New York Times Book Co., 1973); Mary Daly: *Gyn/Ecology: the Metaethics of Radical Feminism* (Boston: Beacon Press, 1978); Sheila Collins: *A Different Heaven and Earth* (Valley Forge, Pa.: Judson Press, 1974); Mary Vetterling-Braggin *et al.*: *Feminism and Philosophy* (Totowa, NJ: Littlefield, Adams and Co., 1977); Rosemary Reuther: *Religion and Sexism* (New York: Simon and Schuster, 1974).

13. For example, in *Beyond Mere Obedience,* Dorothee Sölle describes the life story of a woman who broke many of the conventions of her day and whose life would probably be judged by most to include some unethical acts. Nonetheless, within the context of her total life, she has gone "beyond mere obedience" into a life of freedom, and she expresses some virtues and character that over-ride her particular misdoings.

14. Sheila Collins is particularly emphatic on this point. See *A Different Heaven and Earth, op. cit.,* and "Reflections on the Meaning of Herstory" and "Theology in the Politics of Appalachian Women", in Carol Christ and Judith Plaskow: *Womanspirit Rising.* New York: Harper and Row, 1979.

15. James Cone: *A Black Theology of Liberation.* New York: J. B. Lippincott, 1970. It is not clear whether "black" refers to skin colour necessarily or whether those of like spirit but different skin colour might be "black".

16. See essays by Plaskow, Goldenberg, Washburn, and Christ in *Womanspirit Rising, op. cit.*

17. See essays by Trible, Fiorenza, McLaughlin in *Womanspirit Rising, op. cit.*

Chapter Three
THE PROFESSION AND ITS INTEGRITY

Introduction

When Christians "profess" their faith they commit themselves to God and to God's cause. From *profateri* (to confess, own, acknowledge), *profession* first meant "the declaration, promise, or vow made by one entering a religious order" (*Oxford English Dictionary,* s.v. *profession*). In a religious context the requirement of integrity upon the "professor" is clear and compelling, even if sometimes complex. The term has been secularized, however, and applied to other occupations which require special knowledge or skill. This chapter confronts the reader with two basic questions: first, whether the profession of medicine still declares, promises, or vows anything which would make a requirement of integrity clear and compelling, if sometimes complex; and second, whether and, if so, how the profession of medicine is related to a profession of the Christian faith.

The first question may be framed in a number of different ways: Should the profession of medicine be understood as a value-free collection of skills learned by training and accessible to consumers or as a value-laden form of human activity constituted as much by the ends it seeks as by the skills it uses? Can medical ethics be done by articulating and applying the goods and standards implicit in the profession or only by specifically applying norms learned outside the profession, whether by reason or revelation? Is the expertise and authority of the professional only technical or also, in some sense, moral? Is professional excellence a technical matter or a moral matter as well? Does it make sense for a physician to introduce a moral claim by saying, "As a physician I think . . . "?

The excerpt from Veatch below rejects the claim to a special professional ethic as fallacious and dangerous. The other essays agree in defending a professional ethic which is not simply the application of universal and rational norms to the specialties of medicine. But the agreement that there is a professional ethic does not entail agreement about what it is or about how to describe and defend it. The disagreements extend even to different assessments of the famous Hippocratic Oath and are related in turn to different understandings of the medical tradition and the medical community.

If there is a professional ethic, then the question of the relation of the medical profession to the Christian profession will be as important to those who would reflect theologically about medical ethics as is the question of the relation of an impartial and rational perspective to a Christian perspective (an issue raised in the previous chapter). Thomas Sydenham's eloquent and powerful description of "the doctor" is suggestive of some of the ways a Christian profession nurtured and sustained a medical professional. In Sydenham's remarks there seems to be a powerful identification of the Christian profession and the medical profession, or at least a neat harmony between the declaration a physician makes as a Christian and the declaration a Christian makes as a physician. Other Christian voices have been raised in prophetic protest against medicine and what was taken to be the ethos of physicians: the Christian profession has been set over against the medical profession. Edmund Pellegrino raises the question of the relation of the Christian profession to the medical profession in terms of what is "added," but perhaps the possibility (or necessity) of a creative tension or even transformation should not be overlooked.

Another question here, of course, is the theological resources to be brought to bear on the medical profession. Pellegrino attends especially to the model of Christ's healing ministry. William May attends especially to features of covenant in the biblical tradition. Allen Verhey attends to native senses of gratitude and dependence, of a tragic fault, of responsibility to the transcendent, and suggests that these be informed by the biblical narrative. None of the authors claim to be exhaustive, but their suggestions nevertheless can—and should—be subjected to critical review in terms of their appropriateness to medicine and their adequacy to the Christian profession.

Perhaps Sydenham's "profession" sounds quaint, even naive, today. The medical profession has become considerably more complex, and Christian profession has perhaps become less confident. But those who would search for and live with integrity, while they not only stand in plural communities and traditions but also own, acknowledge, and profess their causes, will celebrate Sydenham's declaration. Perhaps a pleasant harmony of medical profession and Christian profession no longer exists, but it may honor Sydenham to strike the discordant note if integrity with what has been promised or vowed requires it.

Suggestions for Further Reading

Alexander, Leo, M. D. "Medical Science under Dictatorship." *The New England Journal of Medicine* 241 (July 14, 1949): 39-47.

Allen, David F. "The Ethical Responsibility of the Physician: A Judeo-Christian Perspective." *The Yale Journal of Biology and Medicine* 49 (1976): 447-54.

Cassell, Eric. *The Healer's Art.* New York: Lippincott, 1976.

Camenisch, Paul. *Grounding Professional Ethics in a Pluralistic Society.* New York: Haven Publications, 1983.

Campbell, Alastair V. *Professional Care: Its Meaning and Practice.* Philadelphia: Fortress, 1984.

Etziony, M. B. *The Physician's Creed: An Anthology of Medical Prayers, Oaths, and Codes of Ethics Written and Recited by Medical Practitioners Through the Ages.* Springfield, Ill.: Charles C. Thomas, 1973.

Gustafson, James M. "Professions as Callings." *Social Science Review* 5 (December, 1982): 501-15.

Hauerwas, Stanley. "Authority and the Profession of Medicine." In *Responsibility in Health Care,* edited by G. Agich, 83-104. Dordrecht: D. Reidel, 1982.

Jenkins, Daniel T., ed. *The Doctor's Profession.* London: SCM, 1949.

Kass, Leon. "Professing Ethically: On the Place of Ethics in Defining Medicine." *Journal of the American Medical Association (JAMA)* 249 (March 11, 1983): 1305-10.

May, William F. *The Physician's Covenant.* Philadelphia: Westminster, 1983.

Pellegrino, Edmund D., and David C. Thomasma. *A Philosophical Basis of Medical Practice: Toward a Philosophy and Ethics of the Healing Professions.* New York: Oxford University Press, 1981.

12. The Doctor

THOMAS SYDENHAM

It becomes every man who purposes to give himself to the care of others, seriously to consider the four following things:—First, that he must one day give an account to the Supreme Judge of all the lives entrusted to his care. Secondly, that all his skill, and knowledge and energy as they have been given him by God, so they should be exercised for His glory and the good of mankind, and not for mere gain or ambition. Thirdly, and not more beautifully than truly, let him reflect that he has undertaken the care of no mean creature, for, in order that we may estimate the value, the greatness of the human race, the only begotten son of God became himself a man, and thus ennobled it with His divine dignity, and, far more than this, died to redeem it. And, fourthly, that the doctor, being himself a mortal man, should be diligent and tender in relieving his suffering patients, inasmuch as he himself must one day be a like sufferer.

From Edward F. Griffith, ed., *Doctors by Themselves,* 1951. Courtesy of Charles C Thomas, Publisher, Springfield, Illinois.

13.
The Doctor's Oath—and a Christian Swearing It

ALLEN VERHEY

The Hippocratic Oath

I swear by Apollo Physician and Asclepius and Hygeia and Panacea and all the gods and goddesses, making them my witnesses, that I will fulfill according to my ability and judgment this oath and this covenant:

To hold him who has taught me this art as equal to my parents and to live my life in partnership with him, and if he is in need of money to give him a share of mine, and to regard his offspring as equal to my brothers in male lineage and to teach them this art—if they desire to learn it—without fee and covenant; to give a share of precepts and oral instruction and all the other learning to my sons and to the sons of him who has instructed me and to pupils who have signed the covenant and have taken an oath according to the medical law, but to no one else.

I will apply dietetic measures for the benefit of the sick according to my ability and judgment; I will keep them from harm and injustice.

I will neither give a deadly drug to anybody if asked for it, nor will I make a suggestion to this effect. Similarly I will not give to a woman an abortive remedy. In purity and holiness I will guard my life and my art.

I will not use the knife, not even on sufferers from stone, but will withdraw in favor of such men as are engaged in this work.

Whatever house I may visit, I will come for the benefit of the sick, remaining free of all intentional injustice, of all mischief and in particular of sexual relations with both female and male persons, be they free or slaves.

Whatever I may see or hear in the course of the treatment or even outside of the treatment in regard to the life of men, which on no account one must spread abroad, I will keep to myself holding such things shameful to be spoken about.

If I fulfill this oath and do not violate it, may it be granted to me to enjoy life and art, being honored with fame among all men for all time to come; if I transgress it and swear falsely, may the opposite of all this be my lot.[1]

The Oath According to Hippocrates In So Far as a Christian May Swear It

Blessed be God the Father of our Lord Jesus Christ, Who is blessed for ever and ever; I lie not.

I will bring no stain upon the learning of the medical art. Neither will I give poison to anybody though asked to do so, nor will I suggest such a plan. Similarly I will not give treatment to women to cause abortion, treatment neither from above nor from below. But I will teach this art, to those who require to learn it, without grudging and without an indenture. I will use treatment to help the sick according to my ability and judgment. And in purity and in holiness I will guard my art. Into whatsoever houses I enter, I will do so to help the sick, keeping free from all wrongdoing, intentional or unintentional, tending to death or to injury, and from fornication with bond or free, man or woman. Whatsoever in the course of practice I see or hear (or outside my practice in social intercourse) that ought not to be published abroad, I will not divulge, but consider such things to be holy secrets. Now if I keep this oath and break it not, may God be my helper in my life and art, and may I be honoured among all men for all time. If I keep faith, well; but if I forswear myself may the opposite befall me.[2]

The Hippocratic Oath is the most familiar of that long line of oaths, prayers, and codes by which doctors have transmitted an ethos to members of their profession. Indeed, it is sometimes simply called "the doctor's oath." In our age, however, enamored of novelty and confident of its technological powers, familiarity seems to have bred, if not contempt,[3] at least the sort of quaint regard which relegates ancient documents to the historian's museum of curiosities. It is my intention, nevertheless, to suggest that there are lessons to be learned—or relearned—from this oath and its history, lessons which can be instructive concerning a professional ethic for physicians and the possible contributions of theology to that ethic.

The intention ought not be misunderstood. I will not suggest that the Hippocratic Oath is an adequate and comprehensive foundation for a professional ethic today. I will not call upon doctors and moralists concerned with medical ethics to swear it again. I will not

Reprinted with permission from *Linacre Quarterly,* vol. 51, no. 2, pp. 139-58. 850 Elm Grove Road, Elm Grove, WI 53122. Subscription rate: $20 per year; $5 per single issue.

deny that the invocation of Apollo, Asclepius, Hygeia, Panacea, and all the gods and goddesses sounds quaint to modern ears or claim that such an invocation can be made with Christian integrity. I will not deny that the ancient institutions presupposed in the oath for the learning and practice of medicine differ from their contemporary counterparts. And I will not recommend the stipulations of the oath as a code to simplify the address to the dilemmas and quandaries posed by medical practice.

That list of disclaimers, it may easily be observed, involves every part of the oath. It may prompt the question of what is to be salvaged. But the lessons to be gleaned from this ancient document are not to be found in its content so much as in certain features of its history and its method. I want to suggest that there are lessons to be learned (1) from its reformist intention; (2) from its treatment of medicine as a practice with intrinsic goods and standards; and (3) from setting these standards in a context which expressed and evoked an identity and recognized one's dependence upon and indebtedness to a community and to the transcendent. Finally, I want to suggest (4) that there is a lesson for Christians who would contribute to the discussions of bioethics in the early Church's adoption and revision of the doctor's oath. In an age when medicine's powers flourish, but its ethos flounders, the ancient oath may help us to attend to ways of doing medical ethics which are not currently popular. I undertake, therefore, both to describe certain features of the ancient oath and to defend them as having some promise for the contemporary consideration of medical ethics in comparison to certain features of the current literature.

The Reformist Intention

According to Ludwig Edelstein, interpreter of the oath, the Hippocratic Oath was not formulated by the great Hippocrates himself, but by a small group of Pythagorean physicians late in the fourth century B.C. Edelstein observes that the oath was a minority opinion, "a Pythagorean manifesto," written against the stream and intending the reform of medicine.[4]

For centuries before the oath, ancient physicians had provided poison for those whom they could not heal, had counted abortifacients among the tools of their trade, and had been disposed to the use of the knife instead of the less invasive use of dietetics and pharmacology. Moreover, they had sometimes been guilty of injustice and mischief toward their patients, and sometimes quite shamelessly broken confidences.

When the little sect of Pythagoreans set out to reform the condition of medicine, they found no help in the law, which forbade neither suicide nor abortion. They could plainly find no help in the conventional behavior of physicians in antiquity. Nor did they find help in any "philosophical consensus," for, insofar as there was any agreement about these issues, it worked against the Pythagorean position. Platonists, Cynics, and Stoics could honor suicide as a courageous triumph over fate. Aristotelians and Epicureans were much more circumspect, but they did not forbid suicide. And abortion was typically considered essential for a well-ordered state. The arguments between Pythagoreans and other Greek philosophers must have seemed as interminable and as conceptually incommensurable as any contemporary moral argument. The minority status of their opinions, however, did not dissuade the Pythagoreans.

The point is not to defend the oath's absolute prohibitions of abortion and euthanasia and surely not to defend Pythagorean philosophy or the premises it might supply to defend such prohibitions.[5] The point is rather to call attention to this feature of the oath's method and history, that in spite of their minority position, the convictions of this community led them and moved them to reform. They refused to be satisfied with the medicine they saw around them. They refused to reduce medical morality to what the law allowed or what some philosophical consensus determined. They intended the reform of medicine.

The lesson, I suggest, for the contemporary discussions of medical ethics is that some, at least, should take courage to investigate and articulate a medical ethic which may stand at some remove from conventional behavior and attitudes within the profession and which may be based on convictions and standards more particular and profound than legal and contractual obligations or some minimal philosophical consensus. Communities with convictions about what human persons are meant to be and to become, with visions of what it means for embodied persons to flourish and thrive, have an opportunity and vocation to think through the art of medicine from their own perspectives.

The recent literature on medical ethics has not owned such an agenda. Indeed, the moral convictions and visions of particular communities typically have been tolerated and trivialized in the literature. On the one hand, there is an insistence that everyone's moral point of view should be respected. On the other hand, there has been an insistence that the only arguments which may count publicly are those which can be made independently of a distinctive moral point of view. This simultaneous tolerance and trivialization is accomplished by making the autonomy of the agent the highest human good, by making contracts between such autonomous agents the model of human relationships, and by focusing almost exclusively on the procedural question of who should decide.[6] The ancient enterprise of attempting to understand and communicate the intrinsic good of human persons and of some human relationships and activities has been largely abandoned. Attempts to articulate communities' or traditions' address to those ancient questions may be tolerated if the "good" is kept to themselves, relegated resolutely to a "private" arena and, thus, trivialized. It may not even be tolerated if the "good" is announced as "public" good, for then it threatens to restrict and subvert autonomy. Such recent literature on medical ethics has provided—and can provide—only a "thin theory of the good,"[7] only a shriveled and dangerously minimal construal of the moral life in its medical dimensions. We find, in much contemporary medical ethics, for example, a readiness to insist on procedures to protect autonomy but a reticence to provide any advice about the morally proper uses of that autonomy and a dismissal of the idea that physicians should be the ones to give such advice.

The Hippocratic Oath, however, can remind us that the current focus on autonomy and contracts and procedural questions provides only a minimal account of medical morality. It can encourage us to own a fuller vision of medical morality and to seek the reform of medicine in the light of that vision.

The Pythagoreans' reform movement finally triumphed. The oath gradually moved from the status of a counter-cultural manifesto to a historic document which formed and informed the ethos of physicians for centuries. The explanation for this triumph was not any philosophical triumph by the Pythagoreans; their influence, never great, waned. Their reform, however, articulated not just Pythagorean moral premises and conclusions, but standards inherent in medicine when it is seen as a practice with certain intrinsic goods. They situated these standards in a context which provided and formed identity and which recognized dependence and indebtedness to a community and to the transcendent. These standards finally won the support of another minority community, a community which did move to dominance in Western culture—the Christian Church. These features of the oath explain its triumph. They are still instructive and, after more than two millennia, again innovative. They can help form the "fuller vision" of medical morality which may once again call for and sustain the reform of medicine.

Medicine as a Practice

The Pythagoreans began with their own convictions about human flourishing. But one of these convictions concerned the moral significance of the crafts, the arts, the *teknē*.[8] The Pythagoreans honored the arts, especially music and medicine, as having moral and, indeed, ontological significance. Therefore, they did not simply apply Pythagorean premises to morally neutral medical skills; instead, they tried to educe and elucidate the moral significance of the craft, the art, the *teknē* of medicine itself. Because this Pythagorean attitude to the crafts came to be dominant in late philosophical schools, notably the Stoics,[9] the Pythagorean reform of medicine flourished while Pythagorean philosophy waned.

In striking an intriguing contrast to most contemporary literature on medical ethics, which so often picks an ethical theory (whether Mill's or Rawls's or Nozick's or . . .) and applies it to dilemmas faced by medical practitioners, the Pythagorean conviction about the crafts allowed and required one to identify the good implicit in the craft and to articulate the standards coherent with the good of the craft. According to the oath, then, the doctor is obligated not because he is a Pythagorean, but because he is a doctor, and his obligations consist not only of standards based on Pythagorean doctrine but also of standards implicit in medicine.

The oath treats medicine as a craft, an art, a *teknē,* or to use Alasdair MacIntyre's term,[10] as a practice, not simply as a set of technical skills. That is to say, it treats medicine as a form of human activity with goods internal to it and standards of excellence implicit in it, not simply as an assortment of skills which can be made to serve extrinsic goods with merely technological excellence.

The goal of medicine, the good which is intrinsic to the practice, is identified by the oath as "the benefit of the sick." To benefit the sick is not simply the motive for taking up certain ethically neutral skills nor merely an extrinsic end to be accomplished by ethically neutral technical means.[11] It is, rather, the goal of medicine as a practice, and so it governed the physician's use of his skills in diet, drugs, and surgery, and the use of his privileged access to the patient's home and privacy. This intrinsic good entailed standards of professional excellence which could not be reduced to technological excellence.

The pattern is repeated again and again in the oath. Its prohibitions of active euthanasia, of assisting in suicide, and of abortion, for example, were not argued on the basis of Pythagorean premises; they were given as standards of a practice whose goal is to benefit the sick. Because the ends intrinsic to medicine are to heal the sick, to protect and nurture health, to maintain and restore physical well-being, limits could be imposed on the use of skills within the practice. The skills were not to be used to serve alien ends, and the destruction of human life—either the last of it or the first of it—was seen as an alien and conflicting end. The point was not that one would fail to be a good Pythagorean if one violated these standards, although that is true enough, but rather that one would fail to be a good medical practitioner. The good physician is not a mere technician; he is committed by the practice of medicine to certain goods and to certain standards.

The notoriously difficult foreswearing of surgery, even on those who stand to benefit from it, is also founded on the notion of medicine as a practice. Edelstein is probably right in tracing this stipulation to the Pythagorean preference for dietetics and pharmacology as modes of treatment,[12] but the foreswearing in the oath did not appeal to any uncompromising Pythagorean position about either the appetitive and dietetic causes of illness or the defilement of shedding blood. It rather articulated a standard for medical practice whose goal is to benefit the sick: namely, don't attempt what lies beyond your competence. To benefit the sick was not merely a motive, but the good intrinsic to medicine, and to put the patient at risk needlessly—even with the best of intentions—can be seen to violate medicine understood as such a practice. There was, therefore, no universal prohibition of surgery, only the particular prohibition of surgery by those ill-equipped to attempt it. That standard may well have been of particular relevance to Pythagorean physicians, but one need not have been a Pythagorean to accept its wisdom as a standard of practice.

The stipulations concerning decorum are yet another example. They can be readily understood against the background of Pythagorean asceticism and the proverbial "Pythagorean silence,"[13] but, again, the oath presented them not as Pythagorean stipulations, but as standards of medicine understood as a practice. The goal of the practice, "the benefit of the sick," was repeated in this context even as the (necessary) intrusion into the privacy, the homes, of the sick was acknowledged. The physician's access to the intimacies of the patient's body and household and his exposure to the vulnerability of the patient and his household were granted and accepted for the sake of the goal intrinsic to medicine. To use such access for any other end or to make public the vulnerability to which the physician was made privy was seen to subvert the relation of such access and such exposure to the end of medicine. It debased the patient who should be benefitted. It vitiated medicine as a practice and, therefore, the standards prohibiting sexual relations with patients and prohibiting breaches of confidentiality were implicit in medicine as a practice.

These standards could be further explicated,[14] and, if the point of this essay were to treat the oath as a code, then the further explication would be necessary. But that is not the point. It is not my claim that the oath provides an unexceptionable code of conduct. The standards of a practice at any particular time are not immune from criticism. The point is to call attention to this feature of the oath's method, that it construes medicine as a practice. It does not provide a timeless code for medicine, but there are standards of excellence appropriate to and partly definitive of the practice, whose authority must be acknowledged, and there is a good intrinsic to the practice which must be appreciated and allowed to govern the skills and to form and reform the standards. The lesson, I suggest, for the contemporary discussions of medical ethics, is that those who seek the constant reform of medicine should also construe medicine as a practice with implicit goods and standards.

That is a hard but important lesson in a culture as bullish on technology and as pluralistic in values as our own. There is a constant tendency to reduce medicine to a mere—but awesome—collection of techniques that may be made to serve extrinsic goods, themselves often reduced to matters of taste.

The technology of abortion is a telling example. In *Roe v. Wade,* the Court declared that a woman's decision with respect to abortion was a private matter between herself and her physician. It recognized that the moral status of the fetus was controverted, but it held that the fetus is not a *legal* person and so is not entitled to the protection the law extends to persons. It wanted to leave the moral controversy about the status of the fetus within that private arena of the decision a woman and her doctor would make. The court presumed (and suggested by calling the decision to abort a "medical decision") that the professional ethos of physicians would limit abortions, even if abortion were legalized, and it might have been, if there had been a vivid sense of medicine as a practice.[15] The legal license was interpreted by many (both women and physicians) as a moral license and the outcome has been a callous and frightening disregard for fetal life and welfare. The protests—usually applying some extrinsic good or extrinsic standard—have been long and loud and have sometimes exhibited callous disregard for the rights of women with respect to their own bodies and ignored the legitimate controversy about the status of the fetus. The opportunity for medicine to reassert itself as a practice, different from the practice of politics or the marketplace, has almost been lost. But the lesson of the oath is that the attempt is both possible and worthwhile.

The notion of medicine as a practice stands in marked contrast to a good deal of the current literature concerning the professions in general and medicine in particular. Michael Bayles, for example, would reject the normative characteristics of the professions, including medicine.[16] He reduces the professions to skills learned by training and made accessible to consumers. The professions, on this view, are not justified or guided by any intrinsic good but by "the values of a liberal society."[17] Thus, there are no standards implicit in the practice but only "ordinary norms" to be applied in professional contexts.

The problems with such a view are manifold. One is linguistic. "Professional" and "unprofessional" continue to be used evaluatively and, moreover, with respect to excellences not merely technical.

The notion of applying ordinary norms to medical dilemmas is also problematic. It is naive and presumptuous to suppose that a moral philosopher or theologian can boldly put to flight a moral dilemma by expertly wielding a sharp principle or some heavy theory.[18] And how shall we select the "ordinary norms" to apply? Justice is surely relevant, but there is more than one theory of justice. Good ends surely ought to be sought in medicine, too, but shall we use St. Thomas Aquinas or John Stuart Mill to define a good end? The values of society may be important, but none of us, I trust, has forgotten the atrocities committed when Hitler's vision of a "third reich" was applied to medicine.

I am much more comfortable with Bayles's "values of a liberal society" than with Hitler's "third reich," but I am not so much more confident about the practice of politics than the practice of medicine that I would make the professional ethic dependent upon our political ethic. Indeed, I wonder whether a society is truly "liberal" if it tailors the professions to a liberal society's (minimal) vision of the good. A liberal society can be guilty of trivializing ancient wisdom about human flourishing when it renders the professions, including medicine, merely instrumental skills to satisfy consumer wants.

Bayles's application of his "ordinary norms" to medicine leads to minimal moral claims and, because the minimal character of the claims is not acknowledged, to a truncated and distorted medical ethic. There is, for example, no limit to "professional services" when a profession is basically skills accessible to consumers: laetrile, genetic testing for sex determination, plastic surgery to win the Dolly Parton look-alike contest, all become the sphere of the professional-entrepreneur. Immoral clients cannot be refused on the basis of "professional integrity," for there is no such thing. Bayles is aware of the problem posed by clients who would use professional skills for ends which are morally questionable but which do not clearly violate the "ordinary norms," and he presents two options for dealing with such clients. The "no difference" option quite candidly leaves no room for integrity of any kind and renders the professional the "animated tool" of the consumer.[19] The second option permits the physician to refuse services to such clients on the basis of "moral integrity," but this "moral integrity" is represented as strictly personal and private rather than professional.[20]

Bayles's attempt to reduce professional norms to "ordinary norms" applied in a medical context, to give one more example, leads to a minimal and truncated version of the prohibition of sexual intercourse with patients.[21] The ordinary norm he provides, that sexual intercourse requires the free consent of both parties, is itself a dangerously minimal account of sexual ethics. It does provide a justification for the prohibition, but it does not discount either the possibility or the importance of a "professional" justification, that the (necessary) access to the patient's privacy and vulnerability must be guided by and limited to the "good" of medicine and not be used for extrinsic ends (even when they are freely chosen or consented to).

The debate about the crafts, about the professions, is an ancient and an enduring one. The lesson of the oath is that we should not too readily accept the notion of medicine as a collection of skills accessible to consumers. We should not identify our task as simply applying universal and rational norms of conduct to medicine and to the quandaries faced within it.[22]

If the *teknē* of medicine is construed simply in terms of its techniques or skills, learned by training and accessible to consumers, then, of course, it is morally neutral. Skill in pharmacology enables one to be a good healer or a crafty murderer. But if a *teknē* is more than technique, if it has its own goal and its own virtues, then it is hardly morally neutral. Then some moral wisdom about living as a finite body may exist within the practice of medicine and within those communities and traditions which learn and teach medicine as a practice. Then medicine's fragile capacity to resist being co-opted by an alien ideology, even a liberal ideology (not to mention the "third reich"), can be strengthened and nurtured. The lesson of the oath, I suggest, is that for some, at least, the task should be to defend the vision of medicine as a practice while educing and elucidating the goods and standards implicit in that practice.

The Hippocratic Oath had its origins among the Pythagoreans who had the courage to attempt the reform of medicine and the wisdom not merely to apply Pythagorean premises to medicine but to construe it as a practice. It was handed down not as legislation but as a voluntary rule imposing voluntary obedience. Its power to reform was not coercive or simply rationally persuasive; its power to reform was its power to form character and a community which nurtured it. It did not set its standards in a context of legal sanctions or in a context of impartial rationality. It set these standards in a context which expressed and evoked an identity and recognized one's dependence upon and indebtedness to both a community and the transcendent. To those features of the oath we turn next.

Identity, Community, and the Transcendent

The oath, like all oaths and promises, was a performative declaration rather than a descriptive one. It did not just describe reality; it altered it. The one who swore this oath was never the same "one" again. The one swearing this oath adopted more than a set of rules and skills; he or she adopted an identity. The goods and standards of medicine as a practice were owned as one's own and gave shape to integrity with one's identity. Therefore, "physician" was a description not only of what one knew or of what one did or of what one knew how to do, but of who one was. Henceforth, one examined questions of conduct in this role not as an impartial and rational agent, calculating utility sums, say, but as a physician. Integrity with this identity called for the physician to exert himself on behalf of the patient at hand, even the patient-scoundrel at hand, without calculating the greatest good for the greatest number. Indeed, to allow that question, to bear toward the patient the kind of impartial relation which makes it plausible, was to lose one's identity, to forfeit one's integrity.

This feature of the oath calls our attention to the moral significance of "identity." Once again the lesson of the doctor's oath sets a different agenda than the one contemporary medical ethics has generally undertaken. Contemporary medical ethics usually adopts the perspective of impartial rationality, either in the form of utilitarianism or in the form of contract theory.[23] To adopt any such impartial perspective, however, requires the doctor's alienation from his own moral interests and loyalties *qua* physician, from himself and from his special relationship to his patient. Doctors are asked, indeed, obliged, by this perspective to view the project and passion of their practice as though they were outside objective observers.

They are asked by this approach to disown—and for the sake of morality—the goods and standards they possess as their own and which give them their moral character as physicians.[24]

The perspective of impartial rationality is not to be disowned. It can enable conversation between people with different loyalties and the adjudication of conflicting interests, and it can challenge the arbitrary dominance of one perspective over another. To be made to pause occasionally and, for the sake of analysis and judgment, to view things as impartially as we can is not only legitimate, but also salutary. But such an ethic remains minimal at best, and if its minimalism is not acknowledged, it can distort the moral life. Physicians—and patients—cannot consistently live their moral lives like that with any integrity. The Hippocratic Oath calls our attention to the importance of a physician's identity, character, and integrity. Such an approach might recover the importance of performative rituals like swearing an initiatory oath, and it would surely attend not only to the ways in which acts effectively realize ends, but also to the ways in which acts express values and form character.[25]

The oath expressed and evoked an identity, but it was an identity which recognized its dependence upon and indebtedness to a community and the transcendent.

The oath bound one to a community where not only the requisite skills were taught, but where the requisite character and identity were nurtured. The doctor swore to live in fellowship (Gk.: *koinosasthai*) with his teacher, to share a common life with him. He pledged, moreover, to teach the art to his teacher's sons, to his own sons, and to all who wanted to learn not simply the skills, but also the practice. Here was not an autonomous individual practitioner, utilizing his skills for his private good or according to his private vision of the good or as contracted by another to accomplish the other's "good." The doctor who swore the oath stood self-consciously in a community and in a tradition. He acknowledged gratefully his dependence upon this community and tradition, his indebtedness to his teacher, and his responsibility to protect and nurture the practice of medicine.[26]

This section of the oath is often criticized.[27] It is accused of fostering a medical guild where obligations to colleagues take priority over obligations to patients, so that medical incompetence and malpractice are usually covered up and the incompetent and unscrupulous (protected by the guild) do further harm to patients. The charge is a serious one, and the profession's reluctance to discipline its members makes it cogent. The fault is not with the oath, however, but with the corruption of the oath in the absence of a commitment to medicine as a practice. When there is such a commitment, it governs relations with colleagues as well as patients, and protecting and nurturing the practice—both the requisite skills and the requisite character—enable and require communal discipline. The failure of the profession to discipline itself adequately may be traced not to the perspective of the oath but to the dismissal of the perspective of the oath.

Today the training for medicine has shifted to university-based medical schools, which pride themselves on their scientific detachment from questions of value in their dispassionate pursuit of the truth. Such a context can virtually sponsor the construal of medicine as a collection of skills and techniques to be used for extrinsic goods which are not matters of truth but matters of taste.[28] Then there is no community of people committed to a practice and under its standards; there is only the camaraderie of those who have undergone the same arduous routine. Then the profession lacks both a commitment to a practice which makes discipline possible and a genuine enough community to make discipline a nurturing as well as a punishing activity.

The stress on community in the oath can help call our attention to the moral necessity of attending to the institutions, communities, and traditions within which the physician's identity is nurtured. Adding courses in medical ethics taught by philosophers or theologians to the curricula of medical schools may be important, but it is neither essential nor sufficient. Indeed, if such courses are co-opted as token evidence of the moral concern of the institution, or if clinical instructors abdicate the responsibility for difficult decisions to "the moral expert," the results could be counter-productive. It is more important to have teachers chosen and rewarded not only for their excellent skills but also for their excellence in medical practice—chosen and rewarded not only for their ability to teach the skills, but also for the ability to model the practice. The philosopher or theologian may then have an important role as participant in—and midwife for—a continuing dialogue between such teachers and their students about the goods and standards implicit in medicine as a practice. In such a continuing dialogue there will surely be continuing conflicts, but so any living tradition is passed down.

No less important than institutions where doctors are trained are institutions within which they practice and the communities within which they live, including the religious communities. That religious communities might nurture and sustain the identity of physicians is, of course, suggested by the doctor's oath itself. The physician acknowledged his dependence upon and indebtedness to not only the community of doctors, but also the transcendent.

The opening line called all the gods and goddesses as witnesses to this oath, and the last line puts the doctor at the mercy of divine justice. The invocation of the gods and their divine retribution served, of course, to signify the solemnity of the oath and the stringency of the obligations. More than that, however, was accomplished by the oath's piety, by its recognition of our dependence upon and indebtedness to transcendent power which bears down on us and sustains us. A narrative is provided, a narrative which helps inform identity and helps sustain community, a narrative which supports and tests the practice of medicine. The deities named are a lineage. Apollo, the god of truth and light, here invoked as "Apollo Physician," is the father of Asclepius. Asclepius, the father of medicine and the patron of physicians and patients, had two daughters, Hygeia and Panacea, or "Health" and "All-heal," the goddesses of health maintenance and therapy.[29] It is a story of the divine origins and transmission of the work physicians are given and gifted to do. To undertake the work of a physician was to make this story one's own story, to continue it and embody it among human beings. They were not tempted to "play God" or to deny their subordinate role, but they were supported and encouraged in their ministrations by this story. In serving patients in their practice, they continued a narrative that had its beginnings among the gods. They were not tempted to magic by this story,[30] but they were enabled to acknowledge the mystery of healing, the subtle and profound connections of the spirit and the body.[31]

This feature of the oath can remind us of the religious dimensions of medicine and medical morality. It is a hard but important lesson for an age as noisily secular as ours. The oath, I think, is an example of the moral significance of a natural piety, the importance of what Calvin would call a *sensus divinitatis,* the sense of the divine. This natural piety includes the sense of gratitude for the gifts of life and of the world, a sense of dependence upon some reliable, but dimly known order, a sense of some tragic fault in the midst of our world, and a sense of responsibility to the inscrutable power Who stands behind the gifts and the order and Who judges the fault.[32] One can do worse, I think, than name this other wrongly; one could understand (misunderstand) this other as the "enemy" of his own work, as a deluding power, or one could deny or (like so much of the contemporary literature) ignore this other and these senses. The oath adopted neither of those forms of distrust;[33] rather, it set the practice of medicine in the context of a natural piety, in the context of a sense of gratitude, of dependence, of tragedy, and of responsibility to the transcendent. Such a natural piety can still nourish and sustain the physician's calling. Its responsiveness to the transcendent can protect the physician both from the presumption of "playing God" and from the reductionism of plying the trade for hire. It remains part of the fuller vision of medicine.

The Christian's Swearing It

The triumph of the doctor's oath may finally be attributed to the triumph of a new religion in the ancient world. Christianity adopted it as its own, finally presenting it in a Christian form, "The Oath According to Hippocrates In So Far As A Christian May Swear It." There were certain revisions, to be sure, but the continuity of the Christian version with the ancient oath is undeniable. Both the continuity and the revisions are instructive for Christian theologians and communities who take part in the current discussions of bioethics.

First, note the adoption and reiteration of the standards of the Hippocratic Oath. There are some minor variations in the stipulations governing the practice—the operation clause is omitted, even "unintentional" harm (negligence) is forbidden, the prohibition of abortion is amplified—but the similarity is the striking thing. The claim is not that here finally we have a Christian code to be used and applied to current dilemmas. The claim is rather that there is a lesson here for those Christians who would contribute to the conversations about medical ethics. The lesson is that Christian ethics does not disown "natural" morality. It does not construct an ethic *ex nihilo,* out of nothing. It selects and assimilates the "natural" moral wisdom around it in terms of its own truthfulness and in terms of its integrity with the Christian vision. The theologians who would contribute to the conversations about bioethics must first listen attentively and respectfully to "natural" moral wisdom concerning medicine. Then they can speak responsively and responsibly about the adoption and selection of certain standards as coherent with reason, with medicine construed as a practice, and with the Christian vision.

"The Oath In So Far As A Christian May Swear It" offers a second lesson for theologians interested in medical ethics. Note the two obvious changes. The first is that the practice and its standards were set in the context of a Christian identity and of the Christian story. God, the Father of our Lord Jesus Christ, was invoked rather than Apollo *et al.;* the physician cast himself on the mercy of His justice. Once again, the invocation of God and His retribution served not only to signal the solemnity of the oath and the stringency of the obligations, but also to set the physician's identity and practice in the context of a story which has its beginnings with God. This feature was expressed visibly as well. "The Oath In So Far As A Christian May Swear It"—or at least some copies of it—was written in the shape of a cross.[34] The one who swore such an oath adopted the physician's identity as a follower of Christ, "Who took our infirmities and bore our diseases" (Matt. 8:17; cf. Is. 53:4). A Christian identity nurtured, sustained, and shaped the physician's identity for those who took such an oath seriously.

The second obvious change is the reduction of duties to one's teacher. Historically, this change is understandable. Medical instruction had shifted from artisan families and guilds to universities and eventually to faculties of medicine. The Church itself was, for centuries, the nurturing and sustaining institution and community for medicine. It chartered and administered the universities; it dominated the curriculum; its pervasive ethos ruled the professions.[35] Morally, the change was required by setting the oath in the context of the Christian story, for that story makes service the mark of greatness as well as of gratitude. So, it was inevitable that service to the patient was emphasized rather than obligations to teachers. The Christian story of breaking down the barriers that separate people, moreover, made it inevitable that the emphasis shifted from professional elitism to open access to this community of service.

What Is the Lesson Here?

The lesson here is not that we should attempt to reintroduce "Christendom" or even the patterns of medical instruction of that time. Notwithstanding the impossibility of such an attempt, the dominion of the Church was marked by parochialism as well as majesty, by pettiness as well as grandeur, by obscurantism as well as learning. The reformist intention does not lead back to Christendom for either medicine or the Church. There is little hope for a Christian medical ethic that proceeds by way of a theological triumphalism, that claims to have truth, if not captive, at least cornered. The lesson is rather that Christian medical ethics cannot proceed with integrity if it always restricts itself to articulating and defending standards of the practice or certain applications of impartial principles of philosophy or law to medical dilemmas. It is lamentable that so little of the work in medical ethics by Christian theologians candidly and explicitly attends to the Christian story and its bearing on medicine.[36] It is lamentable for the communities of faith out of which these ethicists work, for they want to live in faith, to live in integrity with the identity they have been given and to which they are called. But it is also lamentable for the broader community, for a pluralistic society profits from the candid expression of different perspectives. Candid attention to the theological dimensions of morality could prevent the reduction and distortion of morality to a set of minimal expectations necessary for pluralism and remind all participants in such a culture of broader and more profound questions about what human persons are meant to be and to become. The integrity to think about and talk about the relevance of the Christian story is the second lesson of "The Oath In So Far As A Christian May Swear It."

The first lesson of "The Oath In So Far As A Christian May Swear It" was that Christian ethics does not disown "natural" morality. The Christian story does not force those who own it to disown either medicine as a practice or human rationality. The second lesson of "The Oath In So Far As A Christian May Swear It" is that Christians concerned with medical ethics should have the integrity to set medicine in the context of the Christian story, to form, inform, and reform medicine. The first lesson stands against any premature sectarian stance, against opting prematurely for either a sectarian community or a sectarian medicine.[37] The second lesson stands against any simple identification of a Christian ethic either with universal and rational principles or with a professional ethic, against, for example, sanctifying contract theory by identifying it with "covenant."[38] The task is to transform or, to put it less presumptuously, to qualify[39] a rational ethic and a professional ethic by candid attention to the Christian story.

There will be tensions, of course. With respect to decisions about the refusal of treatment, for example, a universal and rational ethic may emphasize the patient's autonomy, but a professional ethic may emphasize the physician's commitment to the life and health of his or her patient, and a theological ethic may emphasize dispositions formed and informed by a story where the victory over death is a divine victory, not a technological victory, where people need not stand in dread of death, but may not practice hospitality toward it.[40] These tensions and their resolution will require the careful attention of those who make it their task to think about medicine and who care about the Christian story as the story of our life, our whole life.

Finally, it may be observed that theological reflection, even when it is presumptuous enough to talk about "transformation," does not represent an alien imposition upon the practice of medicine. As we have seen, the tradition of medicine as a practice is at home in piety. Loyalty to God, the Father of our Lord Jesus Christ, fulfills and redeems natural piety. The native senses of gratitude and dependence, of a tragic fault in the midst of our world, and of responsibility, are not disowned by a theological approach, but informed and reformed by the Christian story. The current literature on bioethics stands at risk of ignoring that story, of neglecting those resources. Christians have a vocation to identify and articulate the significance of the Christian story for medicine not only because that agenda stands comfortably in an ancient tradition, but also because it will serve both integrity within the Christian community and humanity with medical practice. To renege on this opportunity and vocation will diminish not only the communities of faith, but the art of medicine as well.

Notes

1. Edelstein, Ludwig, "The Hippocratic Oath: Text, Translation and Interpretation," *Ancient Medicine,* ed. by Oswei Temkin and C. Lillian Temkin (Baltimore: Johns Hopkins University Press, 1967), pp. 3-63.

2. Jones, W. H. S., *The Doctor's Oath: An Essay in the History of Medicine* (New York: Cambridge University Press, 1924), pp. 23-25.

3. The attitude of Robert Veatch toward the oath can only be characterized as contempt. He argues that the oath is morally "dangerous." See Robert Veatch, *A Theory of Medical Ethics* (New York: Basic Books, 1981), pp. 18-26, 79-107, and especially 141-169. See also his "The Hippocratic Ethic: Consequentialism, Individualism, and Paternalism," *No Rush to Judgment,* ed. by David Smith and Linda M. Bernstein (Bloomington, Ind.: Poynter Center, 1978), pp. 238-264; "Medical Ethics: Professional or Universal?" *Harvard Theological Review,* 65:4 (Oct., 1972), pp. 531-539; and *Death, Dying, and the Biological Revolution* (New Haven: Yale University Press, 1976), pp. 171, 172. Veatch criticizes both the basis and the content of the oath. The basis is criticized because the oath is based on a special professional ethic rather than on universal rational moral norms. The content is criticized because the oath is construed as consequentialist, individualist, and paternalistic.

4. Edelstein, *op. cit.* I am convinced by Edelstein concerning the Pythagorean origins of oath. Even if it originated in some other community, however, it would still have had the intention to reform ancient medicine, and that is the feature of the oath to which I would call attention.

5. For example, the Pythagorean premise concerning the status of the fetus was supplied by a physiology which took the seed to be clot of brain containing the warm vapors whence came soul and sensation. The Pythagorean asceticism, which justified intercourse only as the necessary condition

for procreation, surely affected their perspective on abortion. See Edelstein, *op. cit.* It is important to observe, however, that the oath, while coherent with Pythagorean doctrines and beliefs (as Edelstein shows), does not simply apply Pythagorean doctrine *to* medicine (as Edelstein presumes to have shown). The oath draws *from* medicine the morality to guide and limit the behavior of physicians. See section 2, "Medicine as a Practice" and reference 8 below.

6. So, for example, Robert Veatch, *A Theory of Medical Ethics.* See the review by Allen Verhey, "Contract—or Covenant?" *Reformed Journal,* 33:9 (Sept., 1983), pp. 23, 24.

7. The phrase, of course, is John Rawls's. See, e.g., *A Theory of Justice* (Cambridge, Mass.: Harvard University Press, 1971), pp. 396ff. The complaint about "the thin theory of the good" in the contemporary literature echoes Daniel Callahan, "Minimalist Ethics," *Hastings Center Report,* 11:6 (Oct., 1981), pp. 19-25.

8. Edelstein recognizes the importance of the Pythagorean attitude toward the crafts (e.g., "The Professional Ethics of the Greek Physician" in his *Ancient Medicine,* pp. 319-348, p. 327), but he fails to recognize that it warrants construing medicine as a practice with intrinsic goods and implicit standards (e.g., ibid., n. 21). The same failure marks Veatch's use of Edelstein (e.g., *A Theory of Medical Ethics,* p. 21).

9. *Precepts* and *On Decorum,* later writings in the Hippocratic corpus, are probably Stoic in origin; see Edelstein, *op. cit.*

10. On the notion of a practice, see Alasdair MacIntyre, *After Virtue* (Notre Dame: University of Notre Dame Press, 1981), pp. 175-178.

11. Veatch's criticism of the oath's "consequentialism" relies heavily on the oath's commitment to "the benefit of the sick." Veatch's understanding of the oath at this point makes "benefit" an extrinsic good and, moreover, renders benefit definable in terms of the physician's (or the patient's) private preferences. I am convinced that this is a misunderstanding. The *teknē* of medicine is not construed in the oath as morally neutral skills accessible to consumers; it is not just a "means" even to health; it is a human activity of inheriting and learning and teaching and applying a wisdom about living with a finite body. See further E. Pellegrino and D. Thomasma, *A Philosophical Basis of Medical Practice* (New York: Oxford University Press, 1981); and Stanley M. Hauerwas, "Authority and the Profession of Medicine" (manuscript). That Veatch misunderstands the oath at this point is obvious when he suggests—quite against the oath's own straightforward prohibition—that the oath's concern for benefit of the patient could permit participation in bringing about the death of an infant (*A Theory of Medical Ethics,* pp. 15-26).

12. Edelstein, "The Hippocratic Oath," *op. cit.,* pp. 21-33.

13. *Ibid.,* pp. 33-39.

14. See especially Leon Kass, "The Hippocratic Oath: Thoughts on Medicine and Ethics," a lecture given on Nov. 12, 1980, in the seminar series sponsored by the program in the Arts and Sciences Basic to Human Biology and Medicine and the American Medical Students' Association, at the University of Chicago.

15. The court's use of Edelstein's study of the Pythagorean origins of the Hippocratic Oath, unfortunately, tended to reinforce the position that extrinsic goods and standards may be applied to medicine but that goods and standards intrinsic to medicine do not exist. At the very time the court laid a heavy burden on physicians by calling abortion a "medical decision," it weakened physicians' resolve and ability to resist this culture's tendency to construe medicine as a set of skills to satisfy consumer wants.

16. Bayles, Michael, *Professional Ethics* (Belmont, Calif.: Wadsworth Publishing Co., 1981). See also Alan Goldman, *The Moral Foundations of Professional Ethics* (Tutowa, N.J.: Rowman and Littlefield, 1980).

17. In Goldman's view, *op. cit.,* the justification and guidance are provided by a modified utilitarianism.

18. See further Arthur L. Caplan, "Ethical Engineers Need Not Apply: The State of Applied Ethics Today," *Science, Technology and Human Values,* 6:33 (Fall, 1980), pp. 24-32.

19. This is, of course, Aristotle's definition of a slave. See Paul Ramsey, *Ethics at the Edges of Life* (New Haven: Yale University Press, 1978), pp. 45, 158.

20. Bayles, *op. cit.,* pp. 52ff.

21. *Ibid.,* p. 21.

22. Veatch, *A Theory of Medical Ethics, op. cit.,* is a case in point.

23. Again, Veatch, *ibid.,* is a case in point.

24. See further Stanley Hauerwas, *Truthfulness and Tragedy: Further Investigations in Christian Ethics* (Notre Dame: University of Notre Dame Press, 1977), pp. 23-25; and Bernard Williams, "A Critique of Utilitarianism," in J. J. C. Smart and Bernard Williams, *Utilitarianism: For and Against* (New York: Cambridge University Press, 1973), pp. 100-118.

25. Childress, James, *Priorities in Biomedical Ethics* (Philadelphia: Westminster Press, 1981), p. 82, citing Max Weber, *Max Weber in Economy and Society,* nicely distinguishes "goal-rational" and "value-rational" conduct.

26. Veatch's charge that the oath is "individualistic" (*A Theory of Medical Ethics,* pp. 154-159, and "The Hippocratic Ethic," pp. 255-259) fails to recognize this communal character of the practice of medicine in the oath. The oath, indeed, seems much more cognizant of the social and historical character of medicine than Veatch himself, for whom independent and autonomous individuals contract for medical services. Veatch's accusation cannot stand; it can, in fact, be turned against Veatch's own position, for it is Veatch's contract model which protects and perpetuates the individualism of modern liberalism and sets medicine in the ethos of the marketplace. Veatch's contract theory may provide a minimal account of medical morality, but unless its minimalism is acknowledged, it can distort medical morality into the most arid form of individualism, quite incapable of nurturing or supporting other than contractual relationships. See further James Childress, "A Masterful Tour: A Response to Robert Veatch," *Journal of Current Social Issues,* 4:12 (Fall, 1975), pp. 20-25.

27. See, e.g., William F. May, "Code and Covenant or Philanthropy and Contract?" in *Ethics in Medicine: Histori-*

cal Perspectives and Contemporary Concerns, ed. by Stanley J. Reiser, Arthur J. Dyck, and William J. Curran (Cambridge, Mass.: MIT Press, 1977), pp. 65-76 (an expanded and revised form of an essay first published in *Hastings Center Report,* 6:5 [Dec., 1975], pp. 29-38).

28. See further William F. May, *Notes on the Ethics of Doctors and Lawyers,* a Poynter Pamphlet (Bloomington, Ind.: Poynter Center, 1977), pp. 16–21; and his "Normative Inquiry and Medical Ethics in Our Colleges and Universities," in *No Rush to Judgment,* pp. 332-361.

29. Kass, *op. cit.*

30. See Edelstein, "Greek Medicine in Its Relation to Religion and Magic," *op. cit.,* pp. 205-246.

31. Kass, *op. cit.*

32. See further James M. Gustafson, "Theocentric Interpretation of Life," *The Christian Century,* July 30-Aug. 6, 1980, p. 758; and *Ethics from a Theocentric Perspective* (Chicago: University Press, 1981), pp. 129-136.

33. See H. R. Niebuhr, *The Responsible Self* (New York: Harper & Row, 1963), pp. 115-118.

34. See facsimiles in W. H. S. Jones, *The Doctor's Oath,* frontispiece and p. 26.

35. May, *Notes on the Ethics, op. cit.,* pp. 16, 17; and "Normative Inquiry," *op. cit.*

36. See James M. Gustafson, "Theology Confronts Technology and the Life Sciences," *Commonweal,* 2:5 (June, 1978), pp. 386-392. See also Stanley Hauerwas, "Can Ethics Be Theological?" *Hastings Center Report,* 5:8 (Oct., 1978), pp. 47, 48. To his credit, Robert Veatch introduces the notion of "covenant" into his *A Theory of Medical Ethics.* Unfortunately, it is unclear how, if at all, the religious significance of covenant affects his understanding of the contract between physician and patient. Indeed, the meaning of "covenant" seems to be reduced to the notion of "contract." For some of the differences between contract and covenant (and for an outstanding example of theological reflection on medical ethics focusing on the notion of covenant), see William May, "Code and Covenant," *op. cit.*

37. Stanley Hauerwas calls for the formation of "a sectarian medicine to be supported by an equally sectarian community" ("Authority and the Profession of Medicine," p. 22).

38. As Robert Veatch, *A Theory of Medical Ethics, op. cit.*

39. See James M. Gustafson, *Can Ethics Be Christian?* p. 173 *et passim.*

40. See further, Allen Verhey, "Christian Community and Identity: What Difference Should They Make to Patients and Physicians Finally?" *Linacre Quarterly,* 52:2 (May, 1985), pp. 149-169.

14. From "Medical Ethics: Professional or Universal?"

ROBERT M. VEATCH

There is an obvious tone of idealism in the claim that the individual layman's inputs into decision-making should be maximized. The professional would rightly claim that this, if carried to extremes, would complicate his task to the point of absurdity. He would have to spend hours explaining the technical details and policy options to each patient. For choices which are ethically trivial and technically complex this is just impossible. The more trivial the value alternatives involved, the less technically complex the choices have to be to make informed decision-making by the layman needlessly wasteful. Laymen are willing to spend more time and money paying professionals to clarify the options for them when the decision involves experimental heart surgery than when it involves which brand of antacid to use. This does not mean, however, that the layman should not be routinely consulted for decisions such as whether to use a generic name drug which should be cheaper but (under present FDA controls) perhaps more variable than the brand name drug.

Nevertheless, the professionals are right. It is logically and logistically impossible to defer every decision to the layman. This does not mean, however, that the decision reverts to the professional in his professional role because of his superior technical skills, his unique set of norms, or his superior ability in reaching ethical judgments. It may revert to him—it must in many cases—but it will revert to him as another human being with no necessarily superior decision-making skills. He may be using the layman's system of values. If he is dedicated, he will try to do so when it does not conflict with his own and will consciously withdraw from the case when it does; but he may be using a system which is quite at odds with the patient's. If the secondary factors of group identification and cultural system of meaning are significant in the decision-making process, the odds may be quite good that it is different from the patient's. When we are dealing in trivialities in medically serious situations such as the brand of compress to use to close a serious

Reprinted with permission of author and publisher, from the *Harvard Theological Review* 65 (1972): 531-59.

arterial wound, the value system conflict may be nearly irrelevant, but we should not overlook the fact that it is still there. A system of decision-making which is rooted in a universal, human ethic may still call on the professional to make many decisions; it certainly will insist that he practice his trade ethically; but the decisions he makes will be made within a universal frame of reference, one which is not unique to the profession he is practicing.

The conclusion to which one is led is that medical ethics must not be thought of as a special "professional ethic" at all, but as a specific application of the universal norms of ethical action. Those traditional and more modern codes of ethics and professional responsibility which are rooted in relativistic norms which cannot be universalized must be distinguished from those which have more universal foundations. The universally rooted principles of medical ethics are extremely important for curbing certain kinds of excesses and hastily-conceived actions. The professional codes of medical ethics, on the other hand, are not only irrelevant—if that were the case we could just ignore them. They are actually dangerous diversions which lead professionals to believe that there is a special type of ethics appropriate for their own professional discipline. Rather, we must first reject the fallacy of generalization of expertise—that expertise about the technical facts of a given area also gives one expertise in the evaluative factor required for decision-making in that area. . . . Special norms or a special process of balancing norms cannot exist for a professional group without collapsing into ethical relativism and particularism. Expertise in ethical decision-making in questions relevant to a profession may reside in certain members of that profession, but other members of that profession may be particularly deficient in that skill, and on balance there is no evidence of a quantum difference in this regard between professionals and laymen. Finally, although professional review committees may be appropriate for certain limited functions, such as protecting the interests of the profession from the gross offenses of certain of its members, without the premises which have just been rejected, there is no theoretical reason for relying on these committees for adjudication of disputes within a professional area. There is some empirical evidence suggesting that they are not particularly effective and may actually be harmful by diverting the attention of other groups which may take up the cases. Let us hope that, if medical ethics is to emerge as an independent discipline, it is a special case of the universal norms of ethical behavior and not as a special professional ethic.

15. Code and Covenant or Philanthropy and Contract?

WILLIAM F. MAY

When it first broke in the news the Summer of 1975, the case of the Marcus twins (gynecologists at a teaching hospital in New York City) posed in vivid circumstances several difficult and illuminating problems in professional ethics; problems which worry both laymen and doctors. The usual analysis of such problems, which appeals to the language of Philanthropy and Contract, boggles at the Marcus case. The categories of Code and Covenant (which are related to Philanthropy and Contract as *genera* to *species*) offer at least the beginnings of solutions to the professional ethical problems embodied in the case.

The Marcus brothers were physicians who, although technically expert (they wrote one of the best current textbooks on gynecology) and professionally and sympathetically involved, allowed themselves to become addicted to barbiturates, to miss appointments, and to offer consultation, diagnosis, and treatment while under the observable influence of drugs. They retained skill and expertise enough, however, to refrain from killing any of their patients. Their colleagues and the institutions in which they worked were slow to blow the whistle on them.

The Marcus case poses ethical problems for the professional. At what point is a doctor who prescribes drugs for himself misusing his technical expertise? At what point does a professional's duty to laymen override his duties to his fellow professionals? At what point does professional courtesy become professional whitewash? Is there a duty to a profession, as distinct from a duty to those individuals who practice the profession and those who benefit from its practice? These problems tend to concern the layman more than the experts in moral philosophy. Professional moralists tend to apply their analytical skills to issues they find intellectually interesting. They tend to solve moral puzzles rather than outline the foundations for professional character. They have produced in recent years elegant work on abortion, euthanasia, organ transplants, scarce medical resources and other sub-

From *Ethics in Medicine: Historical Perspectives and Contemporary Concerns,* ed. Stanley J. Reiser et al. (Cambridge: MIT Press, 1977), pp. 65-76.

jects tantalizing at a theoretical level. The layman meanwhile is concerned with more prosaic questions. He wonders whether the doctor's real loyalty is to the patient or to the guild. Are medical societies, hospitals, and other health agencies ready and willing to weed out incompetent or unscrupulous practitioners? Will the profession find ways of challenging those doctors who order unwarranted surgery, charge fees that always press against the ceiling, play Ping Pong with referrals, process patients through their office with the speed of salts, or commit the sick to the hospital with indecorous haste?

Such blatantly unethical behavior (perhaps its self-evident wrongness explains why the professional moralist seldom attends to it) stirs the layman's anger. The profession seems to belong to an elite, utterly beyond the reach of his criticism. Certainly the physician is beyond serious challenge from the nurse and the social worker. His professional hegemony is well-nigh total over other health professionals. As long as doctors are in scarce supply and badly distributed, they are also beyond the reach of consumer criticism—except through the melodramatic, spotty, random, and sometimes, in its own right, unjust resort to the malpractice suit. For the same reason to date, they have not been seriously limited—except for the demands of paperwork—by outside agencies—the government, Blue Shield, and insurance companies. Under current conditions, the maintenance of professional standards of conduct depends largely on the doctor's own internal sense of professional obligation and on the willingness of the profession to enforce standards of conduct on its members.

This essay on the basis of professional ethics will therefore divide into two questions: why, despite the existence of medical codes and enforcement procedures, is the medical profession reluctant to engage in serious self-criticism? How are the concepts of code and covenant useful in interpreting professional duties and in establishing their obligatory power?

When the *New York Times* first carried its story on the Marcus brothers, it seemed a potentially scandalous reminder that the profession is loath to accept responsibility for professional discipline. The death of the gynecologists exposed both the ineffectualness of the well-intentioned New York Medical Society and the possible lack of zeal of the teaching hospital in protecting patients from two derelict professionals.

As it turned out, the case was not quite so pure an instance of *noblesse néglige* as it first appeared. The New York Hospital did write a letter terminating the services of the gynecologists. (Unfortunately for the reputation of the hospital and the profession, the termination date set in the letter preceded their death only by seventeen days, and, at a stage so far along the road of addiction that the body weight of these six footers at death was 115 and 100 pounds each.) Officials also made the point that the work of professionals is always monitored by colleagues in the hospital but they conceded that such controls would not apply to the Marcus brothers' private practice. In this as in other cases of solo practice, the patient—certainly the unsophisticated patient—is unprotected by the profession from its incompetent or unscrupulous members.

Whatever the final disposition of the Marcus brothers' case, a fundamental problem remains—and grows—that deserves the attention of moralists; that is, the tension in medical ethics between obligations to patients and obligations to one's fellow professionals. The tendency in the profession is to take the latter duties more seriously than the former. Professional ethics has traditionally had two social vectors: one concerned with behavior toward patients or clients; the other, with conduct toward one's colleagues. When concern for colleagues prevails, professional ethics reduces itself to courtesy within a guild. Certain arguable responsibilities to patients (such as informing them about incompetent treatment) are not simply eclipsed, they are professionally denied, that is, they are viewed as a breach of the discretionary bonds that pertain within the guild. Thus an inversion occurs. A report on incompetent or unethical behavior to patients becomes a breach in "professional ethics," that is, a breach in courtesy.

There are many reasons both material and ideological for the reluctance of doctors to engage in professional self-criticism and regulation. First, like any professional group, doctors find themselves in a complex, interlocking network of relations with fellow professionals: they extend favors, incur debts; exchange referrals; intertwine personal histories. The bond with fellow professionals grows, while ties with patients seem transient. Further, any society organized around certain ends tends to generate a sense of community among professional staff members serving those ends. This experience of collegiality becomes an end in its own right and subtly takes precedence over the needs of the population served. Hence criticism gets muted.

Second, professional self-regulation may be even more difficult to achieve in medicine because self-criticism seems somewhat more natural to lawyers and academicians whose work goes on in an adversarial or, at least, a disputatious setting. The doctor, however, has a special role in relation to his patients, quasi-priestly-parental, which seems more severely subverted by criticism. Trust is a very important ingredient in the relationship; criticism seems outside the boundaries of professional behavior.

Third, the doctor's authority, while great, is precarious. The analogy often drawn between the authority of the modern doctor and the traditional power of the parent and priest obscures an important difference between them in the security of their status. The modern doctor's position, while exalted, is inherently less stable. Apotheosized by many of his patients, he is resented bitterly if his hand slips publicly but once. The reason for this instability lies in differing sources to authority. Parents and priests in traditional society derived their authority from sacred powers perceived to be creative, nurturant, and beneficent. Given this positive derivation of power, human defect in the authority figure could be tolerated. The power of good would prevail despite human lapse. The modern doctor's authority, however, is reflexively derived from a grim negativity; that is, from the fear of death. This self-same power of death that exalts him and makes him the most highly paid, the most authoritative, professional in the modern world threatens to bring him low if through his own negligence, unscrupulousness or incompetence, he endangers the life of his patient. Thus while the modern physician enjoys much more prestige and authority than the contemporary teacher or lawyer, his position as a professional is, in one sense, more precarious than theirs. Resentment against him is potentially much greater. Professional self-criticism in academic life or in the law seems like child's play compared with medicine. The slothful teacher deprives me merely of the truth; the negligent lawyer forfeits my money, or, at worst, my freedom; but the incompetent doctor endangers my life. The stakes seem much higher in the case of medicine. The profession is tempted to draw its wagons around in a circle when any of its members are challenged.

Fourth, Americans of all walks of life have a morally healthy suspicion of officiousness. They are loath to press charges against their neighbors or colleagues. They are peculiarly sensitive to the injustice and hypocrisy of those who are zealous about the sliver in their neighbor's eye while unmindful of the beam in their own. Better, then, to comply with moral standards in one's own professional conduct, but, beyond that, to live and let live. It is difficult, after all, to tell the difference between an honest mistake and culpable negligence. Who can know enough about a particular medical case to second-guess the physician in charge? Is it not better to keep one's mouth shut? Must a person be his colleague's keeper?

This revulsion against officiousness deserves sympathy, but it fails to respect fully the special moral situation of the professional. Professionals are those who, on the basis of their special knowledge and competence, claim final right to pass judgment (in professional matters) on colleagues or would-be colleagues. The state honors and supports this right when it establishes licensing procedures under the control of professionals and backs up these procedures by prosecuting imposters and pretenders. In effect, the state sanctions a monopoly (a limitation on the supply of professionals) from which, to be sure, patients profit, but also from which the professional profits—handsomely, financially. If the professional were in fact a free-lance entrepreneur (as the myth would have it) without the protection of the monopoly, he would not fare nearly so well.

Professional accountability therefore cannot be restricted to the question of one's own personal competence; it includes also the question of the competence of the guild. The right to pass judgment on colleagues carries with it the duty so to judge; otherwise doctors profit from a monopoly established by the state without enforcing those standards the need for which alone justified the monopoly. The license to practice is based on the prior license to license. If the license to practice carries with it the duty to practice well, the license to license carries with it the duty to judge and monitor well.

Ethical standards sag and falter when they are no longer accepted as universally binding. The usual test of whether an individual holds an ethical principle to be universally valid is whether he concedes its application not only to others but to himself. No one can make of himself an exception. The famous confrontation between King David and Nathan the prophet was devoted to that point. The king who makes judgments and enforces laws shall live by the law himself.

Today, however, in professional ethics, the test of moral seriousness may depend not simply upon personal compliance with ethical principles, but upon the courage to hold others accountable. Otherwise, the doctor's oath to his patients has yielded to the somewhat tarnished majesty of the guild.

A fifth and final cause for reserve in pressing for disciplinary action is neither exclusively modern nor American. It is prepared for in principle as far back as the Hippocratic Oath. The ancient oath made an important distinction between two sets of obligations: those that pertain to the doctor's treatment of his patients and those he accepts toward his teacher and his teacher's progeny. Obligations to one's fellow professionals flow from an original indebtedness of the student to his teacher; consequently, they acquire a gravity that makes them take precedence over obligations to patients.

To explore this distinction in obligations, we will need to press back into alternative ways of conceptualizing professional ethics and corresponding perceptions of its binding power. For this reason, in the second section of this essay, we will examine certain root terms for interpreting professional obligation, specifically the concepts of code, covenant, philanthropy, and contract. This investigation will take us beyond the somewhat narrower issue of professional discipline with which we began, but it remains a topic to which, in closing, we will need to return.

The Hippocratic Oath is a useful place to begin not only because of its prominence in medicine, but because it forces reflection on the distinction between code and covenant. The oath itself includes three elements: first, codal duties to patients; second, covenantal obligations to colleagues; and, third, the setting of both within the context of an oath to the gods, specifically, the gods of healing.

The duties of a physician toward his patients, as elaborated in the oath, include a series of absolute prohibitions (against performing surgery, assisting patients in attempts at suicide or abortion, breaches in confidentiality, and acts of injustice or mischief toward the patient and his household, including sexual misconduct); more positively, the physician must act always for the benefit of the sick (the chief illustration of which is to apply dietetic measures according to the physician's best judgment and ability), and, more generally, to keep them from harm and injustice.

The second set of obligations, directed to the physician's teacher, his teacher's children and his own, require him to accept full filial responsibilities for his adopted father's personal and financial welfare, and to transmit without fee his art and knowledge to the teacher's progeny, his own, and to other pupils, but only those others who take the oath according to medical law.

In his monograph on the Hippocratic Oath, Ludwig Edelstein characterizes those obligations that a physician undertakes toward his patients as an ethical code and those assumed toward the professional guild and its perpetuation as a covenant. Just why this difference in terminology is appropriate, Edelstein does not say. In my judgment, the chief reason for resorting to the word covenant in describing the second set of obligations is the fact of indebtedness. The doctor may have duties to his patients, but he owes something to his teacher. He is the beneficiary of goods and services received to which his filial services are responsive. This is one of the hallmarks of covenant. Both the Hammurabi Code and the Mosaic Law detail those statutes that will give shape to a civilization; in this respect, they are alike. But the biblical covenant differs in that it places the moral duties of the people within the all-important context of a divine act of deliverance: "I am the Lord thy God who brought thee out of the land of Egypt, the house of bondage." Thus the promises which the people of Israel make at Mt. Sinai to obey the statutes of God are responsive to goods already received. Analogously, in the Hippocratic Oath, the physician undertakes obligations to his teacher and his progeny out of gratitude for services already rendered. It will be one of the contentions of this essay that the development of the practice of modern medicine, for understandable reasons, has tended to reinforce this particular and ancient distinction between code and covenant and opted for code as the ruling ideal in relations to patients, but not with altogether favorable consequences for the moral health of the profession.

The Hippocratic Oath, of course, includes a third element: the vow or religious oath proper, directed to the gods. "I swear by Apollo, the physician, and Aesculapius and health and all-heal and all the Gods and Goddesses that, according to my ability and judgment, I will keep this oath and stipulation." A religious reference appears again in the statement of duties to patients: "In purity and holiness I will guard my life and art"; and the promise-maker finally petitions: "If I fulfill this oath and do not violate it, may it be granted to me to enjoy life and art . . . ; if I transgress it and swear falsely, may the opposite of all this be my lot."

This religious oath, in the literal sense, makes a "professional" out of the man who takes it. He professes or testifies thereby to the power of healing of which his duties to patients and his obligations to his teacher are a specification. Swearing by Apollo and Aesculapius is at the ontological root of his life. He professes those powers by which his own state of being is altered. Henceforth he is a professional, a professor of healing.

It is an intriguing, but not quite resolvable, question as to whether this oath is an ingredient of a covenant or simply a part of the full meaning of a code. In some respects, it is like a covenant. The physician makes a promise which has a reference to the gods from whom the profession of healing is ultimately derived. This religious promise becomes then the basis for that secondary promise or covenant which the physician makes to care for his teacher and for those duties which he undertakes toward his patients. His promise by the gods gives gravity and shape to the whole. Yet in two important respects the oath itself differs from a biblical covenant: it offers no prefatory statement about the actions of the divine to which the human promise is responsive; and, second, its form is such as to deemphasize the responsive nature of the physician's action, for he swears *by* the gods instead of promises *to* the gods to undertake his professional duties.

Similarly, the question can be raised as to whether this religious vow should be interpreted as part of the full meaning of a code, but, to argue this case, the concept of code needs to be expanded to include more than it means currently in the medical profession.

The word "code" in current professional ethics usually has two meanings—depending on the way in which professional duties are mediated. It can refer alternatively to those *unwritten* and habitual modes of behavior that are transmitted chiefly in a clinical setting from generation to generation of physicians or to those *written* codes, beginning with the Hippocratic Oath and concluding with the various AMA codes that have had wide currency in this country. Technical proficiency is the prized ideal in the informal codes of behavior passed on from doctor to doctor; the ideal of philanthropy (that is, the notion of gratuitous service to humankind) looms larger in the more official, engraved tablets of the profession.

Code, however, covers a third form of activity—above and beyond habitual modes of behavior and collections of written statutes—it refers also to special languages, coded messages, and solemn oaths within special groups. It is this third aspect of code which may be most ethically illuminating; for it implies a special initiation, a profession of allegiance, the possession of a key, and a mutual understanding available only to those who have undergone an alteration in their being which privileges them to use the codebook, the vocabulary, and the technical proficiency.

This third dimension of code prompted us to suggest that the religious vow in the Hippocratic Oath might be interpreted in codal as well as covenantal terms. The professional not only enters into a relationship with a patient, a colleague, or a guild, but also makes a *profession* in and through which his being is altered. He recognizes that his subsequent life for good or ill is derived from this profession. Whenever the medical guild fails to recognize this third aspect of code, it reduces itself to the ideal of technical proficiency alone or it tries to elevate itself to the compensatory and ultimately pretentious concept of philanthropy.

The Current Codal Ideal of Technical Proficiency

Both the ideal of technical proficiency and the skills that go with it are transmitted largely in a clinical setting. A code operating in this milieu shapes human behavior in a fashion somewhat similar to habits and rules. A habit, as Peter Winch has pointed out,[1] is a matter of doing the same thing on the same kind of occasion in the same way. A moral rule is distinct from a habit in that the agent in this instance *understands what is meant* by doing the same thing on the same kind of occasion in the same way. Both habits and rules are categorical, universal, and to this degree ahistorical, they do not receive their authority from particular events by which they are authorized or legitimated. They remain operative categorically on all similar occasions. *Never* assist patients in attempts to suicide or abortion, or *never* break a confidence except under certain specified circumstances.

A code is usually categorical and universal in the aforementioned senses but not in the sense that it is binding on any and all groups. Hammurabi's code is obligatory only for particular peoples. Moreover, inner circles within certain societies—whether professional or social groups—develop their special codes of behavior. We think of code words or special codes of behavior among friends, workers in the same company, or professionals within a guild. These codes offer directives not only for the content of action, but also for its form. In its concern with appropriate form, a code, partly understood, moves in the direction of the aesthetic. It becomes less concerned with what is done or why it is done than with how it is done; so reduced, a code becomes preoccupied with matters of style and decorum. Thus medical codes include directives not only on the content of therapeutic action, but also on the fitting style for professional behavior including such matters as dress, discretion in the household, fitting behavior in the hospital, and prohibitions on self-advertisement.

Insofar as a code becomes more exclusively concerned with style, image, and decorum, it runs the danger of detaching itself from its ontological root. Style functions to protect the stylist from the assaults of life (and death) and to preserve him also from any alterations in his own being. This tendency to move ethics in the direction of aesthetics, rather than ontology, is conveniently illustrated in the work of the modern novelist who is most associated with the aesthetic ideal of a code—Ernest Hemingway. The ritual killing of a bull in the short stories and novels of Hemingway offers a paradigm for the professional; the bullfighter symbolizes an ethic in which stylish performance becomes everything: ". . . the bull charged and Villalta charged and just for a moment they became one. Villalta became one with the bull and then it was over" (*In Our Time,* Hemingway). For the Hemingway hero, there is no question of permanent commitments to particular persons, causes, or places. Robert Jordan of *For Whom the Bell Tolls* does not even remember the "cause," "power," or "profession" for which he came to Spain to fight. Once he is absorbed in the ordeal of war, the test of a man is not a cause to which he is committed but his conduct from moment to moment. Life is a matter of eating, drinking, loving, hunting, and dying well; Jordan can no longer "profess" a cause or sustain a long-term commitment; just like Catherine in *A Farewell to Arms,* he must die. Hemingway writes about lovers, briefly joined, but rarely about marriage or the family. Just for a moment, lovers become one and then it is over.

The bullfighter, the wartime lover, the doctor—all alike—must live by a code that eschews involvement; for each there comes a time when the thing is over; matters are terminated by death. At best, one can hope to escape from the pain of time; thus the aesthetic aspires to the timeless. Men must learn to live beautifully, stylishly, fittingly. Discipline is all, according to the aesthetic code. There is a right and a wrong way to do things. And the wrong way usually results from a deficiency in technique or from an excessive preoccupation with one's ego. The bad bullfighter either lacks technique or he lets his ego—through fear or vanity—get in the way of his performance. The conditions of beauty are technical proficiency and a style wholly purified of disruptive preoccupation with oneself. Literally, however, when the critical moment is consummated, it is over, it cannot shape the future. Partners must fall away; only the code remains.

For several reasons, the medical profession has been attracted to the aesthetic ideal of code for its interpretation of its ethics. First, such a code requires one to subordinate the ego to the more technical question of how a thing is done and done well. At its best, the discipline of a code cultivates the aesthetic. It encourages a proficiency that is quietly eloquent. It conjoins the good with the beautiful. Since the technical demands of medicine have become so great, the standards of the guild are largely transmitted by apprenticeship to those whose preeminent skills define the real meaning of the profession. All the rest is a question of disciplining the ego to the point that nervousness, fatigue, faintheartedness, and temptations to self-display (including gross efforts at self-advertisement) have been smoothed away.

A code is additionally attractive in that it does not, in and of itself, encourage personal involvement with the patient; and it helps free the physician of the destructive consequences of that personal involvement. Compassion, in the strictest sense of the term, "suffering with," has its disadvantages in the professional relationship. It will not do to pretend that one is the second person of the Trinity, prepared with every patient to make the sympathetic descent into his suffering, pain, particular form of crucifixion, and hell. It is enough to offer whatever help one can through finely honed services. It is important to remain emotionally free so as to be able to withdraw the self when those services are no longer pertinent, when, as Hemingway says, "it is over." Such is the attraction of the codal ideal of technical proficiency.

The Ideal of a Covenant

A covenant, as opposed to a code, has its roots in specific historical events. Like a code, it may give inclusive shape to behavior, but it always has reference to a specific historical exchange between partners leading to a promissory event. Edelstein was quite right in distinguishing code from covenant in the Hippocratic Oath. Rules governing behavior toward patients have a different ring to them from that fealty which a physician owes to his teacher. Loyalty to one's instructor is founded in a specific historical event—that original transaction in which the student received his knowledge and art. He receives, in effect, a specific gift from his teacher which deserves his life-long loyalty, a gift that he perpetuates in his own right and turn as he offers his art without fee to his teacher's children and his own progeny. Covenant ethics is responsive in character.

In its ancient and most influential form, a covenant usually included the following elements: first, an original experience of gift between the soon-to-be covenanted partners; and, second, a covenant promise based on this original or anticipated exchange of gifts, labors, or services. However, these temporal and contractual elements of a covenant were but two aspects of a tripartite concept: a covenant included not only an involvement with a partner in time, and a responsive contract, but the notion of a change of being; a covenanted people is a people changed utterly by the covenant. This third aspect of covenant is, like the third aspect of the concept code, ontological in nature. The aesthetic code attempts to remove style from time; a contract has a limited duration in time, but a covenant imposes a change on all moments. A mechanic can act under a contract, and then, when not fixing the piston, act without regard to the contract, but a covenanted people is covenanted while eating, sleeping, working, praying, stealing, cheating, healing, or blundering. Paul remarks, in effect, "When you eat, eat to the glory of God, and when you fast, fast to the glory of God, and when you marry, marry to the glory of God, and when you abstain, abstain to the glory of God."[2] When the professional is initiated, he is covenanted, and the physician is a healer when he is healing, and when he is sleeping, when he is practicing, and when he is malpracticing. A covenant changes the shape of the whole life of the covenanted. It changes the totality of the subsequent life of the covenanted in two ways: first, it contains very specific contractual obligations; the law of Moses, and the Talmudic code based on this law, changed the life of the covenanted by specifying not only the way in which God was to be worshipped, but in their methods of stewing kids; a physician contracts not only to do no harm, but specifically to educate free of charge other professionals' kids. However, the covenant changes are not restricted to the codified and specified changes. It alters the covenanted pervasively in his being; at the beginning of the oath, the physician seals himself, and his whole life, to the gods through his profession. This second change is ontological.

The scriptures of ancient Israel are littered with such covenants between men and controlled throughout by that singular covenant which embraces all others. The covenant between God and Israel includes the aforementioned elements: (1) a gift (the deliverance of the people from Egypt); (2) an exchange of promises (at Mt. Sinai); and (3) the shaping of all subsequent life by the promissory event. God "marks the forehead" of the Jews forever, as they respond by accepting an inclusive set of ritual and moral commandments by which they will live. These commands are both specific enough to make the future duties of Israel concrete (e.g., the dietary laws), yet summary enough (e.g., love the Lord thy God with all thy heart . . .) so as to require a fidelity that exceeds any specification.[3]

For some of the reasons already mentioned, the bond of covenant, in the classical period, tended to define and bind together medical colleagues to one another, but it did not figure large in interpreting the relations between the doctor and his patients. The doctor receives his professional life from his teacher; this gift establishes a bond between them and prompts him to assume certain life-long duties not only toward the teacher (and his financial welfare), but toward his children. This symbolic bond with one's teacher acknowledged in the Hippocratic Oath is strengthened in modern professional life by all those exchanges between colleagues to which reference was made in the opening section of this essay—referrals, favors, personal confidences, and collaborative work on cases. Thus loyalty to colleagues is a responsive act for gifts already, and to be, received.

Duties to patients are not similarly interpreted in the medical codes as a responsive act for gifts or services received. This is the essential feature of covenant conspicuously missing in the interpretation of professional duties to patients from the Hippocratic Oath to the modern codes of the AMA. Compensatorily, the profession has tended to elaborate the codal ideal of philanthropy.

Philanthropy versus Covenantal Indebtedness

The medical profession includes in its written codes an ideal that Hemingway never shared and that seldom looms large in the ethic of any self-selected inner group—the ideal of philanthropy. The medical profession proclaims its dedication to the service of mankind. This ideal is implicitly at work in the Hippocratic Oath and the culture out of which it emerged;[4] it continues in the Code of Medical Ethics originally adopted by the American Medical Association at its national convention in 1847 and it is elaborated in contemporary statements of that code.

This ideal of service, in my judgment, succumbs to what might be called the conceit of philanthropy when it is assumed that the professional's commitment to his fellow man is a gratuitous, rather than a responsive or reciprocal, act flowing from his altered state of being. Statements of medical ethics that obscure the doctor's prior indebtedness to the community are tainted with the odor of condescension. The point is obvious if one contrasts the way in which the code of 1847 interprets the obligations of patients and the public to the physician, as opposed to the obligations of the physician to the patient and the public. On this particular question, I see no fundamental change from 1847 to 1957.

Clearly the duties of the patient are founded on what he has received from the doctor:

> The members of the medical profession, upon whom is enjoined the performance of so many important and arduous duties, toward the community, and who are required to make so many sacrifices of comfort, ease, and health, for the welfare of those who avail themselves of their services, certainly have a right to expect and require that their patients should entertain a just sense of the duties which they owe to their medical attendants. (Art. II, Sect. 1, "Obligations of Patients to Their Physicians," Code of Medical Ethics, American Medical Association, May 1847; Chicago: A.M.A. Press, 1897.)

In like manner, the section on the Obligations of the Public to Physicians (Art. II, Sect. 1) emphasizes those many gifts and services which the public has received from the medical profession and which are the basis for its indebtedness to the profession.

> The benefits accruing to the public, directly and indirectly, from the active and unwearied beneficiaries of the profession, are so numerous and important that physicians are justly entitled to the utmost consideration and respect from the community.

But turning to the preamble for the physician's duties to the patient and the public, we find no corresponding section in the code of 1847 (or 1957) which founds the doctor's obligations on those gifts and services which he has received from the community. Thus we are presented with the picture of a relatively self-sufficient monad, who, out of the nobility and generosity of his disposition and the gratuitously accepted conscience of his profession, has taken upon himself the noble life of service. The false posture in all this blurts out in one of the opening sections of the 1847 code. Physicians "should study, also, in their deportment so as to unite tenderness with firmness, and condescension with authority, so as to inspire the minds of their patients with gratitude, respect and confidence."

I do not intend to demean the specific content of those duties which the codes set forth in their statement of the duties of physicians to their patients, but I am critical of the setting or context in which they are placed. Significantly the code refers to the *Duties* of Physicians to their Patients but to the *Obligations* of Patients to their Physicians. The shift from "Duties" to "Obligations" may seem slight, but, in fact, I believe it is a revealing adjustment in language. The AMA thought of the patient and public as *indebted* to the profession for its services but the profession has accepted its *duties* to the patient and public out of noble conscience rather than a reciprocal sense of indebtedness.

Put another way, the medical profession imitates God not so much because it exercises power of life and death over others, but because it does not really think itself beholden, even partially, to anyone for those duties to patients which it lays upon itself. Like God, the profession draws its life from itself alone. Its action is wholly gratuitous.

Now, in fact, the physician is in very considerable debt to the community. The first of these debts is already adumbrated in the original Hippocratic Oath. He is obliged to someone or some group for his education. In ancient times, this led to a special sense of covenant obligation to one's teacher. Under the conditions of modern medical education, this indebtedness is both substantial (far exceeding the social investment in the training of any other professional) and widely distributed (including not only one's teachers but those public monies on the basis of which the medical school, the teaching hospital, and research into disease, are funded).

In view of the fact that many more qualified candidates apply for medical school than can be admitted and many more doctors are needed than the schools can train, the doctor-to-be has a second order of indebtedness for privileges that have almost arbitrarily fallen his way. While the 1847 code refers to the "privileges" of being a doctor it does not specify the social origins of those privileges. Third, and not surprisingly, the codes do not make reference to that extraordinary social largesse that befalls the physician, in payment for services, in a society where need abounds and available personnel is limited. Further, the codes do not concede the indebtedness of the physician to those patients who have offered themselves as subjects for experimentation or as teaching material (either in teaching hospitals or in the early years of practice). Early practice includes, after all, the element of increased risk for patients who lay their bodies on the line as the doctor "practices" on them. The pun in the word but reflects the inevitable social price of training. This indebtedness to the patient was most recently and eloquently acknowledged by Judah Folkman, M.D., of Harvard Medical School in a Class Day Address.

> In the long run, it is better if we come to terms with the uncertainty of medical practice. Once we recognise that all our efforts to relieve suffering might on occasion cause suffering, we are in a position to learn from our mistakes and appreciate the debt we owe our patients for our education. It is a debt which we must repay—it is like tithing.
>
> I doubt that the debt we accumulate can be repaid our patients by trying to reduce the practice of medicine to a forty-hour week or by dissolving the quality of our residency program just because certain groups of residents in the country have refused, through legal tactics, to be on duty more than every fourth or fifth night or any nights at all.
>
> And, it can't be repaid by refusing to see Medicaid patients when the state can't afford to pay for them temporarily.
>
> But we can repay the debt in many ways. We can attend postgraduate courses and seminars, be available to patients at all hours, teach, take recertification examinations; maybe in the future even volunteer for national service; or, most difficult of all, carry out investigation or research.[5]

The physician finally is indebted to his patients not only for a start in his career. He remains unceasingly in their debt in its full course. This continuing reciprocity of need is somewhat obscured for we think of the mature professional as powerful and authoritative rather than needy. He seems to be a self-sufficient virtuoso whose life is derived from his competence while others appear before him in their neediness, exposing their illness, their crimes, or their ignorance, for which the professional, as doctor, lawyer, or teacher, offers remedy.

In fact, however, a reciprocity of giving and receiving is at work in the professional relationship that needs to be acknowledged. In the profession of teaching, for example, the student needs the teacher to assist him in learning, but so also the professor needs his students. They provide him with regular occasion and forum in which to work out what he has to say and to rediscover his subject afresh through the discipline of sharing it with others. Likewise, the doctors needs his patients. No one can watch a physician nervously approach retirement without realizing how much he has needed his patients to be himself.

A covenantal ethics helps acknowledge this full context of need and indebtedness in which professional duties are undertaken and discharged. It also relieves the professional of the temptation and pressure to pretend that he is a demigod exempt from human exigency.

Contract or Covenant

While criticizing the ideal of philanthropy, I have emphasized the elements of exchange, agreement, and reciprocity that mark the professional relationship. This leaves us with the question as to whether the element of the gratuitous should be suppressed altogether in professional ethics. Does the physician merely respond to the social investment in his training, the fees paid for his services, and the terms of an agreement drawn up between himself and his patients, or does some element of the gratuitous remain?

To put this question another way: is covenant simply another name for a contract in which two parties calculate their own best interests and agree upon some joint project in which both derive roughly equivalent benefits for goods contributed by each? If so, this essay would appear to move in the direction of those who would interpret the doctor-patient relationship as a legal agreement and who want, on the whole, to see medical ethics draw closer to medical law.

The notion of the physician as contractor has certain obvious attractions. First, it represents a deliberate break with more authoritarian models (such as priest or parent) for interpreting the role. At the heart of a contract is informed consent rather than blind trust; a contractual understanding of the therapeutic relationship encourages full respect for the dignity of the patient, who has not, because of illness, forfeited his sovereignty as a human being. The notion of a contract includes an exchange of information on the basis of which an agreement is reached and a subsequent exchange of goods (money for services); it also allows for a specification of rights, duties, conditions, and qualifications limiting the agreement. The net effect is to establish some symmetry and mutuality in the relationship between the doctor and patient.

Second, a contract provides for the legal enforcement of its terms—on both parties—and thus offers both parties some protection and recourse under the law for making the other accountable for the agreement.

Finally, a contract does not rely on the pose of philanthropy, the condescension of charity. It presupposes that people are primarily governed by self-interest. When two people enter into a contract, they do so because each sees it to his own advantage. This is true not only of private contracts but also of that primordial social contract in and through which the state came into being. So argued the theorists of the eighteenth century. The state was not established by some heroic act of sacrifice on the part of the gods or men. Rather men entered into the social contract because each found it to his individual advantage. It is better to surrender some liberty and property to the state than to suffer the evils that would beset men apart from its protection. Subsequent enthusiasts about the social instrument of contracts[6] have tended to measure human progress by the degree to which a society is based on contracts rather than status. In the ancient world, the Romans made the most striking advances in extending the areas in which contract rather than custom determined commerce between people. In the modern world, the bourgeoisie extended the instrumentality of contracts farthest into the sphere of economics; the free churches, into the arena of religion. Some educationists today have extended the device into the classroom (as students are encouraged to contract units of work for levels of grade); more recently some women's liberationists would extend it into marriage; and still others would prefer to see it define the professional relationship. The movement, on the whole, has the intention of laicizing authority, legalizing relationships, activating self-interest, and encouraging collaboration.

In my judgment, some of these aims of the contractualists are desirable, but it would be unfortunate if professional ethics were reduced to a commercial contract. First, the notion of contract suppresses the element of gift in human relationships. Earlier I verged on denying the importance of this ingredient in professional relations, when I criticized the medical profession for its conceit of philanthropy, for its self-interpretation as the great giver. In fact, this earlier criticism was not an objection to the notion of gift but to the moral pretension of a profession whenever it pretends to be the exclusive giver. Factually, the professional is also the beneficiary of gifts received. It is unbecoming to adopt the pose of spontaneous generosity when the profession has received so much from the community and from patients, past and present.

But the contractualist approach to professional behavior falls into the opposite error of minimalism. It reduces everything to tit for tat. Do no more for your patients than what the contract calls for. Perform specified services for certain fees and no more. The commercial contract is fitting instrument in the purchase of an appliance, a house, or certain services that can be specified fully in advance of delivery. The existence of a legally enforceable agreement in professional transactions may also be useful to protect the patient or client against the physician or lawyer whose services fall below a minimal standard. But it would be wrong to reduce professional obligation to the specifics of a contract alone.

Professional services in the so-called helping professions are directed to subjects whose needs are in the nature of the case rather unpredictable. The professional deals with the sickness, ills, crimes, needs, and tragedies of humankind. These needs cannot be exhaustively specified in advance for each patient or client. The professions therefore must be ready to cope with the contingent, the unexpected. Calls upon services may be required that exceed those anticipated in a contract or for which compensation may be available in a given case. These services moreover are more likely to be effective in achieving the desired therapeutic result if they are delivered in the context of a fiduciary relationship that the patient or client can really trust.

Contract and covenant, materially considered, seem like first cousins; they both include an exchange and an agreement between parties. But, in spirit, contract and covenant are quite different. Contracts are external; covenants are internal to the parties involved. Contracts are signed to be expediently discharged. Covenants have a gratuitous, growing edge to them that spring from ontological change and are directed to the upbuilding of relationships.

There is a donative element in the upbuilding of covenant—whether it is the covenant of marriage, friendship, or professional relationship. Tit for tat characterizes a commercial transaction, but it does not exhaustively define the vitality of that relationship in which one must serve and draw upon the deeper reserves of another.

This donative element is important not only in the doctor's care of the patient but in other aspects of health care. In a fascinating study of *The Gift Relationship,* the late economist, Richard M. Titmuss, compares the British system of obtaining blood by donations with the American partial reliance on the commercial purchase and sale of blood. The British system obtains more and better blood, without the exploitation of the indigent, which the American system has condoned and which our courts have encouraged when they refused to exempt non-profit blood banks from the antitrust laws. By court definition, blood exchange becomes a commercial transaction in the United States. Titmuss expanded his theme from human blood to social policy by offering a sober criticism of the increased commercialism of American medicine and society at large. Recent court decisions have tended to shift more and more of what had previously been considered as services into the category of commodity transactions with negative consequences he believes for the health of health delivery systems.[7] Hans Jonas has had to reckon with the importance of voluntary sacrifice to the social order in a somewhat comparable essay on "Human Experimentation."[8] Others have done so on the subject of organ transplants.

The kind of minimalism that a contractualist understanding of the professional relationship encourages produces a professional too grudging, too calculating, too lacking in spontaneity, too quickly exhausted to go the second mile with his patients along the road of their distress.

Contract medicine encourages not only minimalism, it also provokes a peculiar kind of maximalism, the name for which is "defensive medicine." Especially under the pressure of malpractice suits, doctors are tempted to order too many examinations and procedures for self-protection. Paradoxically, contractualism simultaneously tempts the doctor to do too little and too much for the patient—too little in that one extends oneself only to the limits of what is specified in the contract, yet, at the same time, too much in that one orders procedures useful in protecting oneself as the contractor even though not fully indicated by the condition of the patient. The link between these apparently contradictory strategies of too little and too much is the emphasis in contractual decisions on self-interest.

Three concluding objections to contractualism can

be stated summarily. Parties to a contract are better able to protect their self-interest to the degree that they are informed about the goods bought and sold. Insofar as contract medicine encourages increased knowledge on the part of the patient, well and good. Nevertheless the physician's knowledge so exceeds that of his patient that the patient's knowledgeability alone is not a satisfactory constraint on the physician's behavior. One must at least, in part, depend upon some internal fiduciary checks which the professional (and his guild) accept.

Another self-regulating mechanism in the traditional contractual relationship is the consumer's freedom to shop and choose among various vendors of services. Certainly this freedom of choice needs to be expanded for the patient by an increase in the number of physicians and paramedical personnel. However, the crisis circumstances under which medical services are often needed and delivered does not always provide the consumer with the kind of leisure or calm required for discretionary judgment. Thus normal marketplace controls cannot be relied upon fully to protect the consumer in dealings with the physician.

For a final reason, medical ethics should not be reduced to the contractual relationship alone. Normally conceived, ethics establishes certain rights and duties that transcend the particulars of a given agreement. The justice of any specific contract may then be measured by these standards. If, however, such rights and duties adhere only to the contract, then a patient might legitimately be persuaded to waive his rights. The contract would solely determine what is required and permissible. An ethical principle should not be waivable (except to give way to a higher ethical principle). Professional ethics should not be so defined as to permit a physician to persuade a patient to waive rights that transcend the particulars of their agreement.

The donative mode seems to provide for a more satisfactory analysis than the philanthropic or the contractual, but it shares their flaws. Analysis based on donative elements suggests that the professional fulfills his contract, lives up to his specified technical code, and then, gratuitously, throws in something extra to sweeten the pot. All of these tools of analysis allow the analyst to evade the uncomfortable and demanding ontological implications of Initiatory Code, Covenant as Chosen, and Profession as transformation. The ontological changes implied in Secret Code, Covenanted People, and Profession of a mystery are complete changes in substance which affect the total life of the professional. A carpenter who contracts to build a chair, when he eats an ice cream cone, does not eat it as a carpenter, nor, when he gets his union card, does he imply that his initiation has changed him utterly, relating him, before everything else, to the mystery of chair making or shellac. A profession of a mystery, in theological terms changes one from damned to saved; in professional terms, from a man who studies medicine, to a man who at all times embodies healing. Malpractice, then, is rather like the sin against the Holy Ghost, uncomfortable for those sinned against, but utterly negating the identity of the sinner. A professional eats to heal, drives to heal, reads to heal, comforts to heal, rebukes to heal, and rests to heal. The transformation is radical, and total. The Hippocratic Oath, under this ontological aspect, can be summarized: *aut medicus aut nihil;* from this moment, I am a healer or I am (literally) nothing. He takes his identity from that which he professes, and that which he professes, to which he is covenanted, whose code he will embody, transcends him and transcends his colleagues.

Transcendence and Covenant

Two characteristics of covenantal ethics have been developed in the course of contrasting it with the ideal of philanthropy and the legal instrument of contracts. As opposed to the ideal of philanthropy that pretends to wholly gratuitous altruism, covenantal ethics places the service of the professional within the full context of goods, gifts, and services received; thus covenantal ethics is responsive. As opposed to the instrument of contract that presupposes agreement reached on the basis of self-interest, covenantal ethics may require one to be available to the covenant partner above and beyond the measure of self-interest; thus covenantal ethics has an element of the gratuitous in it.

We have to reckon now with the potential conflict between these characteristics. Have we developed our notion of covenant too reactively to alternatives without paying attention to the inner consistency of the concept itself? On the one hand, we had cause for suspecting those idealists who founded professional duties on a philanthropic impulse, without so much as acknowledging the sacrifice of others by which their own lives have been nourished. Then we have reasons for drawing back from those legal realists and positivists who would circumscribe professional life entirely within the calculus of commodities bought and sold. But now, brought face to face, these characteristics conflict. Response to debt and gratuitous service seem opposed principles of action.

Perhaps our difficulty results from the fact that we have abstracted the concept of covenant from its original context within the transcendent. The indebtedness of a human being that makes his life—however sacrificial—inescapably responsive cannot be fully appreciated by totaling up the varying sacrifices and investments made by others in his favor. Such sacrifices are there; and it is lacking in honesty not to acknowledge them. But the sense that one is inexhaustibly the object of gift presupposes a more transcendent source of donative activity than the sum of gifts received from others. For the biblical tradition this transcendent was the secret root of every gift between human beings, of which the human order of giving and receiving could only be a sign. Thus the Jewish scriptures enjoin the covenanted people: when you harvest your crops, do not pick your fields too clean. Leave something for the sojourner for you were once sojourners in Egypt. Farmers obedient to this injunction were responsive, but not simply mathematically responsive to gifts received from the Egyptians or from strangers now drifting through their own land. At the same time, their actions could not be construed as wholly gratuitous. Their ethic of service to the needy flowed from Israel's original and continuing state of neediness and indebtedness before God. Thus action which, at a human level, appears gratuitous, in that it is not provoked by a specific gratuity from another human being, at its deepest level is but gift answering to gift. This responsivity is theologically expressed in the New Testament as follows: "In this is love, not that we loved God, but that He loved us . . . if God so loved us, we also ought to love one another." (1 John 4:10-11) In some such way, covenant ethics shies back from the idealist assumption that professional action is and ought to be wholly gratuitous and from the contractualist assumption that it be carefully governed by quotidian self-interest in every exchange.

A transcendent reference may also be important in laying out not only the proper context in which human service takes place but also the specific standards by which it is measured. Earlier we noted some dangers in reducing rights and duties to the terms of a particular contract. We observed the need for a transcendent norm by which contracts are measured (and limited). By the same token, rights and duties cannot be wholly derived from the particulars of a given covenant. What limits ought to be placed on the demands of an excessively dependent patient? At what point does the keeping of one covenant do an injustice to obligations entailed in others? These are questions that warn against a covenantal ethics that sentimentalizes any and all involvements, without reference to a transcendent by which they are both justified and measured.

Further Reflections on Covenant

So far we have discussed those features of a covenant that affect the doctor's conduct toward his patient. The concept of covenant has further consequences for the patient's understanding of his role as patient, for the accountability of health institutions, for the placement of institutional priorities within other national commitments, and, finally, for such collateral problems as truth-telling.

Every model for the doctor-patient relationship establishes not only a certain image of the doctor, but also a specific concept of the patient. The image of the doctor as priest or parent encourages dependency in the patient. The image of the doctor as skillful technician encourages the patient to think of himself as passive host to a disease. The doctor and his technical procedures are the only serious agent in the relationship. The image of the doctor as covenanter or contractor bids the patient to become a more active participant both in the prevention and the healing of disease. He must bring a will-to-live and a will-to-health to the partnership.

Differing views of disease are involved in these differing patterns of relationship to the doctor. Disease today is usually interpreted by the layman as an extraordinary state, discrete and episodic, disjunctive from the ordinary condition of health. Illness is a special time when the doctor is in charge and the layman renounces authority over his life. This view, while psychologically understandable, ignores the build-up, during apparent periods of health, of those pathological conditions that invite the dramatic breakdown when the doctor "takes over."

The cardiovascular accident is a case in point. Horacio Fabrega[9] has urged an interpretation of disease and health that respects more fully the processive rather than the episodic character of both disease and health. This interpretation, I assume, would encourage the doctor to monitor more continuously health and disease than ordinarily occurs today, to share with the patient more fully the information so obtained, and to engage the layperson in a more active collaboration with the doctor in health maintenance.

The concept of covenant has two further advantages for defining the professional relationship, not enjoyed by models such as parent, friend, or technician. First, covenant is not so restrictively personal a term as parent or friend. It reminds the professional community that it is not good enough for the individual doctor to be a good friend or parent to the patient, it is important also that whole institutions—the hospital, the clinic, the professional group—keep covenant with those who seek their assistance and sanctuary. Thus the concept permits a certain broadening of accountability beyond personal agency.

At the same time, however, the notion of covenant also permits one to set professional responsibility for this one human good (health) within social limits. The professional covenant concerning health should be situated within a larger set of covenant obligations that both the doctor and patient have to other institutions and priorities within the society at large. The traditional models for the doctor-patient relationship (parent, friend) tend to establish an exclusivity of relationship that obscures these larger responsibilities. At a time when health needs command $120 billion out of the national budget, one must think about the place that the obligation to the limited human good of health has amongst a whole range of social and personal goods for which men are compacted together as a society.

Although a covenantal ethic has implications for other collateral problems in biomedical ethics, I will restrict myself simply to one final issue that has not been viewed from the perspective of covenant: the question of truth-telling.

Key ingredients in the notion of covenant are promise and fidelity to promise. The philosopher J. I. Austin drew the distinction, now famous, between two kinds of speech: descriptive and performative utterances. In ordinary declarative or descriptive sentences, one describes a given item within the world. (It is raining. The tumor is malignant. The crisis is past.) In performative utterances, one does not merely describe a world; in effect, one alters the world by introducing an ingredient that would not be there apart from the utterance. Promises are such performative utterances. (I, John, take Thee, Mary. We will defend your country in case of attack. I will not abandon you.) To make or to go back on a promise is a very solemn matter precisely because a promise is world-altering.

In the field of medical ethics, the question of truth-telling has tended to be disposed of entirely as a question of descriptive speech. Should the doctor, as technician, tell the patient he has a malignancy or not? If not, may he lie or must he merely withhold the truth?

The distinction between descriptive and performative speech expands the question of the truth-telling in professional life. The doctor, after all, not only tells descriptive truths, he also makes or implies promises. (I will see you next Tuesday. Despite the fact that I cannot cure you, I will not abandon you.) In brief, the moral question for the doctor is not simply a question of telling truths, but of being true to his promises. Conversely, the total situation for the patient includes not only the disease he's got, but also whether others desert him or stand by him in his extremity. The fidelity of others will not eliminate the disease, but it affects mightily the human context in which the disease runs its course. What the doctor has to offer his patient is not simply proficiency but fidelity.

Perhaps more patients could accept the descriptive truth if they experienced the performative truth. Perhaps also they would be more inclined to believe in the doctor's performative utterances if they were not handed false diagnoses or false promises. That is why a cautiously wise medieval physician once advised his colleagues: "Promise only fidelity!"

The Problem of Discipline Revisited

The conclusion of this essay is not that covenantal ethics should be preferred to the exclusion of some of those values best symbolized by code and contract. If we return to the problem of discipline with which we began, we can see that both alternatives have resources for professional self-criticism.

Those who live by a code of technical proficiency have a standard on the basis of which to discipline their peers. The Hemingway novel, especially *The Sun Also Rises,* is quite clear about this. Those who live by a code know how to ostracize deficient peers. Indeed, any "in-group," professional or otherwise, can be quite ruthless about sorting out those who are "quality" and those who do not have the "goods." Medicine is no exception. Ostracism, in the form of discretely refusing to refer patients to a doctor whose competence is suspected, is probably the commonest and most effective form of discipline in the profession today.

Defendents of an ethic based on code might argue further that deficiencies in enforcement today result largely from too strongly developed a sense of covenantal obligations to colleagues and too weakly developed a sense of code. From this perspective, then, covenant is the source of the problem in the profession rather than the basis for its amendment. Covenantal obligation to colleagues inhibits the enforcement of code.

A code alone, however, will not in and of itself solve the problem of professional discipline. It provides only a basis for excluding from one's own inner circles an incompetent physician. But, as Eliot Freidson has pointed out in *Professional Dominance,* under the present system, the incompetent professional, when he is excluded from a given hospital, group practice, or informal circle of referrals, simply moves his practice and finds another circle of people of equal incompetence in which he can function. It will take a much stronger, more active and internal sense of covenant obligation to patients on the part of the profession to enforce standards within the guild beyond local informal patterns of ostracism. In a mobile society with a scarcity of doctors, local ostracism simply hands on problem physicians to other patients elsewhere. It does not address them.

Code patterns of discipline not only fall short of adequate protection for the patient, they also fail to be collegially responsible to the troubled physician. To ostracize may be the lazy way of handling a colleague when it fails altogether to make a first attempt at remedy and to address the physician himself in his difficulty.

At the same time, it would be unfortunate if the indispensable interest and pride of the medical profession in technical proficiency were allowed to lapse out of an expressed preference for a professional ethic based on covenant. Covenant fidelity to the patient remains unrealized if it does not include proficiency. A rather sentimental existentialism unfortunately assumes that it suffices morally for human beings to be "present" to one another. But in crisis, the ill person needs not simply presence but skill, not just personal concern but highly disciplined services targeted on specific needs. Code behavior, handed down from doctor to doctor, is largely concerned with the transmission of technical skills. Covenant ethics, then, must include rather than exclude the interests of the codes.

Neither does this essay conclude with a preference for covenant to the total exclusion of the interests of enforceable contract. While the reduction of medical ethics to contract alone incurs the danger of minimalism, patients ought to have recourse against those physicians who fail to meet minimal standards. They ought not to be dependent entirely upon disciplinary measures undertaken within the profession. There ought to be appeal to the law in cases of malpractice and for breach of contract explicit or implied.

On the other hand, a legal appeal cannot be sustained in the case of an injustice without assistance and testimony from physicians who take their obligations to patients and their profession seriously. If, in such cases, fellow physicians simply herd around and protect their colleague like a wounded elephant, the patient with just cause is not likely to get far. Thus the instrument of contract and other avenues of legal redress can be sustained only by physicians who have a sense of obligation to the patient and the profession. Needless to say, it would be better for all concerned if professional discipline and continuing education were so vigorously pursued within the profession as to cut down drastically on the number of cases that needed to reach the courts.

The author inclines to accept covenant as the most inclusive and satisfying model for framing questions of professional obligation. Covenant fidelity includes the code duty to become technically proficient; it includes the obligation to meet the minimal terms of contract, but it also requires much more. Moreover, this surplus of obligation may be to the final advantage not only of patients but also of colleagues. The Marcus case, or, if not that one, others like it, suggest a failure in covenant responsibilities not only to patients but to troubled colleagues.[10]

Notes

1. *The Idea of a Social Science and its Relation to Philosophy* (New York: Humanities Press, 1958).

2. A paraphrase of Rom. 4:5-8 and 1 Cor. 10:31.

3. The most striking contemporary restatement of an ethic based on covenant is offered by Hemingway's great competitor and contemporary as a novelist—William Faulkner. See especially "Delta Autumn" and "The Bear" and *Intruder in the Dust.*

4. See P. Lain-Entralgo, *Doctor and Patient* (New York: McGraw-Hill, 1969), for his analysis of the classical fusion of *techne* with *philanthropia,* skill in the art of healing combined with a love of mankind defines the good physician.

5. *New York Times,* Op. Ed. Page, June 6, 1975.

6. Sir Henry Sumner Maine, *Ancient Law* (London: Oxford University Press, 1931).

7. Titmuss does not acknowledge that physicians in the United States have helped prepare for this commercialization of medicine by their substantial fees for services (as opposed to salaried professors in the teaching field or salaried health professionals in other countries).

8. See "Philosophical Reflections on Experimenting with Human Subjects," pp. 616-27 below.

9. Horacio Fabrega, Jr., "Concepts of Disease: Logical Features and Social Implications," *Perspectives in Biology and Medicine,* Vol. 15, No. 4, Summer 1972.

10. This is a revised version of an article that first appeared in *The Hastings Center Report* 5 (December 1975): 29-38.

16. Educating the Christian Physician: Being Christian and Being a Physician

EDMUND D. PELLEGRINO

You have the mission of curing sickness but if you do not bring love to the sick bed I do not think medicine will do much good.

Padre Pio

To be truly a physician, even in purely human terms, is to be committed to a noble ideal. To be a Christian physician is to add dimensions of inspiration and aspiration that elevate the ideal immeasurably, for the Christian physician is called to imitate an ineffable model—an incarnate God whose own ministry was inseparable from healing.[1]

No vocation, even healing, is automatically Christian in spirit. Nor does it suffice to be a Christian who is also a physician. Only in the creative fusion of two existential states—being a Christian and being a physician—is it possible to realize the full nobility of the ideal of Christian healing. That fusion and the special obligations it entails are the unique call to which Christians in their study, teaching, and practice of medicine must individually and collectively respond.

Meeting this challenge today is extraordinarily difficult. We are still seeking how best to teach and practice medical humanism of the secular kind.[2] Can we hope then to teach what it means authentically to witness Christ through the profession of medicine? Even those few medical schools under religious auspices have no formal programs for educating Christian physicians. What teaching occurs is largely by example. Christian physicians have allowed the act of healing to become progressively secularized. They, with their patients, tolerate all too readily an ever widening separation of healing from faith and ministry. They even seem apologetic and reticent about being Christian physicians, thus isolating faith from life.

These responses are the predictable result of misunderstanding both the strength and the limitations of the conception of modern medicine as science. The undeniably dramatic and indispensable contributions of scientific methodology to therapeutics foster an understandable hubris. Specific cure for every known illness is the ambitious aim of medical science. The temptation to believe medicine can stand alone is very strong. What, we are asked, can religion add to these wondrous achievements?

Indeed, it is feared that too zealous an adherence to Christian values might lead to a neglect of science, to passivity in the face of illness and death and an inhibition of the free pursuit of biological knowledge. There are dangers, too, it is thought, of using the vulnerable state of the sick person to proselytize. Finally, religion undeniably introduces complex moral questions which unquestionably impede the uninhibited use of medical science to determine humankind's future.

Even the ethics of medicine, which has long had strong religious roots in America and in the West, is being secularized. In a morally pluralistic society it is difficult to find agreements on the resolution of specific medical-moral dilemmas. Competence and legalism rather than ideals of obligation and service have come to dominate professional codes, as the recently proposed revisions of the code of the American Medical Association (AMA) amply attest.[3]

We urgently need a universally accepted reconstruction of our codes of medical morality. Such a reconstruction is not likely, ever again, to be wholly religiously inspired. At best, we can hope for a common substratum of obligations justified philosophically in the nature of the physician-patient relationship.[4] The Christian physician will have to build upon this substratum those higher levels of inspiration and obligation called for by the revelation of the Christian message.

I cite these obstacles because Christian physicians use them as justification for not addressing the issue of how to educate the Christian physician. Yet, the Christian medical teacher who ignores that challenge risks serious hypocrisy which can frustrate the fullness of the student's Christian experience. Such a teacher derogates the enormous power of Christian humanism to reverse the alarming trend of contemporary medicine to become alienated from the humane purposes to which it is ordained. Such a teacher also deprives patients of the healing powers of faith—powers every true Christian must draw upon.

How is the Christian physician to be educated? What is to be taught and how? What is feasible in a secular institution? What more is possible and demanded in a school specifically dedicated to the education of Christian physicians?

I shall address these questions in three stages: first, by examining what it means to be a physician in

---

Reprinted with permission from *Hospital Progress,* August 1979.

purely human terms—the terms of secular humanism; second, by seeing what must be added to the human ideal by being a Christian—the terms of Christian humanism; and, finally, seeing how the educational goal is to be pursued.

Before I examine these three issues, I am compelled in all justice to acknowledge the dedication to high ideals of morality and practice by those Jewish and Moslem persons and nonbelievers who follow their own perceptions of the good physician. They, too, care deeply for their patients as suffering fellow humans. Often enough, they share with Christians a loving care, charity, and concern for those they attend. As a Christian I would surely be out of order trying to define what additional dimensions believing non-Christians bring to being a physician. It is what Christianity specifically brings that must be my concern.

The Physician *qua* Physician—Reason Unaided by Faith

In a series of papers I have tried to define what it means to be a physician on the basis of a philosophical inquiry into the nature of medicine and the physician-patient relationship. I can only summarize my position here.[5]

The act specific to medicine, that which makes it medicine, and thereby distinguishes it from both science and art, is a decision about what is right and good for a particular patient. The central and irreducible concern of medicine is this patient present to us now with this set of needs, arising out of this particular illness. Science is necessary to specify the causes of the patient's illness and to determine what modes of therapy are available, which are effective, and how safe they are. Art is required to assure perfection in carrying out the decision of a skillful examination, operation, or manipulation. But the essence of medicine is neither art nor science—it is the practical decision, taken in the best interest of a particular person, not in the interest of gaining new knowledge, of the good of society, or of the physician's self-interest.

Once we speak of a "right" and "good" action we are squarely in the realm of morals—of what ought to be done. Medicine, therefore, is at its center—the moment of decision making—a moral enterprise. I have construed it in the Aristotelian sense as a practical virtue—a *recta ratio agibilium.*[6] The physician's obligations arise out of two things: (1) In undertaking to treat the patient the physician promises to act in that patient's best interest, that is, to take the right and good healing action; and (2) the physician makes that promise within a special human relationship arising out of the needs of another human being in a state of special vulnerability, the state of illness.

The person who is ill is in a state of compromised or wounded humanity in which, to varying degrees, the distinctly human possibilities of free and rational decision making about self and body are compromised. The person who is ill does not know what is wrong and lacks the skill of self-healing. He or she can decide what is "best" only on the advice of another human being. The physician's act of "profession" implies that he or she will act competently and in the patient's best interest. That act promises as well that the wounded humanity of the ill person will be healed—that information sufficient to make an informed choice will be provided, that the procedures will be competently and safely performed, that the patient's values, his or her assessment of what is worthwhile, rather than the physician's, will be respected.

In purely human terms, leaving religious imperatives aside for the moment, just being a physician imposes obligations of a special character grounded in the fact of illness. The special human vulnerability in that experience demands that the physician's obligations transcend self-interest to a degree not demanded of other professionals. This is why moral dimensions were recognized so early in the history of medicine and explicitly stated in professional codes.

At first, medical morality was simply that of the good craftsman—the ethics of a competent jobsman. In addition, a kind and sympathetic demeanor was required to assure the patient's cooperation and to establish a good reputation. These were the elements of the early Greek notion of philanthropia—not charity or love in the Christian sense.[7] The nobler sentiments often attributed to Greek medicine were later infusions derived from Stoicism and the precepts of the Christian, Jewish, and Moslem religions. Each of these influences modified and then adopted the Hippocratic ethic and code and thus universalized it for physicians in the West.

It was the middle and late Stoics who raised medical morality to the noblest heights attainable by unaided human reason. Scribonius Largus, physician to the Emperor Claudius and a follower of the moral philosophy of Panaetius and Cicero, first introduced the word "profession" in relationship to medicine. He was the first, also, to suggest that the morality of the physician was specifically related to the nature of the "profession" of medicine. Scribonius went so far as to use the words "humanitas," love of humanity, and "misericordia," mercy. These, he argued, were obligations intrinsic to being a physician. Without them, the practitioner could not be a member of the profession and became tantamount to a traitor or deserter.[8]

Some of the later Stoics, like Sarapion and Libanius (in his address to the young physician), go even further. They specifically admonish the physician to treat the patient as a brother. These Stoics saw medicine as a vocation, as Christians do. They derived the obligations of that vocation from the nature of a calling voluntarily assumed. The nobility of these Stoic sentiments is remarkable. They represent the highest expression of what it is to be a physician to which natural reason, unenlightened by revelation, can attain. Admittedly, some of the later of those pagan writers lived in the early years of the Christian era, and it is conceivable that they imbibed some of the Christian community's teachings. Their historical and textual connections with Christianity are presently not established. Whatever their provenance, the lofty ideal of medical morality, propounded by the Stoics, was a distinct advance over Hippocratic ethics. The ideal they fashioned remains a model of medical humanism which still inspires all—religious and nonreligious—who profess to be humanistic healers.

The Religious and the Christian Physician

With so high an ideal created out of the secular humanism of the Stoic philosophy, what more can be added by a religious dimension? Since even the word "love" was used by the later Stoics, is anything more needed? What additional dimension of obligation does any religion add to those required by the act of profession and by the nature of the physician-patient relationship?

First, I must say what I mean by "religion." I refer to any system of belief that derives its justification from some principle, power, or force outside man, which requires of man certain duties not self-generated and which may, or may not, also require certain ritual practices. The difference between religion and nonreligion is an act of faith, or nonfaith, in a power beyond man. This definition is intentionally broad enough to encompass all varieties of belief. It underscores the fundamental distinction between what is required of the physician as physician by secular humanisms and what is added by any religious belief.

The religious believer who unites personal belief to profession incurs all the obligations implicit in Scribonius's Stoic ideal. But the believer must also be faithful to an additional set of values, inspirations, and practices attributable to the transcendental principle in which he or she believes. The shape and meaning of the Stoic ideals of "humanitas" and "misericordia" are, therefore, specifically modulated by the worldview each religion imposes.

For the religious believer, all morality receives its ultimate justification from a source outside and superior to humankind. The religious person cannot hold that morality is self-justifying. Certain obligations are deducible by reason alone, it is true, but the highest display of human moral agency requires adjustments to the demands of a higher principle in which the religious man or woman has made an act of faith.

For the Christian, this higher dimension is revealed in the Gospels of Jesus Christ, whose irruption into human history redeemed humankind, fulfilled the prophets of the Old Testament, and forever altered the meaning of human relationships. All who follow Christ must love God as the Father and all persons as his brothers and sisters. Every incident in the life of Jesus exemplifies Christian love and charity. The Beatitudes teach us directly and explicitly how being a Christian differs from even the highest expressions of morality in the Old Testament or in the best pagan philosophers.

Kierkegaard's question Who is a Christian? must be answered daily by every Christian and every church. The Christian is committed to the special way of love and charity witnessed by Christ. This way must illuminate the Christian's every action and thought. He and she must become partners in Christ's ministry to the world. With the Church, the Christian is called to evangelize, to witness, to teach, and to announce the "good news."

The Christian physician has in Christ a more explicit model of inspiration than do any other professionals except the clergy. Healing was the daily task of Jesus. He healed in body and soul; in him, healing and salvation were one. Healing exemplified his love for persons in the most concrete way. Christ had compassion on the vulnerability of the sick. He knew the meaning of bodily suffering, which he himself tasted to the fullest in the Garden of Gethsemane and on the cross.

For the Christian physician who follows Christ, healing cannot ever be anything other than ministry—it cannot ever be merely science or public service. Healing insofar as medical knowledge allows, the physician must also care for and feel for the sick person, whether or not the medical means to cure are adequate. Christian compassion means "to suffer with" our brothers and sisters in Christ.

The Christian ministry of healing is not reserved only for those who can pay or for the educated, the grateful, the clean, for "our kind" of people, or for those who "help themselves." It must be extended to all who suffer, it must be given with love to all, or it is not Christian. In the authentic Christian physician Christianity is inseparably united with healing.

This inseparability must be manifest alongside scientific competence, complementing and supplementing it. The two need never be in conflict. Yet the Christian physician should acknowledge a personal dependence upon God and recognize the ultimate source of all the wonders science uncovers for the benefit of all. The Christian physician is not afraid to pray with, and for, the patient, to acknowledge God's participation in all healing acts, to look to him when human measures fail, or to help the patient find him. Praying with the patient and the patient's family is not to deny science or even to weaken our zeal for its fullest application. Rather, it is to recognize human limitations, to ask God's blessing on the physician's action, and to place the patient, the physician, and medicine in proper relationship to God. To minimize the physician's hubris is not to derogate science but simply to place it in the order of God's creation as a great good but not a universal ideology supplanting religion and faith.

How many of us who claim to be Christian physicians, or how many institutions which claim to be Christian, could stand the scrutiny of Jesus? How would he respond to our ward rounds, in the office, at the hospital's board meeting, in its business office or emergency room, at its professional staff meeting? It is the very nobility of the ideal of being a Christian physician or a Christian hospital that makes its fulfillment so exquisitely difficult and its failure so scandalous. Who would not wither before the gaze of Christ were he to see our fee setting, our bill collecting, our self-justifying unavailability, our put-down of the ignorant, our subtle transgressions of the dignity and values of our patients, our standardizing, arithmeticizing, pragmatic assembly-line clinics.

Being a Christian physician, therefore, demands much more than even the highest expressions of pagan medical morality as we find it in the writings of Scribonius, Libanius, or Sarapion, or of today's secular humanists. It encompasses their noble ideals but gives them a moral imperative beyond human devising, one which elevates, refines, and reshapes even the loftiest conceptions of human service taught by reason alone. The Christian physician, seeking nothing less than perfection in Christ, cannot ever be satisfied with mere adherence to a secular professional code. Whereas reason may argue for or against abortion, euthanasia, or test-tube babies, the Christian must resolve these dilemmas in the light of what Christian belief teaches. The Christian has constantly to reflect on his or her ministry of healing, not simply as an obligation arising from the nature of a human relationship—as a philosopher would argue the case—but as an obligation of a believer in the redemptive message of Jesus Christ.

For the Catholic Christian, there is the additional dimension of the particular construal the Church places on the message of Christ. The Roman Catholic is a member of a community, the mystical body, which unites all its members in a community of ministry which vitalizes the healing ministry of each individual in it. That community is a source not only of special grace but also of special obligation.

The Catholic Christian, then, works, thinks, and acts within a multileveled matrix—he or she has obligations simply as a physician, then as a physician committed to a religious principle of justification beyond humankind, then as a Christian, and finally, as a Christian of a particular persuasion.

Christian health workers sorely need a common code of Christian medical morality equal to the complex challenges posed by our secular and morally pluralistic society. Such a moral code would first set out the obligations all Christian physicians share because all are followers of Christ. Each denomination could add to this base in modular fashion its specific obligations with respect to the common moral dilemmas about which there may be disagreement. To elaborate such a common code we must first separate and identify our philosophic and theological formulations of medical morality as this essay suggests.

I do not believe that a professional code justified only philosophically will ever suffice to assure those who are ill the dedicated service the physician owes them. Every trend of modern medicine—its exploitation of technology, its institutionalization, bureaucratization, its power to alter man biologically and behaviorally—ultimately accentuates the need for a religious source of morality. A totally adequate medical morality is not derivable from general morality; nor is morality itself fully justifiable on philosophical considerations alone.

What Can Be Taught and How

I have rather laboriously tried to locate the Christian physician in relationship to medical morality because I cannot speak about teaching until I am clear about what is to be taught. What I have tried to show thus far is that we are required to prepare a physician who is both a competent scientist and an authentic Christian healer. We must prepare the student for a Christian ministry grounded simultaneously in professional competence and the manifestation and proclamation of the Christian faith. The medical school that sets such a goal for itself must undertake the spiritual formation of its medical students as vigorously as it does the preparation of its ordained ministers. Professional and technical capability must be inextricably interwoven with Christian witness. To default in either element is to destroy the unity of the idea of the Christian physician.

The problem is compounded enormously by the fact that the world's medical schools are overwhelmingly secular and often openly antipathetic to any notion of religious formation in any form. Even those medical schools under the aegis of Christian and Catholic universities have thus far only indirectly addressed the problem of Christian formation as an institutional policy.

My recommendations must, therefore, be divided into two parts—what can be done in schools under Christian auspices and what can be done in secular institutions. I wish emphatically to underscore that I am not being critical of schools which have not done what I shall outline. I prefer to emphasize what I think can and should be done in a medical school that makes the education of Christian physicians a stated goal. I will focus on the minimal requirements which would have to be met to enable each student to learn what it is to be a Christian physician.

What are the minimal requirements for a medical school under Christian auspices which consciously establishes the teaching of Christian physicians as an institutional objective?

The first, the indispensable, and the most difficult is teaching by example and behavior. What could be simpler or more difficult for each faculty member? What is demanded is that we be Christian ourselves, that we live the ministry of healing every moment of every day. This entails, at the least, exhibiting those levels of concern and obligation I have outlined above as a requisite for the fusion of being Christian and being a physician. If the student is to be convinced of the probity of the Christian ministry of healing, he or she will expect that the search for God and Christ will be taken seriously, that his or her faith will be sustained and deepened, that a concern for justice and mercy is manifest, and that a dedication to religious and moral values enters into each clinical decision. To be authentic as Christian physicians, we teachers must demonstrate that we care for the patient, that we place the patient's needs above our own convenience and comfort, that we wear our authority and knowledge humbly, that we teach, explain, and are patient and sensitive to every nuance of behavior which might introduce even a trace of humiliation for the vulnerable person who is ill. To turn one's back figuratively or actually to a patient even in a single instance undoes hours of lectures about Christian charity and lets in the odor of hypocrisy, which students can detect even in infinitesimal amounts.

The Christian physician must evidence a sense of the inequality of the relationship between one who has knowledge and another who needs that knowledge to be healed; the Christian physician feels the vulnerability, the wounded humanity, the humiliation, the nakedness of body and soul, that illness brings. The Christian feels these things along with the person who is ill. That is what com-passion means. The Christian physician takes every decision, performs every medical act, always aware of this existential meaning of illness.

Ministry is service infused by the invigorating powers of faith, hope, and love. How authentic is that mission if our competence is in any way dubious? How authentic when we hurry the patient or chide or scold or ridicule? How authentic when we rush off to our amusement or recreation or make ourselves "unavailable" at this or that time? How authentic when we justify our fees and our procedures by our needs for a certain style of life or even by the disingenuously inane claim that every other physician does the same?

Those who hope to teach what it is to be a Christian physician must themselves exemplify an impossibly difficult ideal. They must not be discouraged by the perfection of the model they are called upon to imitate—the healing ministry of Christ himself. The teacher is destined forever to fall short of the model. Yet, even in falling short he or she can make the lesson clear by pursuing the goal with conscious purpose, humility, and clear intent to be a Christian.

The Importance of Ethics, Philosophy, Theology

Because of these difficulties, teaching by example must be supplemented by formal instruction in certain cognitive essentials. The student must comprehend the intellectual foundations of Christian practice and morals, especially as they pertain to clinical decision making. Formal teaching in ethics, theology, and philosophy is crucial if the Christian physician is to understand and justify personal clinical decisions, especially the value questions they so often encompass.

I argued above that the medical act is a moral one, that it involves a choice of what ought to be done for a particular patient and that it must be taken in the patient's interest. The Christian physician must, therefore, take account of the patient's values and conscience even when they are opposed to the physician's. The Christian physician must respect the patient's exercise of moral agency, and cannot manipulate, force, or ignore the patient's personal moral choices without becoming less Christian. This demands a careful understanding by the Christian of his or her own value system, and where it does or does not conflict on essential points with the patient's. The Christian is required to know when to disassociate himself or herself kindly, respectfully, and firmly from a particular patient whose definitions of what is right and good violate Christian morality. To try to teach the patient and to justify his or her own stance is important, but the physician must also be prepared to withdraw if the patient's demands violate the physician's Christian conscience.

Important decisions of this kind cannot safely rest on feelings or on someone else's example alone. Each physician must understand his or her conscience, what moral principles are in conflict, and where or where not to compromise. The systematic study of philosophy, theology, and ethics enables the student to locate himself or herself as a Christian with reference to today's increasingly frequent moral dilemmas and conflicts of obligations. Faith and reasoned understanding of that faith are the necessary accouterments of the educated Christian.

The teaching of ethics, philosophy, and theology cannot be left to medical teachers alone, no matter how enlightened or well-intentioned they may be. These courses must be taught as rigorously as the scientific foundations of medicine. They are best taught by professional theologians and philosophers in the clinical setting, by the case method, and related to the concrete dilemmas of medical decision making. A decade of experience in teaching the humanities in American medical schools shows that cooperative teaching by clinicians and humanists is the most effective method.[9]

The Christian physician needs to understand his or her beliefs as an educated person. In treating men and women of all beliefs and persuasions, the physician is called to witness Christianity for all through both intellect and behavior. Theology cannot safely be isolated from medicine, because, as Cardinal Newman pointed out, "Religious truth is not only a portion but a condition of general knowledge. To blot it out is nothing short, if I may so speak, of unravelling the web of university education."[10]

That faith and reason are complementary does not require that science become subservient to theology or that faith replace competence. Every class in anatomy need not be interlarded with readings from the Scriptures, as some seem to suppose. This kind of *reductio ad absurdum* is the easy refuge of the secularist who cannot comprehend that both faith and competence are demanded of the Christian physician.

The formal teaching of theology and ethics does not mean that the physician becomes an amateur theologian or replaces the minister. Nor does it require that theology be used as an instrument of apologetics or of proselytization. To take such advantage of the vulnerability of the sick, even for so good a purpose, is to violate Christian charity and the patient-physician covenant.

Still, the Christian physician is bound to attend to body, mind, and spirit, recognizing needs in all three realms. A theology of illness strengthens both physician and patient to transform the fact of illness into an opportunity for spiritual growth. Religion is a source of meaning and explanation not available to the secular humanist. The student is not taught to usurp the functions of the minister but to encourage and facilitate them, learning to avoid the attractive temptation to which physicians are susceptible, to extend their technical and legal authority at the bedside to include moral and religious questions.

The student must also be taught to be Christian in his or her mode of evangelization in the message taken to the sick and dying. The lines separating facilitation and coercion, persuasion and manipulation, are too fine for advance determination. Every Christian physician must recognize that bodily and spiritual healing are never really separable. Healing is grounded in a human relationship binding one in need and one who professes to help. The freedom of each person in that relationship is crucial to authentic healing.

If the student is to be taught optimally, the formal and informal teaching I have described must be reinforced daily. The medical school and hospital must exhibit a corporate and collective concern for the Christian healing ministry in every function. Its behavior, like that of the individual teacher, must be Christian. All the patients are entitled to charity, mercy, and justice. To be a Christian institution demands of the collectivity who constitute the institution the same behavior as that required of the individual physicians.

Being a Christian institution is even more difficult to accomplish than being a Christian individual. It is much easier to shift responsibility in a corporate entity like a hospital—to do a "Pontius Pilate" act. Who, for example, decides—and how—to resolve the conflicts between fiscal soundness and a patient's needs? Do we treat each other, our workers, and our patients with Christian love and charity? Does the institution concern itself with social justice in health care? Is such care truly available and accessible to all in need? Who is morally responsible for the lack of Christian charity when it occurs? Any hospital that declares itself to be a Christian institution assumes stringent obligations. I have outlined some of these obligations elsewhere for the Catholic hospital.[11]

The same obligation to practice Christian morality binds the medical school. There are ethical obligations which bind all medical schools simply by virtue of their special function in society.[12] Additional obligations are imposed on any medical school under religious or Christian auspices. Without detailing those obligations, it suffices to say that such a school is required to be Christian in its treatment of each of its major constituencies—patients, students, and faculty. At a minimum this must mean teaching students their moral obligations to patients and to society, providing opportunity for their personal spiritual growth, placing the needs of patients above the needs of teaching and research whenever they are in conflict, and responding to the needs of the poor, the afflicted, and the disadvantaged who are under the care of the faculty and students.

Much of the "dehumanization" medical students feel and see in the process of education and staff training would be ameliorated if medical schools were truly Christian in their institutional morality. Yet, there are serious difficulties in establishing any uniform set of principles which might shape the collective behavior of a school's faculty or administration. We need only reflect on the importance of the principles of academic freedom, civil rights, and participatory democracy in our society. How does an institution, medical school, or hospital assure that it is Christian? Does it limit its faculty and staff to Christians? How does it deal with differences between the value systems of those it treats and those who serve it? There are legal issues of constitutionality as well as moral and spiritual issues that are relevant to any attempt to develop a sense of institutional commitment to authentic Christianity.

The difficulties notwithstanding, there is one irreducible principle in this entire discourse. If we are to teach an ideal as lofty as that of the Christian physician, then we must teach and practice everything in the spirit of Christ's own healing ministry. The motto of St. Pius X, "*Instaurare Omnia in Christo,*" is the quintessence of that ministry. No school or hospital will attain full perfection in the practice of that ideal. We are redeemed, but we will never be perfect in this world. We do have an incomparable model to guide us. The model of Christ the Healer transcends even the loftiest sentiments of philosophically derived medical moralities.

The challenge to medical schools and hospitals professedly Christian is being met in many ways by schools under religious auspices. My only message to them is that they must reflect continually, critically, and analytically on whether they are as close to the ideal as they can be. They should ask themselves what Christ might say if he witnessed their daily work.

The Secular Medical School

I leave to the last the problem of teaching in a secular medical school what it is to be a Christian physician. Here we cannot demand institutional commitment of the kind I have outlined. We can only demand what is philosophically justifiable through human reason unilluminated by revelation. These are the obligations derivable from the nature of medicine and of the physician-patient relationship. These are the obligations that derive simply from being an institution of healing or teaching. Even here we need a new, philosophically justifiable medical morality which binds all who profess to heal. The philosophical justifications for medical morality are, I believe, consistent with, but by no means sufficient for, the Christian physician. They serve as a common starting point upon which the higher dimensions of Christian obligation are engrafted.

If a refurbished medical morality is taught in the secular medical schools, that will assure the Christian medical teacher and students a starting point. After that, the students must depend on their own formation as Christians, on the assistance and counseling of Christian faculty members, and on the support of the campus ministry. The formation of associations of Christian faculty and medical students in secular medical schools is a necessity and is already a reality in a number of secular medical schools.

There is, hence, a special and heavy obligation and a special ministry for the Christian faculty member teaching in the secular institution. The teacher has an obligation in charity to meet the special teaching needs of Christian medical students. This includes the obligation to practice the Christian healing ministry for the edification of nonbelievers and members of non-Christian religious institutions as well. The task for the Christian faculty members in a secular institution is difficult and demanding but also most rewarding as I have experienced it in most of my own teaching career.

The Christian medical student in a secular medical school has special obligations. He or she must be a witness to Christianity, must seek his or her own spiritual development, must do the extra reading in ethics, theology, and philosophy, and must seek to work with other Christians to clarify and deepen their idea of what it is to be both true Christian and physician. It is not enough to be one and the other; what is demanded of all—faculty, students, and institutions—is the fusion in the fire of faith and reason of the two existential states of being a physician and being a Christian, a fusion so perfect that we cannot separate curing and healing from ministry and faith.

Christians are different because they are redeemed by Jesus Christ. As the Jews were freed from the slavery of Pharaoh, the Christian has been freed to enjoy the spiritual fullness of the Christian experience of ministry and service.

It is this act of redemption by Christ that imposes a higher morality than human reason alone can devise. Those higher duties transform the practice of medicine into a ministry of healing. Christian medical students, teachers, and practitioners are called to teach these duties to each other by example and concept. Since the model they must imitate is never fully imitable, the task is as difficult as its undertaking is inescapable.

I would like to close with a quotation from Father Thomas Merton, the Cistercian monk who reached out from the solitude of his monastery to engage the most crucial issues of our day:

> The Christian is, I believe, one who abandons an incomplete and imperfect concept of life for a life that is integral, unified and structurally perfect. Yet this entrance into such a life is not the end of the journey but only the beginning.[13]

The inescapable responsibility of Christian teachers of medicine is to start the student on this journey. For the Christian physician, a structurally perfect life is one in which Christian faith and competent practice are indissolubly and perfectly united.

Notes

1. Examples of this fusion of healing and ministry in Christ's life are too familiar to document. In Mark alone, there are some 20. One of the most vivid is the following: "Now when it was evening, and the sun had set, they brought to Him all that were ill and who were possessed. And the whole town had gathered at the door. And He cured many who were afflicted with various diseases, and cast out many devils; and He did not permit them to speak because they knew Him." Mark 1:32-34.

2. E. D. Pellegrino, "Educating the Humanist Physician: An Ancient Ideal Reconsidered," *Journal of the American Medical Association,* March 1974, pp. 1288-1294.

3. This transformation is evident if we compare the detailed presentations of medical morality in the first AMA code in 1848 and the recently proposed revisions (Bruce Nortell, "AMA Judicial Activities," *Journal of the American Medical Association,* April 3, 1978, pp. 1396-1397). The most recent versions are spare, noncommital documents like the testimony of a practiced witness in court, offering a minimum of comment to avoid exposing oneself to further inquiry.

4. E. D. Pellegrino, "The Fact of Illness and the Act of Pro-fession: Some Notes on the Source of Professional Obligation," *Implications of History and Ethics to Medicine Veterinary and Human,* Laurence B. McCullough and James Polk Morris III, eds., Centennial Academic Assembly, Texas A & M U., College Station, 1978, pp. 78-89.

5. E. D. Pellegrino, "The Anatomy of Clinical Judgments," *Philosophy and Medicine,* Vol. VI, D. Reidel, Dordrecht, the Netherlands; Pellegrino, "The Fact of Illness and the Act of Pro-fession: Some Notes on the Source of Professional Obligation."

6. Ibid.

7. I have drawn on the excellent William Osler Oration in the History of Medicine, "The Professional Ethics of the Greek Physician," in L. Edelstein, *Ancient Medicine,* Owsei Temkin and C. Lillian Temkin, eds., The Johns Hopkins Press, Baltimore, 1967, pp. 319-348.

8. Scribonius Largus, *Compositions,* Georgius Helmreich, ed., Lipsiae, 1889.

9. I refer to almost a decade of experience that we in the Institute of Human Values in Medicine have gained with the teaching of the humanities in medical schools. These experiences are detailed in the reports of the Institute for Human Values, Witherspoon Building, Philadelphia.

10. John Henry Newman, "On the Scope and Nature of University Education," introduction by Wilfred Ward, prefatory notes by Herbert Keldany, Everyman's Library, Dutton, New York City, 1965, p. 54.

11. E. D. Pellegrino, "The Catholic Hospital: Options for Survival," *Hospital Progress,* February 1975, pp. 42-52.

12. E. D. Pellegrino, "Philosophy and Ethics of Medical Education," *The Encyclopedia of Bioethics,* Warren T. Reich, ed., Macmillan, Free Press, Riverside, NJ, 1978, pp. 863-869.

13. Thomas Merton, quoted from dust jacket of his book *A Thomas Merton Reader,* Patrick Hart, ed., "The Monastic Journey," Doubleday, Image Books, New York City, 1978, p. 12.

Part II
CONCEPTS IN RELIGION AND MEDICINE

Chapter Four
LIFE AND ITS SANCTITY

Introduction

Advances in medical science and technology have served the good of life. Evidence for that claim is not hard to marshal. Infant mortality rates have dropped; life expectancy has increased; and certain death-dealing childhood diseases have been defeated.

The same advances have confronted us with new choices between life and death, illustrations of which fill this volume: Shall we abort a fetus diagnosed as suffering from a fatal genetic defect? Shall we strive to keep a terminally ill patient alive? Shall we continue the research and development of expensive technological devices for the good of the lives of a few when more goods or more lives might be served by allocating that money and energy elsewhere? Human beings have today a quite remarkable control over life and dying, a control undreamt of not long ago. Accompanying such control, however, is an equally remarkable responsibility.

If people are to take that responsibility seriously, they must think about the nature of life and the appropriate disposition toward it. When confronted with choices of life-or-death significance they are likely to ask themselves what they really believe about "life and its sanctity."

The phrase "life and its sanctity," of course, is not unambiguous. It does not make clear whether all life or only human life is included. It does not make clear whether it is *bios* or *zoe,* biological life or spiritual life, which is due respect. "Sanctity" carries a religious connotation not always welcome to the nonreligious and sometimes adjudged idolatrous by the religious. The deepest ambiguity of all, however, may be that the phrase does not settle the relation of the good of life to other goods. The phrase is open to more than one justification, to more than one interpretation, and so to more than one sort of application. Its ambiguity conspires with its importance to demand reflection about the concept in the context of medical advances.

Reflection about life and its sanctity is at home in all the great religions of the world and surely in Christianity. The Christian scriptures reveal a God who intends life and forbids trespass against it. The traces of this intention are found in creation (see Gen. 2:4b-7), in a rainbow (Gen. 9:1-17), in a commandment (Exod. 20:13), in an empty tomb (John 11:23-26; 1 Cor. 15), and in a vision (Rev. 21:1-8). Christian theologians, however, can give different accounts of life and its sanctity, accounts which bear in different ways on the choices that confront us. The attempt to think both clearly and Christianly about this issue will be served by careful attention to the selections gathered here and by raising certain questions about them.

Some of these questions have been introduced in earlier chapters. For example, the question of the relation of a Christian perspective to an impartial perspective may be raised again by comparing Karl Barth, James Gustafson, and Richard Stith. For Barth, the reverence due life must be seen in Christian perspective, for human dignity is an "alien dignity," a dignity which does not derive from life itself, or from human beings themselves, but from God's dealings with human beings.[1] Roman Catholic thought is as capable as Protestant of articulating this theme of "alien dignity,"[2] but it has typically attended much more self-consciously and confidently to an impartial perspective, a natural-law perspective. So, too, Richard Stith, who appeals to universal moral "intuitions" and defends and explicates the "sanctity of life" as a universal and rational principle.[3]

James Gustafson's essay attends to this quite different question: "In what ways might religious belief qualify the human experience?" What is gained and lost by these different judgments about the relation of theological reflection to "natural" morality? What theological affirmations would be needed to defend one or another of these judgments?

The question of the mode of moral analysis also resurfaces. For example, Barth focuses on the command of God and calls for the obedience of the faithful to the command in the moment. Gustafson explicitly rejects this language in favor of the language of values, dispositions, and intentions. Stith, for his part, rejects in principle the application of the language of values to the meaning of sanctity, and he articulates rules of practice on the basis of this principle. Lewis Smedes starts with the biblical commandment "Thou shalt not kill" and asks what it requires, why it is given, and finally (in a section left out of our collection) how it (with its justification) applies to the ambiguities of human life and death. Which of these models of moral analysis is appropriate? How would such a judgment be formed or defended?

The question to which such self-conscious methodological decisions must finally be addressed is, of course, the meaning of "life and its sanctity." How can and should we think clearly and Christianly about this phrase? How shall we articulate and describe this notion? How shall we defend it? And how shall we begin to apply it? Is it one value among many? Can the value of life come into genuine conflict with other genuine goods? Must we relate these values to one another in ways appropriate to their relation to God's cause(s)? Or must we above all else be sensitive to and obedient to the command of God in our concrete and existential choices about life, formed as we are by God's address? Perhaps we should apply the biblical commandment in ways that are attentive to its biblical context and theological justification, attempting by our obedience to the commandment to be faithful to the God who has revealed his will for human life in Scripture. Or may we take "sanctity of life" as a general principle to be applied along with other general moral norms to formulate particular rules of practice?

These are hard but important questions, the answer to which will determine the way one addresses other hard and important questions, the concrete questions posed by advances in medicine and humanity's unprecedented control over human life and dying.

Notes

1. See also Paul Ramsey, "The Morality of Abortion," in *Life or Death: Ethics and Options,* ed. Daniel H. Labby (Seattle: University of Washington Press, 1968), pp. 60-93; and Helmut Thielicke, "The Doctor as Judge of Who Shall Live and Who Shall Die," in *Who Shall Live?* ed. Kenneth Vaux (Philadelphia: Fortress Press, 1970).

2. Josef Fuchs, *Natural Law* (New York: Sheed and Ward, 1965); Norman St. John-Stevas, *The Right to Life* (New York: Holt, Rinehart and Winston, 1963).

3. One might fruitfully compare the position of Stith with the position Edward Shils develops on the basis, not of Christianity, but of a "deeper, proto-religious 'natural metaphysic' " ("The Sanctity of Life," in *Life or Death: Ethics and Options,* ed. Labby, pp. 2-38; the quote is from p. 9).

Suggestions for Further Reading

Callahan, Daniel. "The Sanctity of Life." In *Updating Life and Death,* edited by Donald R. Cutler, with commentaries by Julian Pleasants, James M. Gustafson, and Henry K. Beecher, 181-250. Boston: Beacon Press, 1969.

Clouser, K. Danner. "The Sanctity of Life: An Analysis of a Concept." *Annals of Internal Medicine* 78 (1973): 119-25.

Crane, Diana. *The Sanctity of Social Life: Physicians' Treatment of Critically Ill Patients.* New York: Russell Sage Foundation, 1975.

Hartt, Julian. "Creation, Creativity, and the Sanctity of Life." *The Journal of Medicine and Philosophy* 4 (December 1979): 418-34.

Ramsey, Paul. "The Sanctity of Life." *Dublin Review* 241 (Spring 1967): 3-21.

Shils, Edward, et al. *Life or Death: Ethics and Options.* Seattle: University of Washington Press, 1968.

Thomasma, David C. *An Apology for the Value of Human Life.* St. Louis: Catholic Health Association of the United States, 1983.

Weber, Leonard J. *Who Shall Live?* New York: Paulist Press, 1976.

17.
Genesis 2:4b–7

In the day that the LORD God made the earth and the heavens, when no plant of the field was yet in the earth and no herb of the field had yet sprung up—for the LORD God had not caused it to rain upon the earth, and there was no man to till the ground; but a mist went up from the earth and watered the whole face of the ground—then the LORD God formed man of dust from the ground, and breathed into his nostrils the breath of life; and man became a living being.

From the Revised Standard Version of the Bible, copyrighted 1946, 1952 © 1971, 1973. Used by permission of the National Council of the Churches of Christ in the U.S.A.

18.
Respect for Life
KARL BARTH

In this title I am borrowing a concept which is adopted and worked out by Albert Schweitzer in the second part of his philosophy of civilisation (*Kultur und Ethik,* 1923, which is essentially a critical history of western ethics) as the "fundamental principle of ethics" and therefore the basis and the measure of all ethics. It cannot be accepted here in this broad sense. Schweitzer's ethics, as he himself describes it, is mystical. In spite of Schiller, life is for him, in its totality as our own life and that of others, "the supreme good," and therefore it is the highest and properly the only lawgiver, and therefore the criterion of all virtue. According to him the first and last word of all ethics is that life must be respected. Its sum is that to preserve and assist life is good, and to destroy and harm it evil (p. 239). It goes without saying that theological ethics cannot accept this. Where Schweitzer places life we see the command of God. Life cannot be for us a supreme principle at all, though it can be a sphere in relation to which ethics has to investigate the content and consequences of God's command. That life should be accepted, treated and preserved with respect is for the moment, however, a suitable formulation of the answer which we must give in this field from the first if not from every standpoint.

So far we have understood obedience to the command of God the Creator as man's freedom for himself and his freedom in the human community. God the Creator calls man to himself and therefore to worship, confession and prayer. He then turns him to his fellowmen and tells him what is and must be essential according to His creative will (in the relation of husband and wife and parents and children) or according to His fatherly disposition (in the relation of near and distant neighbours). Presupposing these first two dimensions of the command and keeping them constantly before our eyes, we now turn to a third. Obedience to the command of God the Creator is also quite simply man's freedom to exist as a living being of this particular, i.e., human structure.

Though it might have seemed logical, we have taken good care not to speak first of this simple and

From Karl Barth, *Church Dogmatics,* III/4, trans. A. T. Mackay et al. (Edinburgh: T&T Clark, 1961), pp. 324–43. Used by permission.

obvious fact. That which constitutes man as man is, of course, his existence in the vertical dimension towards God and in the horizontal towards his fellow-men. Hence he is not first this creature or present as such. He is first for God and his fellow-man, and then and for this reason he exists as this being in accordance with his determination. And his obedience to the command of God must first and supremely be understood as his right action and conduct in relation to God and his fellow-men, and only then and on this basis as his true existence in human life rightly lived as such.

But the command of God does have this third dimension in a very distinct form. As the being of man for God and with his fellow-men includes this particular human structure as a presupposition, so the freedom of man for God in the community includes the freedom for existence as this human creature. Man is also commanded to live, i.e., to live rightly according to the instruction of the command. He always lives, even as a man standing before God and linked to his fellow-men. He is always himself in these relationships. He is so as man, this man, involved as such in a whole complex movement and activity, in which he is of course claimed for God and his fellow-men, but which in itself and as such has its own distinctive content in face of the service of God and fellowship with others, and which by its nature can find only partial expression in movements and activity in the relationships to God and His fellows. If the command of God did not have this special third dimension in which it brings its order into this distinctive but very real and important sphere, we should obviously have here a kind of ethical vacuum in which man's action and abstention would be left to chance or caprice or its own law. In these circumstances his freedom for God and in fellowship would be singularly majestic but also singularly problematic and docetic, hovering over the dark abyss of his multi-coloured vital being rather as the strange, purposeless and inactive spirit of Elohim did over the waters of chaos in Gen. I². Down below and in himself where so much necessarily or arbitrarily stirs and moves, where he desires and loathes, seeks and spurns, demands and does not demand so much that constantly and sometimes ardently interests and claims him, but cannot be rightly and fully viewed and comprehended and defined from the standpoint of the service of God and fellowship with others because it is a matter of his psycho-physical act of being as such, he would have a kind of refuge or holy place with an altar to which he could flee and horns to which he could cling. He would obviously choose, yet would also have no option but to exist there "privately," i.e., without the law, without the duty of obedience, as a neutral abandoned in some sense to chance and caprice. The command, however, as it demands obedience in the first two dimensions, lays hold on the man himself and therefore pierces into the sphere of his humanity as such and therefore into the act of his existence. God is gracious to the man himself, not primarily or exclusively in his relation to God and his fellow-men, but to the man who exists as such in these relations as a living creature created by Him and endowed with a definite structure. Hence his faith and his obedience would not be faith and obedience if, now that the command penetrates to himself, it could be denied or evaded as the command of his Father and Lord, of the God who is gracious to him. This command has a specific dimension in which it also shows itself to be the sanctification of his life as such, as the imperative summons to freedom for human existence. It is in this dimension that we have now to become acquainted with it.

Here we encounter the representatives of various tendencies in philosophical ethics which, according to the different aspects which they usually emphasise, we may more or less correctly describe as eudaemonistic, hedonistic, utilitarian, or, more relevantly, naturalistic or vitalistic ethics. Among them in modern times, Englishmen such as J. S. Mill and Herbert Spencer, Frenchmen like Auguste Comte, Alfred Fouillée and Jean Marie Guyau, and the Germans F. Nietzsche, E. Haeckel and even Albert Schweitzer, have championed such types of ethics. In his initial bent Henri Bergson might also be classed with them, but this is not strictly possible because his natural philosophy did not assume any ethical form. The common element in all these thinkers is their striving for a fundamental orientation of ethics, for a concept of life. It matters little whether this was thought of more in terms of the physical life or the mental, more of the individual or the social, more of the happy or agreeable or the tragic and heroic, more of the will for life or respect for it. Everywhere life itself and as such is regarded as the actual ethical lord, teacher and master of man. As we have just remarked concerning Albert Schweitzer, we can only "encounter" the representatives of this view. In theological ethics the concept of life cannot be given this tyrannical, totalitarian function. But this does not mean that we should avoid it altogether. We cannot command the idealistic rigorism with which W. Herrmann tried to dismiss from ethics as mutely natural and therefore pre-moral the affirmation of the necessity and right of life. On the other hand, it was one of the advantages of the ethics of A. Schlatter, for which he has to thank his thorough independence of the prevailing Kantianism of his time, that in the fourth part of his book, under the peculiar title "Power," he could in his own way take up the ethical concern of the naturalists and bring out the consequences. Precisely when, unlike the naturalists, we understand the moral command strictly and exclusively as that of the God who is also the Creator, we are forced to admit that the man addressed and claimed by Him does not begin at the point where he is distinguished from a purely natural creature. It is a matter of the whole man. We think of Col. 3:17: "And whatsoever ye do in word or deed, do all in the name of the Lord Jesus," and more explicitly 1 Cor. 10:31: "Whether therefore ye eat, or drink, and whatsoever ye do, do all to the glory of God." Insistence on the separation of moral from natural volition and action—and therefore of natural from moral—means that there is no way to ward off the danger that, in so far as the life of man is below that point, however excellent the ethics above it, it is surrendered to a naturalistic ethics of opportunism and expediency. We have to understand the command in its critical and constructive relation to the real action of the real man which as such is always his natural action as well. In all seriousness, therefore, we have to put the question of obedience in this field too.

But what is this simplest element in respect of which we have to ask concerning the command of God, namely, man's existence as such and therefore his life as man? We must first give a brief description and delineation of the sphere which we now enter.

We do well to insist at once that even in this simplest thing we are not dealing with something given and known nor controllable and therefore directly knowable by man. Man assumes that he belongs to himself as he exists in his particularity as a human creature. And from this point he goes on to think that he even exercises a certain though limited power over other life as well, over that of his fellow-men, that of animals and plants and the life generally in which he participates with his own life. But already the first presupposition on which everything else depends is too uncertain, in view of the unmistakeable and many-sided threat to which he himself is exposed, for him to suppose that human life really belongs to him and is thus in the strictest sense his "own." It is on this assumption, however, that he thinks that he can know of himself that he exists, and that he does so as a man; and that he therefore thinks that he can know what human life is, what it means to exist and live as a man, and therefore what life is generally. Yet he does not really know more than certain phenomena which indicate his existence, which seem to distinguish him a human being, and which continually characterise his existence as human—phenomena from which he thinks that he can conclude and know analogically that there is existence and life outside himself, and therefore life in general, and what it is. Even this noetic basis is far too insecure for theological ethics. Our own premises must be as follows.

1. As God addresses man as his Creator and Lord, He acknowledges and reveals, and it is clearly and decisively said to man by Him in a way which cannot be missed but only accepted, that man exists, and that he does so as the creature distinct from Him. If man did not, he could not be the recipient of the Word of God which reaches and speaks to him and which he can hear. If he himself were God, it would not be God's Word as Creator and Lord that he may hear. God's Word as Creator and Lord constitutes as such his knowledge of the reality of his existence in its independence of that of God, and therefore his knowledge that in this reality and independence it does not belong to him because it has been entrusted to him through the free goodness of the One who addresses him. God alone is truly independent. He alone belongs wholly to Himself and lives in and by Himself. Man's creaturely existence as such is not his property; it is a loan. As such it must be held in trust. It is not, therefore, under the control of man. But in the broadest sense it is meant for the service of God. "Know that our God indeed is Lord, And for His glory hath us made, 'Tis wholly on His gracious Word, The life of every man is stayed." This is the simplest information that can be given concerning the fact and meaning of life. Nor is it the result of self-reflection on the part of man. It depends entirely on the fact that God addresses him. It derives from the Word of God as the Word of his Creator and Lord. And implicitly it is the information which is given concerning all other life and the reality and the meaning of life in general.

2. As God addresses man and therefore does not just deal high-handedly with him or rule and control him, as He claims his knowledge and action, He acknowledges and reveals him as a creature which, in virtue of the quickening Spirit who is always God's own Spirit, is in ineffaceable difference, inseparable unity and above all indestructible order, i.e., precedence and subordination, the soul of his body, a creature of perception, thought, desire and volition, a rational being (cf. *C.D.,* III, 2, § 46). To exist as a man in this distinction of soul and body, but also in the unity of these two determinations, is to live in this order. The life-act of man is existence in this differentiated but self-enclosed and self-disposed totality, in derivation and absolute dependence on the free, life-giving act of God Himself, conditioned and sustained always by the fact that God causes it to happen. It is in this sense that human existence is a loan and is to be

held in trust. From its structure as the existence of a rational creature it is clear that it can be understood only as a loan. God alone is truly rational, knowing what He wills and willing what He knows. Creaturely reason as it characterises man's structure cannot as such try to be self-sufficient. And the guarantee that man may take himself seriously in this structure of his being and confidently use his reason is not to be found in the structure itself but in the fact that God addresses him as a rational creature, that He deals with him as such, that He calls him and expects to find in him hearing and obedience. The Word of God decides and reveals that man may never understand himself as merely physical, nor as merely psychical, nor in a mere juxtaposition or higher synthesis of these determinations, but that he must understand himself in this event of his existence as the soul of his body, that he should be in this event, and that this should be his particular human life.

3. As God addresses man, He acknowledges and reveals him as someone, a particular individual, this man. The Word of God not only presupposes a reality different from itself, a life-process, but many specific life-acts. It relates to them all, yet not to a mere totality, but to individual and unique rational creatures. It therefore constitutes as such man's knowledge of the independence of his particular existence in distinction from all other men or creatures. It addresses him in his own life. It holds him directly responsible for this loan and his treatment of it. It confirms him in the particularity of his creatureliness by claiming him in this particularity. This is one of the things bestowed upon him or rather lent to him as a creature. It is not that he possesses himself by being this particular man. The fact that he alone is this individual does not entitle him to make any claims. It is only the mode in which he may be the creature of God and a rational being. God alone is true and self-sufficient, and it is the goodness of God that this particularity, although not self-sufficient, may exist apart from Him in the creaturely world too. There is not the slightest reason, then, to construct or maintain in it a castle of defiance against God or even against other individual life in the creaturely world. Nor may man presume a true and final knowledge who and what he is in his particularity. God knows who and what he may be. God calls him by his name. It must satisfy him to be always the particular creature as which God addresses and thus acknowledges him, and to know himself as such. There can be no doubt, however, that the Word of God, spoken by the divine I to the human Thou, claims the supremely particular hearing and obedience of this specific man, and thus reveals the individuality of his being and life.

4. As God addresses man, He acknowledges, and man is told by Him, that he exists in time, that he is engaged in a movement from a past through a present into a future. The Word of God confirms his life as a being in a succession of different moments. This means that it is a being both in constancy and mutability. In a flux of moments man is always identical with himself. But as such he passes through the flux of moments. The Word of God to him, whether understood as information, question or command, presupposes on the part of the one to whom it is spoken the capacity to hear, answer and obey, i.e., to be *the same* both before and after (e.g., both when the divine question is posed and the answer is given), and to be so *both before and after* (e.g., both when the command is issued and it is obeyed). It constitutes man's knowledge of the reality of the movement in which he exists, of the reality of the fact that his life is temporal, which also means that it is creaturely, and may be known as such by the fact that it is bound to time and can take place only in the succession of beginning and end which are its limits. Unlike the life of God, it is neither free nor eternal. It can be lived only because and as the life of God stands behind it as the true life, the basis and source of life, in which actuality and continuity, constancy and variability, eternity and time are one. Hence it can only be lived and not held fast or possessed. It can only become constantly real in virtue of the free action of the life-giving divine Spirit. It is life as a loan. Yet understood with this reservation and within these limits, it is genuine life and not a mere appearance, made knowable by the drama of man's encounter with the Word of God as real stability in real change and real change in real stability.

5. As God addresses man, it is decided, and man is reassured, that his life possesses a definite origin. He lives his life. He is the soul of his body. He is the living individual. He is the one who moves in time, constant yet changing. The Word of God is not spoken merely to a psycho-physical individual in time which is simply the functioning organ of another author or element in his movement, but to a subject who is himself at all points the author, accomplishing this movement freely, independently and spontaneously. The Word of God, demanding hearing and obedience, presupposes a productive subject, a being capable of making for himself a new beginning with his being, conduct and action (irrespective of his co-existence and connexion with other beings), of planning something new and his very own, corresponding to what he has heard from God and therefore achieved through obedience. The Word of God as it is spoken to man thus constitutes his knowledge of himself as such a

free subject of his life. Otherwise what would be the sense of God speaking to him and not simply disposing of him? Speaking to him, God appeals to his independence. It is a creaturely and therefore not an absolute independence. It cannot in any sense compete with that of God. Hence we cannot say that his life is his own. Together with its independence, it belongs to the One who alone is truly independent. The fact that he himself may and should live his life is one of the things which have been entrusted to him and over which he has no ultimate control and must not try to usurp it. It is from the man who in all his freedom belongs to God that hearing and obedience are demanded. But the fact remains that, as it demands this from him, it discloses and reveals the fact that in his freedom he belongs to God.

6. Yet obviously we cannot fully describe what human existence and life are as such—for they cannot really be considered schematically—without recalling the twofold determination on which they are truly based and by which they are properly characterised as human. We first remember his determination for freedom before God. Life is lent to man under the determination for this freedom. We could not overlook its origin in any of our previous points. Recognisable as such in man's addressability by God, it is real, rational, individual and free existence moving in time as and because it is thus created by God, by the One who has and is all these things properly. Yet it is no less proper to its nature and character as human existence that this origin is also the goal. It does not derive from God in order that it may then have its aim, meaning and purpose in itself or another. It does so with a tendency to return to its place of origin. The Word of God reveals this too. As He addresses him, God calls man to Himself. How could He do this if man's path, as the existentialists imagine, were a random one, uncertain and confused in direction, or if its meaning, purpose and aim were in himself or something else? If God speaks in accordance with His creative will, addressing man concerning that for which He has determined human existence, this means that this existence as such is ordained by its Creator to give Him a hearing and obedience. It is thus from the very outset an existence orientated on His service and praise, on the search for Him and the doing of His will. Life as such thus means to live for the One to whom it belongs and from whom it has been received as a loan. Life, human life, thus hastens as such towards freedom before God, and only *per nefas,* and never according to its own nature, can it depart from this direction or take the opposite one. We must accept the fact that, in respect of this natural direction of his life towards God, man is not its owner and lord. Together with everything else which determines and characterises his life, the fact that it is orientated on God is also and particularly God's creation and loan. But we can understand even human life as such only if we gather, not from speculation but from the event of its confrontation by the Word of God, that it too, without any cooperation of its own but by nature and from the very first, has this vertical direction.

7. The other equally original determination of human existence is that of freedom in fellowship. In every significant and characteristic point life is a possession lent to every man as such, to each in a different way, in a specific time and place, but the same gift to all. To be sure, it is not a collective act. The singularity as well as the spontaneity in which it may be lived militates against such a view. But even its singularity and spontaneity belong to the manner in which it is the same for all. And it is worth noting that these are the two points by which one man recognises another most surely, or at any rate impressively, as someone like himself, namely, by the fact that he is so definitely this man, and lives as man in this distinctive freedom. As he himself acts and reacts specifically and spontaneously as a rational creature, so does also the other. And as the other does, so does he. Human life obviously cannot be lived otherwise than as a life which by its very nature consists in solidarity with those who have also to live it in their own way as it is lent to them. The natural and historical relations in which he stands to them are only the concrete conditions in which this solidarity achieves form, and is visible, and becomes a problem, to him and them. They ensure that this solidarity will not be overlooked and forgotten. But the equality and interrelatedness of all human life consists in its essence and not primarily in these relations. We therefore do not base our knowledge of it on any supposition derived from analogies. They might be unreliable. They can also be evaded. But as God addresses man, He also speaks to him through the solidarity which exists between him and other men. What God says to him applies to him, but to him only as a creature that has others of his kind. For he says it to him as He who is the Creator of each and all men, who as such *mutatis mutandis,* at other times and places, has also addressed, addresses and will address others with a different emphasis, content and commission. However differently and specifically He may thus address each individual, when addressed by Him each recognises himself in the other, and therefore necessarily, compulsorily and definitively, and again as a revelation of His creative will, as a disclosure of a determination which by its very nature is peculiar to human life. Thus the fact that man is determined for fellowship is very far from

being an accident. From this standpoint, human life as such takes place with a view to freedom in fellowship and therefore in the interrelatedness of one man with the other who also in accordance with his place and time can and must live it in all its singularity. Only *per nefas,* and not according to its nature, could it break free from this interrelationship and be lived in opposition to it. Man's life is also to be understood in this respect as God's creation and loan. No power, no possibility of rebellion against God or other men, is given to the individual by the fact that there are so many like him. To the understanding of human life belongs also the insight guaranteed by the Word of God that, again without his own co-operation, it has by nature this horizontal direction.

The question arises whether we ought to have an eighth point on the connexion or even the unity of human life with that of animals and plants and therefore with life generally. In this last and sublimest instance human life would then mean participation in an inclusive and perhaps even a universal life-act, and according to the current theology and philosophy this could be interpreted as the life-act of the created cosmos as such, or as one particular force in the cosmos ("spirit," world-soul, the principle of evolution or dialectical progress or something similar), or as the life-act of God Himself. The realm which we are endeavouring to define would then have its limit at the point where man thinks he recognises more or less closely a similar life to his own or something resembling it. And the ethical question would then have to be answered how ought he to conduct himself as a participant in this inclusive and perhaps even universal event of life.

Now if we were following the way of free speculation, we might think ourselves summoned to think in this direction. But the basis on which we have drawn up our first seven points does not enable us to go on in this way to an eighth. We could no longer speak with the certainty which has been so far possible. For it cannot be maintained that the man addressed by God's Word was spoken to and must recognise himself as a participant in the life of animals and plants or in an almost universal life-act, however interpreted. He may be of the opinion that he should regard this self-understanding as the right one, but it derives from another source and independently of God's Word. He has certainly not gained this personal understanding from his encounter with this Word. For the Word of God is addressed to man. It is an event in his life that it addresses him. That man lives in the cosmos, that he is the neighbour of animals and in a wider sense also the neighbour of plants and their life and all creatures, that his life has something in common with theirs, is not denied in this event but—tacitly—presupposed. Yet it does not follow by any means that the Word is also addressed to all his neighbours in the cosmos in the same way as it is to man. It is not in any sense evident that there exists a corresponding event in what we consider to be their life. We dare not reject this possibility. But equally we dare not affirm it and base the understanding of our human life on this statement. For if through that event in our human life we undoubtedly receive instruction concerning our life and its nature, this is actually limited to our human life, so that strictly what we have to learn about life is in every point relevant with certainty to man alone. We may entertain beautiful and pious thoughts, based sometimes on sensible suppositions and observations, concerning the independent reality of animal and vegetable existence, its rationality, its peculiarity, its relation to time, its spontaneity, its determination for God, its homogeneity with similar beings. But there is one thing we cannot say, namely, that man is addressed by God concerning this existence and its peculiarity, that he is given information about it by the Word of God. Man is not addressed concerning animal and vegetable life, nor life in general, but concerning his own human life. Even in the things which he has in common with animals and plants he is addressed concerning them as elements in human life and not elements in a more or less general life in which he merely participates. Again, we are investigating life as a realm in which the command of God is valid in a particular dimension and form. But the command concerns man and is relevant to his life. How can we know of a command that refers to the life of animals and plants and life generally? Such a command may exist in a hidden form. There is an infinite range of possible but unknown realities in the relation of Creator and creature. We may thus give free rein to our imagination in this field. But we must not maintain that we have any knowledge, namely, that we know a universal, all-inclusive command addressed to all creatures and therefore valid for us. This obviously involves an encroachment of naturalism and evolutionism which we have no reason to support.

We shall thus content ourselves with the seven points in which we have tried to define the realm of life. We are concerned with *theological* ethics and therefore we must adhere to the life which is recognisable in the event of God's Word. And we are concerned with theological *ethics* and therefore we must adhere to the life in relation to which we are asked concerning the good. From both these standpoints we maintain that the sphere of life with which we are concerned here is that of human life. In so doing we do not negate what may also be reality as life of a different and strange type. Neither do we negate the connexion of our human life with this other strange life. Above all, we do not negate the fact of the close relation of animal life with human life. Indeed, it is very forcibly brought out in the biblical saga by the creation of the animal and of man on the same day. We shall have to remember that with human life as our real problem, we must take seriously the problem of animals (and in a certain sense even of plants) as a marginal problem of ethics. We merely deny that any instruction concerning what we have to understand as life, i.e., life under the command of God, is to be expected or received from what we think we know as animal or vegetable life, or from the notion of a life-act in general. We merely state that we have no certain knowledge of the unity of life either in us or outside us. We merely reserve for ourselves the freedom to keep to what we know of life on sure authority.

We thus presuppose the concept of life as defined in this way.

When we ask concerning the command of God on this presupposition, it is tempting to begin with the following consideration. Does not the command always demand specific human decisions, attitudes and acts? Yet, however these actions might be conditioned and directed, there can be no doubt that none of them can become an event without the substratum of a specific life-act. That man is obedient always includes in itself the fact that he lives. Therefore the command, whatever its form, always contains the demand that he should live in his acts, affirming and willing his existence, and doing what is necessary and possible for its preservation and continuation. In some sense it always contains, even if imperceptibly, incidentally or anonymously, the imperative: Thou shalt will to live. A too primitive understanding of this imperative is averted by the fact that to the concept of life—the life that man should will to live—there necessarily belongs his orientation on God and the solidarity in which he is linked with all men. Could we not maintain, then, that wherever and however man is confronted with the Word of God he is always summoned to life in this embracing and solemn sense of the term?

But this tempting and to some extent useful consideration is subject to three difficulties.

1. Human life naturally includes orientation on God and solidarity with similar life. But it is not exhausted by what it is under these supreme and (for its humanity) decisive determinations. According to our first five points, it is always as well a real creaturely existence, psychical and physical by nature and of independent character, a movement in time in the originality of a free act. What is the meaning of the imperative: Thou shalt live, in relation to this other element in life which cannot be directly comprehended under these supreme determinations?

2. The command of God naturally summons man, in accordance with the two supreme determinations of his life, to freedom before God and freedom in fellowship with his fellow-men. But is this all, even from the standpoint of the command? Does it not also summon man to the freedom of existence? And does it really do this only anonymously, in, with and under its other commands? Does not the imperative: Thou shalt will to live, have also its own note, even though it is always heard in harmony? And does not the concept of a corresponding and therefore a good life have also, beyond the right relation of man to God and his fellow-men, a specific content in view of which we must speak of a third specific dimension and form of the command? Is not a special freedom and obedience indicated to man by the fact that as man, as this real, rational, individual, temporal, spontaneously acting and reacting creature, he is called to freedom before God and in fellowship?

3. Is it really true that the command of God in all cases and circumstances contains the imperative that man should will to live? Must not this imperative in some cases at least be formulated in what is from the literal standpoint a very paradoxical sense if it is really to be understood as the command of God? Understood in its most literal sense, it is hardly an unconditional and absolutely valid imperative which as such has necessarily to be included in every form of the divine command. Precisely as the command of God, does it not have a restricted validity, since the God who commands is not only the Lord of life but also the Lord of death? Is it really so unthinkable that, when his command summons man to freedom before Him and fellowship with his fellow-men, it might include a very different imperative, or this imperative in its most paradoxical formulation, to the effect that man should not will to live unconditionally, to spare his life, to preserve it from death, but that he should rather will to stake and surrender it, and perhaps be prepared to die? According to Mk. 8[35] he may save it in so doing, whereas he would lose it if he tried to save it. Is not the peculiarity of the freedom for existence to which man is summoned by God discernible in the fact it might also mean freedom from existence, a superior freedom as opposed to the necessity of having to live and to will to live, the superior freedom of man to be able also to surrender his life, and give it back to God, for the sake of his orientation on God and solidarity with his fellow-men?

If these are real difficulties, the only useful point in

that consideration is that there are forms of the divine command in which there is also silently and implicitly contained the demand that in order to do what he has been ordered man should will and affirm his life. Yet even where it is only an accompanying presupposition this demand still has its own content and character. And it is again the command of God which is issued when it has now independently the content and character of this demand. And again, to the extent that implicitly or explicitly it is the command of God, it is always limited. It is not an absolutely valid demand for the affirmation of life, for the "will to live," but one that exists for the time being, until abrogated, and within the framework of the presuppositions and intentions with which God causes it to be issued.

After this clarification we may attempt a general formulation. The freedom for life to which man is summoned by the command of God is the freedom to treat as a loan both the life of all men with his own and his own with that of all men.

The following points must be made in elucidation of this very general proposition.

First, our purpose in this third section is to understand the extent to which there also exists as such under the command a freedom, i.e., an obedience in respect of human existence.

Secondly, by man's existence, according to the seventh point in our definition of the concept, there is always to be understood both his own life and the similar life of all others. An abstraction between the two is out of the question, as is also an identity, because singularity and spontaneity are just as much essential for the life of man as his solidarity with the life of others. We therefore define the relation between these two elements as a co-existence. With his own life man lives that of all men, and with that of all his own. Under the command of God it is a matter of freedom, i.e., obedience for existence under this twofold definition.

Thirdly, by the command it is also placed in the light of a divine decree. The fact that he lives, and that he does so in this individuality of a rational creature, at this time, in this particular orientation on God and solidarity with others, is something which man cannot create of himself. Nor can he maintain it effectively. Nor can he refashion it when he is no longer alive. He can only accept and live it in the way and within the limits in which it is allotted him by God. He may live by the life-giving Spirit of God.

Fourthly, it is not by an obscure fate or neutral decree, but in receipt of a divine benefit, that he is "alive." The command of God, claiming him as a living person, inscribes upon his heart the fact that, coming wholly from God, it is always (whether recognised or not) an advantage, a good and worthwhile thing, for everyone to be alive. It is not wholly an advantage nor absolutely good and worthwhile. "My flesh and my heart faileth: but God is the strength of my heart, and my portion for ever" (Ps. 73[26]), and: "Thy lovingkindness is better than life" (Ps. 63[3]). But within its limits it is good and worthwhile because the one great opportunity of meeting God and rejoicing in his praise. It must itself be understood—and this anew every morning—as a divine miracle of grace to receive this opportunity of recognising and experiencing the grace of God, and therefore to continue to live. This is true no matter what we may see or not see in life of meaning, hope, success, happiness or even goodness. And wherever we have to deal with a living soul, we have to do *eo ipso* with this divine miracle of grace.

Fifthly, the blessing of life is a divine loan unmerited by man. It must always be regarded as a divine act of trust that man may live. And the basic ethical question in this respect is how man will respond to the trust shown him in the fact that he may do so. Will he recognise and appreciate the value of the gift? Will he realise that it is given him in order that he may use, enjoy and make it fruitful? Will he consider that he does not possess it for ever nor even for long, that used or unused it will melt in his hands and one day will be finally past? Will he handle it as a treasure which does not even belong to him, of which he can dispose only according to the purpose of the One from whom he has it, and therefore not thoughtlessly nor arbitrarily, but remembering that he must finally give an account of his stewardship and use?

Sixthly, and finally, it is a matter of his treatment of this loan. We have seen that it also includes man's spontaneity. But this means his freedom to take on responsibilities, to make resolutions, to carry out decisions, to adopt modes of action, to execute deeds. Human life is to be lived as man's activity, not to be endured and withstood as a mere happening. It is to be accepted and accomplished anew every day. For this purpose, and with the corresponding ability, it is given him as a loan.

This is in the widest sense the particular form and dimension of the divine command in respect of human existence as such. We do not see the wood for the trees if we do not see that from the point of view of Christian theology we have here a particular problem. It is posed by the simple fact that of His own good-pleasure, beyond which we cannot go and which we cannot explain, He who in the biblical message is called God is obviously not interested in the totality of things and beings created by Him, nor in specific beings within this totality, but in man, in this being, who in his distinctive unity of soul and body is in his own time alive through his spirit, in his individuality and freedom and with his orientation on God and solidarity with his kind. Man is obviously at issue when the eternal God, the Creator and Lord of heaven and earth, turns to the creature and is graciously engaged in its preservation and overruling, making Himself the companion of its history. Man is obviously the object of the decree which precedes all existence, of God's eternal election of grace. Man is obviously the partner in the covenant whose institution and fulfilment provides the meaning and centre of all creaturely existence. The fact that God Himself did not become identical with the totality, or with specific beings within it, but with man when He became flesh in Jesus Christ, is the execution of His choice and His decree and the fulfilment of His covenant at the heart and as the meaning of all creaturely existence. God stands by man. To be sure, a cause is at issue in their mutual dealings. God's name is to be hallowed in creation, His kingdom of heaven to come on earth, His will to be done in earth as it is in heaven. The deliverance of man is thus to be accomplished. The unmerited goodness and mercy of God are to come upon him. He is to be called to His service, to be summoned to faith in Him, love for Him and hope in Him. But all this is not to be seen and thought of merely in its reality and objectivity, as if man himself were merely a kind of great X on which God wills to magnify His glory and which is itself to be glorified. Certainly, this is at stake in God's dealings of revelation and grace. But man is not merely the *tabula rasa* on which everything that has been factually and objectively decreed will be inscribed. For in all this it is a particular fact of revelation and grace that man is the central factor, that God deals with him in all these things, that in them all he may be the aim, the object and the partner of the divine action. Everything that God does is glorious, gracious, powerful, unfathomably high and deep, but it is worthy of special consideration that man is so dear and important to Him that He specifically deals with him and receives both man and therefore human life. For also as that aim, object and partner of the divine act, man is as he is the recipient of that loan, as he exists by the divine will and decree under the conditions which constitute his life. He is as the same God who is so mightily concerned for His own glory and man's salvation continually permits and enables him to be, not merely out of concern for His own glory and man's salvation, but in connexion therewith, yet also independently, for his existence. In pursuance of this great cause He continually creates and offers him space to live.

The creation story in Gen. 1 right up to the creation of man is one long account of how God ensured and fashioned this space for man to live on earth. The story of the covenant described in the Old Testament, in indissoluble unity with what takes place and is prepared in it from the strictly spiritual standpoint, is also the history of Israel's conquest of the land by the will of God and its settling in the land by the same faithfulness and goodness—each "under his vine and under his fig-tree." Jesus Christ Himself allowed and commanded His disciples—even before all the other petitions which are materially so much more important and urgent—to pray also for their daily bread. And strikingly the "signs and wonders" by which He attested the kingdom of God come to earth were nearly all genuine aids to life in the simplest sense of the term. Indeed the Old and New Testaments generally have an extraordinary amount to say about such things as man's dwelling, food, drink and sleep, labour and rest, health and sickness, in short about his life and its limitation by death; nor are these statements incidental only, nor overshadowed by the greater and more decisive matters at issue.

We do not forget that the biblical message is concerned with the eternal life of man. In this, God's glory is to be triumphantly and man's salvation fully and definitively manifested. And as distinct from this life it will be eternal in the fact that it is not only lent to man but also given to him as an enduring and inalienable possession, as everlasting life. But even in this new mode it will still be life, and indeed human life. If it is the case that man is to enter into this his new life by the resurrection of the dead, if this entrance and transition take place as this corruptible puts on incorruption and this mortal immortality (1 Cor. 15^{53}), then this eschatological aspect, the limitation of this life by the eternal, does not signify a devaluation but, when it is correctly understood, a proper evaluation even of this corruptible and mortal life. Even in eternal life, however this is to be understood, it will still be a matter of this present temporal life; even in that given life it will still be a matter of this life which is lent. Not even remotely will it then seem as if God has caused man to live this life in vain or as if this life has now perished. The tenet that God holds by man, and therefore in incomprehensible factuality takes a most intimate interest in his puny, transitory and infinitely threatened existence, will not then be called in question. But if this tenet is valid, it is not only not arbitrary but necessary from the standpoint of Christian theology to investigate the range of the divine command for this human existence, and to ask what is meant by freedom, i.e., obedience in this respect. Where there is a particular Gospel, there is also a particular Law. Where God is gracious in a particular way, He wills to sanctify in a particular way. Where a particular purpose of God emerges, there must also be a particular willingness and readiness on the part of man to correspond. But a particular good will of God is in fact revealed in the fact that little man with his existence may in the biblical message stand directly before God and in the centre of all things and occurrence. It is revealed finally and decisively in the fact that the Word became flesh.

We now turn to the specific theme of this first sub-section—respect for life. Those who handle life as a divine loan will above all treat it with respect. Respect is man's astonishment, humility and awe at a fact in which he meets something superior—majesty, dignity, holiness, a mystery which compels him to withdraw and keep his distance, to handle it modestly, circumspectly and carefully. It is the *respicere* of an object in face of which his attitude cannot be left to chance or preference or even clever assessment, but which requires an attitude that is particularly appropriate and authoritatively demanded. This compulsion does not derive from life itself and as such. Life does not itself create this respect. The command of God creates respect for it. When man in faith in God's Word and promise realises how God from eternity has maintained and loved him in his little life, and what He has done for him in time, in this knowledge of human life he is faced by a majestic, dignified and holy fact. In human life itself he meets something superior. He is thus summoned to respect because the living God has distinguished it in this way and taken it to Himself. We may confidently say that the birth of Jesus Christ as such is the revelation of the command as that of respect for life. This reveals the eternal election and love of God. This unmistakeably differentiates human life from everything that is and is done in heaven and earth. This gives it even in the most doubtful form the character of something singular, unique, unrepeatable and irreplaceable. This decides that it is an advantage and something good and worthwhile to be as man. This characterises life as the incomparable and non-recurrent opportunity to praise God. And therefore this makes it an object of respect.

It is really surprising that the Christian Church and Christian theology have not long ago urged more energetically the importance for ethics of so constituent a part of the New Testament message as the fact of the incarnation, instead of resorting, in the vital question why man and human life are to be respected, to all kinds of general religious expressions and to the assertions of non-Christian humanism. The assurances of the latter that the value of human life rests on a law of nature and reason sound quite well. But on this basis they are extremely insubstantial, and it is clear that nature and reason can always be used to prove something very different from respect for man. They also have the disadvantage that by "human life" they understand either his very one-sided intellectual existence, "the infinite value of the human soul," on the one side, or his equally one-sided material existence and prosperity on the other. They have the further drawback of always being bound up with illusory overestimations of his goods, abilities and achievements which can only prove detrimental to the respect which ought really to be paid. And somewhere there obviously lurks the ambiguity that, although reference is made to man, humanity, the dignity of man etc., it is not really man himself who is intended but all sorts of things, ideas, advances and aims which in effect man has only to serve, for which he has only to let himself be used, and for the sake of which he can at any moment be dropped and sacrificed.

In contrast to every other, the respect of life which becomes a command in the recognition of the union of God with humanity in Jesus Christ has an incomparable power and width. For in this recognition it is really commanded with the authority of God Himself and therefore in such a way that there can be no question whatever of disregard as an alternative. Intellectualistic and materialistic one-sidedness in answer to the question what human existence is all about is thus excluded by the grounding of the command in this recognition because the human life in question, the life of the man Jesus, cannot be divided into a psychical or physical but compels us to offer the respect demanded by God to the whole man in his ordered unity of soul and body. The usual overestimations of man and human nature are also excluded, because the distinction of human existence brought about in Jesus Christ is to be seen wholly as grace and therefore only in humility. And finally on the basis of this recognition there can be no question of man's life being secretly honoured again as only the vehicle and exponent of an idea or cause superimposed upon him. For human life itself and as such is seen in the person of the man Jesus to be the matter about which God is concerned and therefore man must also be concerned in His service. In respect of the recognition of the command in the sense which now occupies us the Christian Church and Christian theology have an incomparable weight to throw into the scales. They and they alone know exactly why and in what sense respect for life is demanded from us, and demanded in such a way that there can be no evasions or misunderstandings.

But what does respect for life mean? We have spoken of astonishment, humility, awe, modesty, circumspection and carefulness. Application must now be made to our particular theme. What matters is not something but someone, the real man before God and among his fellows, his individual psychophysical existence, his movement in time, his freedom, his orientation on God and solidarity with others. What matters is that everyone should treat his existence and that of every other human being with respect. For it belongs to God. It is His loan and blessing. And it may be seen to be this in the fact that God Himself has so unequivocally and completely acknowledged it in Jesus Christ. What, then, can be the meaning of respect in relation to this object?

First, it obviously means an adoption of the distance proper in face of a mystery. It is a mystery that I am, and others too, in this human structure and individuality in which we recognise one another as of the same kind, each in his time and freedom, each in his vertical and horizontal orientation. This is indeed an incomprehensible and in relation to ourselves intangible fact, inexhaustible in its factuality and depth and constantly adapted to give us pause. Those who do not know *respicere* in face of it, those who are not startled and do not feel insignificant and incompetent in its presence, those who think they can understand and master and control it, do not know what obedience is. All human life as such is surrounded by a particular solemnity. This is not the solemnity of the divine, nor of the ultimate end of man. Life is only human and therefore created, and eternity as the divinely decreed destiny of man is only an allotted future. But within these limits it is a mystery emphasised and absolutely distinguished by God Himself. As such it must always be honoured with new wonder. Every single point to be observed and pondered is in its own way equally marvellous—and everything is equally marvellous in every human existence. First, then, we have simply to perceive this, and once we have done so we have not at any price to relinquish or even to lose sight of this perception. We must be awake to this need to keep our distance, and always be wakeful as we do so.

But a mere theoretical and aesthetic wonder is not enough. On the contrary, the theoretical and aesthetic wonder which rightly understood forms the presupposition for everything else, must itself have a practical character if it is to be the required respect. And this means that human life must be affirmed and willed by man. We hasten to add that it must be affirmed and willed as his own with that of others and that of others with his own. Egoism and altruism are false antitheses when the question is that of the required will to live. My own life can no more claim my respect than that of others, but neither can that of others. Although they are not the same, but each distinct, the homogeneity and solidarity of all human life is indissoluble. But what is the will to live understood in this sense? Obviously, because to life there also belongs the freedom of this will, it is determination and readiness for action in the direction of its confirmation. That we should spontaneously perceive and affirm the reception of life as a divine loan in its character as a favour shown, a possession entrusted and an opportunity offered to us, is obviously what is expected of us as those who possess it, who are alive. But if this perception and confirmation is our act, it must consist in our making of our life the use prescribed by its nature as seen in these points. What is important is that according to the measure and within the limits of his individuality, and in the time granted to him, each should exist—always in orientation on God and solidarity with others—as this rational creature, attentively, unreservedly and loyally confessing his human existence in willing responsibility to the One to whom he owes it. We cannot live in obedience accidentally, irresolutely, without plan or responsibility. We cannot in obedience let ourselves go or be driven. We cannot and must not seriously tire of life. For it is always an offer waiting for man's will, determination and readiness for action. And it is to be noted that this is real respect for life. In this form as the will to live it is more than passive speculation in face of its mystery. It is the respect which its mystery demands. We really see it as the mystery it is in the fact that we will to live it and accept it responsibly. A life which is not affirmed and willed, which is irresolute, irresponsible and inactive, is necessarily a life without mystery. And against the constant threat of egoism, there is always the safeguard and corrective of recollection that the real human life is the one which is lived in orientation on God and co-ordination with others. The last is particularly important from the practical standpoint. The will to live which is the form of respect for life will always be distinguishable from an inhuman and irreverent will to live contrary to the command, by the fact that it considers the existence and life of others together with its own, and its own together with that of others.

But having considered and said this, we must also show that the commanded respect for life includes an awareness of its limitations. We have already mentioned these. We refer to the creaturely and the eschatological limitations. These cannot diminish respect for life, much less abrogate it. But it is necessarily modified and characterised by the fact that the life to which it is paid has these limitations. As the reverence commanded of man it is not limitless. As such it has within itself its own limitation. Its limitation is the will of God the Creator Himself who commands it, and the horizon which is set for man by the same God with his determination for eternal life. Life is no second God, and therefore the respect due to it cannot rival the reverence owed to God. On the contrary, it is limited by that which God will have from the man who is elected and called by Him. For the life of man belongs to Him. He has granted it to him as a loan. And He decides in what its right use should consist. He also decrees and decides in His command in what man's will to live should at any moment consist or not, and how far it should go or not go as such. And what God will have of man is not simply that he should will to live for himself and in co-existence with others. God can also will to restrict man's will to live for himself and in co-existence with others. He can weaken, break and finally destroy it. He actually does this. And when He does, obedience may not be withheld from Him. As Creator and Lord of life, He has also the right to will and do this, and if He does, then He knows well why it must be so, and in this too He is man's gracious Father. In relation to man, He has much more in mind than what man can see here and now in the fulfilment of his life-act. He has determined him for eternal life, for the life which one day will finally be given him. He is leading him through this life to the other. The respect for life commanded by Him cannot then be made by man a rigid principle, an absolute rule to be fulfilled according to rote. It can only try to assert and maintain itself as the will to live in the one sense understood by man, whether in relation to his own life or that of others. Respect for life, if it is obedience to God's command, will have regard for the free will of the One who has given life as a loan. It will not consist in an absolute will to live, but in a will to live which by God's decree and command, and by *meditatio futurae vitae,* may perhaps in many ways be weakened, broken, relativised and finally destroyed. Being prepared for this, it will move within its appointed limits. It can always be modest. And it will not on this account be any the less respect for life. It will be so in this modesty and in readiness for it. When we come to questions of detail, we shall see how important it is to remember this reservation, or rather this closer definition. Respect for life without this closer definition could be the principle of an idolatry which has nothing whatever to do with Christian obedience.

But this reservation must now be strictly and sharply qualified. This inwardly necessary relativisation of what is required of us as respect for life, this recollection of the freedom of the controlling and commanding God and of eternal life as the limitation of this present life, must not be forgotten for a single moment. But the application of this reservation, the reference to it and the corresponding modesty, cannot have more than the character of an *ultima ratio,* an exceptional case. They arise only on the frontiers of life and therefore of the respect due to it. Hence it is not true that respect for life is alternately commanded and then not commanded us. Neither is it true that alongside the sphere of this respect there is a sphere in which it is not normative, or only partially so. However much what we understand by this respect and therefore by the commanded will to live is limited and relativised by God's free will and man's determination for a future life, this relativisation never means that man is released from this respect. The one God, who is of course the Lord of life and death, the Giver of this life and that which is to come, will in all circumstances and in every conceivable modification demand respect for life. He will never give man liberty to take another view of life, whether his own or that of others. Indifference, wantonness, arbitrariness or anything else opposed to respect cannot even be considered as a commanded or even a permitted attitude. Even the way to these frontiers—the frontiers where respect for life and the will to live can assume in practice very strange and paradoxical forms, where in relation to one's own life and that of others it can only be a matter of that relativised, weakened, broken and even destroyed will to live—will always be a long one which we must take thoughtfully and conscientiously, continually asking and testing whether that *ultima ratio* really applies. The frontiers must not be arbitrarily advanced in any spirit of frivolity or pedantry; they can be only reached in obedience and then respected as such. Recollection of the freedom and the superior wisdom, goodness and controlling power of God, and recollection of the future life, cannot then form a pretext or excuse for attitudes and modes of action in which man may actually evade what is commanded within these limits. They are frontiers which are necessarily set by God, and cannot be claimed as emancipations of man. This will be best understood by those who do not treat respect for life as a principle set up by man. Even on these frontiers they will not see a relaxation of the command or exception to the rule, but only a relaxation of that which they think they should understand and offer as obedience when they accept it as a summons to the will to live. Even here there will be required of them a new and deeper understanding of the will to live, which *ultima ratione* can now take the form of a broken and even destroyed will to live, and, if it be the will of God, must necessarily do so. Yet if it is an obedient and not a frivolous will, if it is not wantoness and self-will, it must always be the will to live, and therefore the practical form of respect for life.

19. The Transcendence of God and the Value of Human Life

JAMES M. GUSTAFSON

Throughout this paper I shall keep in view two general areas of reference, two sources of understanding. One is human experience: of the values of human life, and of valuing. The other is Christian theology, or at least certain affirmations made in the intellectual life of faith which pertain to the valuing of human life. Any discourse which attempts to move between theology and ethics by necessity must keep these two areas and sources in view. If theological principles and affirmations pertain to human moral values, they do so in two ways. Either they are principles and affirmations which include within the divine purposes those purposes which are moral, that is, which stipulate human moral values, ends, rules, etc., or the religious community infers certain moral values, ends, rules, etc., to be consistent, coherent, harmonious, consonant with affirmations about God. If claims are made for transformation, emendation, penetration, alteration, re-orientation of human experience through religious faith, those claims are in principle subject to virtually empirical investigation. There are two pitfalls in the efforts to relate theology and ethics in general which I wish to avoid. On the one hand are the temptations to deduce too much from theological principles for ethics, a pitfall more characteristic of the religious rhetoric of some continental Protestants than of either Roman Catholic or American Protestant theologians, e.g., the claim that what is morally right is determined by the command of God in the moment. On the other hand are the temptations to separate the ethical discourse from the theological, confining the significance of the theological to soteriology, and finding the resources for the ethical only in what (hopefully) all men can accept in common as the human and the moral.

My procedure will be to discuss three general affirmations in an exploratory way, seeking to make clear the relations between Christian belief in the transcendence of God (and the God who is transcendent) and human experience in each. The first is: Human physical life is not of absolute value, but since it is the indispensable condition for human values and valuing

From the *Catholic Theological Society of America Proceedings* 23 (1968). Used by permission.

the burden of proof is always on those who would take it. The second is more complex. Human life has *many values.* Some of these adhere to individuals, others adhere to the relations between persons in interpersonal situations, others adhere to human collectivities, and some adhere to all three. These values are not always in harmony with each other in particular human circumstances. The third is this: Human valuing of others involves several kinds of relations, and several aspects of individual experience; it is no simple single thing either descriptively or normatively.

I. Human Physical Life is not of Absolute Value

Human physical life is not of absolute value. But it is the indispensable condition for human values and valuing, and for its own sake is to be valued. Thus the burden of proof is always on those who would take it. The delicacy of discerning what value is to be given to human physical life under particular circumstances when it is not valued absolutely presents one of the principal practical moral problems men have to face.

H. Richard Niebuhr, in *Radical Monotheism and Western Culture,* stated the broad outlines of the affirmation of the nonabsolute value of all created things from a theological perspective. He closes his chapter, "The Idea of Radical Monotheism," with the following words. "Radical monotheism dethrones all absolutes short of the principle of being itself. At the same time it reverences every relative existent. Its two great mottoes are: 'I am the Lord thy God; thou shalt have no other gods before me' and 'Whatever is, is good.' "[1] The theme is a very familiar one in a great deal of Protestant theology. Kierkegaard wrote about the difficulties of being absolutely related to the absolute, and relatively related to the relative; Paul Tillich's idea of the "protestant principle" functioned to provide men with a point of transcendence from which all finite gods could be assessed with presumed freedom and objectivity.[2] Nothing has been exempted from the edges of this theological sword, including religion (as it is distinguished in Barth, Bonhoeffer, and many followers, from faith). The intentions of many Protestant writers in this vein has been primarily religious and theological; they intend to preserve the majesty of God from confusion with lesser majesties, they intended to make the claim that God alone is worthy of absolute trust and reliance, that is, of absolute faith; they intended to drive men to faith in God by preaching the unworthiness of lesser gods. A few writers have moved on to develop some of the ethical inferences that can be drawn from the theological point; the Niebuhr brothers, for examples, show in part what it means for the political community to confess that God alone is the Lord. It is not unfair, however, to charge almost all of the Protestant giants who perceived the dangers of idolatry with failing to deal with many of the hard cases in which men must judge what the proper reverence is for various relative existents.

Here we see the serious ethical limitations of affirmations of the transcendence of God if the moral inference drawn from it is vaguely the relativity of all things that are not God. A veritable host of conclusions could be drawn from this vagueness. Some of these can be easily listed. 1) Since only God is absolute, all other things are *equally* relative to him and to each other. No one, however, wishes to take this line. 2) Quite different would be this; since the importance of the doctrine of transcendence is to show the majesty and virtual mystery of God, once we see the relativity of all things in relation to him, we have exhausted the theological resources for determining the values of the relativities of life. We are on our own to explore pragmatically the great varieties of human schemes for the ordering of existents in relation to each other: reason, power, utility and other values, and many other things can be brought together in whatever combination to keep life surviving. 3) God, in his absoluteness, had the good sense to foresee the problem of the relativity of all things, and had the good judgment to designate certain persons and institutions with the authority to order the relativities in relation to each other. So men ought to obey these divinely authorized minds and powers, whether ecclesiastical or political. 4) Since man, according to Scripture and his own estimate of himself, is the "highest" being in the created order, all relative things are to be ordered according to his valuations. These empirically might be wrong; but if we can know what man is essentially we can know how normatively all relative things are to be ordered for man's well-being. Which conclusion one accepts will set something of the course he takes in dealing with the question of when human physical life can be taken.

When we turn from theology to human experience, we see that it is not necessary for a person to believe in the transcendence of God in order to affirm the relativity of institutions, religions, morals, physical life, and what have you.[3] Historical and cultural relativism, whatever their intellectual origins might be, are part of the conventional wisdom. And even long before there were tags to put on these notions, men had learned that circumstances of human experience often required them to alter things they professed to be of absolute value, whether these were physical life processes or institutions. "Kill or be killed," the slogan drummed into some of us during the Second World War, has a natural history predating myths of creation. One's own life is to be valued more than the life of the one who attacks, at least under most conditions—if he attacks first, if he has malicious intent, if he seeks to destroy not only one's own life but those of others, if you are under orders to kill him before he kills you in the game of war, etc. But many other things have been valued above human life; the honored legends and narratives of the things men have been willing to die for, all point to the development of human convictions about things to be valued more than physical life itself—justice, liberty of conscience, exemplary witness to a belief, as well as things valued less highly by most people. It is not hard for most men to believe that physical life is not of absolute value, though in the time of assassinations, it is hard to accept the fact that others do not believe it.

How might belief in the transcendence of God qualify, alter, modify, man's understanding of, and response to, the non-absolute human values, and particularly the value of human physical life? If there are theological grounds for accepting the finite values as non-absolute, and if there is experiential grounds for this, in what ways might the religious belief qualify the human experience? I shall not give all the possible answers to these questions, but only some which I deem to be very important.

First, created life is accepted as a gift; it has an author and a source beyond itself, and we and all the other forms of life are dependent on that author and source. Life is given to us; even if man succeeds in creating new physical life, he remains the recipient of a multitude of gifts which make this possible. Thus one could spell out a number of the characteristics of the relationship between man and God which in turn would qualify man's disposition toward the created values around him: man is a *dependent* creature, dependent upon God and upon his fellows—this he remembers in his relationships and responses; man is the recipient of good things which are not of his creation, including his own physical life—this brings a response of *gratitude* both to God and the persons and institutions which sustain the goodness of his life, etc.

Second, since only God is absolute, man must remember his finitude, not to mention his deformed existence. This, as the Protestant theological interpreters of culture remind us, requires that man always be brought under question by himself and by others, that he never absolutize his powers, his acts, his judgments. The requirement, in traditional religious terms, of humility constantly qualifies his tendencies to absolutize the relative.

Third, man is *accountable* to the author and source of life for his use and cultivation of life, including human physical life. He is responsible (in terms of accountable) to God for the ways in which he cares for, preserves, sustains, cultivates, and, in his limited capacity, creates life around him. His disposition is that of the free servant; not servile but acknowledging that his human vocation is under God.

Fourth, in his participation in the created order, man is *responsive* to the *developments and purposes which are being made possible* for him under the power and gifts of life from God. He responds not only to the immediacies of possibilities, but to the course of developments which the transcendent God is making possible and ultimately governing. This fourth brings us to a critical point, in my judgment, in Protestant theologies which most substantiate the first affirmation of this paper. That is, insofar as the transcendent God is the One beyond the Many (H. R. Niebuhr), or the unspeakable ground of being (Tillich), he is peculiarly devoid of meaningful content, and thus man is left almost no substantial theological resources in the determination of the values and purposes which ought to govern his participation in the created order, including his use of human physical life. The human ingenuity left for man to depend on in the absence of theological resources is not to be denigrated; out of reflections on human life man does develop views of the "values" which are human, and which are to be developed and sustained. But the God who is transcendent is not the totally unknown God, and thus there are more resources than man's reflection on his own existence alone.

Since the *sine qua non* of other relative values and of valuing is the existence of human physical life, it is valued and is to be valued with a high priority. To take it is to render it impossible for the other person to experience any values, and for him to contribute to the life of the community in such valued ways as it might be possible to do. Thus, while human physical life is not an absolute value, it is to be preserved unless there are substantial grounds for regarding other values to be of greater significance in the particular circumstances in which judgments are made. Human physical life is the primary gift of God on which all other gifts to man are dependent; this vacuous platitude suddenly becomes cogent when assassin's bullets remove from the human community the values of a great man's life, not only values to himself but to the human community.

II. Human Life has Many Values

Human life has many values. These values are not always in harmony with each other in particular circumstances. Indeed, there is no fixed timeless order of priority of the values of human life which *a priori* determines what ought to occur in all particular circumstances. Put theologically, while God's purposes for man might be summed up in some generalized unitary conception, such as "He wills man's good," man's good is a complex and not simple notion. Indeed, the religious consciousness of Christianity and Judaism has always recognized that God's purposes are multiple and not single in human life. Put in the language of human experience, men have always been aware that human life cannot exist without both freedom and order, without both love and justice, without both peace and freedom or peace and justice, and that these sometimes conflict with each other and with the value of particular human physical lives in particular circumstances.

The God who is transcendent is not a totally unknown God. People who have acknowledged him to be the Lord have historically discerned his activity in the course and purposes of events, in the lives and deeds of particular men, in the responses men have made to each other and to him. They have written accounts of human life in which they have interpreted experience in the light of the purposes of God, the values God confers upon life. They have written in propositional form some of the predicates which they have deduced from the activities of God; God is love, God is just, God is merciful, God is wrathful, God is the creator, God is the redeemer, God is the judge, God is righteous, etc. Many of these accounts and purposes are directly moral in their content; they pertain to what God wills that human life should be if it is in accord with his activities and his purposes, his will in the double sense of what he does and what he requires. To be sure, certain purposes of God are more dominant than others: his redemptive purpose triumphs over his wrath, for example, as Jonah was disappointed to find out. But in particular circumstances the significance of his redemptive purposes might well include his wrath, as religious sentimentalists often fail to see. He is loving, but the forms of his loving are at least as complex as the forms of human loving—sometimes he loves through the provision of an order, a pattern of rules for life, sometimes through spontaneity and boundless mercy, sometimes through the preservation of peace, and sometimes through the break-up of oppressive and unjust peace. Religious men, like others, long to leap to a simple unitive understanding of God's will and purpose, for if they can be true believers in such, they can provide simpler statements of what life in the human world is to be. But the impulse violates both Christian beliefs about the God who is transcendent and the complexity of the life created by him in which his purposes are to be fulfilled. God values many things in human life.

In my judgment, the most current simplification is that God wills the human, a simplification which has ecumenical auspices. The human, it turns out, is either something men are presumed to know intuitively, or it is something which must be spelled out in more rationally defensible terms—which is to open the door to complexity. It may well be that God wills the human, but the human, like the good, is not a simple notion.[4]

The things which human beings value, quite properly, are at least as many, and at least as inconsistent with each other in particular circumstances as are the purposes of God. What common human experience knows about this was depicted philosophically several decades ago by Nicolai Hartmann.[5] Not only is there a plurality of values which are abrasive to each other, but there is a plurality of virtues; indeed, Hartmann wrote about the antinomy of values and of virtues. In his rigorous atheism and his rigorous assertion of the moral autonomy of men, Hartmann painted one of the most awesome pictures of human responsibility I have encountered. One might, however, learn from his phenomenological accounts of moral life without necessarily agreeing with his metaphysics and his anthropology. Human values are many, and many things which men value can be ethically and theologically justified. They do not fall into a neat pattern of priorities which smooths the abrasiveness of particular situations.[6]

Do the Christian beliefs about the God who is transcendent bear any importance upon the choices men make in the ordering of human values in the conduct of life? Or, is one left with a plurality in the transcendent matched by a plurality in the human sphere? In this brief paper I cannot explicate my answers fully. They would, however, take the following line. Since the transcendent God is not a capricious being, man can discern the fundamental directionality of his purposes for human life. There is an orientation, an intention, which sheds its light upon which intentions and values are proper for man. And, as I indicated in the first part of this paper, man is accountable to God, whose purposes can be in part explicated, in the conduct of his affairs. One also receives his knowledge of God's purposes as a gift of light and direction in the conduct of his actions. But this directionality, which can be translated into a generally applicable ordering of human values, does not resolve the conflicts that are bound to be present in the hard cases of moral judgment. Although God is loving, and wills that men shall be loving, love is not *prima facie* consistent with the preservation of human life under all circumstances. If one chooses to say that love is consistent with man's well-being, one has only moved the problem over from one term to the other, without specifying it more carefully.

Further, the transcendence of God has personal meaning only if one has trust in the God who is transcendent, only if there is a gratitude to him, loyalty to him, a sense of obligation to him. Given this faith, then, the religious believer is obligated to seek to discern (not alone, but in the company of the people of God) what the transcendent God's purposes are for the conduct of life with its plurality of human values. But given a measure of plurality of God's purposes, there is no guarantee of man making a risk-proof moral judgment, either in God's or in men's sights. There is no prior guarantee of hitting the mark morally. Given the finitude of men, and the plurality of values discerned in human experience, there is no guarantee *a priori* of moral rectitude in all circumstances. Given man's sin (not explicated here), there is need both for guidance from the communities' beliefs about God, and for the mercy which he grants to all people. The Christian beliefs about the God who is transcendent give guidance in the ordering of life with its plurality of values.

III. Human Valuing

Human valuing is complex and not simple. It involves several kinds of relations, and several aspects of individual experience. A rehearsal of the theories of human valuation is no more possible than a rehearsal of theories of value in this brief paper. To keep the topic manageable I shall confine my discussion to two principal aspects of the experience of valuing. One is valuing things and other persons for their utility, not only for one's own purposes, but for purposes of the human community. The other is valuing things and persons for themselves. My interest in this distinction here is to suggest some of the different characteristics of human responses, and of personhood, which are properly involved in each of these two aspects. The first suggests a mode of life which is largely one of problem-solving, of achievement of specific purposes or ends, and tends to slip into a flat, mechanistic, view of experience. It reduces the sense of awe and wonder. The second suggests a mode of life which is spiritually profound, but tends to slip into the denigration of rationality, of the necessity for specification of ends and means. Both modes of life are advanced under religious auspices; the first is strong in the proposals of those who affirm the advances of technology and urbanization, and share the optimistic spirit that sometimes pervades successful problem solvers. (My personal conviction is that the thinness of such theologically sponsored views is becoming clear with the compounding of human failures and tragedies.) The second is strong in the proposals of radically personalistic Christians, who, in some of their rhetoric, appear to suggest that the organization of persons to be useful to achieve certain ends (particularly in the church) compromises what men are meant to be for each other. The double tendency is not new, of course; one can gain insight into it from reading the theology of St. Augustine, among others from the past.

It would be folly to try to argue that only a belief in the transcendence of God can justify the more personalistic vision of life, with its responses to other persons of awe, wonder, joy, reverence, and profound respect. Certain aspects of contemporary youth culture manifest this kind of valuing while at the same time rebelling against traditional religious beliefs; the relations between young people are "beautiful" in a meaningful way to them. (My son, for example, wrote recently to a friend, "The real world is beautiful, and you are part of it.") The grounds for the fresh appropriation of the Kantian principle that persons are to be treated as ends in themselves and not as means, are more a revulsion against the institutionalization of values of utility which appear to be "dehumanizing" than they are religious beliefs.

I believe it would be equally a folly to argue that no theological support can be given for the instrumental value, the utility value, of persons. If God is intent upon the preservation and cultivation of life, including as it must, men's lives in relation to each other and in relation to the rest of nature, a view of men as functionaries for the achievement of purposes consistent with those larger purposes is proper, and in order. There is an ordering activity in life, with its impositions of duties and obligations, its assignment of tasks and the requirement of their fulfillment, which is part of God's purpose for men.

The general phenomenon of valuing, then, has many aspects, and cannot be reduced to a simple notion, nor be grounded in a simple set of ultimate requirements. In "using" another person one is valuing him for his function in the social economy of life; one values his wife, even, in part for her utility—in providing for the mundane needs of the family (doing laundry, cooking meals, shopping, cleaning the house, etc.) and in fulfilling needs for affection and even sexual gratification. But relations other than utility between persons also include valuing; not all valuing of persons is reducible to utility. To respect another is to acknowledge his value, as is to reverence another, appreciate another, care for another, preserve the life of another, sustain another, love another, honor another. The valuing carried by these notions suggests in each instance an aspect of the value of the other for his own sake, an intrinsic value to the other. These notions suggest aspects of the experience of valuing, and the relationship with the other, which acknowledge the mystery, the autonomy, the value of the existence, of the other. They also suggest that the self, in such valuing, is not simply calculating in a rational way how the other fulfills one's own desires, interests, and needs, or even the interests and needs of the society. Rather they involve the affections, the emotive life of the person.

Belief in the transcendence of God is not a necessary personal condition for proper maintenance of either the utility or the intrinsic values of persons. To claim that it is a necessary condition would be to take on the obligation to prove that those who believe in the transcendence of God are better "valuers" than are those who do not believe. Christian belief in the God who is transcendent, however, does, can, should, and ought to inform and direct the valuing experiences of Christians, and the relations they have with each other and with nature.

To spell this out, I would develop two themes. One is the effect of this belief on the dispositions of the persons who believe it. To accept life as a gift, to acknowledge dependence on God for life, to acknowledge one's finitude and disobedience in humility, would all (if there is some wholeness to the person) predispose one to have respect, reverence, honor, appreciation, and love for others, and for the world. In the life of praise and adoration, of confession and repentance, which are part of the expression of this belief, of the response to the transcendence of God, the affections are nourished, and the dispositions directed toward the responses of respect, honor, appreciation, etc. The calculative rationality of valuations for utility is tempered and impregnated by the sensibilities, dispositions, and affections nourished in religious faith.

The second theme is the effect that the beliefs about the God who is transcendent would have in conditioning the ends and purposes for which the experiences of utilization of others would be directed. Since these ends and purposes can be specified in consistency with the purposes of God who is known in Christian faith, and since ends and purposes which are inconsistent with such knowledge of God would be illicit, the utilization of other persons and of nature would be informed by the affirmations made about the God who is transcendent.

The legitimate claims of Christian thought with reference to God's transcendence and the values of human life could be summarized in the following terms. All created things, including human physical life, are of non-absolute value. Yet as gifts of God they are to be nourished, cared for, protected, developed, etc. The transcendent God is a known God, and the knowledge of his purposes gives direction to the ordering of life's values, but not with such clarity that man is exempted from the responsibility to judge and act in his finite condition. The relation of the believers to God in trust, gratitude, obedience, etc., places upon them the willingness and the obligation to make their orderings of values cohere with God's purposes. It also effects their personal existences; impregnating their affections and intentions, their dispositions and their purposes.

That these explorations require further precision, elaboration, and correction, goes without saying. Their fundamental warrant is this: they maintain the interaction between the positive theological affirmations of the Christian faith on the one hand, and human experience of values and of valuing, on the other.

Notes

1. H. Richard Niebuhr, *Radical Monotheism and Western Culture.* New York: Harper, 1960, p. 37.

2. S. Kierkegaard, *Concluding Unscientific Postscript.* Princeton: Princeton Univ. Press, 1944, pp. 358–68. Paul Tillich, *The Protestant Era.* Chicago: Univ. of Chicago Press, 1948, pp. 161–81.

3. Theologians of various religious persuasions seem to take some pride in the possible historical connection between the belief in God's transcendence and the "secularization" of life, which might be restated "the relativization of all of life" in actual practice. It may make them personally happier to be with the world, but their positive attitude does not in itself resolve the problems of how to differentiate the better and the worse in the secular.

4. I have given some attention to this in two recent articles. See J. M. Gustafson, "Two Approaches to Theological Ethics," *Union Seminary Quarterly Review,* Vol. 23, pp. 337–48, June, 1968, and "New Directions in Moral Theology," *Commonwealth,* Vol. 87: pp. 617–23, Feb. 23, 1968.

5. N. Hartmann, *Ethics,* Vol. II, *Moral Values.* London: G. Allen and Unwin, 1932, esp. pp. 407–43.

6. See J. M. Gustafson, "A Christian Approach to the Ethics of Abortion," *Dublin Review,* No. 514, pp. 346–64, for the way in which this affirmation of plurality affects a particular moral decision and how it is made.

20. Toward Freedom from Value

RICHARD STITH

Introduction

Few would wish for a world where life would always be preserved indefinitely and at all costs, for we feel that life ought sometimes to give way to other human aspirations. At the same time, most of us hold inviolable the life of every individual, regardless of its usefulness for the achievement of our heart's desires.

We have, then, two intuitions: that life must not be destroyed, but that it need not be always preserved; that every person's life is infinitely valuable, but that other things may sometimes be more valuable; that human life has sanctity, but that death may occasionally be welcomed. As we seek to map out even a crooked frontier separating these two sovereign intuitions, we soon learn that each lays claim to perhaps the entire territory of the other, and that neither will remain satisfied for long with those apparently "convenient" compromises represented by distinctions between "active and passive" or "ordinary and extraordinary." If life has infinite value, how can we passively abandon it when its preservation becomes burdensome? Or, if we can indeed abandon it, perhaps it has little value after all, and therefore may be violated. So we discover not only that we cannot easily draw a clear line of separation between our two intuitions, but also that each seeks to annihilate the other.

If we wish to intervene to prevent either side from suffering a total rout, we must begin by finding high ground from which we can describe the proper limits of each. That is, we must develop an appealing and understandable theory of the nature and limits of the prohibition on taking human life.[1]

Here again is our dilemma: if we set the value of life low enough to account for the moral[2] intuition that we need not preserve life at all costs, we have set it too low to account for our other intuition that we ought not to kill no matter what benefits we might gain. On the other hand, if we raise the value of life to the point where no benefits are weighty enough to justify killing, we soon discover that we have committed ourselves to a surely excessive effort to eliminate death. It is my belief that our error here does not lie in valuing "mere" life or "quality" life too highly or too lowly, but rather springs from the ordinary use of the word "value." Is there no other word available? Is there no attitude, besides that of "valuing," which we take to life? I suggest that we already know and name the attitude for which we are searching: "reverence." And we also speak often about the aspect of life which accounts for our attitude of reverence: "sanctity." Unfortunately, life's *sanctity* is ordinarily confounded, or even identified, with its *value*—so that to say that life has sanctity is popularly taken to mean that it has great (or even absolute or infinite) value. Yet it is my contention that sanctity and value are radically different, and that it is precisely thinking in terms of value which obscures and may destroy our sense of the demands of human life. Only by first overthrowing the rulership of value-thought can contemporary man hope to *think* clearly about what he still already knows.

Why not kill? This essay seeks to say what there is about human life[3] as we perceive it which could account for our moral intuition that killing is wrong. In the first part of the essay, it will be argued that the value of life cannot account for the prohibition on killing for two reasons: (1) we often give life such a low "value" that this value alone would be insufficient to preclude permission to kill, and (2) we would not feel killing to be forbidden even if we were to value life infinitely. The value of life, even when made absolute, cannot preclude the taking of life. This is so not because of any defect in life, but because of the impotence of the concept and attitude called valuing. Because all valuing is for a type (or essence), I will argue, it can demand only that a quantity or quality of life exist, but never that a particular person live or be allowed to live. (To debate quantity vs. quality of life is thus *already* depersonalizing, no matter which side one takes.)

Having attacked the notion of valuing and having demonstrated the inadequacy of the attitude we take to life when we value it, in the second part of this essay, I shall describe and distinguish the attitude of reverence, the object of which has sanctity rather than value. Here it will be argued that the sanctity of life primarily demands nonviolation—rather than preservation—of life, and therefore can both forbid the taking of life and coexist with the nonpreservation of life. Thus, both our original intuitions can be affirmed: sanctity makes the individual *matter,* in a way which value does not, and yet does not demand his preservation at all costs.

Dependency, however, raises difficult problems for the meaning of sanctity. If someone's life is dependent upon our actions, is there a difference between causing death and not preserving life? This dilemma is

From *The Jurist* 38 (Winter 1978). Used by permission.

most often currently discussed in the medical context, but it is surely as ancient as the helplessness of every newborn. Its solution, I shall argue, lies not in behavioral but in intentional criteria for actions violative of the sanctity of life.

Finally, some practical consequences of the theory of sanctity will be developed. The demands of sanctity will be described first vis-à-vis medical patients and then as a guide to social and economic planning.

I. The Insufficiency of Value

Not all of us regard killing as always wrong. Most make an exception for self-defense; many do so in cases ranging from war and capital punishment to selective euthanasia. But all of us are *reluctant* to kill. Why?

Perhaps the most frequent answer to this question is "because of the value of life." Indeed, advocates of an absolute prohibition on, say, capital punishment or euthanasia are wont to cite "the *infinite* value of life." And for people used to translating all ethical and policy issues into "value" terminology, these answers are quite understandable. After all, why *would* we protect life unless it had value? And how could the value of life *never* be outweighed unless it were infinite?

Nevertheless, it is my contention here that the value of life cannot adequately explain our reluctance to kill, that some other factor is at work. I shall try to demonstrate this thesis by first showing that even where life's value is clearly insufficient to outweigh other relevant values, we do not kill. Therefore, more than the *value* of life must matter to us. Further, I shall show that even if life had infinite value, this alone could not make killing wrong in many situations where we refrain from killing. And so, again, I conclude that we regard life as having more than value and in subsequent sections will move beyond value in search of the missing element that explains our intuitions.

Sometimes life is not valued highly. For example, many doctors would be willing not to use "extraordinary" measures in order to preserve the lives of persons able to live only a very short time in any event.[4] Such minimal amounts of life are seemingly considered not valuable enough in themselves to require the costs of heroic treatment. Yet at the same time, these physicians are apparently reluctant to kill actively and deliberately in order to avoid equivalent future costs. Why? Do these doctors see something else in life besides its value?

Even a healthy normal life may have insufficient "value" to outweigh other considerations. I am not referring here to the oft-cited case of martyrdom where someone sacrifices his own life for the sake of some noble ideal,[5] but rather, I am speaking of those instances where we value our own *and others'* lives less than comfort and convenience—as is the case with all limitations on "safety." Without a doubt we could individually and collectively live far more safely and so protect life better if we were willing to put up with the accompanying decline in life's "quality."

Nowhere is this fact more obvious than in the question of speed limits. By not drastically lowering the speed limit, our various governments and their constituencies are with statistical *certainty* allowing tens of thousands of violent deaths to occur. Nor do these deaths occur only to those who have chosen to "assume the risk" of driving. Pedestrians and dependents (e.g., children) are also killed; and given our society and economy, even those who "choose" to drive can hardly be said to have much choice in the matter. The simple fact is that thousands upon thousands of innocent and unwilling victims of traffic accidents die each year because our society and government do not want the decline in mobility and in GNP which would be caused by a speed-limit reduction.

And yet my torts teacher, Guido Calabresi, found no takers when he presented to our law school class the hypothetical case of a god who offered us an equivalent increase in societal well-being if we would agree to kill one thousand persons on an altar each year. Why this difference? Why was the class simultaneously willing (albeit with qualms) to let many die in traffic deaths and unwilling to produce the same benefits by the "sacrifice" of a lesser number?[6]

No adequate answer to these questions is possible, I submit, as long as we persist in treating human lives merely as valued objects. The way we regard people, which includes a reluctance to destroy them, has very little analogy to the way we treat that which we value, as we can see again by turning to the "potentiality-actuality" continuum—first in regard to things we value (money and justice, for example) and second in regard to human life.

Now, an object which is valued when we have it (in "actuality"), is also valued when we *could* have it (in "potentiality"). True, we discount the value of the latter by the time, trouble, and uncertainty involved. But we would surely think someone at least confused who were stingy with money that he did not wish to have in the first place. Or again, we would doubt the sincerity of someone who strongly resisted increased injustice and yet also opposed increased justice.

But in an age of individualism and of possible overpopulation, this strange stance seems to be exactly what many people take toward other human beings.

As individuals and as a society, many of us do not wish more children, do not consider them a net value when considering their possible existence. Yet once a child is born (or once it is conceived), killing is for most of us out of the question—even if the child is still "unwanted." This reluctance to destroy that which we never wanted to begin with would border on insanity if we were speaking of something we merely valued. We cannot explain our disinclination to kill by saying simply that we value human life, because sometimes we do not value it and yet are still reluctant to kill.

I have so far argued that life's value is sometimes relatively too low to be sufficient to prevent killing and that we should look elsewhere for reasons not to kill. However, I suspect that at least some of us will not be ready to give up on value this easily. Not knowing what else we may find, some may be appropriately cautious about casting loose from what may seem the only firm mooring for the protection of life. "Should we not," some of us might ask, "find ways instead to increase the value we give to life, even at the cost of a larger population, more respirators, and even more bicycles?"

I want to cut off this last hope in the value of life by arguing that even if we somehow could agree that human life had *infinite* value, we would not necessarily prohibit killing. Only when this has been shown will the inadequacy of value be sufficiently clear to send us in search of a new base on which to anchor the protection of life.

Let us assume, then, for the sake of argument, that human life has infinite value, meaning that a human being is so valuable, of such great worth, that no other kind of entity (thing, relationship, or whatever) or combination of entities can ever be preferable to such a being. In other words, insofar as we choose rationally that which is most valuable, we would *never* choose something else instead of a living human being. Consequently, we would never destroy such a being, no matter what other kinds of benefits we might realize.

But, I submit, we might well destroy such a being for the sake of the *same* kinds of benefits (i.e., human life). Indeed, if we felt that human life were of infinite value, we might well feel morally compelled to kill, whenever such killing would save more lives than those lost.[7] We would promote capital punishment, for example, if it were the only effective means of deterring a greater number of killings. We also would kill a healthy person if his vital organs were needed to save his two ailing siblings.

We might also kill for reasons other than saving life. If life were really of infinite value but our resources were limited, would we not favor those who were most fertile and/or lived longest at least cost? Would we not like some kind of "breeder," put to sleep the fat and the sick to make room for more people to replace them? If every single life had tremendous value, we would want as many as we could afford, for as long as possible, even if this meant destroying those requiring greater care, resources, or space.

Nor would we avoid comparing the lives we valued, and perhaps killing would result. Even if all lives had infinite value, we would have no rational objection to killing whenever an equal *substitute* were available. Even if I valued Austro-Hungarian gold coins infinitely, I would not have any objection to exchanging equivalent coins. So, too, I would not object, say, to killing the newborn if they could be quickly replaced and extra inconvenience compensated for. Moreover, I would actually *prefer* to destroy and replace if the quality of what I have could be in any way improved. Even if I valued those coins infinitely (in that I would give *anything* else to have even one), I no doubt would rather have one without a scratch. Similarly, even though I value every baby infinitely, I would prefer to have one of maximum quality, as long as it is easy to have "defective" ones sent back to their maker and new ones substituted. No value of human life can preclude killing simply to improve life's quality.

These last examples begin to reveal the reason why no amount of *valuing* of human life, not even infinite valuing, can be in harmony with our intuitive regard for life: we think that the *individual* matters, whereas anything which we merely value can be *substituted* for something relevantly identical. In other words, all valuing (in common with many other attitudes) is and must be for *types* (or essences), and not for mere particular examples of such types. No matter how highly I value gold coins, there is no possible reason I would prefer one to another if both partook equally of value-conferring characteristics. If we only *valued* human life, we would likewise treat people as substitutable; since we do not so treat them, we must do more than value them.

Nor can we make do with value by saying that we value the individual examples of the type, rather than the type itself. Such a clarification is no doubt true, in that we do not value some kind of disincarnate type called "human life" any more than I value the abstract type of gold coins. But my point is that as long as the individuals are described as valuable only because they are human beings (i.e., examples of this type), they become substitutable. That is, if I value the set called "individual human beings," I cannot object to the substitution or maximization of the members of this set, even where this involves killing.

Someone might object here that I have misunderstood the way we value human beings; we do not value them merely as examples of the human species, but for their qualities as "unique" persons. Now, although it is certainly commonplace to hear that everyone is unique and therefore valuable, I regard such talk as a meaningful intuition seeking to express itself in meaningless value terminology. For even if people are all unique (which is quite uncertain except in the sense that they are not identical), it seems impossible that we could value them infinitely for their unique characteristics, primarily because the differences are just not so important. I do not care about a stranger in his uniqueness (his never-to-be-repeated fingerprints, or his special facial appearance), but in his humanity. It is only his humanity, in fact, which I know with any degree of certainty, but this knowledge suffices to make me reluctant to kill him. Again, even if all people are unique, we can hypothetically imagine the existence of absolutely identical siblings. Would our reluctance to kill one to save the others be in any degree lessened by their lack of uniqueness? I think not, but obviously something other than valuing their individual or collective uniqueness must be at the root of our reticence. We must somehow explain how the *individual* thus matters to us, in the sense that we are reluctant to kill him even when he is exactly identical to his fellows.

II. The Alternative of Sanctity

What is the moral status of human life? What is there about human life, as we perceive it, which makes us reluctant to destroy it even where we are not interested in producing or preserving it? We have seen that "the value of life" cannot adequately explain our deference to life: Even if human life had an infinite value, *individual* human beings would not necessarily be morally protected. But in fact the value of life is often treated as far less than infinite. *A fortiori* valuing life cannot give it the protection we think it deserves.

We need, therefore, an alternative way to conceptualize our moral recognition of life, a way different from saying "we value life" or "life has value." Before we can even begin to argue about whether or not we *ought* to have the attitudes we have to human life, we must adequately describe the attitudes we *do* have, and "valuing" is not an adequate description.

In particular, we need to explain how we can at once not wish to maximize the quantity (in numbers or years) of life, and yet seek to prevent the killing of every individual simply because he belongs to the type we call "people." We need to find an attitude which is both universally applicable to all human beings and particularly applicable to every individual, making us reluctant to kill even those we do not highly value. We already experience this attitude: I submit that when we contemplate killing someone, our mind does in fact recoil in a way unrelated to any worry about the destruction of something valuable. We feel that we simply ought not to kill, that life is not to be *violated* by us, that life is not entirely subject to our value-judgement and disposal. What name can we give to our regard for life?

Perhaps the first hurdle we must overcome is the modern tendency to identify all affirmative attitudes with some sort of valuing. The world and thought are today assumed to consist entirely of "facts" and "values." Is our reticence about killing due to some empirical fact of life? If not, conventional thought takes it to be a "value-judgement" about life. For such a mind-set, our proof that life cannot be consistently valued sufficiently to prevent killing could be evidence only that our reluctance is irrational and arbitrary.

Against such narrowness, we must show that value-language is a trap and prison of the mind, and that the moral world has a multitude of curious creatures in it—many of whom are at least as fascinating as those two beasts of burden called "fact" and "value."[8]

Our method, then, in the following few pages will be to look at three further attitudes which it is often claimed we take or should take to life: love, respect, and reverence. In each case, we shall first seek phenomenologically to distinguish the given attitude from valuing, in order both to prove that there do exist moral stances other than valuing and to get a better hold on the particular proposed alternative. Then, second, we shall ask whether the suggested attitude is one which would describe adequately our feelings and behavior toward human life.

Love

There is, of course, a loose sense of the word "love" which would seem to apply to many valued objects. I might say that I love steak or horses or diamonds—and mean little more than that I value them.

But love in the full sense in which we say we love God, or a spouse, or a friend, is not normally used for *things,* no matter how highly we value them. We cannot translate all value into love. More surprisingly, the converse is also true: we cannot translate our feelings for those we love into value terminology. "I love my wife" has a very different feel to it than "I value my wife." The latter, of course, seems at first objectionable because of its instrumentalist connotation; one suspects that I care about my wife only because I have some *use* for her. But the antagonism between love and value is even deeper. If anything, it sounds more inappropriate to eschew instrumentalism and to say "I consider my wife to have intrinsic value."

No doubt I can speak of valuing our marriage, but to speak of my wife herself having value seems to demean her—not because of a connotation of instrumental value, but because the very idea of valuing her seems to reduce her to a good or commodity to be prized and even priced. Such an attitude is at least different from, if not incompatible with, love. I appear in some way to have set myself above her and to be evaluating and preferring her, rather than unselfconsciously delighting in her in the way of *eros* and giving myself to her in the way of *agape.* Indeed, to speak solely in value terms of a beloved seems so misguided as to be nearly absurd.

Love is radically different from valuing. Moreover, at least some loves care about the beloved as an *individual,* while valuing regards only types. As we saw earlier, valuing is willing to *exchange,* to accept substitutes of at least equal value. Such willingness is quite appropriate for value since, as we have noted, valuing proceeds from a value-judgement, an evaluation, and it would be silly not to value two entities equally if both were judged to have the same valued characteristics—i.e., to be the same value type. Love, by contrast, is often not willing to accept substitutes, even identical ones. Even if God were to promise me that He would immediately substitute an identical person (or more than one) for my wife if I would let Him take her away, I would refuse. I do not want someone *like* her; I want *her.*

The fact that one cannot give sufficient reasons for one's love is directly related to the fact that one cares about the beloved as an individual and not as a type. If one were to claim that any characteristics of the beloved could fully account for one's love, then one would be saying that anyone else of the same type would be equally loved. But many lovers would not say this. Love can be for particular individuals instead of for types.[9]

Could this love be the alternative to valuing for which we are searching? Could it be that we are reluctant to kill because we love other people, even strangers? Without even beginning to discuss the complex question of whether love precludes killing but allows not preserving life, which the attitude for which we are looking must do, we must reject love. For although love may indeed care for individuals, in a way which valuing does not, this love cannot be extended to all human beings. This is so, not only because such love is too intimate and too scarce a commodity, but also because to universalize it is to destroy its particularity. That is, if we were to love all people simply as people rather than as "John" and "Mary," we would be treating the object of love as a type—i.e., "people." But it is the very non-type caring of love which makes the individual matter. Therefore, we can never fully love individuals simply because they are people. Someone who says he loves people cannot mean love in our sense here and may mean rather in the sense of liking a type.[10] Such "people-liking" may well be no more incompatible with killing individuals than is the people-valuing which we have discussed at length above.

The love alternative, then, will not work, but it has shown at least this much: We are looking for an attitude which finds significance in individuals, but not *only* in individuals—because it must be an attitude which can be for all human beings simply because they are such. We must somehow find a way to respond to this *type* called "people" in a way which nevertheless cares about individual examples of this type.

Respect

Let us look at the *feeling,* similar to admiration and esteem, which we call "respect."[11] In many circumstances, this feeling cannot easily be translated into value-talk.[12] I might tell a judge of my respect for his court, but I would be unlikely to tell him how I valued it. Valuing again seems connected to using, or at least implies congruence with one's desires; the judge is normally not interested in how desirable I find his court's judgements. Just as valuing seemed unloving in regard to a spouse, so here it seems disrespectful in regard to a court. Its evaluative boldness seems necessarily to obscure a court's particular kind of dignity, no matter how highly I finally rank the court in my scale of values.

Nor can we respect just anything we value. I can value diamonds, but do I make sense if I say "I respect diamonds"? The answer is obvious. The important point is not that I am silly or overly materialistic, but that the sentence does not make sense. It would perhaps be wrong of me, but certainly not senseless, to say, "I value diamonds more than anything else in the world." Nor is the problem that diamonds cannot be valued as ends in themselves, or that they are merely desired but not obligatory ends. I can say, "I think diamonds ought to exist for their own sake," or "Everyone has an obligation to produce a maximum number of diamonds." Yet it sounds like gibberish to say, "I respect diamonds." We would be dumb-founded by such a statement during a conversation.

Similarly, we cannot sensibly say, "I respect honor," though certainly many value it. Honor and diamonds just do not seem to be the proper *kind* of object for respect. The same holds for happiness, which has been proposed again and again as the final end of all action. We cannot say, "I respect happiness." Whether or not eudaemonism or hedonism has been refuted is irrelevant here. It certainly is possible to think of happiness as having great value, yet it is not possible even to imagine it as an object of respect.

If someone were to ask us why we could not feel respect for goods of such obviously high value, we might well respond "But they don't *do* anything! How can I say I respect them?" Agency, the ability to act or to participate in action, seems necessary (though not sufficient) for respect. So we can respect intelligence but not good looks, and courage but not honor. We respect not goods or goals, but virtues—not only moral virtues but also what might be called "directed powers."

Moreover, even where the object of valuing appears to be the same as the object of respecting, our stance toward it is quite different. "I value intelligence" has a different feel from "I respect intelligence." The former puts intelligence into my sphere of action and speaks of the preference it has; the latter steps back and accords the virtue of intelligence its own proper sphere of action. The first is a holding and the second a releasing.

Undoubtedly, to respect people means something important other than to value them. In a sense, respect discerns the personhood of human beings as creatures able to persevere powerfully and creatively in their aims. And although this agency is usually discovered in people one-at-a-time, it might be that all human beings are at least potentially capable of some kinds of "virtue" (e.g., moral virtue).[13] If potential virtue is sufficient for respect-worthiness, then perhaps respect is the individual and universal attitude to human life which we are seeking. Or, again, if the human *species* generates respect in us, perhaps this feeling can be appropriate even for individuals in themselves unworthy of respect. In this way, too, respect might be the feeling we seek toward human life.

Without denying the tremendous human importance of respect felt for others (and the even greater importance to human dignity of respect *shown*—i.e., treating people as though they had various virtues even when they may not), we cannot accept respect as an adequate description of our attitude to human life primarily because respect not only does not prevent killing, but it also may even cause it. Someone we respect, after all, may be a friend or an enemy. If he is the latter, then our feeling of respect for his prowess can only increase our determination to act well against him. True, we would do so with appropriate acknowledgement and consideration for his ability, and thus our opposition would not demean him, but it might lead to his destruction. Surely among the greatest epic stories are those in which two heroes seek with all due respect to kill each other.

Reverence

Valuing feels demeaning in contrast to revering, just as it did in contrast to loving and to respecting. The sentence "I value God" seems rather presumptuous and can hardly mean that I revere Him. To talk of valuing art or law, again, is to give them less importance than to speak of reverence for them. Reverence acknowledges a nobility in its object which valuing does not, a quality we may call "sanctity."[14]

The inequality of value and sanctity can be shown in still another way: As with respect, reverence for many objects of value would be nonsensical. Happiness and honor can no more be revered than they can be respected. They are just not the proper *kind* of object for reverence. We do not and cannot revere goods or goals *as such.*[15] Therefore, we cannot revere those entities which can never present themselves to us except as desired goods or goals, and we can revere other entities which we value, such as people, only by seeing them differently than we do when valuing them.

Value is not necessary for sanctity, any more than it is sufficient. One may well not like going to church, yet behave reverentially each Sunday. One might even resent an ugly church while feeling reverence once inside. Reverence, after all, harkens back a bit to its linguistic root of *vereri*—"to fear." There is no necessary correlation between that which we revere and that which we like or value. Consequently, we may well not seek to produce or preserve many objects which partake of sanctity for us—e.g., ugly churches.[16]

Nor does the revered have to have the "virtues" of the respected. I can feel reverence for churches, even if at the same time I do not have a feeling of respect for them (because I regard them as inert objects). Only if I attribute some dynamic qualities to churches in addition to their sanctity can I also feel respect for them. That which we revere does not have to have actional virtues, as did that which we respect.

And unlike love, reverence does not need to fasten *only* upon the individual in order to make him matter. Reverence can be for types, e.g. "churches" or "people." But instead of making and having its types, as does valuing, reverence lets them be. Reverence is reticent and hesitant before that which has sanctity. It seeks to leave room for its object. Above all, it seeks not to violate the object of its concern. But not to violate that which we revere means necessarily not to violate any individual examples of the revered. Because valuing seeks actively to promote its type, it cannot be bothered with individuals, but seeks to use them in furtherance of its goal. Because reverence is a largely passive withdrawing, a "letting be" of its type, it must move back from every individual instance of that type. The only way not to destroy human life is not to destroy *any* human lives.

All valuing seeks to dominate the world. Individual entities as they exist have no significance; what matters is the production and preservation of various valued types. People, facts, matter, the stuff of being become mere resources to be used in the maximization of values. All that exists is expendable, because only the abstractions we have here called "types" count. Even if these types are considered to have intrinsic or infinite value, rather than only an instrumental value, the individual examples of these types (including human beings) are reduced to the status of desired goods and can be destroyed and exchanged at will. No wonder, then, that valuing feels bold and arrogant in contrast to the other attitudes we have examined; a world we only value is a world entirely subject to our evaluation and control.

Reverence, by contrast, eschews domination. It steps back before the "sanctity" of that which is revered, and thus necessarily before every particular which has sanctity. A limit is given to us and to our schemes of domination. We can no longer destroy and rebuild as we wish, but must accept and accommodate being, even the being of individuals. If I revere human life, if I say it has sanctity, then rather than making and controlling it, I acknowledge and defer to it; I let it be. That which has sanctity is beyond the scope of our rightful judgement; even to evaluate it seems presumptuous and wrong. True, I may sometimes (but not necessarily or always) have a kind of attraction to what I revere. But even here my feeling is not the achieving and holding stance which accompanies valuing, but is rather an appreciative awe or delight.

Both universal and individual, both not violative and not necessarily preservative, reverence remedies the deficiencies of valuing, loving, and respecting and provides an adequate concept descriptive of our feelings and behavior toward human life and, in particular, of our reluctance to kill.

Are there no exceptions to the demand that human life not be violated? At first sight it may seem that there is no kind of human killing with which we feel totally at ease, that reverence always shrinks before violence toward human life.

Still, the existence of many traditional permissions to kill must give us pause. The sanctity of life in itself would seem to prohibit capital punishment, for example: Although one can argue that such punishment does not reduce the "value" of life (because by treating the destruction of life as the greatest deterrence and retribution, capital punishment obviously treats life as the greatest good), it clearly does not treat life as something inviolable. So there must be in the minds of ardent supporters of capital punishment some exceptions to the sanctity of human life—perhaps the notion that one voluntarily forfeits one's sanctity by committing a capital crime. Proponents of voluntary euthanasia or assisted suicide would likewise seem to be arguing that one can by choice give up the sanctity of one's own life. Perhaps they are right, although sanctity seems to me something one cannot easily turn off.

But it is at least clear that a low value alone cannot destroy sanctity, cannot create exceptions to reverence for life. Valuing and revering are two separate stances toward the world. One cannot argue from the judgement that a handicapped newborn has a low value life to the conclusion that his life has no sanctity and may be taken. (Nor, of course, can one make the opposite argument that because his life has sanctity it has a high or infinite value, and so an indefinite amount of resources must be expended in keeping him alive.) Moreover, there seems no obvious way to "balance" a life's low value against its sanctity; being entirely different creatures, value and sanctity have no common scale (such as "usefulness" or "satisfaction") by which they could be weighed against each other. We return to a much more specific discussion of practical policy toward life below. Here our only point is to say that the sanctity of life creates at least a prima facie demand not to kill anyone, and that the mere fact that life sometimes lacks highly valued qualities cannot create an exception to this demand.

The same point should be noted with regard to respect and virtue: Because we can revere that which we do not respect, the fact alone that a coward does not call forth respect in everyone cannot prove that everyone does not or should not feel reverence for his life. Human life may have sanctity even when it is neither valued nor respected.

Is the moral significance of the sanctity of life exhausted by a rule forbidding killing? Does reverence for life demand only that we not kill? It would seem not. Rather, the sanctity of life is a foundation, perhaps the only foundation, for all ethical principles which make individual people a matter of moral significance.

All moral attitudes which, like valuing, *demand* something must be indifferent as between individual examples of that which they seek. Only an attitude, such as reverence, which seeks to *respond* to something necessarily has regard for every individual example of the object of its concern. Only a responding can make individuals even have "reality," in the full sense of that which must necessarily be accepted and taken into account in planning how to use the things of the world. Now the word given to individuals who have this reality, who have a final and fundamental moral significance, is "persons." Reverence, by requiring the nonviolation of human life, raises in the soft clay of value the hard rocks of persons. We can *recognize* persons, we can distinguish and make each one matter, not only in spite of the fact that they are all identical *qua* human but because of this fact. Because we revere people's lives, we cannot care only about their quantity or quality; we are suddenly aware of them as individuals who cannot be sacrificed to the whole.

What does the sanctity of human life then entail, besides not killing? The answer to this question may be: everything. All interpersonal morality and all human rights may be derivable from the sanctity of life. For that which has sanctity must be seen as always also an end in itself. Our deference to it prevents us from using it in any destructive way. Metaphorically, we are forced to leave a "space" around persons, not unlike the empty and unused space in churches, within which they can manifest themselves. "Rights" demarcate this space: The necessary supports for personal integrity, such as health, acquire a derivative sanctity which demands their nonviolation. And reverence is not indifferent to personal flourishing in this space, but in service and in delight waits for human fulfillment.

Unfortunately, the attempt to construct an entire moral system founded solely on sanctity is beyond the hope of this article. And it may well be that there are other appropriate objects of reverence (such as nature, truth, or beauty) whose sanctity is not derived from that of human life. Yet even if the sanctity of life could not stand alone, it could provide an invaluable basis for other moral principles. Justice, in particular, requires as its necessary starting point the identification of those *to whom* one must be just. It needs both to know the type on which it is to operate, i.e., human life, and to separate this type into persons. It needs to operate on individuals, but in a world of pure value, individuals cannot easily matter. Reverence for human life lets justice know where to start, lets it know for whom to ready its tools of equal regard.

Perhaps such explanation of the significance of life's sanctity seems overly abstract. Let us then speak frankly of some of the direct effects which a rule against killing may have on our moral life.

Without the sanctity of life, justice is a sham. If we must be fair to the interests of everyone existing, but need not let them remain existing, we effectively undercut all demands of justice. If we must relieve the oppressed unless we kill them, then we will probably choose the latter and easier way. The idea of justice to the weak might never even occur to us if we could get rid of others, instead of having to deal with them, when they get in our way. That justice must be founded on the inviolability of the individual is so obvious it would not be worth stating were it not sometimes overlooked in the way we treat the handicapped. On the one hand, we have today a great awareness of our responsibility for just treatment of those dependent on us as evidenced, for example, by frequent declarations of child and handicapped rights. But on the other hand, we have the "common practice" of infanticide of handicapped newborns.[17] We seem to take a schizophrenic attitude toward these dependent people: we insist that we must treat them justly if they are around, but that we may make sure they die when they first arrive. I submit that the latter allowance must in the long run either destroy the rights even of the older handicapped or else convert these very rights to a pressure to kill them while they are young.

Similarly, the demand for a universal high "quality of life" masks a monstrous choice unless it is accompanied by the recognition of life's sanctity. For there are two ways to ensure that everyone living has a high quality of life: raise the quality of all lives, or eliminate those of low quality. Without the sanctity of life to exclude the less arduous second alternative, any increase in the urgency or degree of the quality of life demanded may lead to mass killing. Achieving top quality life may be felt too expensive, drawn-out, and problematic a process, and death may be found preferable. Already this seems the plight of the "defective" newborn, but unless at some point the quality-of-life ethic is supplemented by the sanctity of life, no one with any quality deficiency can be secure. Without sanctity, we are all likely to be aided only when and to the extent that aid is cheaper than poison. Whether our "defects" are physical or mental, economic or educational, only sanctity can ensure that others see these lacks as reasons to help us rather than to destroy us.

Lastly, the sanctity of life grants us an appreciation of the dignity and meaning of the human condition which we could not otherwise have. This fact was brought home to me last year when I spoke to a meeting of an association of parents of retarded children. During my speech, I had gingerly expressed sympathy for the "burdens" of such children. Afterwards a number of parents came up to me to say that they did not think of their children as "burdens"; they were just "their children," although they did have needs others did not.

Yet surely, I thought, any parent deciding whether or not to let such a newborn child die would perceive these burdens. And then I realized that these people were *not* making such choices. For them, their children were a *given,* something they simply accepted and, indeed (as I later saw), came to delight in.

Now this prochild attitude is possible, I submit, because the sanctity of life not only does not correspond to life's value but also tends to exclude a consideration of its value. Valuing is preferring; preferring is choosing. All valuation implies the possibility of an alternative to the thing valued. But here there is no occasion to compare the child's existence with its nonexistence, and to come up with the feeling that it is a burden, because the sanctity of life excludes the possibility of killing the child.

Would we be likely to call these children "vegetables," or otherwise to denigrate them, if we accepted them and sought to help them? I think not. Yet if we saw killing as an option, could we avoid comparison and evaluation?[18] To allow killing leads us to evaluate and so to "devaluate" those whom we might kill, even if we do not do so. To eliminate the option of killing does not so much cause handicapped life to be given an erroneously high "value" as place it beyond all evaluation and valuing. Handicapped lives become not merely valued, highly or lowly, but appear as the given objects of appreciation and delight.

Sanctity, in sum, by asserting the reality and importance of the individual makes possible or at least facilitates all attitudes which focus on particular persons.[19] It overthrows the depersonalizing tyranny of value, and presents others insistently to us. We must then take them into account and perhaps respond with delight, compassion, justice, or respect. Without the sanctity of human life, could even love long survive? Would it make any sense at all, say, to love a handicapped newborn if he were thought of only as a defective human-type specimen? But if we revere him first, perhaps we will come also to love him.

III. "Do Not Act or Fail to Act in Order to Have Someone Die"

Taking as data our usual feelings and behavior toward human life, we have sought to give them a name. We have focused on the curious fact that we often do not desire human life as a good or goal, and yet are deferentially reluctant to violate it in general or in its individual examples. "Valuing" was rejected as a name for this stance, primarily because such a bifurcated regard for valued objects would be irrational. Exploring more deeply, we also discovered that valuing seems improperly demeaning to human life and this fact likewise demanded an alternative to value. At the same time, love, respect, and reverence were examined; of these, reverence matched up best with the way we treat human life. Reverence does not treat life as a desired good to be achieved (as valuing would), but rather bows before the sanctity of human life, refusing to destroy any individual people (as valuing would not).

What behavior results from reverence for life? What pattern of actions is compatible both with the demand to accept life and with the permission not to achieve or maintain it? How can we both not act destructively against life and also not prolong it indefinitely?

The simplest answer to these questions is no doubt that we must not ourselves cause death, but also need not preserve life. The inviolability of life gets interpreted in a kind of spatial metaphor, so that as long as we do not "trespass" upon life we have not violated it, even though at the same time we do not come to its rescue when we see it threatened. In other words, we may not "kill," but may "allow to die"; we may not "actively" terminate life, but may "passively" stand back and let it end. Life, in this view, set limits to our action, but not to our inaction.

Now we shall see shortly that this concept of the demands of life is quite inadequate, but we should first recognize that it is clearly founded upon more than life's value. It seeks reverently to step back before life, not to violate it. No moral theory based solely upon the *value* of life could explain such behavior; to distinguish a causing and an allowing which have the same valued (or disvalued) consequences for life would be highly irrational.

Therefore, we can already conclude that all valid criticism even of these crude distinctions must take into account the attitude of reverence out of which they may arise. That is, no one can validly be driven to support active killing simply because he believes that passive letting die is permissible. To make such a distinction, he may be operating out of a sense of life's sanctity. He is against active killing because it clearly violates life; he approves of passive letting die because he *thinks* it does not. If one argues that he is inconsistent in the way he *values* life, one has missed his point. If one argues that the active-passive distinctions themselves are meaningless, then one forces him to reevaluate his approval of letting die, rather than his disapproval of killing.

Put generally, the common moral allowance of lethal inaction, omission, passivity and the like cannot be used as a persuasive moral precedent for active killing. No refutation of the distinction between these two types of behavior can justify the latter, because the very reason the former is allowed is that it is thought to be distinguishable from the latter.

With all this said, we must nevertheless insist upon the inadequacy of all interpretations of reverence for life solely as "not causing death." Such an approach would work only if the meaning of "cause" were clear and if the intention of the moral agent were irrelevant to reverence. However, neither of these propositions is true: Causal terminology is highly elastic, and reverence involves an *attitude* of deference as well as nonviolative *behavior* toward life.

All conditions "but for" which a given death would not have occurred are necessary causes of death. Yet few are sufficient causes of death. My driving a car today may well be the *sine qua non* precondition of someone else's death. At the same time, my firing a bullet at someone would not cause his death if he were wearing a bullet-proof vest. If the sanctity of life precluded all necessary causes of death, it would prohibit the automobile; if it demanded only that no person act in a way sufficient to cause death, shooting people in the chest would not violate that sanctity.

Of course, death is far more *likely* in the latter than in the former case. Could we simply say that we must not act in such a way that we make death highly probable for others? Unfortunately, no. If I carefully hide a vial of poison in a tree, hoping that some child will find it and drink it, I have surely violated the sanctity of life even if it is extraordinarily unlikely that my wish will be fulfilled. But at the same time, few would condemn me equally for voting not to lower the speed limit to 20 m.p.h., or for giving my dying aunt requested pain-killing medication, even where these actions probably or even certainly will cause death.

The difficulty in causal terminology is even clearer if we move to the situation of *dependency,* whether another person needs my help to survive. If I fail to feed my child, I can be simultaneously and correctly said to have "caused her death" and to have "let her die." The "no trespassing" metaphor for the sanctity of life does not work here. We live in constant interaction with others; human life is not like some holy altar which we could refrain from touching at all. Indeed, "not touching" may itself violate life. That is, as long as anyone in any way depends upon my actions (a most frequent occurrence), then any omission by me may be as much a necessary or sufficient cause of death as an action could be. To say that dependent persons need not be helped is to say that we may cause their death by omission just as surely as we cause the death of independent persons by action. Yet requiring of us that we never omit any treatment where this omission tends to result in death is equivalent to requiring that we never cease any treatment which preserves life—something which our reverent intuition tells us is not demanded by life's sanctity. Causal terminology either permits killing or demands preserving life. But both are intuitively wrong. Therefore, such terminology is inadequate.[20]

Moreover, regardless of whether or not a particular action is labeled a "cause," I seem a trickster if I aim effectively to bring about someone's death, but claim not to have violated the sanctity of life. If I let my child run in the street hoping that she will be run over, I have killed her even if I could be said not to have "caused" her death. If I fail to give my wife the medicine she needs to survive, in order to collect her insurance, again I cannot honestly claim to abide by the sanctity of life, even if her disease is officially listed as the "cause" of death. Both our idea of morality, which focuses on the intention of the moral agent, and reverence for life itself, which is an inner deference to the sanctity of life before it is an outer step back, seem to preclude my intent to bring about another's death by the clever use of inaction to produce a lethal situation under my control.

Should we then throw out the use of the word "cause" in explaining the demands of sanctity, and substitute the word "intent"? I do not think so. "Not causing death" is too fundamental a human response to ignore. But the word "intent" itself has a causal content: I cannot be said to place my pen in my pocket with the intent that it reach the moon unless I have posited some causal connection between my pocket and the moon. And at the same time, our analysis has been frustrated by our inability to label the morally significant causes of death. Could we not use *intent* to identify *cause?* Could we not say that an action or omission causes death if it is intended to result in death and does so? The vial of poison may be far less dangerous than my car, but I *intend* it, *wish* it to kill children. Therefore, placing it in the tree is contrary to the sanctity of life even if driving is not.

In other words: if I see myself wishing for someone's death and choosing means which I hope will bring about his death, then I have acted against the sanctity of life even if the means chosen consist only in a passive withholding of life supports. More concisely, the practical rule resulting from life's sanctity is the following: *"Do not act or fail to act in order to have someone die."*

Again, let me emphasize that we have not claimed that the sanctity of life is absolute; if it is not, then clearly no rules derived from it can be absolute. This rule would then be only a *prima facie* one, with some exceptions. However, we have not here discovered any exceptions. No one I know of has explained convincingly how life can lose sanctity or how sanctity can be weighed, say, against value. And in any event, description of the operation and limits of this rule is simpler if we state it without exceptions, and we shall adopt this simpler treatment in the rest of this essay.

Perhaps the most troublesome aspect of this rule is not what it prohibits, but what it permits. Purposely bringing about someone's death surely seems to violate the sanctity of life however it is accomplished. But we may well feel that knowingly causing someone's death, even if his death is not desired, also shows a lack of reverence for life. If I fail to give my wife her medicine simply out of laziness rather than out of malice, knowing, however, that she will die as a result, have I not killed her? If I shoot a burglar in the head, is my action in accord with reverence for his life, even if I only wish to stop him from stealing my watch and hope by some miracle that he survives? In other words, is intent here only a matter of purpose (the "in order to" in the rule formulated above), or is it also a matter of "foreseeable consequences"?

It seems to me that there may be at least some sets of foreseeable consequences which are so bound up with our desired goals that they cannot be morally separated. Can I blow up a fat man stuck in the entrance to a cave, wishing only that the cave be opened and not that he be killed? I think not. But still our rule may stand, because if I do intend consequences bound up tightly with my immediate desires, I am held back by the rule. Perhaps the scope of protection afforded by the sanctity of life varies from person to person; some people may sincerely feel themselves wishing for certain foreseeable consequences of their actions while others sincerely do not. Reverence for life could still be said to require that we not act or fail to act with lethal intent. Besides, we are not here claiming that reverence for life means *only* not acting in order to bring about death, but rather that it means *at least* not so intending death. It may mean more, or it may not.

Moreover, I think that the force of this objection to the permissiveness of our rule is greatly diminished by pointing out that a given consequence of an action or omission does not automatically become moral merely because it is not prohibited by this particular rule. We are clearly responsible for all the foreseen and foreseeable results of our moral decisions. But our responsibility may be formulated in terms other than those involving reverence for life alone. Do love and familial obligation allow me to put my laziness ahead of my wife's life? I should think not, even if I in no way can be said to wish her to die. May I shoot a burglar in a fashion obviously likely to result in his death? Justice and prudence might condemn me, even if reverence did not. May we leave a worker trapped in a coal mine as long as we do not *wish* for his death? Surely human sympathy, as well as economic justice, demand that we save him, even if neglecting him is not intentional murder. In other words, our rule is intended to be supplemented by other moral norms, based perhaps on justice, sympathy, and charity. It says only, for example, that I may not fail to give alms to a beggar hoping that he will die.[21] It does not say that I may withhold alms hoping to buy a chocolate sundae. Surely I ought to help him, or at least do my fair share to meet a societal obligation to help him, if his death is otherwise imminent. But unless I ignore him out of a death wish, out of malice against his life, I have not clearly shown a lack of reverence for life.

Perhaps the prime contrast between valuing and revering is that the first seeks to preserve its object while the second need not. The first controls, the second does not. Our maxim prohibiting an antilife intention, but permitting unintended effects harmful to life, is an application of reverence to the complexity of causation and of human dependency which is quite in keeping with the noncontrolling ethos of the principle applied.

"Do not act or fail to act in order to have someone die" both liberates and disciplines us. It frees us from the idea that life is so precious that it must receive priority in all our hopes and plans. It tells us that as long as we never wish for someone's death and act on this wish, we may strive for things other than life. Life is revered while the good life is pursued. Yet the maxim also keeps us away from the countermistake of thinking that because death is sometimes acceptable, human lives may be taken for the sake of noble aims. By making sense of our intuition that life must not be destroyed but need not be preserved, it keeps us off the slippery slope to the dangerous moral abyss where human life is as expendable as the individual things we value.

IV. Applications of the Maxim

Much more investigation needs to be done into the implications of the sanctity of human life. We have in this article described at length only a "nonviolation" requirement of reverence for life, and have specified only the minimal maxim "Do not act or fail to act in order to have someone die." The sanctity of human life surely grounds behavior other than this alone, just as the sanctity of churches demands more than not intentionally vandalizing them. Nevertheless, in an effort to provide as much help as possible in matters of life and death, we shall now seek to understand some ethical consequences of the sanctity of life, as we have so far discerned it, in two areas: medical care and public policy.

The Ethics of Medical Care

A tripartite decision procedure (in all cases where death of the patient is a possibility) would seem adequately to adhere to the maxim developed above.

First of all, medical choices must be for the sake of something other than death. According to our maxim, we may never choose to act or not to act in order to bring about death. Therefore, if we assume that all choices are motivated, there must be some end other than death motivating our choice of treatment. Now, this requirement is not particularly onerous. Other ends are almost always present as possible motivating factors. But it does mean that the hypothetical "costless" patient, whose continued existence was no burden at all to himself or to anyone else, could not be gratuitously dispatched because of, say, the low value or quality of his life. We must always be acting *for* something else, not simply *against* life. And this means also, for example, that a parent or doctor caring for a handicapped newborn could not act or fail to act in any degree out of an elitist desire to put an end to such a life because it is undignified or embarrassing. Wherever a death wish is operative in a decision not to care for a newborn, the decision violates the sanctity of life.

Second, that for the sake of which the decision is made may never be something which can be obtained only by means of the patient's death. I cannot say, for example, "I didn't pull the plug to kill him, but only to collect his insurance" (or ". . . to collect his heart"). Since there is no way I can collect the insurance unless he dies, and since I know death is a necessary means to my end, I do intend death in pulling the plug. The point seems obvious in this case, but it can be more subtle. For example, it might well be in keeping with our maxim for the parents of a handicapped child to refuse a life-saving operation which is so expensive that it would economically ruin the family; here it is quite possible that the parents are still hoping and praying that their child will live. But it would not be permissible to refuse a life-saving operation because the expenses of bringing up the surviving child would be too great; here the parents are in fact wishing for the death of the child. Note that in both cases, the motivation for refusal of the operation is to save money, and the almost certain consequence is death. Nevertheless, there is an important moral difference between them. Only in the second case are the costs the parents seek to avoid the "costs of continued life" (rather than only "costs of the operation"); only in the second case are the money benefits the "benefits of death" (rather than only the "benefits of not operating"). Only in the second case do the parents omit the operation *in order* to have death occur.

Third, our maxim must never be applied alone, must always be used together with other moral norms. We must never assume that a particular action or omission is permissible simply because it is not done in order to have someone die. Social justice, contract, sympathy, charity and all the relevant norms of a complex moral universe must be at least tacitly considered before fatal damage is done. So, for example, besides not seeking to get rid of burdensome newborns, one should also not unjustly neglect them, especially where such neglect is likely lethal.

Pope Pius XII, in his oft-quoted medical address of November 24, 1957, seems to address himself to this third point. He there declares that only failure to provide the "ordinary" means of support would constitute what we have here called "neglect." "Extraordinary" supports would go beyond what justice and charity demand, and so they need not be provided:

> "Natural reason and Christian morals say that man (and whoever is entrusted with the task of taking care of his fellowman) has the right and the duty in case of serious illness to take the necessary treatment for the preservation of life and health. This duty that one has toward himself, toward God, toward the human community, and in most cases toward certain determined persons, derives from well ordered charity, from submission to the Creator, from social justice and even from strict justice, as well as from devotion toward one's family.
>
> "But normally one is held to use only ordinary means—according to circumstances of persons, places, times, and culture—that is to say, means that do not involve any grave burden for oneself or another."[22]

The Pope's permission here to withhold extraordinary life supports is, I suggest, misinterpreted if it is taken to mean that supports may be withheld *in order* to have someone die. Note that he does not even directly mention the sanctity of life in his above enumeration of the norms governing withholding of care. Apparently, he is taking for granted that no actual attack on life is involved, and therefore he considers only the moral principles governing the extent of affirmative duties of care. Indeed, he later adds that even the withholding of extraordinary means (specifically, resuscitation attempts) is subject to two additional norms, both directly relevant to our concept of the sanctity of life:

> Even when it causes the arrest of circulation, the interruption of attempts at resuscitation is never more than an indirect cause of the cessation of life, and one must apply in this case the principle of double effect and of *'voluntarium in causa'.*[23]

Double effect and *voluntarium in causa* are roughly equivalent to the maxim of intention developed in this essay.[24] What the Pope seems to be saying is that if life supports involve extraordinary hardship, then justice *et al.* do not require that they be given—provided, of course, that the intention of the omission is to avoid the hardship rather than to achieve death.

The simple "ordinary-extraordinary" distinction is no doubt a useful rule of thumb, which normally would sufficiently protect life. It is quite unlikely that one would omit the ordinary means of life (e.g., food) unless one's purpose were to kill; and it is quite likely that extraordinary means would be omitted to avoid hardship to the patient or to others. Nevertheless, ordinary means *might* be withheld from a patient without an operative death wish by the physician (e.g., out of deference to the patient's wishes). Similarly, extraordinary means *might* be withheld in order to have a dependent patient die. So, if one treats the papal distinction as authority, one should always point out that even extraordinary care must not be withheld in order to have death occur.

Are these guidelines unduly restrictive? On the contrary, they are at once a protection for the patient and a freedom for those caring for him. The patient knows that he will not be purposely violated in his weakness, though he must also modestly acknowledge that his welfare is not the center of the moral universe. The physician knows that he is free to seek the good of the patient, of his family, and of all others affected, without the fear of death as the ultimate evil—as long as he never wishes for death and acts on this wish. He might, in my opinion, accede to the family's wish to care for a handicapped child at home rather than at the hospital, even if he thought this meant certain death for the child. His goal here might well be to provide a more loving environment for the child, and a wish for death might be far from his mind. Or, as already suggested, he could discontinue a necessary life-saving treatment at the request of a competent patient, having in mind only respect for the patient's autonomy and not a desire for the patient's death. He could, perhaps, inject a dose of morphine into a dying patient, where no other pain-killer were available, even though he knew that the dose were sufficiently high eventually to cause death. He would be acting to relieve suffering, not to achieve death, and would not be disappointed if the patient survived. Or he could disconnect "unnatural" or "undignified" life supports from a comatose patient, out of deference to aesthetic sensibilities, as long as no intent to achieve death were present and no injustice or other wrong were being done.

"Quality of life" criteria might be relevant to such decisions. The fact that a dying patient has at best only a short and/or comatose existence left could be taken into account in deciding whether further burdens on patient, family, medical personnel, and society are worthwhile. Additional resuscitations might seem to do little good where the patient could at best gain only a few hours more of possible unconscious life; and avoiding pointless draining of the hospital staff and perhaps physical abuse of the patient (e.g., broken ribs) might seem a sufficient reason not to resuscitate. In other words, the low benefits to be gained by treatment could be considered as well as the costs to be avoided. Where the sum were negative, the treatment might be discontinued in order to save these costs rather than in order to achieve death.

However, we must again emphasize that this calculus is subject to two very important strictures. First of all, in this cost-benefit weighing neither the "costs of life" nor the "benefits of death" can have any place whatsoever. It is one thing to discontinue a procedure which is a burden and is doing little good; it is quite another to terminate a life which is itself thought burdensome. Second, justice and other moral norms must be brought into play. If parents refuse an expensive operation on their handicapped newborn because they do not want to waste their resources on what their doctor calls a "defective," they are not clearly failing to revere life. They are not trying to kill him, just to save money. Nevertheless, although such a parental decision is not the moral equivalent of murder, it does seem to me quite probably a violation of familial obligation, and a gross injustice if not by the parents then by the society which does not fairly share this financial burden. In not falsely calling such calculated neglect murder, we do not and must not forget the callous selfishness which may motivate our abandonment of those who depend on us for their lives. Here again the sanctity of life must be considered not alone, but as the undergirding of justice. Without the sanctity of life, talk of justice is a sham because we can eliminate those with a claim on us. But without justice, lethal discrimination is easy. Both are necessary. Sanctity must guarantee that individual persons are recognized and not destroyed, and then justice must ensure that all persons are treated fairly.[25]

The Ethics of Public Policy

A similar procedure would be applicable to political decision-making.

First, the sanctity of life would preclude any policy choices, whether by action or omission, done in order to bring about death. Most obviously, capital punishment would not be permissible, unless some relevant exception to life's sanctity exists. Its immediate purpose is without a doubt the taking of human life. But more subtle uses of death would likewise be disallowed. We could not individually or collectively withhold food from drought-stricken foreigners, even if they are our enemies, if our purpose is to have them decimated. We also could not allow famine in order to "teach a lesson" to other countries about the benefits of birth control. One cannot judge the morality of private or governmental actions only by their effects; it is not that we must never allow anyone to die around the world, but rather that we cannot make death a goal of our programs or nonprograms.

And even where death is not obviously a goal, we must be very careful not to include in our cost-benefit calculations any of the "costs of life" or the "benefits of death," because if we do we are unavoidably intending the deaths necessary to eliminate such costs or to achieve such benefits. So, for example, as far as our maxim is concerned, it would seem permissible to leave the speed limit at 55 m.p.h. in order to maintain economic efficiency, even knowing that thousands of persons will thus be killed. We do not here desire their deaths, and may even impose safety requirements to minimize the number of fatal accidents. Death is acquiesced in rather than hoped for. However, it would be impermissible to include in a cost-benefit analysis of various suggested speed limits items such as savings on Social Security benefits as the old are killed or the net economic gain by the elimination of other "marginal" members of society, i.e., members whose consumption is expected to be greater than their production (such as the chronically unemployed). This point cannot be overemphasized, because an advancing medical technology and an increasing marginal population may soon force difficult decisions upon us. Even though these "benefits of death" are real, they must be ignored in policy-making. We must simply shut our eyes to such benefits, out of regard for the sanctity of life, in policy-making for highways, hospitals, and the care of the dependent—at home and abroad. Analysts must, when necessary, submit "inaccurate" figures on the total costs and benefits of various proposed policy options, in order not to allow the benefits of death to have any weight in public planning.[26]

Lastly, and as always, we must never think only of life's sanctity. A high speed limit may be imprudent or unjust even if not irreverent to life. Do pleasure and profit outweigh the enormous violence of traffic deaths? We cannot honestly avoid this question simply by pointing out that we are sorry about these deaths, are looking for means to prevent them, and are compensating those who survive them.

We can speak clearly about the ways we act toward other people only if we do not force all morality into value-talk, but allow words such as "sanctity" to develop an independent resonance. The ethical norms developed in this essay are the echoes of sanctity, and, as such, are meant to be taken seriously. Yet words are prior to echoes, and first of all is freedom of value-free speech.

Acknowledgment. The generous assistance of the St. Louis University School of Medicine made possible this article.

Notes

1. By "life" or "human life" I mean "living humans." This meaning, I take it, is that most commonly understood in speaking of the value or sanctity of human life. To "value human life" thus means to "value people"—except that the first phrase focuses upon those valued as simply alive, while the second pulls us away from the question of life or death and toward the complexities of social existence. Put another way, human life is the foundation which all people have in common; to value life is thus to value people simply because of this foundation rather than because of their maturity, personality, or whatever. A newborn baby is perhaps the clearest example of naked human life.

By contrast, I do not in this essay take seriously the frequent way of speaking which treats life as a thing which may be "given to" or "taken from" someone. For an organism, to live is to *exist.* The idea that existence (life) is a separate entity which can be added to or subtracted from a person seems to me a worthy subject for reflection, but only indirectly and confusedly applicable to the question of whether or not we may destroy people. When I here say "taking human life," I mean eliminating it, not removing it.

2. Except where otherwise stated, this essay deals entirely with morality, and with the moral underpinning of law, rather than with law itself.

3. Implicit here is that there is phenomenologically something *about life* which makes us reluctant to kill. We do not refrain from killing *only* out of obedience to a disincarnate moral rule not to kill, whether that rule derived from God or from ourselves. We genuinely care about not harming people, and therefore are already reluctant to destroy them prior to explicit reflection upon God's commands or upon the moral rules which we personally would like everyone to follow.

Furthermore, we do not feel such rules themselves to be arbitrary or to have a status no higher than our desires. Rightly or wrongly, we feel that they are an expression of human dignity rather than *only* of formalized self-interest or will. In this essay, I argue that this dignity cannot be called "value."

4. See the 1973 A.M.A. statement condemning intentional mercy killing but allowing cessation of extraordinary life support, reprinted and criticized for inconsistency in the important article by J. Rachels, "Active and Passive Euthanasia," *New England Journal of Medicine* 292:2 (January 9, 1975), pp. 78-80. Rachels in turn has been criticized (rightly, in my opinion) by T. Sullivan for misunderstanding the A.M.A. position. See "Active and Passive Euthanasia: An Impertinent Distinction?" in *The Human Life Review,* Vol. III, No. 3, pp. 40-46 (Summer 1977). Sullivan's distinctions are similar, but not identical, to those developed below.

5. Nor am I here or elsewhere in this essay thinking of intentional suicide. The primary method of this essay (placing human life before us, and asking our attitude toward it) is simply not easily adaptable to an examination of self-killing. Perhaps our conclusions are nevertheless applicable to suicide: See the powerful attempt by Germain Grisez to grapple with suicide within a project in many ways similar to that of this essay in "Suicide and Euthanasia," *Death, Dying and Euthanasia,* edited by D. Horan and D. Mall (Washington: University Publications of America, 1977), pp. 742-817.

6. For Calabresi's own explanation of this kind of discrepancy, which differs from my own, see "Reflections on Medical Experimentation in Humans," *Daedalus,* Vol. 98, No. 2 (Spring, 1969), pp. 387-405.

7. Note that I am here assuming only that life has an infinite *exchange* value, i.e., that we would exchange an infinite amount of anything else for one life. If one life were taken to provide infinite *satisfaction,* then we might be indifferent between preserving one life or many. Such infinite satisfaction-value would be even less able to prevent killing than would infinite exchange value, for although it would refute the claim that we ought to kill one person to save 2 or 50 (by affirming that one person has as much value as 50), it would also be indifferent to killing 50 to save one—i.e., it would affirm that no value would thus be lost.

8. Further political and historical studies would be of immense help in a struggle for liberation from value, perhaps along the lines suggested by Karl Mannheim in *Ideology and Utopia* (New York: Harcourt, Brace and World, 1936), p. 82:

> ... [T]he fact that we speak about social and cultural life in terms of values is itself an attitude peculiar to our time. The notion arose and was diffused from economics, where the conscious choice between values was the starting point of theory. This idea of value was later transferred to the ethical, aesthetic, and religious spheres, which brought about a distortion in the description of the real behavior of the human being in these spheres. Nothing could be more wrong than to describe the real attitude of the individual when enjoying a work of art quite unreflectively, or when acting according to ethical patterns inculcated in him since childhood, in terms of conscious choice between values.

9. A particular entity is distinguished not by *what* it is but by *where* it is in space-time. I can think abstractly of a table, but I cannot think of, say, the third identical table I am about to build unless I mentally insert it into space-time and imagine it existing sequentially with the first two. Only if they have differing space-time coordinates can two entities of the same type be distinguished. Only if they so exist, consequently, can they be *thought* of as particular individuals; the mind otherwise knows only quantity and quality, not particulars.

Put another way, one might say that "location" is part of the essence of an individual. In searching for a way of thinking which can respect the individuality of people, we are thus looking for a mode of thought which can take such location seriously.

10. The religious person, however, may mean that he loves God, that God loves all persons individually, and that he thus indirectly loves all those loved by his Beloved as individuals. This alternative to valuing is not insignificant, but its exploration here would take us too far from the common realm of philosophy and phenomenology.

11. The word "respect" is also used for actions which may be quite unconnected to *feeling* respect. So, for example, one might "act respectfully" in church, even though one felt reverence rather than respect. Or one might treat an authority with respect, even though one felt only fear. Or one might respect someone's rights, in the sense simply of not violating them, while feeling nothing at all or even contempt for them. Our concern here is to describe only the feeling we call respect, not the many actions we call by the same name.

12. Certainly value requires more to be treated as a component of respect and a measure of human dignity, as happens in Marvin Kohl's "Voluntary Beneficent Euthanasia," in *Beneficent Euthanasia* (Buffalo: Prometheus Books, 1975), p. 133.

13. So Michael Polanyi, in *The Tacit Dimension* (Garden City: Doubleday, 1966), pp. 51-52 writes:

> "... [H]owever greatly we may love an animal, there is an emotion which no animal can evoke and which is commonly directed toward our fellow men. I have said that at the highest level of personhood we meet man's moral sense, guided by the firmament of his standards. Even when this appears absent, its mere possibility is sufficient to demand our respect.
>
> "[B]oth this moral sense and our respect for it presuppose an obedience to commands accepted in defiance of the immemorial scheme of self-preservation which had dominated the evolutionary process up to this point."

Kant, too, makes the capacity for moral action a basis for respect for humanity, although he sometimes appears to be thinking of a feeling more akin to what is below called "reverence," rather than to what is here called respect. See, e.g., *Critique of Practical Reason* (Indianapolis: Liberal Arts Press, 1956), pp. 99 ff.

14. D. Callahan, in *Abortion: Law, Choice, and Morality* (New York: Macmillan, 1970), may be correct about some of the behavioral consequences of the sanctity of life, but he and others he cites (e.g., Gustafson at p. 325) too quickly assume that sanctity can be only a kind of value. He simply asserts that "when we speak of 'the sanctity of life,' we are . . . speaking of . . . the value we attach to human life" (p. 326). Daniel Maguire, too, despite his seeming awareness of the nature of sanctity, seems to equate it with value. *Death by Choice* (New York: Schocken Books, 1974), pp. 92-93, 156-157.

15. The sanctity of life may, however, be to some degree analogous to the "sanctity" of goods which are owned by another. We leave such goods alone, or feel numinously uneasy with them if we steal them, not because we value them *or* disvalue them, but simply because they are not properly within our control. Note that such "sanctity" necessarily has a transcendent origin: a book is more than a mere book if it is someone else's book. God's ownership of life could be the explanation of *this* kind of sanctity, or there might be a better explanation. In any event, our experience of human life seems not identical to our rather more cool and uncaring deference to the property of others. The sanctity of life may be thus not reducible to the sanctity of property, even of divine property.

16. Churches are used here as a familiar example of that which appears to have sanctity. However, sanctity need not be found only in religious contexts. A history of art teacher has told me of a recent sale of a large piece of land in which buyer and seller quarreled over who should pay the enormous costs of removing certain unsaleable monumental sculptures which neither party wanted or valued. Clearly the simplest and cheapest solution would have been to destroy the sculptures and cart away the pieces. But "the sanctity of art" made this impossible. At the same time, the low value of the works of art justified doing little or nothing to preserve them from gradual destruction by the weather.

17. Robertson, "Involuntary Euthanasia for Defective Newborns: A Legal Analysis," 27 Stanford L. Rev. 213, 214 (1975). Robertson is speaking primarily of passive (or "negative") euthanasia; but see *Pediatric News,* February, 1977, for a report of the 1974 Sonoma Conference on neonatal ethics where 17 out of 20 panelists approved the possible use of active (or "positive") intervention to end the life of a presumably handicapped infant. Most graphic is the documentary film "Who Should Survive?" produced by the Kennedy Foundation in 1971, in which a mongoloid newborn is intentionally let die by his parents and the hospital staff.

18. See David Mall's analysis of human objectification in his essay "Death and the Rhetoric of Unknowing," in *Death, Dying, and Euthanasia, op. cit.,* pp. 659-661.

19. Such tremendous functional significance cannot, of course, justify a personal or societal belief in the sanctity of life. If one "believes" in life's sanctity only because such a belief is useful, then one in fact is only *pretending* to believe—and this pretense will be dropped in private at any time, and in public whenever it becomes too costly. Only if we believe that life *really* has sanctity can we reap the full benefits of this belief.

20. That is, it is inadequate unless one adopts and uses highly conventional definitions of "cause." So, for example, one could say that only the omission of a pre-existing duty can "cause" death. But then one must develop a full description of all prior duties to others before one can make sense of a requirement not to cause death. Such a prerequisite does not seem in keeping with the immediacy of the demand for reverence for life and seems difficult or impossible to fulfill in the area of morality. But cf. the excellent application of this data to the conventions of legal causation in G. Fletcher, *Prolonging Life,* 42 Wash. L. Rev., 999-1016 (1967).

21. Note that such a hope would be joined here with an attempt to effectuate it. A *mere* hope for someone's death, which is not the motive for an action or an omission, might not be precluded by reverence for life.

22. "The Prolongation of Life," reprinted in *Death, Dying and Euthanasia, op. cit.,* pp. 283-284.

23. *Ibid.,* p. 286.

24. For a summary of the meaning of these terms in traditional Catholic moral theology, see T. O'Donnell, *Morals in Medicine* (Westminster: Newman Press, 1960), pp. 39-44.

25. Adequately to develop the proper medical-legal applications of this moral rule would require an additional article. Nevertheless, a few remarks can be made on its legal usefulness and limits.

Because of the extremely subjective nature of the "in order to," it may well be that our legal institutions are unsuited to the full enforcement of the maxim. Even so, the maxim could be a legislative guide in that lawmakers could ask themselves whether or not a proposed legal rule would make it *easy* for those with lethal intent to be successful. "Death with dignity" legislation could be carefully limited to ensure that it is at least *likely* that treatment withdrawals occur to achieve dignity rather than to achieve death. "Proxy" or "substitute" decisions (especially by interested parties) for an incompetent patient could, for example, be strictly limited, in keeping with fiduciary principles. The "trustee" for the patient's life should have far less freedom to refuse life-saving treatment than the patient himself would have, in order to avoid the possibility of the patient being taken advantage of.

But the idea of "specific intent" is not entirely unheard of in our law. It has had a place in the criminal law (see e.g., Rollin M. Perkins, *Criminal Law,* Second Edition (Mineola, New York: Foundation Press, 1969, pp. 762-764) and in recent constitutional law dealing with the intent to segregate (see *Village of Arlington Heights v. Metropolitan Housing Development Corporation,* 97 S.Ct. 555, 563-566 [1977]). Enacting into law a prohibition on the withdrawal of even "extraordinary" or "undignified" life-supports with the specific intent to end life, could serve the salutary function of clarifying and guiding medical decisions, even if because of evidentiary obstacles the laws were seldom if ever enforced. To omit such a prohibition could promote the misunderstanding that the more dependent a person becomes, the less sanctity his life has.

Yet there can never be full legal-moral congruence. The law can never forbid all omissions designed to cause death, but only lethal omissions of a prior legal duty. Law would over-extend itself if it were to prohibit, say, failure to give money to beggars with the secret intent that they die. And, too, it might be appropriate legally, by way of excuse rather than of justification, to allow intentional killing *in extremis* (e.g., lifeboat cannibalism) and/or to show mercy for merciful motives. For all these reasons, our maxim seems most appropriately considered only a guide for law making, rather than an absolute legal rule.

26. Cost-benefit analysts, in other words, must go beyond a pluralistic willingness to have their findings considered only one factor, along with morality and other influences, in policy decisions. If the "benefits of death" are to have zero weight in such decisions, but if other costs and benefits are to be taken into account, then the proposed "inaccurate" figures must at some point be made available. See M. W. Jones-Lee, *The Value of Life: An Economic Analysis* (Chicago: University of Chicago Press, 1976), pp. 3ff for a discussion of the pluralistic or "restricted" theory of policy decision. Mr. Jones also provides an excellent review of the literature on value of life vs. value of safety which is sensitive at various points to the possibility that some people's lives might be found to have a net negative economic value under those modes of analysis which do not rely entirely on gross output measurement, e.g. pp. 33, 43–46.

21.
Respect for Human Life: "Thou Shalt Not Kill"

LEWIS B. SMEDES

The Lord God declares his devotion to the earthly life of his human creatures by commanding us not to destroy it. Most people still believe what the command tells them, that every person is a gift of God, to himself and for his neighbor, a gift not to be abused by murdering hands. But there is a deep irony to our assent to the Sixth Commandment. For we are members of a race that habitually slaughters its own children. We honor those who kill, as long as they kill our enemies. We allow children far away to die of hunger while our own children gorge themselves. We prepare for nuclear holocaust, as if it were our human destiny to perform one ultimate ritual of atomic genocide. And yet we still nod a yes to the sound of the trumpet blaring the message from ancient Sinai: "Thou shall not kill." We affirm the word and yet we know it is an alien message in our world.

In its austere generality this commandment spreads a protective moral shield around every person's life. To God, human beings are dear, be they friend or enemy, productive or dependent, elect or reprobate. No quality or lack of it can disqualify anyone from taking shelter under the moral command of respect for human life.

Yet, we must look carefully at this commandment and the life it means for us to respect if we want a clue to what God expects from us in the conflicts of this life. After all, "Thou shalt not kill" was spoken on a planet where things are badly out of kilter, where some people mean others much harm, and where it seems sometimes as though the only way to rescue life is to destroy the lives of enemies who kill. And the Sixth Commandment speaks to us of life's sacredness while we care for the shrunken bodies of persons who, in terminal exhaustion, call with feeble passion for death. The ambiguities in the human family, the loose ends and tragic contradictions, compel us to linger over this commandment awhile to find out whether this simplest and strongest prohibition against killing really means that no human being may ever preside over the death of another.

What did the ancient Hebrews hear this word from

From Lewis B. Smedes, *Mere Morality* (Grand Rapids: Eerdmans, 1982), pp. 99–110. Used by permission.

the God of life say? What did it tell them? What does it tell us now? Is it an affirmation of life against all assaults on it? Or is it a narrow legal indictment of private, cold-blooded murder? We must ask also why God should have given the command. What is there about even the least of human beings that makes their lives so precious? After all, do we not all burn out sooner than later, like a blade of tender grass in a drought? In the third place, we must ask about modern kinds of killing that many civilized human beings seem all too ready to live with—suicide, capital punishment, abortion, and the decision of mercy to let people die.

I. What Does the Sixth Commandment Tell Us to Do?

A. Killing and Murder

It is sometimes suggested that this commandment should be rendered in English as "Thou shalt not murder"—a prohibition, then, only of private killings which society cannot tolerate, not a word against killing in general.

Indeed, "murder" is not an unreasonable way to translate the Hebrew verb in the command; but it is not the only way. The verb is *rasah,* which the Hebrews usually used when a private citizen killed a personal enemy. The Hebrews had other words that covered the whole gamut of taking life—community stonings, private stabbings, and most every other act of mayhem. The commandment could have used one of these other words to make an inclusive indictment against taking human life. As a matter of fact, however, *rasah* is used at least once for capital punishment (Num. 35:30) and also for accidental manslaughter (Deut. 4:41-43; Josh. 20:3). From a textual point of view, we do not have a clear case for limiting the commandment to private killings, or murder.[1]

The average citizen in ancient Israel probably thought that God was referring only to the private killings we call murder. Israel itself had a ritual for killing people by throwing stones on them—for offenses which would provoke little more than a frown in most modern societies. And who has not heard of Israel's holy massacres against the inhabitants of Canaan? Since God thus seemed to encourage the government of Israel to kill, modern readers often assume that his command against killing was aimed only at vicious violence among private citizens.

If the command meant to prohibit only private murder, God would not be much concerned with the protection of human beings from slaughter. His concern would be only with the blood-shedding arrogance of the individual criminal, while the state would have a blank check for human blood. But is it likely that God would allow open season on the state's enemies? Nobody wants police to shoot shoplifters, executioners to test their equipment on political opponents, or nations to make war to avenge an insult. The killing of human beings shakes the moral structure of life to its foundation, whether the killer is an officer of the state or a psychopathic thug. If the state kills a human being, the burden of proof is on its head. Not even the holy wars of Israel could be justified simply on the ground that a pious man was the anointed head of state. Governments like individuals are set under the command of God: Thou shalt not kill. And, because governments have so much more power than individuals, the word against killing must be directed to them even more urgently.

Limit this commandment to "murder" and it becomes a pale tautology. "Murder," after all, means any killing that society considers immoral, so the commandment would come down to the truism that "immoral killing is immoral." Nor can we paraphrase the commandment, "Thou shalt not kill illegally." Who could believe that legality is the test of God's will for human life? It was legal for Hitler to kill six million Jews and illegal for a German citizen to kill Hitler. We must assume, it seems to me, that God's manifesto of respect for his creaturely human beings is an endorsement of every person's right to exist before his Lord and with his neighbor. The text allows it; common sense requires it.

The story of the Old Testament is full of people who deserved to die. The enemy, God's enemy above all, lost his right to live. "So perish all thine enemies," rhapsodizes Deborah the judge, recalling the spike Jael pounded into Sisera's head (Judg. 5:31). Philistines, Assyrians, Egyptians—all of them enemies of the Lord and his people—forfeited the sacred protection of life. Fellow Hebrews, too—adulterers, homosexuals, abusers of parents, along with killers—were morally killable. Not everyone was protected by the Sixth Commandment.

People whose lives were marked for killing were, however, exceptions to the rule. Even in the early stages of Israel's moral history, people forfeited their right to life only by some specific and grievous offense. They could be killed only *in spite of* their humanity. The list of capital offenses may have been long, but it was nevertheless a list of exceptions to the primeval rule that everyone who bore God's image in his soul had a right to live (Gen. 9:6). The burden of proof, by implication, was on the Lord for allowing the killing. The historians of Israel were content, at least, to leave with God the justification for its own slaughters of the children of men.

B. Killing Animals

The acrid stench of burnt flesh in the temple air suggested that the Sixth Commandment was indifferent to animal life. To a casual observer, the precincts of the holy place smelled like an ordinary slaughter house. If killing was common in sacred places, do we not have a strong signal of divine disregard for the value of animal life? Or is there another message in the bleating of the slaughtered lamb?

Animals were sacrificed, to be sure, but a sacrifice was a costly price for human sin. It was not a trivial exchange, but a tragic drama. Set askew by sin, the world could not be put right without a ritual of life-giving. That God accepted the death of an animal to atone for human sin was a signal, not of his cruelty, but of how highly he esteemed the life of an animal.

Animals, after all, were God's possessions; the cattle on the thousand hills are his, and he cares for them. "The earth is full of thy creatures. . . . These all look to thee, to give them their food in due season" (Ps. 104:24, 27). No wonder that the sight of Nineveh's cattle helped move the Almighty to spare that violent city (Jonah 3:11). He allowed humans to eat meat, but only by a specific ordinance, as if animal slaughter for human consumption should never be taken for granted (Gen. 9:3). And when an animal killed a person, it was treated as a moral offender (Gen. 9:5). The animals of the world are, like human beings, embraced in the reconciliation of the world. They are part of the "all things" that are to be reconciled (cf. Col. 1:20). The wolf and the lamb will snuggle in warm intimacy to share *shalom* in the city of God (Isa. 11:6ff.; 65:25). For now, it may be, as Karl Barth says, that the screams of butchered beasts are minor sounds in the groans and travails of an unredeemed creation (Rom. 8:17), a signal that life is terribly at odds with itself.

If we cannot demonstrate that the Sixth Commandment protects animal life, can we at least assume that it calls us to great care with animal life? If we are forbidden to destroy the earthly, animal life of a human person, are we not called to reconsider our easy slaughter of beasts? Can we justify turning butchery into a major industry? Can we justify breeding cattle by the millions only to kill them out of lust for red meat? And is mass slaughter of grainfed cows not more dubious if it decreases the amount of protein available to hungry people around the world? An imaginative hearing of the Sixth Commandment may place a question mark behind our moral right to a life-style whose centerpiece is the beef steak.

C. Supporting Life

The letter of this commandment asks us only to "live and let live," hardly a summons to heroic moral sacrifice. True, if everyone merely kept his hands off his neighbor's throat, life in our ravaged world would at least have a chance. But fulfilled in love this commandment requires much more. We have not read its real demands unless we hear in it God's will for us to do all we can to protect our neighbor's human life and help it flourish. If we read the commandment as Jesus did, it becomes the law of life that gives flesh and blood to love.[2]

As the law of life, the commandment sends every person toward any neighbor in the human community who needs help to keep life going. It compels us to get food to hungry children—by all means available to us. It requires us to find free medical care for elderly people who cannot afford to buy it. It demands that we assist, not hinder, the development of the unborn toward fuller human existence. Wherever a person needs a hand to help him keep body and soul together, the moral law compels us to reach out with ours.

The law of love moves us to other people simply because they are there, living human beings whose only claim on us is their need for our help to stay alive. They are God's creatures whom he wants to exist along with us, who prize life as much as we do, but who stake a claim on us no matter what benefit or burden their life will add to ours. Never mind that there are so many of them that you need to choose which ones will stay alive because of your help. Never mind the end that always comes to your energy, time, and money. You will have to figure out a way to choose between your neighbors. The point here is only that love will not let us listen to the commandment against killing except as a call for helping our neighbor live. The law is positive and limitless. Pushed by its compelling majesty into the vicinity of neighbors who need us, we will have to pray for discernment, gather the facts, calculate the odds, and then answer our neighbor's right to life while others in this homicidal world ignore him.

II. Why Is It Wrong to Kill?

Most people do not need a special revelation to persuade them that it is wrong to kill another person. As Paul puts it (Rom. 2:14f.), the law of respect for human life is written on their "hearts." It is an intuition—a reason of the heart stronger than most reasons of the mind. Materialists who think that a human being is an exquisitely refined network of physical molecules nevertheless admit that we need very special reasons to justify the killing of any human being. Even a Mafia hit man persuades himself that he is only a kind of "social worker" whose vocation is to eliminate the unworthy. But it is not as if ordinary people are likely to shoot each other in the streets over the price of a theater ticket unless they share a biblical view of the meaning of life.

It may, on the other hand, be true that in times of great testing, one's attitude toward killing a human being will be settled by his fundamental beliefs about what a human life is in terms of its ultimate relationship. So we do well to look more closely at the reasons supporting the divine command.

Faith assumes that what God asks *of* us is also good *for* us, precisely because what he asks matches his original design for our lives. Faith also nudges us to look for signals of that design. If there is a design that determines duty, we ought to be able to see at least some hints of it. A few facets of the human life we all share, which we see in the total biblical picture of humanness, make it clear why God would lay it down as a primal obligation for every human being: Thou shalt not kill.

A. The Sacredness of Persons

Why should human creatures be the one species on earth God declares morally unkillable? The simplest reason is that human beings are persons, and their sacredness as persons puts them off limits to killers. But sacredness is a difficult quality to define. Perhaps it is most easily described by pointing to what it does to people: it inspires *reverence.* Sacredness is a holy specialness that signals people to stand off. Karl Barth had a fine eye for this sort of awe and respect:

> Respect is man's astonishment, humility, and awe . . . at majesty, dignity, holiness, a mystery which compels him to withdraw, and keep his distance, to handle it modestly, circumspectly, and carefully.

When you feel this reverence-like respect while facing another human being, you have found his or her sacred personhood, the quality that makes him or her unkillable.

I think I would rather speak of the sacredness of persons than of the sanctity of life. Not that I do not feel the power of Albert Schweitzer's "reverence for life"; and I know that some of the best arguments against taking any human life are based on the sanctity of life. Who does not tremble now and then at the awful mystery of that vital drive within, which pushes people beyond their limits to love, to grow, and now and then to feel the springs of joy within? How can one never feel reverence for the force of life inside of oneself, threatening in its flimsy unpredictability but reassuring in its vibrant persistency? But Barth warns us against letting this abstract energy or *élan vital* get a tyrannical moral hold on us. Better, for believers anyway, to remember that while God breathes the breath of life into all things living, it is persons whom he loves as his children.

We should then speak of persons—of thinking, feeling, believing creatures—who are indeed alive, but who are always something more than and different from the life they embody. Sacredness belongs to individual creatures who have names, like John Perkins or Doris Dekker. Human life therefore is not to be killed only in the sense that it surfaces through a particular person. As a moral principle, being "pro-person" seems preferable to being merely "pro-life."

What is it, then, that sets a person so absolutely apart from the other marvelous creatures for whom we care? Why may it sometimes be right to shoot a noble thoroughbred or chop down a majestic redwood tree but never to lay killing hands on a dancing child or a crippled athlete?

We could, I suppose, say that the proper study of mankind's value is man himself. And we could then sing Shakespearean doxologies to the noble work of art a woman is, splendid in her faculties, exquisite in intellect, delicate in the ways of loving. We could count the ways in which she excels all creatures and say that, in sum, she alone is worthy of being declared forever unkillable. But if we are honest, we must counter Shakespeare's eulogy on humankind with a Dostoevskian plunge into the darkness of man's soul and acknowledge the legion of demons that compete for control of his ambivalent will.

If we rest our case for the sacredness of persons on our diagnosis of human character, we could be persuaded of our own divinity and our own depravity. A little lower than the angels, we are only a cubit higher than the demons; and we have no clear signal that of all creatures on earth the one who sings of love and plans for war is the only inviolable, untouchable, unkillable creature among them.

We must see every person as someone who lives each moment in relationship with God. We need to see the religious connection if we want to recognize the essence of human sacredness. The concrete person, beautiful or ugly, productive or idle, smart or stupid, is the one whom God made, whom God loves, whose life is in God's hands, and for whom his Son died on the cross. This is the person who walks humbly on the earth as the image and likeness of the Creator who made him. We do not have to agree about what particular feature marks him as God's image—intellect, creativity, or maybe sexuality. In any case, he is, with all his gifts and in spite of all his sins, the sacred person among all other valuable living creatures.

Looking at persons with a believing eye, we may see the advantage of thinking of the *sacredness* rather than of the *value* of persons—at least in this setting. Of course persons have enormous value; God prizes them above all the earth. We mentioned this when we argued earlier that God's love knows the lovableness of his loved ones. But now we are talking about why a mere human being has no right to take the life of another person. If we calculate value at this point, we are tempted to make comparisons. Some people are more valuable to society than others; they make better toys or better tools. Others are not much to look at and not much fun to have about, and they drain our energy and cash besides. And who knows whether a horse who wins the Triple Crown might not be more valuable than a pimp who keeps a stable of prostitutes? If we rate our neighbors on a sliding scale of usefulness, we may lose our hold on the deepest reason for their right to live. Better, then, to respect every person as a sacred being whose presence in life provides the basic reason for saying: Thou shalt not kill.[3]

When I focus on the sacredness of persons, rather than on the value of life, I can respond more fruitfully to questions of life and death in the dilemmas that confront us in this broken world. The "value of life" traps us into an abstract absolutism that cannot match the obscurities of reality. If I am aware of every person's sacred inviolability, however, I am still compelled to walk into every situation where a human life is in the crucible with a directive that life be prolonged and nourished where possible. At the same time, I have to face the specific question of whether or not a sacred person is actually present in the life that is in my hands.

To accept the sacredness of persons as the reason for the command against murderous meddling is also to be aware that we need, within the Christian community, a consensus about how to recognize a person when we see him or her. If we are caring for a live body through whose lungs we are forcing oxygen and through whose veins we are pumping warm blood, we may be sustaining life without a person. And we cannot believe there is a divine mandate to force bodies to stay alive with our marvelous machines. If we are caring for someone on the edge of personal life, without a future of any personal relationship, without a hope of ever being a person in actual living ways, we are probably not mandated to say to that marginal person: "You may die when we get good and ready to let you die." Or, again, when we are confronted with a fetal life whose future is going to be both monstrously difficult and tragically brief, the sheer existence of life need not determine the morality of abortion. I am not making a pro-abortion statement here. I am only saying that it is more compelling, helpful, and relevant to recognize not value of life but sacredness of personhood as the reason it is wrong to kill a human being.

B. The Authority of God

Again and again the Bible pictures our lives as nestled in the creative hands of a sovereign Lord. He knits together our inward parts in our mother's womb (Ps. 139:13). He keeps us alive moment by moment, breathing life into us, so that when he holds his breath, we die (Ps. 104:29). He sweeps us away as we forget our dreams of last night, and this is our death (Ps. 90:5). When we survive accidents, it is because "our God is a God of salvation and to God, the Lord, belongs escape from death" (Ps. 68:20). He is above us, around us, under us, and in us: "in him we live and move and have our being" (Acts 17:28). He has sovereign right to determine our end because he in fact is the one who gives life and takes it away: man's "days are determined, and the number of his months is with thee, and thou hast appointed his bounds that he cannot pass" (Job 14:5).

God alone has the right to take life away, because he is the one who authors it in the first place. To end another person's life is to violate this basic premise. If there is a right time for any person to die, God alone may decide what it is. So it should be, for he is sovereign. The basis for the Sixth Commandment lies not so much in the sacredness of human beings as in God's creative authority.

God's unique authority to determine the ending of human life is a strong theological reason for our duty to respect and not to destroy it. But for the most part God shares his authority with us when he makes us caretakers for one another. He lets us decide whether a human being shall appear on earth by giving us discretion over conception. He gives us the right to stave death off, if we can, with medicines and machines. At both ends of life's line, he lets us collaborate. Does he also give us responsibility for death in those awesome moments when we have the power to let someone die? Does God share his authority with us to the extent that we have not only the power but the right to decide that we need not put our life-coercing contrivances in the way of his death? Divine authority over human life is a powerful reason not to kill. But his magnanimous way of sharing authority indicates that we may sometimes be responsible to act in ways that determine death itself.

C. The Community of Care-Taking

"Am I my brother's keeper?" asked Cain when he murdered Abel. The silence of God was an eloquent Yes. Cain had violated his role as brother and caretaker. In this context the phrase "right to life" is appropriate. We belong to a community of God-like persons, which flourishes only as long as each of us trusts the other to care for his life as a neighbor. Killing destroys community as much as it destroys an individual. Calvin saw the communal reason for the commandment: the Lord, he said, has "bound mankind together by a certain unity," and it is out of this bonding that the obligation comes to man "to concern himself with the safety of all."[4] Because our life is gained only in community, our neighbor has no right to assault it but has an obligation to protect and nourish it, for we are, as Paul put it, "members one of another" (Eph. 4:25).

D. The Givenness of Life

In moments of joy, when we are glad to be alive, we experience life as a gift. Now and then we feel the reality of being held up in life by a power beyond our control and we feel gratitude, which is the essence of joy. This is something different from the right to life. When we sense life as a gift, we do not so much feel a right to protection against assault as we feel a gratitude for what is given. It is simply a feeling of one's creatureliness, the anxiety of hovering over the cliff of nonbeing followed by the joy of being lifted by divine power into new heights of being. It is the feeling of being given life instead of having had to earn it.

There are paradoxes in the notion of life as a gift. Life is a gift we had to accept; none of us was in a position to choose not to be born. And it is strange even to think of our own lives as a gift to ourselves. But anyone who has deeply felt dependence on God knows that, while paradoxical, it is not nonsense: every person's life is God's gift to himself or herself. "What is given is not ours to dispose of as if we created it, not ours . . . to mutilate, wantonly destroy, and to deprive others of. Rather, if life is given in grace . . . we are to care for it and share it graciously."[5]

The gift of life can also turn very sour. This is the second paradox. Life is always a gift; but it can become an almost unbearable burden. A person may be more than ready to let God have his gift back again; indeed, he may give it to him with respectful resignation. Others, whose job it is to care for such a person, may feel bound to force him to bear the gift of life beyond the time when nature calls for release. Are we scorning the gift of life when we let nature release the person who has to bear it? To feel life as a gift is a power to rejoice in it and nourish it. But when we sense that life is a terrible burden, do others have the duty to force us to bear it beyond the span that nature itself dictates?

In the biblical world the Sixth Commandment is rooted in the reality of what persons are in relationship to God and to each other. God's creative love gives them a sacredness. In their relationship with God, they are meant to accept his sovereignty over their lives. In their relationship to one another, they are meant to care for their neighbor's life, to honor the right he has to respect, and to protect his life within the human fellowship. And as possessors of the "grace of life" they are expected to rejoice in this precious gift, which is their birthright as creatures.

For the believer, these theological reasons for the commandment provide a powerful motive for obedient response to it. For believers hear the solemn summons of the Sixth Commandment as a call to the law of their own being. Not that biblical believers alone will contend strongly for other people's right to life; and if good reasons do not always inspire a great commitment, inferior reasons may inspire a heroic one. But when believers do show profound respect for life, they do so with profound reason.

Notes

1. Brevard Childs gives a handy survey of the textual arguments; *The Book of Exodus* (Philadelphia: Westminster, 1974), pp. 419ff. When you consider the textual arguments for "kill" or "murder," the case for "neither of them is completely beyond doubt," says Stamm, concluding that the matter is basically one for Christian ethics to resolve; *The Ten Commandments in Recent Research,* pp. 98ff.

2. The Sixth Commandment, Calvin writes, requires that "if we find anything of use to us in serving our neighbors' lives, faithfully to employ it; if there is anything that makes for their peace, to see to it; if anything harmful, to ward it off; if they are in danger, to lend a hand" (*Institutes,* II.viii.37). It was common sense which taught Calvin that the sparse negative implied this rich affirmative. If the command forbids A, it must require the opposite of A; and since helping someone live is the opposite of causing them to die, the command against killing must require that we help people live. It is the logic in Jesus' word that the whole law "hangs on" love.

3. Since a person's sacred right to live without assault from his neighbor is most deeply embedded in a relationship with God, we must face up to three issues. Here we can do little more than point to the tip of the theological iceberg.

If a person's sacredness depends on a relationship with God, what of those who do not believe in God? To put it as crudely as possible: do the damned have as much right to life as the saved? The answer to this must be clear: persons are in the image of God because God made them so, not because they *admit* to being God's image. Persons are sacred not because they love God but because God loves them. The universal human right to life derives not from belief that God is the Creator, but from the fact that God is Creator. Hence, the personhood of every man and woman, boy and girl, is sacred because God is related to every person on earth and all bear within them the reason why God forbids killing people. It is as wrong to kill an infidel as it is to kill a saint.

The second question is much more difficult, both to state and to answer it. Perhaps we can put it this way: is there something sacred about a person, as he lives and breathes in the company of men and women? Or is he sacred *only* in that God's love is set on him? Is a person's sacredness built-in or is his sacredness a kind of add-on because he walks in God's presence? A man married to a brilliant and famous woman could feel that he gets his own worth as a shadow trailing at the heels of his illustrious wife; but she loves him, so he swallows his pride and enjoys his borrowed dignity. Worried that mere human beings would claim a sacredness all their own, some theologians have allowed them only a borrowed dignity, what Helmut Thielicke calls an "alien dignity," not theirs at all, but God's, lent to them because he loves them. The image of God, writes Thielicke, "is not an attribute of man himself . . . but an attribute of the relationship in which he stands" (*Theological Ethics,* I, 180).

The notion of "alien dignity" raises doubts about what God actually made when he created human beings. Did he create real persons who were truly his image or not? When he looked on his male and female images and called them very good, was he seeing only a mirror of himself, or did he see real persons before him, different from himself, yet endowed with features that were (and are) God-like in their glory? It seems clear that God relates to human beings as he does because they are splendid creatures to be in relationship with. It is not as though they get only a borrowed splendor as shadows of God. God relates to a real being, the person walking and talking on earth, a little lower than the angels (Psalm 8), a marvelous creation, superb even in his fallen misery.

Of course, we exist as persons only through the love of God. And there is no way for any person to exist except in a relationship with God. We are always God-related beings, whether we enjoy the relationship or despise and deny it. So we do get our sacredness, in the deepest sense, from our being God's loved ones. But the fact is that God relates to a somebody, not a shadow; he loves someone wonderful whom his love created. The Jesuit Josef Fuchs comes closer to truth than evangelical personalism does: "God's love creates its object—man. He is truly and in himself . . . the image of God's glory which God embraces in his love"; *Natural Law* (New York: Sheed and Ward, 1965), p. 63. On this basis, the Lord God declares to all human neighbors: You shall not kill this splendid personal creature of mine, my fallen image, my estranged partner, the one for whom my Son died.

The third question is this: if a person's holy right to live is finally rooted in God, can atheists recognize that right? Is the deepest reason for the commandment against killing hidden from the eyes of unbelievers? The issue here is not whether the track record of believers on respect for life has been noticeably better than that of unbelievers, but whether the person who denies God can share the believer's *reasons* for respecting human life.

One experience we all seem to have is a deep sense of our own right to life. I need no theological argument to bolster my belief that my neighbor ought not shoot me in cold blood; my unbelieving neighbor has the same strong sense about his own right to live. And ordinary unbelievers are usually ready to grant me a right to be left alone with my throat uncut. What, then, is the difference between my unbelieving friend's respect for my life and my respect for his? I suspect that the unbeliever sees signals of sacredness in every person; he has a feel for the mystery of a person, even though he does not have the faith to see its ground in God. "It is believed to be sacred not because . . . of a transcendent creator from whom life comes: It is believed to be sacred because it is life"; Edward Shils, cited by Daniel Callahan in *Abortion: Law, Choice, and Morality* (New York: Macmillan, 1970), p. 313. Thanks to the grace of God which has kept human life from losing all its self-evident sacredness, the unbeliever can share the believer's respect for persons' right to life. The unbeliever has, at least, a strong hunch that an ordinary person's life is sacred. The wonder is not so much that believers and unbelievers can share a respect; the wonder is that all of us violate it as often as we do.

4. *Institutes,* II.viii.37.

5. James Gustafson, *Theology and Christian Ethics* (Philadelphia: Pilgrim Press, 1974), p. 170.

Chapter Five
HEALTH AND HEALING

Introduction

What do we do when we distinguish health from illness? More than one thing, it seems. First we indicate an attitude toward a condition; we approve of health and show our disapproval of disease. Second we assign responsibility. Ill persons are relieved of certain responsibilities but are expected to seek a physician, who will be responsible for their care. A third thing we do is sanction certain patterns for dealing with a condition: hospitalization, confinement, avoidance, quarantine, etc. Therefore the way we define health is important; our definition will guide certain evaluations, determine certain responsibilities, and even suggest the appropriateness of certain responses. Definitions of health turn out to be important because in doing the defining, we must explore the relationship of health to other human goods; the relationship of health and responsibility, both of individuals and of the medical profession; and the relationship of health and those conventional modes of treating and coping with illness.

Let us examine first the relationship of health to other human values. If we define health as a state of "complete physical, mental and social well-being" (the World Health Organization's [in]famous definition), we appear to make health and human flourishing equivalent. If we do that, we lose the capacity to weigh the good of health against other human goods. If we lose that capacity, we are unable to understand Paul's words in 2 Corinthians cited below. Paul evidently thought of health as a good but not the only good and certainly not the greatest good. Note that he does not belittle his suffering by negating it either as a mere external affliction that does not affect the inner person or as an illusion that has no reality. His contentment is not mere resignation but participation in Christ and his suffering, his weakness for the sake of God's cause in the world. Compare this to how the other authors relate health and other human values! And how should we?

The second question is the relationship of health and responsibility. We often think of illness, not only as the opposite of health, but as a result of some accident or fate, a matter over which we have no control. The sudden fever of children, the appendicitis attack, the injury inflicted by a tornado—these all seem like paradigm cases of the loss of health. When we become ill, we adopt the sick role. Part of that role is an exemption from our usual responsibilities while we assume the responsibility of trying to become well.

LeRoy Walters, however, argues that this model of relating health and individual responsibility may need to be modified. He points out that we are far more responsible for the condition of our health than we usually recognize. As C. S. Lewis's little "Scrap" makes clear, if we abuse our bodies with alcohol or tobacco, we have no one to blame but ourselves when we suffer from cirrhosis of the liver or lung disease. While it may be true that we are not responsible for all illness from which we suffer, we are responsible for much of it.

Perhaps the clearest way to highlight that responsibility is to define health as a virtue, as Ivan Illich does. Indeed, Illich argues that in the name of the health of the body, we ought to constrain physicians. He points out that modern medicine is often the cause of unhealthy conditions for the patient and that we have to learn to protect ourselves from iatrogenic disease by limiting the physician's work. If we make health a virtue, however, do we blame the sick for their illness? If we blame them, does that mean that we have less responsibility to care for them and to try to restore them to health? How do we relate the ill person's responsibility for becoming ill and getting well again to our responsibilities for caring for her?

Any analysis of health and responsibility which focuses solely upon individuals will turn out to be faulty, for there are social conditions which cause individual illness. Factories which emit poisonous fumes, plants which dump their waste products into rivers which supply drinking water, poverty which makes proper prenatal care inaccessible—these are all causes of illness over which the individual may have little control. This is not to say that other persons do not have responsibility for the creation of such conditions; but it is to point out that the responsible agent and the affected person may not be one and the same. How should we relate individual health and collective or societal responsibility to each other, in terms of both becoming ill and becoming well again.

The question of the relation between health and responsibility has a particular importance for health care givers. Daniel Callahan's objections to the WHO definition include his claim that the result of such broad definitions is that physicians are given too much responsibility. In brief, the physician becomes the caretaker of complete human well-being. Paul Tillich, however, offers another very broad concept of health, one which ranges from the physical and chemical processes of a body to the spiritual and historical processes of a culture. He both justifies and limits the responsibility of a particular healing while calling for a cooperation among healers. The question is, Is Tillich's broad concept of health susceptible to Callahan's critique on the question of responsibility? Is the strength of Tillich's position, that it enables and requires a physician to be attentive to the whole person and not just to the chemical and biological processes of the body, also its weakness, in that it opens the door for an illegitimate expansion of the physician's role? Can we define health in such a way as to restrict and restrain the responsibilities of physicians while at the same time calling upon them to care for the whole person? How should we relate health and the responsibility of physicians?

Finally, the issue of the relationship of health and the conventional models of coping with and treating illness needs to be considered. If we define health too broadly, we tend to want to treat social problems and spiritual problems and deviancy and crime and numerous other problems on the medical model; but should we? And if the answer is no, then how can we appropriately restrict the medical model *and* attend to other ways of ministering to the sick? How can we both restrict the applicability of the medical model and also avoid compartmentalizing the care of the whole person? Can we define health to allow analytic precision, scientific medicine, and the expression of the interrelatedness of life? And can we nurture physicians who care for the whole person through their care of the body?

Suggestions for Further Reading

Beckman, Richard J., and Steven J. Nerheim. *Toward a Healing Ministry: Exploring and Implementing a Congregational Ministry.* Minneapolis: Augsburg, 1985.

Calian, C. S. "Theological and Scientific Understandings of Health." *Hospital Progress* 59 (Dec. 1978): 45-47, 61-62.

Caplan, Arthur L., H. Tristram Engelhardt, Jr., and James J. McCartney, eds. *Concepts of Health and Disease: Interdisciplinary Perspectives.* Reading, Mass.: Addison-Wesley, 1981.

Dubos, Rene. *Mirage of Health.* Garden City, N.Y.: Doubleday, 1959.

Hiltner, Seward. "The Bible Speaks to the Health of Man." In *Dialogue in Medicine and Theology,* edited by Dale White. Nashville: Abingdon, 1968.

Illich, Ivan. *Medical Nemesis: The Expropriation of Health.* New York: Pantheon, 1975.

Kelsey, M. T. *Healing and Christianity.* New York: Harper and Row, 1973.

Marty, Martin E. *Health and Medicine in the Lutheran Tradition: Being Well.* New York: Crossroad, 1982.

McCormick, Richard A. *Health and Medicine in the Catholic Tradition.* New York: Crossroad, 1984.

Seybold, Klaus, and Ulrich B. Mueller. *Sickness and Healing,* trans. by Douglas Stott. Nashville: Abingdon, 1978.

Vaux, Kenneth. *Health and Medicine in the Reformed Tradition: Promise, Providence, and Care.* New York: Crossroad, 1984.

22.
2 Corinthians 12:7–10

To keep me from being too elated by the abundance of revelations, a thorn was given me in the flesh, a messenger of Satan, to harass me, to keep me from being too elated. Three times I besought the Lord about this, that it should leave me; but he said to me, "My grace is sufficient for you, for my power is made perfect in weakness." I will all the more gladly boast of my weaknesses, that the power of Christ may rest upon me. For the sake of Christ, then, I am content with weaknesses, insults, hardships, persecutions, and calamities; for when I am weak, then I am strong.

23.
Sickness and Illusion

KARL BARTH

We have so far accepted the fact that man has the strength to be as man, that he can will and affirm it as such, and that he can therefore will and adopt the corresponding measures of this will in the sphere of his vital functions of soul and body. We have understood disease as merely the weakness opposed to this strength, as that which is not to be willed but contested in the will to live, as the shadow which recedes as it were before health and the will for health. This is one aspect of the matter. But there are two very different aspects, and we must now try to explain what the will to be healthy is in relation to them. We may begin by saying generally that sickness is not an illusion, even though there is such a thing as illusory sickness and therefore those who are ill only in their imagination. . . .

If we see the problem of psychical and physical health and sickness properly in its unity, and this unity itself from a higher standpoint, i.e., in the light of the question of the strength or weakness to be as man, we can only regard and treat the victim of imaginary ailments as one who is really very ill, although not in the way that he thinks. We certainly cannot ridicule him, or find in him support for the general proposition that all sickness is an illusion. Sickness is no illusion, whether in relation to the opposing will to live in the true and secondary sense, or objectively as a different condition from the real strength to be as man and the freedom of secondary vital forces, or in relation to God as the Creator of human life and the will to live.

The tenet that sickness is an illusion is the basic negative proposition which in the seventies of the last century the American Mary Baker Eddy said that she did not lay down but "discovered" through the authoritative inspiration of a book now regarded as canonical, namely, *Christian Science.* What was at first a small group of adherents has since spread to all parts of the world in the form of religious societies which are particularly popular among the upper and middle classes and more especially among women. Karl Holl has depicted and done it almost too much justice in a careful study entitled "Scientismus" (*Ges. Aufs. z. Kgsch.,* III, 1928, p. 460 f.). The positive basis of this teaching is that God is the only reality, that he is Spirit and that the whole creation is only a reflection of his spiritual essence. Apart from God there are only powers, which in reality are only thoughts. All matter as such represents a mere appearance, and the same is true of all such associated features as sin, sickness, evil and death. Man as the image of God always was and is and shall be perfect. Everything that contradicts this perfection is in reality only an illusion and misunderstanding rooted in the forgetfulness of God, which in turn evokes fear. And fear is the true basis of all illness; indeed, it is actually illness itself. For fear creates a picture of illness which then falls externally upon the body. "You maintain that an ulcer is painful; but that is impossible, for matter without mind is not painful. The ulcer merely reveals by inflammation and swelling an appearance of pain, and this appearance is called an ulcer." The true and psychical man is not touched by it. He is only as it were enveloped in a mist and has disappeared from consciousness. Evil is unreal. "Take away fear, and at the same time you have also removed the soil on which sickness thrives." Jesus was and is the embodiment of truth which scatters and breaks through the mist of these false appearances. The power bestowed and the task presented by Him consist in recognising that God is Spirit and that man belongs to Him and is eternally at one with the God who is Spirit. It thus consists in freeing oneself from the false appearances of sin (which even Mrs. Eddy puts first), sickness and death. For death, too, is only man's "disappearance from our level of consciousness." Supremely, this power and task are identical with prayer, in which everything evil really subsides into nothingness. Any other measures, and especially the well-meant action of the doctor, are a sin against the first commandment. Medical diagnosis, which Mrs. Eddy regards as particularly evil, is replaced by "mind-reading," which is possible at a great distance and in which the thought images which dominate the sufferer are noted. Medical treatment is supplanted by prayer, in which it can only be a matter of acknowledging the cure already effected by God, of understanding His completed work and of initiating it in the patient. The "healer"—the name given to the active members of the Christian Science Association—is not then to rouse and fortify the will of others through his own, but simply to make a free path in the sufferer for the divine operation. "Call to mind the presence of health and the fact of harmonious existence, until the body corresponds to the normal condition of health and harmony."

This doctrine has several features which remind us of the message of the New Testament, and which are of course derived from it: the recognition of fear as the basic evil in man's relation to God; an unconditional trust in the efficacy of prayer; and bold reference to a work already completed by God. But these are all devalued by the fact that they are related to a view which has nothing to do with that of the New Testament but in the light of it can only be described as utterly false. The fact that Christian Science can undoubtedly point to successes in healing—as well as to disastrous failures—cannot of itself commend it to Christians. As is well-known, the magicians of Pharaoh could do quite a number of things. And the concession that Karl Holl (*loc. cit.,* p. 477) is willing to make, namely, that its positive presupposition at least is correct, is one which cannot really be made to it. God is indeed the basis of all reality. But He is not the only reality. As Creator and Redeemer He loves a reality which is different from Himself, which depends upon Him, yet which is not merely a reflection nor the sum of His powers and thoughts, but which has in face of Him an independent and distinctive nature and is the subject of its own history, participating in its own perfection and subjected to its own weakness. As the coming of the kingdom, the incarnation of the Word and the death and resurrection of Jesus Christ in His true humanity are not just an appearance, so it is with man in general, whether in his nature or perversion, in his psychical being or his physical, in his divine likeness or his sin and transgression. It is because Mrs. Eddy did not understand this that sin, evil and death—in conquest of which Jesus Christ did not "disappear from our level of consciousness" but actually died on the cross—are for her mere "appearances" of human thinking, and redemption is only the act of man in which he submerges himself in God and leads a life submerged in God in order that God may work in him, putting an end to those "appearances" or thought images and bringing to light the perfection of psychical essence which was never lost, the presence of health and the fact of harmonious being. On this point we can only say that both the Old and New Testaments regard not only God and man, not only sin, evil and death and their conquest, but also sickness in a different light. They certainly do not see it as an illusion, and its conquest as the dispelling of this illusion. Whether Christian Science is really "science" need not occupy us here. But there can be no doubt that it is not "Christian" science.

Sickness is real. Certainly, as an encroachment on the life which God has created, it is not real in the same way as God is. In what sense, then, is it real? We shall take up this point in a moment, but we may begin by simply observing that if man, even the sick man, is really healthy in the strength which he still has and can still exert to be as man, then the weakness which opposes this strength is not as such an appearance but is effective and real, so that his will for health already meets a hard "object" in this primary and essential sense. But the same is also true of the impairing of his psychical and physical powers which takes place in illness. His transition from health to sickness, the resistance which illness offers to his health, the effort and trouble which it costs if he or the doctor adopts the appropriate measures against it, the obstinacy with which it maintains itself in spite of all these measures, the triumphs which it can enjoy in spite of them—these are not all plays of the imagination, but real events in the real history of the real man. And the will to live as the will for health is a serious act of obedience to a serious command of God because man is not dealing with a fake or imaginary opponent but with an enemy which is in some sense real. Yet the question arises what kind of reality this is. And we must try to explain this if we are to understand more deeply and seriously what the will to be healthy really means and does not mean. Again, however, two different aspects open up before us.

The one aspect which dominates the field in the Old and New Testament Scriptures, and which has always to be remembered first materially, is the one in which sickness is a forerunner and messenger of death, and indeed of death as the judgment of God and the merited subjection of man to the power of nothingness in virtue of his sin. From this standpoint, sickness like death itself is unnatural and disorderly. It is an element in the rebellion of chaos against God's creation. It is an act and declaration of the devil and demons. To be sure, it is no less bound to God and dependent on Him than the creature which He created. Indeed, it is impotent in relation to him in a double way. For like sin and death it is neither good nor is it willed and created by God at all, but is real, effective, powerful and menacing only as part of that which He has negated, of His kingdom on the left hand, and therefore with its nullity. But in accordance with the will of God and under His reign it is necessarily dangerous—as the forerunner and messenger of death, the executor of God's final sentence—to the man who has fallen from God and become His enemy.

What does health mean as the power to be as man, and what do the vital functions of soul and body mean as the sphere for the exercise of this strength, if sickness is this reality, if it is an element and sign of the power of the chaos threatening creation on the one hand, and on the other an element and sign of God's righteous wrath and judgment, in short, an element and sign of the objective corruption which is related and corresponds to human sin and from which there is no deliverance apart from the mercy of God in Jesus Christ? . . .

What does health mean from this standpoint, and what is the meaning of the will to be healthy in the primary and secondary senses in which we have hitherto understood it?

The following consideration suggests itself. When seen in this way, sickness is a superior power in relation to which there can be no question at all of health or the will to be healthy. What is man with his health and will for health in face of the invasion of the realm of death to which he himself has deliberately opened the defences? What is he in face of the divine judgment by which he is overtaken in this assault? What can he do in this situation? What can the whole field of ethics tell him in these circumstances? What is there left to will? Strength to be as man? Psycho-physical powers? Is it not almost grotesque from this standpoint to try even to think of a human determination, let alone of human measures, along the lines considered? Are not faith and prayer the only real possibilities in face of this reality of sickness?

But this whole consideration is only defeatist thinking, and not at all Christian. It overlooks the fact that the command of God is not withdrawn but still in force, namely, that man must will to live and not die, to be healthy and not to be sick, and to exercise and not neglect his strength to be as man and the remaining psycho-physical forces which he has for this purpose, and thus to maintain himself. This command has not been revoked even for sinful man forfeited to the judgment of God, and it is not for him to counter God with speculations whether obedience to it is possible or offers any prospects. Unquestioning obedience is his only option if he is not to bring himself into greater condemnation. Again, this consideration overlooks the fact that the realm of death which afflicts man in the form of sickness, although God has given it power and it serves as an instrument of His righteous judgment, is opposed to His good will as Creator and has existence and power only under His mighty No. To capitulate before it, to allow it to take its course, can never be obedience but only disobedience towards God. In harmony with the will of God, what man ought to will in face of this whole realm on the left hand, and therefore in face of sickness, can only be final resistance. Again and supremely, this consideration overlooks the fact that God Himself is not only Judge but faithful, gracious and patient in His righteous judgment, that He Himself has already marched against that realm on the left, and that He has overcome and bound its forces and therefore those of sickness in Jesus Christ and His sacrifice, by which the destroyer was himself brought to destruction. Those who know this, and therefore that they are already helped in this matter, can only reply to the faithfulness of God with a new unfaithfulness if they try to fold their hands and sigh and ask what help there is or what more they can will. Within the modest limits in which this is still possible they must will what God has already willed and indeed definitely fulfilled in Jesus Christ concerning sickness and that whole kingdom on the left hand. With God they must say No to it without asking what the result will be or how much or little it will help themselves or others, without enquiring whether it is not rather feeble and even ridiculous to march into action in accordance with this No. A little resolution, will and action in face of that realm and therefore against sickness is better than a whole ocean of pretended Christian humility which is really perhaps the mistaken and perverted humility of the devil and demons.

There is, of course, a right deduction to be drawn from the fact that sickness is real in this sense, i.e., as an element and sign of the power of chaos and nothingness, and therefore as an element and sign of the judgment of God falling on man. The right deduction is that all resistance to sickness, all human willing of the strength to be as man, all human affirmation, cultivation and promotion of the vital forces of body and soul, is necessarily in vain if God is not God; if He does not live, speak, act and make Himself responsible for man; if this whole cause is not first and supremely His own cause; if His is not the judgment on man from which we cannot escape; if His is not the grace which is the meaning of this judgment; and above all if His is not the judgment on the destroyer and destruction itself which by reason of man's sin can have a little space, but which can have only the space allowed and allotted by God, and in relation to which God is absolute Lord and conclusive Victor. Without or even against God there is, of course, nothing that man can will in this matter. And if faith in Him and prayer to Him cannot be a refuge for weak-willed and defeatist Christians who are lazy, cowardly and resigned in face of His and their enemy, we must also say with the same certainty that if the conflict enjoined upon man in this matter is to be meaningful, faith in Him and prayer to Him must never be lost sight of as its *conditio sine qua non,* but continually realised as the true power of the will required of man in this affair. They cannot replace what is to be modestly, soberly and circumspectly, but energetically, willed and done by man. They cannot replace his determination to exercise his little strength to be as man, and thereby to maintain himself. They cannot replace hygiene, sport and medicine, or the social struggle for better living conditions for all. But in all these things they must be the orientation on the command of God which summons man inexorably, and with no possible conditions, to will and action. They must be the orientation on the righteous judgment of God in recognition of which man constantly discovers, and again without murmuring or surrender, the limitation of his willing and doing and its consequences. Above all, they must be the orientation on the inexhaustible consolation of the promise, on true and effective encouragement by the One who as the Creator of life primarily espouses this as His own cause, and fights and has already conquered for us in the whole glory of His mercy and omnipotence. It is true that without Him, without the orientation on Him, all ethics, all human willing and doing, can only be futile and impotent in relation to the superiority of evil which opposes us also in the form of sickness; and worse still, that it can only be rebellion against the judgment of God and therefore increase its severity. But it is also true, and even more so, that human willing and acting with God, and in orientation on Him, and with faith and prayer to Him, whatever the outcome, has the promise which man cannot lack, and the fulfilment of which he will soon see, if he will simply obey without speculation. Those who take up this struggle obediently are already healthy in the fact that they do so, and theirs is no empty desire when they will to maintain or regain their health. . . .

But the fact is undeniable that sickness has also another aspect. For health, like life in general, is not an eternal but a temporal and therefore a limited possession. It is entrusted to man, but it does not belong to him. It is to be affirmed and willed by man as a gift from God, yet not in itself and absolutely, but in the manner and compass in which He gives it.

We have defined health as the power to be as man exercised in the powers of the vital functions of soul and body. And we have defined sickness as the impairing of this power, as crippling and hampering weakness. We have seen that in the antithesis, contrast and conflict of these two determinations of human life we have to do with a real event in the existence of the real man. And we have first attempted to evaluate this event from the angle from which it presents itself as the collision of normal being, as willed, created and ordered by God, with its negation, so that it is brought under the threat of abnormality and even destruction. On this view it can be understood only as man's encounter with the realm of death and therefore the experience of God's judgment. We have been able to describe the required human attitude, the will to live and to be healthy, only in terms of the resistance and conflict of faith and prayer appealing to the grace and gracious power of God. And if we have now to draw attention to another aspect of the same matter, there can be no question—we are irresistibly prevented by the biblical witness concerning health and sickness—of looking away again from this first aspect or even trying to relativise or weaken it. Sickness is one of the elements in the situation of man as he has fallen victim to nothingness through his transgression, as he is thus referred wholly to the mercy of God, but as he is summoned by this reference to hope and courage and conflict. Not a single word of what we have said in this connexion can be retracted or even limited. It must not be lost sight of or forgotten in whatever we may have to add.

What is there to be added? Simply that, quite apart from his transgression, quite apart from his abandonment to the power of nothingness, and quite apart from the consequent visitation of God's judgment upon him, the life of man, and therefore his health as the strength to be as man in the exercise of the powers of all his vital functions of life, is a life which even according to God's good will as Creator, and therefore normally and naturally, begins and ends and is therefore limited. Man does not possess the power to be as man in the same way as God has His power to be as God, nor does he have power over his vital functions as God has His power as Creator, Ruler and merciful Deliverer of His creature. It does not belong to him to be and to live as God. Rather, he may see the goodness of God the Creator in the fact that to his life and strength and powers a specific space is allotted, i.e., a limited span. He may and should exercise them in it and not in the field of the unlimited. They are adapted for it, for development and application within it. Within its confines he may and should be as man in their possession and exercise. Within its confines he stands before God, and at the limit of this span God is mightily for him and is his hope. Just because it is limited, it is a kind of natural and normal confirmation of the fact that by God's free grace man may live through Him and for Him, with the commission to be as man in accordance with the measure of his strength and powers, but not under the intolerable destiny of having to give sense, duration and completeness to his existence by his own exertions and achievements, and therefore in obvious exclusion of the view that he must and may and can by his own strength and powers eternally maintain, assert and confirm himself, attaining for himself his own dignity and honour. The eternal God Himself guarantees all this, and tells him that He does so by giving him a life that is temporal and therefore limited. In this way it always remains in His hand both in its majesty and in its littleness. In itself and as such this fact cannot be an object of complaint, protest or rebellion, nor can the fact that man must make the concrete discovery that his life and therefore his health and strength and powers are not an unlimited reality, but that he is impeded in their possession and exercise, that weakness is real as well as strength, that there is destruction as well as construction, obstruction as well as development. This is all the more terrible because it is just from this direction that we find ourselves threatened by death and judgment. But is it really surprising and shocking in itself? The life of man, his commission, and his strength to fulfil it, are not limited accidentally but by God, and therefore not to his destruction but to his salvation. Inevitably, then, he always in some way comes up concretely against this boundary of his life. Inevitably he must grow old and decline. Inevitably he must concretely encounter his Creator and Lord and therefore God's omnipotence and mercy. But is it merely a question of necessity? In the correct sense, is it not true to say that, no less than in his unimpeded movement within these confines, this is also a possibility. May it not be that genuine freedom to live can and must be concretely realised in the fact that in the impeding and impairing of his life he is shown that neither his life nor he himself is in his own hand, but that he is in God's hand, that he is surrounded by Him on all sides, that he is referred wholly to Him, but also that he is reliably upheld by Him? Does not this freedom begin at the very point where we are confronted by the hard actuality of the insight that "Christ will be our consolation"? But what if sickness as the concrete form of weakness, of destruction, of the impairing of his strength and powers, of growing old and declining, is the hard actuality which ushers in this genuinely liberating insight? What if it is not only the forerunner and messenger of death and judgment, but also, concealed under this form, the witness to God's creative goodness, the forerunner and messenger of the eternal life which God has allotted and promised to the man who is graciously preserved and guided by Him within the confines of his time?

24.
A Scrap

C. S. LEWIS

'You are always dragging me down,' said I to my Body. 'Dragging *you* down!' replied my Body. 'Well I like that! Who taught me to like tobacco and alcohol? You, of course, with your idiotic adolescent idea of being "grown-up". My palate loathed both at first: but you would have your way. Who put an end to all those angry and revengeful thoughts last night? Me, of course, by insisting on going to sleep. Who does his best to keep you from talking too much and eating too much by giving you dry throats and headaches and indigestion? Eh?' 'And what about sex?' said I. 'Yes, what about it?' retorted the Body. 'If you and your wretched imagination would leave me alone I'd give you no trouble. That's Soul all over; you give me orders and then blame me for carrying them out.'

25.
In Search of Health

LEROY WALTERS

In the past, "health" seemed to be a relatively simple and straightforward concept. However, in recent years increasing controversy has surrounded that concept. To illustrate, here are two quotations. The first is taken from a 1973 article by Peter Sedgwick, a British social scientist:

> All departments of nature below the level of mankind are exempt both from disease and from treatment. The blight that strikes at corn or at potatoes is a human invention, for if man wished to cultivate parasites rather than potatoes (or corn) there would be no "blight" but simply the necessary foddering of the parasite-crop. Animals do not have diseases either, prior to the presence of man in a meaningful relation with them. . . . Outside the significance that man voluntarily attached to certain conditions, there are no illnesses or diseases in nature.

The second quotation appears in the preamble to the constitution of the World Health Organization (WHO): "Health is a state of complete physical, mental and social well-being and not merely the absence of disease or infirmity."

Three questions are raised by these quotations. First, how broadly should the concept of health be construed or applied? Second, is health a natural norm or an arbitrary label? And third, is health to be considered a minimum, a maximum, or something in between, some sort of golden mean?

It is easy for the concept of health to become so broad that it ends up as virtually the equivalent of happiness—or even salvation. This breadth is one of the problems of the WHO definition. If one enjoys "a state of complete physical, mental, and social well-being," what else remains to be enjoyed? For the sake of clarity and simplicity I will consider only the health of bodies, not that of minds or of whole societies. Thus, I will accept only the first aspect of the WHO definition: health is a state of "physical well-being."

With this narrowed definition it is then possible to assert that (physical) health is a natural norm and not merely an artificial construct. In the mental health field mere social deviancy is often labeled as mental illness. In the realm of physical health, however, I think there will be a broad consensus on what is or is not healthy. A deer or a person riddled with cancer is unhealthy, as is the shattered victim of a serious auto accident. On the positive side, we have relatively clear concepts of healthy athletes and even healthy squirrels.

The WHO definition would require that health be a maximum: *complete* physical well-being and not merely the absence of disease or infirmity. In my view, this definition requires too much. Complete physical well-being sounds like an ideal which few of us are likely ever to attain. On the other hand, a bare minimum of well-being seems inadequate to satisfy our concept of health. Therefore, I suggest that we regard physical health as a kind of mean. In other words, health is functional normality or, in the words of Leon R. Kass, "the well-working of the [physical] organism as a whole."

I

Although it is generally assumed that medical care has contributed significantly to the health of human beings, that contribution is frequently overrated. According to Victor Fuchs, a health economist at Stanford University, it was not until well into the 20th century that the average patient had a better than 50-50 chance of being helped by the average physician.

During the past 200 years most of the change in longevity has been due to a reduction in death rates at early ages. "Normal" life expectancy has lengthened very little: for example, between 1900 and 1970 the average life expectancy of persons who reached the age of 65 increased by only one and one-half years.

Much of the improvement in health during the 19th and 20th centuries—especially prior to the mid-1930s—is attributable to better nutrition, falling birth rates, rising living standards, and public health measures: primarily the chlorination of water, the pasteurization of milk, and indoor plumbing. Consider, for example, the case of the "pneumonia-diarrhea" complex. During the 19th century infants and children frequently caught infections which led to chronic diarrhea; the diarrhea in turn often weakened the children's resistance so severely that they became ill with pneumonia and died. In New York city, deaths from this syndrome fell about 80 per cent between 1900 and 1930—this before the advent of antibiotics (statistics from *Who Shall Live?,* by Victor R. Fuchs [Basic Books, 1974]).

It must in fairness be conceded that since 1935 medicine *has* contributed significantly to health, particularly the health of infants and children. Antibiotics and vaccines have been developed for the control of diphtheria, typhoid fever, polio, measles, influenza and certain types of pneumonia. This record of success in the conquest of infectious diseases has sometimes been called the "Golden Age of Medicine."

In dealing with the chronic diseases of adults, however, medicine has not been able to achieve similar increases in life expectancy. Intractable chronic diseases are some of the major killers of our time: heart disease, cancer, stroke. Many of the medical measures used in "treating" them are only palliative; some are also highly expensive. Kidney dialysis, for example, costs approximately $30,000 per year and does nothing to improve the patient's underlying disease. And there is always the possibility that medical care will do harm as well as good: through the side-effects of radiation, drug reactions, infections contracted in hospitals, or the aftereffects of surgery.

In sum, with the exception of antibiotics and vaccines—especially in the case of infants and children—medical care has not made as significant a contribution to health as is sometimes supposed. Indeed, modern medicine has made only slight progress toward the conquest of chronic diseases.

II

In several recent publications on the quest for health there has been a rather decisive shift away from the search for medical cures and toward the issue of personal responsibility for one's own health status. One way into this issue has been to consider the major causes of death in persons 15–24 years of age. Among white males, the five leading causes of death are, in order, motor accidents, other accidents, suicide, cancer and homicide. Only one of these five is a disease, strictly defined.

Dean Lester Breslow and his colleagues at the UCLA School of Public Health have recently completed a series of studies investigating correlations between health practices and physical health status. Inductively, these researchers have discovered seven "rules" which seem to correlate very well with both general healthiness and longevity:

1. Don't smoke cigarettes.
2. Get seven or eight hours of sleep each night.
3. Eat breakfast.
4. Keep your weight down.
5. Drink moderately.
6. Exercise daily.

7. Don't eat between meals.

The Breslow group reports some startling findings in connection with these rules. The physical health status of individuals over 75 who have followed all the rules is about the same as that of people aged 35-44 who observe fewer than three. A person who adheres to at least six of the seven rules has at age 45 a life expectancy 11 years longer than someone who has followed fewer than four. And we may note in passing that "visit your doctor regularly" does not appear on the list!

A further illustration: Victor Fuchs, in *Who Shall Live?,* recounts "The Tale of Two States," Utah and Nevada. Of course, not all Nevadans live in Las Vegas, and not all residents of Utah are abstemious Mormons. But these two adjacent states, with similar income levels and similar numbers of physicians and hospital beds per capita, are at opposite ends of the spectrum in average health status. Adult death rates for Nevada are generally 40-50 per cent higher than for Utah. Deaths resulting from cirrhosis of the liver and lung cancer among males in their 30s are almost *seven* times as high in Nevada as in Utah.

The upshot of all these statistics would seem to be that our life style may have more of an impact on our dying from certain diseases than all the most modern techniques of medical care. Thus, rather than asserting that health is a right, we may need to concede that, at least in certain respects, health is a duty.

Several caveats are in order, lest we overstate the case. Debilitating and even lethal genetic diseases do exist, and a change of life style usually cannot improve the health status of persons suffering from such diseases. There are also environmental determinants of health; e.g., toxic substances in the air, which cannot be controlled by those who are victims of their effects. However, for most of us there remains a significant realm in which our own voluntary behavior and life style have a direct and substantial impact on our personal health status.

III

At the level of public policy, we are faced with a number of difficult questions. How much of the nation's "health" dollar should go into the medical-care sector, and how much should be invested in building tennis courts and jogging tracks or in ensuring adequate nutrition for children? Then, within the medical-care sector, what type of health programs should receive highest priority: ones for crisis medicine, like kidney dialysis, or health-maintenance and preventive-medicine programs?

Another dilemma involves who should pay health-care costs which arise from the patient's own negligence or overexuberant style of life. This problem will become even more serious if a comprehensive program of national health insurance is ever enacted. In the words of one wry commentator: "Utah may be unwilling to pay for the sins of Nevada."

There are also dilemmas to be faced at a more personal level. Physical health is important, and a certain minimum level of health is essential to achieving any other goals in life. Yet there may be times when the benefit of health comes squarely into conflict with other important values—such as responding to friends or working to attain excellence or being faithful to one's Christian commitment.

To illustrate how this conflict may arise, let me cite a few autobiographical lines from a letter of an early Christian missionary, the Apostle Paul:

> Five times the Jews have given me the thirty-nine strokes; three times I have been beaten with rods; once I was stoned; three times I have been shipwrecked, and for twenty-four hours I was adrift on the open sea. I have been constantly on the road; I have met dangers from rivers, dangers from robbers, dangers from my fellow-countrymen, dangers from foreigners, dangers in towns, dangers in the country, dangers at sea, dangers from false friends. I have toiled and drudged, I have often gone without sleep; hungry and thirsty, I have often gone fasting; and I have suffered from cold and exposure. [II Cor. 11:24-27, NEB]

By his own admission, Paul was guilty of violating at least two of the seven rules for good health: he did not always get seven or eight hours' sleep per night, and on occasion he probably skipped breakfast.

So we are left with a paradox. Bodily health is an important value, and we have a duty to promote our own health. Yet there may be times when other important values—like friendship, or excellence, or fidelity to one's Christian commitment—should take precedence over the quest for health.

26.
Health as a Virtue

IVAN ILLICH

Health designates a process of adaptation. It is not the result of instinct, but of an autonomous yet culturally shaped reaction to socially created reality. It designates the ability to adapt to changing environments, to growing up and to aging, to healing when damaged, to suffering, and to the peaceful expectation of death. Health embraces the future as well, and therefore includes anguish and the inner resources to live with it.

Health designates a process by which each person is responsible, but only in part responsible to others. To be responsible may mean two things. A man is responsible for what he has done, and responsible to another person or group. Only when he feels subjectively responsible or answerable to another person will the consequences of his failure be not criticism, censure, or punishment but regret, remorse, and true repentance.[1] The consequent states of grief and distress are marks of recovery and healing, and are phenomenologically something entirely different from guilt feelings. Health is a task, and as such is not comparable to the physiological balance of beasts. Success in this personal task is in large part the result of the self-awareness, self-discipline, and inner resources by which each person regulates his own daily rhythm and actions, his diet, and his sexual activity. Knowledge encompassing desirable activities, competent performance, the commitment to enhance health in others—these are all learned from the example of peers or elders. These personal activities are shaped and conditioned by the culture in which the individual grows up: patterns of work and leisure, of celebration and sleep, of production and preparation of food and drink, of family relations and politics. Long-tested health patterns that fit a geographic area and a certain technical situation depend to a large extent on long-lasting political autonomy. They depend on the spread of responsibility for healthy habits and for the sociobiological environment. That is, they depend on the dynamic stability of a culture.

The level of public health corresponds to the degree to which the means and responsibility for coping with illness are distributed among the total population. This ability to cope can be enhanced but never replaced by medical intervention or by the hygienic characteristics of the environment. That society which can reduce professional intervention to the minimum will provide the best conditions for health. The greater the potential for autonomous adaptation to self, to others, and to the environment, the less management of adaptation will be needed or tolerated.

A world of optimal and widespread health is obviously a world of minimal and only occasional medical intervention. Healthy people are those who live in healthy homes on a healthy diet in an environment equally fit for birth, growth, healing, and dying; they are sustained by a culture that enhances the conscious acceptance of limits to population, of aging, of incomplete recovery and ever-imminent death. Healthy people need minimal bureaucratic interference to mate, give birth, share the human condition, and die.

Man's consciously lived fragility, individuality, and relatedness make the experience of pain, of sickness, and of death an integral part of his life. The ability to cope with this trio autonomously is fundamental to his health. As he becomes dependent on the management of his intimacy, he renounces his autonomy and his health *must* decline. The true miracle of modern medicine is diabolical. It consists in making not only individuals but whole populations survive on inhumanly low levels of personal health. Medical nemesis is the negative feedback of a social organization that set out to improve and equalize the opportunity for each man to cope in autonomy and ended by destroying it.

Note

1. Alfred Schultz, "Some Equivocations in the Notion of Responsibility," in *Collected Papers,* vol. 2, *Studies in Social Theory* (The Hague: Nijhoff, 1964), pp. 274-6.

27.
The Meaning of Health

PAUL TILLICH

The difficulty and the challenge of the meaning of health is that in order to speak of health, one must speak of all dimensions of life which are united in man. And no one can be an expert in all of them. But confronting this challenge is the destiny of the philosopher and the theologian, insofar as they should envisage the whole of life. In any case, only a limited part of the immense problem can be covered.

A Logical Consideration

The title is not "the concept of health," but "the meaning of health." Concepts are defined by subsumption to a more embracing concept; meanings are defined by being brought into configuration with other meanings. This method is in many cases more adequate and not less scientific than the method of subsumption. In our case, it is definitely adequate for a very fundamental reason. Health is not an element in the description of man's essential nature—his *eidos* or *ide,* as Plato would say; his created nature, as theology would express it. Health is not a part of man or a function of man, as are blood circulation, metabolism, hearing, breathing. Health is a meaningful term only in confrontation with its opposite—disease. And disease contains a partial negation of the essential nature of man. Conversely, in order to understand disease, one must know the essential nature of man as well as the possible distortions of it. In contemporary language one would say that health and disease are existentialist concepts. They do not grasp something of man's essential nature; certainly they presuppose this nature and the knowledge of it; but they add a new element, the possibility and reality of its distortion. Health and disease are very good examples of existentialist concepts. Like theology, medicine always did unite essentialist and existentialist elements in its thought. Therefore, psychotherapy, especially in its psychoanalytic form, and existentialism have influenced each other profoundly in the last 50 years; and the idea of an existentialist psychotherapy is only a confirmation and systematization of an actual situation.

From *Perspectives in Biology and Medicine* 5 (Autumn 1961). Used by permission of the estate of Paul Tillich.

The Basic Dialectics of Life Processes

Life processes include two basic elements: self-identity and self-alteration. A centered and balanced living whole goes beyond itself, separates itself partly from its unity, but in doing so it tries to preserve its identity and to return in its separated parts to itself. Going out from one's self and returning to one's self characterizes life under all dimensions, from the structure of the atom to the growth of the plant, to the movement of the animal, to the creativity of the mind, to the dynamics of historical groups. One can call this dialectics of life processes because it implies contrasting movements, a *yes* and a *no,* as in a searching conversation. And all dialectical thought is nothing but a mirror of such life processes.

The contrast between self-identity and self-alteration produces two dangers for every living being. The first is to lose one's self in going beyond one's self and not being able to return to one's self. This happens if special processes separate themselves from the whole and produce dispersion into too many directions, a wrong kind of growth, a loss of the uniting center. In all these cases (which are represented by particular bodily and mental diseases and personal disintegrations) the self-identity is threatened and often completely lost (change of personality and memory).

In reaction to the awareness of this danger, the opposite danger appears. Afraid to lose one's identity, one is unable to go out from one's self into self-alteration. Perhaps one has attempted it, but after having been frustrated, one retreats to a limited form of existence in which the self-identity on a reduced basis is preserved; and it is not only preserved, it is compulsively defended as in most cases of psychoneurosis.

If we ask how it can be explained that the dialectics of life processes are interrupted and how its flux is stopped, we may name three main causes: accidents, intrusions, imbalances. A consideration of these would lead deeply into the philosophy of life, and especially of medicine; we can only point to some characteristics of these causes of disease, as well as to their common cause. They are rooted in what I call the ambiguity of life and of all its processes. Ambiguity means that in every creative process of life, a destructive trend is implied; in every integrating process of life, a disintegrating trend; in every process toward the sublime, a profanizing trend. These ambiguities of life produce the concrete causes of disease. The ambiguities of encounter of being with being make destructive accidents unavoidable, be it bodily injuries or psychological traumata.

The ambiguities of assimilation of elements of the surrounding world—in food, breathing, communication—make unavoidable the destructive intrusions of strange bodies, as in bodily or mental infections; the ambiguities of growth, that is, bodily growth or the development of one's spiritual potentialities, make unavoidable the appearance of imbalances. Generally speaking, disease is a symptom of the universal ambiguity of life. Life must risk itself in order to win itself, but in the risking it may lose itself. A life which does not risk disease—even in the highest forms of the life of the spirit—is a poor life, as is shown, for instance, by the hypochondriac or the conformist.

Health, Disease, and Healing Under the Different Dimensions of Life

When I spoke of dimensions of life, there was implied a rejection of the phrase "levels of life." This must now be made explicit. Man should not be considered as a composite of several levels, such as body, soul, spirit, but as a multidimensional unity. I use the metaphor "dimension" in order to indicate that the different qualities of life in man are present within each other and do not lie alongside or above each other. One can expediently, but not necessarily, distinguish the physical, the chemical, the biological, the psychological, the mental, and the historical dimensions. Different distinctions as well as more particular ones are quite possible. What is important, however, is to see that they do not lie alongside, but within each other, as in the metaphor "dimension" the dimensional lines cross each other in one point.

This point, in our consideration, is man. He is multidimensional unity; all dimensions, distinguishable in experienced life, cross in him. In every dimension of life, all dimensions are potentially or actually present. In the atom only one of them is actual. In man all of them are actually present; he does not consist of levels of being, but he is a unity which unites all dimensions. This doctrine stands against the dualistic theory which sees man as composed of soul and body; or body and mind; or body, soul, and spirit, etc. Man is one, uniting within himself all dimensions of life—an insight which we partly owe to the recent developments of medicine, especially psychiatry.

As confirmation of this idea, one may refer to "psychosomatic" medicine. But although this is not incorrect, one should not forget that a hyphen between "psycho" and "somatic" represents the statement of a problem and not a solution.

The multidimensional unity of life in man calls for a multidimensional concept of health, of disease, and of healing, but in such a way that it becomes obvious that in each dimension all the others are present.

I shall follow the series of dimensions as indicated before and in each case show the meaning of health and disease and the function of healing as determined by the ideas of health and disease in what one could call a philosophy of life in medical terms.

Mechanical Dimension

Under the predominance of the physical dimension, health is the adequate functioning of all the particular parts of man. Disease is the non-functioning of these parts because of incidents, infections, and imbalances. Healing, then, is the removal of the diseased parts or their mechanical replacement: surgery. The prevalence of surgery since the Renaissance is based on an image of man (classically formulated by Descartes) which views him as a well-functioning body-machine, the disabled parts of which are removed or replaced so that after successful surgery, health means the functioning of the machine with reduced or artificially strengthened force. Analogies to bodily surgery in the other dimensions can be found, for instance, in the removal of elements in the psychological makeup of a person by psychotherapeutic methods. The patient is healed but reduced in power of being. A conspicuous case in which bodily surgery and psychological reduction are united is lobotomy, the total being reduced to a rather low functioning, but in some respect being healed. And under the dimension of the spirit, there can also be found an analogy in the moral and educational repressing of vital trends which have become infected or imbalanced, and dangerous for the whole. But such healing of the person is surgery; its healing is reduction of the power of being.

Chemical Dimension

There is no bodily surgery which does not consider the chemical processes in the body that is operated on. Health in this dimension is the balance of chemical substances and processes in a living organism. Here, reduction by sedatives and increase by adding stimulating substances to the organism are equally important. But it is not full healing in either case. The present drug-medicine fashion puts before us a profound problem. If it is possible to determine the self-altering as well as the self-preserving life processes in a living being from the dimension of chemism, what does this mean for the dimensions of the psychological, the spiritual, and the historical? In answering this, one must realize that even if we imagined the total determination of individuals on this basis as possible, the question would remain: What about the chemism of those who determine the chemical composition of others? Who decides? Here the dimension of health in the social-historical structure—with its presuppositions of spirit, morality, culture, and religion—appears in the health idea of the "brave new world." In this idea of human health, self-alteration is reduced to a minimum and life dries up.

Biological Dimension

Disregarding these extremes, which are threats on the horizon of our life, we must consider the biological dimension in which the balance is achieved between self-alteration and self-preservation. This is done by acts in which the total organism in its relation to environment and world is the object of healing, as for instance through rest, awakening of interest, increased movement, change of food and climate, etc. This is well expressed in the word "recreation," which indicates that the created vitality was stopped either in its power of going out beyond itself or in its power of returning to itself. Either the life processes had been reduced to routine existence or they were excited by the innumerable stimuli of daily life. Here a new dimension appears. The attempt to recreate life in the biological dimension demands the inclusion of the problem of health in the dimension of self-awareness—the psychological.

Psychological Dimension

Health in the dimension of self-awareness shows the dialectical structure of life processes most clearly. The processes of psychological growth demand self-alteration in every moment—in receiving reality, in mastering it, in being united with parts of it, in changing it, etc. But in all this a risk is involved, and this accounts for the reluctance to take all these encountered pieces of reality into one's centered self; thus the desire to withdraw into a limited reality becomes effective. One is afraid of going out and one defends compulsively the limited place to which one has retired. Something went wrong in the process of pushing ahead. And now a reduced health is unconsciously produced. The reduced health of the neurotic is the limited health he is able to reach—but reality makes him aware of the dangers of his limitation and so he wants to overcome the limits with the help of the analyst. If in reaching some degree of liberation, reality shows itself to him irrefutably, the question arises whether the neurotic can face reality. Often he can, sometimes he cannot; and it is left to the judgment of the healer whether he shall even try to heal if the result is so ambiguous.

We can compare the causes of psychological diseases with the causes of bodily diseases. Traumatic experiences stand in analogy to accidents (and are sometimes caused by accidents) and are the intrusion of forces which remain alongside the centered self as strange elements which are not taken into the center. Healing means helping to make somebody aware of these inhibitions of the outgoing processes and accepting the fact of limited health, because if it is accepted, its compulsory form is undercut and openness for pushing ahead becomes possible. Then, of course, the danger arises that the outgoing process may become so uninhibited that the return is stopped and self-identity is destroyed.

Spiritual Dimension

Again we are in the situation that we have separated the dimension of self-awareness from the dimension of spirit ("spirit," with a small *s* designating the life in meanings and values inherent in morality, culture, and religion). In these three functions of the spirit, the problem of health receives another depth and breadth, which then, conversely, is decisive for all the preceding dimensions. Morality is the self-actualization of the person in his centered encounter with the other person. This act is the basis of life in the dimension of the spirit. It is not the subjection to a law from God or man, but it is the actualization of what we potentially are, of our created nature. Its distortion in the line of outgoing is legalistic repression of parts of our being. Its distortion in the line of self-identity as a person is the lawless explosion of all possibilities.

Here the psychotherapeutic problem becomes the moral problem of the person and his self-actualization. And healing is the power of overcoming both distortions. But the healing of the spirit is not possible by good will, because the good will is just that which needs healing. In order to be healed, the spirit must be grasped by something which transcends it, which is not strange to it, but within which is the fulfillment of its potentialities. It is called "Spirit" (with a capital *S*). Spirit is the presence of what concerns us ultimately, the ground of our being and meaning. This is the intention of religion but it is not identical with religion. For as a function of the human spirit and as a realm of human activities, religion also stands under the dialectics of all life and under its ambiguities and, because its claims are higher, is even more profound than the others. Religious health is the state of being grasped by the Spirit, namely the Divine Presence, enabling us to transcend our religion and to return to it in the same experience. Unhealthy religion is the state of being enslaved—socially or personally—by a concrete religious system, producing bigotry, fanaticism, inordinate self-destructive ecstasy, dogmatism, ritualism. But neither is it healthy if in the breakthrough out of all this one loses the identity of a personal and communal religious center.

It must be added here that the healing power of the Spiritual Presence is far removed from the magic practice of "faith-healing." There *is* such a thing, a magic force from man to man. And without doubt the magic influence of the healer on the patient or of the patient upon himself is an element in most forms of healing. (Magic: the impact of one unconscious power upon another one.) But this is not the healing power of being centered in the universal, the divine center.

Here again the question arises how the healing helper, in most cases the minister or priest, can judge (like the psychoanalyst) whether the self-restriction to a religion of limited health (accepting authority, relying on a conversion experience) should be accepted or revealed in its limitation; and the same question arises in a well-established remoteness from a concrete religion. When is conversion required for Spiritual health?

Historical Dimension

When dealing with the cultural function in the light of the idea of health, we are driven to the last of the dimensions of life, the historical. The decisive question here is: To what degree is personal health possible in a society which is not a "sane society" (Erich Fromm)? "By creating a sane society" is an inadequate answer: first, because it disregards the ambiguities of historical existence which can be conquered only fragmentarily; second, because it overlooks the fact that without personal health in the leading groups, no social health is possible (the communist society). The cultural situation of a society has the same dialectics—the inhibition against pushing forward or the impossibility of returning to a guiding set of symbols. The unsolved situation in this respect is partly the result, partly the cause of the lack of health in all the other dimensions. But this goes beyond our limited subject.

Healing, Separated and United

The road through the many dimensions, and the meaning of health within them, has shown (1) that the dialectics of life processes are the same under each dimension; (2) that in each of them the others are presupposed; (3) that there is always a fulfilling and a reducing idea of health; (4) that complete healing includes healing under all dimensions.

This raises the question of the justification of limited healing. Human finitude makes particular healing necessary. The hurt finger requires surgical or chemical help, the physically healthy neurotic requires psychotherapeutic help. There are special helpers and healing methods called for under every dimension. But this independence of particular ideas of health and healing is limited by the mutual within-each-otherness of the dimensions. This is partly untrue to the human situation and leads to a phenomenon I would call "unhealthy health." It comes about if healing under one dimension is successful but does not take into consideration the other dimensions in which health is lacking or even imperilled by the particular healing. Successful surgery may produce a psychological trauma; effective drugs may calm down an uneasy conscience and preserve a moral deficiency; the well-trained, athletic body may contain a neurotic personality; the healed patient of the analyst may be sick through a lack of an ultimate meaning of his life; the conformist's average life may be sick through inhibited self-alteration; the converted Christian may suffer under repressions which produce fanaticism and may explode in lawless forms; the sane society may be the place where the pressure of the principles of its sanity may produce psychological and biological disruptions by the desire for creative insanity.

Particular healing is unavoidable, but it has the tendency to provoke diseases in another realm.

Thus, it is important for healers always to cooperate in every healing situation. This requirement was embodied in the ideal of the *soter*, the saviour (precisely, "the healer") who makes healthy and whole. The word has been applied to medical men, to gods of healing, to great rulers, to divine-human mediators. They all were considered to be healers. But the ideal was the *one* healer, the saviour, whose healing powers indicate the coming of the new eon. This is the background of the New Testament accounts of healing, which should not be taken as miracle stories, but as stories pointing to the universal healer.

This mythological symbol, which was applied to the man Jesus, shows the unity of the religious and the medical most clearly. And if salvation is understood in the sense of healing, there is no conflict between the religious and the medical, but the most intimate relation. Only a theology which has forgotten this relation, and sees salvation as the elevation of the individual to a heavenly place, can come into conflict with medicine. And only a medicine which denies the non-biological dimensions of life in their significance for the biological dimension (including its physical and chemical conditions) can come into conflict with theology. But an understanding of the differences as well as the mutual within-each-otherness of the dimensions can remove the conflict and create an intensive collaboration of helpers in all dimensions of health and healing.

The concept of health cannot be defined without

relation to its opposite—disease. But this is not only a matter of definition. In reality, health is not health without the essential possibility and the existential reality of disease. In this sense, health is disease conquered, as eternally the positive is positive by conquering the negative. This is the deepest theological significance of medicine.

28. The WHO Definition of 'Health'

DANIEL CALLAHAN

There is not much that can be called fun and games in medicine, perhaps because unlike other sports it is the only one in which everyone, participant and spectator, eventually gets killed playing. In the meantime, one of the grandest games is that version of king-of-the-hill where the aim of all players is to upset the World Health Organization (WHO) definition of "health." That definition, in case anyone could possibly forget it, is, "Health is a state of complete physical, mental, and social well-being and not merely the absence of disease or infirmity." Fair game, indeed. Yet somehow, defying all comers, the WHO definition endures, though literally every other aspirant to the crown has managed to knock it off the hill at least once. One possible reason for its presence is that it provides such an irresistible straw man; few there are who can resist attacking it in the opening paragraphs of papers designed to move on to more profound reflections.

But there is another possible reason which deserves some exploration, however unsettling the implications. It may just be that the WHO definition has more than a grain of truth in it, of a kind which is as profoundly frustrating as it is enticingly attractive. At the very least it is a definition which implies that there is some intrinsic relationship between the good of the body and the good of the self. The attractiveness of this relationship is obvious: it thwarts any movement toward a dualism of self and body, a dualism which in any event immediately breaks down when one drops a brick on one's toe; and it impels the analyst to work toward a conception of health which in the end is resistant to clear and distinct categories, closer to the felt experience. All that, naturally, is very frustrating. It seems simply impossible to devise a concept of health which is rich enough to be nutritious and yet not so rich as to be indigestible.

One common objection to the WHO definition is, in effect, an assault upon any and all attempts to specify the meaning of very general concepts. Who can possibly define words as vague as "health," a venture as foolish as trying to define "peace," "justice," "happi-

From the *Hastings Center Studies* 1, no. 3 (1973): 77-87. Used by permission of the publisher and the author.

ness," and other systematically ambiguous notions? To this objection the "pragmatic" clinicians (as they often call themselves) add that, anyway, it is utterly unnecessary to know what "health" means in order to treat a patient running a high temperature. Not only that, it is also a harmful distraction to clutter medical judgment with philosophical puzzles.

Unfortunately for this line of argument, it is impossible to talk or think at all without employing general concepts; without them, cognition and language are impossible. More damagingly, it is rarely difficult to discover, with a bit of probing, that even the most "pragmatic" judgment (whatever *that* is) presupposes some general values and orientations, all of which can be translated into definitions of terms as general as "health" and "happiness." A failure to discern the operative underlying values, the conceptions of reality upon which they are based, and the definitions they entail, sets the stage for unexamined conduct and, beyond that, positive harm both to patients and to medicine in general.

But if these objections to any and all attempts to specify the meaning of "health" are common enough, the most specific complaint about the WHO definition is that its very generality, and particularly its association of health and general well-being as a positive ideal, has given rise to a variety of evils. Among them are the cultural tendency to define all social problems, from war to crime in the streets, as "health" problems; the blurring of lines of responsibility between and among the professions, and between the medical profession and the political order; the implicit denial of human freedom which results when failures to achieve social well-being are defined as forms of "sickness," somehow to be treated by medical means; and the general debasement of language which ensues upon the casual habit of labeling everyone from Adolf Hitler to student radicals to the brat next door as "sick." In short, the problem with the WHO definition is not that it represents an attempt to propose a general definition, but it is simply a bad one.

That is a valid line of objection, provided one can spell out in some detail just how the definition can or does entail some harmful consequences. Two lines of attack are possible against putatively hazardous social definitions of significant general concepts. One is by pointing out that the definition does not encompass all that a concept has commonly been taken to mean, either historically or at present, that it is a partial definition only. The task then is to come up with a fuller definition, one less subject to misuse. But there is still another way of objecting to socially significant definitions, and that is by pointing out some baneful effects of definitions generally accepted as adequate. Many of the objections to the WHO definition fall in the latter category, building upon the important insight that definitions of crucially important terms with a wide public use have ethical, social, and political implications; defining general terms is not an abstract exercise but a way of shaping the world metaphysically and structuring the world politically.

Wittgenstein's aphorism, "don't look for the meaning, look for the use," is pertinent here. The ethical problem in defining the concept of "health" is to determine what the implications are of the various uses to which a concept of "health" can be put. We might well agree that there are some uses of "health" which will produce socially harmful results. To carry Wittgenstein a step further, "don't look for the uses, look for the abuses." We might, then, examine some of the real or possible abuses to which the WHO definition leads, recognizing all the while that what we may term an "abuse" will itself rest upon some perceived *positive* good or value.

Historical Origin & Context

Before that task is undertaken, however, it is helpful to understand the historical origin and social context of the WHO definition. If abuses of that definition have developed, their seeds may be looked for in its earliest manifestations.

The World Health Organization came into existence between 1946 and 1948 as one of the first major activities of the United Nations. As an outcome of earlier work, an Interim Commission to establish the WHO sponsored an International Health Conference in New York in June and July of 1946. At that Conference, representatives of 61 nations signed the Constitution of the WHO, the very first clause of which presented the now famous definition of "health." The animating spirit behind the formation of the WHO was the belief that the improvement of world health would make an important contribution to world peace; health and peace were seen as inseparable. Just why this belief gained ground is not clear from the historical record of the WHO. While there have been many historical explanations of the origin of World War II, a lack of world health has not been prominent among them; nor, for that matter, did the early supporters of the WHO claim that the Second World War or any other war might have been averted had there been better health. More to the point, perhaps, was the conviction that health was intimately related to economic and cultural welfare; in turn, that welfare, so it was assumed, had a direct bearing on future peace. No less important was a fervent faith in the possibilities of medical science to achieve world health, enhanced by the development of powerful antibiotics and pesticides during the war.

A number of memorandums submitted to a spring 1946 Technical Preparatory Committee meeting of the WHO capture the flavor of the period. The Yugoslavian memorandum noted that "health is a prerequisite to freedom from want, to social security and happiness." France stated that "there cannot be any material security, social security, or well-being for individuals or nations without health . . . the full responsibility of a free man can only be assumed by healthy individuals . . . the spread of proper notions of hygiene among populations tends to improve the level of health and hence to increase their working power and raise their standard of living. . . . " The United States contended that "international cooperation and joint action in the furtherance of all matters pertaining to health will raise the standards of living, will promote the freedom, the dignity, and the happiness of all peoples of the world."

In addition to those themes, perhaps the most significant initiative taken by the organizers of the WHO was to include mental health as part of its working definition. In its memorandum, Great Britain stated that "it should be clear that health includes mental health," but it was Dr. Brock Chisholm, soon to become the first director of the WHO, who personified what Dr. Chisholm himself called the "visionary" view of health. During the meeting of the Technical Preparatory Committee he argued that: "The world is sick and the ills are due to the perversion of man; his inability to live with himself. The microbe is not the enemy; science is sufficiently advanced to cope with it were it not for the barriers of superstition, ignorance, religious intolerance, misery and poverty. . . . These psychological evils must be understood in order that a remedy might be prescribed, and the scope of the task before the Committee therefore knows no bounds."

In Dr. Chisholm's statement, put very succinctly, are all of those elements of the WHO definition which led eventually to its criticism: defining all the problems of the world as "sickness," affirming that science would be sufficient to cope with the causes of physical disease, asserting that only anachronistic attitudes stood in the way of a cure of both physical and psychological ills, and declaring that the cause of health can tolerate no limitations. To say that Dr. Chisholm's "vision" was grandiose is to understate the matter. Even allowing for hyperbole, it is clear that the stage was being set for a conception of "health" which would encompass literally every element and item of human happiness. One can hardly be surprised, given such a vision, that our ways of talking about "health" have become all but meaningless. Even though I believe the definition is not without its important insights, it is well to observe why, in part, we are so muddled at present about "health."

Health & Happiness

Let us examine some of the principal objections to the WHO definition in more detail. One of them is that, by including the notion of "social well-being" under its rubric, it turns the enduring problem of human happiness into one more medical problem, to be dealt with by scientific means. That is surely an objectionable feature, if only because there exists no evidence whatever that medicine has anything more than a partial grasp of the sources of human misery. Despite Dr. Chisholm's optimism, medicine has not even found ways of dealing with more than a fraction of the whole range of physical diseases; campaigns, after all, are still being mounted against cancer and heart disease. Nor is there any special reason to think that future forays against those and other common diseases will bear rapid fruits. People will continue to die of disease for a long time to come, probably forever.

But perhaps, then, in the psychological and psychiatric sciences some progress has been made against what Dr. Chisholm called the "psychological ills," which lead to wars, hostility, and aggression? To be sure, there are many interesting psychological theories to be found about these "ills," and a few techniques which can, with some individuals, reduce or eliminate anti-social behavior. But so far as I can see, despite the mental health movement and the rise of the psychological sciences, war and human hostility are as much with us as ever. Quite apart from philosophical objections to the WHO definition, there was no empirical basis for the unbounded optimism which lay behind it at the time of its inception, and little has happened since to lend its limitless aspiration any firm support.

Common sense alone makes evident the fact that the absence of "disease or infirmity" by no means guarantees "social well-being." In one sense, those who drafted the WHO definition seem well aware of that. Isn't the whole point of their definition to show the inadequacy of negative definitions? But in another sense, it may be doubted that they really did grasp that point. For the third principle enunciated in the WHO Constitution says that, "the health of all peoples is fundamental to the attainment of peace and security. . . . " Why is it fundamental, at least to peace? The worst wars of the 20th century have been waged by countries with very high standards of health, by nations with superior life-expectancies for individuals and with comparatively low infant mortality rates. The greatest present threats to world peace come in great part (though not entirely) from developed countries, those which have combatted disease and illness most effectively. There seems to be no historical correlation whatever between health and peace, and that is true even if one includes "mental health."

How are human beings to achieve happiness? That is the final and fundamental question. Obviously illness, whether mental or physical, makes happiness less possible in most cases. But that is only because they are only one symptom of a more basic restriction, that of human finitude, which sees infinite human desires constantly thwarted by the limitations of reality. "Complete" well-being might, conceivably, be attainable, but under one condition only: that people ceased expecting much from life. That does not seem about to happen. On the contrary, medical and psychological progress have been more than outstripped by rising demands and expectations. What is so odd about that, if it is indeed true that human desires are infinite? Whatever the answer to the question of human happiness, there is no particular reason to believe that medicine can do anything more than make a modest, finite contribution.

Another objection to the WHO definition is that, by implication, it makes the medical profession the gate-keeper for happiness and social well-being. Or if not exactly the gate-keeper (since political and economic support will be needed from sources other than medical), then the final magic-healer of human misery. Pushed far enough, the whole idea is absurd, and it is not necessary to believe that the organizers of the WHO would, if pressed, have been willing to go quite that far. But even if one pushes the pretension a little way, considerable fantasy results. The mental health movement is the best example, casting the psychological professional in the role of high priest.

At its humble best, that movement can do considerable good; people do suffer from psychological disabilities and there are some effective ways of helping them. But it would be sheer folly to believe that all, or even the most important, social evils stem from bad mental health: political injustice, economic scarcity, food shortages, unfavorable physical environments, have a far greater historical claim as sources of a failure to achieve "social well-being." To retort that all or most of these troubles can, nonetheless, be seen finally as symptoms of bad mental health is, at best, self-serving and, at worst, just plain foolish.

A significant part of the objection that the WHO definition places, at least by implication, too much power and authority in the hands of the medical profession, need not be based on a fear of that power as such. There is no reason to think that the world would be any worse off if health professionals made all decisions than if any other group did; and no reason to think it would be any better off. That is not a very important point. More significant is that cultural development which, in its skepticism about "traditional" ways of solving social problems, would seek a technological and specifically a medical solution for human ills of all kinds. There is at least a hint in early WHO discussions that, since politicians and diplomats have failed in maintaining world peace, a more expert group should take over, armed with the scientific skills necessary to set things right; it is science which is best able to vanquish that old Enlightenment bogeyman, "superstition." More concretely, such an ideology has the practical effect of blurring the lines of appropriate authority and responsibility. If all problems—political, economic and social—reduce to matters of "health," then there ceases to be any ways to determine who should be responsible for what.

The Tyranny of Health

The problem of responsibility has at least two faces. One is that of a tendency to turn all problems of "social well-being" over to the medical professional, most pronounced in the instance of the incarceration of a large group of criminals in mental institutions rather than prisons. The abuses, both medical and legal, of that practice are, fortunately, now beginning to receive the attention they deserve, even if little corrective action has yet been taken. (Counterbalancing that development, however, are others, where some are seeking more "effective" ways of bringing science to bear on criminal behavior.)

The other face of the problem of responsibility is that of the way in which those who are sick, or purportedly sick, are to be evaluated in terms of their freedom and responsibility. Siegler and Osmond elsewhere in this issue discuss the "sick role," a leading feature of which is the ascription of blamelessness, of non-responsibility, to those who contract illness. There is no reason to object to this kind of ascription in many instances—one can hardly blame someone for contracting kidney disease—but, obviously enough, matters get out of hand when all physical, mental, and communal disorders are put under the heading of "sickness," and all sufferers (all of us, in the end) placed in the blameless "sick role." Not only are the concepts of "sickness" and "illness" drained of all content, it also becomes impossible to ascribe any freedom or responsibility to those caught up in the throes of sickness. The whole world is sick, and no one is responsible any longer for anything. That is determinism gone mad, a rather odd outcome of a development which began with attempts to bring unbenighted "reason" and free self-determination to bear for the release of the helpless captives of superstition and ignorance.

The final and most telling objection to the WHO definition has less to do with the definition itself than with one of its natural historical consequences. Thomas Szasz has been the most eloquent (and most single-minded) critic of that sleight-of-hand which has seen the concept of health moved from the medical to the moral arena. What can no longer be done in the name of "morality" can now be done in the name of "health": human beings labeled, incarcerated, and dismissed for their failure to toe the line of "normalcy" and "sanity."

At first glance, this analysis of the present situation might seem to be totally at odds with the tendency to put everyone in the blame-free "sick role." Actually, there is a fine, probably indistinguishable, line separating these two positions. For as soon as one treats all human disorders—war, crime, social unrest—as forms of illness, then one turns health into a normative concept, that which human beings must and ought to have if they are to live in peace with themselves and others. Health is no longer an optional matter, but the golden key to the relief of human misery. We *must* be well or we will all perish. "Health" can and must be imposed; there can be no room for the luxury of freedom when so much is at stake. Of course the matter is rarely put so bluntly, but it is to Szasz's great credit that he has discerned what actually happens when "health" is allowed to gain the cultural clout which morality once had. (That he carries the whole business too far in his embracing of the most extreme moral individualism is another story, which cannot be dealt with here.) Something is seriously amiss when the "right" to have healthy children is turned into a further right for children not to be born defective, and from there into an obligation not to bring unhealthy children into the world as a way of respecting the right of those children to health! Nor is everything altogether lucid when abortion decisions are made a matter of "medical judgment" (see *Roe vs. Wade*); when decisions to provide psychoactive drugs for the relief of the ordinary stress of living are defined as no less "medical judgment"; when patients are not allowed to die with dignity because of medical indications that they can, come what may, be kept alive; when prisoners, without their consent, are subjected to aversive conditioning to improve their mental health.

Abuses of Language

In running through the litany of criticisms which have been directed at the WHO definition of "health," and what seem to have been some of its long-term implications and consequences, I might well be accused of beating a dead horse. My only defense is to assert, first, that the spirit of the WHO definition is by no means dead either in medicine or society. In fact, because of the usual cultural lag which requires many years for new ideas to gain wide social currency, it is only now coming into its own on a broad scale. (Everyone now talks about everybody and everything, from Watergate to Billy Graham to trash in the streets, as "sick.") Second, I believe that we are now in the midst of a nascent (if not actual) crisis about how "health" ought properly to be understood, with much dependent upon what conception of health emerges in the near future.

If the ideology which underlies the WHO definition has proved to contain many muddled and hazardous ingredients, it is not at all evident what should take its place. The virtue of the WHO definition is that it tried to place health in the broadest human context. Yet the assumption behind the main criticisms of the WHO definition seem perfectly valid. Those assumptions can be characterized as follows: 1) health is only a part of life, and the achievement of health only a part of the achievement of happiness; 2) medicine's role, however important, is limited; it can neither solve nor even cope with the great majority of social, political, and cultural problems; 3) human freedom and responsibility must be recognized, and any tendency to place all deviant, devilish, or displeasing human beings into the blameless sick-role must be resisted; 4) while it is good for human beings to be healthy, medicine is not morality; except in very limited contexts (plagues and epidemics) "medical judgment" should not be allowed to become moral judgment; to be healthy is not to be righteous; 5) it is important to keep clear and distinct the different roles of different professions, with a clearly circumscribed role for medicine, limited to those domains of life where the contribution of medicine is appropriate. Medicine can save some lives; it cannot save the life of society.

These assumptions, and the criticisms of the WHO definition which spring from them, have some important implications for the use of the words "health," "illness," "sick," and the like. It will be counted an abuse of language if the word "sick" is applied to all individual and communal problems, if all unacceptable conduct is spoken of in the language of medical pathologies, if moral issues and moral judgments are translated into the language of "health," if the lines of authority, responsibility, and expertise are so blurred that the health profession is allowed to pre-empt the rights and responsibilities of others by re-defining them in its own professional language.

Abuses of that kind have no possibility of being curbed in the absence of a definition of health which does not contain some intrinsic elements of limitation—that is, unless there is a definition which, when abused, is self-evidently *seen* as abused by those who know what health means. Unfortunately, it is in the nature of general definitions that they do not circumscribe their own meaning (or even explain it) and contain no built-in safeguards against misuse, e.g., our "peace with honor" in Southeast Asia—"peace," "honor"? Moreover, for a certain class of concepts—peace, honor, happiness, for example—it is difficult to keep them free in ordinary usage from a normative content. In our own usage, it would make no sense to talk of them in a way which implied they are not desirable or are merely neutral: by well-ingrained social custom (resting no doubt on some basic features of human nature) health, peace, and happiness are both desired and desirable—good. For those and other reasons, it is perfectly plausible to say the cultural task of defining terms, and settling on appropriate and inappropriate usages, is far more than a matter of getting our dictionary entries right. It is nothing less than a way of deciding what should be valued, how life should be understood, and what principles should guide individual and social conduct.

Health is not just a term to be defined. Intuitively, if we have lived at all, it is something we seek and value. We may not set the highest value on health—other goods may be valued as well—but it would strike me as incomprehensible should someone say that health was a matter of utter indifference to him; we would well doubt either his sanity or his maturity. The cultural problem, then, may be put this way. The acceptable range of uses of the term "health" should, at the minimum, capture the normative element in the concept as traditionally understood while, at the maximum, incorporating the insight (stemming from criticisms of the WHO definition) that the term "health" is abused if it becomes synonymous with virtue, social tranquility, and ultimate happiness. Since there are no instruction manuals available on how one would go about reaching a goal of that sort, I will offer no advice on the subject. I have the horrible suspicion, as a matter of fact, that people either have a decent intuitive sense on such matters (reflected in the way they use language) or they do not; and if they do not, little can be done to instruct them. One is left with the pious hope that, somehow, over a long period of time, things will change.

In Defense of WHO

Now that simply might be the end of the story, assuming some agreement can be reached that the WHO definition of "health" is plainly bad, full of snares, delusions, and false norms. But I am left uncomfortable with such a flat, simple conclusion. The nagging point about the definition is that, in badly put ways, it was probably on to something. It certainly recognized, however inchoately, that it is difficult to talk meaningfully of health solely in terms of "the absence of disease or infirmity." As a purely logical point, one must ask about what positive state of affairs disease and infirmity are an absence of—absent from what? One is left with the tautological proposition that health is the absence of non-health, a less than illuminating revelation. Could it not be said, though, that at least intuitively everyone knows what health is by means of the experiential contrast posed by states of illness and disease; that is, even if I cannot define health in any positive sense, I can surely know when I am sick (pain, high fever, etc.) and compare that condition with my previous states which contained no such conditions? Thus one could, in some recognizable sense, speak of illness as a deviation from a norm, even if it is not possible to specify that norm with any clarity.

But there are some problems with this approach, for all of its commonsense appeal. Sociologically, it is well known that what may be accounted sickness in one culture may not be so interpreted in another; one culture's (person's) deviation from the norm may not necessarily be another culture's (person's) deviation. In this as in other matters, commonsense intuition may be nothing but a reflection of different cultural and personal evaluations. In addition, there can be and usually are serious disputes about how great a deviation from the (unspecified) norm is necessary before the terms "sickness" and "illness" become appropriate. Am I to be put in the sick role because of my nagging case of itching athlete's foot, or must my toes start dropping off before I can so qualify? All general concepts have their borderline cases, and normally they need pose no real problems for the applicability of the concepts for the run of instances. But where "health" and "illness" are concerned, the number of borderline cases can be enormous, affected by age, attitudinal and cultural factors. Worse still, the fact that people can be afflicted by disease (even fatally afflicted) well before the manifestation of any overt symptoms is enough to discredit the adequacy of intuitions based on how one happens to feel at any given moment.

A number of these problems might be resolved by distinguishing between health as a norm and as an ideal. As a norm, it could be possible to speak in terms of deviation from some statistical standards, particularly if these standards were couched not only in terms of organic function but also in terms of behavioral functioning. Thus someone would be called "healthy" if his heart, lungs, kidneys (etc.) functioned at a certain level of efficiency and efficacy, if he was not suffering physical pain, and if his body was free of those pathological conditions which even if undetected or undetectable could impair organic function and eventually cause pain. There could still be dispute about what should count as a "pathological" condition, but at least it would be possible to draw up a large checklist of items subject to "scientific measurement"; then, having gone through that checklist in a physical exam, and passing all the tests, one could be pronounced "healthy." Neat, clean, simple.

All of this might be possible in a static culture, which ours is not. The problem is that any notion of a statistical norm will be superintended by some kind of ideal. Why, in the first place, should anyone care at all how his organs are functioning, much less how well they do so? There must be some reason for that, a reason which goes beyond theoretical interest in statistical distributions. Could it possibly be because certain departures from the norm carry with them unpleasant states, which few are likely to call "good": pain, discrimination, unhappiness? I would guess so. In the second place, why should society have any interest whatever in the way the organs of its citizens function? There must also be some reason for that, very possibly the insight that the organ functioning of individuals has some aggregate social implications. In our culture at least (and in every other culture I have ever heard of) it is simply impossible, finally, to draw any sharp distinction between conceptions of the human good and what are accounted significant and negatively evaluated deviations from statistical norms.

That is the whole point of saying, in defense of the WHO definition of health, that it discerned the intimate connection between the good of the body and the good of the self, not only the individual self but the social community of selves. No individual and no society would (save for speculative, scientific reasons only) have any interest whatever in the condition of human organs and bodies were it not for the obvious fact that those conditions can have an enormous impact on the whole of human life. People do, it has been noticed, die; and they die because something has gone wrong with their bodies. This can be annoying, especially if one would, at the moment of death, prefer to be busy doing other things. Consider two commonplace occurrences. The first I have alluded to already: dropping a heavy brick on one's foot. So far as I know, there is no culture where the pain which that event occasions is considered a good in itself. Why is that? Because (I presume) the pain which results can not only make it difficult or impossible to walk for a time but also because the pain, if intense enough, makes it impossible to think about anything else (or think at all) or to relate to anything or anyone other than the pain. For a time, I am "not myself" and that simply because my body is making such excessive demands on my attention that nothing is possible to me except to howl. I cannot, in sum, dissociate my "body" from my "self" in that situation; my self is my body and my body is my pain.

The other occurrence is no less commonplace. It is the assertion the old often make to the young, however great the psychological, economic, or other miseries of the latter: "at least you've got your health." They are saying in so many words that, if one is healthy, then there is some room for hope, some possibility of human recovery; and even more they are saying that, without good health, nothing is possible, however favorable the other conditions of life may be. Again, it is impossible to dissociate good of body and good of self. Put more formally, if health is not a sufficient condition for happiness, it is a necessary condition. At that very fundamental level, then, any sharp distinction between the good of bodies and the good of persons dissolves.

Are we not forced, therefore, to say that, if the complete absence of health (i.e., death) means the complete absence of self, then any diminishment of health must represent, correspondingly, a diminishment of self? That does not follow, for unless a disease or infirmity is severe, it may represent only a minor annoyance, diminishing our selfhood not a whit. And while it will not do to be overly sentimental about such things, it is probably the case that disease or infirmity can, in some cases, increase one's sense of selfhood (which is no reason to urge disease upon people for its possibly psychological benefits). The frequent reports of those who have recovered from a serious illness that it made them appreciate life in a far more intense way than they previously had are not to be dismissed (though one wishes an easier way could be found).

Modest Conclusions

Two conclusions may be drawn. The first is that some minimal level of health is necessary if there is to be any possibility of human happiness. Only in exceptional circumstances can the good of self be long maintained in the absence of the good of the body. The second conclusion, however, is that one can be healthy without being in a state of "complete physical, mental, and social well-being." That conclusion can be justified in two ways: (a) because some degree of disease and infirmity is perfectly compatible with mental and social well-being; and (b) because it is doubtful that there ever was, or ever could be, more than a transient state of "complete physical, mental, and social well-being," for individuals or societies; that's just not the way life is or could be. Its attractiveness as an ideal is vitiated by its practical impossibility of realization. Worse than that, it positively misleads, for health becomes a goal of such all-consuming importance that it simply begs to be thwarted in its realization. The demands which the word "complete" entails set the stage for the worst false consciousness of all: the demand that life deliver perfection. Practically speaking, this demand has led, in the field of health, to a constant escalation of expectation and requirement, never ending, never satisfied.

What, then, would be a good definition of "health"? I was afraid someone was going to ask me that question. I suggest we settle on the following: "health is a state of physical well-being." That state need not be "complete," but it must be at least adequate, i.e., without significant impairment of function. It also need not encompass "mental" well-being; one can be healthy yet anxious, well yet depressed. And it surely ought not to encompass "social well-being," except insofar as that well-being will be impaired by the presence of large-scale, serious physical infirmities. Of course my definition is vague, but it would take some very fancy semantic footwork for it to be socially misused; that brat next door could not be called "sick" except when he is running a fever. This definition would not, though, preclude all social use of the language of "pathology" for other than physical disease. The image of a physically well body is a powerful one and, used carefully, it can be suggestive of the kind of wholeness and adequacy of function one might hope to see in other areas of life.

Chapter Six
DEATH AND ITS (IN)DIGNITY

Introduction

If life has been sanctified, what of death? If life is for all people under the power of God, is death the limit to that power? Is death a sign that there is an alien power in our world? Is death the enemy or a friend? Is it simply a sign of our powerlessness? God's powerlessness? Is death "natural," dying a part of living? Our concept of what death is naturally affects our disposition toward it. Should we fear it? Welcome it? Accept it? Fight it? May we pray for it? May we complain to God in the face of it? Does death have dignity as a necessary and welcome limit to living, or is death an indignity, an affront to human worth and human hope?

The first thing that should be observed about these questions is how little they are discussed in our culture. William May points out that there appears to be a conspiracy of silence in our culture on the subject of death; even the churches are silent. But if the churches were to speak, what should they say?

Paul Ramsey has some suggestions. He argues that death itself is an indignity, something alien to human beings, something to be resisted; and he rejects any understanding of death which regards it as first and foremost "natural" to human beings. On this point Robert Morison disagrees; he argues in direct opposition to Ramsey that death is simply a "fact of life," natural, integral to the human life cycle rather than alien to it. Leon Kass follows this up and argues that it is good for us that we die, that the fact of death gives us an opportunity to give some point or purpose to our lives. William May accepts that death can so influence life but cautions that the awareness of death may well stir people to frenetic activity in an attempt to distinguish themselves before their own life is extinguished.

Christian Scripture raises questions for us about how we ought to understand death. Paul claimed that "the wages of sin is death!" (Rom 5:32). In his view, death comes from Adam and life from Jesus. Does Paul then give us a way in which we might understand the phrase, "the indignity of death"? Is death an indignity for those who are destined ultimately for life?

Our awareness of death changes how we think we ought to approach any discussion of the issue. Human beings know that they will die: death is not simply something that happens in the world but something that will happen to *me.* This opens up the possibility that we ought to approach death differently from how we approach the external problems that confront us simply because we inevitably participate in this. If death is not a problem that can be solved but rather a mystery that must be lived with and confronted, then we would do well to formulate a provisional stance toward it rather than merely to assume that it is something that we can understand exhaustively.

William May points out that whether death is natural or not, it is an event which inspires awe and terror in many people in our culture. He raises questions not only about the way in which death is treated in our society but also about how Christians fail to witness to what they believe: that death is not the final word about human life. May suggests that Christians often act as though they were abandoned in death, as though the power of the love of God were defeated here. He points to the typical Christian funeral service as evidence for this.

Yet even if one affirms with May that God rules even in death, indeed, that finally death is defeated, there are important questions still to be addressed. Is this affirmation to be expressed in terms of resurrection of the body or immortality of the soul? If resurrection, as May argues, what does this mean?

Beyond these questions is another question, "What difference do these different beliefs make in practice—when we act for and upon the dying person?" Do they in fact change anything for the dying person? What about for the medical personnel who care for the dying? Do they alter what means and methods we might recommend in caring for the dying? As we shall see, many authors have questions to raise about the inappropriate use of technology as a means for forestalling death. As we shall also see, however, there are vigorous disagreements over what is appropriate and inappropriate; and these disagreements are related to different perspectives on the visage of death and different responses to its power.

A central difference that arises in the readings here concerns differences on the question of the amount of control one ought to have over one's dying. Morison seems to equate dying with dignity with dying in control of one's death. This raises the question of whether it is always necessary to have control in order to have human dignity. What are the assumptions of the claim that one gains dignity as one gains control of events? William May asserts that one of the things that happens in medical settings is that we find ourselves not in control. We have lost control both to those who are caring for us and to the machines that they use in that care. May suggests that the reality of this loss of control ought to remind us of the futility of seeking control in all aspects of our lives. The important question for us is, Is this claim correct, or should we seek the control that Morison finds central to human dignity?

It should be clear by now that one of the important topics of discussion under the question of control and dignity is the use of medical technology. But that technology is not a simple instrument of control by physicians over patients. Indeed, the very technology which is often criticized as inhumane because it leads to a loss of individual control may serve as an instrument of grace, in that it may serve life. One of the most difficult questions in front of us concerns how we might use this technology as a servant of life rather than as an instrument designed solely to avoid and delay death. Our disposition toward death is critical as we approach that question.

Suggestions for Further Reading

Aries, Philippe. *Western Attitudes Toward Death: From the Middle Ages to the Present,* translated by Patricia M. Ranum. Baltimore: Johns Hopkins University Press, 1974.

Bailey, Lloyd R., Sr. *Biblical Perspectives on Death.* Philadelphia: Fortress, 1979.

Cleary, Francis X., S.J. "On Death and After Life: A Biblical Reflection," *Hospital Progress* (Dec. 1975): 40–44.

Congdon, Howard K. *The Pursuit of Death.* Nashville: Abingdon, 1977.

Cullmann, Oscar. "Immortality of the Soul or Resurrection of the Dead." In *Immortality and Resurrection,* edited by Krister Stendahl. New York: Macmillan, 1965.

Jüngel, Eberhard. *Death: The Riddle and the Mystery.* Philadelphia: Westminster, 1974.

Kübler-Ross, Elisabeth. *Death and Dying.* New York: Macmillan, 1969.

Steinfels, Peter, and Robert M. Veatch, eds. *Death Inside Out.* New York: Harper and Row, 1975.

Tolstoy, Leo. *The Death of Ivan Ilyich.* Translated by Lynn Solotaroff. New York: Bantam, 1981.

Westphal, Merold. *God, Guilt, and Death.* Bloomington, Ind.: Indiana University Press, 1984.

Williams, Bernard. "The Makropulos Case: Reflections on the Tedium of Immortality." Paper in *Problems of the Self,* 82–100. Cambridge: Cambridge University Press, 1973.

29.
Psalm 88

O LORD, my God, I call for help by day;
  I cry out in the night before thee.
Let my prayer come before thee,
  incline thy ear to my cry!

For my soul is full of troubles,
  and my life draws near to Sheol.
I am reckoned among those who go down to the Pit;
  I am a man who has no strength,
like one forsaken among the dead,
  like the slain that lie in the grave,
like those whom thou dost remember no more,
  for they are cut off from thy hand.
Thou hast put me in the depths of the Pit,
  in the regions dark and deep.
Thy wrath lies heavy upon me,
  and thou dost overwhelm me with
    all thy waves. *Selah*
Thou hast caused my companions to shun me;
  thou hast made me a thing of horror to them.
I am shut in so that I cannot escape;
  my eye grows dim through sorrow.
Every day I call upon thee, O LORD;
  I spread out my hands to thee.
Dost thou work wonders for the dead?
  Do the shades rise up to praise thee? *Selah*
Is thy steadfast love declared in the grave,
  or thy faithfulness in Abaddon?
Are thy wonders known in the darkness,
  or thy saving help in the land of forgetfulness?

But I, O LORD, cry to thee;
  in the morning my prayer comes before thee.
O LORD, why dost thou cast me off?
  Why dost thou hide thy face from me?
Afflicted and close to death from my youth up,
  I suffer thy terrors; I am helpless.
Thy wrath has swept over me;
  thy dread assaults destroy me.
They surround me like a flood all day long;
  they close in upon me together.
Thou hast caused lover and friend to shun me;
  my companions are in darkness.

---

30. The Sacral Power of Death in Contemporary Experience

WILLIAM F. MAY

Theological reflection on the subject of death usually has an air of unreality because it has no contact with death as it is actually experienced by men in its sacral power. This is especially true of theology in an age that likes to think of itself as secular without remainder. Presumably there are no religious realities left to contend with. Men are relatively self-sufficient and autonomous, blessedly free of the incubus of religion in all its forms. The gospel has only to address itself to a world-come-of-age, commanded and populated by secular men.

Theologians of the secular persuasion may be right when they attempt to free the gospel from its earlier, uncritical ties with religion, but they are wrong when they assume that religion is dead. While religions, in the sense of official historical traditions, may indeed have entered a period of decline, the experience of the sacred is still very much with us. Nowhere is this more apparent than in the contemporary experience of death. . . .

Death in Its Religious Reality

Pastors rarely approach the gravely ill without noticing immediately the evasions and the brave lies that encircle the dying. Doctors often refuse to inform the patient of his true condition in the case of a terminal illness. Needless to say, most families cooperate readily with the doctor and his instructions.

A heavy silence surrounds death. I believe that this painful reticence has a source more profound than our childlike submission to the advice of a doctor. For the instructions of a doctor would not hold for a minute if men felt they had recourse in their words and actions against death. In fact, where else except from the dying has the doctor himself learned his reticence? He has seen too many men avoid asking the big question about their illness. Or he has heard them ask the question without being certain that they really wanted an answer.

Despite some charges to the contrary (which I will discuss later), I do not think of the doctor as the villain of the piece in this conspiracy of silence. Silence has its origin in the awesomeness of death itself. Just as the Jew, out of respect for the awesomeness of God, would not pronounce the name of Jahweh, so we find it difficult to bring the word *death* to our lips in the presence of its power. This is so because we are at a loss as to how to proceed on the far side of this word. Our philosophies and our moralities desert us. They retreat and leave us wordless. Their rhetoric, which seemed so suitable on other occasions, suddenly loses its power, and we may well wonder whether our words themselves are not caught up in a massive, verbose, uneasy flight from death, while we are left with nothing to say, except to "say it with flowers."

Without provision against death, our rituals and ceremonies are characterized by a powerful flight from its presence. This is a phenomenon that has already received savage treatment at the hands of satirists in the Anglo-Saxon world: Aldous Huxley, *After Many a Summer;* Muriel Spark, *Memento Mori;* Evelyn Waugh, *The Loved One;* and most recently, Jessica Mitford, *The American Way of Death.* Interestingly enough, all are English writers, and three of the four focus on the American attitude toward death. They are wrong, however, when they suggest that Americans believe in a triumph of technology over death by virtue of which they reduce death to the incidental or the unreal. Rites are evasive not because Americans react to death as trivial or incidental but because they feel an inner sense of bankruptcy before it. The attempts at evasion and concealment are pathetic rather than casual. The doctor's substitute diagnoses and vague replies and the undertaker's allusions to the "loved one" or to the "beautiful memory picture" reflect a culture in which men sense their own poverty before this event.

Men evade death because they recognize in the event an immensity that towers above their resources for handling it. In effect, death (or the reality that brings it) is recognized as some sort of sacred power that confounds the efforts of man to master it. James Joyce uses a particularly gloomy expression to convey this sense of death as sacred power in *Ulysses—"Dio Boia"*—the "Hangman God." Joyce happens to import the phrase into English literature from the Italian, but the reality of which he speaks crosses national boundaries—death recognized as the power before which all human efforts are ineffectual longings to no avail; death admitted as the reality that may have inspired philosophers to meditate but brings these meditations to their conclusion, that may have crowned the hero or martyr with renown but eventually drags into oblivion even those whom it has lifted up; death

From *Social Research* 39 (Autumn 1972). Used by permission of the publisher and the author.

honored as the power that unravels every human community, taking those fervent little intersections of human want—husband and wife, lovers, father and son—and eventually forcing all these intersecting lines to honor its presence with the rigid parallels of the graveyard.

So understood, death is not merely a biological incident that ends human life. It reaches into the course of life, gripping the human heart with love, fear, hope, worry, and flight, long before the end itself is reached. Whenever the concert is over, the meal is digested, or the career turns barren in one's hands, a man experiences the quiet, disturbing fall from life to death. Because death is more than the incident of biological demise, it is difficult to do justice to its scope without falling into parody of the psalmist's sense of the omnipresence of God. For the power that brings death besets men on every side. It drives men from behind as they flee into frenetic activities—the pursuit of career, virtuosity, or the display of some glory—hoping to escape their metaphysical solitude by outlining themselves against a dark background. It confronts men frontally as they mount their battles against their threatening enemies, whether that enemy happens to be soldier, competition, or sibling. It lies in wait and ambushes from the side—the young, the high-minded, and the frivolous—with the unexpectedness of a clipping at a football game. It stirs beneath human life in the profoundest of pleasures, as it touches with melancholy the marriage bed or as it ladens with guilt the relations between the generations. And at night, it settles down from above and breathes gently within men who are weary with all other forms of fleeing, fighting, and sidestepping death and who long now for sleep and the surcease of care.

If, in some such fashion, men experience death as a religious reality, then one might expect the language of religion to describe most appropriately man's primordial attitude toward the onslaught of the event. This is in fact the language that Joyce chooses in the opening passage of the *Dubliners.* A young boy—friend to a dying priest—muses on the word "paralysis," and offers therein a fine description of religious awe. " 'Paralysis' . . . it sounded to me like the name of some maleficent and sinful being. It filled me with fear and yet I longed to be near it and to look upon its deadly work."[1] Joyce's description captures beautifully that ambivalence of spirit that the phenomenologists of religion have recognized in all religious feeling and which they have variously termed: "awe," "dread," "astonishment," "wonder," or "amazement." A peculiar ambivalence, a strange vibration, a sort of motionless motion obtains in the religious man, an attentiveness somewhat akin to the attention that a hummingbird gives to a flower, when its wings beat furiously and yet it hovers at the spot. This is the way men relate to death in its dreadful reality.

The analysis has uncovered so far two basic responses to the event of death in contemporary culture: concealment and obsession. Only the category of the sacred explains their connection. Men are tempted to conceal death or to hold themselves enthralled before it only because they recognize death as an overmastering power before which all other responses are unavailing.

Geoffrey Gorer, the English sociologist, in his essay "The Pornography of Death,"[2] brings together the phenomena of obsession and concealment by appeal to the religious category of *taboo.* On the one hand, death is a taboo subject, the unmentionable event; on the other hand, death (and violence) is an obsession at every level of our culture. Gorer finds the solution to this oddity in a comparison with the Victorian attitude toward sex. A prudish culture in which personal sexual life is a taboo subject is also likely to develop simultaneously a pornographic obsession with sex. In contemporary culture, argues Gorer, the personal event of death has replaced sex as a taboo subject: Death has replaced copulation and birth as the unmentionable. At the same time, an obsession with violence has dominated our age. Concealment and obsession go together in the same culture.

The chief feature of pornography, of course, is an obsession with the sex-act abstracted from its normal human emotion which is love; the pornography of death therefore is an obsession with death abstracted from its natural human emotion which is grief. For the sake of his thesis Gorer might be altogether satisfied with the development of the James Bond movie. When the sexual act is abstracted from love it becomes somewhat repetitive and dull; therefore, pornographic literature rescues its readers from boredom by filling the fantasy with the sex-act performed in an endless variety of ways, each more elaborate or intense than the last. Interest is removed altogether from love to the technology of the act itself. Correspondingly, when death is abstracted from grief the same restless elaboration of technology occurs. It is difficult to maintain interest in the subject of death unless violence is done in a variety of ways. Thus technicians in violence have to equip James Bond with the ultimate in a death-dealing car that surpasses with exquisite ingenuity the death-dealing instruments that General Motors has already put on the road. And the makers of the movie *Thunderball* bring both lines of pornography to their absurd conclusion, inasmuch as lovemaking and murdering are somehow managed underwater.

The fascination with death in pornography and the concealment of death in the liturgies of polite society are both rooted in religious feeling. It is a religious enthrallment with death that eventuates in the strategies of helpless evasion in the homelike atmosphere of the funeral parlor and in the pornographic experimentations of the entertainment industry.

The traditional belief in the immortality of the soul does not seem to provide men with a sense of resource against the threat of death. In this respect the consciousness of the twentieth century has undergone a radical break with the recent Western past. Christian theologians from the Church Fathers through the Reformers of the sixteenth century held to a doctrine of the immortality of the soul. This doctrine was continued in an altered form by many theologians and philosophers (particularly those of idealist persuasion) in the eighteenth through the late nineteenth century. But today the situation has changed. Naturalists among the philosophers dismiss the doctrine of the immortality of the soul as just so much idealistic vaporing. Psychoanalysts interpret the longing for immortality as a perpetuation of infantile desires. Social critics have condemned the doctrine for its encouragement of an attitude of otherworldly indifference to social ills. Existentialists have opposed the doctrine because it distracts a man from his most essential task as an authentic human being: the appropriation of his own finitude and mortality. Even modern Biblical scholars have rejected the doctrine as they usually distinguish today between the primitive Christian hope of the resurrection of the body and the Hellenic-idealist doctrine of the immortality of the soul.

This is not to say that a belief in the immortality of the soul has had no hold upon modern men. The idealist tradition has had its defenders in Germany, England, America, and France. Dualists of the stripe of Unamuno have tried to reckon with the heart's longing for eternal life, along with the mind's crushing sense of death. Even existentialists, such as Marcel, have made appeal to the existence of a beloved community that transcends the empirical order of death. Finally, and somewhat less grandly, the ordinary man likes to think of himself as immortal, or at least, invulnerable. Tolstoy has observed[3] that the passion for finding out the "cause" of someone else's death is a way of satisfying oneself that the other fellow died accidentally or fortuitously by virtue of special circumstances affecting him (but not me). This shabby impulse, however, is hardly a serious expression of the traditional confidence in the immortality of the soul. Rather it is the hedonist's inveterate bargaining for a little more time in which to dawdle over just one more last cigarette.

Despite traces of contemporary belief in the immortality of the soul, the minister is ill advised to rely on it in the presence of death. Nowhere is the bankruptcy of the doctrine so evident as in a certain type of Protestant funeral service in which the minister strains to give the impression that the person "lives on" in the trappings of the service itself. The minister disastrously seeks to "personalize" the service, not by simple reference to the name and biography of the deceased, but by including his alleged favorite hymns, poems, prayers, and songs. We are supposed to have the impression that we are in the presence of a kind of *aurora borealis* of the dead man's personality, shimmering miraculously in the darkest hour of grief. Instead, however, the minister gives the sad impression that he has a repertory of three or four such "personalized" services, designed like Sears Roebuck seat covers to fit any and all makes and models of cars. Its ill-fitting imposition upon the dead man only reminds us ever so forcibly and comfortlessly that he is, indeed, dead.

Theological Reflection on Death

The attempt to cover up death in the funeral service is an unmitigated disaster for the church, preceded and prepared for by the church's failure to reckon with death in its own preaching and pastoral life. Many persons have said that they have never heard their minister take up frontally in a sermon the question of their own dying. This state of affairs, once again, is not entirely the fault of the professional. People tend to expect from the church service an hour's relief from the demons that plague them in the course of the week. In this atmosphere sermons on death would seem intrusive and unsettling. Better to avoid them and protect this hour from everything that jangles the nerves—even though the service comes to an end and the demons must be faced once again on Monday, fully intact, unexorcized, and screeching. The melancholic effect of this arrangement is that the church offers a temporary sanctuary, a momentary respite, from one's secret apprehensions about death, but inevitably they take over once again, without so much as a candid word of comfort intervening.

To preach about death is absolutely essential if Christians are to preach with joy. Otherwise they speak with the profound melancholy of men who have separated the church from the graveyard. They make the practical assumption that there are two Lords. First, there is the Lord of the Sabbath, the God who presides over the affairs of cheerful Philistines while they are still thriving and in good health. Then there is a second Lord, a Dark Power about whom one never speaks, the Lord of highway wrecks, hospitals, and graveyards who handles everything in the end. Under these circumstances, there can be no doubt as to which of the two Lords is the more commanding power. The death-bringer God already encroaches upon the sanctuary itself, inasmuch as people gathered there are so unsettled as to refuse to hear of his name.

The Christian faith, however, does not speak of two parallel Lords. The Lord of the church is not ruler of a surface kingdom. His dominion is nothing if it does not go at least six feet deep. The church affirms the one Lord who went down into the grave, fought a battle with the power of death, and by his own death brought death to an end. For this reason the church must be unafraid to speak of death. It is compelled to speak of death as the servant of Jesus Christ, the Crucified and Risen Savior, who has freed men from the power of the Unmentionable One.

But even when the church speaks about the subject, does the church evade it? Is theological reflection on the subject of death itself a method of circumlocution? Existentialism, after all, from Kierkegaard to Heidegger, has made men sensitive to the way in which objective discourse on the subject of death may be a way of escaping from one's own personal destiny as a creature who dies. Camus has condemned Christian thought on the subject of death for placing, in effect, theological screens before the eyes of the condemned.[4] Apparently the Christian hope of eternal life only serves to divert attention away from the stark conditions of life in the flesh. "The order of the world is shaped by death," says one of the heroes of *The Plague.*[5]

At the outset, then, by way of reply, it must be argued that Christian reflection, far from screening death from view actually tears away the screens and forces men to look at death and to look toward their own dying. This is the unavoidable focus of a faith that has to reckon with the factual dying of its Savior. Even if men wanted to avoid death, they cannot if they look toward such a savior. In fact, he exposes the flimsiness of the partitions that men raise in order not to have to consider death. The purpose of this comment is not to outdo the existentialist in pessimism but to lay the only sure basis for Christian hope, a hope that is not based on screens, mirrors, or sentiment. It is based on the good news that men do not have to go beyond Jesus for a knowledge of death in its fullest scope; death is not an additional realm alongside of Jesus terrorizing men from the side.

Death in Jesus

In the light of Jesus Christ it is possible to explore the scope of death as it threatens a man in his three most fundamental identities as a human being. Death threatens a man's identity with his flesh, with his community, and with his God. (Insofar as the doctrine of the immortality of the soul abstracted the question of future life from these three fundamental identities, it tended to offer an impoverished if not ghostly sense of future existence.)

A man is clearly identified with his flesh. He is not a ghost. The body is more important to his identity than words to a poet. He both controls his world and savors his world, and reveals himself to others, in and through the living flesh. Part of the terror of death is that it threatens a man with a loss of identity with his flesh, an identity which is essential to him in at least these three ways.

First, man's flesh is the means to his control of his world. Except as he uses his flesh instrumentally (feet for walking, hands for working, tongue for talking), he could not relate to the world by way of mastery and control. When death therefore threatens to separate him from his flesh, it threatens him first with a comprehensive loss of possession and control of his universe. Death meets him as the dispossessor (Luke 12:15–21), even though he retaliates as best he can against his loss of control with an assortment of insurance policies. Quite shrewdly the medieval moralists saw a special connection between the capital sin of avarice and old age. Avarice is the special sin in which a man focuses his life on his possessions. The closer a man gets to the time of his dispossession, the more fiercely he clings to what he has and the more suspicion he feels toward all those who would dispossess him with indecorous haste.

Second, a man's flesh is more than instrumental, it is also the site for the disclosure of the world to him, the world which he will never be able to reduce to property but which is there for the savoring. Except as flesh is sensitive, susceptible, and vulnerable, a man could not be open to the world as it pours in upon him in a wild profusion of colors, sounds, and feelings. He could not fall under the spell of powers that both enchant and terrify him. When death therefore threatens to separate him from flesh it threatens also to separate him from the propertyless creation, the world which he may not control but which is his for the beholding in ritual, art, and daily routine.[6]

Third, flesh is more than instrumental and more than sensitive to the world; it is also revelatory. A man reveals himself to his neighbor in and through the living flesh. He is inseparable from his countenance, gestures, and the physical details of his speech. Part of the terror of death, then, is that it threatens him with a loss of his revelatory power. The dreadfulness of the corpse lies in its claim to be the body of the person, while it is wholly unrevealing of the person. What was once so expressive of the human soul has suddenly become a mask.

We have referred to the *threat* of separation from the flesh in each case not only because a man can anticipate it before it occurs, but also because this separation does not occur all at once. It is shocking to encounter a young man who is dying and recognize a spirit that is still alive with its original power and promise while the flesh abandons it. Or again it is possible to look upon the aged whose spirits have long since absented themselves while their bodies persist so mindlessly alive.

Part of the melancholy of this loss of identity is that no frontal assault can be launched against it. The fear of death only intensifies insofar as a man plunges deeper into his possessions as a way of securing himself against the day of his dispossession, or gives himself over to the frenetic carnivals of a death-ridden age as a way of savoring his world, or takes daily inventory of his physical appearance in the quiet ceremonies before the morning mirror.

Death not only threatens a man with separation from the flesh; it also tears him away from his community. This threat has already been anticipated in the discussion of the revelatory power of the flesh. Death means the unraveling of human community. It divides husband and wife, father and son, and lovers from one another. Not even the child is exempt from this threat. In demanding the reassurance of a voice, the touch of a hand at bedtime, he shows that he knows all the essential issues involved in a sleep that is early practice in dying. Death threatens all men with final separation, exclusion, and oblivion. And again, this threat is operative beforehand, as the fear of oblivion can prompt men to force their way into the society of others in ways which are ultimately self-isolating.

But death also threatens men with separation from God. This is the terror of death that men have never fully faced because they have never wholly honored the presence of God. But it is the terror of which all others are but prologue and sign. Men fear separation from their flesh because they know life in and through their flesh. They fear separation from community because they know life in and through their community. But what are these compared with separation from God, who is the source of life in the flesh and life in the community? This question remains partly rhetorical for all men inasmuch as they do not know fully what they ask. But it was the last question on the lips of the One whom Christians worship and adore in his cry of abandonment from the cross.

Jesus knew death in all its dimensions. The creed puts it: He "suffered under Pontius Pilate, was crucified, dead and buried; he descended into Hell." His death, like others, meant separation from the flesh. The narratives are utterly factual in detail about his ordeal in the flesh. He suffered dispossession: the king with no subjects, the teacher with no pupils, the healer who bleeds. He suffered severance from the world, reduced as it was to a sop of vinegar, the darkness of the sixth hour, and a spear in the side; and he, like all other men before and after him, suffered the final conclusion of his life in the unrevealing corpse.

His death meant also separation from community. One can see this separation at work beforehand in the persecution of the high priest, the ambiguities of the Roman governor, the fickleness of the crowds, the betrayal of Judas, the cowardice of Peter, and the sleepiness of followers in Gethsemane. It was consummated in his burial when he, like all other men, was removed from sight.

Finally Jesus experienced what men know only through him: separation from God. The Son of God cries out, "My God, my God, why hast thou forsaken me?" The Son of God descends into the region that stands under the naked terror of the absence of God and stands fast there for every man.

Because the Son of God has done this, the Christian cannot be content simply to tell horror stories about the ravaging power of death. If in looking toward Jesus, he looks toward death in its full terror and power, so also he looks toward the Savior who exposes death in its ultimate powerlessness. No final power remains to death, if death itself has become the event in which Jesus exposes the powerfulness of God's love. Death can still menace, but it can no longer make good on its threats. In Jesus' death, God, flesh, and community are indissolubly met in self-expending love. For this reason, it is no longer necessary to stare in the mirror, worrying about the defeat of one's flesh, or to plunge into communities, worried about exclusion at their hands, or to lift up one's eyes to heaven, attempting in a blind fury of good works to force the presence of God. For the Savior who is identified, soul and body, with men in his descent is the one who remains their Lord in his ascent, to bring men new life—bodily, together, in the presence of God.

Life in Jesus

Usually when a man asks the question of eternal life, he wonders simply whether he will continue to live beyond the grave. Putting the question this way, he assumes that a human being can be separated from his ties with his flesh, community, and God. This is the assumption by virtue of which the doctrine of the immortality of the soul, in some of its versions, actually led to an impoverishment of the notion of eternal life. Eternal life, in effect, became an eternalization of death, as the soul projected itself endlessly into the future—deprived of everything that formerly made it jubilant with life. Cut off from its ties with its flesh, community, and God, the soul so imagined is spectral and wraith-like. Its daydreams about the future have turned into ghoul-ridden nightmares.

The Risen Christ, however, cuts through the nonsense of these daydreams about eternity with the sharp actuality of his life. He is not ghoulishly divested of a body; on the contrary, he shows himself to his disciples, his flesh still bearing the marks of his crucifixion. He is not banished from community like a spook (whose appearance always causes men to scatter and run); on the contrary, his appearance among men is such as to establish and nourish human community. Neither is he grievously separated from God; the account of his resurrection is followed by the acknowledgment of his ascension. This testimony to the ascension of Christ excludes the fantasy of a ghostly Savior drifting in the nether world between God and men. His proximity to God, in turn ("at the right hand of the Father"), is at the basis of his power to create a full-bodied life for his community among men.

Correspondingly, the eternal life that Jesus imparts to men is neither spectral nor rootless. Jesus extends to men the specific hope of future life in the body. "We wait for adoption as sons, the redemption of our bodies" (Rom. 8:23). Wholly consistent with this promise of a glorified body is the apostolic assurance of a new heaven and a new earth to which the body gives access. Man is not destined to live on perpetually in the tedium of a worldless "I." Neither however will he live on in isolation from his fellow. Jesus imparts eternal life to him through a community. As Ephesians puts it, "God . . . made us alive together in Christ" (2:4, 5). The word "together" in the passage does not convey the incidental bit of intelligence that others beside oneself are involved in the resurrection, as though men were like strangers, temporarily herded together to receive a fortune from a benefactor whom each knew in his private way. Rather God creates in the community of disciples a freedom for each other that would not be there except through participation in his life.

Finally eternal life means bodily life, together, in the *presence* of God. Resurrection means intimacy with God. Jesus says to the thief on the cross, "Today you will be with me in paradise." (Luke 23:43) The Christian hope is not simply for a deathless, endless life in which relations between a man, his body, and his neighbor have been set in order. To center hope on a perfected world alone is eschatological atheism. If God exists, eternal life cannot be defined apart from his presence. Without him the perfection of this world would be like the sterile order of a house that a woman kept immaculate for no other end than its own tidiness, as though she did not desire the presence of her husband. In the humblest of marriages the vital presence of the husband belongs to the joy of the house, so the presence of God fills out the joy of heaven.

Eternal life is the future destiny of man, but participation in this life is not reserved to the future alone. Just as death is not simply an event at the end of life but overtakes men by way of fear, worry, and disease in the present moment, so also the resurrection is not an event wholly reserved for the other side of the grave. Men can live now in the power of the resurrection. Surely the martyr faced death with hope in his heart for the future glory, yet he did so in the present enabling power of the resurrection. Otherwise the fullness of God fills only the future, fills only the far side, powerless finally to redeem the present and powerless to sustain men in the agony of dying itself. Men can look forward to the coming ages of his kindness toward them because he stands with them already on this side of the grave.

The fact of the resurrection of Christ, however, does not mean that the Christian is altogether removed from the experience of natural grief and sorrow. Were it otherwise, the Christian should be able to face his own death without a tremor, and he should be able to walk confidently into the sickroom, contending with its silence by "talking up" a victory that has not yet, apparently, reached the ears of those who await an imminent defeat. This is a professional Christian cheerfulness, a grisly boy-scoutism, for which there is no justification in Scripture. The apostle Paul expressed himself carefully: Only "when this corruptible *shall* have put on incorruption . . . *shall* there come to pass the saying that is written, Death is swallowed up in victory" (I Cor. 15:54, italics added). The Christian knows grief in this life. He is not granted on this side of the grave a pure, steadfast, confident, and transparent sense of his limits—or the limits of his neighbor—before God. He tastes of eternal life in Christ, but not a life that removes him from death and the sting of death. The work of death is still very much evident in the inner and the outer man. Death remains the last enemy. Not until the gift of life beyond the limit has been granted to man is it possible for him to say wholeheartedly:

> O Death, where is thy victory?
> O Death, where is thy sting?

This does not mean, however, that nothing of importance has occurred. Although the Christian does not yet know an eternal life without death, he has reckoned in Christ with an eternal life under the conditions of death, that permits him to live hopefully in the crisis of his neighbor's death and his own. This is the basis for the witness of the church to the dying.

The Church's Behavior Toward the Dying

Let it be said at the outset that the church cannot act as though it possesses something that the dying lack. A demoralizing feature of illness for any patient is the condescending cheerfulness of nurses and friends, whose very display of good health reminds the mortally ill that they are about to be dispossessed of their world. The church cannot behave in such a way as to add yet another possession, i.e., Christian hope, that distinguishes the Christian from the unbeliever or the sorely tried believer who is mortally ill.

This consideration, however, produces an oddity. Does the Christian somehow have to assume the *unreality* of the resurrection in order to avoid removing himself from his fellowman? Must he ignore the resurrection so as not to appear like a self-assured Christ-dispenser in the sickroom? Does he find himself saying, in effect, that the resurrection has taken place but that its fruits are a long way off for all of us and therefore nothing has occurred that need disturb the humanity of my response to your illness and imminent death?

Actually, the reverse is the case. It is precisely in the absence of a sense of the resurrection that the Christian is tempted to think solely in terms of those possessions he has to offer the sick. He makes the painful assumption that he must be a God-producer, a Christ-dispenser, or a religious magician in the sickroom. Failing miserably, of course, at all these roles, he feels keenly his poverty. He makes a lame effort to produce the decisive and healing word, only to stutter and to fall silent. In the absence of a sense of resurrection he feels the terrifying lack of a gift between himself and the dying, a frightening gulf of silence between them. He is inclined therefore with every healthy fiber of his being to shy away from the dying to avoid his own poverty.

The resurrection of Christ frees a man for approach to the dying not because it arms him with a possession to give, but because it frees him from all this worry and confusion about possessions. Christ is already the decisive gift between the living and the dying, the mediator between them. There is no need to produce Christ in the sickroom when he is already there in advance of a man's approach. The Christian is mercifully free, therefore, to offer whatever secondary gifts he can—of anxiety, suffering, money, words, friendship, and hope—letting them be, wherever possible, signs of a divine love which they do not produce.

The Church's Witness and Separation from the Flesh

It is angelism to assume that the sole witness of the church to the dying and the bereaved is the testimony of theology alone. A ministry to the flesh is a true and valid ministry. It need not be supposed that Christian witness is invariably something more than this. Admittedly the apparatus of medicine—doctors, nurses, and sanitary hospitals—can function as a shield behind which the larger community of health protects itself from contact with the dying. But this need not be the case. There is no reason why the machinery of modern medicine—awesome and impersonal though it is—may not yet serve human purposes and therefore function as a sign of a life that exceeds its own powers to heal. To do this, however, some sensitivity must be shown toward the several crises that a man experiences in his flesh.

It was noted earlier that sickness and death involve a traumatic loss of control over one's world. A man who has brutally exploited his body as an instrument of aggression against his world suddenly suffers a heart attack. The very flesh through which he exercised mastery suddenly explodes from within. He is helpless in the hands of others, unable even to control disturbing noises down the hall. Under these circumstances the apparatus of medicine can be frightening; it demonstrates to him his helplessness and therefore reminds him of the poverty of all his attempts to solve the problem of his existence through mastery alone. The machinery of medicine thus assumes the terrifying shape of a parable of judgment. It brings his past life to nought. At the same time, however, the apparatus of medicine can be a testimony to grace. It does after all serve the body; and in this it can be a mute sign of the Lord whose mastery took the form of life-giving and life-comforting service. Seen in this light, it is the special task of the church not to ignore the work of medicine as a sub-Christian activity but to accompany and to criticize it in such a way as to help it to serve this end of service.

The second crisis for the flesh is the loss of the world in its uncontrolled splendor and diversity. A toothache has a way of reducing the world to itself. Unfortunately, the apparatus of medicine, dedicated as it is to the medical recovery of the patient, presents the hospitalized patient with a functional but blank and abstract environment, devoid of the irrelevant details that make up a truly human existence. (Yeats once registered his complaint against the scientific formula H_2O by observing, "I like a little seaweed in my definition of water.") Many European hospitals admirably manage to maintain gardens as part of their grounds. A functionally irrelevant expense, perhaps, in an institution dedicated to treating and discharging people as fast as it can, but some patients, after all, are discharged for burial, and it is well to maintain a sign for them of a world that has not shrunk to the final abstraction of their irremediable pain.

The third crisis for the flesh is the imminent loss of its revelatory power. The falterings of the body in old age increasingly prevent it from being expressive of the soul in its full dignity. There is warrant here for a sensitive ministry to the body in its infirmities which extends to the humblest of details in the daily routines of eating and cleansing. Upon death, moreover, there is warrant for a funeral service in which the body is not treated as a disposable cartridge to be thrown away like garbage. This argument for a fitting disposal of the remains, however, is hardly an apology for present-day funeral practice. Quite the contrary, it opens the way for an even more savage criticism of these practices. Precisely because the body has been (and will be) what it is only by the power of God to glorify it, it cannot become in Christian practice a lewd object of the mortician's craft. It is one thing for the mortician to minimize the violence done to the body by death, but it is quite another thing for him to impose upon the deceased the suggestion of a character other than its own. Only too often today Uncle John is not allowed to die. He must be prettied up with rouge on his cheeks and his casket opened so that his friends can see his face forced into a smile. Poor Uncle John never smiled in his life, but now he does—beatifically. It is not only the beautification of Uncle John, but his beatification that one attempts to achieve. The church won't canonize him but the mortician will. One is supposed to go to the funeral parlor, look on the face of the corpse, and say about Uncle John, "Doesn't he look natural?" which, of course, is the one thing he does not look. Let death be death. There is no reason to add to its hideousness by mocking the inability of the dead to reveal themselves.

The Witness of the Church and Separation from Community

One of the most devastating features of terminal illness is the fear of abandonment.[7] Sickness has already isolated the patient from his normal identity in the community: Strong and authoritative, he is now relatively helpless; gregarious by nature, he suddenly finds friends exhausting. Ironically the very apparatus by which the community ministers to his physical need isolates him further. The modern hospital segregates the sick and the dying from their normal human resources. One doctor has observed that in an Arabian village a grandmother dies in the midst of her children and grandchildren, cows and donkeys. But our high level of technological developments leads simply to dying a death appropriate to one's disease—in the heart ward or the cancer ward.[8]

Most desolating of all is the breakdown of communication between the dying patient, the doctor, and the nearest of kin. Substitute diagnoses are sometimes justified on the grounds that they establish an emotional equilibrium (homeostasis) essential to the health and comfort of the patient, but this justification ignores the fact that evasiveness can itself be emotionally disturbing. It is demoralizing for everybody concerned to get stuck with a lie, because, once told, life tends to organize itself around it. Even when the lie isn't working, even when it produces the anguish of suspicion, isolation, and uncertainty, the doctor may rely on it to keep his own relation to the patient in a state of equilibrium. Homeostasis, in other words, is a problem not only for the patient but also for the doctor and for the family. The family also grows accustomed to the explanation and enmeshes itself more deeply in the demands of make-believe. It seems too late for everybody concerned to recover an authentic relationship to the event. Isolated by evasion and lies, the patient is driven out of community before his time. He has forced upon him a premature burial. While trying to avoid the fact of death, the community actually reeks of death, for it has already excluded him.

It would be wrong, however, to make the doctor the scapegoat here and therefore to underestimate woefully the problems of sharing the truth. This was the mistake of a group of psychiatrists in the previously referred to study of *Death and Dying: Attitudes of Patient and Doctor.*[9] The psychiatrists reported that 69 to 90 percent of physicians (depending on the specific study) were not in favor of informing the patient in cases of mortal illness. Meanwhile on the basis of their own interviews with patients, the psychiatrists reported that approximately 82 percent of patients in terminal cases actually wanted to be informed of their true condition. Several psychiatrists explained this discrepancy between the apparent desire of patients and the actual performance of doctors by appeal to the psychological defects of doctors or to faults in their training: (1) they are more afraid of death than other professional groups; (2) they shy away from dealing with chronic and terminal cases because such cases are a blow to the doctor's professional self-esteem; (3) they receive inadequate preparation in medical school for coping with the problem of handling terminal cases.

Doubtless, all these observations are valid in given instances, but I found the psychiatrists breathtakingly naïve in the evidence they accepted as proof that patients really want to know the truth. First, it is not clear that patients are so willing to talk about the possibility—or the inevitability—of their own death *with their own doctor,* as the percentages reported by the psychiatrists in their interviews with patients would indicate. Dr. Samuel Feder indirectly admitted this fact when he observed that "all . . . patients, when they were asked to see me as a 'new doctor,' reacted with great anxiety."[10] All but two of the patients, however, were delighted to discover that he was "only" a psychiatrist. He admits that this was a unique experience for him as a psychiatrist. Obviously patients were glad that "he was not one of those other doctors—those other doctors being the bearers of bad tidings."

Dr. Feder interpreted these anxiety reactions as proof that people knew that they were going to die. Therefore the doctors had no excuse for avoiding the subject. I interpret them, however, as proof that these people were frightened of hearing just this verdict from their own doctors. The doctor in charge is less approachable on this subject precisely because he is the keeper of desolate truths. By the same token, the psychiatrist is more accessible since he brings no final verdict. If this analysis is correct, then the doctor's reticence to discuss the subject cannot be written off solely as a question of his own fear of death or his oversensitive, professional self-esteem. The sacral dimensions of death are too awesome to admit of easy professional solution. The problem of isolation cannot be solved by handing out truth like pills since the truth itself can have a disturbing and an isolating effect.

Yet there are ways in which people can reach out to one another in word and actions and maintain some measure of solidarity before the overwhelming event of death. It would be pretentious to outline these ways since they are not fully given to men except in the concrete case. Nevertheless it is possible to clarify (and perhaps even to clear the way of) certain obstacles that men face in their behavior toward the dying. They divide very simply into those of word and deed.

The Problem of Words

Perhaps we are especially inhibited in our talk with the dying because the alternatives in language seem so poor. There are several types of discourse available to us: (1) direct, immediate, blunt talk; (2) circumlocution or double-talk; (3) silence (which can be, of course, a mode of sharing, but oftentimes, is a way of evading); and (4) discourse that proceeds by way of indirection.

Too often we assume (especially as Americans) that the only form of truth-telling is direct, immediate, blunt talk. Such talk seems to be the only alternative to evasive silence or circumlocution. On the subject of sex, for example, we assume that the only alternative to the repressions of a Victorian age is the tiresome, gabby explicit discussion of sex we impose upon the adolescent from junior high forward. So also on the subject of death we assume that truth-telling requires something approaching the seminar in loquacity. But obviously gabby bluntness in the presence of one dying is wholly inappropriate. It reckons in no way with the solemnity of the event. To plead for the explicit discussion of diagnosis or prognosis with every patient in clinical detail would be foolhardy. But the alternative to blunt talk need not be double-talk, a condescending cheerfulness, or a frightening silence. There is such a thing as *indirect* discourse in both love and death.

Perhaps examples of what I mean by indirection will suffice. One doctor reports that many patients instinctively brought up the question of their own death in an indirect form. Some asked him, for example, whether he thought they should buy a house, marry, or have plastic surgery done to their face. The doctor realized that the answer, "Yes, surely, go ahead— " in a big, cheerful voice was an evasion. Meanwhile the answer, "No," was a summary reply which would have made further discussion impossible. He found it important however to convey to them somehow that he recognized the importance of the question. From that point on, it was possible to discuss their uncertainties, anxieties, and fears. Some kind of sharing could take place. It was not necessary to dwell on the subject for long; after its acknowledgment it was possible to proceed to the details of daily life without the change of subject seeming an evasion.

Indirection may be achieved in another way. Although it may be too overbearing to approach the subject of death frontally under the immediate pressure of its presence, a kind of indirection can be achieved if death is discussed in advance of a crisis. The minister who suddenly feels like a tongue-tied irrelevancy in the sickroom gets what he deserves if he has not worked through the problem with his people in a series of sermons or in work sessions with lay groups. Words too blunt and inappropriate in the crisis itself may, if spoken earlier, provide an indirect basis for sharing burdens.

The language of indirection is appropriate behavior because, as it has been argued throughout, death is a sacred event. For the most part, toward the sacred the most fitting relation is indirect. The Jew did not attempt to look straight on Jahweh's face. A direct, immediate, casual confrontation was impossible. But avoidance of God's presence was not the only alternative. It was given to the Jew to hold his ground before his Lord in a relation that was genuine but indirect. So also, it is not necessary to dwell directly on the subject of death interminably or to avoid it by a condescending cheerfulness wholly inappropriate to the event. It is possible for two human beings to acknowledge death, be it ever so indirectly, and to hold their ground before it until they are parted.

The Problem of Action

Deeds are no easier to come by than words in extremity. Everyone grows uneasy. When nothing is left to be done toward the dying, a man is inclined to pay his respects, look at his watch, and fish out an excuse that fetches him home. Perhaps, however, our discomfort stems partly from a view of action somewhat inappropriate to overwhelming events. T. S. Eliot once said that there are two types of problems we face in life. In one case, the appropriate question is: what are we going to do about it? In the other case: how do we behave toward it? The deeper problems in life are of the latter kind.

But unfortunately as Americans, and especially as Americans in those professions that get tinged with a slight messianic pretension—medicine and the ministry—we are used to tackling problems in terms of the first question, and are left somewhat bereft, therefore, when that question is inappropriate to the crisis. If all we can say is, What are we going to do about it?, then the dying indeed (and our own death) is a fatal blow to professional self-esteem. But this is not the only question we can ask ourselves in crisis. In extremity it may not be possible to do something about a tragedy, but this inability need not altogether disable our behavior toward it.

The Witness of the Church and the Threat of Separation from God

Since this is the threat in which the name of God appears, it is assumed that the special witness of the church in this case is theology. It may indeed be theology—but neither invariably nor exclusively so and certainly not theology conceived as a series of truths that provide men with access to God while putting them at a comforting distance from the sting of death. Such a theology, while trying to screen death from view, would only succeed in shielding men from the presence of God. For who is God as the Christian knows him? He is the God and Father of Jesus Christ, crucified and risen from the dead. Possessed by Jesus Christ, the church is not removed from the sting of existence come to an end. Rather it lives by a concrete existence that cuts into death with all the power of God's love to make death itself the very instance of that love. Because this is the case, the church cannot shield death from view without seeking—foolishly—to place theological screens before the eyes of the redeemed.

The witness of the church to the presence of God is not always direct and verbal. This fact has already been anticipated in our discussion of death. Just as an authentic acknowledgment of death can take place within the limits of indirect discourse, so also an authentic witness to Jesus Christ can occur without the inevitable footnote giving reference to his name. The Christian sense of the presence of God can express itself indirectly in the way in which the Christian responds to other levels of crisis. The calm with which he offers friendship in crisis may count for more than theological virtuosity in testifying to God's presence. The worry with which he offers advice will reveal more than the advice itself when he is really stricken with a sense of God's absence. But even in the case of failure he cannot, with Christian consistency, take his failure too seriously. God is the ultimate presence in death, whether men succeed in testifying to him or not. Neither life, nor death, nor the failure of Christians, will be able to separate men from the love of God. This is the message of Rom. 8 and the substance of Christian witness. When the church fails by its words and deeds to make this witness to the dying, let the dying among her members be brave enough to make this witness to the church.

Notes

1. James Joyce, *The Dubliners* (New York: The Modern Library), p. 7.

2. Reprinted as an appendix in his book, *Death, Grief, and Mourning* (Garden City, N.Y.: Doubleday & Co., 1965).

3. Leo Tolstoy, *The Death of Ivan Ilyitch* (New York: Boni and Liveright), p. 8. See also Sigmund Freud, "Thoughts for the Times on War and Death," Collected Papers, Vol. IV, 1915, trans. Joan Riviere (London: The Hogarth Press, 1925), p. 305.

4. "In Italian museums are sometimes found little painted screens that the priest used to hold in front of the face of condemned men to hide the scaffold from them." Albert Camus, *The Myth of Sisyphus and Other Essays.*

5. Albert Camus, *The Plague,* trans. Stewart Gilbert (London: Hamish Hamilton, 1948), p. 123.

6. Karl Rahner has argued that the severance of a man from his flesh may mean not the loss of a world but rather a release of the soul from the more restricted world it knows in the flesh to an all-cosmic relationship that transcends the limitations of life within the province of a body. Even so Rahner must admit that this eventuality, if it be our destiny, is precisely the future which death, in its darkness, obscures. As we know it now, death threatens to separate us from the flesh and so banish us from that site through which the world is disclosed. See Karl Rahner, *On the Theology of Death,* pp. 29 ff.

7. "The dying patient faces emotional problems of great magnitude, including fear of death itself, fear of the ordeal of dying and the devastating fear of abandonment." See Ruth D. Abrams, M.S., "The Patient with Cancer—His Changing Pattern of Communication," *New England Journal of Medicine,* Vol. 274, No. 6, p. 320.

8. Bryant M. Wedge, in discussion at the conclusion of a symposium on *Death and Dying: Attitudes of Patient and Doctor,* sponsored by the Group for the Advancement of Psychiatry, Symposium No. 11, Vol. V.

9. See especially the essay by Herman Feifel, "The Function of Attitudes Toward Death," Ch. V in *Death and Dying: Attitudes of Patient and Doctor,* pp. 633-37.

10. Samuel L. Feder, "Attitudes of Patients with Advanced Malignancy," Chap. III in *Death and Dying: Attitudes of Patient and Doctor,* pp. 614-20.

31. The Indignity of 'Death with Dignity'

PAUL RAMSEY

Never one am I to use an ordinary title when an extraordinary one will do as well! Besides, I mean to suggest that there is an additional insult besides death itself heaped upon the dying by our ordinary talk about "death with dignity." Sometimes that is said even to be a human "right"; and what should a decent citizen do but insist on enjoying his rights? That might be his duty (if there is any such right), to the commonwealth, to the human race or some other collective entity; or at least, embracing that "right" and dying rationally would exhibit a proper respect for the going concept of a rational man. So "The Indignity of Death" would not suffice for my purposes, even though all I shall say depends on understanding the contradiction death poses to the unique worth of an individual human life.

The genesis of the following reflections may be worth noting. A few years ago,[1] I embraced what I characterized as the oldest morality there is (no "new morality") concerning responsibility toward the dying: the acceptance of death, stopping our medical interventions for all sorts of good, human reasons, *only* companying with the dying in their final passage. Then suddenly it appeared that altogether too many people were agreeing with me. That caused qualms. As a Southerner born addicted to lost causes, it seemed I now was caught up in a triumphal social trend. As a controversialist in ethics, I found agreement from too many sides. As a generally happy prophet of the doom facing the modern age, unless there is a sea-change in norms of action, it was clear from these premises that anything divers people agree to must necessarily be superficial if not wrong.

Today, when divers people draw the same warm blanket of "allowing to die" or "death with dignity" close up around their shoulders against the dread of that cold night, their various feet are showing. Exposed beneath our growing agreement to that "philosophy of death and dying" may be significantly different "philosophies of life"; and in the present age that agreement may reveal that these interpretations of human life are increasingly mundane, naturalistic,

From the *Hastings Center Studies* 2 (May 1974): 47-62. Used by permission of the publisher and the author.

antihumanistic when measured by *any* genuinely "humanistic" esteem for the individual human being.

These "philosophical" ingredients of any view of death and dying I want to make prominent by speaking of "The Indignity of 'Death with Dignity'." Whatever practical agreement there may be, or "guidelines" proposed to govern contemporary choice or practice, these are bound to be dehumanizing unless at the same time we bring to bear great summit points and sources of insight in mankind's understanding of mankind (be it Christian or other religious humanism, or religiously-dependent but not explicitly religious humanism, or, if it is possible, a true humanism that is neither systematically nor historically dependent on any religious outlook).

Death with Dignity Ideologies

There is nobility and dignity in caring for the dying, but not in dying itself. "To be a therapist to a dying patient makes us aware of the uniqueness of each individual in this vast sea of humanity."[2] It is more correct to say that a therapist brings to the event, from some other source, an awareness of the uniqueness, the once-for-allness of an individual life-span as part of an "outlook" and "on-look" upon the vast sea of humanity. In any case, that is the reflected glory and dignity of caring for the dying, that we are or become aware of the unique life here ending. The humanity of such human caring is apt to be more sensitive and mature if we do not lightly suppose that it is an easy thing to convey dignity to the dying. That certainly cannot be done simply by withdrawing tubes and stopping respirators or not thumping hearts. At most, those omissions can only be prelude to companying with the dying in their final passage, if we are fortunate enough to share with them—they in moderate comfort—those interchanges that are in accord with the dignity and nobility of mankind. Still, however noble the manifestations of caring called for, however unique the individual life, we finally must come to the reality of death, and must ask, what can possibly be the meaning of "death with dignity"?

At most we convey only the liberty to die with human dignity; we can provide some of the necessary but not sufficient conditions. If the dying die with a degree of nobility it will be mostly their doing in doing their own dying. I fancy their task was easier when death as a human event meant that special note was taken of the last words of the dying—even humorous ones, as in the case of the Roman Emperor who said as he expired, "I Deify." A human countenance may be discerned in death accepted with serenity. So also there is a human countenance behind death with defiance. "Do not go gentle into that good night," wrote Dylan Thomas. "Old age should rage and burn against the close of day; Rage Rage against the dying of the light." But the human countenance has been removed from most modern understandings of death.

We do not begin to keep human community with the dying if we interpose between them and us most of the current notions of "death with dignity." Rather do we draw closer to them if and only if our conception of "dying with dignity" encompasses—nakedly and without dilution—the final indignity of death itself, whether accepted or raged against. So I think it may be profitable to explore "the indignity of 'death with dignity'." "Good death" (euthanasia) like "Good grief!" is ultimately a contradiction in terms, even if superficially, and before we reach the heart of the matter, there are distinctions to be made; even if, that is to say, the predicate "good" still is applicable in both cases in contrast to worse ways to die and worse ways to grieve or not to grieve.

"Death is simply a part of life," we are told, as a first move to persuade us to accept the ideology of the entire dignity of dying with dignity. A singularly unpersuasive proposition, since we are not told what sort of part of life death is. Disease, injury, congenital defects are also a part of life, and as well murder, rapine, and pillage.[3] Yet there is no campaign for accepting or doing those things with dignity. Nor, for that matter, for the contemporary mentality which would enshrine "death with dignity" is there an equal emphasis on "suffering with dignity," suffering as a "natural" part of life, etc. All those things, it seems, are enemies and violations of human nobility while death is not, or (with a few changes) need not be. Doctors did not invent the fact that death is an enemy, although they may sometimes use disproportionate means to avoid final surrender. Neither did they invent the fact that pain and suffering are enemies and often indignities, although suffering accepted may also be ennobling or may manifest the nobility of the human spirit of any ordinary person.

But, then, it is said, death is an evolutionary necessity and in that further sense a part of life not to be denied. Socially and biologically, one generation follows another. So there must be death, else social history would have no room for creative novelty and planet earth would be glutted with humankind. True enough, no doubt, from the point of view of evolution (which—so far—never dies). But the man who is dying happens not to be evolution. He is a part of evolution, no doubt: but not to the whole extent of his being or his dying. A crucial testimony to the individual's transcendence over the species is man's problem and his dis-ease in dying. Death is a natural fact of life, yet no man dies "naturally," nor do we have occasions in which to practice doing so in order to learn how. Not unless the pursuit of philosophy is a practice of dying (as Plato's *Phaedo* teaches); and that I take to be an understanding of the human being we moderns do not mean to embrace when we embrace "death with dignity."

It is small consolation to tell mortal men that as long as you are, the death you contribute to evolution is not yet; and when death is, you are not—so why fear death? That is the modern equivalent to the recipe offered by the ancient Epicureans (and some Stoics) to undercut fear of death and devotion to the gods: as long as you are, death is not; when death is, you are not; there's never a direct encounter between you and death; so why dread death? Indeed, contrary to modern parlance, those ancient philosophers declared that death is *not a part of life;* so, why worry?

So "death is not a part of life" is another declaration designed to quiet fear of death. This can be better understood in terms of a terse comment by Wittgenstein: "Our life has no limit in just the way in which our visual field has no limit."[4] We cannot see beyond the boundary of our visual field; it is more correct to say that beyond the boundary of our visual field *we do not see.* Not only so. Also, we do not see the boundary, the limit itself. There is no seeable bound to the visual field. *Death is not a part of life* in the same way that the boundary is not a part of our visual field. Commenting on this remark by Wittgenstein, James Van Evra writes: "Pressing the analogy, then, if my life has no end in *just the way* that my visual field has no limit, then it must be in the sense that I can have no experience of death, conceived as the complete cessation of experience and thought. That is, if life is considered to be a series of experiences and thoughts, then it is impossible for me to experience death, for to experience something is to be alive, and hence is to be inside the bound formed by death."[5] This is why death itself steadfastly resists conceptualization.

Still, I think the disanalogy ought also to be pressed, against both ancient and contemporary analytical philosophers. That notion of death as a limit makes use of a visual or spatial metaphor. Good basketball players are often men naturally endowed with an unusually wide visual field; this is true, for example, of Bill Bradley. Perhaps basketball players, among other things, strive to enlarge their visual fields, or their habitual use of what powers of sight they have, if that is possible. But ordinarily, everyone of us is perfectly happy within the unseeable limits of sight's reach.

Transfer this notion of death as a limit from space to time as the form of human perception, from sight to an individual's inward desire, effort and hope, and I suggest that one gets a different result. Then death as the temporal limit of a life-span is something we live toward. That limit still can never be experienced or conceptualized; indeed death is *never* a part of life. Moreover, neither is the boundary. Still it is a limit we conative human beings know we live *up against* during our life-spans. We do not live toward or up against the side-limits of our visual-span. Instead, within that acceptable visual limit (and other limits as well) as channels we live toward yet another limit which is death.

Nor is the following analogy for death as a limit of much help in deepening understanding. ". . . The importance of the limit and virtually *all* of its significance," writes Van Evra, "derives from the fact that the limit serves as an ordering device"—just as absolute zero serves for ordering a series; it is not *just* a limit, although nothing can exist at such a temperature. The analogy is valid so far as it suggests that we conceive of death not in itself but as it bears on us while still alive. As I shall suggest below, death teaches us to "number our days."

But that may not be its only ordering function for conative creatures. Having placed death "out of our league" by showing that it is not a "something," or never a part of life, and while understanding awareness of death as awareness of a limit bearing upon us only while still alive, one ought not forthwith to conclude that this understanding of it "exonerates death as the purported snake in our garden." Death as a limit can disorder no less than order the series. Only a disembodied reason can say, as Van Evra does, that "the bound, not being a member of the series, cannot defile it. The series is what it is, happy or unhappy, good or bad, quite independently of any bound as such." An Erik Erikson knows better than that when writing of the "despair and often unconscious fear of death" which results when "the one and only life cycle is not accepted as the ultimate life." Despair, he observes, "expresses the feeling that the time is short, too short for the attempt to start another life and to try out alternate roads to integrity."[6]

It is the temporal flight of the series that is grievous (not death as an evil "something" within life's span to be balanced, optimistically or pessimistically, against other things that are good). The reminder that death is *not a part of life,* or that it is only a boundary never encountered, is an ancient recipe that can only increase the threat of death on any profound understanding of human life. The dread of death is the dread of oblivion, of there being only empty room in one's stead. Kübler-

Ross writes that for the dying, death means the loss of every loved one, total loss of everything that constituted the self in its world, separation from every experience, even from future possible, replacing experiences—nothingness beyond. Therefore, life is a time-intensive activity and not only a goods-intensive or quality-intensive activity. No matter how many "goods" we store up in barns, like the man in Jesus' parable we know that this night our soul may be required of us (Luke 12:13-21). No matter what "quality of life" our lives have, we must take into account the opportunity-costs of used time. Death means the conquest of the time of our lives—even though we never experience the experience of the nothingness which is natural death.

"Awareness of dying" means awareness of *that;* and awareness of that constitutes an experience of ultimate indignity in and to the awareness of the self who is dying.

We are often reminded of Koheleth's litany: "For everything there is a season, and a time for every matter under heaven: a time to be born and a time to die; a time to plant, and a time to pluck up what is planted," etc. (Eccles. 3:1,2). Across those words of the narrator of Ecclesiastes the view gains entrance that only an "untimely" death should be regretted or mourned. Yet we know better how to specify an untimely death than to define or describe a "timely" one. The author of Genesis tells us that, at 180 years of age, the patriarch Isaac "breathed his last; and he died and was gathered to his people, old and full of years . . . " (Gen. 35:29). Even in face of sacred Scripture, we are permitted to wonder what Isaac thought about it; whether he too knew how to apply the category "fullness of years" *to himself* and agreed his death was nothing but timely.

We do Koheleth one better and say that death cannot only be timely; it may also be "beautiful." Whether such an opinion is to be ascribed to David Hendin or not (a "fact of life" man he surely is, who also unambiguously subtitled his chapter on euthanasia "Let There Be Death"),[7] that opinion seems to be the outlook of the legislator and physician, Walter Sackett, Jr., who proposed the Florida "Death with Dignity" Statute. All his mature life his philosophy has been, "Death, like birth, is glorious—let it come easy."[8] Such was by no means Koheleth's opinion when he wrote (and *wrote* beautifully) about a time to be born and a time to die. Dr. Sackett also suggests that up to 90 percent of the 1,800 patients in state hospitals for the mentally retarded should be allowed to die. Five billion dollars could be saved in the next half century if the state's mongoloids were permitted to succumb to pneumonia, a disease to which they are highly susceptible.[9] I suggest that the physician in Dr. Sackett has atrophied. He has become a public functionary, treating taxpayers' pocketbooks under the general anesthesia of a continuous daytime soap opera entitled "Death Can Be Beautiful!"

"Death for an older person should be a beautiful event. There is beauty in birth, growth, fullness of life and then, equally so, in the tapering off and final end. There are analogies all about us. What is more beautiful than the spring budding of small leaves; then the fully-leaved tree in summer; and then in the beautiful brightly colored autumn leaves gliding gracefully to the ground? So it is with humans." Those are words from a study document on Euthanasia drafted by the Council for Christian Social Action of the United Church of Christ in 1972. An astonishing footnote at this point states that "the naturalness of dying" is suggested in funeral services when the minister says "God has called" the deceased, or says he has "gone to his reward," recites the "dust to dust" passage, or notes that the deceased led a full life or ran a full course!

Before that statement was adopted by that Council on Feb. 17, 1973, more orthodox wording was inserted: "Transformation from life on earth to life in the hereafter of the Lord is a fulfillment. The acceptance of death is our witness to faith in the resurrection of Jesus Christ (Rom. 8). We can rejoice." The subdued words "we can rejoice" indicate a conviction that *something* has been subdued. The words "acceptance of death" takes the whole matter out of the context of romantic naturalism and sets it in a proper religious context—based on the particular Christian tenet that death is a conquered enemy, to be accepted in the name of its Conqueror. More than a relic of the nature mysticism that was so luxuriant in the original paragraph, however, remains in the words, "Death for an older person should be a beautiful event. There is beauty in birth, growth, fullness of life and then, *equally so,* in the tapering off and final end." (Italics added.) I know no Christian teaching that assures us that our "final end" is "equally" beautiful as birth, growth and fullness of life. Moreover, if revelation disclosed any such thing it would be contrary to reason and to the human reality and experience of death. The views of our "pre-death morticians" are simply discordant with the experienced reality they attempt to beautify. So, in her recent book, Marya Mannes writes "the name of the oratorio is euthanasia." And her statement "dying is merely suspension within a mystery," seems calculated to induce vertigo in face of a fascinating abyss in prospect.[10]

No exception can be taken to one line in the letter people are being encouraged to write and sign by the

Euthanasia Societies of Great Britain and America. That line states: "I do not fear death as much as I fear the indignity of deterioration, dependence and hopeless pain." Such an exercise in analyzing *comparative indignities* should be given approval. But in the preceding sentence the letter states: "Death is as much a reality as birth, growth, maturity, and old age—it is the one certainty." That logically leaves open the question what sort of "reality," what sort of "certainty," death is. But by placing death on a parity with birth, growth, maturity—and old age in many of its aspects—the letter beautifies death by association. To be written long before death when one is thinking "generally" (i.e. "rationally"?) about the topic, the letter tempts us to suppose that men can think generally about their own deaths. Hendin observes in another connection that "there is barely any relation between what people think that they think about death and the way they actually feel about it when it must be faced."[11] Then it may be that "the heart has its reasons that reason cannot know" (Pascal)—beforehand—and among those "reasons," I suggest, will be an apprehension of the ultimate (noncomparative) indignity of death. Talk about death as a fact or a reality seasonally recurring in life with birth or planting, maturity and growth, may after all not be very rational. It smacks more of whistling before the darkness descends, and an attempt to brainwash one's contemporaries to accept a very feeble philosophy of life and death.

Birth and death (our *terminus a quo* and our *terminus ad quem*) are not to be equated with any of the qualities or experiences, the grandeur and the misery, in between, which constitute "parts" of our lives. While we live toward death and can encompass our own dying in awareness, no one in the same way is aware of his own birth. We know that we were born in the same way we know *that* we die. Explanations of whence we came do not establish conscious contact with our individual origin; and among explanations, that God called us from the womb out of nothing is as good as any other; and better than most. But awareness of dying is quite another matter. That we may have, but not awareness of our births. And while awareness of birth might conceivably be the great original individuating experience (if we had it), among the race of men it is awareness of dying that is uniquely individuating. To encompass one's own death in the living and dying of one's life is more of a task than it is a part of life. And there is something of indignity to be faced when engaging in that final act of life. Members of the caring human community (doctors, nurses, family) are apt to keep closer company with the dying if we acknowledge the loss of all worth by the loss of him in whom inhered all worth in his world. Yet ordinary men may sometimes nobly suffer the ignobility of death.

By way of contrast with the "A Living Will" framed by the Euthanasia Society, the Judicial Council of the AMA in its recent action on the physician and the dying patient had before it two similar letters. One was composed by the Connecticut Delegation:

To my Family, my Physician,
my Clergyman, my Lawyer—

> If the time comes when I can no longer actively take part in decisions for my own future, I wish this statement to stand as the testament of my wishes. If there is no reasonable expectation of my recovery from physical or mental and spiritual disability, I, ..., request that I be allowed to die and not be kept alive by artificial means or heroic measures. I ask also that drugs be mercifully administered to me for terminal suffering even if in relieving pain they may hasten the moment of death. I value life and the dignity of life, so that I am not asking that my life be directly taken, but that my dying not be unreasonably prolonged nor the dignity of life be destroyed. This request is made, after careful reflection, while I am in good health and spirits. Although this document is not legally binding, you who care for me will, I hope, feel morally bound to take it into account. I recognize that it places a heavy burden of responsibility upon you, and it is with the intention of sharing this responsibility that this statement is made.

A second letter had been composed by a physician to express his own wishes, in quite simple language:

To my Family, To my Physician—

> Should the occasion arise in my lifetime when death is imminent and a decision is to be made about the nature and the extent of the care to be given to me and I am not able at that time to express my desires, let this statement serve to express my deep, sincere, and considered wish and hope that my physician will administer to me simple, ordinary medical treatment. I ask that he not administer heroic, extraordinary, expensive, or useless medical care or treatment which in the final analysis will merely delay, not change, the ultimate outcome of my terminal condition.

A comparison of these declarations with "A Living Will" circulated by the Euthanasia Society reveals the following signal differences: neither of the AMA submissions engages in any superfluous calculus of "comparative indignities";[12] neither associates the reality of death with such things as birth or maturation; both allow death to be simply what it is in human experience; both are in a general sense "pro-life" statements, in that death is neither reified as one fact among others nor beautified even comparatively.[13]

Everyone concerned takes the wrong turn in trying either to "thing-ify" death or to beautify it. The dying have at least this advantage, that in these projects for dehumanizing death by naturalizing it the dying finally cannot succeed, and death makes its threatening visage known to them before ever there are any societal or evolutionary replacement values or the everlasting arms or Abraham's bosom to rest on. Death means *finis,* not in itself *telos.* Certainly not a telos to be engineered, or to be accomplished by reducing both human life and death to the level of natural events.

"Thing-ifying" death reaches its highest pitch in the stated preference of many people in the present age for *sudden* death,[14] for death from unanticipated internal collapse, from the abrupt intrusion of violent outside forces, from some chance occurrence due to the natural law governing the operation of automobiles. While for a comparative calculus of indignities sudden *unknowing* death may be preferred to suffering knowingly or unknowingly the indignity of deterioration, abject dependence, and hopeless pain, how ought we to assess in human terms the present-day absolute (noncomparative) preference for sudden death? Nothing reveals more the meaning we assign to human "dignity" than the view that sudden death, death as an eruptive natural event, could be a prismatic case of death with dignity or at least one without indignity. Human society seems about to rise to the moral level of the "humane" societies in their treatment of animals. What is the principled difference between their view and ours about the meaning of dying "humanely"? By way of contrast, consider the prayer in the Anglican prayer book: "From perils by night and perils by day, perils by land and perils by sea, and *from sudden death,* Lord, deliver us." Such a petition bespeaks an age in which dying with dignity was a gift and a task (*Gabe und Aufgabe*), a liberty to encompass dying as a final act among the actions of life, to enfold awareness of dying as an ingredient into awareness of one's self dying as the finale of the self's relationships in this life to God or to fellowman—in any case to everything that was worthy.

Man Knows that He Dies

Before letting Koheleth's "a time to be born and a time to die" creep as a gloss into *our* texts, perhaps we ought to pay more attention to the outlook on life and death expressed in the enchantment and frail beauty of those words,[15] and ask whether that philosophy can possibly be a proper foundation for the practice of medicine or for the exercise of the most sensitive care for the dying.

That litany on the times for every matter under heaven concludes with the words, "What gain has the worker from his toil?" (Eccles. 3:9). In general, the author of Ecclesiastes voices an unrelieved pessimism. He has "seen everything that is done under the sun," in season and out of season. It is altogether "an unhappy business that God has given to the sons of men to be busy with"—this birthing and dying, planting and uprooting; "all is vanity and seeking after wind" (Eccles. 1:3b, 14). So, he writes with words of strongest revulsion, "I hated life, because what is done under the sun was grievous to me"; "I hated all my toil and gave myself up to despair . . . " (Eccles. 2:17, 18a, 20).

After that comes the litany "for everything there is a season"—proving, as Kierkegaard said, that a poet is a man whose heart is full of pain but whose lips are so formed that when he gives utterance to that pain he makes beautiful sounds. Koheleth knew, as later did Nietzsche, that the eternal recurrence of birth and death and all things else was simply "the spirit of melancholy" unrelieved, even though there is nothing else to believe since God died.[16] (The Pope knows: he was at the bedside.)

"Death with dignity" because death is a "part" of life, one only of its seasonal realities? If so, then the acceptable death of all flesh means death with the same signal indignity that brackets the whole of life and its striving. Dying is worth as much as the rest; it is no more fruitless.

"For the fate of the sons of men and the fate of the beasts is the same; as one dies so dies the other. They all have the same breath, and man has no advantage over the beasts; for all is vanity" (Eccles. 3:19). "Death with dignity" or death a part of life based on an equilibration of the death of a man with the death of a dog? I think that is not a concept to be chosen as the foundation of modern medicine, even though both dogs and men are enabled to die "humanely."

Or to go deeper still: "death with dignity" because the dead are better off than the living? "I thought the dead who are already dead," Koheleth writes in unrelieved sorrow over existence, "more fortunate than the living who are still alive; and better than both is he who has not yet been, and has not seen the evil deeds that are done under the sun" (Eccles. 4:2,3). Thus the book of Ecclesiastes is the source of the famous interchange between two pessimistic philosophers, each trying to exceed the other in gloom: First philosopher: More blessed are the dead than the living. Second philosopher: Yes, what you say is true; but more blessed still are those who have never been born. First philosopher: Yes, wretched life; but few there be who attain to that condition!

But Koheleth thinks he knows some who have attained to the blessed goal of disentrapment from the cycles in which there is a time for every matter under heaven. " . . . An untimely birth [a miscarriage] is better off [than a living man], for it [a miscarriage] comes into vanity and goes into darkness, and in darkness its name is covered; moreover it has not seen the sun or known anything; yet it finds rest rather than he [the living]" (Eccles. 6:3b,4,5). So we might say that death can have its cosmic dignity if untormented by officious physicians, because the dying go to the darkness, to Limbo where nameless miscarriages dwell, having never seen the sun or known anything. Thus, if dying with dignity as a part of life's natural, undulating seasons seems not to be a thought with much consolation in it (being roughly equivalent to the indignity besetting everything men do and every other natural time), still the dying may find rest as part of cosmic order, from which, once upon a time, the race of men arose to do the unhappy business God has given them to be busy with, and to which peaceful darkness the dying return.

Hardly a conception that explains the rise of Western medicine, the energy of its care of the dying, or its war against the indignity of suffering and death—or a conception on which to base its reformation! Dylan Thomas' words were directed against such notions: "The wise men at their end know dark is right,/Because their words had forked no lightning."

There is finally in Ecclesiastes, however, a deeper strand than those which locate men living and dying as simply parts of some malignly or benignly neglectful natural or cosmic order. From these more surface outlooks, the unambiguous injunction follows: Be a part; let there be death—in its time and place, of course (whatever that means). Expressing a deeper strand, however, Koheleth seems to say: Let the natural or cosmic order be whatever it is; men are different. His practical advice is: Be what you are, in human awareness apart and not a part. Within this deeper understanding of the transcendent, threatened nobility of a human life, the uniqueness of the individual human subject, there is ground for awareness of death as an indignity yet freedom to encompass it with dignity.

Now it is that Koheleth reverses the previous judgments he decreed over all he had seen under the sun. Before, the vale of the sunless not-knowing of a miscarriage having its name covered by darkness seemed preferable to living; and all man's works a seeking after wind. So, of course, there was "a time for dying." But now Koheleth writes, " . . . there is no work or thought or knowledge or wisdom in Sheol, to which you are going" (Eccles. 9:10b). While the fate of the sons of men and the fate of the beasts are the same, still "a living dog is better than a dead lion"; and to be a living man is better than either, because of what Koheleth means by "living." "He who is joined with all the living has hope" (Eccles. 9:4), and that is hardly a way to describe dogs or lions. Koheleth, however, identifies the grandeur of man not so much with hope as with awareness, even awareness of dying, and the misery of man with the indignity of dying of which he, in his nobility, is aware. "For the living know that they will die," he writes, "but the dead know nothing . . . " (Eccles. 9:5). Before, the dead or those who never lived had superiority; now, it is the living who are superior precisely by virtue of their awareness of dying and of its indignity to the knowing human spirit.

Therefore, I suggest that Koheleth probed the human condition to a depth to which more than twenty centuries later Blaise Pascal came. "Man is but a reed, the feeblest in nature, but he is a thinking reed. . . . A vapour, a drop of water, is sufficient to slay him. But were the universe to crush him, man would still be nobler than that which kills him, for *he knows that he dies,* while the universe knows nothing of the advantage it has over him. Thus our whole dignity consists in thought."[17] (Italics added.)

So the grandeur and misery of man are fused together in the human reality and experience of death. To deny the indignity of death requires that the dignity of man be refused also. The more acceptable in itself death is, the less the worth or uniqueness ascribed to the dying life.

True Humanism and the Dread of Death

I always write as the ethicist I am, namely, a Christian ethicist, and not as some hypothetical common denominator. On common concrete problems I, of course, try to elaborate analysis at the point or on a terrain where there may be convergence of vectors that began in other ethical outlooks and onlooks. Still one should not pant for agreement as the hart pants for the waterbrooks, lest the substance of one's ethics dissolve into vapidity. So in this section I want, among other things, to exhibit some of the meaning of "Christian humanism" in regard to death and dying, in the confidence that this will prove tolerable to my colleagues for a time, if not finally instructive to them.

In this connection, there are two counterpoised verses in the First Epistle of St. John that are worth pondering. The first reads: "Perfect love casts out fear" (which being interpreted means: Perfect care of the dying casts out fear of one's own death or rejection of their dying because of fear of ours). The second verse reads: "Where fear is, love is not perfected" (which being interpreted means: Where fear of death and dying remains, medical and human care of the dying is not perfected). That states nothing so much as the enduring dubiety and ambiguity of any mortal man's care of another through his dying. At the same time there is here applied without modification a standard for unflinching care of a dying fellowman, or short of that of any fellow mortal any time. That standard is cut to the measure of the perfection in benevolence believed to be that of our Father in Heaven in his dealings with mankind. So there is "faith-ing" in an ultimate righteousness beyond the perceptible human condition presupposed by those verses that immediately have to do simply with loving and caring.

Whatever non-Christians may think about the *theology* here entailed, or about similar foundations in any religious ethics, I ask that the notation upon or penetration of the human condition be attended to. Where and insofar as fear is, love and care for the dying cannot be perfected in moral agents or the helping professions. The religious traditions have one way of addressing that problematic. In the modern age the problematic itself is avoided by various forms and degrees of denial of the tragedy of death which proceeds first to reduce the unique worth and once-for-all-ness of the individual life-span that dies.

Perhaps one can apprehend the threat posed to the dignity of man (i.e. in an easy and ready dignifying of death) by many modern viewpoints, especially those dominating the scientific community, and their superficial equivalents in our culture generally, by bringing into view three states of consciousness in the Western past.

The burden of the Hebrew Scriptures was man's obedience or disobedience to covenant, to Torah. Thus sin was the problem, and death came in only as a subordinate theme; and, as one focus for the problematic of the human condition, this was a late development. In contrast, righteousness and disobedience (sin) was a subordinate theme in Greek religion. The central theme of Greek religious thought and practice was the problem of death—a problem whose solution was found either by initiation into religious cults that promised to extricate the soul from its corruptible shroud or by belief in the native power of the soul to outlast any number of bodies. Alongside these, death was at the heart of the pathos of life depicted in Greek tragical drama, against which, and against the flaws of finitude in general, the major character manifested his heroic transcendence. So sin was determinative for the Hebrew consciousness; death for the Greek consciousness.

Consciousness III was Christianity, and by this, sin and death were tied together in Western man's awareness of personal existence. These two foci of man's misery and of his need for redemption—sin and death—were inseparably fused. This new dimension of man's awareness of himself was originally probed most profoundly by St. Paul's Letter to the Romans (5-7). Those opaque reflections, I opine, were once understood not so much by the intellect as along the pulses of ordinary people in great numbers, in taverns and market places; and it represents a cultural breakdown without parallel that these reflections are scarcely understandable to the greatest intelligences today. A simple night school lesson in them may be gained by simply pondering a while the two verses quoted above from St. John's Epistle.

The point is that according to the Christian saga the Messiah did not come to bring boors into culture. Nor did he bear epilepsy or psychosomatic disorders to gain victory over them in the flesh before the interventions of psychoneurosurgery. Rather is he said to have been born *mortal* flesh to gain for us a foretaste of victory over sin and death where those twin enemies had taken up apparently secure citadel.

Again, the point for our purposes is not to be drawn into agreement or disagreement with those theological affirmations, and it is certainly not to be tempted into endless speculation about an after-life. Crucial instead is to attend to the notation on the human condition implied in all that. Death is an enemy even if it is the last enemy to be fully conquered in the Fulfillment, the eschaton; meanwhile, the sting of death is sin. Such was the new consciousness-raising that Christianity brought into the Western world. And the question is whether in doing so it has not grasped some important experiential human realities better than most philosophies, whether it was not attuned to essential ingredients of the human condition vis-a-vis death—whatever the truth or falsity of its theological address to that condition.

The foregoing, I grant, may be an oversimplification; and I am aware of needed corrections more in the case of Hebrew humanism than in the case of Greek humanism. The New Testament word, "He will wipe away every tear from their eyes, and death shall be no more, neither shall there be mourning nor crying nor pain any more, for the former things have passed away" (Rev. 21:3,4), has its parallel in the Hebrew Bible: "He will swallow up death forever, and the Lord God will wipe away tears from all faces . . . " (Isa. 25:8). Again, since contemplating the Lord God may be too much for us, I ask only that we attend to the doctrine of death implied in these passages: it is an enemy, surely, and not simply an acceptable part of the natural order of things. And the connection between dread of death and sin, made most prominent in Christian consciousness, was nowhere better stated than in Ecclesiastes: "This is the root of the evil in all that happens under the sun, that one fate comes to all. Therefore, men's minds are filled with evil and there is madness in their hearts while they live, for they know that afterward—they are off to the dead!"

One can, indeed, ponder that verse about the source of all evil in the apprehended evil of death together with another verse in Ecclesiastes which reads: "Teach us so to number our days that we may apply our hearts unto wisdom." The first says that death is an evil evil: it is experienced as a threatening limit that begets evil. The second says that death is a good evil: that experience also begets good. Without death, and death perceived as a threat, we would also have no reason to "number our days" so as to ransom the time allotted us, to receive life as a precious gift, to drink the wine of gladness in toast to every successive present moment. Instead, life would be an endless boredom and boring because endless; there would be no reason to probe its depths while there is still time. Some there are who number their days so as to apply their hearts unto eating, drinking and being merry—for tomorrow we die. Some there are who number their days so as to apply their hearts unto wisdom—for tomorrow we die. Both are life-spans enhanced in importance and in individuation under the stimulus of the perceived evil of death. Knowledge of human good or of human evil that is in the slightest degree above the level of the wild beasts of the field is enhanced because of death, the horizon of human existence. So, debarment from access to the tree of life was on the horizon and a sequence of the events in the Garden of Paradise; the temptation in eating the fruit of the tree of knowledge of good and evil was because that seemed a way for mortal creatures to become like gods. The punishment of that is said to have been death; and no governor uses as a penalty something that anyone can simply choose to believe to be a good or simply receive as a neutral or dignified, even ennobling, part of life. So I say death may be a good evil or an evil evil, but it is perceived as an evil or experienced indignity in either case. Existential anxiety or general anxiety (distinguishable from particular fears or removable anxieties) means anxiety over death toward which we live. That paradoxically, as Reinhold Niebuhr said, is the source of all human creativity and of all human sinfulness.

Of course, the sages of old could and did engage in a calculus of comparative indignities. "O death, your sentence is welcome," wrote Ben Sira, "to a man worn out with age, worried about everything, disaffected and beyond endurance" (Ecclus. 41:2,3). Still death was a "sentence," not a natural event acceptable in itself. Moreover, not every man grows old gracefully in the Psalms; instead, one complains:

> Take pity on me, Yahweh,
> I am in trouble now.
> Grief wastes away my eye,
> My throat, my inmost parts.
> For my life is worn out with sorrow,
> My years with sighs;
> My strength yields under misery,
> My bones are wasting away.
> To every one of my oppressors
> I am contemptible,
> Loathsome to my neighbors,
> To my friends a thing of fear.
> Those who see me in the street
> Hurry past me.
> I am forgotten, as good as dead, in their hearts,
> Something discarded. (Ps. 31:9-12)

What else is to be expected if it be true that the madness in men's hearts while they live, and the root of all evil in all that happens under the sun, lies in the simple fact that every man consciously lives toward his own death, knowing that afterward he too is off to the dead? Where fear is—fear of the properly dreadful—love and care for the dying cannot be perfected.

Unless one has some grounds for respecting the shadow of death upon every human countenance—grounds more ultimate than perceptible realities—then it makes good sense as a policy of life simply to try to outlast one's neighbors. One can, for example, *generalize,* and so attenuate our neighbors' irreplaceability. "If I must grieve whenever the bell tolls," writes Carey McWilliams, "I am never bereft: some of my kinsmen will remain. Indeed, I need not grieve much—even, lest I suggest some preference among my brethren, should not grieve much—for each loss is small compared to what remains."[18] But that solace, we know, is denied the dead who have lost everything making for worth in this their world. Realistic love for another irreplaceable, noninterchangeable individual human being means, as Unamuno wrote, care for another "doomed soul."

In this setting, let us now bring into consideration some empirical findings that in this day are commonly supposed to be more confirmatory than wisdom meditated from the heart.

In the second year anatomy course, medical students clothe with "gallows humor" their encounter with the cadaver which once was a human being alive. That defense is not to be despised; nor does it necessarily indicate socialization in shallowness on the students' part. Even when dealing with the remains of the long since dead, there is special tension involved—if I mistook not a recent address by Renée Fox—when performing investigatory medical actions involving the face, the hands, and the genitalia. This thing-in-the-world that was once a man alive we still encounter as once a communicating being, not quite as an object of research or instruction. Face and hands, yes; but why the genitalia? Those reactions must seem incongruous to a resolutely biologizing age. For a beginning of an explanation, one might take up the expression "carnal knowledge"—which was the best thing about the movie bearing that title—and behind that go to the expression "carnal *conversation,*" an old, legal term for adultery, and back of both to the Biblical word "knew" in "And Adam *knew* his wife and begat. . . . " Here we have an entire anthropology impacted in a word, not a squeamish euphemism. In short, in those reactions of medical students can be discerned a sensed relic of the human being bodily experiencing and communicating, and the body itself uniquely speaking.

Notably, however, there's no "gallows humor" used when doing or observing one's first autopsy, or in the emergency room when a D.O.A. (Dead on Arrival) is brought in with his skull cleaved open. With regard to the "newly dead" we come as close as we possibly can to experiencing the incommensurable contrast between life and death. Yet those sequential realities—life and death—here juxtaposed never *meet* in direct encounter. So we never have an impression or experience of the measure and meaning of the two different worlds before which we stand in the autopsy and the emergency room. A cadaver has over time become almost a thing-in-the-world from which to gain knowledge of the human body. While *there* a little humor helps, to go about acquiring medical knowledge from autopsies requires a different sort of inward effort to face down or live with our near-experience of the boundary of life and death. The cleavage in the brain may be quite enough and more than enough to *explain* rationally why this man was D.O.A. But, I suggest, there can be no gash deep enough, no physical event destructive enough to account for the felt difference between life and death that we face here. The physician or medical student may be a confirmed materialist. For him the material explanation of this death may be quite sufficient rationally. Still the heart has its reasons that the reason knows not of; and, I suggest, the awakening of these feelings of awe and dread should not be repressed in anyone whose calling is to the human dignity of caring for the dying.

In any case, from these empirical observations, if they be true, let us return to a great example of theological anthropology in order to try to comprehend why death was thought to be the assault of an enemy. According to some readings, Christians in all ages should be going about bestowing the gift of immortality on one another posthaste. A distinguished Catholic physician, beset by what he regarded as the incorrigible problems of medical ethics today, once shook his head in my presence and wondered out loud why the people who most believe in an afterlife should have established so many hospitals! That seems to require explanation, at least as against silly interpretations of "otherworldliness." The answer is that none of the facts or outlooks cited ever denied the reality of death, or affirmed that death ever presents a friendly face (except comparatively). The explanation lies in the vicinity of Christian anthropology and the Biblical view that death is an enemy. That foundation of Western medicine ought not lightly to be discarded, even if we need to enliven again the sense that there are limits to man's struggle against that alien power.

Far from the otherworldliness or body-soul dualism with which he is often charged, St. Augustine went so far as to say that "the body is not an extraneous ornament or aid, but a part of man's very nature."[19] Upon that understanding of the human being, Augustine could then express a quite realistic account of "the dying process":

> Wherefore, as regards bodily death, that is, the separation of the soul from the body, it is good to none while it is being endured by those whom we say are in the article of death [dying]. For the very violence with which the body and soul are wrenched asunder, which in the living are conjoined and closely intertwined, brings with it a harsh experience, jarring horribly on nature as long as it continues, till there comes a total loss of sensation, which arose from the very interpenetration of flesh and spirit.[20]

From this Augustine correctly concludes: "Wherefore death is indeed . . . good to none while it is actually suffered, and while it is subduing the dying to its power. . . . " His ultimate justifications attenuate not at all the harshness of that alien power's triumph. Death, he only says, is "meritoriously endured for the sake of winning what *is* good. And regarding what happens after death, it is no absurdity to say that death is good to the good, and evil to the evil."[21] But that is not to say that death as endured in this life, or as life's terminus, is itself in any way good. He even goes so far as to say:

> For though there can be no manner of doubt that the souls of the just and holy lead lives in peaceful rest, yet so much better would it be for them to be alive in healthy, well-conditioned bodies, that even those who hold the tenet that it is most blessed to be quit of every kind of body, condemn this opinion in spite of themselves.[22]

Thus, for Biblical or later Christian anthropology, the only possible form which human life in any true and proper sense can take here or hereafter is "somatic." That is the Pauline word; we today say "psychosomatic." Therefore, for Christian theology death may be a "conquered enemy"; still it was in the natural order—and as long as the generations of mankind endure will remain—an enemy still. To pretend otherwise adds insult to injury—or, at least, carelessness.

There are two ways, so far as I can see, to reduce the dreadful visage of death to a level of inherently acceptable indifference. One way is to subscribe to an interpretation of "bodily life" that reduces it to an acceptable level of indifference to the person long before his dying. That—if anyone can believe it today, or if it is not a false account of human nature—was the way taken by Plato in his idealized account of the death of Socrates. (It should be remembered that we know not whether Socrates' hands trembled as he yet bravely drank the hemlock, no more than we know how Isaac experienced dying when "fullness of years" came upon him. Secondary accounts of these matters are fairly untrustworthy.)

Plato's dialogue *The Phaedo* may not "work" as a proof of the immortality of the soul. Still it decisively raises the question of immortality by its thorough representation of the incommensurability between mental processes and bodily processes. Few philosophers today accept the demonstration of the mind's power to outlast bodies because the mind itself is not material, or because the mind "plays" the body like a musician the lyre. But most of them are still wrestling with the mind-body problem, and many speak of two separate languages, a language for mental events isomorphic with our language for brain events. That's rather like saying the same thing as Socrates (Plato) while claiming to have gone beyond him (Søren Kierkegaard).

I cite *The Phaedo* for another purpose: to manifest one way to render death incomparably welcomed. Those who most have mature manhood in exercise—the lovers of wisdom—have desired death and dying all their life long, in the sense that they seek "in every sort of way to dissever the soul from the communion of the body"; "thought is best when the mind is gathered into herself and none of these things trouble her—neither sounds nor sights nor pain nor any pleasure—when she takes leave of the body. . . . " That life is best and has nothing to fear that has "the habit of the soul gathering and collecting herself into herself from all sides out of the body." (Feminists, note the pronouns.)

Granted, Socrates' insight is valid concerning the self's transcendence, when he says: "I am inclined to think that these muscles and bones of mine would have gone off long ago to Megara and Boeotia—by the dog, they would, if they had been moved only by their own idea of what was best. . . . " Still Crito had a point, when he feared that the impending dread event had more to do with "the same Socrates who has been talking and conducting the argument" than Socrates is represented to have believed. To fear the loss of Socrates, Crito had not to fancy, as Socrates charged, "that I am the other Socrates whom he will soon see, a dead body." Crito had only to apprehend, however faintly, that there is not an entire otherness between those two Socrates *now,* in this living being; that there was unity between, let us say, Socrates the conductor of arguments and Socrates the gesticulator or the man who stretched *himself* because his muscles and bones grew weary from confinement.

The other way to reduce the dreadful visage of death is to subscribe to a philosophy of "human life" that reduces the stature, the worth, and the irreplaceable uniqueness of the individual person (long before his dying) to a level of acceptable transiency or interchangeability. True, modern culture is going this way. But there have been other and better ways of stipulating that the image of death across the human countenance is no shadow. One was that of Aristotelian philosophy. According to its form-matter distinction, reason, the formal principle, is definitive of essential humanity. That is universal, eternal as logic. Matter, however, is the individuating factor. So when a man who bears a particular name dies, only the individuation disintegrates—to provide matter for other forms. Humanity goes on in other instances. Anything unique or precious about mankind is not individual. There are parallels to this outlook in Eastern religions and philosophies, in which the individual has only transiency, and should seek only that, disappearing in the Fulfillment into the Divine pool.

These then are two ways of denying the dread of death. Whenever these two escapes are *simultaneously* rejected—i.e., if the "bodily life" is neither an ornament nor a drag but a part of man's very nature; and if the "personal life" of an individual in his unique life-span is accorded unrepeatable, noninterchangeable value—then it is that Death the Enemy again comes into view. Conquered or Unconquerable. A true humanism and the dread of death seem to be dependent variables. I suggest that it is better to have the indignity of death on our hands and in our outlooks than to "dignify" it in either of these two possible ways. Then we ought to be much more circumspect in speaking of death with dignity, and hesitant to—I almost said—thrust that upon the dying! Surely, a proper care for them needs not only to know the pain of dying which human agency may hold at bay, but also care needs to acknowledge that there is grief over death which no human agency can alleviate.

Notes

1. Paul Ramsey, "On (Only) Caring for the Dying," *The Patient as Person* (New Haven: Yale University Press, 1971).
2. Elisabeth Kübler-Ross, *On Death and Dying* (New York: Macmillan, 1969), p. 247.
3. Schopenhauer's characterization of human history: if you've read one page, you've read it all.
4. Wittgenstein, *Tractatus,* 6.4311.
5. James Van Evra, "On Death as a Limit," *Analysis* 31 [5] (April, 1971), 170-76.
6. Erik Erikson, "Identity and the Life Cycle," *Psychological Issues,* I, [1] (New York: International University Press, 1959).
7. David Hendin, *Death as a Fact of Life* (New York: W. W. Norton, 1973).
8. Reported in *ibid.,* p. 89.
9. *The Florida Times-Union,* Jacksonville, Fla., Jan. 11, 1973.
10. Marya Mannes, *Last Rights* (New York: William Morrow, 1973), p. 6 (cf. 80, 133).
11. Hendin, *Death as a Fact of Life,* p. 103.
12. What, after all, is the point of promoting, as if it were a line of reasoning, observations such as that said to be inscribed on W. C. Field's tombstone: "On the whole I'd rather be here than in Philadelphia"?
13. I may add that while the House of Delegates did not endorse any particular form to express an individual's wishes relating prospectively to his final illness, it recognized that individuals have a right to express them. While it encouraged physicians to discuss such matters with patients and attend to their wishes, the House nevertheless maintained a place for the conscience and judgment of a physician in determining indicated treatment. It did not subsume every consideration under the rubric of the patient's right to refuse treatment (or to have refused treatment). That sole action-guide can find no medical or logical reason for distinguishing, in physician actions, between the dying and those who simply have a terminal illness (or have this "dying life," Augustine's description of all of us). It would also entail a belief that wishing or autonomous choice makes the moral difference between life and death decisions which then are to be imposed on the physician-technician; and that, to say the least, is an ethics that can find no place for either reason or sensibility.
14. Cf. the report of a Swedish survey by Gunnar Biörck, M.D., in *Archives of Internal Medicine,* October, 1973; news report in *The New York Times,* Oct. 31, 1973.
15. In the whole literature on death and dying, there is no more misquoted sentence, or statement taken out of context, than Koheleth's "time to be born and a time to die"—unless it be "Nor strive officiously to keep alive." The latter line is from an ironic poem by the nineteenth century poet Arthur Hugh Clough, entitled "The Latest Decalogue":

> Thou shalt not kill; but need'st not strive
> Officiously to keep alive.
> Do not adultery commit;
> Advantage rarely comes of it:
> Thou shalt not steal; an empty feat,
> When it's so lucrative to cheat:
> Bear not false witness; let the lie
> Have time on its own wings to fly:
> Thou shall not covet; but tradition
> Approves all forms of competition.
> The sum of all is, thou shalt love
> If anybody, God above:
> At any rate, shalt never labor
> More than thyself to love thy neighbor.

16. Nietzsche, *Thus Spake Zarathustra,* especially XLVI and LXVI.
17. Pascal, *Pensées,* p. 347.
18. Wilson Carey McWilliams, *The Idea of Fraternity in America* (Berkeley: University of California Press, 1973), p. 48.
19. Augustine, *City of God,* Book I, Chapter XIII.
20. *Ibid.,* Book XIII, Chapter VI.
21. *Ibid.,* Book XIII, Chapter VIII.
22. *Ibid.,* Book XIII, Chapter XIX.

32. The Last Poem: The Dignity of the Inevitable and Necessary

ROBERT S. MORISON

Paul Ramsey suggests that anyone unable to speak as a Christian ethicist must do so as some "hypothetical common denominator." Maybe so, but for the present I will think of myself as a latter-day (not very animistic) pagan. I will also remind you that I tend to look upon death as a process and therefore regard the phrase "*death* with dignity" as essentially equivalent to "*dying* with dignity." Paul Ramsey's paper seems to follow no consistent line on this issue. Sometimes he seems to be talking simply about dying and how to do it or be helped to do it. At other times, he rages with Dylan Thomas about death as an arbitrary, wholly unacceptable event descending from God-knows-where to take away one's own very special and unique gift of life. I will try to talk separately and successively about these two views although I recognize that in between these extremes are a number of other interpretations and nuances that must be neglected for the present.

Undignified Prolongation of Life

In the first place, then, let us talk about the process of dying and whether or not it can be carried out with dignity. I take it that it is this question that most occupies those numerous individuals who are proposing an increasing flood of legislation, composing letters of intent to their physicians, or simply appearing on television programs under the title "Death with Dignity."

To approach the subject somewhat from the back door, I will start by saying that, together with a number of other people, I hold that at a certain stage in the process of dying, it is basically *un*dignified to continue casting desperately about for this or that potion, philter, or device to prolong some minor sign of life, after all reasonable chance for the reappearance of its major attributes has disappeared. Admittedly, this is an instinctive, possibly purely pagan reaction on my part. I simply find something offensive about this frantic search for some last remedy, some magic wire to hook up merely to postpone the inevitable.

From the *Hastings Center Studies* 2 (May 1974): 63-66. Used by permission of the publisher and the author.

Actually, as Paul Ramsey would agree, his behavior and mine would ordinarily differ very little at the bedside of such a patient. What goes on in our heads may, however, be quite different. To put the difference in its most extreme form: He might be saying to himself "Death is an undignified matter at best, and I feel that the appropriate treatment for this stage of this patient's illness is to withdraw active efforts to prolong life and thus allow God to decide, unimpeded by human intervention, how to get this undignified business over with as quickly as possible. Even if I give the patient some morphine to ease his pain, and even though I know that this will slow his respiration and reduce his interest in coughing, I will in no way be causing his death because this is simply a secondary or incidental effect of my actions."

I might be saying to myself, on the other hand: "To be candid about it, the trajectory of this patient's life has now reached its final stage of decline. Virtually everything that once made his life a pleasure to himself, a delight to his friends, and an asset to society has now disappeared, never to return. All that remain are the least dignified of his interchanges with the environment, and even these in their least dignified form. I am sure from previous conversations that this man would not wish to remain in this subhuman condition, and I will therefore withdraw all treatments that would prolong life and continue only those that will prevent restlessness and pain, fully recognizing that such measures will also hasten the end. By thus fulfilling the wishes of my friend and patient, I restore to him the dignity of controlling, to the extent possible, the circumstances under which he returns to an inanimate state."

There is an implicit indignity in the conception of the meaning of human life revealed by overvigorous efforts to maintain its outward, visible, and entirely trivial signs. It is not breathing, urinating, and defecating that makes a human being important even when he can do these things by himself. How much greater is the indignity when all these things must be done for him, and he can do nothing else. Not only have means thus been converted into ends; the very means themselves have become artificial. It is simply an insult to the very idea of humanity to equate it with these mechanically maintained appearances.

The Examined Death

Clearly, then, the omission of what are so oddly referred to as *heroic* means can spare us at least in part from death with indignity. Does such restraint at the same time convert the process into death *with dignity,* or are we simply left with a blank sheet of paper, a soul wandering about in limbo perhaps, free of the ultimate indignity but unable to attain dignity?

Here Paul Ramsey himself may inadvertently have given us a clue to improving matters. In the first place, he speaks with contempt of those who wish for sudden death. His grounds are that, to be appreciated, death must be experienced, if not indeed thought carefully about in advance. He quotes with approval Pascal's observation that man's nobility lies in the fact that he knows that he dies. He also notes that the Book of Common Prayer includes sudden death among various other perils from which the Lord is especially petitioned to deliver us. Obviously, the pagan will agree, and it is in just this spirit that latter-day pagans are thinking about their deaths well in advance. Indeed, against all current custom and in some discordance with existing legislation, they are endeavoring to prepare not only themselves, but their friends and physicians, to cooperate with them in their wish to face death with dignity.

A particularly interesting example of divine cooperation with the human desire not to die suddenly and unprepared, but only after calm reflection in one's study is provided by the pagan philosopher Seneca in his comment on the suicide of Cato the Younger.

In it he quotes Cato as scorning to die in hand-to-hand combat (as two of his young officers had chosen to die) on the grounds that "it were as ignoble to beg death from any man as to beg life." He then goes on to describe the deliberation with which he arranged for the escape of his followers, spent an evening in his usual studies, and then attempted suicide by stabbing himself in the abdomen. He did not die immediately and apparently was attended by a surgeon who sutured the wound, which Cato tore open at the next opportunity. This double effort causes Seneca to make the following memorable comment:

> His virtue was held in check and called back that it might display itself in a harder role; for to seek death needs not so great a soul as to reseek it. Surely the gods looked with pleasure upon their pupil as he made his escape by so glorious and memorable an end! Death consecrates those whose end even those who fear must praise.

It seems from what we have said so far that Ramsey, with his respect for Pascal, and I, with my respect for Seneca, are really not so far apart on the possibility of carrying out the final process of dying with dignity.

We turn, then, to the contention that the very fact of death, the inevitability that the individual human life must always end, is an indignity in some sort of universal sense.

I am not sure that I fully understand Ramsey's bitter hostility against those who, on the contrary, attempt to see a certain dignity in death as an inevitable, indeed as an essential, part of life as we know it. I shall begin my comment, however, with an attempt to establish a positive case for the view and then to go on to comment on some of Paul Ramsey's strictures about Koheleth, the Preacher.

In the first place, let me say that I find something basically undignified in a failure to accept the inevitable logic or the empirically demonstrable structure of the natural world. Whatever else may be said about him, Dostoievski's antihero in "Notes from the Underground," who rails against the fact that two plus two make four, is not a *dignified* figure. Conversely, for most of us, Job gains in dignity when he finally accepts the way that God has decided to run things. Much the same spirit activated Milton when he intoned, "Just are the ways of God and justifiable to man." Seneca wrote his little essay on Providence in part to "reconcile" a friend to the ways of God. Such individuals seem far closer to my conception of what is meant by human dignity than Paul Ramsey's curious choice of Dylan Thomas, whom he commends for raging "against the close of day."

Biological Necessities

In other papers and presentations I have often stressed the basic biological necessities that set up a constant tension between the individual man and his society. In his recent book, *The Tyranny of Survival,* Daniel Callahan has reviewed the same evidence in connection with his discussion of the generally pessimistic thoughts expressed by Freud in *Civilization and Its Discontents.* Incidentally, the German title is somewhat to be preferred—*Das Unbehagen in der Kultur*—since, following Spengler and others, one tends to think of civilization as a relatively late human development, whereas "the uneasiness of culture" dates back to man's earliest days as a human being.

After all, Freud is not really concerned with such modern discontents as waiting in line for some gasoline, but with the much more profound sacrifices every human being must make because he is at the same time an individual and a member of society. Much of man's basic physiology is designed to ensure his survival in strictly individual terms. He eats, he drinks, he fights or runs away at the command and with the help of this complex, highly individual apparatus. Many of these activities are accompanied by intense subjective experiences and drives. Nevertheless, his survival equally depends upon his interactions with his group, tribe, society, or *Kultur.* As Freud and many others pointed out, this dependence on the group demands certain painful sacrifices as an individual, but, as Willard Gaylin recently remarked, "Not everyone finds these sacrifices as painful as Freud did since we are also provided with additional physiological machinery which helps bind us to others and gives us at least some pleasure in doing something for them."

It is, of course, well known that in other animals reproductive behavior from courting to weaning is under rather strict endocrine and genetically determined nervous control. It is probable that human beings cannot entirely escape this, although the learned or cultural element is much larger, as La Rochefoucauld recognized when he remarked that few people would fall in love if they hadn't read about it. However determined, man's social interdependence is a fact, and he derives from it satisfaction, as well as pain. Sometimes, perhaps more often than not, the pain and the satisfaction are closely intermingled. The limiting case may be that of the young man, so often praised by both poet and politician, who lays down his life for his country.

But in a larger and deeper sense, every human death is ultimately for the good of the group. It is, at least in biological terms, the most fundamental of creative acts. For an audience such as this, it is scarcely necessary to review all the facts that attest to the role of selective death in the evolutionary process. It must be equally, or perhaps even more, obvious that cultural evolution also relies on death not only to select the "fittest," but simply to make room and to give more opportunity for the bearers of new ideas and novel life styles. If Ponce de León and his colleagues had ever found the Fountain of Eternal Youth, it would have soon shown itself a pool of stagnation.

Discontent, or the slightly more uncomfortable German *Unbehagen,* may be rather weak words to describe the obligation to die, as well as to sublimate for one's culture. Indeed, it is possible to find not only dignity, but a certain grandeur in the concept. To rage with Dylan Thomas and other rebellious Celts at the injustice of it all, is to rage at the very process which made one a human being in the first place. It is all these things that the pagan biologist has in mind when he says that death is part, parcel, and process of life and not some absurd event tacked on at the end out of divine spite or, worse still, as a punishment for sin.

Indeed, it is in their reading of the book of Genesis that the pagan finds it hardest to follow the Christians. The idea that death was laid upon us as a punishment for original sin is so foreign to the pagan biologist that he must make a constant effort to remind himself that other people really do believe it, and that it is this belief that colors so much of their thinking on other issues.

It is not that we do not believe in sin, because of course many of us do, and we all believe in death. We simply don't see much connection between the two. Furthermore, the whole business of being saved from sin by having salvation bestowed on us in the twinkling of an eye in the form of immortality seems bizarre in the extreme. But perhaps this is another story.

The "Preacher" comes much closer to the biological position and is even regarded by some as a pagan himself. At any rate, in words which even Paul Ramsey has to admit have a certain beauty, he reflects helpfully on the cyclical and seasonal character of life. It seems clear from the context that he regarded these regularities as "fitting and proper." What made him sad and pessimistic was not the regularity of sowing and reaping, but the inexplicable *ir*regularities and perversities within the system—the fact that the race was not always to the swift or riches to the wise, but that time and chance happens to them all—in other words, there ain't no justice under the sun. Also and furthermore, men tend to look for the wrong things. All these human failings bothered the Preacher, but I see nothing in his remarks to suggest that he found indignity in death. Indeed, he mentions death only very rarely, most notably in Chapter 7, where he says,

> A good name is better than precious ointment and the day of death than the day of one's birth. It is better to go into the house of mourning than to go into the house of mirth. . . . The heart of the wise is in the house of mourning, but the heart of the fool is in the house of mirth.

Good Grief

Incidentally, this passage may also serve as a text for commenting on Paul Ramsey's summary dismissal of "good grief" as a contradiction in terms. Even in its simplest terms, grief is recognized by every physician and by such nonprivy counselors as Ann Landers as not only a good, but the best therapy. Indeed, the inability to experience grief is the sign of the worst of all human detachments—pathognomonic, as we doctors would say, of schizophrenia.

Like every other good thing, the Greeks had a word for it: *catharsis.* What, indeed, are the tragedies of the house of Atreus but exercises in good grief? Not very long ago, some of us gained wisdom by entering into the house of mourning with Creon and Eurydice on Public Television while fools twisted their dials to the houses of mirth.

In the midst of his discussion of the Preacher, Paul Ramsey admits, citing Kierkegaard, that the Preacher was a poet and that as a poet his heart was full of pain but his lips were so formed that when he gives utterance to that pain he makes beautiful sounds. Alfred Kazin put the matter more succinctly when he said that art is the fusion of suffering with form. One might pursue the thought a little further and observe that "Death with Dignity" is simply the title of the last poem, in which the end of life is given its proper form. But perhaps this is a view that appeals only to pagans and stoics, who sometimes seem to have regarded the whole business of life as the study of how to give form and dignity to suffering.

33.
Averting One's Eyes, or Facing the Music?— On Dignity and Death

LEON R. KASS

This paper is dedicated to the memory of Gerhard Emil Otto Meyer, teacher and friend, who died at the age of seventy in December, 1973, three weeks after completing a thirty-six-year career in undergraduate teaching at the University of Chicago. He lived the way he thought he should, and the way he thought he should coincided with the way he wanted. He will remain for many of us a touchstone of human dignity.

The thesis of Paul Ramsey's paper "The Indignity of 'Death with Dignity' " is that current campaigns to naturalize, romanticize, beautify, or dignify death—which he collects together as campaigns for "death with dignity"—heap added insults and indignities upon dying people. This thesis rests on two foundations. First, Ramsey believes that many adherents of "death with dignity" have an impoverished and shrunken view of the meaning and dignity of human life which, in turn, leads them to an impoverished and insensitive view of the meaning of death for dying individuals and their near ones. Second, Ramsey believes that death itself—even an easy and painless death coming in old age to a human being who has lived a worthy and happy life—is inherently an indignity, and one which cannot be overcome or even mitigated. There are then two themes—"The Indignity of 'Death with Dignity,' " and "The Indignity of Death"—and the first theme rests upon the second, as Ramsey himself admits, discussing his title in his opening paragraph: "So 'The Indignity of Death' would not suffice for my purposes, even though *all* I shall say *depends* on understanding the contradiction death poses to the unique worth of an individual human life." (Emphasis added.)

This commentary will deal almost exclusively with the question of the "indignity of death." My purpose is to expose some of the roots of Ramsey's argument and thus to open up and join on some questions that need further and more serious attention. I shall also point to some alternative ways of thinking about our subject, though I am fully aware that I discuss none of them adequately, and perhaps some of them even

From the *Hastings Center Studies* 2 (May 1974): 67-80. Used by permission of the publisher and the author.

incorrectly. Though I hesitate to start a quarrel I am unable to finish, I hope others may profit from this beginning.

I hesitate to make public my sharp disagreement with Ramsey on this matter because I happen to share some of his concerns regarding our current and future practices toward the dying. I worry that the accelerating drive to compensate for previous excessive denial and avoidance of death may, on an equally distant swing, lead us past the sensible mean to a weakened respect for life. I see a real danger that the combination of our general zeal to rectify wrongs all at once, our swelling and not unjustified revulsion at some results of senseless (but also of sensible) efforts to prolong life at all costs, our delight in debunking myths and in shedding taboos, our prejudices against the old and "useless," and, in some cases, our simply crass and selfish interests, sometimes masquerading as compassion, may lead to grave excesses. I am therefore reluctant to give any comfort to the insensitively zealous by attacking one of their most articulate and intelligent critics. Yet if close attention be paid, it will be seen that my criticism of Ramsey's principles contains a criticism also of some of those he confronts.

For yet more personal reasons do I hesitate to present the following comments. While much of the early part of his paper is a punch and jab critique of the fuzzy opinions of others, Ramsey later reveals that it is by the light and with the fists of a Christian teaching that he has been in combat. Am I not foolish to engage this Goliath of a Christian thinker and pugilist, and on the very subject of his profoundest beliefs? My task is made yet more difficult because I respect and admire this Christian gentleman, owe much of my current career to his encouragement, and regard him as my friend. Yet I think he might not mind—and I hope not merely feel the need to turn the other cheek—if I proceed in the spirit of a remark made by a wise man of old, who, faced with a similar dilemma but with a far more imposing challenge than mine, said:

> Yet it would perhaps seem to be better and even necessary, for the sake of safeguarding the truth, even to destroy the things of our own, especially as we are lovers of wisdom; for while both are dear, it is fitting to prefer the truth.

The Title

The same wise man has also said, "The beginning is more than half the whole." Let me begin then at the beginning, with the title: "The Indignity of 'Death with Dignity.' " This is a clever, paradoxical, and hence enticing title. We do not yet know what it means, and therefore, whether as a proposition it is true. But it serves immediately to raise questions about the meaning of the phrase "death with dignity" and about the possibilities and limits of such a death, whatever the phrase turns out to mean. More radically, it points to questions about the meaning of *"dignity,"* about the existence of *"human dignity,"* and about whether and how any such dignity is attained or lost, conferred or withdrawn.

This preference for the extraordinary use of words—a confessed addiction of the author—is, however, a risky business generally, and here in particular. Though it can dramatically call attention to a question hitherto relatively ignored, extraordinary usage can distort the terms in which the question is posed and discussed. An extraordinary title may indeed succeed in prolonging the life of a question but only at the price of reducing or disfiguring its character—and also—if ignorance may be said to be one form of "suffering"—of prolonging suffering. This, as I will try to show, is here the case. Would that Ramsey had adhered to his own medico-moral teaching about eschewing extraordinary means.

The difficulty to which I refer concerns the nature of human dignity and the relation of death to any such dignity. The opinions which lie behind my critique are that dignity is something that belongs to a human being and is displayed in the way he lives, and hence something not easily taken away from him; therefore, that death is, at the very least, neutral with respect to dignity; that, further, human mortality may even be the necessary condition for the display of at least *some* aspects of a human being's dignity; and, finally, that human dignity is more dependent on the exercise of those generic human qualities rather than on those things which make him Ramsey and me Kass. These individuating differences may be pleasing and may make life more "interesting," but there is more dignity in our common effort to understand each other and to understand the meaning of human life, or in our parallel efforts to live fully human lives, than in any of our unique, distinctive, and idiosyncratic features.[1]

Before proceeding to the discussion, we need to disentangle the questions and clarify some terms.

What is the Question?

The slogan "death with dignity," whatever its difficulties, stands partly for the proposition: "There are more and less dignified ways to face death or to die."

Ramsey and I would agree with this proposition, and so, I think, should anyone; numerous examples could be cited that would draw common assent. The *possibility* of dying with dignity can be diminished, undermined, or even eliminated by many things in many ways, for example, by coma or senility, unbearable pain, madness, sudden death, denial, depravity, ignorance, cowardice, isolation, destitution, as well as by excessive and impersonal medical and technological intervention—and even, as Ramsey rightly points out, by the imposition of a false or exploitative or insensitive or shallow doctrine of "death with dignity."

On this last point, the primary surface theme and target of Ramsey's paper, I hasten to add my agreement. Ramsey and I agree, on the one hand, that excessive efforts to prolong life and the impersonal institutional arrangements and callous treatments these efforts tend to foster can be an affront to dying patients, their families and friends, indeed, to all of us. But Ramsey and I also agree, on the other hand, that it can be equally insensitive and insulting to do battle with these excesses under a slogan that implies that dignity will reign if only we can push back officious doctors, machinery, and hospital administrators. Moreover, I suspect that Ramsey might even agree with me in holding that an inadequate or partial notion of human dignity informs both the excessive efforts to prolong life *and* some of the current efforts to curb these excesses.

A death with dignity—which may turn out to be something rare or uncommon, even under the best of circumstances, like a life with dignity, on which a death with dignity may most often depend[2]—entails more than the absence of external indignities. Dignity in the face of death cannot be given or conferred from the outside—at least not by other men—but requires a dignity of soul in the human being who faces it. This, despite the many claims to the contrary, neither the partisans of "death with dignity" nor the myriad servants of mankind, from the Department of Welfare to departments of medicine or psychiatry, can supply—though they can, perhaps, offer some assistance. On these matters I think Ramsey and I agree, and we need no longer tarry over them, except perhaps to note a useful distinction. Crudely speaking, we might say that the *possibility* of a humanly dignified facing of death can be destroyed from without (and, of course, from within), but the *actualization* of that possibility depends largely on the soul, the character, the bearing of the dying man himself—i.e., on things *within.* This distinction may bear also on the later and more crucial question of whether it is true that *death as such* is an "ultimate indignity" or an indignity at all—i.e., whether there is truth in this proposition which Ramsey admits is the one on which *all* he has to say depends.

But first, what is meant here by "death"? "Death," as Ramsey uses the term in this paper, suffers from frequent personification and reification: "Death is an enemy," "Death means the conquest of the time of our lives," "The dreadful visage of death," "The shadow of death on every human countenance," and "The sting of death is sin," to cite but a few examples. More serious and confusing is Ramsey's failure to distinguish among (1) the state of *"being" dead,* i.e., of nonbeing, (2) the "final" *transition,* whether process or event,[3] between the state of being alive and the state of being dead, (3) the process, often drawn out, of *"being dying,"* to borrow from Cassell,[4] and (4) *the fact of human mortality,* of human finitude. All of these Ramsey calls simply "death." Yet it is the fourth sense, "death" as *mortality,* that Ramsey must mean when he speaks of the "contradiction *death* poses to the unique worth of an individual human life." Thus Ramsey's "The Indignity of Death" I take to mean "The Indignity of Human Mortality."

From this clarification, two others follow. First, we are not here talking about the dignity or indignity of *premature* death or *painful* death or *violent* death or *untimely* death, that is, of the death of a young child by drowning or of an elderly widow with disseminated cancer or of a middle-aged President killed by an assassin or of a composer in the midst of writing his greatest symphony. We are talking only about the fact that we must die. Indeed, another way of stating Ramsey's claim is to say that there is no such thing as a timely death, as a death in season, because the "contradiction" of our mortality means that there never is a right time to die. Second, if mortality is an indignity, so are aging and senescence. The waning of the light, no less than its inevitable extinction, must come under Ramsey's charge of "indignity," as must everything which diminishes or jeopardizes human vitality and ripeness.

A second cause of confusion, as perplexing as his imprecision in the use of the term "death," is Ramsey's frequent weaving back and forth between (1) a subjective perspective on a *particular* "death" in its "individuality"—including some identified particular "deaths"—and its implications for the dying man, his loved ones, or a disinterested observer, and (2) an objective perspective on human mortality itself, and on the implications for each of us as human beings of the fact that death is (in this sense) a necessary and inescapable condition of human life.

Now Ramsey's paper is, admittedly, presented in the context of current discussions of "allowing to die" and "medical mercy killings"; his remarks are therefore addressed to people who will think less about human mortality in general and more about how to care for particular dying human beings. Were he writing mainly to the philosophical and theological questions he might have written differently. Yet never before, even when addressing practical men and their practical problems, have I known Ramsey to detach himself from the normative questions—to the annoyance of some and the delight of others, including myself. Though he enjoys good anecdotes and can conjure cases better than most, the particular cases are for the sake of the generic and, ultimately, the normative. He usually would be the first to call attention to the difference between what men *do* and what they *should do*—even men like Isaac and Socrates about whom he here fishes for empirical evidence that they acted other than we know. Thus, I invite him to join me in his usual question: How *should* Socrates or Isaac or Ramsey or Kass or any human being regard—now and when we are dying—the fact that we must each and all die? Who *should* we take as our model: Socrates, his wife, Crito, Ivan Ilych, Joan of Arc, Dr. Sackett, a Kamikaze pilot, Dylan Thomas' old man, Isaac upon the altar or at the end of his days, Achilles facing Hector, Shakespeare's Caesar or Brutus or Antony or Cleopatra, the Eskimo elder walking off to freeze, or Zarathustra? We may not be able to emulate fully our model, either now or in the face of our own "being dying," but this in no way detracts from the importance of the question. On the contrary, we may find our own stance toward our mortality, now and then, *improved* as a result of thinking through the truth about the questions, "How should we regard the fact that we must die?" "Is our mortality an indignity?"

To be sure, this question may be dealt with differently—or even ignored—by different people. The doctor, the death-bed confessor, the general, and the philosopher may, and perhaps must, adopt different perspectives, according to their different works. Yet there can be and usually are prevailing opinions and outlooks which inform these perspectives. Further, there may even be a *truth* about these matters which might be in conflict with these prevailing opinions, and which, if we could discern or approach it, could conceivably reform and improve these opinions, or at least free us from certain harmful superstitions. (Do we not implicitly, even if unwittingly, make just such assumptions when we engage in serious discussion about this—or any subject?) But, on the other hand—and here I at least must pause—it is possible that certain opinions, even so-called superstitions, may be more beneficial than the unvarnished truth or than that portion of the truth which may be accessible to us. This, I submit, may be the case here.

Let us consider what course we should follow on the assumption that there is a tension between "the true" and "the useful." Are we and should we be interested in fostering opinions which could possibly be popularly embraced and which could give comfort and solace, regardless of whether or not they are true? Or are we and should we be interested in pursuing the truth, allowing the chips to fall where they may?

Ramsey and I agree, I think, at least in this instance, on the superiority of the latter course, though we may soon thereafter part company on where to look in our pursuit of what is true. And since we have not yet shown that the truth about death is deadly, or is likely to be, I am willing to venture to inquire into what is true about the meaning of the fact that human beings die and the relationship of this fact to the dignity of human life.

Formally, there are at least three positions on our question about the dignity or indignity of death itself: (1) That men must die is inherently an indignity or an affront to human dignity which cannot be overcome, no matter how dignified one's stance toward death; (2) That men must die is inherently part of human dignity; and (3) That men must die is neutral with respect to dignity, dignity or indignity in dying, as in living, depending only on the actions of the human being involved. These formal alternatives stated, we can make no material progress toward an answer unless and until we know what we mean by dignity. The failure to provide an analytic of "dignity" is, I hold, a major weakness in Ramsey's paper. Had he explored this question I suspect—and I will try to show why—he would have been sorry he saddled himself with these terms.

Toward an Analytic of Dignity

The English word "dignity" derives from the Latin *dignitas,* which, according to the *White and Riddle Latin-English Dictionary,* means (1) a being worthy, worthiness, merit, desert, (2) dignity, greatness, grandeur, authority, rank, and (3) (of inanimate things) worth, value, excellence. The noun is cognate with the adjective *dignus* (the root *DIC,* related to the Sanskrit *DIC* and the Greek *DEIK,* means "to bring to light," "to show," "to point out"), literally, "pointed out" or "shown," and hence, "worthy" or "deserving" (of persons), and "suitable," "fitting," "becoming," or "proper" (of things).

"Dignity," in the *Oxford English Dictionary,* is said to have eight meanings, the four relevant ones I reproduce here: (1) The quality of being worthy or honourable; worthiness, worth, nobleness, excellence (for instance, "The real dignity of a man lies not in what he *has,* but in what he *is,*" or "The dignity of this act was worth the audience of kings"); (2) Honourable or high estate, position, or estimation; honour; degree of estimation, rank (for instance, "Stones, though in dignitie of nature inferior to plants," or "Clay and clay differs in dignity, whose dust is both alike"); (3) An honourable office, rank, or title; a high official or titular position (for instance, "He . . . distributed the civil and military dignities among his favorites and followers"); (4) Nobility or befitting elevation of aspect, manner, or style; becoming or fit stateliness, gravity (for instance, "A dignity of dress adorns the Great").

The central notion, in both Latin and English, is that of worthiness, elevation, honor, nobility, height—in short, of excellence. In all its meanings, it is a term of distinction: dignity is not something which, like a navel or a nervous system, is to be expected or to be found in every living human being. Dignity is, in principle, aristocratic—this is inescapable, quite apart from however one might specify the *content* of excellence or distinction.

Certain qualifications should be noted. First, honor and rank are, of course, problematic. Though they are meant to be signs of worth, they often depend more on those who bestow them than on those who receive them. For example, the lasting honor and glory of Achilles depends on the greatness of Homer, that of Pericles on Thucydides and Plutarch. More generally, the worth and tastes and opinions of the bestowers will be decisive for determining what is honored. Esteem is given not always for excellence, and excellence is not always esteemed. Esteem and honor can be withdrawn, whereas dignity, in the sense of worthiness, excellence, and nobility, is something not easily taken from a man. Nevertheless, despite elements of relativity and the possibilities of error, the simple fact that human beings do bestow praise and blame, and *point out* by these means examples of worthiness, acknowledges the existence of various human excellences that bring themselves to light. This is also attested to by the great pains men often take to bring their judgments of worthiness in line with some standards of what is indeed noble and excellent.

Second, one can, of course, seek to democratize the principle; one can argue that "excellence," "being worthy" is a property of *all* human beings, say, for example, in comparison with animals or plants, or with machines that may perform certain tasks as well as human beings. This, I take it, is what is meant by "*human* dignity." This is also what is implied when it is asserted that much of the terminal treatment of dying patients is dehumanizing, or that attachments to catheters, pacemakers, monitors, respirators, suction tubes, intravenous tubes, and oxygen masks destroy or hide the human countenance and thereby insult the dignity of the dying. This view is not without some merit. Yet on further examination this universal attribution of dignity to human beings pays tribute to human potentiality, to the *possibilities* for human excellence. The human countenance is expressive of the presence of the human soul and of the possibilities of its excellences. *Full* dignity, or dignity properly so-called, would depend on the *realization* of these possibilities.

Moreover, to speak of dignity as predicable of all human beings, say in contrast to animals, is to tie dignity to those distinctively human features of human animals, such as thought, image-making, the sense of beauty, freedom, friendship, and the moral life, and not the mere presence of life itself. *Among* human beings, there would still be, on any such material principle, distinctions to be made—unless one evacuates the meaning of the term, and the predicate "dignity" is held to add nothing to "born of woman." Thus even if one were to accept the rather attenuated notion of dignity implied in Pascal's "Our whole dignity consists in thought" (by which he means preeminently self-consciousness and awareness of mortality), one would have to wonder about the relative ranking of those who think more and less, that is, are more or less self-conscious. Or, to take another possible ground of human dignity, while each human being can be said to have a moral life in that everyone faces moral choices, *dignity* would seem to depend on having a *good* moral life, that is, on choosing well. Clearly, we do not want to say that there is dignity—or much dignity—in the life of a paid killer, a slave-dealer, or a prostitute, or that they compare in dignity with Gandhi, Abraham Lincoln, or Joan of Arc. And is there not more dignity in courage than in cowardice, in moderation than in self-indulgence, in righteousness than in wickedness?[5]

A brief look at *indignity,* again from the *Oxford English Dictionary.* "Indignity" is "any action toward another which manifests contempt for him," "an offense against personal dignity," "incivility," "unmerited contemptuous treatment," in short, an *affront.*

It is important to note that dignity, in the sense of worth and worthiness, is not precisely or even mainly the opposite of indignity. Dignity does not consist merely in the absence of indignity, and indignity is not itself merely the absence of dignity. Dignity and indignity seem to be two separate "things," each of which one can "possess" more or less or not at all.

Thus, the more accurate meaning of "death with dignity," when used as a slogan against excessive medical intervention, is really "death without further or additional indignity."

Death and Dignity

Without *further* or *additional* indignity? Additional to what? To death itself? We have come at last to our question. In what sense can death (mortality) be an indignity? Is it an "action toward another"—and if so, whose? Or "an offense against personal dignity" or "unmerited contemptuous treatment" or an affront? I think not. Only if dignity were synonymous or coextensive with life itself could we even begin to make such a case.[6]

And yet, though merely to live is not yet to live excellently or with dignity, to die is to put an end to all further possibility of dignity. Human life is a necessary condition of there being any human dignity, and one ought—even on this ground alone—to respect it and respect it highly. My previous argument appears to need some qualification. Could we not call death or mortality "an indignity" because it "destroys" or limits the conditions of dignity, even though the conditions as such—life—are not by themselves sufficient to produce dignity or worthiness? (Here we may have an analogy to the distinction drawn above in my discussion of more and less dignified ways to die, where it was noted that "external" conditions could make a so-called "dignified death" difficult if not impossible.) Could it be said, then, that death is in this sense "the ultimate indignity," just as murder is perhaps the ultimate personal crime—ultimate precisely because, by destroying the foundations, it makes impossible the entire edifice, right up to the crown?

I think not. Death *may* be a great evil, but it should not be considered *in itself* an "indignity."[7] I offer several suggestions that might be developed into full-blown arguments. *First,* looking to our common sense ways of speaking and feeling, for all that we may fear death, we do not react as if death were an indignity to Picasso or Stravinsky or DeGaulle, each of whom died full of days after a rich and worthy life. We may miss them, but do we regard their death as an affront to them? Do we even regard it as an evil?

Second, as many instances of heroism or martyrdom show, death can be for some human beings the occasion for the display of dignity, indeed of their greatest dignity, for example, in the laying down of one's life for one's friend, one's country, or one's beliefs. Far from undermining their worth, their death—like the life it terminates—is a necessary condition for their display of dignity. Consider, for example, the Athenians eulogized by Thucydides' Pericles in the famous Funeral Oration:

> Thus choosing to die resisting, rather than to live submitting, they fled only from dishonor, but met danger face to face, and after one brief moment, while at the summit of their fortune, escaped, not from their fear, but from their glory. . . .
>
> Comfort, therefore, not condolence, is what I have to offer to the parents of the dead who may be here. Numberless are the chances to which, as they know, the life of man is subject; but fortunate indeed are they who draw for their lot a death so glorious as that which has caused your mourning, and to whom life has been so exactly measured as to terminate in the happiness in which it has been passed.[8]

And this need not only be true of heroes. Take the case of Tolstoi's unheroic Ivan Ilych. It has been argued that with the insight the dying Ilych gets into the meaninglessness of his (former) life,

> the man grows far beyond himself in the last hours of his life; he attains an inner greatness which retroactively hallows all of his previous life—in spite of its apparent futility—and makes it meaningful. . . . Not only the sacrifice of one's life can give life meaning; life can reach nobility even as it founders on the rocks.[9]

Though I think the claim made here for Ivan Ilych is excessive, the general point is worth pondering.

Third, to expand this point, it has been argued that human mortality is a necessary spur, throughout all of one's life, to the pursuit of excellence and the acquisition of dignity, and that immortal life, even without senescence, could not be lived with seriousness or with passion.[10] Ramsey himself notes that without death "life would be an endless boredom, and boring because endless; there would be no reason to probe its depths while there is still time." And so, when Ramsey says that "death may be a good evil," I think he means to acknowledge the importance of mortality for at least some aspects of human worthiness. I myself have doubts about the full adequacy of this view, and seriously question the notion of human life as "living-toward-death." In this connection, I suggest we consider the alternative outlooks implied either in the life of Socrates, as Plato presents it, or in the possibly apocryphal story about St. Francis who, while in the garden planting onions, was asked, "What would you do if you learned that you were to die tomorrow?" and who supposedly answered, "I would continue planting onions." And yet, if we consider the statesman, the warrior, the athlete, the painter, the poet, the actor, the architect, the teacher, or the lover, we can see the importance of not having world enough and time.

Fourth, as Hans Jonas has pointed out, death may not only be the necessary spur to our numbering our days, but also the condition of the possibility of renewed life and youth and hope:

> With their ever new beginning, with all their foolishness and fumbling, it is the young that ever renew and thus keep alive the sense of wonder, of relevance, of the unconditional, of ultimate commitment, which (let us be frank) goes to sleep in us as we grow older and tired. It is the young, not the old, that are ready to give their life, to die for a cause[11]—

and I would add, it is the cycle of birth answering death that brings the ever renewable possibility of a concern for excellence and dignity.

Death as Natural

Yet I think I would emphasize a fifth and final reason why death cannot be regarded as an indignity, or I might even add, as an ultimate evil. I return, without romanticism but with a sober appreciation of what I think is true, to the fact that *death is natural and necessary and inextricably tied to life.* To live is to be mortal; death is the necessary price for life. To decline and to die are necessary parts of the *life cycle,* whether fully and *consciously* experienced or not. (I admit freely that "one's own nonbeing" cannot be experienced—it is an impossibility—though I am not certain that it cannot be imagined.) Already Aristotle notes that living things have in themselves a principle of growth *and decay.* Decay and decline are not "affronts from outside," but are natural processes *built into* the principle that causes life.

Ramsey's personification of death is at least partly responsible for his failure to appreciate this point. "Death is an enemy," and his other personifications all treat "death" as an external agent. Ramsey is thus easily led to the view that death is always an assault from outside, and even when timely, so-to-speak "violent." Even his more neutral formulations of "living-toward-death" and "living toward a limit" also externalize mortality and fail to acknowledge the degree to which that limit is set within.

Modern biology has in no fundamental way altered Aristotle's view; the maximum life-span of a species is governed from within, the result of processes that are genetically determined—that is, natural—and encoded in the genome that "contains the information" for the other processes of life. How can death be an indignity if it is the natural and necessary accompaniment of life itself? When we "buy" life we "buy" death. Is there thus not even some indignity—some childish desire to cheat, or to eat one's life and keep it—in the suggestion that death is a contradiction to the *worth* of a human life? Is there really dignity in attempting the impossible or in railing against the inevitable? Is there not more dignity in facing up to such things and in facing them nobly and bravely? Consider the following passages from Aristotle's *Ethics.* After acknowledging that "death is the most terrible of all things; for it is the end, and nothing is thought to be any longer either good or bad for the dead," Aristotle concludes his discussion of courage:

> Death and wounds will be painful to the brave man and against his will, but he will face them because it is noble to do so or because it is base not to do so. And the more he is possessed of virtue in its entirety and the happier he is, the more he will be pained at the thought of death; for life is best worth living for such a man, and he is knowingly losing the greatest goods, and this is painful. But he is none the less brave, and perhaps all the more so, because he chooses noble deeds of war at that cost.[12]

Against the view that mortality is a "part of life" Ramsey has urged that "disease, injury, congenital defects are also a part of life, and as well murder, rapine, and pillage." But are any of these as natural, necessary, and inextricably bound up with life as are death or decay? The closest case would be disease; but whereas both disease and decline have "natural" causes, much disease is caused at least in part by external agency, and the body responds to disease by "attempting" to heal itself, to make itself healthy, to make itself whole. In this sense, disease is *fought* by nature working within, whereas decline is *produced* by nature working within. This is, of course, oversimplified and crude, but nevertheless adequate enough to suggest that, unlike all those other things which *occur* in life, decline and death are a *part* of life, an integral part which cannot be extruded without destroying the whole.

Against this view Ramsey has also urged the empirical argument that although "death is a natural fact of life yet no man dies 'naturally,' nor do we have occasions in which to 'practice' doing so in order to learn how." Maybe most men don't, but some men do. Maybe not always eagerly—if that is what he means by "naturally"—but often willingly, or at least not unwillingly. And if he means by "naturally" something like "spontaneously" or "not without training," it is simply not true that there is *no* occasion to practice doing so; there is more occasion to practice dying—indeed, a nightly occasion—than to practice childbearing or child-rearing.

There are many things which human beings do "by nature," by virtue of capacities and possibilities that are inborn in them as human beings, but which nevertheless require training and habituation. Man is by nature an animal that speaks, but each one of us must be taught a language. According to Aristotle, man is by nature a *polis*-animal, that is, an animal that lives in cities, yet he also adds that the man who *discovered* the *polis* was a great benefactor of mankind. More generally, habit is regarded as a kind of second nature; and while our habits do not come to us "naturally," at birth, still our *capacity to form habits,* and good habits, is itself inborn. And while it is true that, unlike speech and the civic and philosophical lives it makes possible, death is not an end or purpose of human life (*telos*) but merely its termination (*finis*), it is nevertheless possible for us to educate ourselves about the role and meaning of mortality, and thereby to habituate our sentiments and feelings, so that we may live properly before it, without undue fear or anxiety. For this, more important than the experience of sleeping may be the experience of the lives and deaths of those who have gone before, whether in fact or in myth, experience accessible to us if we study the lives of some great human beings and if we carefully read and think about the great literature of our tradition. And even if we have not studied, and even if we never saw anyone die, we could still, in principle, learn something about how *we ought* to stand toward death—and not only how most of us do—if we reflect on the fact that we were once not here and that we will again not be here, and that this is the way things are and must be. If we are really to eschew whistling in the dark, let us come fully into the light and see nature as it is.

Ramsey's paper fails to give nature her due. Though what nature is is a great mystery and a long question, she deserves more respect than Ramsey gives her. He complains that certain modern "interpretations of human life are increasingly mundane, naturalistic, antihumanistic when measured by *any* genuinely 'humanistic' esteem for the individual human being." Here we come close to fundamentals. Ultimately, though not in this paper, we shall have to ask whether the "esteem" for the "individual human being" is tied first and most to what is *individuated* or to what is *human*—that is, generic—about that *particular* human being. Ramsey speaks briefly to this question, and nods to Aristotle, at the end of his paper. But he presents little if any argument. He intimates that there are few adherents of Plato and Aristotle around today, as if that constituted a valid argument against them, and concludes, why I do not know, that *"a true humanism and the dread of death seem to be dependent variables."* (Emphasis added.) A true humanism or a true humanitarianism? In either case, does he mean "true," or merely "more comforting"? And he adds, again I know not why, "I suggest that it is better to have the indignity of death on our hands and in our outlooks than to 'dignify' it in either of these two possible ways." Why and how *better?* But I digress—this is for another day.

For the present, I note from the above passage only how Ramsey has demoted the world and nature, and thereby also man insofar as he is (merely) natural and worldly. What are the opposites of "mundane, naturalistic, antihumanistic," if not "other-worldly, unnaturalistic, humanistic"?

To the First Things and the Origin of Death

Ramsey's critique of a view of death as natural and hence acceptable is a critique which rests not on his reason but in his faith. He speaks as if the really *proper* condition for a being such as man is immortality, that man fell to a merely mortal, merely natural condition. He speaks as if man had a chance for immortality but squandered it. (That Ramsey is not a pessimist stems from his unstated belief that men—though not as worldly men—have not really lost immortality.) Notice where dignity lies on Ramsey's view of nature and man. Man, the mortal sinner, has only an alien dignity bestowed upon him by God, who out of His infinite love became man and was crucified, and who thus redeems man and offers him salvation from sin and the conquest of death. Ramsey's view of death as an indignity rests upon his belief in "the Fall of Man," as recounted in Genesis, but not called "the Fall of Man" in Genesis, or, as far as I know, anywhere else in the Hebrew tradition. (I checked the latest edition of the *Encyclopedia Judaica* and found between Falkowitsch, Joel Baerisch, and Falticeni, Rumania, only Fall River, Massachusetts.)

This may perhaps be an appropriate place to mention that I have serious questions about the adequacy of Ramsey's treatment of the Hebrew sources or tradition on this topic. It is a simplification, and I think a gross distortion, to say as he does that "sin was determinative for the Hebrew consciousness" (so too, "death for the Greek consciousness"). Even at this simplistic formulaic level, what about "covenant" or "sanctification" or "love of God"? Also, Ramsey's interpretation of Ecclesiastes is at variance in some important respects with the few Hebrew commentators I have read,[13] and I myself would dispute whether the book shows "an unrelieved pessimism," and whether "the practical advice" of Koheleth isn't more akin to "Live joyously; do not toil in vain or seek wisdom," than to Ramsey's formulation, "Be what you are, in human awareness apart and not a part," which makes Koheleth too much like Pascal to be Koheleth. And, concerning the critical passage, "Everything has its appointed time," etc. (Eccles. 3:1-9), while it is clear from the overall context that these lofty verses do not constitute simply a paean of praise but also something of a complaint, it seems that the complaint is for man's ignorance of God's purpose in arranging things thus, rather than for change and death. The real "conclusion" of the litany may not be "What profit then has the worker in his toil?" (Eccles. 3:9), but rather the sequel:

> I know the concern which God has given men to be afflicted with. Everything He has made proper in its due time, and He has also placed the love of the world in men's hearts, except that they may not discover the work God has done from beginning to end.
>
> I know that there is no other good in life but to be happy while one lives. Indeed, every man who eats, drinks and enjoys happiness in his work—that is the gift of God. I know that whatever God does remains forever—to it one cannot add and from it one cannot subtract, for God has so arranged matters that men should fear Him. What has been, already exists, and what is still to be, has already been, and God always seeks to repeat what has gone by.[14]

In any event, the Book of Ecclesiastes is perplexing and resists simple formulation and I am not yet prepared to say much more than I think the matter needs more study. There are numerous problems of exegesis and interpretation, not to speak of difficulties caused by translators who have tried to "improve" upon the original. I understand too that there has long been controversy about the Jewishness of this Jewish book, and that it is probably not the best source for the many Jewish teachings on the subject of death.

A better one may be the minor and late Talmudic tractate "Mourning" (generally referred to by its euphemistic title *Semahot,* "Rejoicings"; that it is a minor tractate, compared with major tractates on Benedictions or Sabbath or Marriage or property damage and personal injury or sacrifices, may say something about the place of death in Jewish thought). From here comes the following passage on the theme of timely and untimely death:

> Whosoever dies before he is fifty has been cut down before his time.
>
> At the age of fifty-two: this is the death of Samuel the Ramathite.
>
> At the age of sixty: this is the death of which Scripture speaks, for it is said: *Thou shalt come to thy grave in ripe age, like a shock of corn cometh in its season.* (Job 5:26)
>
> At the age of seventy: this is the death of divine love, for it is said: *The days of our years are threescore and ten.* (Ps. 90:10)
>
> At the age of eighty: this is the death of 'strength,' for it is said: *Or even by reason of strength fourscore years.* (Ps. 90:10)
>
> Similarly, Barzillai said to David: *I am this day fourscore years old, can I discern between good and bad?* (2 Sam. 19:36)
>
> After this, life is anguish.

Let me return with Paul Ramsey to the Garden of Eden. Ramsey, ultimately, cannot accept the view that death is "natural," because he follows the teaching about original sin and its wage: "Wherefore, as by one man sin entered into the world, and death by sin; and so death passed upon all men, for that all have sinned" (Rom. 5:12). To be sure, there is Hebrew Biblical support for this view, and one strand of Jewish thought also attributes man's mortality to disobedience (but probably more to each man's disobedience than to Adam's), grounding this view on Genesis 3: 22-24. But the most traditional Jewish view on the necessity of death traces not to the expulsion from the Garden, and not even to disobedience. Death is held to be part of the order of the world since creation. God made man from the dust of the earth, and to dust he must return (Gen. 2:7 and 3:19). Even the account of Genesis 1, with the creation of two sexes and the first commandment to "Be fruitful and multiply, and replenish the earth," already implies the "creation" of mortality. At the completion of creation of the world God saw "everything He had made, and behold, it was very good." The sage Rabbi Meir commenting on this verse says, "it was very good, that is 'death was good,' " which comment Maimonides later cites approvingly in a section of *The Guide of the Perplexed,* which, at least on the surface, teaches that *everything which is is good:* "Even the existence of this inferior matter, whose manner of being it is to be a concomitant of privation entailing death and all evils, all this is also *good* in view of the perpetuity of generation and the permanence of being through succession."[15]

This last passage permits me to open up a question

that goes beyond the dignity or indignity of death. Is death an evil or a good, or a good *evil* or an evil *good?* The passage from Maimonides, while acknowledging that death is an evil (or, at least, is to be grouped with "all evils"), asserts death to be a good. As already noted, Ramsey has made an analogous concession, stating that *awareness* of death can be the cause of a virtuous life if it teaches us to number our days. But for Ramsey, the genus of mortality is ineradicably *evil,* even though for some of us it may be a good evil: "So I say death may be a good evil or an evil evil, but it is perceived as an evil or experienced indignity in either case." In contrast, Maimonides and Rabbi Meir seem to say that death is an evil good. This latter view seems to me correct. The following are some elements of an argument.

First, even though an evil, death is and ought to be preferred to some greater evils. If to lay down one's life under some circumstances is noble, and to continue to live under others is base, then death cannot be an ultimate or worst evil. This does not yet show, of course, that death is a good.

Second, mortality is an evil for the individual—though an evil that is, I repeat, part and parcel of the good which is his life, or more precisely, of the bittersweet bargain which is mortal life, as well as, perhaps, the mother of certain strivings toward the good and the beautiful—but it is necessary for the group, be the group defined as the political community or the species. Death is necessary not just in the sense of "unavoidable," which it is also for the individual, but in the sense of "indispensable." Mortality, like taxation, is both certain *and indispensable* for the common good, and the common good is, needless to say, a good from which each individual benefits.

Third, the evil which death is for us as individuals—for instance, in the sense of the earlier passage from Aristotle in which he calls death the most terrible of all things—becomes good because of generation, continuity, and renewal, that is, "in view of the perpetuity of generation and the permanence of being through succession." The secret is to transcend one's selfish attachments and to shun the view which preaches the "dread of death" as "the dread of oblivion, of there being only empty room in one's stead." Rather one should harken to transmission and regeneration, and to the view which sees in death the presence of one's children and one's grandchildren in one's stead.

Finally, I add an empirical test of Ramsey's view. If death is indeed an irreducible evil, then he should, it seems to me, be willing *in principle* (that is, setting aside other compelling arguments about boredom and about the possible disrupting social consequences) to embrace current biochemical research which aims to retard the process of aging and greatly extend our life expectancy. On *his* principles, were he to find the fountain of youth, he should drink. But knowing Ramsey's other writings, I suspect he would, on principle, refuse. His heart may know the reasons why he should not drink and why, indeed, "There is a time to be born and a time to die," but his reason's reasons—at least those given in this paper—would not tell him or us why not.

To pull together some threads, though there is no Biblical word for "nature," it seems that we can say that death, on the Jewish view, no less than on the Aristotelian or the modern scientific view, is "natural" or "proper to a man." The Christian view—or at least Paul Ramsey's view of the Christian view, which he seems to rest largely on the teachings of St. Paul—disputes this. There are, of course, other Christian views. For example, with St. Thomas Aquinas' efforts to hold together Aristotelian nature and the Gospels, "death as natural" and "Nature as a standard" acquired a permanent place in Christian thought. But whether it is really possible to reconcile Aristotle's elevated nature and natural death with the Pauline view of nature as base and death as the wages of sin I do not know.

These are matters about which I am largely ignorant. I raise these points only to suggest that the "true humanism" dependent on the "dread of death" may turn out to be only one variety of Christian humanism—or rather humanitarianism—though, nevertheless, still possibly true. Also, it is possible that the hyphen needs to be removed from the Judaeo-Christian traditions, at least on this fundamental matter.

But however true the metaphor of the Garden of Eden may be for displaying man's inherent moral weakness or for making intelligible the presence of suffering in the world, can we regard the story as *literally* true? What is the truth about nature and man's place in it? Is nature the prison to which man has fallen or the home out of which he has risen? And more specifically, what is the truth about the origins of human mortality?

We cannot honestly think about the origin of mortal man without facing up to the theory of evolution. In part, Ramsey should be pleased by this move. For never has there been a scientist whose theory so resonates with what Ramsey claims to be the Christian outlook on the world as Darwin: Evolution by natural selection; everything is sin and separation—albeit the only sin is the failure to be fruitful and multiply. Whether the "special theory of evolution," that is, the theory of natural selection, can fully account for the rise of man, or mutation for the appearance of large evolutionary novelties, is a long question. But that man has not always been, and was not specially created *as he now is,* is beyond dispute. Man never was immortal or capable of bodily immortality. He is mortal because his prehuman ancestors were mortal, because each living being is and has always been mortal. He has come to be as a result of birth and death, emerging gradually, via other living forms, out of potentialities that must have been present even in pre-animate matter. That there should be life at all is the greatest "miracle" and wonder, and that through a process blind but perhaps not dumb an intelligent being came to be who considers where he comes from and how he is to live, who sees beauty in nature and who imitates it in his works, who is capable of so much that is excellent—and also so much that is base—here lies a being and a process with dignity.

In Darwin's view, this rise of man and the higher animals was the result of selective death. Here is how he concludes *The Origin of Species:*

> Thus, from the war of nature, from famine and death, the most exalted object which we are capable of conceiving, namely, the production of the higher animals, directly follows. There is grandeur in this view of life, with its several powers, having been originally breathed into a few forms or into one; and that, whilst this planet has gone cycling on according to the fixed law of gravity, from so simple a beginning endless forms most beautiful and most wonderful have been, and are being, evolved.[16]

To the Last Things?

And yet, to come back a little bit toward Ramsey, and to restore the ecumenical spirit, I must add this final qualification. We now know that "the perpetuity of generation and the permanence of being through succession," which enabled Maimonides to deem death a good, is itself not guaranteed, neither by theory nor in practice. Evolution merely means change, not necessarily "progress," and extinction of species is the general rule. If the death of the individual is an evil for him and a loss to his survivors, the death or extinction of the human species would be far more than that. Man is, regardless of how he came to be, the only being which, though only a part of the whole, can think of, appreciate, and care for the whole. The extinction of man would rob the world of its dignity.

Given our current predicaments, for which we are ourselves largely to blame, perhaps we should begin to pray that there is indeed a providential hand that will not let it happen.

Notes

1. Indeed, I would suggest that Ramsey's predicament of finding himself in bed with too many partners may stem in part from the fact that both he and they give too much emphasis to "uniqueness," to the subjective, to the individual human soul in its "individuation." Could it be that the stress on the "unique worth of the individual" connects together the mainstream of today's secular thought and its severed theological source, from which Paul Ramsey still takes his watering?

2. Consider Cephalus' answer to Socrates' question about whether old age is a hard time of life. See Plato, *Republic* 1. trans. by Allan Bloom (New York: Basic Books, 1968), p. 5:

> "'By Zeus, I shall tell you just how it looks to me, Socrates,' he said. 'Some of us who are about the same age often meet together and keep up the old proverb. Now then, when they meet, most of the members of our group lament, longing for the pleasures of youth and reminiscing about sex, about drinking bouts, and feasts and all that goes with things of that sort; they take it hard as though they were deprived of something very important and had then lived well but are now not even alive. Some also bewail the abuse that old age receives from relatives, and in this key they sing a refrain about all the evils old age has caused them. But, Socrates, in my opinion these men do not put their fingers on the cause. For, if this were the cause, I too would have suffered these same things insofar as they depend on old age and so would everyone else who has come to this point in life. . . . But of these things and of those that concern relatives, there is one certain cause: not old age, Socrates, but the character of the human beings. If they are balanced and good-tempered, even old age is only moderately troublesome; if they are not, then both age, Socrates, and youth alike turn out to be hard for that sort.'"

3. Robert S. Morison, "Death: Process or Event?" *Science* 173 (August, 1971), 694-98; and Leon R. Kass, "Death as an Event: A Commentary on Robert Morison," *Science* 173 (August, 1971), 698-702.

4. Eric J. Cassell, "Being and Becoming Dead," *Social Research* 39 (Autumn, 1972), 528-42.

5. This is not necessarily to say that one should treat other people, including those who eschew dignity, as if they lacked it. This is a separable question. It may indeed be salutary to treat people on the basis of their capacities to live humanly, despite even great falling short or even willful self-degradation. Yet this would, in the moral sphere at least, require that we expect and demand of people that they behave worthily. One cannot, without self-contradiction, both attribute moral dignity to everyone and then excuse a man's crimes and moral failings by blaming them on his toilet training, his poverty, or "The System." Moral dignity without the presumption of responsibility and accountability is impossible, and to assert it is ludicrous.

6. Ramsey in fact adopts a view very close to this, in locating dignity in the once-and-for-all, never-to-be-repeated, unique living-toward-death that is, for him, the "definition" of a human life. Man's *worldly* dignity, for Ramsey, stems from the perceived threat of death which, he implies, is ever present with every man so long as he lives. This strikes me as a most misanthropic view of dignity. Moreover, death, which Ramsey claims to be an ultimate indignity, paradoxically emerges on his own view as the "great individualizer," and hence as the source of all worldly dignity. (I am indebted to William F. May for this last insight.)

7. As the above analysis of the relation between "dignity" and "indignity" suggests, to show that mortality is not an indignity would say nothing about whether it is "beautiful" or "full of dignity"; for these excessive claims I hold no brief.

8. *The Complete Writings of Thucydides: The Peloponnesian War,* trans. by Richard Crawley, Modern Library Edition (New York: Random House, 1934), pp. 107-08.

9. Viktor E. Frankl, *The Doctor and the Soul* (New York: Vintage Books, 1973), p. 106.

10. See, for example, Eric J. Cassell, "Death and the Physician," *Commentary,* June, 1969, pp. 73-79.

11. Hans Jonas, "Contemporary Problems in Ethics From a Jewish Perspective," *Journal of Central Conference of American Rabbis* (January, 1968), 27-39; reprinted in *Judaism and Ethics,* ed. by D. J. Silver (New York: Ktav Publishing Company, 1970).

12. W. D. Ross translation.

13. See, for example, Robert Gordis, *Koheleth: The Man and His World: A Study of Ecclesiastes* (New York: Schocken, 1967) and *Midrash Rabbah Ecclesiastes,* trans. by Rev. A. Cohen (London: Soncino Press, 1961). Consider, as one example, how differently from Ramsey one Midrash interprets the verse, "A good name is better than precious oil, and the day of death better than the day of birth" (7:1):

"When a person is born all rejoice; when he dies all weep. It should not be so; but when a person is born there should be no rejoicing over him, because it is not known in what class he will stand by reason of his actions, whether righteous or wicked, good or bad. When he dies, however, there is cause for rejoicing if he departs with a good name and leaves the world in peace. It is as if there were two ocean-going ships, one leaving the harbor and the other entering it. As the one sailed out of the harbor all rejoiced, but none displayed any joy over the one which was entering the harbor. A shrewd man was there and he said to the people, 'I take the opposite view to you. There is no cause to rejoice over the ship which is leaving the harbor because nobody knows what will be its plight, what seas and storms it may encounter; but when it enters the harbor all have occasion to rejoice since it has come in safely.' Similarly, when a person dies all should rejoice and offer thanks that he departed from the world with a good name and in peace. That is what Solomon said, *And the day of death [is better] than the day of one's birth.*

14. Trans. by Robert Gordis, in Gordis, *The Wisdom of Ecclesiastes* (New York: Behrman House, 1945).

15. Maimonides, *The Guide of the Perplexed,* trans. by Shlomo Pines, Vol. III (Chicago: Univ. of Chicago Press, 1963), Chap. 10.

16. For those who may wonder about the adequacy of Darwin's views about the ultimate origin of life, and for those who think the above passage is meant to support a quarrel between science and religion, it is perhaps worth noting that, beginning with the second and continuing through the sixth and last edition of the *Origin,* that is, long after there would be any need to appease religious objectors, Darwin inserted "by the Creator" into the above passage, between "breathed" and "into."

Chapter Seven
NATURE AND ITS MASTERY

Introduction

The report of some new scientific or medical breakthrough is likely to be greeted by both shouts of celebration and cries of alarm. The reasons for this may be many, but surely one of them is that people have different dispositions toward nature and its mastery. Some see in the new power to intervene purposefully in natural processes the possibility and the promise of doing genuine good; they, of course, will celebrate human mastery over nature. Others see in the new power the pride that sets us over and against nature rather than in it, and they complain and warn that nature will yet master presumptuous humanity.

There are reasons for people's different dispositions toward nature, and some of them at least are religious reasons, reasons formed by a response to God and informed by reflection about God's relations to human beings and to the nature on which they depend and try to master.

Such reflection is frequently founded on Scripture and can in fact be found already in Scripture. See, for example, Genesis 1:27-28:

> So God created man in his own image, in the image of God he created him; male and female he created them. And God blessed them, and God said to them, "Be fruitful and multiply, and fill the earth and subdue it; and have dominion over the fish of the sea and over the birds of the air and over every living thing that moves upon the earth."

This verse has frequently served as a sort of proof text for those who would celebrate human dominion or mastery over nature.[1] The historical and canonical context of these words, however, may affect the way they shape our disposition toward nature and its mastery. If they were originally written (as many biblical scholars claim) to a people exiled to Babylon, powerless and hopeless according to the ordinary canons of judgment, then they were words of hope and promise. But what was blessing in one historical context may become curse in another—in the twentieth century with its technological power and pride, for example—or at least so say some who are more suspicious of technology.

The canonical context may also remind us of other dispositions toward nature. The world of nature was seen not just in terms of regularity and law-governed order (it is worth noting, however, that there is some of this, e.g., Eccles. 1:5-7) but also as a witness to the glory of God (e.g., Ps. 19:1ff.). Scriptural reflection about man's relation to nature does contain a celebration of human mastery of nature (for an example of this, see Job's dramatic account of the technological powers of human beings in Job 28). But Scripture also gives accounts of the intimate bonding of human beings with nature, in creation (signaled by the common root of *'adam,* man, and *'adamah,* earth), in the Fall, and decisively in the visions of renewal and shalom (e.g., Isa. 11:6-9; Rom. 8:18-25). The ambiguity found in Scripture may reflect the ambiguities of nature and its mastery; and faithfulness to Scripture in our reflection may mean the recognition of those same ambiguities. A staphylococcus infection is not considered good, or even benign, simply because it is a part of nature; in fact, the natural processes of the body move quickly to identify and counter staph. Medical intervention may be necessary when the natural defenses are unsuccessful, but effective intervention must not only destroy the staph but also respect and sustain the body's natural systems.

Near Eastern idolatry was the background for a good deal of biblical reflection on nature and the appropriate disposition toward it. Ba'al was an ancient god of fertility who, it was believed, controlled the fertility of both field and wombs and whose name means "master." The people of God were constantly warned in Scripture against such idolatry, and those warnings surely contributed to the desacralization of nature which prepared the way for a technological mastery of nature. Today, however, one may ask whether there is not a new idol, a new object of ultimate loyalty and trust, a new thing on which human beings found their hopes: technology. Daniel Callahan raises that question in a profound way in his essay included below.

To recognize ambiguities is important, but it is not all that can be done or ought to be accomplished in reflection about nature and its mastery. The essays collected here raise a number of important questions. One such question is how to understand technology. Is technology basically a tool box with which to build the sort of world human beings already want, or is it fundamentally power, not just of human beings over nature but of some people over other people?

Another question is the relation of technology to man's inner nature. C. S. Lewis warns of "the abolition of man"; Karl Rahner and Joseph Fletcher argue that human nature is essentially creative and free, and marked by technological control.

Finally, the question of the relation of technology and values must be considered. Are technological innovations simply a function of our values, ways to achieve what we already want, or do they shape our values as well? Worth pausing over is Callahan's observation that some technologies have become socially enforced after being initially introduced as a way of increasing our options. Which values or principles should we attempt to apply to technology, and how should we apply them? Are there objective moral norms of the sort Lewis refers to as the "Tao" which can be used to limit and guide research and technology? Or should we calculate the consequences and then direct innovation to the greatest good for the greatest number? Fletcher identifies his focus on consequences and benefits with love, and Rahner also appeals to love as one limit and guide for the technological shaping of the future—but do they mean the same thing by "love"? If not, is one more faithful to the narrative within which and in terms of which Christians understand love? James Childress attends to consequences but also to the distribution of the harms and benefits of technology and to the distinction between "goal-rational" and "value-rational" types of action.

Many concrete decisions about technology will remain deeply ambiguous, for the question of our right relation to nature is a complex one—complex because we are related not only to nature but to each other and not only to each other but to God who has ordered and redeemed it and us.

Notes

1. Lynn White, Jr., "The Historical Roots of our Ecological Crisis," *Science* 155 (March 10, 1967): 1203-7.

Suggestions for Further Reading

Anderson, Bernhard W. "Human Dominion over Nature." In *Biblical Studies in Contemporary Thought,* edited by Miriam Wood. Somerville, Mass.: Green Hadden, 1975.

Ellul, Jacques. *The Technological Society.* Translated by John Wilkinson. New York: Knopf, 1965.

Geyer, Alan. "The EST Complex at MIT: The Ecumenical-Scientific-Technological Complex." *Ecumenical Review,* Oct. 1979, 372-80.

Gustafson, James M. "Christian Attitudes Toward a Technological Society." *Theology Today,* July 1959, 173-87.

Illich, Ivan D. "Technology and Conviviality." In *To Create a Different Future,* edited by Kenneth Vaux. New York: Friendship Press, 1972.

Jonas, Hans. "Technology and Responsibilities: Reflections on the New Tasks of Ethics." In *Philosophical Essays.* Englewood Cliffs, N.J.: Prentice-Hall, 1974.

Shinn, Roger, ed. *Faith and Science in an Unjust World: Report of the World Council of Churches' Conference on Faith, Science and the Future.* Vol. I. Philadelphia: Fortress, 1980.

Teich, Albert H., ed. *Technology and Man's Future.* 2d ed. New York: St. Martin's, 1977.

Walters, LeRoy. "Technology Assessment and Genetics." *Theological Studies* 33 (1972): 666-83.

34.
Ode on a Plastic Stapes

CHAD WALSH

for Dr. Rufus C. Morrow, surgeon

What God hath joined together man has put
Asunder. The stapes of my middle ear
Rests in some surgical kitchen midden.
Good riddance to an otosclerotic pest.
And welcome to the vibrant plastic guest
That shivers at each noise to let me hear.

What would the theologians make of this?
The bone God gave me petered out and failed.
But God made people, too. One of them sawed
A dead bone off and put a new one in.
I hear now through a storebought plastic pin.
Where God's hand shook, his creature's skill availed.

Dig where they bury me and you will find
A skeleton of bone perfected in plastic.
Gleam down the buried years, synthetic bone,
Await the judgment of the Resurrection,
The shining glory or the sharp correction
When calendars and clocks read chiliastic.

Will my old stapes rise, expel my plastic?
Do I own or do I merely borrow?
God is no divorce court judge. What man
Hath joined together, he will not put asunder.
Praise God who made the man who wrought this
  wonder,
Praise God, give thanks tomorrow and tomorrow.

From Chad Walsh, *The End of Nature* (Chicago: Swallow Press, 1969). Copyright 1969 by Chad Walsh. Used by permission.

35.
The Abolition of Man

C. S. LEWIS

It came burning hot into my mind, whatever he said and however he flattered, when he got me home to his house, he would sell me for a slave.

Bunyan

'Man's conquest of Nature' is an expression often used to describe the progress of applied science. 'Man has Nature whacked' said someone to a friend of mine not long ago. In their context the words had a certain tragic beauty, for the speaker was dying of tuberculosis. 'No matter,' he said, 'I know I'm one of the casualties. Of course there are casualties on the winning as well as on the losing side. But that doesn't alter the fact that it is winning.' I have chosen this story as my point of departure in order to make it clear that I do not wish to disparage all that is really beneficial in the process described as 'Man's conquest,' much less all the real devotion and self-sacrifice that has gone to make it possible. But having done so I must proceed to analyse this conception a little more closely. In what sense is Man the possessor of increasing power over Nature?

Let us consider three typical examples: the aeroplane, the wireless, and the contraceptive. In a civilized community, in peace-time, anyone who can pay for them may use these things. But it cannot strictly be said that when he does so he is exercising his own proper or individual power over Nature. If I pay you to carry me, I am not therefore myself a strong man. Any or all of the three things I have mentioned can be withheld from some men by other men—by those who sell, or those who allow the sale, or those who own the sources of production, or those who make the goods. What we call Man's power is, in reality, a power possessed by some men which they may, or may not, allow other men to profit by. Again, as regards the powers manifested in the aeroplane or the wireless, Man is as much the patient or subject as the possessor, since he is the target both for bombs and for propaganda. And as regards contraceptives, there is a paradoxical, negative sense in which all possible future generations are the patients or subjects of a power wielded by those already alive. By contracep-

From C. S. Lewis, *The Abolition of Man* (London: William Collins Sons & Co. Ltd., 1946). Used by permission.

tion simply, they are denied existence; by contraception used as a means of selective breeding, they are, without their concurring voice, made to be what one generation, for its own reasons, may choose to prefer. From this point of view, what we call Man's power over Nature turns out to be a power exercised by some men over other men with Nature as its instrument.

It is, of course, a commonplace to complain that men have hitherto used badly, and against their fellows, the powers that science has given them. But that is not the point I am trying to make. I am not speaking of particular corruptions and abuses which an increase of moral virtue would cure: I am considering what the thing called 'Man's power over Nature' must always and essentially be. No doubt, the picture could be modified by public ownership of raw materials and factories and public control of scientific research. But unless we have a world state this will still mean the power of one nation over others. And even within the world state or the nation it will mean (in principle) the power of majorities over minorities, and (in the concrete) of a government over the people. And all long-term exercises of power, especially in breeding, must mean the power of earlier generations over later ones.

The latter point is not always sufficiently emphasized, because those who write on social matters have not yet learned to imitate the physicists by always including Time among the dimensions. In order to understand fully what Man's power over Nature, and therefore the power of some men over other men, really means, we must picture the race extended in time from the date of its emergence to that of its extinction. Each generation exercises power over its successors: and each, in so far as it modifies the environment bequeathed to it and rebels against tradition, resists and limits the power of its predecessors. This modifies the picture which is sometimes painted of a progressive emancipation from tradition and a progressive control of natural processes resulting in a continual increase of human power. In reality, of course, if any one age really attains, by eugenics and scientific education, the power to make its descendants what it pleases, all men who live after it are the patients of that power. They are weaker, not stronger: for though we may have put wonderful machines in their hands we have preordained how they are to use them. And if, as is almost certain, the age which had thus attained maximum power over posterity were also the age most emancipated from tradition, it would be engaged in reducing the power of its predecessors almost as drastically as that of its successors. And we must also remember that, quite apart from this, the later a generation comes—the nearer it lives to that date at which the species becomes extinct—the less power it will have in the forward direction, because its subjects will be so few. There is therefore no question of a power vested in the race as a whole steadily growing as long as the race survives. The last men, far from being the heirs of power, will be of all men most subject to the dead hand of the great planners and conditioners and will themselves exercise least power upon the future. The real picture is that of one dominant age—let us suppose the hundredth century A.D.—which resists all previous ages most successfully and dominates all subsequent ages most irresistibly, and thus is the real master of the human species. But even within this master generation (itself an infinitesimal minority of the species) the power will be exercised by a minority smaller still. Man's conquest of Nature, if the dreams of some scientific planners are realized, means the rule of a few hundreds of men over billions upon billions of men. There neither is nor can be any simple increase of power on Man's side. Each new power won *by* man is a power *over* man as well. Each advance leaves him weaker as well as stronger. In every victory, besides being the general who triumphs, he is also the prisoner who follows the triumphal car.

I am not yet considering whether the total result of such ambivalent victories is a good thing or a bad. I am only making clear what Man's conquest of Nature really means and especially that final stage in the conquest, which, perhaps, is not far off. The final stage is come when Man by eugenics, by pre-natal conditioning, and by an education and propaganda based on a perfect applied psychology, has obtained full control over himself. *Human* nature will be the last part of Nature to surrender to Man. The battle will then be won. We shall have 'taken the thread of life out of the hand of Clotho' and be henceforth free to make our species whatever we wish it to be. The battle will indeed be won. But who, precisely, will have won it?

For the power of Man to make himself what he pleases means, as we have seen, the power of some men to make other men what *they* please. In all ages, no doubt, nurture and instruction have, in some sense, attempted to exercise this power. But the situation to which we must look forward will be novel in two respects. In the first place, the power will be enormously increased. Hitherto the plans of educationalists have achieved very little of what they attempted and indeed, when we read them—how Plato would have every infant 'a bastard nursed in a bureau,' and Elyot would have the boy see no men before the age of seven and, after that, no women,[1] and how Locke wants children to have leaky shoes and no turn for poetry[2]—we may well thank the beneficent obstinacy of real mothers, real nurses, and (above all) real children for preserving the human race in such sanity as it still possesses. But the man-moulders of the new age will be armed with the powers of an omnicompetent state and an irresistible scientific technique: we shall get at last a race of conditioners who really can cut out all posterity in what shape they please. The second difference is even more important. In the older systems both the kind of man the teachers wished to produce and their motives for producing him were prescribed by the *Tao**—a norm to which the teachers themselves were subject and from which they claimed no liberty to depart. They did not cut men to some pattern they had chosen. They handed on what they had received: they initiated the young neophyte into the mystery of humanity which over-arched him and them alike. It was but old birds teaching young birds to fly. This will be changed. Values are now mere natural phenomena. Judgements of value are to be produced in the pupil as part of the conditioning. Whatever *Tao* there is will be the product, not the motive, of education. The conditioners have been emancipated from all that. It is one more part of Nature which they have conquered. The ultimate springs of human action are no longer, for them, something given. They have surrendered—like electricity: it is the function of the Conditioners to control, not to obey them. They know how to *produce* conscience and decide what kind of conscience they will produce. They themselves are outside, above. For we are assuming the last stage of Man's struggle with Nature. The final victory has been won. Human nature has been conquered—and, of course, has conquered, in whatever sense those words may now bear.

The Conditioners, then, are to choose what kind of artificial *Tao* they will, for their own good reasons, produce in the Human race. They are the motivators, the creators of motives. But how are they going to be motivated themselves? For a time, perhaps, by survivals, within their own minds, of the old 'natural' *Tao.* Thus at first they may look upon themselves as servants and guardians of humanity and conceive that they have a 'duty' to do it 'good.' But it is only by confusion that they can remain in this state. They recognize the concept of duty as the result of certain processes which they can now control. Their victory has consisted precisely in emerging from the state in which they were acted upon by those processes to the state in which they use them as tools. One of the things they now have to decide is whether they will, or will not, so condition the rest of us that we can go on having the old idea of duty and the old reactions to it. How can duty help them to decide that? Duty itself is up for trial: it cannot also be the judge. And 'good' fares no better. They know quite well how to produce a dozen different conceptions of good in us. The question is which, if any, they should produce. No conception of good can help them to decide. It is absurd to fix on one of the things they are comparing and make it the standard of comparison.

To some it will appear that I am inventing a factitious difficulty for my Conditioners. Other, more simple-minded, critics may ask 'Why should you suppose they will be such bad men?' But I am not supposing them to be bad men. They are, rather, not men (in the old sense) at all. They are, if you like, men who have sacrificed their own share in traditional humanity in order to devote themselves to the task of deciding what 'Humanity' shall henceforth mean. 'Good' and 'bad,' applied to them, are words without content: for it is from them that the content of these words is henceforward to be derived. Nor is their difficulty factitious. We might suppose that it was possible to say 'After all, most of us want more or less the same things—food and drink and sexual intercourse, amusement, art, science, and the longest possible life for individuals and for the species. Let them simply say, This is what we happen to like, and go on to condition men in the way most likely to produce it. Where's the trouble?' But this will not answer. In the first place, it is false that we all really like the same things. But even if we did, what motive is to impel the Conditioners to scorn delights and live laborious days in order that we, and posterity, may have what we like? Their duty? But that is only the *Tao,* which they may decide to impose on us, but which cannot be valid for them. If they accept it, then they are no longer the makers of conscience but still its subjects, and their final conquest over Nature has not really happened. The preservation of the species? But why should the species be preserved? One of the questions before them is whether this feeling for posterity (they know well how it is produced) shall be continued or not. However far they go back, or down, they can find no ground to stand on. Every motive they try to act on becomes at once a *petitio.* It is not that they are bad men. They are not men at all. Stepping outside the *Tao,* they have stepped into the void. Nor are their subjects necessarily unhappy men. They are not men at all: they are artefacts. Man's final conquest has proved to be the abolition of Man.

Yet the Conditioners will act. When I said just now

*What Lewis calls the *Tao* is "the doctrine of objective value, the belief that certain attitudes are really true, and others really false, to the kind of thing the universe is and the kinds of things we are." *The Abolition of Man* (New York: Macmillan, 1962), p. 29.—Ed.

that all motives fail them, I should have said all motives except one. All motives that claim any validity other than that of their felt emotional weight at a given moment have failed them. Everything except the *sic volo, sic jubeo* has been explained away. But what never claimed objectivity cannot be destroyed by subjectivism. The impulse to scratch when I itch or to pull to pieces when I am inquisitive is immune from the solvent which is fatal to my justice, or honour, or care for posterity. When all that says 'it is good' has been debunked, what says 'I want' remains. It cannot be exploded or 'seen through' because it never had any pretensions. The Conditioners, therefore, must come to be motivated simply by their own pleasure. I am not here speaking of the corrupting influence of power nor expressing the fear that under it our Conditioners will degenerate. The very words *corrupt* and *degenerate* imply a doctrine of value and are therefore meaningless in this context. My point is that those who stand outside all judgements of value cannot have any ground for preferring one of their own impulses to another except the emotional strength of that impulse. We may legitimately hope that among the impulses which arise in minds thus emptied of all 'rational' or 'spiritual' motives, some will be benevolent. I am very doubtful myself whether the benevolent impulses, stripped of that preference and encouragement which the *Tao* teaches us to give them and left to their merely natural strength and frequency as psychological events, will have much influence. I am very doubtful whether history shows us one example of a man who, having stepped outside traditional morality and attained power, has used that power benevolently. I am inclined to think that the Conditioners will hate the conditioned. Though regarding as an illusion the artificial conscience which they produce in us their subjects, they will yet perceive that it creates in us an illusion of meaning for our lives which compares favourably with the futility of their own: and they will envy us as eunuchs envy men. But I do not insist on this, for it is mere conjecture. What is not conjecture is that our hope even of a 'conditioned' happiness rests on what is ordinarily called 'chance'—the chance that benevolent impulses may on the whole predominate in our Conditioners. For without the judgement 'Benevolence is good'—that is, without re-entering the *Tao*—they can have no ground for promoting or stabilizing their benevolent impulses rather than any others. By the logic of their position they must just take their impulses as they come, from chance. And Chance here means Nature. It is from heredity, digestion, the weather, and the association of ideas, that the motives of the Conditioners will spring. Their extreme rationalism, by 'seeing through' all 'rational' motives, leaves them creatures of wholly irrational behaviour. If you will not obey the *Tao,* or else commit suicide, obedience to impulse (and therefore, in the long run, to mere 'nature') is the only course left open.

At the moment, then, of Man's victory over Nature, we find the whole human race subjected to some individual men, and those individuals subjected to that in themselves which is purely 'natural'—to their irrational impulses. Nature, untrammelled by values, rules the Conditioners and, through them, all humanity. Man's conquest of Nature turns out, in the moment of its consummation, to be Nature's conquest of Man. Every victory we seemed to win has led us, step by step, to this conclusion. All Nature's apparent reverses have been but tactical withdrawals. We thought we were beating her back when she was luring us on. What looked to us like hands held up in surrender was really the opening of arms to enfold us for ever. If the fully planned and conditioned world (with its *Tao* a mere product of the planning) comes into existence, Nature will be troubled no more by the restive species that rose in revolt against her so many millions of years ago, will be vexed no longer by its chatter of truth and mercy and beauty and happiness. *Ferum victorem cepit:* and if the eugenics are efficient enough there will be no second revolt, but all snug beneath the Conditioners, and the Conditioners beneath her, till the moon falls or the sun grows cold.

My point may be clearer to some if it is put in a different form. Nature is a word of varying meanings, which can best be understood if we consider its various opposites. The Natural is the opposite of the Artificial, the Civil, the Human, the Spiritual, and the Supernatural. The Artificial does not now concern us. If we take the rest of the list of opposites, however, I think we can get a rough idea of what men have meant by Nature and what it is they oppose to her. Nature seems to be the spatial and temporal, as distinct from what is less fully so or not so at all. She seems to be the world of quantity, as against the world of quality: of objects as against consciousness: of the bound, as against the wholly or partially autonomous: of that which knows no values as against that which both has and perceives value: of efficient causes (or, in some modern systems, of no causality at all) as against final causes. Now I take it that when we understand a thing analytically and then dominate and use it for our own convenience we reduce it to the level of 'Nature' in the sense that we suspend our judgements of value about it, ignore its final cause (if any), and treat it in terms of quantity. This repression of elements in what would otherwise be our total reaction to it is sometimes very noticeable and even painful: something has to be overcome before we can cut up a dead man or a live animal in a dissecting room. These objects *resist* the movement of the mind whereby we thrust them into the world of mere Nature. But in other instances too, a similar price is exacted for our analytical knowledge and manipulative power, even if we have ceased to count it. We do not look at trees either as Dryads or as beautiful objects while we cut them into beams: the first man who did so may have felt the price keenly, and the bleeding trees in Virgil and Spenser may be far-off echoes of that primeval sense of impiety. The stars lost their divinity as astronomy developed, and the Dying God has no place in chemical agriculture. To many, no doubt, this process is simply the gradual discovery that the real world is different from what we expected, and the old opposition to Galileo or to 'bodysnatchers' is simply obscurantism. But that is not the whole story. It is not the greatest of modern scientists who feel most sure that the object, stripped of its qualitative properties and reduced to mere quantity, is wholly real. Little scientists, and little unscientific followers of science, may think so. The great minds know very well that the object, so treated, is an artificial abstraction, that something of its reality has been lost.

From this point of view the conquest of Nature appears in a new light. We reduce things to mere Nature *in order that* we may 'conquer' them. We are always conquering Nature, because 'Nature' is the name for what we have, to some extent, conquered. The price of conquest is to treat a thing as mere Nature. Every conquest over Nature increases her domain. The stars do not become Nature till we can weigh and measure them: the soul does not become Nature till we can psycho-analyse her. The wresting of powers *from* Nature is also the surrendering of things *to* Nature. As long as this process stops short of the final stage we may well hold that the gain outweighs the loss. But as soon as we take the final step of reducing our own species to the level of mere Nature, the whole process is stultified, for this time the being who stood to gain and the being who has been sacrificed are one and the same. This is one of the many instances where to carry a principle to what seems its logical conclusion produces absurdity. It is like the famous Irishman who found that a certain kind of stove reduced his fuel bill by half and thence concluded that two stoves of the same kind would enable him to warm his house with no fuel at all. It is the magician's bargain: give up our soul, get power in return. But once our souls, that is, our selves, have been given up, the power thus conferred will not belong to us. We shall in fact be the slaves and puppets of that to which we have given our souls. It is in Man's power to treat himself as a mere 'natural object' and his own judgements of value as raw material for scientific manipulation to alter at will. The objection to his doing so does not lie in the fact that this point of view (like one's first day in a dissecting room) is painful and shocking till we grow used to it. The pain and the shock are at most a warning and a symptom. The real objection is that if man chooses to treat himself as raw material, raw material he will be: not raw material to be manipulated, as he fondly imagined, by himself, but by mere appetite, that is, mere Nature, in the person of his dehumanized Conditioners.

We have been trying, like Lear, to have it both ways: to lay down our human prerogative and yet at the same time to retain it. It is impossible. Either we are rational spirit obliged for ever to obey the absolute values of the *Tao,* or else we are mere nature to be kneaded and cut into new shapes for the pleasures of masters who must, by hypothesis, have no motive but their own 'natural' impulses. Only the *Tao* provides a common human law of action which can over-arch rulers and ruled alike. A dogmatic belief in objective value is necessary to the very idea of a rule which is not tyranny or an obedience which is not slavery.

I am not here thinking solely, perhaps not even chiefly, of those who are our public enemies at the moment. The process which, if not checked, will abolish Man, goes on apace among Communists and Democrats no less than among Fascists. The methods may (at first) differ in brutality. But many a mild-eyed scientist in pince-nez, many a popular dramatist, many an amateur philosopher in our midst, means in the long run just the same as the Nazi rulers of Germany. Traditional values are to be 'debunked' and mankind to be cut out into some fresh shape at the will (which must, by hypothesis, be an arbitrary will) of some few lucky people in one lucky generation which has learned how to do it. The belief that we can invent 'ideologies' at pleasure, and the consequent treatment of mankind as mere ὕλη, specimens, preparations, begins to affect our very language. Once we killed bad men: now we liquidate unsocial elements. Virtue has become *integration* and diligence *dynamism,* and boys likely to be worthy of a commission are 'potential officer material.' Most wonderful of all, the virtues of thrift and temperance, and even of ordinary intelligence, are *sales-resistance.*

The true significance of what is going on has been concealed by the use of the abstraction Man. Not that the word Man is necessarily a pure abstraction. In the *Tao* itself, as long as we remain within it, we find the concrete reality in which to participate is to be truly human: the real common will and common reason of humanity, alive, and growing like a tree, and branching out, as the situation varies, into ever new beauties and dignities of application. While we speak from within the *Tao* we can speak of Man having power over himself in a sense truly analogous to an individual's self-control. But the moment we step outside and regard the *Tao* as a mere subjective product, this possibility has disappeared. What is now common to all men is a mere abstract universal, an H.C.F., and Man's conquest of himself means simply the rule of the Conditioners over the conditioned human material, the world of post-humanity which, some knowingly and some unknowingly, nearly all men in all nations are at present labouring to produce.

Nothing I can say will prevent some people from describing this lecture as an attack on science. I deny the charge, of course: and real Natural Philosophers (there are some now alive) will perceive that in defending value I defend *inter alia* the value of knowledge, which must die like every other when its roots in the *Tao* are cut. But I can go further than that. I even suggest that from Science herself the cure might come. I have described as a 'magician's bargain' that process whereby man surrenders object after object, and finally himself, to Nature in return for power. And I meant what I said. The fact that the scientist has succeeded where the magician failed has put such a wide contrast between them in popular thought that the real story of the birth of Science is misunderstood. You will even find people who write about the sixteenth century as if Magic were a medieval survival and Science the new thing that came in to sweep it away. Those who have studied the period know better. There was very little magic in the Middle Ages: the sixteenth and seventeenth centuries are the high noon of magic. The serious magical endeavour and the serious scientific endeavour are twins: one was sickly and died, the other strong and throve. But they were twins. They were born of the same impulse. I allow that some (certainly not all) of the early scientists were actuated by a pure love of knowledge. But if we consider the temper of that age as a whole we can discern the impulse of which I speak. There is something which unites magic and applied science while separating both from the 'wisdom' of earlier ages. For the wise men of old the cardinal problem had been how to conform the soul to reality, and the solution had been knowledge, self-discipline, and virtue. For magic and applied science alike the problem is how to subdue reality to the wishes of men: the solution is a technique; and both, in the practice of this technique, are ready to do things hitherto regarded as disgusting and impious—such as digging up and mutilating the dead. If we compare the chief trumpeter of the new era (Bacon) with Marlowe's Faustus, the similarity is striking. You will read in some critics that Faustus has a thirst for knowledge. In reality, he hardly mentions it. It is not truth he wants from his devils, but gold and guns and girls. 'All things that move between the quiet poles shall be at his command' and 'a sound magician is a mighty god.'[3] In the same spirit Bacon condemns those who value knowledge as an end in itself: this, for him, is to use as a mistress for pleasure what ought to be a spouse for fruit.[4] The true object is to extend Man's power to the performance of all things possible. He rejects magic because it does not work,[5] but his goal is that of the magician. In Paracelsus the characters of magician and scientist are combined. No doubt those who really founded modern science were usually those whose love of truth exceeded their love of power; in every mixed movement the efficacy comes from the good elements not from the bad. But the presence of the bad elements is not irrelevant to the direction the efficacy takes. It might be going too far to say that the modern scientific movement was tainted from its birth: but I think it would be true to say that it was born in an unhealthy neighbourhood and at an inauspicious hour. Its triumphs may have been too rapid and purchased at too high a price: reconsideration, and something like repentance, may be required.

Is it, then, possible to imagine a new Natural Philosophy, continually conscious that the 'natural object' produced by analysis and abstraction is not reality but only a view, and always correcting the abstraction? I hardly know what I am asking for. I hear rumours that Goethe's approach to nature deserves fuller consideration—that even Dr. Steiner may have seen something that orthodox researchers have missed. The regenerate science which I have in mind would not do even to minerals and vegetables what modern science threatens to do to man himself. When it explained it would not explain away. When it spoke of the parts it would remember the whole. While studying the *It* it would not lose what Martin Buber calls the *Thou*-situation. The analogy between the *Tao* of Man and the instincts of an animal species would mean for it new light cast on the unknown thing, Instinct, by the only known reality of conscience and not a reduction of conscience to the category of Instinct. Its followers would not be free with the words *only* and *merely*. In a word, it would conquer Nature without being at the same time conquered by her and buy knowledge at a lower cost than that of life.

Perhaps I am asking impossibilities. Perhaps, in the nature of things, analytical understanding must always be a basilisk which kills what it sees and only sees by killing. But if the scientists themselves cannot arrest this process before it reaches the common Reason and kills that too, then someone else must arrest it. What I most fear is the reply that I am 'only one more' obscurantist, that this barrier, like all previous barriers set up against the advance of science, can be safely passed. Such a reply springs from the fatal serialism of the modern imagination—the image of infinite unilinear progression which so haunts our minds. Because we have to use numbers so much we tend to think of every process as if it must be like the numeral series, where every step, to all eternity, is the same kind of step as the one before. I implore you to remember the Irishman and his two stoves. There are progressions in which the last step is *sui generis*—incommensurable with the others—and in which to go the whole way is to undo all the labour of your previous journey. To reduce the *Tao* to a mere natural product is a step of that kind. Up to that point, the kind of explanation which explains things away may give us something, though at a heavy cost. But you cannot go on 'explaining away' for ever: you will find that you have explained explanation itself away. You cannot go on 'seeing through' things for ever. The whole point of seeing through something is to see something through it. It is good that the window should be transparent, because the street or garden beyond it is opaque. How if you saw through the garden too? It is no use trying to 'see through' first principles. If you see through everything, then everything is transparent. But a wholly transparent world is an invisible world. To 'see through' all things is the same as not to see.

Notes

1. *The Boke Named the Governour,* I. iv: 'Al men except physitions only shulde be excluded and kepte out of the norisery.' I. VI: 'After that a childe is come to seuen yeres of age . . . the most sure counsaile is to withdrawe him from all company of women.'

2. *Some Thoughts concerning Education,* § 7: 'I will also advise his *Feet to be wash'd* every Day in cold Water, and to have his Shoes so thin that they might leak and *let in Water,* whenever he comes near it.' § 174: 'If he have a poetick vein, 'tis to me the strangest thing in the World that the Father should desire or suffer it to be cherished or improved. Methinks the Parents should labour to have it stifled and suppressed as much as may be.' Yet Locke is one of our most sensible writers on education.

3. *Dr. Faustus,* 77-90.

4. *Advancement of Learning,* Bk. I (p. 60 in Ellis and Spedding, 1905; p. 35 in Everyman Edn.).

5. *Filum Labyrinthi,* i.

36. Technological Devices in Medical Care

JOSEPH FLETCHER

A mass circulation magazine recently ran a two-page advertisement by General Electric which showed an eight-year-old boy at play in the fields. The ad explained how an implanted pacemaker maintains a 92 per minute beat in Brian Coe's heart. The caption read, "This boy's heart runs on batteries." Such devices are at work in patients from six-month-old girls to ninety-four-year-old men. "Helping people live longer," said the advertisement, "is progress of the most important kind."

The Terms and Ideas We Use

When we submit technological devices to ethical analysis, we need first to be clear about what we mean by "technological" and what we mean by a "device." Too often, I think, we use the concept of technology in a narrow way, doing less than justice to its practitioners and their triumphs. In the popular image, for example, the term "technology" usually connotes a gadget, a mechanical tool or arrangement of some kind. Indeed, the common error is precisely to conceive of technology as a matter of mechanics. And the same is true of devices—they are thought of as more or less ingeniously "devised" mechanical tools or arrangements. But this mechanical model is far from adequate for the ethical evaluation of technology as it plays its part (an increasingly essential part) in medical care.

Arnold Toynbee has spoken of "technology's relentless progress," and it is my own belief that technology, with its often revolutionary innovations in how we do things, is the source or cause of the most pressing problems of ethics. Either it poses perennial problems of good and evil in significantly new forms, or it confronts us with new problems of conscience, new in the sense that they are unanticipated and often even seemingly bizarre. This happens in medicine fully as much as in industry or war or communications or any other field. In a moment we shall have occasion to look at some typical examples.

But first, there are various ways to think technology. Another word for it could be "techniquery." It is indeed a matter of devices or of "devising" ways and means. It is at bottom a matter of process, innovation, method. Nevertheless, technology is far more than merely ingenious. It is a knowledgeable combination of information and skill, of know-what (science) and know-how (technology). In its bluntest definition, it is applied science. It is the scientifically disciplined and sophisticated invention of devices to serve the ends or goals or "goods" we cherish. In medicine these ends are health and life and psychophysical well-being. As a matter of means and ends, therefore, technology is of the greatest direct ethical concern. Perhaps the best definition is Webster's: "the totality of the means employed to provide objects necessary for human sustenance and comfort."[1]

But let me repeat: technology—perhaps especially in medicine—is far from being a matter of mechanics only. The "hardware" is less important than the "software." In medicine, the systems engineering of technology is not only mechanical but also chemical, biological, physical, psychological, and surgical. Hyperbaric chambers put chemistry and physics to use in crisis surgery. The use of hormones to regulate both primary and secondary sexual conditions is an example of how almost all of these disciplines may be harnessed together by medicine. Even surgery is involved in some cases, for example, in transexual alterations. A cardiology device such as a blood-pressure sensor or tiny electronic monitoring device, so small (five one-hundredths of an inch) that it can be injected into an artery with a hypodermic needle and then maneuvered into a ventricle to send signals to a recording machine in an intensive care unit, is obviously a union of physics, biology, and surgery. And a left-ventricle assist-device, especially if it is of synthetic or plastic material (such as DuPont's Lycra) adds chemistry to the team. Artificial insemination, "one of the best kept secrets in American medicine," is another example of how technology in medicine entails psychology, physiology, biology, and often also physics and mechanics, as in the centrifugal collection of sperm for homologous inseminations to overcome a husband's low sperm count. Or a battery and tiny transmitter may be mounted on a pessary to signal temperature changes following ovulation in order to assist in overcoming sterility, or to make the rhythm "method" more accurate, or even to give some control over the sex of offspring. All resuscitation techniques for the drowned or frozen, for cardiac arrest, cardiovascular lesions, spontaneous hypoglycemia, and the like, involve technologies of a multidisciplinary kind.

In this context it is worth remembering that cybernetics itself is a conflation of biology (especially brain physiology) and communications theory, automatic control mechanics (especially feedback), mathematics, and logic. Strange as it may seem, physicians in this era need to be good engineers as well. Much of the work on medical-surgical technology—for example, in heart, lung, and limb renewals, replacements, and supportive prosthetics (so-called cyborg medicine)—has come from people who are both. I think in this connection of Nikolai Amasov of the Kiev Institute of Thoracic Surgery, and Mikhail Bykhovsky of the cybernetics laboratory in the Vishnesky Institute of Surgery in the Soviet Union.[2] They have their counterparts in America, Europe, and around the world.

The Influence of Technology

Technology by this date is fully in service to medicine. As a matter of fact, it is changing more than just man's environment and his tools: it is changing man himself. Hence our recent more mature and scientific interest in ecology. "Once men start down the technological road," says Roger Revelle, "they cannot turn back. Once they have bitten into the fruit of the tree of knowledge, there can be no return to Eden."[3] As I put it sometime ago at the Mayo medical center, we have reached the end of the age of innocence, that is, of ignorance, and the end of ignorance means the end of alibis and excuses.[4]

Every widening or deepening of our knowledge of reality and our control of its forces adds to our ethical problems; knowledge and control are the ingredients of both freedom and responsibility. Less and less are we the helpless and therefore nonmoral victims of whatever life happens to bring to us—and by "life" here I mean not only circumstances but the vital principle of biological life itself. Knowledge and virtue have always been coupled, as by Confucius and Socrates—an association recently reexamined by the English biologist C. H. Waddington in his essay *The Ethical Animal,*[5] and by Rene Dubos in *Adapting Man.*[6]

As Pascal thought, the problem of ethics is *"travailler à bien penser,"* "to work hard at good thinking." Not feeling or guessing, but thinking and knowing. "Let us," he said, "strive to think well—therein is the principle of morality."[7] And Kant called ethics "practical reason." In this spirit we can say that the heart of the problems of medical ethics is the science and technology at stake in them, along with a willingness to see our values and goals in the fresh light of fresh developments, and even to add to or abstract from them as the data suggest. I would be the first to echo the opinion of J. Robert Oppenheimer, who said, "I believe the strength and soundness of Christian sensibility, the meaning of love and charity, have changed the world at least as much as technological developments." But, as Oppenheimer suggests, I want to insist that it is in love working with technology, not in love alone, that we find the key to human hopes.

Biology is the great new realm of technological change, and medicine is its chief beneficiary. After the First World War our cultural emphasis lay on the social and behavioral sciences. Then it shifted at the time of the Second World War to the physical sciences, due in the main to new frontiers in nuclear research. But by the sixties the greatest excitement was being found in the biological sciences. Of what was once called "pure biology" there is little left in these days of biochemistry, psychobiology, biophysics, microbiology, bionautics, and the like.

It was "only yesterday" that so much started to happen in biology. Jean Rostand tells us how Viguier only a few decades ago made fun of what he called the "chemical citizens, the sons of Madame Sea-Urchin and Monsieur Chloride of Magnesium," but now we speak calmly of the solitary generation of creatures by artificial parthenogenesis, and of diploid rather than sexual reproduction.[8] Ancient alchemy dreamed of the "creation" of life, and now—at least theoretically in a scientific sense—it is possible, given Kornberg's partial success in first producing a synthetic virus containing DNA, the basic substance of all life, and then in getting it to reproduce itself in a living cell.

The momentum of our scientific-technical development is hard to grasp—and nowhere more so than in medicine. By leaps and bounds it proceeds, in invention (finding new methods), in innovation (introducing new methods into use), and in diffusion (spreading their use). Lots of it comes like serendipity, unexpected profit in side effects. After all, we need to remember, Roentgen had no real idea what he was doing when all of a sudden he saw the skeleton of his own hand. And it has been said that if all the wisest medical people in 1890 had been asked to suggest the next important invention, none would have mentioned the X ray.

I have two dictionaries in my study, and while I still prefer the 1913 Webster for literary purposes, I have to rely upon a 1967 edition because the old one of half a century ago has almost none of the language of present-day technological discourse. This is a hundredfold truer of medical dictionaries. For example, the intrauterine devices have reopened the question whether conception is accomplished at fertilization or at nidation. They have also reopened the definition of abortion: Does it cover direct interference with the development of a preuterine or unimplanted zygote? Or only of uterine material?

More substantially than the words we use, our knowledge and data are mounting so fast that although we have a hundred times as much to know as in 1900, by A.D. 2000 there will be a thousand times as much. There is a tremendous explosion of information, investigation, and publication, and our archival and bibliographic methods are already antiquated in spite of computerized retrieval. In fact, specialties are so fractured by the knowledge expansion that a "generalist" nowadays is just what a specialist was only a couple of decades ago.

As a consequence of this complexity, medicine turns more and more to computerized diagnosis. A LINC (Laboratory Instrument Computer) quickly does what a clinical interview takes hours to do. For example, the answer to such a question as "Have you ever had hives?" triggers the LINC to go on to maybe four hundred queries about related allergies, whereas doctors would never think of them all. This multiphasic screening will mean the revelation of hidden diseases cybernetically. As things stand now, for every cervical cancer diagnosed, dozens go undetected, and so with diabetes, and so on. And as computers (especially analog) get more complicated they will probably find heretofore unsuspected and undescribed diseases and maladies. Even in isolated communities physicians could connect by telephone landlines to central computers—like a central catalogue for bibliographic inquiries from libraries—and get diagnoses in fifteen seconds over teletype. This is what the combination of "hardware" and "software" in technology can do. Names like Pasteur, Lister, Roentgen, and the Curies will, of course, have their successors in the technological age, but far more will be achieved corporately and by team work without any hero mystique, because of technology's built-in process of interdependence or collective achievement.

The Ethical Problems Posed

The picture of what has happened in the technology of medicine and paramedical care fills us, ambivalently, with fear and confidence, assurance and doubt—both as to the facts themselves and as to the value-meaning of the facts, their ethical significances. For example, how are we to regard the prospect of human hibernation for short periods (hours or days) and later for longer periods (months or years), as cryonics develops from its present uses as "deep freeze" for surgical purposes? What will the surgical use of laser beams ultimately entail (besides the dangers of the so-called death ray)? Genetic control of the basic human constitution by microbiological manipulation of "code" material, DNA and RNA, is at hand. Is there any cause to be squeamish or chary about using techniques for cosmetic changes of human features, figure, complexion, skin color, and even physique? Or the more radical technology of chemotherapy in controlling fatigue, relaxation, alertness, mood, sleep, personality, perception, and fantasies? Lurking behind all such questioning is the factor of control: We wonder whether we may establish and exercise management of the very essentials of personal identity and existence. The question really is not whether we can but whether we should. We can do it, but the ethical question is: Ought we to?

Chemotherapy is far less challenging morally than the immediate or prospective manipulations of psychopharmacology, for example, in changing the chemical composition of the nervous system, its neurons and chemical transmitters of impulses, or than the chemical control and improvement of memory and learning (even, theoretically, programmed dreams). The very concepts of choice, chance, self, and rationality, so central to classical or traditional reasoning, may have to be altered or even "reconceptualized."

Take the notion of "identity," a notion so prominent in the current rhetoric of psychology, especially under the influence of Erikson's thesis about the identity crisis. Given the present and future trends in cyborg medicine, one may well ask: Who is it that functions physiologically with borrowed or artificial veins and arteries (whether synthetic or plastic), bone structures, prosthetic devices, cardiac implants—including even donated aortas or whole hearts—audio and visual aids, manipulators and pedipulators, donated kidneys, or artificial dialysis for kidney function, artificial kidneys and hearts powered by isotopic energy, and many other technological devices, logically ending in a sort of *ultima ratio* with transplanted brains?

Who is the child born as a result of predetermined sex, germinal selection, genetic control, and artificial mutations—and after birth modified not only by cyborg technology but by chemical and electronic means, for example, by effective appetite controls and weight controls, electric brain stimulation by electrodes and surgical subcuts, endocrine alterations, and the like?

For just as we once reached the point at which diabetics could regulate the sugar in their blood systems, so we will have autocontrol of mood and intelligence. Who, then, is who? How will we think of it when theoretical brain transplants become operational? As they say, today's "science fiction" is tomorrow's science.

Who *is* the recipient patient—is he the preoperative person or the donor? This kind of basic conceptual question, like the one about when and what is death, will inevitably change not only the language but also the mental constructs with which we think about moral values, ethical responsibility, and even the very notion of the moral agent himself.

What are our licit or morally justifiable choices, initiatives, and purposes as we employ the technology of medicine? What are the values we should seek or preserve—such as freedom from pain, health, euphoria, even life itself—and in what order of relative desirability are we to rank them? What comes first as the *summum bonum,* in the sense that, if necessary, all else is to be subordinated or sacrificed? Life? Self-image? Personal survival? Social welfare? In the conventional wisdom nearly all such questions have been almost ignored, or their answers complacently assumed. But technology has a way of undermining conventions, of changing the world, and with it our values and priorities.

The Problem of Control

As I remarked earlier, my own opinion is that, morally, the heart of the matter is control. The question is whether human beings may choose or make the conditions of life, health, and death. (I am sure that death control, as in direct or indirect euthanasia, is as much a part of modern medicine as birth control and health control are.) The key to control, however, is initiative. True control of life puts the initiative in man's hands; that is, it is a matter of choice. Nothing not chosen has ethical importance. Babies born by chance rather than choice may be precious, but their birth is amoral if not actually immoral. A patient who dies in personality-blotting suffering, or after personality is gone and irretrievable, may be an object of compassion, but his actual dying is nonmoral and his own relationship to it is either amoral or immoral, as is that of his medical servants as well.

What we do when we can do it, by our own choice, initiative, and purposiveness, is moral action—either right or wrong, as the case may be. If we refuse to do what we can when we can, on the ground that we may not or ought not to take the initiative, this is nonmoral and antiethical—I would even add "subhuman," because truly human acts are moral, that is, free and responsible. For example, not to take the initiative by using a Bennett valve and mask in a case of respiratory failure on the operating table might in a concrete situation be a responsible decision to let the patient go. Such a decision might, for example, be made for a nonagenarian patient with grievously metastasized cancer. But *never* to revive artificially a patient whose respiration fails would be immoral, that is, it would be a refusal to exercise initiative and choice. It would be irresponsible and therefore immoral.

A great deal of ethical reasoning in the past has been of this immoral kind—arguing against initiative and human control on grounds that it is allegedly "unnatural" or "against nature." That kind of ethics simply cannot survive in a technological civilization. "Nature" and "human nature" are no more fixed and finished than any of the other concepts moralists like to posit. In Catholic moral theology it used to be held that we are only tenants of our bodies, that we may not alter them because we have only their usufruct, not their dominion. As stewards, not proprietors, of our bodies we have charge only of the *bene esse,* not of the *esse.* Hence, no mutilation was morally justified, except to preserve life. This ruled out donations of organs such as kidneys and ovaries, as well as free decision for or against the new transformations possible as a result of scientific and technical development. But that old morality of nature is being superseded, happily, by a new morality of love. What this means, for example, is that those who have courage will gladly risk the sacrifice of one of their kidneys for a friend, thus deliberately reducing their own survival quotient by half; or that a nun who has embraced the vocation of childlessness will eagerly donate an ovary to a sterile patient.

The new morality of situation ethics has little patience with those who object in principle to heart transplants from cadaveric donors. Such a position has been taken by Dr. Werner Forssmann, chief surgeon at the Düsseldorf Evangelical Hospital and Nobel prize winner in medicine for 1956. In commenting on Christian Barnard's successful transplants in South Africa, he said such transplants are morally dangerous because they involve a third person, the donor, as well as the doctor and the recipient patient, and because they offend against the medical rule *nil nacere,* "hurt nothing." There is a danger, of course, that surgeons will sacrifice the chances of one patient for the sake of the other, that this will lead, for example, to executing criminals in order to get vital organs, and to an inequitable tendency to select recipients on the basis of wealth, personal friendship, or politics. On the other hand, most Catholic moralists already say that "it is morally permissible to transfer parts from a corpse to a living person,"[9] and in Dr. Barnard's interview with the pope no objections were voiced. I am myself convinced that we must stick to the maxim of most moralists, *abusus non tollit usum,* "the abuse of the thing does not bar its use." As Raymond Queneau once said, "The people who whine about naughty robots and inhuman machinery have never proved anything except their own lack of imagination and fear of liberty."[10] As the old saw put it, "conscience" gets a lot of credit that belongs to cold feet.

Dr. Forssmann also believes that it was wrong to put a pig's liver in a dying woman in Buenos Aires—presumably on the ground that heterografts or xenogenic (i.e., interspecific) transplants are "unnatural." By this logic we would, for example, have to give up the transplantation of monkeys' thymus glands into cancerous patients' thighs in an effort to let the antibodies help in the struggle against the neoplasm. This will be a hard kind of classicism to maintain as immunosuppressive techniques overcome the rejection reaction, and as better antigen typing and tissue preservation are developed.[11] It is a matter of time, that is all, until herds of animals are raised directly for human spare parts—cows, swine, chimpanzees, and the like. Already, barely on the threshold of transplant technique, we have only a sad short-supply of paired organs (livers, lungs, hearts) for postmortem donation, and of nonpaired organs (kidneys, ovaries, testes) for pre- or postmortem donation. Even if we could discourage the present subethical practice of burying or burning (cremating) precious vital organs—here is immorality ritualized—there still would be a need for interspecific supplies.

One of the ethical issues at stake, then, is whether any procedure or process is, as such, to be proscribed as always wrong for some intrinsic reason. A hundred years ago dissection of human bodies was forbidden, so that grave robber and medical student meant the same thing; yet all that is gone by now—a mythology demythologized. For some people abortion is still held to be immoral in all cases except when necessary to preserve the life and/or health of a patient. But unlike this absolutism (really a mystique) of the old morality, the new morality decides the right or the wrong of medical treatments relatively, according to the factors in each situation. If, for example, there is at least a 25 percent chance that a PKU child (phenylketonuric) will be born of a union of PKU heterozygotes, producing a retarded child, why not abort? Especially if normal children can be adopted or conceived by artificial insemination from a donor? Why submit to the cruel workings of subhuman, physical nature? Technology by its very principle and method substitutes human control for nature's control—and holds, indeed, that control is a word appropriate only to the moral decisions of people and inappropriate to the determinism of mindless processes. As a writer in the *British Medical Journal* once put it very simply, "Each case must be judged on its merits." . . .

"Playing God"

At this point somebody always cries, "You are playing God!" I think the only honest and constructive reply is, "Yes, we are." This is part of the meaning of the Bible's creation and "fall" myths. By gaining know-what and know-how we become responsible, by eating the fruit of the tree of knowledge we make ourselves "like God"—whose superiority is threatened by man's inquiry and invention. But that old, primitive God is dead, that God of the gaps, the God whose majesty and power derived from man's ignorance. That God was God because of human ignorance and fear, and he has been dying by inches with the advance of human knowledge and the control over life and death which knowledge brings to man. In the matter of human knowledge we are indeed "playing the God of the gaps." If such achievements as ectogenetic reproduction, genetic control, and the production (not creation) of life in a test tube shakes anybody's faith, then his God is only one that plugs up the gaps in his knowledge, a hypothesis of ignorance. If we have to say goodbye to God because science solves the mysteries of life and technology gives us control of life, then our God is only a doomed idol.

What we need then is a new God. It is better to believe in God as creator, the creative principle behind all the workings of nature and of human achievement. He is as much the will and the love behind a test tube as behind "natural phenomena." This God can be worshiped as the other no longer can. After all, as Eric Ambler once said, "If there is such a thing as a super-human law, it is administered with subhuman inefficiency."[12]

We must get rid of that obsolete theodicy which imagines that God is not only the cause but the builder of nature and its works, and not only the builder but the manager—so that it is God himself who is the efficient as well as the final cause of earthquake and fire, of life and death, with the logical inference that "interference with nature" (which is precisely what medicine and technology are) is "playing God." That God is dead.

As I have expressed it in the *Atlantic Monthly,* in an article about neonatal defects such as the Down's syndrome, "The belief that God is at work directly or indirectly in all natural phenomena is a form of animism or simple pantheism. If we took it really seriously, all science, including medicine, would die away because we would be afraid to 'dissect God' or tamper with His activity. Such beliefs are a hopelessly primitive kind of God-thought and God-talk, but they hang on long after theologians generally have bid them good-bye."[13]

Some decisions are less radically problematic, although equally statistical. For example, we debate whether it is wise to give mass smallpox vaccinations, since postvaccinal encephalitis is fairly common whereas the risk of getting smallpox, at least in industrially mature societies, is not great. How shall we figure the probabilities? Here, it seems to me, the differential consideration is that the risk of getting smallpox is low precisely because of the preventive practice of mass vaccination. But it is not a simple moral question, comparable to "doing all we can for the patient" in clinical medicine.

We are pursued by ambivalences as much as by ambiguities. For example, diabetics were in mortal danger until we found the insulin treatment, yet they still could not risk pregnancy and childbirth. Now we can deliver them safely, but with what result? The result is an increase in diabetes, the spread of a genetic defect. There is always a risk of cancer to kidney recipients from cancerous donors. Synthetics have unexpected side effects, as was found with Chloromycetin (chlorophenicol) which has been connected with leukemia and aplastic anemia. Artificial hearts fueled with isotopic energy may spread radiation. But will that be any worse, or more lethal, than smog, water pollution, air pollution, and highway traffic? After a few years the danger to the cyborg himself can be serious; for example, leukemia may result. If only two or three more years of life are possible, is it worth the trouble and expense of a cardiac substitute? If a patient says, "No, I don't want it," is that suicide? As hemodialysis improves it will foreseeably increase the incidence of suicide, because patients will weary of it all. If a man has been deterioratively paralyzed by a massive stroke and wants to give his heart to a much younger wife because hers is failing, is that suicide? Or is it an act of sacrificial love, realized by technology?

A Serious Conclusion

The Faustian question plagues some people when they discuss technology and morality; it takes possession of them and inhibits them—for example, Jacques Ellul.[14] Will man's growing power over his life and world be his undoing? Like Faust, is he selling his soul for knowledge, power, and riches; and are these things nothing more than what Sorokin called "sensate" values?[15] Or, to vary the figure, are we too Promethean, stealing the fire from heaven and the gods—to our own mortal danger?

Jean Rostand is right to warn us, "Let us not give ourselves the airs of demigods, or even of demiurges, when we have only been petty magicians."[16] We do not want to be trapped by a Promethean intoxication, or in a bad bargain of Faustian proportions. And we must not suppose that know-how, as in technology, is of itself enough to show us what is good or worth seeking. On the contrary, we must guard against what Veblen called "the trained incapacity of the specialist," his inability to consider what lies outside his expertise. Perhaps the correct model for modern medicine, in its partnership with the engineers and biologists, is the space probe program of the National Aeronautics and Space Administration in which the design and fabrication of hardware and the operations system are all subjected to a careful testing of their impact on the astronauts themselves, the human needs at stake. Good science (which is itself an ethical phrase) unites facts and values. As Lawrence Granberg has put it, "The very language of our most basic science, quantum mechanics, is the language of expectation and of probability amplitudes."[17]

Kant said two things filled him with awe: the starry heavens above and the moral law within.[18] If, by the first, he meant a sincere humility before the order and power of nature, we can agree; but not if he meant simply acceptance of nature without human interference or manipulation. As to the moral imperative, the "oughtness" of human beings, if he meant the sense of obligation and aspiration, especially to and for human welfare, we can go along with Kant, but not if by "law" he meant ethical rules, or final or universal or "natural" prescriptions of right and wrong regardless of changing needs and situations. There are no hard and fast rules, no fixed norms, no moral recipes.

Dr. Delford Stickel at Duke's medical center has declared that situation ethics, as I have formulated it, "provides a useful and helpful frame of reference within which to deal with the moral aspects" of medical problems, and that it "can foster a quality of responsibility which is in keeping with the best traditions of Western medicine."[19] Let me add, then, that we can only have a choice between three methods of moral decision-making: (1) moral absolutism, (2) anomic indifference, and (3) pragmatic situation ethics.

The first, absolutist ethics, has been the traditional method. Life and death are regarded as a divine monopoly, dependent on the will of God—either directly by special providence or indirectly through delegated processes of nature, presumably including such devices as sexual passion, menstrual cycles, senescence, gangrene, melanoma, and heart failure. On this view it has been wrong to try to be "equal with God" by exerting birth and death control, to say nothing of our many forms of health control.

The second method, the anomic and indifferent (acedic) one, is unconcerned about whether medical control is good or evil. It looks upon such questions as "adiaphora," morally neutral. On this basis we could be eager either to push technology or to restrain it without regard to right-wrong questions, merely accepting human controls as self-validating and *sui justificatis.*

The third alternative, situation ethics, finds technology neither good nor evil in and of itself. Its standard of the good is human well-being; and technology at any place, in any time, of any form, is therefore right or wrong according to whether it detracts or contributes to the good, that is, human need.

This morality finds life good sometimes, and death good sometimes—depending on the situation, on the case or the context. Life is not good in itself, nor is death evil as such. Drugs and prosthetics and transplants, all forms of medical techniquery, are subject to the same ethical contingency. The question to ask about any technological device is not what is right or which one is good, but *when* are they right and *when* are they good. The answer is never prefabricated, in heaven or on earth. The decision lies with us. The age of innocence is gone. We have eaten the apple, the fruit of the tree of knowledge.

Katherine Mansfield once said, "At the end, truth is the only thing worth having; it's more thrilling than love, more joyful and more passionate." She was mistaken. Truth is sought for love's sake, not for its own sake. And love is for people—patients, neighbors, family and friends, fellow human beings.

Notes

1. *Webster's Seventh New Collegiate Dictionary* (Springfield, Mass.: G. & C. Merriam Company, 1967).
2. See Y. Saparina, *Cybernetics Within Us,* trans. V. Talmy (Moscow: Peace Publishers, 1966).
3. *Boston Globe,* 1 January 1967.
4. See Joseph Fletcher, "Medicine's Scientific Developments and Ethical Problems," in *Dialogue in Medicine and Theology,* ed. Dale White (Nashville: Abingdon Press, 1968), pp. 103-33.
5. C. H. Waddington, *The Ethical Animal* (Chicago: University of Chicago Press, 1960).
6. Rene Dubos, *Adapting Man* (New Haven: Yale University Press, 1965).
7. H. F. Stewart, ed., *Blaise Pascal's Pensées* (New York: Pantheon, 1950), p. 83.
8. Jean Rostand, *Can Man Be Modified?* trans. Jonathan Griffin (New York: Basic Books, 1959), p. 11.
9. See, e.g., Robert White, M.D., and Charles Curran, Th.D., "The Morality of Human Transplants," *The Sign* (March 1968), pp. 19-30.

10. Rostand, *op. cit.,* p. 62.

11. Rejection may be solved by studying how mothers for nine months avoid rejecting the fetus which consists of foreign or alien tissue! The secret might well be in the placenta. (In all animal life, even the lowly earthworm, the rejection mechanism occurs.)

12. Eric Ambler, *A Coffin for Dimitrios* (New York: Dell, 1939), p. 9.

13. Bernard Bard and Joseph Fletcher, "The Right to Die," *Atlantic Monthly* 221, no. 4 (April 1968): 64.

14. See Jacques Ellul, *The Technological Society* (New York: Knopf, 1967), esp. pp. 428-36.

15. See Pitirim A. Sorokin, *Social and Cultural Dynamics* (New York: American Book Co., 1937).

16. Rostand, *op. cit.,* p. 25.

17. Lawrence Granberg, unpublished paper in the physics department at the University of Virginia, Charlottesville, Virginia.

18. Emmanuel Kant, *Critique of Practical Reason,* trans. T. K. Abbott (London: Longmans Green & Co., 1923), p. 260.

19. Delford L. Stickel, M.D., "Ethical and Moral Aspects of Transplantation," *Monographs in the Surgical Sciences* (Baltimore: Williams and Wilkins, 1966), 3, no. 4: 292.

37. Science: Limits and Prohibitions

DANIEL CALLAHAN

The special power of Sigmund Freud's contribution to the analysis of "civilization and its discontents" lay in his unwillingness to engage in easy talk of liberation, to raise the question of altruism and its widening drive for community in the most tentative way only, and to reserve his most probing dissection for those deepest of human pathologies which stand in the way of happiness. If there is ever to be, to use Philip Rieff's term, a "science of limits" for technology, Freud's sober, anti-visionary spirit provides a healthy starting point. The question is not so much what should be done with technology, and what goods should be sought, but what boundaries should not be transgressed in the process. Yet to speak of "boundaries" in the full sense of the term is to recognize the importance of Freud's stress on the "cultural superego," which establishes psychological limits deep within the unconscious of entire societies. The route to a rational and humane technology is through the culture's unconscious, where its ultimate premises and values lie hidden from sight.

There are at least two reasons why a science of technological limits is needed. First, limits need to be set to the boundless hopes and expectations, constantly escalating, which technology has engendered. Advanced technology has promised transcendence of the human condition. That is a false promise, incapable of fulfillment. Human desires are infinite and cannot be achieved by the finite means of technology.

Second, a science of technological limits is necessary in order that the social pathologies resulting from technology can be controlled. These pathologies can be introduced either by attempts to impose new technologies, or by attempts to correct the harms wrought by technology through the introduction of sanctions against those who, not having introduced the technology in the first place, are supposed to compensate personally for its extant hazards. While technology can and does cure, save and free, it can also become the vehicle for the introduction of new repressions in society, both because it provides ever more precise methods of controlling human behavior and also because fear in the face of its excesses can

From *The Hastings Center Report* 3 (November 1973): 5-7. Used by permission of the publisher and the author.

engender social terrorism as a defensive, corrective response.

Yet the temptation to a casual, irrational, anti-technological spirit must be resisted. The most important perception is to understand and accept the fact that man is a technological animal. It makes no sense to talk of *Homo sapiens* without technology or to distinguish man from technology. A science of technological limits cannot be built upon hostility to technology, which has always turned out historically to be self-defeating, setting the stage for a new spiral of unrestricted expectations. Together with the cultural, political, philosophical and religious systems which the human race has developed, science and technology can take their place among the greatest of human achievements.

To speak of "limits" at all is to introduce a dour note in the face of those achievements, yet one which should be embraced in all its rigor. I mean by a "science of limits" a system of prohibitions, denials and interdictions which establishes the limits of technological aggressiveness, hopes and mandates. The word "No" perfectly sums up what I mean by a limit—a boundary point beyond which one should not go. Technological development has been subject both to a tyranny of individualism and a tyranny of survival; neither knows how to say No. Individualism does not know how to deny anything to the private self. The cult of survival does not know how to say No to the needs of the community and the species.

A science of limits must, as a minimal demand, be able to establish the legitimacy of prohibitions, repressions and interdictions in the use of technology. The first required interdiction is a sharp dampening of the unchecked and uncorrected technological imagination. This dampening should take its point of departure from the biological reality principle that, however much human beings need technology, it cannot provide the full measure of human happiness, and will in fact lead to misery if, in a lust for infinite possibility, the reality principle is set aside even for a moment. This is essentially a task for the cultural super-ego, which could curb the desire for technological infinity and transcendence by scaling down the emotional and visionary demands made upon technology in the first place—by putting in their place a sense of radical finiteness, even a sense of guilt for demanding too much.

I do not want to be misunderstood. I am not proposing that we cease the careful rational analysis of the possibilities, good and bad, of new technologies; far more of that kind of analysis is needed. I am only proposing that we not continue to be caught in a cultural situation in which, our technological imagination out of hand, we are then forced to make judgments on technological givens which in a more prudent society might not have been present at all. Only a cultural super-ego imbued with an innate skepticism toward technological infinity, a spontaneous sobriety in the face of futuristic scenarios which would lure us into unrealistic hopes, and a healthy repugnance toward those who would, by the siren song of happiness and plenty, lure us away from our doubts and inhibitions, will suffice.

The second interdiction must take its rise from a social reality principle. By that principle I mean the inherent resistance that groups and populations initially and ordinarily feel toward efforts to force new technologies upon them, or toward bearing socially imposed penalties in order to control technology. The history of technology shows that specific developments are almost always justified on the ground that they will increase freedom of choice and maximize voluntary options. That same history, however, also shows how short-lived the new freedoms are. Specified choices—usually in the name of a "responsible" use of freedom—quickly make the new options mandatory, either by law, economic force or social custom. When horses were still available, the automobile was introduced as an optional, alternative mode of transportation; that choice is now gone. Genetic counseling was originally hailed as a means of giving people the freedom to choose the avoidance of a defective child, if they wanted to avail themselves of that option. But signs are already present that they will in the future be considered socially irresponsible if they do not make use of their "free" choice to choose against bearing defective children.

The repetition of the historical pattern which sees free choices quickly become mandatory suggests a modest wisdom: assume, in trying to judge the benefits and harms of any new technology, that its use will eventually become a socially enforced requirement. And assume, as well, that if there are some hazardous by-products from the technology, everyone will be forced to pay for them, however innocent they may have been in introducing them.

The second interdiction, then, must be a prohibition of careless meddling in social orders and structures by technologists and, beyond that, a refusal to believe that the answer to the derangements of society is technological. There is no reason whatever to assume that all problems can be solved by technological solutions, and no reason to assume either that it is even good to seek a technological answer. It is precisely these assumptions which need to be denied. As matters now stand, nothing is allowed to compete with technology, so deeply ingrained is the tendency to give it the first crack at any serious issue.

Moreover, there is no reason to presume that technological advances must be taken advantage of once they are available. The most noxious combination is the joining of technological possibility with demands for survival. Survival obsessions wipe out choices and options—that is their power and why they are invoked. When survival and technology join hands, a technological imperative is introduced: the technology must be used.

The third interdiction springs from a psychological reality principle. By that principle I mean the fact that human beings are not at all likely to give up their attempts to find happiness through technology. The new burst of technological fervor, already foreshadowed in the marriage of psychological technology to counterculture mysticism and communitarianism, shows that people are not disillusioned with technology, despite superficial indications of an anti-technological mood. But if people will not cease to hope for happiness through technology, how can they be expected to impose upon themselves the restrictions necessary to ground their hopes in reality and thus limit them? In one way only. There must be deeply imbedded in the cultural super-ego the profound perception that violent reactions against technology carry within them the seeds of a subsequent collapse once again in the face of the seductions of technology. That has been the historical rhythm of the matter, where the juxtaposition of the fundamental human need for technology and the harms wrought by technology present a dilemma which cannot and will not be resolved.

The third interdiction, necessary in light of the psychological reality principle of technology, is that there must be an intuitive censorship of visions of a non-technological society. The only possibility of a check to an over-investment of hope in technology is, paradoxically, the existence of checks against an overinvestment of hopes in non-technology. Needed is a scaling down of technology and a rational control of it—neither its deification nor its denial. Interdictions against an infinitizing of technological promise, impossible of fulfillment, will become feasible only when the extremes of hope and despair have been once and for all excluded.

No substitute for technology has yet been found for the primary human business of facilitating adaptation and preservation; and no one urged to give up technology can fail to miss that fact. Nor has any substitute been found for the economic strength which technological societies provide. The irreversibility of technology—whatever the theory of the matter, that is the historical reality—poses the most important obstacle to its management. Since people cannot go back on technology, they find themselves impelled to go forward, to avoid returning to that which lies behind them, and to seek that which technology has yet to deliver—and will not deliver. A limit to *always* going forward is needed; when to go forward and when not to is the question.

The only possible hope for the development of an interdictory cultural super-ego lies in a shift from viewing technology as a vehicle for saving and satisfying individuals, to one which roots its values in the needs of the community: basic health and economic needs, the sustaining of viable educational institutions, the preservation of natural resources, clean air and water, and a cultural life which provides physical and aesthetic enrichment.

Naturally, even to suggest a list of this kind—noncontroversial enough on its face—does not take us far toward determining what a sufficient *level* of these goods would be. The fact that technological societies work from a very high baseline of desires and expectations, perceived as "necessities," poses the most stubborn difficulty. The main work of an interdictory cultural super-ego would be to lower the base-line of expectation and demand, neutralizing the sense of restlessness, unrequited desire, and obsessive attempts to achieve still more happiness through technology that are the marks of advanced industrial societies. A downward shift in demand can emerge only from a social rather than an individual ethic.

The most difficult task in creating a rational social ethic which can win support and dig itself into the cultural super-ego is that of finding the proper balance between the rights of individuals and those of the community. Societies and historical circumstances differ, and for just that reason there is no possibility of abstractly establishing the proper balance for every community at every given moment in time. In technological societies, the individualistic demands made upon technology can have the effect of creating a false sense of scarcity. If every individual wants everything, and believes he or she has a right to it as a necessary condition of personal self-realization, then scarcity becomes psychologically endemic, with every person so affected living under a constantly perceived threat of degradation or annihilation.

It is much easier to proclaim the need for community-centered rather than individual-centered thinking than to work through the ethical difficulties this stance engenders. Once the community (or the species) has been given moral preeminence, there can be a very rapid descent to persecution and tyranny in the name of the common good. Is there any middle ground between an unlimited individualism, which can generate terror, and an unlimited regard for the community, which can generate no less terror? Only in two ways: by establishing upper limits to what individuals can demand and expect, and internal restraints on the harm a community may do to individuals in the name of its own welfare.

Lacking an instinct for limitations and prohibitions, society has at present no real way to judge and control technology. When intrinsic limits are denied, and every proposal for a limit subjected to tests which no prohibition could pass, then all possibility for rational communal behavior ceases. The stage is then set for force to be applied.

The greatest need Freud saw was that of reconciling human beings to civilization. The individualism underlying technology has made that task more difficult than ever. Technology has given the private person illusory arms with which to better fight off civilization and its repressive demands. The possibility of altruism, which Freud defined as an impulse to merge with others in the community, is ever hard pressed; egoism drives us in another direction.

The individual will always have to bargain with society and with nature. Technology has made a better bargain possible. But that possibility is constantly threatened by the demand for a perfect bargain. That will never be possible. That insight is the foundation of a science of limits.

38.
The Experiment with Man

KARL RAHNER

1. Christian Cool-Headedness in the Face of Man's Future

Man is fundamentally 'operable' and legitimately so. If this proposition, which we shall elucidate directly, is assumed, the first thing which the theologian must say to himself, to Christians and to the Church is that one is not to take fright at this self-manipulation of man. Of course possibilities of self-manipulation are becoming apparent today which are immoral and unworthy of man, and which may indicate a 'Fall' on the part of society. And we shall refer to the Christian's and the Church's duty to have the courage to oppose with utter resoluteness those kinds of self-manipulation which are the most recent forms of barbarity, slavery, the totalitarian annihilation of personality and formation of a monochrome society.

But it would only be symptomatic of a cowardly and comfortable conservatism hiding behind misunderstood Christian ideals and maxims if at the outset one were to simply condemn the approaching age of self-manipulation as such; to break out into lyrical laments on the theme of degrading barbarity, the cold, technological rationalism, the destruction of what is 'natural', the rationalisation of love, the heathenist lack of understanding in the face of illness, suffering, death, poverty, the levelled-down mass society, the end of history in a faceless fellahin society without a history, etc. Although we are unable to produce a concrete picture of the life of society and mankind in the year 2000, although we must take radical catastrophes and threats to man's existence into account, against which a Christian will have to fight with the greatest determination, tomorrow's world will be different from that of today. And in this coming world man will be the one who, both as an individual and as a society, plans, controls and manipulates himself to a degree which was previously both undreamed-of and impracticable. He *must* do so; he can do no other if he wishes to exist on the Earth side by side with many thousand millions of other human beings. He must *want* to be 'operable' man, even though the extent and the right way of carrying out this self-manipulation

---

From Karl Rahner, *Theological Investigations,* vol. 9, trans. Graham Harrison (New York: Crossroad, 1972), pp. 210–23. Used by permission.

are still largely obscure, and although it is apparent that the Anglo-Saxon and Communist prophets of this future self-manipulation are themselves able to give only very vague details of this future. For whether one proclaims, with Huxley, that man's goal and future is pure 'fulfilment and self-expression', or says, with Elisabeth Mann Borghese, that at least everyone will have time to devote himself to what is true, good and beautiful; or whether one exalts the classless society where abilities, achievements and needs all finally coincide and where a common peace reigns in equality, freedom from illness, self-alienation and oppression—all these aims are highly abstract, imprecise and *uninspiring* too.

But it is true: the future of man's self-manipulation has begun. And the Christian has no reason to enter this future as a hell on Earth nor as an earthly Kingdom of God. Jubilation or lamentation would both run counter to the Christian's cool-headedness. For the Christian, both he himself and his world always remain (as long as history lasts) a world of creation, of sin, of the promise of judgment and blessing, in a unity which he himself can never dissolve.

2. Self-Determination as the Nature and Task of Man's Freedom as Understood by Christianity

According to Christian anthropology man really is the being who manipulates himself. Naturally, on account of the genuine historicity of his being and of his apprehension of truth, this fact has entered even into the Christian's awareness of faith in a quite new and penetrating way. But this fact, to which he is called at this present time and which confronts him as something new, can be recognised and accepted by him all the same as his very own, as the truth of old which has always been his and which gives itself to him anew in this form—if he accepts it.

According to a Christian understanding, man, as the being who is free in relation to God, is in a most radical way empowered to do what he wills with himself, freely able to align himself towards his own ultimate goal. He is able so to determine and dispose of himself that two absolutely different final destinations become possible: man in absolute salvation and man in the absolute loss of salvation. For what happens to a man in death and judgment (to use the language of the Catechism) is not an external gratuitous action upon him, a reaction to his previous dealings, but the manifestation of the naked reality of his own ultimate goal, with which he has identified himself. It is certainly the case that this absolutely inescapable transcendental self-determination occurs in dialogue with or against God; certainly its precondition is what we know as free creation and free grace; it is assuredly a freedom which knows itself to be continually exposed to the intractable nature of its situation, and thus knows that in all its activity it is also unavoidably passive. But this does not alter the fact—which is a commonplace to the Christian—that freedom is the power to determine oneself to an absolutely irreversible final state, that what a man will be for all eternity is what he has made himself. Man is the one whose freedom is laid upon him as a burden; this freedom is creative and what it creates is man himself in his final state, so that the beginning of this history of man's divinely appointed freedom—man's 'essence' as we say—is not an intangible something, essentially permanent and complete, but the commission and power which enable him to be free to determine himself to his ultimate final state.

In a correctly developed ontology of the subject and his dealings, as opposed to the 'thing' and its 'activity' (which unfortunately is taken for the most part as a model for the 'activity' of the genuine subject), it could be made plainer that in an anthropology based on a really Christian philosophy, a man's free action—which, in affecting the world, determines himself too—must not be imagined as an external epiphenomenon sustained on the surface of a substantial essence which itself remains untouched, but becomes part of the innermost determination of this essence itself. In contradistinction to 'things' which are always complete and which are moved from one mode of completion to another and thus are at the same time always in a final state and yet never ultimate, man begins his existence as the being who is radically open and incomplete. When his essence *is* complete it is as he himself has freely created it.

3. Self-Manipulation as a New Manifestation in Our Time of Man's Essential Freedom

What is new in this issue is therefore not that man is *faber sui ipsius,* but that this fundamental constitution of man is manifested historically today in a totally new way. Today for the first time man's possibility of transcendental self-manipulation irreversibly takes on a clear and historically categorical form. I.e. until now man's genuine, radical self-manipulation (which is a constant factor, creating eternity) was operative almost exclusively in the field of contemplative metaphysical knowledge, knowledge in faith and moral action in reference to God. Therefore as soon as it arose, it disappeared, so to speak, into the mystery of God. This was all the more the case since the categorical and tangible aspect of this contemplation and moral practice (which was naturally always present) is constantly equivocal: it can be either genuine free action or the mere product of intramundane material causality. As mere equivocal objectifications they are therefore incapable of furnishing man automatically with a clear view of his own free self-manipulation. Now, however, man's transcendental self-manipulation has been clearly manifested, even if from the theological point of view it remains ultimately ambivalent.

No longer does man create himself merely as a moral and theoretical being under God, but as an earthly, corporeal and historical being. Passive biological evolution is being extended, at least to an initial degree, by an active evolution of civilisation. But the latter is not only external and supplementary: it is actually continuing its own biological evolution. This self-manipulation is not only carried out unconsciously, as was the case almost exclusively in the past, but deliberately planned, programmed and controlled. Man no longer makes himself merely with reference to eternity but with reference to history itself as such.

In this way, however, what he has always been now comes to light. What he has always been at the root of his transcendental spiritual and intellectual essence as a free being now extends its influence to his psyche and his physical and social existence, and is made manifest expressly in these dimensions. To a certain degree his ultimate essence has broken through to the outer regions of his existence. To a larger, more comprehensive, radical and tangible extent man has become what, according to the Christian understanding, he *is:* the free being who has been handed over to himself.

Here we have not space to show how this modern man not only *corresponds* to Christianity's fundamental understanding of man but also how the historical breakthrough from theory to practice, from self-awareness to self-actualisation was essentially a *product* of Christianity, however much many Christians opposed this emancipating movement of history. For this possibility, which has arisen from modern rationality, science and technology, has grown historically because according to Christianity the world and nature are not something intangible, numinous and brooding in which man humbly experiences himself as hidden, but something finite, non-numinous and created; as a real partner of the God of the 'other world' man can and must stand over against *this* world as its lord.

4. The Question of the Normative Essence, the 'Nature' of Man

It will be immediately apparent from what has been said that, as a result of this material and categorial self-manipulation—which has now become possible and which in the future will embrace a wide range of possibilities—theology is faced anew with the question of man's essence. For according to Christian theology man in his freedom can act contrary to his nature in an absurd and self-contradictory way. Ontologically and existentially this latter possibility is not of the same order, nor is it radically possible to the same extent, as action which *is* consonant with man's nature (a fact which must never be forgotten), but it *is* possible: the ambivalence of moral freedom in its potential for good or ill is reproduced in the categorial self-manipulation of man, even though it is not reproduced univocally and homogeneously (which needs to be considered in much greater depth) but only reflects this radical ambivalence in a partial and inconclusive manner. Consequently in the dimension of categorial self-manipulation the good is never as 'good' and the evil is never as radically evil as in the dimension of fundamental transcendental freedom.

But since a Catholic and Christian anthropology, on account of the *whole* man's unity and vocation to salvation, can never accept an absolute separation of the ethics of man's inner disposition from the ethics of his external actions and practical norms, the question arises as to *which* 'nature' of man must be the guide for man's categorial self-manipulation, lest he be put in a situation of radical, destructive self-contradiction. Although this question could never have been simply nonexistent, it was never put before men and Christians so clearly and urgently and in such a pointed manner prior to this historical age of self-manipulation.

This question arises from an apparent dilemma: if the 'essence' of man is taken in a purely transcendental and theological sense to be the personal spirit which, in freedom and radical self-possession, is confronted with the absolute mystery of God (as the One Who communicates Himself in love), and if this essence were *nothing else,* it seems initially at least as though—in the biological, physical, social and institutional dimensions—man's categorial self-manipulation would be unable to come into really serious conflict with his nature, or at most only in peripheral areas. For all practical considerations categorial self-manipulation would be thus irrelevant to the ethical and religious field. However, if one regards the nature of man as being everything which is on the one hand empirically observable and on the other hand not shown to be 'nonessential' as a result of the biological, psychological and other changes which happen to man apart from his reflex self-manipulation, man's categorial self-manipulation would have no morally legitimate object. At most it could gently reinforce the unmanipulated changes of 'nature'; it could not set itself any aims concerning the formation of man which had not already been set by 'nature' without man's assistance. But in this case the fundamental legitimacy of this categorial self-manipulation would itself be called in question and, in fact, denied. And that again is not admissible, if we understand it as a manifestation of that transcendental self-manipulation which—be it noted—has several very radically differing possibilities at its disposal, even in the area of what is morally good.

Formulating the dilemma here in such an abstract way was unavoidable. Ultimately, of course, it can only be an *apparent* dilemma, although it seems to call in question either the nature of man and the knowledge of this nature, or man's categorial self-manipulation, conceived as a fundamental possibility and task. (However, one has only to consider the well-known—too well-known—problem of biochemical birth-control, for instance, to see clearly what is meant. We cannot enter into this special issue here, but however it ought to be dealt with in principle, there can be no doubt that in recent decades traditional text-book moral theology has often used a concept of 'nature' ('natural', 'according to nature') which ignores the fact that, although man has an essential nature which he must respect in all his dealings, man himself is a being who forms and moulds his own nature through culture, i.e. in this case through self-manipulation, and he may not simply presuppose his nature as a categorial, fixed quantity.)

In any case, as a result of man's categorial self-manipulation, today's theology has been presented with the pressing task of finding out just what this nature of man is which forms the horizon and limitations even of self-manipulation. Difficult and painful changes may be expected in this area. For in questions of concrete morality people have often spoken with reference to a condition of man which, though currently existent, was not of his essence; which, though stable until recently, has now been drawn into the changes involved in man's controlling of himself. Too often it has been said, for instance: this or that is contrary to the nature of private property, of money; contrary to the 'nature' of woman, the nature of the family; contrary to the natural function of a biological organ, etc., whereas in reality it was a question of a variable and relative quantity *within* man's constant nature.

We cannot devote any more space here to this complex question of the nature of man which lies at the bottom of the metaphysical and moral natural law, how it appears in a historically conditioned concrete form and yet can be recognised for what it is, how the possibility of knowledge of metaphysical essence is compatible with an inescapable historical conditioning of this knowledge, and how the theoretical and operative knowledge of man's essence form a fundamental and yet variable unity. We are only concerned with ascertaining what problems theology is presented with as a result of categorial self-manipulation. But in this connection we may make one further observation: nowadays the moralist often says (and practically speaking he is thoroughly justified in doing so) that a situation has now arisen in which man must learn that he *must* not and *ought* not to do everything he *is able* to do. At the same time the hard-headed sceptic will generally retort that on the whole one cannot expect man to *stop* doing what he *can* do, and that since man can do infinitely more than heretofore, what he does will be immeasurably more terrible and destructive. However correct these observations of the moralist and the pessimistic sceptic may be, two things must be added.

In the first place, if the radical ontological difference between good and evil is understood, i.e. if it is comprehended that evil is ultimately the absurdity of desiring what is impossible (because it has neither being nor meaning), then in the last analysis there is nothing which man is really able to do and yet *may not* do; and conversely, what he really *can* do, he *ought* to do without hesitation. The moralist who is really close to life, therefore, would have to show modern man that, wherever he ought not to act, it is ultimately pointless, even today, to do so (i.e. in a categorial and intramundane sense too).

Secondly, because man's creaturely and finite freedom is co-determined by that which it presupposes, which exerts its influence particularly in this very categorial area of freedom (and hence of self-manipulation), biological, psychological and sociological laws can be apprehended and accepted which, without vitiating the freedom of self-manipulation, act to a certain extent like regulating systems and in the long run and on the whole stop this self-manipulation from going off the path into an absurdity contrary to man's essence. As a few crude examples: every lie gradually reduces itself *ad absurdum;* where there are few children they become all of a sudden interesting and desirable again; the man who is too concerned with his own health becomes ill; when something new, which was fiercely striven for, is attained, it loses its impetus, becomes of necessity old and thus slowly abolishes itself; it is not only lemmings who jump into the sea when they become too numerous.

This is by no means an excuse for *laissez faire* and it gives no guarantee against a catastrophe, but it does constitute a consolation and an exhortation not to be too anxious. Apparently the 'essence' varies around a constant, innermost centre. And the *whole* essence consists of this centre together with the essential variations and aberrations and the attempts to express this constant essence in a new way. This applies to self-manipulation too. Especially since in this case, wherever the moralist believes he has located 'objective' self-manipulation running counter to man's essence and must combat it, he must be continually aware that it is only 'objectively' so; often and to a large extent—according to his own basic conviction—such instances, on a social and not merely individual scale, do not imply a genuine subjective state of sin before God. Objectively they belong to the same category as those instances where subhuman, 'innocent' nature permits itself to produce monstrous, aberrant things leading into biological and other culs-de-sac. Even aberrant categorial self-manipulation, seeming to spring from a really transcendental freedom *vis-à-vis* God, can be an ultimately harmless experiment on the part of nature, experimenting and slowly trying to bring forth what the genuine future holds in promise. This may be the case even where it seems as though it is only using man's intelligence and freedom for its own purposes, exercising its own essence and not man's free essence as such.

5. The Seriousness of Irreversible Historical Decisions

Having said all this we must not minimise the importance of the historical process involved in the initiation of man's self-manipulation. We are warned against this by a particular theological topic of Christian anthropology, which has probably never before been taken into account in this context, namely, the dogma of Original Sin. We cannot give a full account here of its actual content, but we merely draw attention to one of its particular principal aspects which is of significance in interpreting theologically the coming large-scale manipulation of mankind. The 'Fall' was actually the first act of self-manipulation by mankind even if its context was essentially the dimension of religious, transcendental self-determination before God, and even if we leave open the question as to how far it had categorially tangible consequences, delivering man up not only to his own nature alone, which could conceivably be guiltless. But in this case of self-manipulation *sui generis* there is one thing which is an indubitable element of the dogma: the act had irreversible consequences, it inaugurated a process and mankind cannot get back beyond the beginning of that process. All future human history is ineradicably determined by this situation of guilt so long as history itself lasts. Although redemption embraces this fact of human history and ultimately sets its mark upon it, it does not abolish it.

In turn this implies the principle that even at the stage of self-manipulation mankind continues on its one-way, irreversible historical course. Where a collective self-manipulation on the part of the totality of mankind is concerned, it is at least in principle the case that an about-turn is simply no longer possible, even if the way is kept open to the most diverse future possibilities. For people unconsciously connect the idea of self-manipulation with the notion that it can do anything whatsoever *and can continue to do anything;* that every false manipulation can be rectified, at least in succeeding generations (and the self-manipulation ideologists are very little concerned for the individual living at any one time; he is only treated as material to be expended for the sake of the more distant future). However, the dogma of Original Sin warns us against this illusion; history will remain a one-way process in the future too; it will continue under the law incurred by its guilty beginning, involving death, futility, contradiction and suffering (however much the *forms* of the latter may change), such that no self-manipulation on the part of mankind can abolish this law. (Yet the Church and theologians must beware of thinking that they already know precisely what concrete forms this irreversible beginning will assume in the future; they must beware of prophesying that the poor, wars, TB, the class struggles, etc., will be perpetuated in their classical forms for all time.) Furthermore it may be that the projected large-scale manipulation of mankind will have irreversible and irreparable consequences which no further self-manipulation will be able to change. Such conceivable irreversible consequences cannot reverse the definitive victory, through Christ, of God's self-communicating dealings with mankind. But neither does this mean that mankind can experiment upon itself freely without fear of irreparable consequences. So long as mankind exists with its vocation to salvation, history (including the history of man taking himself in his own hands) remains a one-way street. Man's self-manipulation must not be thought of according to the model of a limited laboratory experiment where, for the most part, isolated processes can be performed and reversed at will.

6. Planning the Future and the Absolute Future of Man

Christianity is the religion of the absolute future. However, at the same time it stands in a quite definite and unique relation to the categorial self-manipulation of man and mankind. It is very difficult to define the highly differentiated relationship between anticipating the absolute, eschatologically occurring future in faith and theological hope on the one hand, and anticipating the intramundane future by means of planning and active self-manipulation on the other hand. So far this particular chapter of a Christian theology of history and the world has been almost totally neglected; consequently it is impossible here to give an account of it and thus provide a theological context within which man's active self-manipulation can be really theologically understood. At this point we can only make a few modest observations. We say that Christianity is the religion of the absolute future to the extent in the first place that God is not only 'above us' as the ground and horizon of history, but 'in front of us' as our own future, our destination, sustaining history as its future. For Christianity acknowledges the absolute, infinite God who is superior to the world, a radical and infinite mystery, as the God who in free grace communicates himself in his absolute mystery as its innermost principle and ultimate future, who sustains and drives history as his genuinely most intimate concern, not only distinguishing himself from it as its creator.

Secondly we say that man's ultimate design for the future, which God has destined for him and authorised, does not aim at what can be planned and executed out of the multiple possibilities of the plural world, but has already overtaken all such intramundane designs for the future, criticising them and unmasking them in their appearance of absoluteness, and thus (as we shall see) *confirming* them.

All human planning, every active human self-realisation involving the manipulation of a plurality of factors, is embraced by the fact (which can be neither planned nor manipulated) of the infinite mystery manifesting itself to us as love, which we experience and call God. Man is not only concerned with what he can *do* in the future; he experiences something which is not 'done' at all, but which is his destiny, the infinity of absolute reality, which is love. According to Christianity's experience of absolute future in Jesus Christ, the arrival of this future occurs essentially in the act of death. It occurs in this way and in no other; life is not thereby devalued, because in order to be able to die one must genuinely have lived life. But one only reaches the absolute future by way of death's zero hour, not because the former is death's gift, not because it could be calculated to be impossible in any other way, but because, beyond all deduction, absolute love was pleased to triumph in its greatest defeat.

If now this absolute future, confessed in hope by Christianity and to which the Christian, in planning his existence, opens himself, is related to the design for the future which is manifested and executed in the self-manipulation of mankind today (and it does not make any difference whether it is in a Western or Eastern form, in an explicit collectivism or one which is in practice so), the following brief remarks at least may be made:

7. Shaping the Future as a Christian Task

In the first place man's active intramundane self-planning in self-manipulation has fundamentally a positive relationship to man's openness to the absolute future in faith and hope. However 'secular' man's active self-manipulation is and remains (i.e. not positively deducible from the Christian design for existence as it is expressed in its ecclesial and verbal form), yet it must not be understood as an 'interim activity' (which, when pursued morally, receives a heavenly reward) lasting until the absolute future, the 'Kingdom of God' finally arrives in God's self-communication. But in its irreducible positive and negative duality it constitutes the necessary medium and historical form by which man is to embrace that 'openness' which is both active and passive, forming the precondition for the arrival of the absolute future.

Basically Christianity has always known and proclaimed this in teaching that, *inter alia,* the love of one's neighbour is the form and medium of the love of God and that this love must really be action and not ideology or the mere inclination of the affections. Only it must be borne in mind that, as a necessary medium for the love of God (and not merely as a secondary by-product of it), this active intercommunication can no longer be realised merely in the private interpersonal sphere involving each man and his 'neighbour'. Even if a person rejects a 'collectivism' in the pejorative sense of the word, he cannot and must not overlook the fact that mankind today must of necessity realise higher levels and forms of social existence (and has actually already begun to do so) if each person is to really and truly affirm every other person's existence. Mankind is beginning to enter upon a post-individualistic phase of its history. This new phase brings with it new changes and dangers to the genuine, unique personality and dignity of the individual. It must not annihilate this individuality, but actually provide it with a greater area of genuine freedom.

This means, however, that loving intercommunication itself takes on a new form; now it can and must be also a servant of the new forms of man's social existence, a servant of humanity. For now 'humanity' no longer exists merely as an idea, as an ideology, but begins to exist as a concrete reality. If 'society' is a reality in a quite new way, if it is slowly and inevitably reconstructing itself on quite new lines, it can be in a totally new way a partner in this task of loving one's fellows, which is the form and medium of that love in hope and faith through which the absolute future 'arrives'. Understood in this way, however, the love of others must *will* and *co-operate* in these higher achievements of society and humanity *as they are and must be in today's particular form:* i.e. mankind's self-manipulation with a view to the future.

Of course, the love of one's neighbour itself cannot provide the material principle from which to conclude the concrete aim and methods of this intramundane self-manipulation of mankind. The aim and methods remain secular, like the bread which in earlier times was given in love to the poor man lest he should starve. Nevertheless, mankind's active self-manipulation today and tomorrow can and must be the concrete, active expression of the love of one's fellows, making possible the 'openness' to God's absolute future, even if it cannot itself bring about this absolute future. As the religion of the absolute future, Christianity is and must be the religion which sends man into the world to act.

8. Death as the Permanent Door to the Absolute Future

At the same time, however, Christianity warns self-manipulating man that, in his movement towards the God who is in front of him, he is obliged to pass through death's zero hour. It is strange how little man's death and the death of history is talked about today in the customary future utopias. Death is pushed to one side; what is talked about is a kind of super welfare state with little work, a great deal of automation, the elimination of illness, long life, complete equality of the sexes—their differences having been almost smoothed out; a society in which all internal and external conflicts have been eradicated by genetic and pharmacological manipulation and social training, where the altruistic instincts of insect-like state-builders are formed, where history, steered by a few wise men, has been actually brought to a standstill in a high-level euphoric fellahin existence. One has the impression that it could be a horribly boring existence: the ash of unchallenged equality and security, spread homogeneously over the fire of life, could either smother the fire or else have the effect of making it suddenly burst out at some point as a mass madness trying to break out of a deathly equality and security. Death and the readiness to die, which is what keeps life 'alive' in this aeon, and which alone is the door of eternal life, is being pushed to one side.

We have already emphasised the fact that the concrete forms of death, futility, suffering and pain do not authorise a conservative defence of the particular forms of death and conflict which currently set their mark on man's situation. Especially since this kind of pseudo-Christian defence, which was and is all too common, is mostly put forward by those who have to suffer least in this regard. There is naturally little point in the rich man extolling the blessings of poverty and the person in power in society praising the value of humility. It remains true, however, that self-manipulation and all its concrete and utopian aims are constantly subject to the law of death—which can be neither disposed of nor manipulated. And this experience of death (in this comprehensive sense) arises from the experience of self-manipulation itself. For every plan, every pre-set and pre-calculated system gives rise to new elements which were *not* planned and *not* scheduled, because it is constructed of pre-existing elements which can never be adequately penetrated and categorised. By definition, an absolute and absolutely transparent system, functioning without friction, could only be constructed by another one standing outside it; even a machine capable of learning and adapting itself can only do this within a finite area, so long as it is not identical with the universe.

And so long as man is a being of absolute transcendence, he observes all this in terror; he can only 'alter' it by anticipating it in a formal and empty manner in the world of theory. In actual practice he cannot alter it, however much of a concretely practicable nature may still lie ahead of him as an intramundane future which *can* be manipulated. He sees his limitation; namely, those things which *cannot* be manipulated, and death, *his* death, rising up out of the very midst of the things which *can* be manipulated. And he will always be asking whether this unfathomable thing which surrounds him is the void of absolute absurdity or the infinitude of the mystery of love, the absolute future which is reached through death, so that only by accepting it can man really discover and 'invent' himself. (This is always possible, even where categorial self-manipulation is in its infancy, and it remains the highest priority even where the latter has made the kind of progress which is inconceivable at present.)

This death is not only the zero hour through which the individual must pass on his way to the absolute future, but also the zero hour for mankind as a whole. If we like, we can demythologise the end of all history as proclaimed by Christianity. No stars need fall from heaven: it can be the end as a result of genocide; it can be a social end (as a result of atom bombs, for instance); a physical end in a world catastrophe; it could be (who can know for sure?—the Christian must take even absurdity into account) that mankind might actually regress biologically to the level of a technically intelligent and self-domesticated aboriginal herd or an insect-state without the pain of transcendence, history and the dialogue with God. I.e. it might extinguish itself by collective suicide, even if it were to continue to exist at the biological level. A Christian theology of history basically need not take fright at such an idea in itself (any more than at the idea of individual suicide or self-induced stultification), for it knows that the history of men always ultimately arrives at God, whether in salvation or judgment, or else it simply ceases to be the history of spiritual persons at all.

Man exists in an immediate relationship with God only by moving towards the future in front of him, but consequently he exists in this way *always,* at every moment of his individual and collective history. And this immediacy is always mediated by death, which keeps history alive for as long as there are men. For this reason too the celebration of the death of the Lord is the solemn anticipation of the arrival of the absolute future, and cannot be replaced by any festive proclamation concerning man's self-manipulation.

39. The Art of Technology Assessment

JAMES F. CHILDRESS

Technology, Assessment, and Control

"It was the best of times, it was the worst of times, it was the age of wisdom, it was the age of foolishness." These words, which Charles Dickens uses for the French Revolution in *A Tale of Two Cities,* could easily apply to our discourse about technology. Positive and negative superlatives abound. We are quick to applaud or to disapprove. Rarely do we grasp the ambiguity of technology and the necessity of subtle and nuanced evaluations. Our public policies will not be responsible until we grasp this ambiguity and deal with it in relation to moral principles and values.

In the late 1950s and early 1960s, many commentators declared that the modern world had lost interest in, or the capacity to answer, big questions such as the meaning of life and the goals of our institutions. Social scientists such as Daniel Bell announced the "end of ideology," philosophers such as Peter Laslett observed that "political philosophy is dead," and theologians such as Harvey Cox noted the decline of religion. According to Cox, the secular city was emerging, and its inhabitants would be pragmatic and profane, interested only in what will work in this world. All these interpretations converged: individuals and communities are no longer interested in, or able to deal with, ideology, metaphysics, and mystery.[1] Some interpreters even went so far as to say that the important issues are merely technical and can be handled by the technicians or experts. President Kennedy expressed this viewpoint in the early '60s, when he held that the real issue today is the management of industrial society—a problem of ways and means, not of ideology. As he put it, "the fact of the matter is that most of the problems, or at least many of them, that we now face are technical problems, are administrative problems [requiring] . . . very sophisticated judgments which do not lend themselves to the great sort of 'passionate movements' which have stirred this country so often in the past."[2]

The obituaries for ideology, social and political philosophy, and religion were premature—as the events

From James F. Childress, *Priorities in Biomedical Ethics* (Philadelphia: Westminster Press, 1981), pp. 98-118. Used by permission.

of the last twenty years have demonstrated. In the rapid growth of various religious communities and in the conflicts over civil rights, the war in Vietnam, abortion, and technology, it became clear that interest in the big questions was only dormant or overlooked in the rush to embrace new trends.

For the most part, those who wrote the obituaries for meaning and value in the modern world were quite sanguine about technological society and the technocrats who would run it without worrying about larger perspectives. But while they praised technological man, others such as Jacques Ellul viewed him with distrust and disdain.[3] However, their debates lacked subtlety and discrimination largely because the protechnologists and the antitechnologists tended to agree that the issue was technology as such (or at least modern technology as such). As a result, they obscured the importance of assessing and controlling particular technologies.

Unfortunately, these global perspectives endure. Two examples can be found in recent books. In *The Republic of Technology: Reflections on Our Future Community,* Daniel Boorstin, the Librarian of Congress, connects the growth of technology with the (alleged) decline of ideology: "Technology dilutes and dissolves ideology. . . . More than any other modern people we have been free of the curse of ideology."[4] Holding that we are most human when we are making and using tools, Boorstin is enthusiastic about technology as such.

An example of a global perspective that is negative toward technology (at least within one area of medicine) is Stanley Reiser's *Medicine and the Reign of Technology.* Reiser, a historian of medicine, traces the development of various diagnostic technologies such as the stethoscope and concludes that they have increasingly alienated physicians from patients. Because they provide external, objective signs, the physician no longer relies on his own personal contact with the patient for diagnosis. Thus, the physician concentrates on the measurable aspects of illness rather than on human factors. "Accuracy, efficiency, and security are purchased at a high price," Reiser contends, "when that price is impersonal medical care and undermining the physician's belief in his own medical powers." The physician, he says, must rebel against this "reign of technology."[5]

It is interesting that both Boorstin and Reiser choose "political" metaphors and images when they discuss technology: "republic," "reign," and "rebellion." And despite their different responses to technology, both appear to hold a form of technological determinism, either hard or soft. Technology determines social relationships, for example, between patient and physician. Not only are there problems with this determinism which makes technology an independent variable, but it is not accurate or helpful to approach technology as such, to offer global praise or blame. More precise and discriminate judgments are required if we are to reap the benefits and avoid the evils of particular technologies. One attempt in the last fifteen years to provide a way to control technologies through public policy is *technology assessment.* I want to examine the art of technology assessment, its possibilities and its limitations.

For our purposes, "technology" can be defined as the "systematic application of scientific knowledge and technical skills for the control of matter, energy, etc., for practical purposes."[6] I shall concentrate on biomedical technologies: the technologies (techniques, drugs, equipment, and procedures) used by professionals in delivering medical care. Examples include insulin, the totally implantable artificial heart, kidney dialysis, CAT scanners, and in vitro fertilization.

We assess technologies in order to be able to "control" them responsibly through our public policies.[7] Public policy is a purposive course or pattern of action or inaction by government officials. Public policies designed to "control" technologies may operate in many different ways. The most typical and common controls are the allocation of funds (e.g., the decision to give research on cancer priority) and regulation or prohibition (e.g., the prohibition of the use of Laetrile). But it is also possible to permit and even to fund a technology while trying to control its side effects through other measures.

Control cannot be properly directed without an assessment of technology. The phrase "technology assessment" was apparently first used in 1966 by Philip Yeager, counsel for the House Committee on Science and Astronautics, in a report by the House Subcommittee on Science, Research and Development chaired by Congressman Emilio Q. Dadderio (D-Conn.), later the first head of the Office of Technology Assessment. Basically, technology assessment is a comprehensive approach, considering all the possible or probable consequences, intended and unintended effects, of a technology on society. It is thus multidisciplinary and interdisciplinary.

Against some interpreters and practitioners of technology assessment, I would argue that it is "an art form," not a science.[8] As an art form, it is basically the work of imagination which is indispensable for judgment-making. All sorts of methods can be used, and technology assessment should not be identified with any particular methods. Before policy makers had access to systems analysts, and the like, they consulted astrologers, and, on the whole, Hannah

Arendt once suggested, it would be better if they still consulted astrologers! I want to show that technology assessment can be more than a narrow technique and that, as a broad approach, drawing on several different methods, it is an indispensable art.

Theological Convictions

Technology assessments will draw on theological (or quasi-theological) convictions as well as on moral principles and values. Before turning to the latter, I want to indicate how general theological convictions provide perspectives on and engender attitudes toward technology, often through perspectives on and attitudes toward nature.[9] It should be noted that Christian (and Jewish) convictions reflect certain tensions which may be creative or destructive.

On the one hand, the Christian tradition affirms the goodness of creation, holding that nature is not an enemy to be assaulted. On the other hand, it also leads to what Max Weber called "the disenchantment of the world" or "the rationalization of the world."[10] Its stress on God's transcendence tends to exclude spirits in nature who need to be approached with awe, and it thus frees nature for man's dominion.

Another tension can be seen in the distinction between sovereignty over nature and stewardship of nature. Although the Christian tradition has sometimes engendered (or at least supported) attitudes of human sovereignty over nature,[11] its dominant theme is human stewardship, deputyship, or trusteeship. While the sovereign is not accountable, the trustee is accountable to God and for what happens to nature. Human action takes place within a context in which humans are ultimately responsible to God as the sovereign Lord of life, Creator, Preserver, and Redeemer. Within this perspective of trusteeship, we cannot be satisfied with a short-term view of responsibility. For example, there is penultimate responsibility to and for future generations; it is not legitimate to slight this responsibility by asking, What has posterity ever done for us? And there is penultimate responsibility to and for nonhuman nature, not only because "nature bats last"!

Some theological critics reject the image of stewardship or trusteeship because it involves *dominium terrae.* But it is irresponsible to neglect or to repudiate human control over nature. The issue is not control (technology) but, rather, the ends, effects, and means of control (technology). This control is not total or unlimited; it is not absolute dominion. It is limited and constrained by nature itself, by moral principles and rules, and by ultimate loyalty and responsibility to God. It is not necessary or desirable to conceive these limits and constraints in terms of "rights" (e.g., rights of trees) as though we can imagine moral requirements only when we can invoke rights. However important rights are—and they are very important—we can conceive moral limits on our control of nature without appealing to them.

The ends of *dominium terrae* are also subject to criticism. If there is a hierarchy of interests, and if human interests are dominant, they should not be construed narrowly—for example, in terms of material goods. Nor should they exclude the goods of nature which are not reducible to human interests. Theologically, the propensity of human beings to construe their interests narrowly and to exclude nonhuman interests or goods is explained in terms of sin. Because humanity is fallen, its control over nature will frequently be misdirected and even destructive. In addition, as we will see when we discuss process later, procedures and mechanisms for reducing the effects of sin are indispensable; even though they cannot eradicate sin, they can lessen its destructiveness.

According to some theological critics, the image of stewardship or trusteeship is also suspect because it appears to separate human beings and nonhuman nature. To be sure, this image depends on a distinction between humanity and nature, but it does not imply an invidious separation. Humanity is part of nature. But, created in the image of God, it is a distinctive, even unique, part of nature. In addition, there may be a hierarchy of value with humanity at the apex. However much we need to emphasize the continuity between humanity and nature, discontinuity, at least as distinction, is still evident and important. Even as part of nature, humanity can still be a steward and trustee for nature.

Furthermore, to distinguish humanity and nature is not to deny their interdependence. Humanity should recognize its solidarity, its community of interests, with nature, because what affects nonhuman nature also affects humanity. It is not necessary or desirable, however, to focus on oneness or organic harmony or to develop a process theology in order to support an adequate ethic. It is possible, for example, to develop adequate limits on human control over nature from a perspective of conflict between humanity and nature in a fallen world. As Gerhard Liedke argues, such a perspective would hold that nonhuman nature is more than material, for, at the very least, it is a rival partner in a conflict. And it needs protection to ensure its participation as an equal in this conflict.[12] Furthermore, recognizing nature in this way is compatible with an attitude of awe and wonder that supports limits on human control over nature.

Although general theological (or quasi-theological)

convictions provide perspectives and engender attitudes, they are not by themselves sufficient for the assessment of technologies. For such a task, we need an ethical bridgework or framework to connect these convictions, perspectives, and attitudes with judgments about technologies. Such a bridgework or framework will consist, in part, of general principles and values. But theological convictions, along with the perspectives they provide and the attitudes they engender, do not merely serve as warrants for moral principles and values. They also shape interpretations of situations to which we apply principles and values. Consider, for example, beliefs about death in debates about technologies to prolong and extend life. If a society views death as an enemy, always to be opposed, it will be inclined to provide funds to develop life-prolonging and life-extending technologies and to use them even when the expected quality of life is poor. An adequate critique would thus include convictions, perspectives, and attitudes that shape interpretations of situations, as well as moral principles and values.

Because it is not possible here to establish all the important connections between theological convictions, moral principles and values, and interpretations of situations, I shall assume several principles and values in order to trace their implications for the assessment of technologies.[13] Unless a single principle or value is accepted as overriding, conflicts and dilemmas are inevitable. As Guido Calabresi and Philip Bobbitt emphasize in *Tragic Choices,* tragedy is largely a cultural phenomenon: it depends on the principles and values of the individual or the society.[14] This point was underlined during a 1979 visit to the People's Republic of China with an interdisciplinary and interprofessional delegation interested in ethics, public policy, and health care. Frequently members of our delegation asked Chinese policy makers, health care professionals, and others how they handle some of our "problems" such as refusal of treatment. The most common response was: "That's not a problem here. It doesn't exist here." Sometimes this response reflected the stage of technological development; often, however, it reflected the unimportance of some Western principles and values such as autonomy, privacy (for which there is no Chinese word), and other ingredients of individualism.[15]

Principles and Values in Technology Assessment

I now want to indicate how technology assessment might proceed and, in particular, what principles and values it ought to consider. Nothing in its logic requires that it be as narrow as it sometimes is. Its practitioners need not be what John Stuart Mill called "one-eyed men" attending only to the "business" side of life.[16]

1. Any technology assessment depends to a great extent on the principle of proportionality—proportion between the probable good and bad effects of technologies. This principle is expressed in various methods used to assess technologies, for example, cost-benefit analysis and risk-benefit analysis, which are only "new names for very old ways of thinking" (as William James said of pragmatism). They represent attempts to systematize, formalize, and frequently to quantify what we ordinarily do. For example, outside Canton, patients in a commune hospital formed their own risk-benefit analysis of traditional Chinese herbal medicine and Western medicine, both of which were available. They said, "Chinese medicine might not help you, but it won't hurt you; Western medicine might help you, but it also might hurt you."

I shall concentrate on *risk* and *benefit,* viewing risk as one sort of cost, i.e., cost as threat to safety, health, and life. The terms "risk" and "benefit" are perhaps not the best. Risk includes both amount or magnitude of harm and probability of harm. When we juxtapose benefit and risk, we are likewise interested in the magnitude and probability of benefit. It would be more accurate then to say that we need to balance the probability and magnitude of harm and the probability and magnitude of benefit. But since that expression is too cumbersome, I will use the common formulation of *risk-benefit analysis.*

Risk-benefit analysis involves what has been called "statistical morality."[17] Risks are everywhere, and one major question is how far we are willing to go in order to reduce the risks of premature mortality, morbidity, and trauma. Let us concentrate on mortality and ask the troubling question: How much is it worth to save a life (really to postpone death since lives are never really saved)? Or what is the value of a life? Consider the controversy over the Pinto. Apparently in 1973 Ford officials decided not to install a safety device that would prevent damage to the Pinto's gasoline tank in rear-end collisions. According to some reports, this device would have cost eleven dollars per vehicle or 137 million dollars for the whole production run. It is not accurate to say that Ford valued human life at eleven dollars. Rather, using a figure of approximately $200,000 per life, it concluded that the safety device should not be used because its costs outweighed its benefits.[18]

Economists propose two different ways to determine the value of life.[19] First, discounted future earnings. This approach tends to give priority to young adult white males. Thus a program to encourage motorcyclists to wear helmets would be selected over a cervical cancer program. Second, a willingness to pay. The question is not how much we would be willing to pay in order to avoid certain death, but how much we would be willing to pay to reduce the risk of death. How is willingness to pay determined? By finding out how much all those who are affected would be willing to pay, summing up the individual amounts, and then dividing by the anticipated number of deaths prevented. While it might be possible to study actual behavior (e.g., in the workplace), one promising approach uses opinion polls to determine, for example, how much a community would be willing to pay in taxes for a technology that would reduce the chances of death after a heart attack.

Although it may be impossible to avoid valuing lives (at least implicitly) in technology assessment, criticisms abound. Religious critics contend that life has infinite or absolute value. But their criticism is not serious insofar as it is directed against policies that do not do everything possible to reduce the risk of death. Judaism and Christianity, to take two examples, do not hold that life is an absolute value, superior to all other values. Both traditions honor martyrs who refuse to value life more highly than other goods such as obedience to the divine will. Furthermore, there is a difference between negative and positive duties, and the duty not to kill is more stringent than the duty to save lives.

Other critics hold that it is immoral to put a value on life. But we all have life plans and risk budgets.[20] Our life plans consist of aims, ends, and values, and our risk budgets indicate the risks to our health and survival we are willing to accept in order to realize some other goods. Health and survival are conditional, not final, values. A society might justly choose to put more of its budget into goods other than health and survival, as I argued in *Priorities in Biomedical Ethics.* Such a choice may be more political, i.e., to be resolved through the political process in terms of the community's values, or even aesthetic. One way to make this choice is to determine a community's willingness to pay for different goods.

An extension of these religious and moral objections opposes the calculation of consequences. Utilitarianism has sometimes been depicted as "ethics in cold blood." But, as I will argue later, consequences are always morally relevant even if they are not always morally decisive. This objection to calculation of consequences may simply be an objection to doing self-consciously and openly what we have to do. For example, Steven Rhoads argues that we should do a little dissembling since to put a public value on life would shock the community and perhaps lead to callousness.[21] In effect, he offers consequentialist grounds for not openly pursuing consequentialism.

These various objections to valuing lives do not hold. For the most part, they are not even aimed at the right targets. And it would be useful for us as individuals and members of a community to ask how much we are willing to spend to reduce the risk of death (in brief, to put a value on life).

It is obvious that value considerations determine what counts as benefit and what counts as harm. They also determine how much particular benefits and harms count, how much weight they should have in the calculation. An adequate risk-benefit analysis needs to keep in play a wide range of values to identify, weigh, and balance benefits and harms. Analysts tend to prefer the hard, quantifiable variables, rather than the soft variables that are less susceptible to quantification. But a "narrow" cost- or risk-benefit analysis fails to convey the richness of our moral values and principles.

2. Value considerations not only shape our perceptions of benefits and harms, they also "dictate the manner in which uncertainty as to the potential adverse consequences will be resolved."[22] To some analysts, the absence of evidence that harm will result is taken as evidence that the harm will not result, and so forth. The resolution of uncertainty, then, will reflect the value judgments of the analyst, whether he uses his own values or reflects the society's values. Description and evaluation cannot be separated even in the determination of the probability of harm because of "opposing dispositions or outlooks toward the future" such as confidence and hope or fear and anxiety.[23]

In the face of uncertainty, a procedural suggestion seems justified.[24] In the past, technology has been presumed innocent until proven guilty. ("Guilt" and "innocence" are used metaphorically to refer to risk-benefit analysis.) But in the light of our experiences in the last twenty years, we cannot be satisfied with this approach: we should, perhaps, presume that technology is guilty until proven innocent. The burden of proof and of going forward should be placed on the advocates of a technology who hold that its benefits will outweigh its harms. Such a shift in the *onus probandi* would not signal opposition to technological development. It would only indicate that we have not been sufficiently attentive to the harmful side effects and second-order consequences in technological development and that we intend to correct this deficiency.

A version of this procedure is mandated for the Food and Drug Administration, which cannot approve drugs for use outside research until they have been shown to be safe and efficacious. In effect, research may go forward (within the limits sketched in Chapter 3 of my *Priorities in Biomedical Ethics* [Philadelphia: Westminster, 1981], "Human Subjects in Research"), research may even be funded (in accord with priorities sketched in Chapter 4 of the same book, "Allocating Health Care Resources"), but let's not introduce a technology until we have determined with a reasonable degree of assurance that its probable benefits will outweigh its probable harms. This procedure will not harass or arrest technology.

3. It is not sufficient for a technology to have a favorable risk-benefit ratio; its proponents should also show that its risk-benefit ratio is more favorable than alternative technologies or even no technology at all. For example, if both X and Y have favorable risk-benefit ratios, they may not be equally acceptable if Y's ratio is more favorable. Many critics of technology call on society to consider alternative technologies, particularly technologies that emphasize the values of smallness and the integrity of person, community, and nature.[25] To a great extent, the issue is again the range of values that should be invoked for risk-benefit analysis.

4. We should seek to minimize risks even by *some* reduction in the probability and amount of the benefit we seek, if that is the only way to minimize the risks. Because we have duties to do no harm and to benefit others, we are responsible for balancing harms and benefits in an imperfect world. But, *ceteris paribus,* the principle of not harming others (including imposing risks) takes priority over the principle of benefiting others; thus, we should minimize risks even at some reduction in the magnitude and/or probability of the benefit. Although this principle is sound, it is difficult to specify how far we should go to minimize risks short of making it impossible to realize the benefit we seek.

5. In the long run, "the reversibility of an action should . . . be counted as a major benefit; its irreversibility a major cost."[26] Thus, reversibility of a technology and its effects should be preferred over irreversibility. Why should reversibility have this privileged position? Surely, if we could realize the ideal social order on earth, we would prefer that it be irreversible and imperishable. But precisely because of the *uncertainties* about probabilities and magnitudes of benefits and harms, we should be particularly cautious about technologies with apparently irreversible effects. The "preservation of future options" is an important goal, and it requires, for example, special concern about the destruction of an animal species and about nuclear waste.

Let me summarize these points about the principle of proportionality, the first consideration in technology assessment. We should balance the probabilities and amounts of benefits and harms. Value considerations will influence all aspects of the balance, including what counts as benefits and harms, how much they count, and how uncertainty is to be resolved. If lives are valued in public policy by determining how much people are willing to pay, the process of valuing lives is not inherently objectionable and may even be illuminating. Procedurally, the advocates of a technology should demonstrate its innocence before it is implemented and should show that its risk-benefit ratio is more favorable than any alternative technologies. We should minimize risks even when we reduce (within limits) the probability and amount of benefit. Finally, reversibility is a benefit, irreversibility a cost.

Limiting Principles

Many flaws in contemporary technology assessments can be traced to the perspective of utilitarianism—the moral, social, and political doctrine that acts and policies are to be judged by their consequences and effects. It is an end-result view of life. After my praise for the principle of proportionality, the reader may wonder whether I am not at least a "closet utilitarian." After all, isn't the principle of proportionality roughly what the utilitarians mean by the principle of utility—maximizing net benefit relative to harm? Any adequate moral, social, or political theory must include the principle of proportionality or the principle of utility. In a world that is not ideal, it is impossible always to do good and to avoid harm. Often doing good produces at least the risk of harm. The principle of proportionality or utility requires that we weigh and balance these benefits and harms when they come into conflict and that we try to produce a net benefit (or, when considering only bad states of affairs, the best of the alternatives). Whatever we call this principle, it is required by any adequate morality.

But we can accept the principle of proportionality or utility without accepting utilitarianism, which may be stated more sharply as the doctrine that right and wrong are determined *only* by the consequences of acts or policies. It makes the utility the *only* principle (act-utilitarianism) or the *primary* principle (rule-utilitarianism). And it distorts many technology assessments by restricting the range of relevant moral considerations. In particular, it concentrates on aggregative rather than distributive matters and it ignores other moral limits such as "rights" (which it frequently translates into "interests").

Utilitarian assessors sum up the interests of various individuals and groups to be affected by the technology, and they use this summation to determine our policy toward that technology. Although they may take account of wider and wider ranges of impacts and interests, they frequently overlook how burdens and harms are distributed. "Acceptable level of risk" of a technology, for example, should not be considered only in terms of the summed-up interests of the society. Principles of justice require that we consider the distribution of risks and benefits.

This issue can be sharpened by an examination of four possible patterns of distribution of risks and benefits. (1) The risks and benefits may fall on the same party. For example, in most therapy, the patient bears the major risks and stands to gain the major benefits. (2) One party may bear the risks, while another party gains the benefits. For example, in nontherapeutic research, the subject bears risks, while others in the future will gain the benefits. Or we may gain the benefits of some technologies that will adversely affect future generations. (3) Both parties may bear the risks, while only one party gains the benefits. For example, a nuclear-powered artificial heart would benefit the user but would impose risks on other parties as well as on the user. (4) Both parties may gain the benefits, while only one party bears the risks. For example, persons in the vicinity of a nuclear power plant may bear significantly greater risks than other persons who also benefit from the plant. These patterns suggest the importance of considerations of distributive justice. As an Advisory Committee on the Biological Effects of Ionizing Radiations reports:

> For medical radiation, as well as for certain uses of radiation in energy production, the problem of balancing benefits and costs is complicated by issues of ethics and discrimination. As an example, increased years of life expectation or increased economic productivity can be a useful measure of health benefit in some contexts. If, however, these parameters are used to balance the benefit-cost equation against the elderly with limited life expectancy or those with limited productivity, important values of society will have been overlooked.[27]

Utilitarianism in technology assessment often fails to take account of other limits because of its particular view of rationality. Max Weber drew classic distinctions between types of social action: "goal-rational" (*zweckrational*), "value-rational" (*wertrational*), affective, and traditional types of action. For our purposes, the first two, which I introduced in Chapter 4 of *Priorities in Biomedical Ethics,* are the most important. Value-rational conduct involves "a conscious belief in the absolute value of some ethical, aesthetic, religious, or other form of behaviour, entirely for its own sake and independently of any prospects of external success."[28] Goal-rational conduct involves reasoning about means to ends. It is a form of "instrumental rationality," involving the choice of effective (and efficient) means to given ends. It has been dominant not only in technology but also in technology assessment. By stressing limits, I have tried to include another type of rationality that may modify instrumental rationality by setting boundaries and constraints on the pursuit of goals.

Instrumental rationality tends to exclude value-rational considerations because they do not fit easily into the schema of means and ends. Just as I suggested about policies of the allocation of resources, we might choose policies toward technologies not because they *achieve* certain goals, but because they *express* certain values. They are expressive, symbolic, or representative. This range of considerations frequently involves *gestures,* not only *tasks.* For example, we might approach nature to make it serve our needs, or to express a certain attitude toward or relationship with it. As Laurence Tribe indicates, technology assessors typically ask what are society's current values regarding nature and they treat nonhuman life merely in relation to those values. But suppose society asked seriously, How should we value nature, including wildlife? And suppose the society came to the conclusion that it should treat nature with respect. Although this conclusion would not necessarily imply that the society would never give human interests priority over nature, "the very process of according nature a fraternal rather than an exploited role would shape the community's identity and at least arguably alter its moral character." As Tribe suggests, the decision maker's own identity might be at stake, for in choosing policies toward technologies, "the decision-maker chooses not merely how to achieve his ends but what they are to be and who he is to become."[29] Who are we and who shall we be? These are considerations of agent-morality that do and should influence our technology assessments.

Process

One critical issue in technology assessment is often overlooked: process. Process is largely a matter of who should decide—that is, who should make the assessment, and how. It is possible to argue that technology assessors do not overlook process. Rather, they judge processes by their results. They ask whether particular processes "pay off" in producing the best possible outcomes—that is, the best possible predictions, evaluations, and controls of technology. When this judgment of processes by their results is combined with the view that we should judge technologies by their predicted consequences for human interests, as measured by preferences, there is one obvious conclusion: the *experts* should make the assessment. This viewpoint simply perpetuates the myth of the end of ideology even while trying to control technology.

Its critics are numerous and vocal. Many of them are concerned with processes of evaluation and decision-making in some independence of their results. In technology assessment, the demand for public participation has become widespread and has encouraged the language of "participatory technology."[30] The World Council of Churches Church and Society Conference on "Faith, Science and the Future" at the Massachusetts Institute of Technology in July 1979 emphasized "a just, participatory and sustainable society." As the general secretary of the WCC, Philip Potter, put it in his address at the MIT conference, "a just and sustainable society is impossible without a society which is participatory." He continued:

> In the present situation of science and technology, they are not really participatory, or rather they are forced to be biased on the side of those who wield economic and political power. There is little sign that they are on the side of the oppressed, the deprived and the marginalized, or simply the people.[31]

It is no exaggeration to claim that "the central issue in technology assessment concerns democratic theory."[32] Involving the public, and especially the individuals and groups affected by the technology, expresses the value of equal concern and respect. It should be built not so much on anticipated results as on the right to treatment as an equal.[33] Processes of public participation in technology assessment are essential to embody this right to treatment as an equal, as one whose wishes, choices, and actions count. In addition, fairness, a principle derived from the principle of equal concern and respect, applies to specific procedures that may be used for public participation (e.g., adversary hearings and public forums). These values and principles are independent of the results of the procedures and processes.

Emphasizing that technology requires a "new ethics of long-range responsibility," Hans Jonas notes the "insufficiency of representative government to meet the new demands on its normal principles and by its normal mechanics."[34] In a lighter vein, H. L. Mencken once said, "I do not believe in democracy, but I admit that it provides the only really amusing form of government ever endured by mankind." He went on to describe democracy as "government by orgy," an orgy of public opinion. Obviously, it is necessary to devise procedures and mechanisms that can both satisfy independent principles and values and sustain effective and disciplined public participation in technology assessment. The creation of such procedures and mechanisms may presuppose that we transcend interest-group liberalism.

Temporal Perspective

As currently practiced, technology assessment tends to "find opportunities for making judgments and taking action only at those points in which a new development in technology occurs."[35] Why? Perhaps because the utilitarianism back of much technology assessment is forward-looking, or because many assessors believe that what we now have is good, or because they believe that we cannot undo what has already been done. Whatever the reason, technology assessment for the most part predicts and evaluates for the future and is less interested in the evaluation of technologies already developed. Langdon Winner argues that we need not only "technology assessment" but also "technology criticism," which can look at the past and the present as well as the future, which can look at long-term trends of technological development as well as at particular technologies, and which can look at the society as well as at the technologies it produces.[36]

Winner's concerns are legitimate, but technology assessment, properly understood, can encompass them. It should be an ongoing process, dealing not only with the introduction of a technology but also with its impact as it is implemented. For example, there was no systematic assessment of the technology of renal dialysis in the 1950s and 1960s, but it has received careful scrutiny since its introduction, widespread use, and funding by the Government. While it is difficult to make adjustments once societal momentum has reached a certain point, we have learned and are continuing to learn from the experience with dialysis, and our experience may improve our policies in other areas. Among the numerous questions that remain about dialysis are whether it is worth the cost (already over one billion dollars a year), whether the money could have been spent better elsewhere, and whether we are able to cope with the successes of technologies (e.g., prolongation of life vs. quality of life of dialysis patients). Nevertheless, our struggle with these questions, and others, may illuminate present and future technology assessments.

Another point needs to be made about temporal orientation. Historical perspective may bring a cautionary tone to discussions of technology assessment. In a fine essay, entitled "Technology Assessment from the Stance of a Medieval Historian," Lynn White, Jr., directs our attention away from the easily measured factors to what he calls the "imponderables" and insists that technology assessment requires "cultural analysis" since the impact of a technology is filtered through the culture and the society.[37] Among his several case studies is alcohol, which was distilled from wine as a pharmaceutical at Salerno, the site of Europe's most famous medical school. How, he asks, could anyone have offered an assessment of alcohol in the twelfth century? Alcohol was praised in medieval literature as a pharmaceutical with beneficial effects for chronic headaches, stomach trouble, cancer, arthritis, sterility, falling or graying hair, and bad breath. It was supposed to be good for people who had a "cold temperament." But then widespread drunkenness and disorder became problems. To shorten the history, we have problems of traffic deaths and cirrhosis of the liver. White observes, "A study group eight centuries ago, equipped with entire foresight, would have failed at an assessment of alcohol as we today fail."

Although White's point is not always clear, it appears to be that technologies touch on many aspects of life (e.g., psychological and sociological factors) that cannot be determined with great precision. What will happen in the interactions between technologies and society, culture, and psyches is an "imponderable." His lesson is salutary. History is ironic, and we can only be modest about (*a*) our ability to *predict* effects, (*b*) our ability to *assess* effects, and (*c*) our ability to *control* effects. It is true, as a character in *Death Trap* puts it, that "nothing recedes like success." While modesty is in order because our abilities are indeed limited, we have no choice but to try to predict, to assess, and to control in the light of moral principles and values.[38]

Notes

1. See Harvey Cox, *The Secular City* (Macmillan Co., 1965); Daniel Bell, *The End of Ideology* (Free Press of Glencoe, 1960), especially "An Epilogue: The End of Ideology in the West"; and Peter Laslett (ed.), *Philosophy, Politics and Society,* First Series (Oxford: Basil Blackwell, Publisher, 1957), "Introduction."

2. Arthur Schlesinger, Jr., *A Thousand Days* (Houghton Mifflin Co., 1965), p. 644. See also William Lee Miller, *Of Thee, Nevertheless, I Sing* (Harcourt Brace Jovanovich, 1975), pp. 78-95. These themes were prominent in President Kennedy's commencement speech at Yale University in 1962.

3. Jacques Ellul, *The Technological Society,* tr. from the French by John Wilkinson (Vintage Books, 1964).

4. Daniel J. Boorstin, *The Republic of Technology: Reflections on Our Future Community* (Harper & Row, 1978).

5. Stanley Joel Reiser, *Medicine and the Reign of Technology* (Cambridge University Press, 1978).

6. This definition is a modification of the definition offered in *Assessing Biomedical Technologies: An Inquiry Into the Nature of the Process,* by the Committee on the Life Sciences and Social Policy, National Research Council (Washington, D.C.: National Academy of Sciences, 1975), p. 1.

7. The term "control" is anathema to many critics of contemporary society and technology, perhaps especially in religious contexts; some critics have retreated into the private sphere because technology appears to be out of control or because the issues are thought to be cultural rather than political. For a valuable discussion of "autonomous technology," see Langdon Winner, *Autonomous Technology: Technics-out-of-Control as a Theme in Political Thought* (MIT Press, 1977).

8. Joseph F. Coates, "The Identification and Selection of Candidates and Priorities for Technology Assessment," *Technology Assessment,* Vol. 2, No. 2 (1974), p. 78. For an overview of technology assessment, see LeRoy Walters, "Technology Assessment," in Reich (ed.), *Encyclopedia of Bioethics,* Vol. 4, pp. 1650-1654.

9. See James M. Gustafson, *The Contributions of Theology to Medical Ethics,* The 1975 Pere Marquette Theology Lecture (Marquette University Press, 1975). In a critique of most, if not all, theological approaches to technology and the life sciences, Gustafson castigates casuists and moralists for their myopia and prophetic theologians for their inability to deal with specifics. See James M. Gustafson, "Theology Confronts Technology and the Life Sciences," *Commonweal,* June 16, 1978, pp. 386-392.

10. Weber drew the phrase "disenchantment of the world" (*Entzauberung der Welt*) from Friedrich Schiller. See Max Weber, *The Protestant Ethic and the Spirit of Capitalism,* tr. by Talcott Parsons (Charles Scribner's Sons, 1958), esp. pp. 105 and 221-222, fn. 19, and H. H. Gerth and C. Wright Mills (eds.), *From Max Weber: Essays in Sociology* (Oxford University Press, 1958), p. 51.

11. Lynn White, Jr., "The Historical Roots of Our Ecologic Crisis," *Science,* March 10, 1967.

12. Gerhard Liedke, "Solidarity in Conflict," in *Faith and Science in an Unjust World: Report of the World Council of Churches' Conference on Faith, Science and the Future,* Vol. 1, Plenary Presentations, ed. by Roger Shinn (Fortress Press, 1980), pp. 73-80. In contrast, Charles Birch's presentation in the same volume stresses oneness and harmony and calls for a process theology ("Nature, Humanity and God in Ecological Perspective," pp. 62-73).

13. For some of these principles, see Beauchamp and Childress, *Principles of Biomedical Ethics.*

14. Calabresi and Bobbitt, *Tragic Choices.*

15. See James F. Childress, "Reflections on Socialist

Ethics," and H. Tristram Engelhardt, Jr., "Bioethical Issues in Contemporary China," *The Kennedy Institute Quarterly Report,* Fall 1979, pp. 11-14 and 4-6.

16. Mill, "Bentham," in Warnock (ed.), *Utilitarianism, On Liberty, Essay on Bentham,* pp. 92 and 105.

17. Warren Weaver, "Statistical Morality," *Christianity and Crisis,* Jan. 23, 1961, pp. 210-215. In Chapter 4 of *Priorities in Biomedical Ethics* (Westminster Press, 1981), I introduced Thomas Schelling's idea of "statistical lives." For a fuller analysis of risk, see James F. Childress, "Risk," in Reich (ed.), *Encyclopedia of Bioethics,* Vol. 4, pp. 1516-1522.

18. For a discussion, see George I. Mavrodes, "The Morality of Chances: Weighing the Cost of Auto Safety," *The Reformed Journal,* March 1980, pp. 12-15.

19. See Steven E. Rhoads (ed.), *Valuing Life: Public Policy Dilemmas* (Westview Press, 1980), especially his chapter "How Much Should We Spend to Save a Life?" pp. 285-311. His formulations have shaped this paragraph.

20. These are Charles Fried's terms as introduced in the chapter 4 of James Childress, *Priorities in Biomedical Ethics.*

21. Rhoads, "How Much Should We Spend to Save a Life?" pp. 305-306.

22. Harold P. Green, "The Risk-Benefit Calculus in Safety Determinations," *George Washington Law Review,* Vol. 43 (1975), p. 799.

23. James M. Gustafson, "Basic Ethical Issues in the Biomedical Fields," *Soundings,* Summer 1970, p. 153.

24. National Academy of Sciences, Panel on Technology Assessment, *Technology: Processes of Assessment and Choice.* Report to the Committee on Science and Astronautics, U.S. House of Representatives, July 1969 (Washington, D.C.: Government Printing Office, 1969), pp. 33-39.

25. For a defense of "intermediate technologies," see E. F. Schumacher, *Small Is Beautiful* (Harper & Row, 1973); for a defense of "alternative technology," see David Dickson, *The Politics of Alternative Technology* (Universe Books, 1975). For a critique of these movements, see Witold Rybczynski, *Paper Heroes: A Review of Appropriate Technology* (Doubleday & Co., 1980).

26. National Academy of Sciences, *Technology: Processes of Assessment and Choice,* p. 32.

27. Advisory Committee on the Biological Effects of Ionizing Radiations, National Research Council, *Considerations of Health Benefit-Cost Analysis for Activities Involving Ionizing Radiation Exposure and Alternatives* (Washington, D.C.: National Academy of Sciences, 1977), p. 150.

28. Weber, *Max Weber on Law in Economy and Society,* p. 1. It should also be obvious from my argument that I believe that it is both possible and desirable to have rational deliberation about the ends that are chosen. They are not merely arbitrary. Yet, as I suggested in Chapter 4 of *Priorities in Biomedical Ethics,* the selection of some ends is mainly political or even aesthetic.

29. Laurence Tribe, "Technology Assessment and the Fourth Discontinuity: The Limits of Instrumental Rationality," *Southern California Law Review,* June 1973, pp. 657, 634-635. See also Laurence Tribe, "Policy Science: Analysis or Ideology," *Philosophy and Public Affairs,* Fall 1972, pp. 66-110. Tribe's discussion has been important for this chapter, especially for this paragraph and the previous one. For another critique of the assumptions of much technology assessment, see Carroll Pursell, "Belling the Cat, Critique of Technology Assessment," *Lex et Scientia,* Oct.-Dec. 1974, pp. 130-145.

30. See James D. Carroll, "Participatory Technology," *Science,* Vol. 171 (1971), pp. 647-653.

31. Philip Potter, "Science and Technology: Why Are the Churches Concerned?" in *Faith and Science in an Unjust World,* Vol. 1, Plenary Presentations, pp. 26-27. For the reports and recommendations, see *Faith and Science in an Unjust World,* Vol. 2, ed. by Paul Abrecht (Fortress Press, 1980). For a critical analysis of the conference, see Alan Geyer, "The EST Complex at MIT: The Ecumenical-Scientific-Technological Complex," *Ecumenical Review,* October 1979, pp. 372-380, and other essays in that issue (e.g., those by Ian Barbour and Ole Jensen).

32. Harold P. Green, "Cost-Risk-Benefit Assessment and the Law: Introduction and Perspective," *George Washington Law Review,* August 1977, p. 908.

33. For the principle of equal concern and respect, see Ronald Dworkin, *Taking Rights Seriously.*

34. Hans Jonas, "Technology and Responsibility: Reflections on the New Tasks of Ethics," *Philosophical Essays: From Ancient Creed to Technological Man* (Prentice-Hall, 1974), pp. 18-19.

35. Langdon Winner, "On Criticizing Technology," in Albert H. Teich (ed.), *Technology and Man's Future,* 2d ed. (St. Martin's Press, 1977).

36. *Ibid.*

37. Lynn White, Jr., "Technology Assessment from the Stance of a Medieval Historian," *Medieval Religion and Technology: Collected Essays* (University of California Press, 1978), pp. 261-276.

38. This chapter originated in a lecture for a Conference on the Technological Society and the Individual sponsored by the Program on Social and Political Thought at the University of Virginia in 1978. It was subsequently delivered in modified form at Whitworth College (1979), at a symposium on Religious Belief in the Age of Science and Technology sponsored by the Religion Club of the University of Virginia (1980), at Earlham School of Religion as one of the 1980 Willson Lectures, and at Miami University (Ohio) as one of the 1980 Wickenden Lectures. It has been strengthened by various comments and suggestions I received in these settings. I am particularly grateful to Dante Germino who, alas, will not be satisfied that I have answered his criticisms.

Chapter Eight
CARE OF PATIENTS AND THEIR SUFFERING

Introduction

Medical personnel confront suffering on a daily basis. How does a medicine shaped by Christian convictions understand suffering? What stance does it take toward it? One of the great temptations is to deny the seriousness of suffering, and Christians are, perhaps, especially tempted to negate suffering as a mere external and "earthly" reality in the enthusiastic flight to another and better world. If we can deny the reality of suffering, we somehow feel more comfortable ourselves. But this sort of "Gnostic" dualism was called a heresy early in the church's history.

If the first temptation is avoided, a second awaits us. It is easy and comfortable to think of suffering as constituted solely by physical pain. If Bradley Hanson is to be believed, that is not the experience of the sufferer; and if the Christian tradition is to be believed, the external person, the body, is never quite so neatly separated from the inner person. But while the Christian tradition of an embodied soul or ensouled body may keep us from either denying suffering or reducing it to physical pain, what does it contribute positively to our understanding of suffering and to our response to it?

Perhaps it can nurture the truthfulness and humility necessary to see suffering honestly. That is no small contribution by itself, but surely it is the place to start. Humility is necessary because we can never really know another person's suffering. Pain crowds out a full awareness of the surrounding world for those who are suffering, yet they become aware at the same time that others do not know what they are experiencing. Consequently, sufferers often feel isolated precisely at the time when human contact is most needed. Pain relief alone is thus a necessary but incomplete response to suffering; the resultant alienation must be addressed as well. There is a further problem for the sufferer. Those who care for them are tempted to categorize suffering and to deny that there is an element of suffering which is singular, which cannot be experienced by anyone else. These individual differences in suffering may be difficult for others to notice. Nevertheless, David Smith points out, these individual differences must be attended to by the caretakers of the suffering person.

Humility is also necessary because suffering makes it clear to all that its victims are not in control of the world. The consequences of this for the person suffering are, or should be, obvious. There is a sense of powerlessness, not simply in the face of this suffering, but in the face of meaningful action in the world. And there are consequences for those who care for the suffering as well. They are tempted to shun the suffering because they stand as a sign of the brokenness of the world. That is why truthfulness is so important a contribution. Without a truthful acknowledgment of the brokenness of the world, caregivers are tempted to remove all traces of the pain and suffering, even if that finally requires the removal of the sufferers. Arthur McGill has pointed out that this is done because our culture holds a dualistic conception of humanity and suffering. If suffering is present, humanity must be absent. To maintain humanity, suffering must be fought at all costs, even if it means large doses of anesthetizing drugs. In that fashion, one does not have to witness the suffering. But notice that under this scenario it is not the comfort of the sufferer which is at stake, but the comfort and peace of mind of the caretaker.

If Hanson and McGill are correct, we must take pains to resist the responses of denial and withdrawal. What the sufferers need to know is that they are not isolated from human contact, that they are not forgotten by the world, that even if the suffering cannot be relieved there will be someone present to be with them. Note that this recommendation does not solve the problem of suffering; it simply gives advice to us in our response to the sufferer.

This section takes us to the heart of some of the reasons why we have medicine and how we understand the point and purpose of medicine. Those who argue that medicine is for the care of ill persons are usually making two points. First, medicine is not simply for the cure of disease; it is for persons. Second, as much as we are all enthralled with the advances of modern medicine, which do in fact cure us, we must remember that there are many unhealthy states of the body for which there is no cure and that as successful as medicine has been, we will still die someday. Where there is no longer the possibility of cure, all of us need care.

But if all need care, what should be said about the givers of care. In our society, caregiving is often organized—in some cases organized into professions. Recently, there has been much written about professions, and the very idea of being a professional has come under suspicion. One of the things most suspect is the claim that professionals care for their clients and that the clients ought therefore to be grateful to their caregivers. What is argued in response is first of all that professionals need their clients both for their income and also because caring for them fills an important personal need for the professional. The second response is that care can become a way for the professional to dominate the client. The clients are already vulnerable because of illness or some other need, and now, in addition, they are asked to submit to the demands of the professional because he "cares." It is no wonder that the concept of care is approached with some suspicion.

Stanley Hauerwas argues that respect for the other must be an integral part of care if the other is not to be tyrannized. But, according to Hauerwas, respect is only a minimum and we should attempt to go beyond it. This might lead us to the graceful caring of Alastair Campbell, a caring in which the client can participate. This caring provides a clue for how to approach suffering for at least one of our authors.

The fact of suffering traditionally has raised a number of questions for Christians. The first is, Why is there suffering at all? Is it something that human beings deserve? Is it something that simply strikes us, good and bad alike? Alternatively, does suffering have any point, or is it part of the world that has no reason, point, or purpose? If we think of it as deserved, should we seek a reason for *this* particular suffering. If we think of it as having a point, should we attempt to draw the point out of all of our suffering?

Christians obviously are not the first people to try to understand suffering. They are heirs of traditions of discourse like those found in the book of Job. There Job protests against his "friends" and "comforters" that his suffering is undeserved. In what follows, the arguments of his friends may be destroyed, but his accusations of God come to nought in confrontation with the God of the whirlwind. Job bears witness by his suffering that righteousness does not mean freedom from suffering. Perhaps that was the point of Job's suffering, but does all suffering have a point? How does one say that the suffering of a child burn victim has a point? "For whom?" we ask. What possibly could the point be?

David Smith suggests in fact that the only thing Christians should say about suffering is that God suffers with us. That is the meaning of the cross. For Smith, suffering is not a problem to be solved; it is a human reality to be shared. If so, medicine may be more important as a gesture of care in the midst of suffering than as a promise of a technological triumph over suffering.

Suggestions for Further Reading

Campbell, Alastair V. *Professional Care.* Philadelphia: Fortress, 1984.

Dougherty, Flavian, C.P. *The Meaning of Human Suffering.* New York: Human Sciences Press, 1982.

Dyck, Arthur J. *On Human Care.* New York: Abingdon, 1977.

Farrar, Austin. *Love Almighty and Ills Unlimited.* New York: Doubleday, 1961.

Hauerwas, Stanley. "Reflections on Suffering, Death and Medicine." *Ethics in Science and Medicine* 6 (1979): 229-237.

——. *Suffering Presence: Theological Reflections on Medicine, the Mentally Handicapped, and the Church.* Notre Dame, Ind.: University of Notre Dame Press, 1986.

McGill, Arthur C. *Suffering: A Test of Theological Method.* Philadelphia: Westminster, 1982.

Nouwen, Henri. *The Wounded Healer.* Garden City, N.Y.: Doubleday, 1972.

Ramsey, Paul. *The Patient as Person: Explorations in Medical Ethics.* New Haven: Yale University Press, 1970.

Ricoeur, Paul. *The Symbolism of Evil.* Boston: Beacon Press, 1967.

Soelle, Dorothee. *Suffering.* Translated by Everett Kalin. Philadelphia: Fortress, 1975.

40.
School of Suffering

BRADLEY HANSON

The School of Suffering has a demanding curriculum that includes practical experience as well as thinking and reading. The practical requirement makes this school different from any humanly designed institution of higher learning, for most of its students have not requested entrance. Admission usually happens to one rather than is sought. Yet once one becomes a student in the School of Suffering, one finds that it has a distinguished faculty.

My own recent illness thrust me into the school and although I am not a biblical scholar, I was impelled to seek out one of its greatest teachers, the apostle Paul, and to especially ponder his Second Epistle to the Corinthians. I found that Paul has four major lessons on suffering. His first two lessons cast light on my experience of suffering and in turn were confirmed and illuminated by that experience. His third lesson is rather advanced for me, and I have only begun to comprehend it. The fourth is well beyond me, and I can do little more than identify it.

I

Paul's first lesson is that the sufferer is not forgotten, because God cares and often expresses his caring through the comfort given by other people. I learned this the hard way over a period of about four months when I endured increasing pain. I learned to distinguish between levels of pain. At the lowest level is an ache. While it is a bother, if one becomes engaged in something the ache is forgotten. The next level is a mild pain, sharper and more noticeable than an ache. Yet again if one becomes fully involved in some activity or conversation, the mild pain is forgotten. As the level of pain increases, the pain occupies more and more of one's consciousness. At the upper limit pain crowds out awareness of anything else; this is excruciating pain. A notch below is what I came to call intense pain, in which pain occupies nearly all of one's awareness; other things are noticed only as peripheral and subordinate to the pain. One cannot forget about intense pain. As the weeks passed the visits of intense pain came more often and lasted longer.

One result of the pain was that I was pushed to the margins of life. Many things that I enjoyed had to be given up—playing football with my sons, attending a concert or a play, spending an evening in conversation with friends, and the enjoyable activities that remained became clouded by pain. Life became dull and uninteresting as it took all available energy just to get through the day's minimum duties.

Not only is existence on the margins of life flat, it tends to be lonely. My friends and associates were at the center, and I felt increasingly like a crippled child left on the sidelines while other children play a game. Adding to the sense of loneliness was a certain privacy about my experience of physical pain. Much suffering has a communal character. When a family member dies, the survivors share their common grief. When a minority endures discrimination, they have many common elements in their experience. But few of the people around me knew first hand what it was to endure chronic intense pain. There are many who suffer like this, with no one near who fully understands their plight. Whatever the particular circumstances, being pushed to the margins of life in some form or other is nevertheless a universal feature of human suffering.

It is precisely because all genuine suffering includes psychological and social dimensions as well as the physical, that comfort from others is so terribly important. The sufferer longs to be assured that others care, and that others are striving to relieve the suffering. To feel abandoned, alone in one's suffering, would crush the sufferer with an unbearable burden.

The powerful need for this assurance was brought home to me late one night in September. I awoke as usual about 2 a.m. with intense pain. Usually it had lasted 30–45 minutes, but this night it kept on and on. After about two hours I began to cry, not a gentle weeping but great gasps. I felt unable to stand up to the pain any longer, and I cried out in anguish at being overwhelmed. My cries were also a call to my wife that I needed her. She awoke and held and stroked me. The pain did not cease for some time, but her presence made it more tolerable.

A few days later Paul's words caught my eye, "But God, who comforts the downcast, comforted us by the coming of Titus . . . " (II Cor. 7:6 RSV). When Paul speaks of comfort, he uses it against the Old Testament background in which comfort includes deliverance as well as tender stroking (e.g. Isaiah 40:1,2). The news that the Corinthian church had taken Paul's severe letter well delivered him from his anxiety; but first he mentions that the mere arrival of his friend and associate Titus was a comfort.

From *Dialog* 20 (Winter 1981): 39-45. Used by permission.

Paul sees this ordinary series of events in theological perspective. The arrival of his friend with good news encourages Paul who has been afflicted with anxieties and conflicts in his work; but it is ultimately God who has comforted him through Titus. "But God, who comforts the downcast, comforted us by the coming of Titus." Thus for Paul the aid that one human being gives to another is a human transaction grounded in and manifesting the character of God, "The Father of mercies and God of all comforts" (II Cor. 1:3).

When strong and privileged socially concerned Christians hear that God comforts sufferers through other people, they are likely to hear only a call to be active in relieving the suffering of others, but that is not what *sufferers* need to hear. To issue such an ethical challenge to those who suffer is to increase their trouble by laying another burden on them. The strong and privileged are able to give, the sufferer needs first of all to receive. So Paul's first word to those Corinthian Christians who endure sufferings with him is to bless "The God and Father of our Lord Jesus Christ, the Father of mercies and God of all comfort, who comforts us in all our afflictions . . . " (II Cor. 1:3,4). If those who suffer are to interpret the meaning of their suffering within the Christian perspective, they need to know they are not abandoned in their suffering. Others care, and God cares. This word of comfort rather than a word of moral challenge is the first lesson in learning the Pauline meaning of suffering.

II

Paul's second lesson is that those who have received comfort from God in their suffering are called to give comfort to other sufferers, for God "comforts us in all our affliction, so that we may be able to comfort those who are in any affliction . . . " (II Cor. 1:3,4). Paul's "so that" expresses purpose.

Of course, Paul's audience and his own situation shape what he says. Paul speaks as a man who has endured much affliction yet has lived through it all; and his audience are Christians in Corinth and the province of Achaia who also were no strangers to suffering. Paul does not consider those whose suffering is such that they do not live through it or fail to receive comfort in their suffering. He considers only those cases in which people are able to learn something from their suffering. He also is not speaking to non-sufferers, even though they might be eager to help those less fortunate. The admission fee to this particular lesson on suffering is high—it requires suffering, for comfort is received only in suffering. It is sufferers who are given comfort "so that" they may comfort others.

It is true that Paul's "we" in II Cor. 1:3-11 refers primarily to himself, but the plural "we" likely indicates that the pattern of affliction and comfort so dramatically exemplified in the apostle's existence has wider application. He certainly does not set himself totally apart from the Corinthians whom he also recognizes as sharing in comfort and suffering.

So Christians who have been comforted in their suffering may affirm as part of its meaning that their experience of suffering and comfort includes God's call to comfort others and that the experience itself equips them to do it. There is a psychological aspect to this, because someone who has experienced a certain kind of affliction is peculiarly equipped to help others with that affliction. Having known poverty first hand can enable one to more fully understand the plight of the poor and to bring genuine comfort. To be sure, deliverance from suffering often requires also the technical knowledge of a physician or economic changes on a broad front. Still direct experience of suffering and comfort gives a depth and sensitivity to compassion which is irreplaceable in the total effort to comfort the afflicted.

The truth of this lesson began to dawn on me one night shortly before entering the hospital. My wife was helping me use a heatlamp, and we began to talk about the meaning of my suffering. I had to admit that the most prominent feature of the suffering up to this point had been its emptiness of purpose. There had been no goal which I could affirm and strive for, except to fight against the pain and seek healing. The suffering itself was an experience of passivity, of being acted upon by negative forces beyond my control. The pain was a harsh reminder of the blind physical roots of life, an irrational reminder without purpose. I felt kinship with the insect accustomed to living in the supportive environment of black soil suddenly turned on its back in the sun, legs moving helplessly. The brute physical reality of pain was devoid of meaning. The only glimmer of meaning I could own at this time was that I now felt much greater sympathy for others who had to suffer, especially those who had to endure chronic pain without hope of relief.

Upon further reflection after my suffering was over, I came to see that the scope of "suffering with others" should not be unduly extended by overdramatized portrayals of the Christian life, which picture the concerned Christian as suffering with the afflicted. There are tendencies toward this sort of rhetoric in Dorothee Soelle's book *Suffering.*

There are at least three distinct ways for Christians to bring comfort through sharing in the suffering of others. One way is to have concern and sympathy for those who suffer and to express it in some concrete way. Such active compassion is an expression of love for neighbor. Paul's collection for the needy in Jerusalem appealed to this sort of compassion.

Another way to bring comfort by sharing in the sufferings of others is by enduring the same suffering they do (e.g. to starve with the starving). Very infrequently would one choose to suffer with others in this way and only when it would serve some constructive end.

A third way to share in the suffering of others is through profound identification with them. Paul does not define suffering for us; but a good definition is that a person is suffering when being acted upon in such a way that the person wishes strongly that his or her state were different.[1] If the sun is shining on one during a hot summer's day walk, one is uncomfortable but not suffering. If one were forced to walk 20 miles in scorching heat, one would suffer. The wish that one's state were otherwise would be very powerful indeed. Using this definition, to suffer with another would mean that the other's suffering would have such a deep impact on a person that one would fervently wish that the other's state (and one's own) would be changed. Parents who agonize over the serious illness of their child genuinely suffer; their anxiety causes them to lose sleep, to weep, etc. To suffer with another in this way requires a profound identification with that other person; the other's welfare is intimately linked with one's own.

While Christians frequently exhibit active concern for others in affliction, they seldom actually suffer with them. This should be honestly recognized. When there was mass starvation recently in Cambodia, I prayed for them and sent contributions through Oxfam and church. This and other manifestations of compassion are good, but it is not suffering.

A final comment about receiving comfort in order to comfort others. It would be reading too much into Paul to infer from this lesson that God *sends* suffering in order to build character. That pedagogical view of suffering may or may not be true, but Paul does not consider such a question of justification for suffering. He begins with the fact of suffering and comfort, and says that God sends *comfort* at least in part so that those who are comforted may be able to comfort others.

Paul also sees this principle of "comforting as one has been comforted" in theological depth, for Christians are to comfort others "with the comfort with which we ourselves are comforted by God" (II Cor. 1:4). This brings us back to the foundation of Paul's first lesson—the ultimate source of comfort is not our own skill or personality but God's compassion for His creatures.

III

The third Pauline lesson is that suffering Christians share in the suffering of Christ. I found this to be the most difficult lesson to understand and appropriate. Two obstacles stood in the way.

I encountered the first obstacle when I read Second Corinthians while in the hospital. When I first read Paul's list of his own sufferings in II Cor. 11:23-29, I felt that my own affliction from pain did not qualify as suffering that shares in the suffering of Christ. Paul mentions sufferings from persecution as a Christian missionary—he was imprisoned, beaten, lashed, and stoned. He also speaks of hardships that came with being a traveling missionary—the dangers of first century travel, hunger, and cold. On top of all that was the anxiety he felt as an apostle for all the churches.

My suffering found no place among those listed by Paul. I was not persecuted for the faith. About the only hazard I faced in carrying out my vocation as a professor of religion was a loss of muscle tone from sedentary work. And while some Christians can confess to anxiety over the church, I could not recall losing any sleep for that reason. If only persecution, hardship, and anxiety for the faith could count as sharing in the sufferings of Christ, then I, and by far most American Christians, were left out.

Later, after serious study of Paul's thought, two things led me to include myself as having shared in Christ's suffering. One is that Paul refers to two personal afflictions which were very likely physical. In II Cor. 1:8 he mentions "the affliction we experienced in Asia" which brought him very near death. And in II Cor. 12:7 he alludes to his "thorn." Although Paul never tells us exactly what either of these were, the bulk of commentators think that the indications make physical afflictions the best guess.

The second reason is that Paul does not set himself totally apart from other Christians, for he says that they are comforted when they "patiently endure the same sufferings that we suffer" (II Cor. 1:6). It could hardly be literally true that they experienced the same sufferings as the well-traveled apostle. It is likely that other Christians at Corinth underwent some persecution, especially the Jewish Christians, but such opposition most likely focused on Paul as the instigator of changes (Acts 18:12-17). While the disciplic pattern of suffering/death and resurrection is most vividly evident in the apostle's life, still he recognizes its presence in the more ordinary lives of other Christians as well.

It is very doubtful that Paul meant to set strict boundaries to what sort of sufferings share in the sufferings of Christ. The specific afflictions he cites from his own experience are merely examples, and even these examples are varied, including anxiety, illness, and physical disability. It seems likely that Paul would agree with I Peter 4:12–19 that suffering as a murderer or wrongdoer would not count, but he opens the circle beyond the persecution cited by Peter to include any innocent suffering. Thus those Christians whose more settled circumstances do not expose them to persecution and hardship for the faith will still at times have sufferings which bring them to share in the sufferings of Christ.

Having surmounted the first obstacle, another still loomed ahead: What does it *mean* to share in Christ's sufferings? A number of commentators think that at least part of what Paul means is connected with his beliefs about the end times. C. K. Barrett points out that there was a Jewish notion of the "sufferings of the Messiah" which did not mean that the Messiah himself would suffer but that the age of the Messiah would be a time of tribulation prior to eternal bliss. Paul probably believed that Jesus had taken most of this end-time tribulation upon himself, yet in the brief time remaining before the end some of this messianic suffering had "overflowed to" Jesus' followers. "For as we share abundantly in Christ's sufferings" (II Cor. 1:5) is perhaps better rendered, "... as the sufferings of Christ overflow to us."[2]

If these commentators are correct, there is the question what this can mean for us today. When Paul believed that the Christians of his time were living in the last days, the idea of sharing in the end-time woes with Christ lent drama and rich meaning to their suffering. It might have given a sense of high privilege to be among this chosen band. But what happens after 1900 years have elapsed and belief in the imminent end has waned? Most of the power in this interpretation of suffering is lost.

Of course, it is not impossible to view the course of human history in Paul's framework if one lengthens the end time considerably, but it is difficult not to lose the vibrancy of that belief unless one believes this nearly 2000-year end-time era is about to close. Jehovah's Witnesses, Seventh Day Adventists, and dispensationalist minded Christians can resonate to this interpretation of sharing in Christ's suffering, but it leaves me unmoved. For me, and I suspect for most mainline church-goers, its power has been dissipated by the passage of time and numerous failed prophecies of when the end would come. We simply do not approach each day thinking this might be the day when Christ returns.

The more important and durable meaning of sharing in Christ's suffering depends on Paul's conception of the relationship between Christ and believers as expressed in the terms "Body of Christ" and "in Christ." Considerable historical study is required to grasp what Paul might have meant with these expressions, for they are many-leveled metaphors. Eduard Schweizer's discussions of these terms are a happy contrast to numerous murky treatments of Paul's mysticism. Much of what Schweizer says can be grouped under three heads.

First, Schweizer says that when Paul speaks of the body of Christ and being in Christ, he is following the Jewish way of thinking in terms of spheres, in which there are certain places or spheres where God's lordship is experienced more directly than in other places, e.g. the temple. Such a sphere of life could bear the stamp of a man such as Abraham, Jacob, or Moses. When Paul speaks of the church as the body of Christ, he is speaking of the place or sphere bearing the stamp of Christ.[3]

Secondly, "body of Christ" has several rich overtones which make it especially suitable as a metaphor for the community/sphere in which Christ's stamp is manifest. One level of its meaning is always the historical body of Christ sacrificed on the cross. In Paul's day this reminder that God expressed His love for people supremely in that physical realm counteracted common Hellenistic tendencies to escape from the physical world into some pure spiritual realm. For Christians the body is the appropriate place and means for meeting and serving others. By extension the Christian community is also appropriately called the body of Christ, because in this down to earth sphere people are accepted by God on the basis of Christ's bodily sacrifice and are called to obedient service. Life in this community bears the stamp of Christ. "Life in the body of Christ is identical with life 'in Christ.' "[4]

Thirdly, Schweizer says that the expressions "body of Christ" and "in Christ" are also part of Paul's translation of Jesus' call to discipleship for a Hellenistic audience. When Jesus called Matthew and others to be his disciples, it meant to come with him as he traveled from place to place, but after the resurrection that sort of accompaniment was no longer possible. Discipleship to Christ needed reinterpretation. Paul translated Jesus' call to discipleship into spatial images readily understandable to the Hellenistic mind already accustomed to calling a social group a "body" and to thinking in Platonic and Stoic fashion of the world as the body in which God dwells as its soul. It was not a great step for them to think of the Christian community as the body in which Christ dwells.[5]

What had special appeal to the Hellenistic audience was to say that following Christ would mean being glorified with him and elevated above the trials of this physical world; but to say only this would have falsified the account of Christian discipleship. Paul had to say that following Christ also means obedience to Him in daily life with its defeats as well as its victories. Indeed, following the crucified Christ means that his disciples cannot expect to be delivered from the ills of life; their way will also include suffering and death.

I think the idea of discipleship is the key to a contemporary interpretation of how Christians share in Christ's suffering. My own experience of suffering suggests how the relationship of lord and disciple can be understood to involve participation in the Lord's suffering. There were a few people who shared by suffering to the extent that they suffered with me; above all it was my wife, to a lesser extent my children and parents. There were friends and other relatives who were concerned and sympathetic to my situation, yet could hardly be said to suffer with me. What seems to account for the difference between the sympathizers and the fellow sufferers is that those who suffered with me were so closely identified with me that I was included in their sense of self; their own identity as persons was closely intertwined with me as husband, father, or son.

There is a useful analogy here to the believer's participation in the sufferings of Christ, although the basis of the participation is the relationship of disciple to lord rather than husband and wife, father and children, son and parents. The identity of the disciple is inseparably linked with the lord, and the identity of the lord with his disciples ("Saul, Saul, why do you persecute me?" Acts 9:4). Christ's relationship with his disciples belongs to his very being as Christ; he cannot be Christ all by himself. The relationship of disciples with Christ is also constitutive of their being; they cannot be Christians apart from identifying with Christ as their lord.

The relationship of Christ with his disciples is asymmetrical, for the relationship rests on his choosing them while it is their secondary place to respond to the lord's call. Therefore the sufferings of Christians are also Christ's sufferings fundamentally because Christ identifies himself so closely with his church. If a concerned parent hurts when the child hurts, how much more does Christ share in the suffering of his people. So our sufferings are his primarily because he makes them his. He wills to include us in his own being as Christ the lord.

Secondarily, disciples of Christ are called to recognize that suffering is an integral part of Christian discipleship. If they hope to be glorified with Christ, they should also expect to share in his suffering by following the way that includes suffering. To identify with the crucified one as lord is to include in one's own self-definition the expectation of suffering. When the son of a Nigerian territorial ruler came to medical school in the United States, he refused to do some dirty work expected of beginning medical students in the hospital. That lay outside his self-definition, and he was prepared to drop out of university rather than do that menial work. Suffering does not lie outside the self-definition of Christians.

Because the disciple's identity is dependent upon that of the lord, the disciple's sufferings are not just his or her own but are a sharing in the lord's suffering. That is to say, the disciple's identity is patterned after the lord's identity. So when the disciple of Christ suffers, it is not simply sharing in a common human experience as it is when one laughs or plays; it is more importantly a sharing in the specific way of Jesus Christ.

Not every path of discipleship follows that way. Suffering cannot be ignored, but one after another religious leaders point a way out of it, and suffering is usually regarded as a sign that disciples are failing to follow their leader. Jesus Christ leads his disciples more deeply into suffering, for he himself went into the depths of suffering before the resurrection. Thus while suffering comes to every human being, Christians can believe that their suffering is not alien to their relationship to Christ, but an integral part of it. Even as Christ shares in their suffering by virtue of his identification with his church, so also Christians share in his suffering by following his way.

I have found that this Pauline lesson is not as easily appropriated as the first two. To be sure, I take comfort in the thought that Christ has so closely identified himself with the community of believers that he makes their suffering his own. That is a reassuring expression of God's love for me. But the idea that suffering is an integral part of Christian discipleship is contradictory to human inclinations. I am very much like that African medical student who refused to do menial work. I shy away from including suffering in my self-definition.

My tendency is to assume that it is my *right* to be healthy, to be able to run, to have good eyesight and hearing, to have the normal functioning of all my limbs and organs. I believe it is my right to be happy, and I become enraged at any violation of these rights. Thus I deny my creatureliness, for I assume that God (or 'life') owes me happiness as though the cosmic order were established by some grand social compact like a club or nation. I do not want to admit that as a creature, whatever I have has been given to me. Certainly health and happiness are goods which I should seek, but there is no cosmic bill of rights which guarantees that I should have them.

Just as Paul's lesson goes against our denial of creaturely limits, so it also goes against our tendency to deny being disciples of Christ. I definitely think of myself as a "Christian" or a "believer in Jesus Christ." I realize that when those terms are properly understood, they include discipleship, but my inclination is not to understand myself as one who is called to obediently follow the way of Christ, a characteristic basic to discipleship. I am more interested in what comfort Christ can give to me than in the summons to follow him. So I tend to ignore the call to take up my cross and follow him even when the cross has knocked me flat on my back. The resistance to being a disciple is strong.

Christ did not claim any right to a happy normal life (not even equality with God was a thing to be grasped). He accepted God's call to service and followed it through suffering and death. "A disciple is not above his teacher." So Christians need to include suffering in their self-definition. Not that they should welcome affliction or go looking for it, but there should be a recognition that suffering is both an inevitable risk for human creatures and an integral element in Christian discipleship.

Because my resistance to discipleship is so strong, I have barely opened the book on this lesson. Yet in an elementary way I have found that suffering brings lord and disciple into closer fellowship. I am drawn closer to Christ as I more fully appreciate the nature of the sufferings that he endured. The sheer physical pain must have been excruciating and prolonged. Scholars often downplay this because it is not unique to Jesus, but having known extended intense pain myself, I marvel at anyone voluntarily undergoing great pain. Adding to Jesus' suffering was the sense of abandonment by most disciples. And depending on the interpretation of Jesus' words, "My God, my God, why hast thou forsaken me?" most terrifying of all may have been abandonment by God and apparently meaningless suffering. Since my illness, I have felt a bond with anyone who suffers pain or illness. I am even drawn closer to Christ, for in some sense he suffered for me.

Being drawn closer to the suffering Christ has revealed that discipleship is a fulfilling relationship of deeper fellowship between lord and disciple. In this relationship the disciple finds fulfillment in surprising ways. There has been a glimpse of the truth that through following the lord's way of suffering, my own true identity is being fashioned, for it is mysteriously intertwined with Christ.

IV

Yet another lesson that Paul teaches about suffering is that it has the potential for being a means through which God's power can be revealed to others. Paul accepted his thorn in the flesh when told, "My grace is sufficient for you, for my power is made perfect in weakness" (II Cor. 12:9). Besides whatever else it means that God's power is made perfect in weakness, it means that the divine power is especially evident when the human vessel is weak (II Cor. 4:7). God's power is more apparent when his will is accomplished in and through one who lacks the human power of strength, beauty, wealth, etc. So Paul gladly boasts of the weaknesses evident in his own sufferings, because through them God's power is plainly revealed to others.

This too is a teaching difficult to appropriate, and it may be that it does not have as wide application as the previous lessons. It seems presumptuous to regard one's own affliction as a vehicle for God's revelation except when circumstances clearly warrant it. I know of nothing in my own suffering that made it a means for divine revelation to others. One cannot assume that one's suffering is automatically being used in this way, but one can certainly pray that God will so use it and one can seek to be open to the grace that will make that possible. If it turns out that one's suffering becomes a medium of revelation to others, that is grounds for seeing yet another profound meaning in one's suffering.

V

Very likely Paul has other lessons on suffering, but these are enough for one term. Learning Paul's lessons is not easy, because the required involvement in suffering is a very high tuition to pay for the School of Suffering. Yet more than enough suffering will come to every Christian over a lifetime even without choosing it, so it is good that Christians can draw upon Paul's insights. When we can affirm for ourselves some of his rich meaning in suffering, then we too can paradoxically rejoice in our suffering at the same time that we long for deliverance.

Notes

1. Cf. David R. Mason, "Some Abstract, Yet Crucial, Thoughts About Suffering," *Dialog,* Vol. 16 (Spring, 1977), pp. 94-96.
2. C. K. Barrett, *A Commentary on the Second Epistle to the Corinthians* (New York: Harper & Row, 1973), pp. 61, 62.
3. Eduard Schweizer, *Jesus* (Richmond: John Knox, 1971), p. 110.
4. *Ibid.,* p. 113.
5. Eduard Schweizer, *Lordship and Discipleship* (London: SCM, 1960), pp. 104-113.

41. Suffering, Medicine, and Christian Theology

DAVID H. SMITH

I. Suffering

If we are to make a proposal about what suffering is, it is helpful to consider the complex relationship between suffering and pain. A prisoner being tortured to extract secrets suffers, but it does not follow that the presence of pain is either a necessary or a sufficient condition for the presence of suffering. It would seem strange to think of someone who experiences only minor pain as suffering; the annoyances of cramping shoes, a small boil, and a scratch are painful, but it would be bizarre to describe their subject as suffering. In order to cause suffering, then, pain must be of a certain intensity: it cannot be trivial.

Furthermore, not every serious pain is a cause of suffering. When a wound is cauterized or an abscess lanced, there may be intense pain, but there is no suffering. Decapitation may be painful, but if we abstract from the anticipation of the event, we do not think its victim suffers. The reason is that suffering involves pain that lasts for a while; it must have a kind of *duration.* That is, if our perceptions were discontinuous, if they did not involve memory and anticipation, we could not suffer. Suffering involves a sense of the continuity of the self in time. Our pain must be recalled or expected for us to be able to speak of suffering. Intense pain of some duration seems to be a sufficient condition for the existence of suffering.

But it is not a necessary condition because people can suffer without being in pain. When someone worries about the health of a parent, grieves over the death of a child, or has professional hopes smashed, we rightly say that that person suffers. There is a metaphorical quality to our usage here, for our paradigmatic experiences of suffering are physical and one function of an assertion of "psychic" suffering is to suggest that the hurt is just as serious as physical suffering. Nevertheless, *suffering* can denote experiences that are not directly associated with physical pain.

This paper was part of a Hastings Center research group project on Death, Suffering, and Well-Being. The project was supported in part by the Arthur Vining Davis Foundations. Used by permission of the Hastings Center and the author.

Thus far I think I have described the way we use the word suffering. I now wish to propose, consistent with this usage, that for suffering to occur, there must be a subject who can comprehend or interpret his experience. Austin Farrar puts it well: "We never know a naked pain, we always take it as a *something*—as a thorn, as a sharp intruder, as a danger, as a cruelty, an outrage. . . . Our manner of taking it is human; it is colored through and through with the habit of thought."[1] The peculiar characteristic of suffering, as opposed to pain or simple disappointment, is that the cause of the discomfort is perceived by us in a special way, as an assault on or a threat to our world. The thorn or intruder, the cruelty or outrage cause us to suffer because they suggest to us a lack of order or control.

In other words, we suffer because we have a perspective on the world that can be threatened by events. Precisely because people's perspectives differ, causes of suffering are diverse, and they have changed over time. They vary from person to person. A way of life that was comfortable to a medieval monk or a Tudor servant would cause me suffering, as would the luxuries of a Jet Set existence. Skin blemishes and unattractive clothes cause suffering to a teenager that is as genuine as professional failure or bursitis to a middle-aged parent. The common core in the experience of suffering is always the same, however. Suffering is associated with a disruption in the coherence and order that I perceive in the world.

Promising as this general line of thought may be, it is probably too general. For suffering is not strictly an intellectual matter, and one can imagine some pretty abstract debates about the structure of the cosmos. In order for the assault or disruption to cause me suffering, I must perceive it as affecting me. This is clearly the case in physical suffering which occurs when the body that I identify with experiences pain of the sorts I have previously described. (It may well be that some kinds of suffering can be relieved if the sufferer is able to dissociate his self from his body.) Moreover, we identify with things other than our body—with other persons, causes, and groups, with a past and with a future. The death of a given person will cause me to suffer insofar as that person had been a part of my world, a part of my understanding of myself. My self is the summation of my various identifications; when the self so constituted is harmed, then it suffers.

Suffering is a kind of identity crisis. It represents a threat to the self. It often involves pain; it disrupts the control the self exerts over its world. A threat to the identity of the self is a necessary and sufficient condition for the existence of suffering.

My proposal implies that unconscious suffering is not really a possibility. This may run counter to some of our common usages, as, for instance, when we say, "He suffers from an inability to see his own limitations." If this is construed to mean simply, "He is deficient because he has no perspective on himself," then our usage of *suffer* in the original sentence is a counterexample to my proposal. It is not clear that this is correct. The original sentence may mean to express the more subtle idea that "He is suffering because he cannot acknowledge his limits," and, if so, it can be reconciled with my proposal. But I concede that we rightly use the word *suffering* in contexts where my attempt at a consistent and narrow definition does not fit.

The area of misfits is fairly broad. We say that a child "suffers from malnutrition," and we do not need to ask the child any questions about diet or food supply in order to learn whether we have made a sensible assertion. The reason we speak in this way is that we assume a common core of experiences that would, we think, cause anyone to suffer. We cannot imagine a human being who would not suffer from the amputation of a limb without anesthesia, from starvation, or from being burned at the stake. Similarly, it is hard to imagine a person who would not suffer at the death of a child, or betrayal by a lover. There are certain physical experiences, some abandonments and betrayals, some disappointments that we cannot imagine to be free of suffering. We almost think that people *ought* to suffer when they have these experiences—that if they do not they are sick or depraved. These are the kinds of sufferings represented in the book of Job, and appropriately so, as they seem inextricably bound up with human life as we know it. The basis of our imputation of suffering in these senses is a kind of soft notion of rationality. We are assuming that anyone whose consciousness is rational must suffer in such and such circumstances.

There are contexts in which it is appropriate to speak in this way, but it is important to bear in mind the specificity and pluralism involved in suffering: Suffering is fundamentally a threat to my identity, my loyalties, my sense of self; things that so threaten one person do not necessarily threaten another. I may suffer every time I take off in an airplane; others may find spelunking intolerable.

To summarize: In the narrow and precise sense we must speak of the suffering of a specific person. Here our discussion must focus on the individual: his or her identity and particular threats to it. In a more general but important sense, however, we can speak of things (prototypically, traumas to the body) that would threaten anybody—that would cause anyone to suffer. Medical practice oriented toward relief of suffering must be aware of both levels and the distinction between them: the sufferings of this particular patient are different from those events in the world that, so far as we can tell, will cause suffering to anyone.

II. Traditional Theodicies

Reflection about suffering has often led Western Christian writers to speculate about the problem of evil, and their ideas are in many ways instructive for our thought about the problem—instructive in their omissions as well as their claims. I mention omissions at the outset, for it is well to note the cliché that suffering (in the sense of pain, disappointment and fear) often has not been the core problem addressed by Christian theodicies. Rather, those arguments characteristically address the question of the existence of *moral evil* or sin. A preoccupation with suffering as we ordinarily understand that term is much more characteristic of Buddhism, for what Siddhartha offers is a path out of dukkha: the imperfections, hurts, and sufferings of existence. Christian theodicies in contrast, even modern versions, focus on sin and a person's need for redemption from its effects. Thus, in order to get to the inevitable question of physical evil and suffering, they have to establish a connection between the kind of evil with which they are most concerned (sin) and various "derivative" forms of evil (suffering and death). Attempts to establish this linkage are at least as old as the narrative of the Fall in Genesis, and I do not mean to deny their instructiveness, as I hope the following will make clear. Still, it is important to remember that a characteristic concern of many Western theodicies is somewhat beside our point.

John Hick has clearly delineated two types of Christian theodicy.[2] The dominant Augustinian tradition was picked up by the medieval church and Aquinas. It controls in the thought of both Luther and Calvin and has been resurrected in modern dress by Karl Barth in the twentieth century. The general lines of this theodicy are familiar and clear enough. Evil is seen as the product of a primordial fall by heretofore perfect creatures (either angels or humans). The evils of the real world are fundamentally punitive for that "original" crime. How could an omnipotent and good God have allowed this to happen? This is the narrow question of theodicy and it is, as Henry David Aiken once remarked,[3] a function of the "monotheistic syndrome," i.e., it is easily avoidable if one is willing to alter one's beliefs so as to accept a finite god, make God's goodness equivocal, or deny the reality of evil.

The common Western response to this problem is the so-called "free will defense" in which the characteristic Western preoccupation with freedom is ascribed to the deity. God wanted, so the argument goes, to create beings in his own image. They must, therefore, be free. Had he created them without the possibility of sinning, they would not have been free. Nor would they really have been free if, predictably saints, they had only had the *abstract* possibility of choosing an evil alternative. A range of ancillary problems inevitably comes up: What is the origin of the evil impulse in the original being(s)? Did God know and in some sense predestine the Fall? If so, does he predestine redemption as well? Why should God will a creation involving a range of seemingly dysfunctional beings? Interesting as these issues are, I have neither time nor ability to pursue them.

What is central to our purpose is to note that in terms of the Augustinian tradition (as delineated by Hick), suffering is always in some sense of the word *deserved.* It may not be deserved by the sufferer per se, but if not, then it is deserved by someone: Adam, all humankind, relatives. Thus a conception of vicarious or substitutionary suffering is central to this view. Related to this understanding of suffering is a conception of God as a judge and, obviously, a conception of the relationship between persons and God as being fundamentally juridical. God is assumed to be the all-just, all-powerful monarch who treats his human subjects according to their deserts.

I do not mean to suggest that there is no truth in this view, for it expresses some things that are very important. Suffering is sometimes deserved, and people do suffer for the sins of others. Those are often unhappy facts, but they are facts nevertheless. Still, this whole tradition runs into two problems. First, so far as our observation carries us, it clearly represents an overgeneralization. It is grotesque to say that a child deserves an early, painful death, or to imply that anything anyone has ever done could merit such a torture and waste in the eyes of a good God. Second, this common perception is reinforced by the New Testament which offers portraits of a God who has other attributes, and other forms of relationship with persons, besides those modeled on a forensic basis. Thus other theodicies have been attempted.

Hick himself constructs what he calls an Irenaean tradition that germinated in the thought of the second-century Gaulish theologian and has been more systematically developed by "liberal" theologians beginning with Schleiermacher in the nineteenth century. In Hick's reconstruction of this view the theological distinction between the "image" and the "likeness" of God is crucial. Persons are made in God's image, but they must perfect themselves as moral agents in order to live in God's likeness. The Fall is not a key doctrine, either in a literal or metaphorical sense. The germ of truth in the Genesis account is its testimony to the present imperfection of human nature. Evil is necessary as an obstacle to be overcome. The world is a vale of "soul-making" in which moral personality can develop. For this development to occur, persons must be free: able to choose between good and evil, able to make mistaken judgments about that which is good. This means that they must live at a certain "epistemic distance" from God, related to him only by faith. They need space in which to grow into his likeness.

Therefore, on this view, suffering serves a fundamentally pedagogical function. As weights, obstacle courses, and calisthenics are necessary for the development of the physical self, so pain, regret, and disappointment enable the formation of a vigorous, virtuous character. The world is a kind of gymnasium or classroom, and God is the ultimate nondirective teacher, creating an environment in which genuinely self-directed learning and growth can occur. God's ultimate responsibility for evil is admitted "up front," but this does not discredit him. There is a sense, indeed a time, in which this evil will be seen to have been worth the suffering. (With Kant, Hick postulates immortality.) Thus Hick is able, in his own way, to affirm the famous "O Felix Culpa" (O Blessed Fall), for without moral struggle there could be no moral virtuosity, indeed no character at all.

This modification of the Western Christian tradition of theodicy is instructive. It rests on the affirmation of a truth known to all: that people can grow as they suffer. But this view faces a special problem in the extraordinarily large and dysfunctional amount of suffering in the world. Nondirective instruction is always rather inefficient, and it would seem that God is unusually bumbling within the context of the Irenaean system. Moral personality is as often broken by suffering as it is created by it, and the unobserved sufferings and deaths of millions of persons are very hard to vindicate. If one is going to save the hypothesis by an assumption of immortality, it is hard to see why this solution was not invoked in the first place and a great deal of discussion avoided.

These theodicies, then, attempt to "justify the ways of God to man." They are answers to the question of why evil should exist. As such, their great relevance to our purpose lies in the fact that we often assume that an understanding of the purpose of something will help us know how to respond to and/or control that thing. If I know why my dog is barking, my chances of making her stop are increased. We tend to think that if we know why people suffer, we will be aided in our response to their suffering.

The connection is not altogether logical, but I think that we can see an affinity between the two theodicies just discussed and our own responses to suffering. The Augustinian tradition suggests that it is appropriate for suffering to exist as a punishment. The natural ethical inference is that suffering that is *deserved* is appropriate; undeserved suffering should not exist and should be fought. The medical result would be to suggest that it is more important to treat infectious diseases and the results of natural disasters and genuine accidents than to treat forms of suffering that people in some sense bring on themselves. Desert might be related to habitual behavior (like smoking or drinking), carelessness (as in the accident prone), environmental practices, or social habits.

In contrast, the Irenaean tradition's claim that suffering's role in the world is pedagogical plausibly leads to the idea that our major concern should be with *pointless* suffering. Pain that causes me to move away from destruction, disappointment from which I learn to redirect my energies—those forms of suffering can be said to have a point. Although they may be ameliorated, they do not require us to bring out the heavy artillery. Those guns should be brought to bear on the suffering that serves no good purpose: pain, unhappiness, or guilt that enervates and simply destroys. We should grow ourselves as we alleviate the pointless sufferings of others, rather than trying to create the morally unchallenging and therefore unnourishing world that would exist if persons never suffered at all. Were we to adopt this paradigm we would find ourselves constantly making judgments about the "value" of a specific form of suffering. Will it be good for my friend to endure that? Can he learn from the experience?

In fact there are social contexts in which reasoning of this sort is important and appropriate. Most human relationships include components of judgment and justice, of concern for the education and growth of another person. I see no reason to assume that medical relationships should be exempted completely from this generalization. Notions of desert and personal growth are legitimate ingredients in a physician's care for a patient. The problem is that these models of the cause and alleviation of suffering are grossly *insufficient.* They tend to hedge our concern for suffering in ways that are ultimately implausible. One does not have to be very sophisticated to know just how ambiguous a notion "desert" is, and it is very pretentious to presume to judge which hardships will benefit another human being. Perhaps the monotheistic God of the Western traditions can make such judgments, but human power to do so is distinctly limited.

If we push this problem to the theological level, we

can say that both of these theodicies are excessively moralistic. Each assumes that the nub of the problem of evil is to be found in the choices of free human beings. Evil exists as a punishment for a wrong choice or as an opportunity for the correct one. Persons were or will be perfect moral agents. The result is ultimately a rather Promethean attitude toward evil, one we should expect to associate with a culture that has always been politically and environmentally activistic. These theodicies assume that suffering and evil are "sometime things," that there was or will be a time in which people did not or will not suffer in virtue of their morality. Suffering could have been or will be stopped.

This is their great mistake, for suffering is an experience or event that suggests that the self's purposes, or the rules it lives by, are no longer valid. The vision and the assumptions upon which moral identity has been based are just what suffering challenges.[4] Suffering persons are not morally autonomous persons; they are lost and confused. Small consolation is received when appeal is made to some hypothesized purpose of the deity; bereaved parents may be incredulous or destroyed by references to guilt or desert. If human existence were the self-controlled and rational thing these theodicies presume it to be *au fond,* then suffering as we know it would not exist. Moral evil would exist, but not suffering, for our very sense of self or identity would never be called in question. The kinds of experience that a writer about suffering must discuss, then, are just those kinds of experiences that are not addressed by these traditional Western theodicies.

III. Sketch of an Alternative

A more interesting religious approach to this question begins with acknowledgment that suffering raises not so much the question of purpose or guilt, but the question of identity. Genuine suffering is something that appears to me as purposeless, a violation of the principles or rules that had constituted myself and my world. If my prior interpretive framework were adequate to handle it, it would not really be suffering. At such a time the subject is not in charge. He is trying to cope, to respond. He has to reassess who he is, what he stands for, before he can take up the ethical and philosophical question of theodicy. That is, we have to turn to the *theology* of suffering.

Fundamentally, there are two possible responses to the crisis of selfhood that suffering provokes. One kind of response involves an attempt to secure the self against invasion, assault, and attack. We look for areas or territory in which we can be secure and powerful. This leads to a preoccupation with our own independence, as commitments or alliances always limit or bind a self and make it vulnerable. For the independent self, the only real powers beyond the self that are acknowledged are powers that are seen as a threat, and the only kinds of relationships with other persons that are comfortable are those that are distant and superficial or those in which the self is in charge—as parent, teacher, or physician. (We do not like to be children, pupils, or patients.)

In his book *Suffering: A Test of Theological Method,*[5] Arthur McGill pointed out the relationship between this response to suffering and the Arian (from Arius, the fourth-century Christian writer) view of God. For Arius, God's identity is a mirror of the independent self just described. God is "unbegotten and unbegetting." His power is unshared and his individuality uncompromised. While he does relate himself beneficently to the world, this relationship ultimately has no effect upon him. God is the great king par excellence. Jesus, therefore, can not be his equal but must be construed to be his close confidant. God could never suffer; his junior colleague or child certainly can.

McGill notes that a major segment of the Christian movement (led by Athanasius) rejected this understanding of God. For them God's identity and power were associated with his giving himself, his involvement with the world, rather than with his independence. Their idea was that in the Incarnation God surrendered independence, bound himself to the world and in doing so made himself vulnerable. Thus the incredible debates about the status of Jesus in the fourth century were not "a furor over a diphthong" as Gibbon would have it but concerned the very nature of God. In insisting that the Son was of the same identity as the Father the Athanasians were claiming that God himself suffers, that true selfhood involves vulnerability to suffering.

On these terms God is not primarily the cause of suffering—by sending it as punishment or training. Rather, God is the true *subject* of suffering, the paradigmatic and quintessential sufferer. The whole idea of Christology is that suffering is a "moment in divinity."[6] The symbol of Christ on the cross is the characteristically Christian datum in the debate about suffering, and theory construction is temporally and epistemically secondary. Thus prior to theological speculations about atonement, about the Fall, or about the value of suffering there is a simple insight: whatever and whoever else he may be, at least we can be sure of this about God: he suffers with us; we do not suffer alone. Christian art and literature through the ages dwell on the suffering of Christ because it was comforting. Why? Because in his suffering the Christian is identified with God: "When you suffer, *your sufferings are God's sufferings,* not his external work, not his external penalty, not the fruit of his neglect, but identically his own personal woe. In you God himself suffers, precisely as you do. . . ."[7]

The Christological symbolism, in other words, suggests two things: identification of the absolute power in the cosmos with suffering persons and illustration of the optimal response to suffering. Suffering accepted by God suggests that suffering is eternal, unlikely to disappear. And someone whose identity is formed by acceptance of this fact finds it possible to identify with the sufferings of others. That is the cause of God.

Human selves modeled on this image would be very different from those preoccupied with independence and power over their own turf. They would see suffering as inseparable from their being, for they would seek identity in loyalties to others. The commitments those loyalties involve inevitably involve vulnerability. This begins with identification of themselves with their own imperfect bodies and includes their friendships, marriages, children, and jobs. Living *in* those identities means living with suffering. Thus distinctions between deserved and undeserved, purposeless and purposeful suffering must always strike the Christian as, at best, provisional. The disciple seems left in the dilemma of Thidwick the Big Hearted Moose,[8] trying to do everything for everybody.

We can, however, put the issue in another way. We can ask, "whose suffering" rather than "which suffering." Answers to this question abound in Christian traditions. Aquinas answered it with the development of an *ordo caritatis,* a set of priorities among neighbors. The Protestant Reformers rejected this strategy and developed theories of the peculiar calling of this or that Christian. Rather than attempt to go through those debates here, I shall simply assume that there are significant differences among persons with regard to their vulnerability, or openness, to my help. I can do more (and more important) things for some people than for others.

In his discussion of this question, Aquinas explicitly argues that a person can do the most for himself, that he is his own best friend. I should like to note my ambivalence about this claim. But it is true, I think, that through choice or chance we find ourselves in special, specific relationships in which distinctive opportunities to respond to suffering present themselves. Of course I refer to our various social roles: professor, physician, parent, child. And I contend that those roles are constitutive of special duties to alleviate suffering. I have unusually great responsibilities for the disappointments of my students, the grief of my child. Their suffering has a special claim on me.

I hold no brief for exclusivity: there are things that others can do for my child that I cannot—precisely because they are others. And I certainly have duties outside my "station." I only contend for a general matter of priority. If that is given, it may be that our response to suffering need not be indiscriminate when moralism is given up. Our ultimate principle of selection is, however, the moral *proximity* of other persons.

IV. Conclusions

Let me close by trying to draw together some conclusions from these reflections.

1. Suffering is not an intrinsic good but the occasion for moral action on the parts of self or others. We can imagine a past or future fictitious world in which people did not suffer and that world would be, in a sense, better than the world we know. The problem with this line of thought, however, is that it is too unrealistic to be relevant. The world all persons have lived in and, so far as we can judge, will always live in will contain suffering. That suffering is intrinsically, although not absolutely, bad.

2. Nevertheless, we would say that someone who lacked the capacity to suffer was defective. This follows from the theory of suffering I tried to advance in the opening sections, when I contended that suffering involves a threat to one's identity. If human power to control the world is limited, it follows that identities will always be threatened. The only way to be free from suffering would be to become a "hollow man" lacking in cares or loyalties—even to one's own body—cares or loyalties that could be called into question. The retreat from commitment so characteristic of much of our society is a flight from suffering and a mimicking of the Arian, uninvolved God.

3. By calling a person's identity into question, suffering can be the occasion for moral growth. Thus, we find that most people we respect are people who have suffered in one way or another. But it is important not to draw fallacious inferences from this fact, for moral growth can occur without suffering—through education, imagination, and argument—and suffering can destroy persons as well as helping them to grow. Thus, suffering is not necessarily an instrumental good.

4. One kind of intellectual response to the crisis of selfhood produced by suffering could be called a response of "domestication." In this response, characteristic of the Augustinian and Irenaean theodicies, a purpose or rationale for suffering is discovered and

suffering is thus accommodated to the previously formulated, autonomy-centered world view. (It may be that this response of domestication is characteristic of nontheistic or nonmonotheistic thought as well, although I have not here tried to advance that claim.) In addition to the strictly theological and/or metaphysical puzzles such maneuvers engender, they inevitably have two problems: (i) Suffering is a situation in which the self is not its own master, not in control. Thus it is bizarre to explain suffering in terms of the self's past or future hypothesized powerfulness and agency. Suffering reveals a fundamental powerlessness. (ii) Explaining suffering as those theodicies do suggests plausibly that some kinds of sufferings (those that are deserved, those with a point) are relatively tolerable. I think that we find such a conclusion oversimple.

5. Christianity has often contended that openness to suffering is an inevitable component of an identity of loyalty to the suffering God. The Christian takes the name of God and receives His identity in community. This unique identity or loyalty is as open as any other to betrayal; the Christian who suffers may become apostate. But this is the issue that suffering raises for the Christian conscience: discipleship or infidelity. One can accept the basic identity or one can give it up; it is contradictory to accept it and deny the truth of its foundation.

6. A physician who adopted some variation of this stance would see the practice of medicine as a form of ministry to the suffering. Since suffering is a crisis of the self and not, in the last analysis, of the body, medical practice would ultimately focus on the patient as person rather than as tissue. This would imply that it is fundamental for a doctor to respect the integrity of patients: the loyalties, the interpretive frameworks that are the core of the patient's being. Medical practice should be directed to the health of suffering human beings. Furthermore, as William May has often argued,[9] a health professional whose identity was formed in this way would be forced to acknowledge his or her own indebtedness. The doctor is not like the Arian God but dependent—on his patients, family, teachers, colleagues, and the general public. Physicians have special relationships to their patients, ones in which they can learn as well as give.

7. Perhaps it is a confession of failure, but I note in conclusion that if these reflections are plausible they may imply that the concept of suffering is of limited relevance to a public debate about health care policy. For I have said that everyone suffers—to be a self is to suffer—and that attempts to discriminate among types of suffering are often inappropriate. Thus I am unconvinced that we will find ourselves able to draw meaningful lines between the suffering caused by arthritis and manic depressive illness, between the heartache of divorce and that of the loss of a child. The concept of suffering offers us no universal, clear, and "hard" policy guidelines.

At the same time, as I have conceded above and at the outset, we can speak of those kinds of experiences that cause anyone to suffer and then argue that those anguishing pains and bereavements ought to have high priority claims on our resources. Reasonable people can come to some consensus about this. But that consensus will need to be supplemented with a focus on two questions: What kinds of needs *can* we meet, and how can we meet them *justly.* I am not sure what else we can do, this side of the eschaton.[10]

Notes

1. Austin Farrar, *Love Almighty and Ills Unlimited* (New York: Doubleday and Company, 1961), p. 95.

2. Hick, *Evil and the God of Love,* rev. ed. (San Francisco: Harper and Row, 1978).

3. Aiken, *Reason and Conduct: New Bearings in Moral Philosophy* (New York: Alfred A. Knopf, 1962), pp. 171f.

4. See H. Richard Niebuhr, *The Responsible Self* (New York: Harper and Row, 1963), pp. 58-60.

5. McGill, *Suffering: A Test of Theological Method* (Philadelphia: The Geneva Press, 1967).

6. Paul Ricoeur, *The Symbolism of Evil* (Boston: Beacon Press, 1967), p. 328.

7. Josiah Royce, "The Problem of Job," in *The Basic Writings of Josiah Royce,* ed. John J. McDermott (Chicago: University of Chicago Press, 1969), II:843.

8. William F. May (personal communication).

9. May, "Code and Covenant or Philanthropy and Contract?" in *The Hastings Center Report* 5 (December 1975); see pp. 83-96 above.

10. In addition to the comments made by several members of the Hastings Center research group on Death, Suffering and Well-Being, I have been greatly helped by colleages in the Religious Studies Department at Indiana and by members of a NEH Seminar "Selected Topics in Bioethics" that met in Bloomington in 1981-82.

42. Care

STANLEY HAUERWAS

The Ambiguity of "Care"

Care and medicine have become closely identified, if not synonymous, in the minds of many. For example, medicine, nursing, and other health-related activities are often referred to as "caring professions." Or "care" is used to indicate that someone is receiving medical aid, e.g.: "She is getting the best care possible." But it is not clear why we associate medicine with care except as we think of both care and medicine as appropriate responses to people in distress.

On analysis, care proves to be an extremely ambiguous notion. We sometimes use "care" to indicate an attitude, feeling, or state of mind about a person or state of circumstance—"I really care for Judy," or "Everyone ought to care for the outdoors." To say that I care for X is, therefore, very similar to saying I like X, except "to care" may denote a stronger intention "to pay particular attention to."

"Care" is also used in a manner that does not involve any attitude, but rather is a correlative to someone's having a certain skill. For example, we say that a mechanic cares for our car not because he likes our car, but because he possesses a technical ability that is necessary to be able to repair a car. He cares for our car because we have established a particular relationship with him, namely, we pay him for his service.

Both senses of care require further specification to determine for what or how one ought to care. "Care" is a context-dependent term, i.e., it carries no particular meaning apart from the context in which it is used. Thus to say that "we ought to care about X or Y" does little more than to remind us that certain kinds of attitudes or skills are appropriate in certain contexts. "Care," like the word "good," is a notion that is incomplete because its significance depends on further specification in relation to particular roles, principles, expectations, or institutions.[1]

The reason "care" seems so appropriate to medical and health-related activities is that these activities involve both senses of care. For example, the doctor is expected to care for his patients because he has a responsibility to have a positive attitude toward securing their well-being. But doctors are also expected to have the skills that give them the ability to "take care" of their patients beyond simply "caring" for them. But as I will suggest below, it is by no means clear how these senses of care are interrelated or specified in contemporary medicine.

Moral Ambiguity of "Medical Care"

The identification of medicine with care seems to be based on the assumption that we owe it to someone to pay special attention to them because they are in particular need or trouble. However, when used in this manner the moral force of care is ambiguous. For it is not clear if care as an attitude and care as a skill are both required and, if they are, on what grounds. For example, we normally think that it is a good thing to care for people in need, but we do not generally assume that it is a moral obligation to do so; that someone may know how to repair cars does not mean that he is obligated to repair our car. Do the skills that doctors possess mean that they are morally obligated to care, and if so, why?

Hans Mayeroff has suggested that to care for someone, "I must know many things. I must know, for example, who the other is, what his powers and limitations are."[2] But in the case of injury or illness we normally assume that the need to maintain basic physical integrity clearly sets the context for the kind of care appropriate. Moreover, because physical need is prerequisite for all other activities we assume that if persons with such need can be helped they should be helped. Thus, while we have no obligation to help some to have a better running car than others, we may feel we should care for them through the office of medicine if it is necessary to maintain their physical existence.

Thus the language of "care" when used in a medical context may assume that, because doctors have the training and skill to care for our physical integrity, they have an obligation to care for those in distress. Care and medicine are closely identified because many of the skills associated with medicine are correlative or even necessary for our most basic human needs. But it does not follow from our assumption that medicine is such a basic form of care that doctors are morally required to provide their service. Such a conclusion must be based on further argument that involves issues that cannot be settled simply by deter-

---

mining whether medicine is or is not a way to "care." Moreover, even if it can be shown that it is a good thing to try to care for someone through the means of medicine, it does not follow that we always ought to do so by these means.

It may well be that we should care for the injured or the ill, but it is by no means clear that medicine offers the best or only way to care for them. Whether the "care" that medicine can provide should be provided will depend on the kind and extent of the medical skill that has been developed. For example, are we required to provide all the "medical care" that is technically possible to someone suffering from kidney disease? Such questions are not meant to deny that medicine may be a basic form of care, but they do make clear that, even if that is the case, whether such care should be provided remains open to decision by doctor and patient.

Paul Ramsey, however, has argued that "care" is not meant to provide a basis for judgment for specific actions in the medical context. Rather, "care" is the "source of all particular obligations and one's court of final appeal for deciding the features of actions and practices that makes what we do right or wrong in any context."[3] Ramsey suggests that this sense of care generates basic rules of practice that embody the physician's commitment to the "preciousness of life." Indeed, it is Ramsey's contention that such an ethics of care provides the basis for a professional ethic that consists in: "(1) rules constitutive of medical care, e.g. the consent requirement, the prohibition of direct killing, and randomizing life-and-death decisions to insure equality of access to sparse resources, which are always binding; (2) directives to cure and save life which true care sometimes suspends and replaces by comfort and dignity for the dying; (3) balancing situational decisions, such as to operate or not to operate, or to use this or that research protocol."[4] However, as we shall see below, many doubt if "care" in itself can generate the kind of ethic Ramsey thinks it implies.

Medical Care as Personal Care

The emphasis on care as a morally significant notion for medicine often serves as a way to stress that patients have needs that are other than "strictly medical." It is not enough for physicians to provide the best technological care available; they also have a responsibility to treat the patient as a "whole person."[5] The demand for a more humane practice of medicine is not a call for the physician to be personally concerned about the patient over and above what he or she can do for the patient medically, but rather it is to remind physicians that their responsibility is to treat not a disease or a medical problem but the person who is subject to the disease or injury. In other words, care and compassion for the patient are not just something nice for the physician to have beyond his responsibilities as a physician, but such personal care is an integral component for the practice of good clinical medicine.

To care in this manner means that the physician must have the capacity to share in the pain and anguish of those who seek help from him. It means that the physician must "have some understanding of what sickness means to another person, together with a readiness to help and to see the situation as the patient does. Compassion demands that the physician be so disposed that his every action and word will be rooted in respect for the person he is serving."[6] Such care should not be confused with pity, condescension, or paternalism. Rather it is to respect the uniqueness of each patient by helping the patient to make those choices that are best for him or her.

Though most assume the physician should "care" in this compassionate or personal manner, the matter is not quite as straightforward as it seems. For, while few deny the medical importance of empathy for the physician's treatment of the patient, it cannot be forgotten that competent care is equally important. "Which would you rather have—warm, compassionate care to usher you into the next world, or cool scientific care to pull you back to this one?"[7] It is, of course, hoped that this rhetorical question does not present a genuine alternative, since good medicine should combine both.[8] The problem for doctors and patients alike is "how the priceless personal equation can be retained in the face of the constantly expanding arsenal of knowledge and inexorable trend toward mass production in medicine no less than in other fields. For, to be true to his calling, a doctor must always complement his expertise with his understanding and view the patient as a whole person rather than merely the sum of his symptoms."[9]

It is important to note, however, that what it means for anyone to care for the "whole person" remains ambiguous. The problem of the kind of personal care the physician should give the patient is not just occasioned by the increasingly sophisticated technology or the demand of justice to try to extend the physician's skill to as many as possible. But it is not clear that care of the "whole person" simply means to treat patients with empathy or compassion. Indeed, it may well be that to treat someone impersonally is a way of caring, especially if we remember that respect is an important aspect of all care. For, if respect is missing, the physician's concern for the patient, even with the best will, can too easily become paternalistic manipulation. For example, the respect due the patient may perhaps mean that the physician must allow the patient not to choose to be "cared" for medically. Open-heart surgery may help many, but that does not mean that the physician has grounds for urging all his patients to undergo such surgery.

Care and the Primacy of the Patient's Interest

The importance of understanding "care" in terms of respect is the basis of Paul Ramsey's suggestion that "care" is the term that best expresses "the ultimate requirement or standard or warrant binding in all cases upon the helping and healing profession."[10] That the physician must "care" does not mean just that the patient should be given personal care, but that the physician has a commitment to each individual patient that is not and cannot be overridden by any other consideration. Care or respect for the patient, therefore, carries the substantive commitment that no patient should be cared for as a means for the betterment of others without his or her consent. In the language of normative ethics this means that the requirement of the physician to care for each individual patient is a basic deontological commitment that cannot be overridden by any considerations including teleological ones, e.g., the physician must continue to give care to the aged even though by ignoring them he might be able to serve more patients. Such a commitment sets the primary task of medical ethics, according to Ramsey, which is to reconcile the welfare of the individual with the welfare of mankind when both must be served.[11]

Even if it is generally accepted that a physician may have an overriding commitment to each patient in his care, medicine and its practitioners face issues that such a commitment does not resolve. Such grounds make problematic the commitment of public health medicine to "care" for a "patient" that may be a city, state, or country. For example, does the commitment to care for the individual patient mean physicians should not recommend everyone be inoculated against an illness because they know that a few will die from the inoculation itself?

The commitment to care for the individual patient is certainly an important and perhaps even crucial commitment for medical ethics. The problem is that such a commitment, in itself, is not sufficient to show how we should care in such complex matters as the just allocation of scarce medical resources.[12] Nor is it sufficient to determine the ethical guidelines as to how we should think about the use of statistical lives, random clinical trials, and the risks that are inherent in the development and practice of normal medicine. Because of these kinds of problems some argue that the kind of "care" offered by medicine cannot be limited to the needs of the individual patient.

Even if "care" is so limited, many questions remain unanswered about what form such "care" should take. For it is often unclear what it means for the doctor to act or to refrain from acting in the patient's interest. The definition of the patient's "interest" that is important to guide the physician depends on the definition of health, which is itself in need of clarification. "The concept of good health implies a concept of the good life, and the goodness of life includes a large number of other factors besides simply its length."[13] But without a more detailed or concrete sense of what those "factors" should be, and what kind of particular responsibility medicine has for sustaining and enhancing them, there can be little consensus about what kind of "care" the physician is obligated to give the patient. Indeed, some have recently argued that there is no readily apparent moral position or philosophy that can provide the moral direction that medicine necessarily requires.[14]

It is often assumed that for a physician to care for a patient means that he should try to cure the patient. To confuse care with cure often results in the cruel abandonment of the dying, as we assume we can no longer care for them if we cannot cure them. Moreover, it may be that some patients are subjected to attempts to cure them in a manner that is antithetical to caring for them. For example, to encourage some patients to undergo surgery that only sustains but does not enhance their lives may be incompatible with care. Ironically the technological power of modern medicine raises the question whether it is not often the best way to care for the patient by refraining from doing what medically we have the skill and power to do. This kind of issue makes many decisions in neonatal care today particularly agonizing.[15]

The problem of the relation between caring and curing is perhaps most clearly, but by no means exclusively, illustrated in relation to how we deal with the dying. For example, even though Ramsey argues that medical care as a moral institution can never act directly to take the life of a terminal patient, there comes a time when to respect life means *only* to care for the dying. This means we must be ready to be with the dying, to comfort them, to assure we will not desert them, but at the same time we will not oppose their death. This means that the requirement to care and to save life is not always to be applied strictly in medical practice. "Care never ceases; yet care, never ceasing, has no duty to do the impossible or useless."[16]

Ramsey, therefore, seems to indicate that the "care" that is incumbent on doctors does not involve simply their medical skills, but the moral skill to be present with those who are suffering. However, it is not clear why the doctor's role involves such a skill. To be sure, communities should provide someone to "only care for the dying," but there is no reason to think the doctor has any different obligation from those of any of us in this respect. It may be, however, that because of their experience in dealing with the sick and the dying doctors have learned better how to care for them, that is, to be with them, better than most of us.

Care, Respect, and Truth-Telling

If care is not equivalent to cure, then the question of what kind of care is due the patient remains open. While no general notion of "care" can be given to account for every kind of medical context, it is clear that a fundamental respect for the patient is required in all medical care. This is often difficult in the medical context because the patient's helplessness and suffering often seem to require that the independence of the patient be qualified in order to "help" the patient. But the inequity of power in such helping situations should but remind us that care for another must be done in a manner that his integrity is not violated.[17] To care for another is to help him maintain or establish an independent existence, which means to help him care for something or someone else. It also means to help the person to care for himself and become responsive to his own need to care and be responsible for his life.[18]

Charles Fried, therefore, suggests that, whatever else care may involve, it must provide the conditions for the maintenance of the patient's lucidity, autonomy, fidelity, and humanity.[19] Lucidity requires that the patient know all the relevant details about the situation in which he finds himself. Autonomy means that, even if a patient is fully informed but does not wish to undergo the therapy recommended by the physician, he cannot be forced to do so. For a person's autonomy to be respected requires that he be allowed to dispose himself according to the life plan and conception he has chosen.

Fidelity requires that we meet the justified expectations that develop from our dealing with one another. Such expectations are often not articulated, but they are not any less significant because they are implicit. Not to meet such expectations is a form of deceit of which lying is but the most dramatic example. The notion of humanity, while admittedly vague, requires that a person should be treated in a manner that does justice to his particular wishes and desires. A person may have no right to be treated affirmatively, but once we are in a significant relationship, our wants, needs, and vulnerabilities should not be ignored. Simply being treated honestly and with autonomy is not sufficient. We should also be noticed.[20]

Assumed in this account of "care" is the importance of telling the patient the truth about his condition. For to withhold the truth is to fail to respect his status as a moral agent capable of being lucid, autonomous, and faithful. Put positively, to care for a patient means that he is to be treated in a manner that assumes that he or she is capable of acting in a morally responsible way. Concretely this means that the simple fact that we are dying does not release us from being held morally responsible for how we die. Moreover, if the patient is unwilling to know the truth about his condition, that does not mean his family or the physician has the right to withhold the truth. However, the importance of the patient's knowing the truth does not mean that he or she must be told the truth bluntly or without feeling. Rather, part of what it means to be truthful in the context of medical ethics is that the truth be spoken to a patient in a skillful, kind, and caring manner.

Conclusion

Care often appears to be a more important regulative notion for determining the moral basis and direction of health-related activities than is morally justified. Care, however, is a significant notion that reminds us that medicine serves as one of the ways we can help others maintain basic physical and psychological integrity. Moreover, care directs our attention to the concrete patient in need without subjecting him or her to manipulation for the good of others. However, it is important that the care given the patient be based on the respect due each of us, well or ill, for otherwise our attempts to care can lead to sentimental or paternalistic perversions.

Notes

1. Julius Kovesi, *Moral Notions: Studies in Philosophical Psychology,* ed. R. F. Holland (New York: Humanities Press, 1967), 124.

2. Milton Mayeroff, *On Caring,* World Perspectives, vol. 43, ed. Ruth Nanda Anshen (New York: Harper & Row, 1971), 13.

3. Paul Ramsey, "Conceptual Foundations for an Ethics of Medical Care: A Response," in *Ethics and Health Policy,* ed. Robert M. Veatch and Roy Branson (Cambridge: Ballinger Pub. Co., 1976), 47.
4. Ibid., 51.
5. See W. Walter Menninger, "'Caring' as Part of Health Care Quality," *Journal of the American Medical Association* 234 (1975): 836–37.
6. Edmund D. Pellegrino, "Educating the Humanist Physician: An Ancient Ideal Reconsidered," *Journal of the American Medical Association* 227 (1974): 1289.
7. Selig Greenberg, *The Quality of Mercy: A Report on the Critical Condition of Hospital and Medical Care in America* (New York: Atheneum, 1971), 205–6.
8. Eric Cassell, "Preliminary Explorations of Thinking in Medicine," *Ethics in Science and Medicine* 2 (1975): 2.
9. Greenberg, *The Quality of Mercy,* 206.
10. Paul Ramsey, "The Nature of Medical Ethics," in *The Teaching of Medical Ethics,* National Conference on the Teaching of Medical Ethics Sponsored by the Institute of Society, Ethics and the Life Sciences and Columbia University, College of Physicians and Surgeons, June 1–3, 1972, ed. Robert M. Veatch, Willard Gaylin, and Councilman Morgan (Hastings-on-Hudson, N.Y.: Hastings Center Publications, 1973), 20.
11. Paul Ramsey, *The Patient as Person: Explorations in Medical Ethics* (New Haven: Yale University Press, 1970), xiv.
12. Charles Fried, *An Anatomy of Values: Problems of Personal and Social Choice* (Cambridge: Harvard University Press, 1970), 183–207.
13. Charles Fried, *Medical Experimentation: Personal Integrity and Social Policy,* Clinical Studies, A North-Holland Frontier Series, vol. 5, ed. A. G. Bearn, D. A. K. Black, and H. H. Hyatt (New York: North-Holland, 1974), 150.
14. Alasdair MacIntyre, "How Virtues Become Vices: Values, Medicine and Social Context," in *Evaluation and Explanation in the Biomedical Sciences,* Proceedings of the First Trans-Disciplinary Symposium on Philosophy and Medicine, Held at Galveston, May 9–11, 1974, ed. H. Tristram Engelhardt, Jr., and Stuart F. Spicker, *Philosophy and Medicine,* vol. 1 (Dordrecht, the Netherlands and Boston: D. Reidel, 1975), 97–111.
15. Stanley Hauerwas, "The Demands and Limits of Care: Ethical Reflections on the Moral Dilemma of Neonatal Intensive Care," *American Journal of the Medical Sciences* 269 (1975): 222–36.
16. Ramsey, "The Nature of Medical Ethics," 24; idem, *The Patient as Person,* 124–32.
17. Mayeroff, *On Caring,* 17; James Bruce Nelson, *Human Medicine: Ethical Perspectives on New Medical Issues* (Minneapolis: Augsburg, 1973), 29–30.
18. Mayeroff, *On Caring,* 10–11.
19. Fried, *Medical Experimentation,* 101–4.
20. Ibid., 103.

43.
Caring and Being Cared For

ALASTAIR V. CAMPBELL

Just as the person who comes to me needs me for help, I need him to express my ability to give help.
James Hillman[1]

The first enters wearing the neon armour
Of virtue
Ceaselessly firing all-purpose smiles
At everyone present
She destroys hope
In the breasts of the sick
Who realize instantly
That they are incapable of surmounting
Her ferocious goodwill
Charles Causley, 'Ten Types of Hospital Visitor'[2]

Love means willingness to participate in the being of the other at the cost of suffering, and with the expectation of mutual enrichment, criticism and growth.
D. Day Williams[3]

I am of the opinion that the relationship between the helper and the helped has a transcendent aspect, suggesting not just knowledge but also the 'foolishness of faith', leading to a sacramental understanding of caring. By 'sacrament' we may understand an outward and physical sign, usually conveyed in bodily action (washing, feeding, anointing, touching), of a reality which eludes rational description. Now we must look more closely at this idea. Is it possible to see a theological dimension in caring, one which is other than the 'rhetoric of self-advancement' with which professions often surround themselves?

In exploring this question I shall consider first the advantages and disadvantages of describing a professional relationship in terms of 'covenant' rather than of 'contract'. I shall identify two features of the conventional relationship which appear to give it a special character: faithfulness and spontaneity. Despite these special features, however, covenants (like contracts) also have a necessary element of exchange. I shall therefore explore the mutuality (or reciprocity) of the covenantal relationship, which needs emphasiz-

From Alastair V. Campbell, *Professional Care* (Philadelphia: Fortress Press, 1984). Copyright © 1984 by Alastair V. Campbell. Used by permission of Fortress Press.

ing to avoid the dangers of paternalism and overzealous helping. This will take us from the idea of covenant to the idea of grace, especially as this expresses itself in bodily forms of caring.

1. Contract and Covenant

In his writings on medical ethics, the moral theologian, Paul Ramsey, expresses powerfully the idea that the professional relationship is to be viewed in terms of the biblical concept of covenant. In the Preface to the *Patient as Person* he writes:

> We are born within covenants of life with life. By nature, choice, or need we live with our fellow men in roles or relations. Therefore we must ask, What is the meaning of the *faithfulness* of one human being to another in every one of these relations?[4]

Ramsey goes on to state that in discussing medical ethics he will 'not be embarrassed to use as an interpretative principle the biblical norm of fidelity to covenant'.[5] We should notice, however, that Ramsey's move from the social nature of human beings to his 'interpretative principle' of fidelity to covenant is by no means the simple step he seems to imply. He appears to be canvassing presuppositions about fidelity, without showing why these are especially appropriate to professional helping relationships. If we are to speak of covenants in professional relationships, then we must explain why contracts are not enough, why fidelity is essential. This issue is explored with some care by William F. May in a paper entitled, 'Code, Covenant, Contract or Philanthropy'.[6] The discussion which follows is based largely on May's exposition.

We should note first that there are considerable *similarities* between contracts and covenants. Both entail an agreement between parties which imposes mutual obligations. The biblical covenants might be summed up in the formula: 'If you obey me, you will be my chosen people' (Exod. 19.5), and in the Old Testament we find God continually lamenting his people's broken promises. May describes covenant and contract as 'first cousins', but he goes on to argue that although they have material similarities, they differ radically *in spirit.* Contracts define a precise set of relationships, and, if these are correctly observed, then the contractual obligation is fully discharged. But covenants 'have a gratuitous, growing edge to them that nourishes rather than limits relationships'.[7] We see this in the development of the idea of covenant in the Old Testament: God's steadfast love constantly attempts to win back his people (Jer. 30); despite Israel's unfaithfulness, her lover still seeks her out (Hosea 2.19–23); God is angry at being betrayed, but his anger will not endure for ever (Hosea 11.8–9). Moreover, while contracts imply no more than a *quid pro quo,* covenants contain an element of promise which resists precise specification. The calculation of whether both parties have equal opportunity for gain is alien to the spirit of covenants, but it is central to the concept of a just contract. There is also a communal aspect to covenants. Whereas contracts are typically between two parties, each of whom is regarded as an individual with certain rights to be safeguarded, covenants often define communal relations, a set of interlocking obligations binding a whole group or nation in a common cause. Finally, covenants begin with a gratuitous act, a gift, and this element of spontaneous giving characterizes the continuing relationship.

It might appear that covenant is the more adequate concept for describing the relationship between client and professional helper, but we must avoid too hasty a conclusion on this point. The notion of contract, with its emphasis on mutual advantage, equal obligation and clearly specified criteria for breach of the agreement, has much to commend it. A contractual approach can protect the clients of professionals against paternalism and exploitation. If the obligations of doctors, nurses and social workers are left ill-defined, then it is very difficult for people to know whether they have grounds for complaint. The air of mystery which surrounds professional work can be used to conceal serious error, inadequate standards of work and outright fraud. Moreover, the notion of exchange serves to remind the people who consult professionals that they too have obligations and that they cannot expect continuing help if they refuse to respect the helper's judgement or if they make unreasonable demands.

On the other hand, the contractual relationship appears to give insufficient weight to certain features of professional care. Firstly, those who need the help of a doctor, nurse or social worker are rarely in the position of buyers on the open market, who can protect their interests on the principle, *caveat emptor* ('Let the buyer beware'). Illness and worry impair people's judgement and may encourage them to make hasty and ill-considered attempts to gain help. They must rely on offers of help which are genuinely concerned for their welfare, not merely attempts to gain maximum financial or other advantage for the 'seller' of help. Secondly, the person seeking help is rarely sufficiently well informed about the problem to be able to specify precisely what is expected from the 'seller' of services. A 'contract' can be defined in only the vaguest of terms and the client must rely largely on professional expertise to specify precisely what should be done to help. Thirdly, a contractual approach may encourage both 'minimalism' and 'defensive over-treatment' by professionals. In minimalism the client is given only as much as is economically worthwhile for the professional to offer. In defensive over-treatment professionals protect their own interests by an excess of treatment in order to safeguard themselves against lawsuits. In neither case is the interest of the client paramount.

We may conclude that by encouraging a view of helping relationships as covenants rather than contracts we may avoid the calculation of the more and the less, based solely on self-interest, which leads to the neglect of the true welfare of clients. The professional has a commitment to people, which is not limitless certainly, but which promises more active concern and open-ended helpfulness than the restrictive language of contract implies. Ramsey may, therefore, be correct in describing the professional helping relationship as one of 'covenantal fidelity.'

2. Reciprocity

The Need to be Needed

There are, however, considerable dangers in too fervent a support for the concept of fidelity, if this is taken to imply a kind of saintlike condescension by the professional, a heroic dedication to the needy with no thought of reward. We have already observed that contract and covenant are 'first cousins' and, although there is an element of gratuitousness in covenant, there is also reciprocity. Both parties to a covenant are recipients of gifts; neither is just a selfless giver. It is not simply that the professional helper makes a living out of being helpful to others, though this should never be overlooked. There are also more subtle rewards. The choice of a career of caring for people in need presumably stems from some needs in the helper, which gain satisfaction when one's working life is spent in an encounter with illness or social disability. The needy person obviously needs to be helped: but that help most likely comes from someone who needs to be needed. Unless we recognize the element of personal need leading people into professional caring, we shall fail to see how damaging some forms of over-commitment can be. One thinks of the 'ferocious goodwill' of Charles Causley's first type of hospital visitor, which 'destroys hope in the breasts of the sick'. The detachment or emotional neutrality of professionals is meant to protect people against such dangerous dedication. As William May puts it: 'It will not do to pretend to be the second person of the Trinity, prepared to make with every patient the sympathetic descent into his suffering. . . . It is important to remain emotionally free so as to be able to withdraw the self when [one's] services are no longer pertinent.'[8]

James Hillman has described in *Insearch* the influence of archetypal symbols of healing and salvation on modern helpers' conceptions of their task. Ancient symbols, suggests Hillman, are often combined with early experiences in which the theme of rescue is prominent, for example, the helpless child who must be saved from a wicked parent.[9] Such unconscious motivations inflate the importance of the help offered to cosmic dimensions, and make a constant supply of needy people a psychic necessity. The *need* to be helpful becomes an insistent *demand* to be perpetually rescuing people. In an article entitled 'The Helping Personality' Hugh Eadie has made some similar observations, based on his research into the health of Scottish clergy. He describes people so anxious to be loving that they continually feel guilty at falling short of the impossible ideal that they have set themselves.[10]

The picture we get from such writings suggests, rather paradoxically, that the truly needy person in some helping relationships may well be the helper. Sick and disadvantaged people are sought out to fill an inner loneliness. Here is how the poet Paris Leary portrays such a person, a priest whose good works bring him admiration and gratitude, but no assuagement of his own needs:

> 'He's frightfully good at coping', Andrew said,
> 'though arthritis makes him snap a bit.
> But he's got all the gen on rules of life,
> and everyone at Bart's, of course, adores him.
> The clergy house is a sort of Coventry-
> cum-hospital . . .
>   He's frightfully good
> at coping, you know. They all end up here.' . . .
> Stiff in the chair which grows and grows around
>   him
> he sits as the dull shilling burns away.
> 'Andrew', he whispers. He cries, 'Andrew', crying
> for young Andrew and the dozens, dozens . . . [11]

Gratitude

The disturbing element in such need-driven caring is that it undermines the spontaneity and gratuitousness which characterizes a covenant relationship. The over-committed helper appears to eschew all personal comfort and private interest in the name of service to others. The reality, however, is often quite other. The hidden rewards are so great that this seeming selflessness is a form of self-assertion, which seeks to deny the reciprocity in all acts of caring and to keep the helper firmly in the ranks of the strong and the need-free.

Three inter-related ideas—gift, gratitude and grace—can help to give a different perspective on this issue. We may restore reciprocity to helping relationships if we emphasize gratitude in the *helper* as well as the helped. This gratitude stems from the experience of receiving gifts, which made the giving of care possible. The Christian belief in calling or vocation expresses this in terms of *charisma,* an ability one possesses as a result of God's grace, not through any personal merit. Those who work in the 'caring professions' are the recipients of such *charismata.* They have gifts of intelligence and personality which enable them to practise a profession in a skilled and effective manner. Their work gives them a sense of fulfilment, of putting to use that which they have been given, and thus of expressing themselves in helping others. So professional care becomes a response to gifts, an act of gratitude, which has its own reward, rather than an act of grudging labour seeking some other satisfaction.

Moreover, part of the reward in such work is the personal character of the relationships which it creates. Using gifts for caring is productive of more gifts from those who are cared for. Frequently the patients of doctors and nurses feel a deep sense of gratitude or indebtedness for the help they have received and they want to express this in monetary or material terms. But the professional, who is aware of how much he or she gains in support, enlightenment and personal development from helping others, may well feel a greater indebtedness. It is often more blessed to care than to be cared for; and the ability to care is frequently made possible by the understanding and sensitivity of the needy person. Such reciprocity suffuses the relationship of caring with a spontaneity, with a sense of grace which enriches carer and cared-for alike.

3. The Grace of Caring and Being Cared For

A closer examination of grace in caring requires an exploration of the relationship between grace and gracefulness. We feel cared for when *our* need is recognized and when the help which is offered does not overwhelm us but gently restores our strength at a pace which allows us to feel part of the movement to recovery. Conversely, a care which imposes itself on us, forcing a conformity to someone else's ideas of what we need, merely makes us feel more helpless and vulnerable. The experience of being cared for, rather than being 'managed', is summed up in the adjective 'graceful'. Graceful care refers to something which is not offered by anxious people trying to earn love, but by sensitive people who release us from bonds of our own making in spontaneous and often surprising ways. The gracefulness in caring is as closely connected to bodily expression as it is to an intellectual understanding or emotional awareness. The body gracefully offers and gracefully receives, in harmony with thought and feeling. Here especially spontaneity (or lack of it) is seen.

By way of illustration of this theme we may consider two quite unusual stories from the New Testament accounts of the ministry of Jesus, each concerned with an overtly physical form of caring—the anointing of the body with oil or ointment. A notable feature of both stories is that they portray women ministering to Jesus, against voices of protest from the male company who witness the events.

Anointing by a 'Sinful' Woman

The first story (Luke 7.36-50) describes how a woman 'who lived a sinful life' washed Jesus' feet with her tears, dried them with her hair, kissed them and anointed them with perfume. The sensuous detail in the story may well underline the sense of freedom she feels from the exploitation of her own body in the past. Stressing the idea of gratitude in the woman's actions, Jesus tells the parable of the man who owed little and the man who owed much and concludes, 'whoever has been forgiven little, shows only a little love'. These words of understanding are apparently matched by the physical responses of Jesus. He accepts the woman's tender caresses, despite the disapproval of his host. He gives care by receiving care and he does so in a graceful, bodily way.[12]

The sensuous aspect of such anointing is one which has been given too little attention, because of a tendency to confuse sensuousness with sensuality. Sensuousness is an acceptance and celebration of our senses: sensuality the exploitation of them. Anointing is sensuous, but not necessarily sensual, because it provides comfort and relaxation to a strained or tired body, restoring the person's sense of being 'at home' in the body and renewing mobility and strength. These features may underlie the ancient practice of anointing the sick which is commended elsewhere in the Bible (James 5.14f.), and they are to be seen in the physical care which doctors and nurses provide for bedridden patients. Such acts are genuinely caring when they are gracefully administered, that is to say, carried out in a way which is appropriately sensuous, with a tender respect for the disabled person.

Anointing for Burial

The second story (Mark 14.3-9 and parallels) describes the anointing of the head of Jesus by an unnamed woman. The perfume she uses is so costly that some of the onlookers protest at the extravagance. The reply of Jesus makes his awareness of his own need very plain. He does not deny the needs of the poor, but he praises the act because it ministers to him as he approaches an inevitable death. Here is a care which sees *his* need and he is grateful for it. Elisabeth Moltmann-Wendel comments on the implications of this story for an understanding of Jesus' humanity:

> This Jesus needs people. He is not the solitary hero. He is not so sovereign that he can do without his neighbour . . . The luxurious anointing comes from the comforting proximity of women: a delight, enjoyment, pleasure in a solitude that is becoming increasingly painful.[13]

The connection between anointing and death is perhaps as important as its sensuous connotations. The embalming of dead bodies or the use of ointments to delay and conceal putrefaction is an acknowledgement of our fleshly nature. At our death we may receive this last service of others, the gentle and respectful handling of our 'mortal remains'. So in moments of weakness in our lives, the person who cares gracefully for us is like the unnamed woman, acknowledging and helping us to accept our mortality. Much is communicated and shared in the simplest of bodily ministrations.

Sexuality and Gracefulness

We have now seen two examples in which women respond to Jesus' bodily needs. In discussing sexual stereotypes in chapter 3 of *Professional Care: Its Meaning and Practice,* I made the point that while women should not be relegated to merely a subordinate, 'handmaiden', role they do in fact show a greater interest than men in responding to the emotional needs of others. It is perhaps not surprising, then, that in the gospels it is women who are the ministers to Jesus, while the male disciples misunderstand him, fall asleep, or deny him at his time of greatest need. It is the women who offer a costly caring, though the men might equally be capable of it. It is the women whose bodily care gives comfort to Jesus, while the men struggle for places of honour.

Ideally such graceful caring should be accessible to men and women alike. But it is clear that (whether because of nature or nurture) men find it difficult to offer and receive care in a physical way, perhaps fearing that their masculinity will be under threat or that their action or reaction will be interpreted as a sexual advance. The psychoanalyst Ian D. Suttie has written of the 'taboo on tenderness' and he draws attention to the phenomena of male societies or brotherhoods which seem to be attempting to give covert expression to the prohibited feelings of tenderness in men. Suttie believes that there is a primal need to give and receive bodily expressions of tenderness. The caressing of companionship, Suttie argues, is earlier in human development and ultimately more important than sexual arousal. The need to be touched, held and nurtured is with us from the very beginning to the very end of life.[14]

There is something very basic, then, in the experience of being cared for. Each of us knew it in the tender embrace of our mother—that is our first (and perhaps our most important) bodily awareness of grace. All human acts of caring mediate a grace which knows and sustains the person as the mother knows and nurtures the child. Yet these acts must also be appropriate to the situation in which care is required. For the professional person, offering care to a wide variety of people within the context of specific needs, there can rarely (if ever) be the closeness and constancy of a mother's love. This would be inappropriate in most circumstances and would lose sight of the autonomy and coping capacity of the person helped. But although (as I have suggested throughout *Professional Care*) the love of professional care is a *moderated* one, and so should not be confused with the more intimate forms of love we receive from parent or friend, there remains the important element of gracefulness in caring, whose similarity to maternal tenderness and sexual intimacy must not be overlooked. The covenantful relationship, which promotes trust and mutuality, requires bodily mediation in order for its true value to be appropriated by helped and helper alike. The 'sacrament' of caring is the use of the physical closeness of bodies to a therapeutic end, the overcoming of weakness and the restoration of hope which another human presence makes possible.

4. Brotherliness, Companionship and Hopefulness in Caring

We are now in a position to look to the images of caring which I used in previous chapters of my book to epitomize the relationships of each professional group surveyed, and to see their sacramental character, that is to say, the way in which their physical nature mediates a transcendent love.

We note that an essential aspect of the medical relationship is the use of knowledge to restore bodily integrity, to welcome back the stranger into the human community and to challenge the health-denying features of contemporary society. This 'brotherly' or 'sisterly' work of medicine is sacramental in character because no physical explanation in terms of disease-eradication or restoration of function can do full justice to its aims. Medical practice deals with living, self-conscious social beings, not merely with isolated parts of organisms. When genuine care is offered to patients (many of whom can have no hope of physical recovery) only the startling imagery of Edwin Muir's 'Christ the recrucified'[15] can portray the message which this care represents. The consistent attention which a humane doctor offers a damaged fellow human being reveals a vision behind the Cross to the young wood in a green corner of Eden. (This can certainly become *hubris,* that vying with God to which medical practice is so prone, and it may lead to a 'heroic' medicine which denies our mortality, but it need not be arrogance of this kind.) A caring response to someone who may soon die creates and discovers the value which cannot be destroyed. It refuses to discard the person because the organism is decaying. This is the secular sacrament of medical care.

In a similar way, the companionship of nursing care provides through physical means a transcendent encouragement which can lead to recovery or to an acceptance of the irremediable. The nurse's actions are, as we have already observed, reminiscent of the mother's care of an infant. The most basic activities of eating, sleeping, excretion and ensuring bodily comfort generally become part of the nurse's concern when a person is seriously ill. In addition, the presence of the nurse is as important to the anxious patient as is the mother's to the frightened child. The nurse often becomes the interpreter to the patient of matters which are perhaps only half understood or half heard when first communicated by the doctor. These features of the nursing relationship make the care which nurses offer their patients an especially powerful means for good or ill. The nurse as companion possesses that gracefulness which we have identified at the heart of caring. There is a sensitivity in companionship which shares without invading privacy and which helps in the other's journey without attempting to dominate and create crippling dependency. When such sensitivity is lacking all the unhelpful features of idealization, demeaning maternalism and stigmatization of unpopular patients which were discussed earlier make nursing care into a health-denying force. But the nurse who offers companionship to patients, even those who seem incapable of much reaction or positive response, embodies the value-creating love, which (to recall Muir's poem once more) helps the tormented wood to cure its hurt. The physical act points to a transcendent reality. The sacramental element is the loyalty of simple care.

Finally, in social work, the gracefulness of caring is found in a stalwart commitment to personal and communal renewal. (Judas a child once more at his mother's knee?) Of the three professions surveyed, social work appears most removed from the physical, most caught in verbalization without concomitant practical action. No doubt this explains the virulence of the debate about the nature of social work and especially about whether radical political change can be one of its objectives. But if we resist the polarization of the personal and the political we may begin to discern the sacramental aspect of social work.

In chapter 4 of *Professional Care* I described the 'dimensions of hope' in the social-work relationship. More than any other profession (except perhaps the clerical profession, which is not under discussion in this volume) social work is obliged to see people 'four-dimensionally'. Precisely because they offer no physical treatment—indeed, rarely any kind of bodily contact—social workers are prevented from relying on one method of helping to the exclusion of the complexities of the client's life and special context. This is evident from the history of social work, which reveals perpetual disenchantment with the favoured method of the previous generation. First the Poor Law and 'welfare worker' image, with its emphasis on handing out material benefits, had to be discarded; then psychoanalytically influenced casework, with its predilection for self-determination and insight, was revealed as masking social injustice; then advocacy for client's rights was challenged as insufficiently radical in its political involvement; now we find questioning about whether politically radical social work can honestly claim to be social work at all, and whether the emerging emphasis on systems theory and change-agency is too managerial and manipulative. Of course, social work is not unique in this tendency to have a succession of fashionable theories, but the range of theory and the rapidity of change is unusual and it reveals the elusive character of social-work action.

How then may a sacramental significance be found in so diverse and ill-defined an activity? I attempt to answer this question in the final chapter of *Professional Care,* in which I attempt to describe a theological image of 'the politics of love'. Provisionally, however, we may recall the theme of hope based on four-dimensional perception. The social worker's care is one which enriches the client's self-perception and the perception of the client by others through patient and persistent emphasis on complexity and change. Thus social work care is a sacrament of the future, a set of actions which mediate hope for individuals, families and neighbourhoods simply by refusing to dismiss them as inadequate, beyond remedy, better forgotten. This insistence on hopeful, multidimensional perception means that there can be no split between individual and society in social work. Any attempt to insulate the political from the personal merely results in an impoverishment of one's understanding of the person. Social work heralds more forcefully than the other professions, the signs of the times in which an uncaring society brings not only the sad harvest of broken people but also, unless there is change and renewal, its own destruction.

Notes

1. J. Hillman, *Insearch* (Hodder and Stoughton 1967), p. 13.

2. *Oxford Book of Contemporary Verse,* 1945–1980, chosen by D.J. Enright (Oxford U.P. 1980), p. 81.

3. D.D. Williams, *The Spirit and the Forms of Love* (Nisbet 1968), p. 288.

4. P. Ramsey, *The Patient as Person* (Yale U.P. 1970), p. xii, author's emphasis.

5. Ibid.

6. W.F. May, 'Code, Covenant, Contract or Philanthropy', in *The Hastings Center Report,* vol. 5 (December 1975), pp. 29–38. Although this refers specifically to medicine, May's ideas can be applied more widely. See also his recent publication, *Physician's Covenant: Images of the Healer in Medical Ethics* (Westminster Press 1983).

7. W.F. May, 'Code, Covenant, Contract or Philanthropy', p. 34.

8. Ibid., p. 30.

9. Hillman, op. cit., ch. 1.

10. H.A. Eadie, 'The Helping Personality', *Contact,* 49 (Summer 1975), pp. 2–17.

11. Excerpts from 'He's frightfully good at coping' by Paris Leary from *Poets of Today,* VII (New York, Scribner, 1960).

12. No doubt this is an interpretation of the text, which may be reading more into it than is justified. Yet the striking physical descriptions in this story can scarcely be ignored. As in other similar stories, the actions are as important as the words which accompany them. It is unfortunate that subsequent tradition has put the emphasis on the woman's sinfulness and (through a confusion with Mary Magdalene, who is mentioned in the subsequent chapter) has created 'maudlin' associations of a weeping penitent woman saved from sexual sin. This is more the attitude of the Pharisee than that of Jesus!

13. E. Moltmann-Wendel, *The Women Around Jesus* (SCM 1982), p. 102.

14. See I.D. Suttie, *The Origins of Love and Hate* (Kegan Paul, Trench and Trubner 1935), ch.6. A striking example of such care is described in John Steinbeck's *Grapes of Wrath,* when a young mother suckles a weak, dying old man.

15. See Muir's poem "The Transfiguration," *Collected Poems of Edwin Muir* (Faber and Faber 1963), p. 200.

Chapter Nine
RESPECT FOR PERSONS AND THEIR AGENCY

Introduction

If there is one topic that marks off post-World War II discussions of medical ethics from earlier discussions, it is that of autonomy. Although it is not always clear what a particular author means by the term, even a cursory glance at the literature of medical ethics makes it clear that autonomy is a central idea.

At first glance, it might be difficult to discern what is at stake in this discussion for Christians. After all, autonomy might be a way for persons to claim independence—first from fellow human beings and second from God. If that is what is at stake, then the idea of autonomy would appear to be at odds with some conceptions of the Christian faith.

For some thinkers, autonomy does stand in tension with any form of relationship. Autonomy means, among other things, the right to will what one will without attention to one's relationships, one's communities, and even one's past. Only the agreements into which one has freely entered or the basic rights of others to their autonomy can stand as limits to the expression of one's autonomy.

But that understanding of autonomy does not make clear all that is at stake in the discussion. A historical perspective might be helpful here. What are the factors which have led to the call for respect for autonomy in medicine in our day and time? They seem to be four. First, physicians performed experiments on people without their consent. This happened in this country as well as abroad. Second, physicians performed putatively therapeutic procedures upon patients "for their own good" without their consent. Third, certain features of modern medicine are depersonalizing. Technological medicine often makes it difficult to see the patient as a fellow human being. The patient is simply a part of nature and thus is not unique. Fourth, through the use of science and technology, physicians have gained an enormous amount of power. Just as the cries for reform in earlier times against the unchecked power of kings and priests led to discussions of individual rights, so today's response to the power of physicians is a call for respect for the autonomy of patients.

But freedom for a Christian can mean more than freedom from the depersonalizing power of technology and the uncaring care of the professional. This is not to argue that these are unimportant, but they may not be all that is at stake. If Karl Rahner is correct, the real freedom of human beings is to be found in one's decision for God. Rahner insists that in our whole life we must be treated as free; and that includes that part of our life in which we are dying. He argues that threats to the agency of the dying are in fact threats to this possibility of decision for God. We have to decide whether Rahner is correct when he claims that if we do not recognize freedom for the dying, we deny the dying an opportunity to make their life whole.

There is possibly an additional issue here for those who are sick but not dying. One of the real injuries of illness is that people lose a sense of their own agency. In illness we often cannot bend either the external world or our own body to our purposes. We are helpless before the ministrations of others. If they will respect our wishes, however, then there remains, even for the ill, a sense of personal agency and autonomy. What we see is that the term *autonomy* is referred to in slightly different ways. There is the autonomy of the patient which may be the goal of medical care, the autonomy of the patient understood as a constraint upon the power of medicine, and the respect for autonomy which should be a basic attitude of the health care provider, or so say autonomy's defenders.

But what is the relationship between autonomy and other values? Do other values limit autonomy? James Gustafson claims that respect for persons demands more than simply respecting the autonomy of others; we must also respect their social relations and their biological natures. If we agree with Gustafson that respecting persons ought to mean more than simply assenting to their wishes, how does that help us in situations of conflict? Do we respect a pregnant Jehovah's Witness who wishes to undergo surgery without receiving blood when we know that to do so threatens the life of the fetus? What if, in addition, the patient is a mother of a young child? Do we override, if necessary, the mother's wishes on the grounds that she owes it to her child to remain alive? There are other values in our society which are in tension with respect for autonomy. If we agree with the defenders of autonomy, the bonds of relationships not freely chosen do not count. If we disagree with them, we appear to be attacking personal liberty.

If we think that other values are necessary, we must ask the question, "What is necessary to be an autonomous person?" The law may answer, "The person must be competent." Generally, this means that the person must be of sound mind and, perhaps, of a certain minimum age. For example, people are usually not considered competent to drive an automobile if they have not reached the age of sixteen.

Moralists might want to add the requirement that whatever values or principles the person acts upon, they should be the person's, and not those of a pressure group, a peer group, or some other agency external to that person. That is to say, one's actions must be in conformity with one's own freely held view of the world. Usually this principle is used to criticize authoritarian regimes and agencies; yet it can be used to criticize any activity which does not proceed from views adopted as one's own.

But that leaves open the question about one's views of the world. Even in a pluralistic society, there surely are views we do not want people to act upon, even if they are competent and hold the particular view as their own. The view that it is permissible to enslave people of African descent would be one such view. This means that the question of the truth of the view that one holds as one's own is still an important issue.

Even when there is agreement that the wishes of the person ought to be respected, there is still a problem of determining who is a person. If one assumes that respect for autonomy applies only to persons the question is, "How do I know that I am taking care of a person?" Some authors assume that there are tests to determine whether a patient is a person—to be a person one must have a certain minimal level of IQ or be at a certain level of development. As we shall see in the discussion of abortion, for some authors almost everything hinges upon the question of whether the fetus is a person.

For others, the above approach is mistaken. The issues seem to be twofold. First, what is the purpose of our use of the term *person?* Is the purpose to distinguish some human beings from other human beings? Or is the point to distinguish human beings from other animals? Until we are clear about the purposes of our use of the term, we cannot begin to discuss the criteria of personhood.

Second, is it true that physicians are using the term *person* the same way that moral philosophers and theologians sometimes use the term? Might it not be the case that medical personnel are interested in the relationships of the patient and not the question of personhood? Is this approach defensible? If so, on what grounds? The articles in this section will raise these questions.

Finally, if it is reasonable to claim that the relationships surrounding the patient are primary, are we then back where we started in the discussion of autonomy, trying to decide when, if ever, the wishes of an autonomous person ought to be respected? That question is especially important when those wishes might be destructive of relationships. In the readings which follow, you will be asked to think carefully about these and similar questions.

Suggestions for Further Reading

Carlton, Wendy. *In Our Professional Opinion . . . : The Primacy of Clinical Judgment Over Moral Choice.* Notre Dame, Ind.: University of Notre Dame Press, 1978.

Childress, James F. *Who Should Decide? Paternalism in Health Care.* New York: Oxford University Press, 1982.

Dyck, Arthur J. *On Human Care.* Nashville: Abingdon, 1977.

Lammers, Stephen E. "Autonomy and Informed Consent." In *Respect and Care in Medical Ethics,* edited by David H. Smith. Lanham, Md.: University Press of America, 1984.

Lebacqz, Karen. *Professional Ethics: Power and Paradox.* Nashville: Abingdon, 1985.

Reich, Warren. "Toward a Theory of Autonomy and Informed Consent." In *Annual of the Society of Christian Ethics, 1982,* edited by Larry Rasmussen, 191-215.

Thomasma, David C. *An Apology for the Value of Human Life.* St. Louis: The Catholic Health Association of the United States, 1983.

Veatch, Robert M. *A Theory of Medical Ethics.* New York: Basic Books, 1981.

44.
Four Indicators of Humanhood—The Enquiry Matures

JOSEPH F. FLETCHER

Jean Rostand describes a meeting of French Catholic intellectuals; they spoke of a prosecution for infanticide following the thalidomide disaster of the Sixties.[1] Morvan Lebesque: "After centuries of morality, we still cannot answer questions like those raised by the trial in Liege. Should malformed babies be killed? Where does man begin?" Father Jolif: "No one knows what man is any longer."

That is the situation, exactly. Whether or not we ever knew in the past what man is, in the sense of having a consensus about it, we do not know now. To realize this, make only a quick scan of the wild confusion and variety on the subject gathered together by Erich Fromm and Ramon Xirau in their historical compendium.[2]

First There Was One

Yet it is this question, how we are to define the *humanum,* which lies at the base of all serious talk about the quality of life. We cannot appraise quality or enumerate human values if we cannot first say what a human being is. The *Hastings Center Report* (November 1972) published a shortened version of an essay of mine in which I made a stab at this problem, under the title "Indicators of Humanhood: A Tentative Profile of Man."[3]

In substance I contended that the acute question is what is a *person;* that rights (such as survival) attach only to persons; that out of some twenty criteria one (neocortical function) is the cardinal or hominizing trait upon which all the other human traits hinge; and then I invited those concerned to add or subtract, agree or disagree as they may. This was intended to keep the investigation going forward, and it worked; the issue has been vigorously discussed pro and con.

What crystals have precipitated? Without trying to explore them in any detail, as each of them deserves to be, four different traits have been nominated to date as the singular *esse* of humanness; neocortical function, self-consciousness, relational ability, and happiness—the last being included more in a light than a heavy vein. Various additional criteria of the optimal or *bene esse* kind are mentioned in a growing correspondence, but no argument *against* any one of them has been offered; e.g., one correspondent (Robert Morison) wants concern for the meek and dependent stipulated under my eighth trait, "concern for others."

But on the question which one of the optimal traits and capabilities is the *sine qua non,* the essential one without which no combination of the others can add up to humanhood, there are now four contenders in the running. It should be noted at the outset that of the four discrete cardinal criteria thus far entered, none of them is mutually exclusive of any of the others, any more than the optimal indicators are (sense of time, curiosity, ideomorphous identity, obligation, reason-feeling balance, self-control, changeability, etc.). The decisive question therefore appears to be about precondition. Which one of these traits, if any, is required for the presence of the others? To answer this is to find *the* criterion among the criteria.

Now There Are Four

I. Michael Tooley of Stanford contends that the real precondition to "having a serious right to life" or to being the kind of moral entity we call a person, as in the Sixteenth Amendment sense, is subjectivity or self-awareness (no. 2 in my original list). He called it "the self-consciousness requirement."[4] As he points out, fetuses and infants lack that requirement. Machines have no consciousness at all, and therefore may be sacrificed in a competing values situation. Animals are probably not self-conscious, although a few pet lovers claim they are. Once a growing baby's neurological "switchboard" gets hooked up, allowing consciousness of self to emerge, he or she is a person. (Mind is, as Dubos points out, a verb—not a noun; it is not something given but acquired, a process rather than an event.[5] It is what the mind does, not what it is.) So runs Tooley's thesis.

II. Richard McCormick of the Kennedy Center for Bioethics at Georgetown University, on another tack, says "the meaning, substance, and consummation of life is found in human relationships," so that when we try to make quality of life judgments ("and we must"), as in cases of diseased or defective newborns, "life is a value to be preserved only insofar as it contains some potentiality for human relationships."[6] On this basis anencephalics certainly, and idiots probably, lack personal status, with a consequent lack of claim upon rights. If you lack what he calls "the relational potential" (what I call "the capability to

---

From *The Hastings Center Report* 4 (December 1975): 4-7. Used by permission of the publisher and the author.

relate to others," no. 7) you cannot be human. "If that potential is simply nonexistent or would be utterly submerged and undeveloped in the mere struggle to survive, that life has achieved its potential" and we need not save it from death's approach.

III. When a pediatrician at the Texas Medical Center (Houston), whose work takes her daily into a service for retarded children, heard me at a grand rounds expound my suggestion that minimal intelligence or cerebral function is the essential factor in being human, she rejected it: "I know a little four-year-old boy, certainly 20 minus or an idiot on any measurement scale and untrainable, but just the same he is a human being and nobody is going to tell me different. He is happy and that makes him human, as human as you or I." By "human" she meant morally, not only biologically. She described the child's affectionate responses to caresses and his constant euphoria. I thought of my neighbor's kitten and recalled the euphoria symptom as happiness without any reason for it, and I remembered Huxley's *Brave New World* where everybody was happy on drugs—except the rebellious intellectuals. I asked her if she really meant to say that euphoria qualifies us for humanhood. I took her silence to be an affirmative answer.

IV. As far as I can yet see, I will stand by my own thesis or hypothesis that neocortical function is the key to humanness, the essential trait, the human *sine qua non.* The point is that without the synthesizing function of the cerebral cortex (without thought or mind), whether before it is present or with its end, the person is nonexistent no matter how much the individual's brain stem and mid-brain may continue to provide feelings and regulate autonomic physical functions. To be truly Homo sapiens we must be sapient, however minimally. Only this trait or capability is necessary to *all* of the other traits which go into the fullness of humanness. Therefore this indicator, neocortical function, is the first-order requirement and the key to the definition of a human being. As Robert Williams of the University Medical Center (Seattle) puts it, "Without mentation the body is of no significant use."[7]

THE ORIGINAL
INDICATORS OF HUMANHOOD:
A TENTATIVE PROFILE OF MAN

Positive Human Criteria

1. Minimal intelligence
2. Self-awareness
3. Self-control
4. A sense of time
5. A sense of futurity
6. A sense of the past
7. The capability to relate to others
8. Concern for others
9. Communication
10. Control of existence
11. Curiosity
12. Change and changeability
13. Balance of rationality and feeling
14. Idiosyncrasy
15. Neo-cortical function

Negative Human Criteria

1. Man is not non- or anti-artificial
2. Man is not essentially parental
3. Man is not essentially sexual
4. Man is not a bundle of rights
5. Man is not a worshiper

Discussion Goes On

This search for a *shared* view of humanness, a consensus, may not find a happy ending. James Gustafson's (University of Chicago Divinity School) skepticism about reaching agreement has now been graduated into skepticism also about applying whatever criterion we might agree to.[8] He thinks now that "intuitive elements, grounded on beliefs and profound feelings," would color our judgments seriously. More sharply, Rostand warns us (p. 66) that looking for a single trait is "a temptation for the fanatics—and there are always fanatics everywhere—to think that his adversary is less human than himself because he lacks some mental or spiritual quality." In scientific and medical circles I find that a *biological* definition is thought to be feasible, but not a list of moral or psychological traits—to say nothing of picking out only one cardinal trait subsumed in all the rest.

One slant on the problem is to deny the problem itself, not as insoluble but as specious (no pun intended). For example, William May of Catholic University, trying to justify the prohibition of abortion, objects to "the thought of Fletcher, Tooley, and those who would agree with them" that membership in a *species* is of no moral significance.[9] He argues that we are human by virtue of what we are (our species), not what we achieve or do. A member of the biological species is, as such, a human being. Thus, we would be human if we have opposable thumbs, are capable of face-to-face coitus and have a brain weighing 1400 grams, whether a particular brain functions cerebrally or not. (I put in the thumbs and coitus to exclude elephants, whales and dolphins, the only other species having brains as big or bigger than man's.) In this reasoning the term "human" slides back and forth between meaning sometimes the biological, sometimes the moral or personal, thus combining the fallacy of ambiguity with the fallacy of ostensive definition. ("He has opposable thumbs, therefore he is a person.")

Tristram Engelhardt of the Texas Medical Branch (Galveston) takes a different path; he renounces not the need to define humanhood but the attempt to single out any one crucial or essential indicator.[10] Instead, he is synoptic in the same manner that René Dubos has so superbly shown us in *Man Adapting* and *So Human an Animal.* Engelhardt distinguishes the biological from personal life but follows a multifactorial, non-univocal line. Indeed, he points precisely to the traits elected in all three of the major univocal definitions discussed here; together they compose his own—cerebral function, self-consciousness, and relationship or the societal dimension. Yet it is difficult, studying his language, not to believe that he gives cerebral function the determinative place, as when he says that "for a person to be embodied and present in the world he must be conscious in it," but follows that up by adding, "The brain is the singular focus of the embodiment of the mind, and in its absence man as a person is absent" (p. 21).

Being careful in all this is supremely important. Leonard Weber of Detroit urges "caution in adopting a neocortical definition of death" because this is tantamount to a definition of personhood, although he doesn't throw it out of court. He further asks us to make sure "the biological is not being under-valued as a component of human life."[11] On both scores I agree. I take "caution" to mean carefulness, which is always in order, and I certainly want to affirm our physical side, since why even talk of cerebral function apart from a cerebrum? "Mind is meat" may be too crass, but I agree that it contains a vital truth.

Rapprochement?

To Tooley and McCormick I would want to say, "You are on sound ground, so far.' Of all the optimal traits of a full and authentic human life, I am inclined with you to give top importance to awareness of self (Tooley's cardinal and my optimal trait no. 2) and to the capacity for interpersonal and social relations (McCormick's cardinal and my optimal traits no. 7 and no. 8)." But I still want to reason that *their* key indicators are only factors at all because of *my* key criterion—cerebral function. Is this not an issue to be carefully weighed?

Rizzo and Yonder of Canisius College, Buffalo, have argued the case for the neocortical definition.[12] Their conclusion is that "when there is incontrovertible evidence of neocortical death, the human life has ceased." To Professor Tooley and Father McCormick I would say, "Neocortical death means that both self-consciousness and other-orientedness are gone, whereas neither non-self-consciousness nor inability to relate to others means the end of neocortical activity." Just remember amnesia victims when self-consciousness is proposed as the key; just remember radically autistic and schizophrenic patients when the relational key is proposed. The amnesiac has lost his identity, his selfhood, and the psychotic is still *thinking,* no matter how falsely and in what disorder. On these grounds we cannot declare that such individuals are no longer persons, just as we cannot do so at some levels of mental retardation. Only irreversible coma or a decerebrate state is ground for such a serious determination. It seems that possibly the neocortical key is more conservative than some observers of the ethical debate suppose.

The importance of self-awareness is obvious. Abraham Maslow has taught this generation that much. Being able to recognize and respond to others is of the greatest importance to being truly human, as Gordon Allport's interpersonalism made plain. But as Julius Korein, the New York University neurologist, tells us, "Basic to the definition of the death of an individual is identification of the irreversible destruction of that critical component of the system which represents the essence of the person," and that essence, he says, is "cerebral death."[13] The "vegetable" patient, no matter how many spontaneous vital functions may be continuing, is dead, a nonperson, but not at the point he appears to be incapable of self-perception or of relational affect—only when neurologic diagnosis determines that cerebral function has ended permanently.

The non-neocortical theories (or paraneocortical) fall because they do not account for all cases. "Neocortical death," on the other hand, *necessarily* covers all other criteria, because they are by definition impossible criteria when neocortical function is gone. The key trait must be one that covers all cases, no matter how infrequently they are seen clinically. Incidentally but not unimportantly, the neocortical indicator is *medically* determinable, whereas Tooley's and McCormick's are not.

If it proves that very many ethicists feel these issues about a sound hypothesis for the *humanum* are crucial, those whose training has been in the humanities will need the help and advice of psychiatrists, psychologists, neurologists and brain specialists, to teach us the limiting principles involved and expedite our discussion.

Notes

1. J. Rostand, *Humanly Possible: A Biologist's Notes on the Future of Mankind,* trans. by L. Blair (New York: Saturday Review Press, 1973), p. 8.
2. E. Fromm and R. Xirau, *The Nature of Man* (New York: Macmillan, 1968).
3. The full text is "Medicine and the Nature of Man," in *The Teaching of Medical Ethics,* ed. by R. M. Veatch, W. Gaylin and C. Morgan (Hastings-on-Hudson, N.Y.: Institute of Society, Ethics and the Life Sciences, 1973), pp. 47–58. It appeared also in *Science, Medicine and Man* I (1973), 93–102.
4. M. Tooley, "Abortion and Infanticide," *Philosophy and Public Affairs* 2 (Fall, 1972), 37–65.
5. R. Dubos, *Man Adapting* (New Haven: Yale University Press, 1965), p. 7n.
6. R. A. McCormick, "To Save or Let Die: The Dilemma of Modern Medicine," *Journal of the American Medical Association* 229 (July 8, 1974), 172–76.
7. R. H. Williams, *To Live and To Die* (New York: Springer-Verlag, 1974), p. 18.
8. J. M. Gustafson, "Basic Ethical Issues in the Bio-Medical Fields," *Soundings* 53 (1970), 177; and "Mongolism, Parental Desires, and the Right to Live," *Perspectives in Biology and Medicine* 16 (Summer, 1973), 529–57.
9. W. May, "The Morality of Abortion," *Catholic Medical Quarterly* 26 (July, 1974), 116–28.
10. H. T. Engelhardt, Jr., "The Beginnings of Personhood: Philosophical Considerations," *Perkins* (School of Theology) *Journal* 27 (1973), 20–27.
11. L. J. Weber, "Human Death or Neocortical Death: The Ethical Context," *Linacre Quarterly* 41 (May, 1974), 106–13.
12. R. F. Rizzo and J. M. Yonder, "Definition and Criteria of Clinical Death," *Linacre Quarterly* 40 (November, 1973), 223–33.
13. J. Korein, "On Cerebral, Brain, and Systemic Death," *Current Concepts of Cerebrovascular Disease* 8 (May–June, 1973), 9.

45. Must a Patient Be a Person to Be a Patient? Or, My Uncle Charlie Is Not Much of a Person But He Is Still My Uncle Charlie

STANLEY HAUERWAS

As a Protestant teaching at a Catholic university, I continue to learn about problems I had no idea even existed. For example, recently I was called down for referring to Catholics as "Roman Catholics." I had been working on the assumption that a Catholic was a Roman Catholic; however, it was pointed out to me that this phrase appeared only with the beginning of the English reformation in order to distinguish a Roman from an Anglo-Catholic. A Catholic is not Roman, as my Irish Catholic friend emphatically reminded me, but is more properly thought of simply as a Catholic.

I recount this tale because I think it has something to do with the issue I want to raise for our consideration. For we tend to think that most of our descriptions, the way we individuate action, have a long and honored history that can be tampered with only with great hesitation. Often, however, the supposed tradition is a recent innovation that may be as misleading as it is helpful.

That is what I think may be happening with the emphasis on whether someone is or is not a "person" when this is used to determine whether or what kind of medical care a patient should receive. In the literature of past medical ethics the notion of "person" does not seem to have played a prominent role in deciding how medicine should or should not be used vis-à-vis a particular patient. Why is it then that we suddenly seem so concerned with the question of whether someone is a person? It is my hunch we have much to learn from this phenomenon as it is an indication, not that our philosophy of medicine or medical ethics is in good shape, but rather that it is in deep trouble. For it is my thesis that we are trying to put forward "person" as a regulative notion to direct our health care as substitute for what only a substantive community and story can do.

From *Connecticut Medicine* 39 (December 1975). Copyright 1975, *Connecticut Medicine.*

However, before trying to defend this thesis, let me first illustrate how the notion of "person" is being used in relation to some of the recent issues of medical ethics. Paul Ramsey in his book, *The Patient as Person,* [1] uses the notion of person to protect the individual patient against the temptation, especially in experimental medicine, to use one patient for the good of another or society. According to Ramsey, the major issue of medical ethics is how to reconcile the welfare of the individual with the welfare of mankind when both must be served. Ramsey argues that it is necessary to emphasize the personhood of the patient in order to remind the doctor or the experimenter that his first responsibility is to his immediate patient, not mankind or even the patient's family. Thus Ramsey's emphasis on "person" is an attempt to provide the basis for what he takes to be the central ethical commitment of medicine, namely, that no man will be used as a means for the good of another. Medicine can serve mankind only as it does so through serving the individual patient.

Without the presumption of the inviolability of the "person," Ramsey thinks that we would have no basis for "informed consent" as the controlling criteria for medical therapy and experimentation. Moreover, it is only on this basis that doctors rightly see that their task is not to cure diseases, but rather to cure the person who happens to be subject to a disease. Thus, the notion of "person" functions for Ramsey as a Kantian or deontological check on what he suspects is the utilitarian bias of modern medicine.

However, the notion of "person" plays quite a different function in other literature dealing with medical ethics. In these contexts, "person" is not used primarily as a protective notion, but rather as a permissive notion that takes the moral heat off certain quandaries raised by modern medicine. It is felt if we can say with some assuredness that X, Y or Z is not a person, then our responsibility is not the same as it is to those who bear this august title.

Of course, the issue where this is most prominent is abortion. Is the fetus a human person? Supposedly on that question hang all the law and the prophets of the morality of abortion. For if it can be shown that the fetus is not a person, as indeed I think it can be shown, then the right to the care and protection that modern medicine can provide is not due to the fetus. Indeed, the technological skill of medicine can be used to destroy such life, for its status is of no special human concern since it lacks the attribute of "personhood."

Or, for example, the issue of *when* one is a person is raised to help settle when it is morally appropriate to withdraw care from the dying. If it can be shown, for example, that a patient has moved from the status of being a person to a non-person, then it seems that many of the difficult decisions surrounding what kind and the extent of care that should be given to the dying becomes moot. For the aid that medicine can bring is directed at persons, not at the mere continuation of our bodily life. (Since I will not develop it further, however, it is worth mentioning that this view assumes a rather extreme dualism between being a person and the bodily life necessary to provide the conditions for being a person.)[2]

Or, finally, there are the issues of what kind of care should be given to defective or deformed infants in order to keep them alive. For example, Joseph Fletcher has argued that any individual who falls below the 40 I.Q. mark in a Stanford-Binet test is "Questionably a person," and if you score 20 or below you are not a person.[3] Or Michael Tooley has argued young infants, indeed, are not "persons" and, therefore, do not bear the rights necessary to make infanticide a morally questionable practice.[4] Whether, or what kind, of medical care should be given to children is determined by whether children are able to meet the demands of being a person. You may give them life-sustaining care, but in doing so you are acting strictly from the motive of charity since nothing obligates you to do so.

As I suggested at the first, I find all this rather odd, not because some of the conclusions reached by such reasoning may be against my own moral opinions, or because they entail practices that seem counter-intuitive (e.g., infanticide), but rather because I think this use of "person" tends to do violence to our language. For example, it is only seldom that we have occasion to think of ourselves as "persons"—when asked to identify myself, I do not think that I am a person, but I am Stanley Hauerwas, teacher, husband, father or, ultimately, a Texan. Nor do I often have the occasion to think of others as persons. I do sometimes say, "Now that Joe is one hell of a fine person," but so used, "person" carries no special status beyond the naming of a role. If I still lived in Texas, I would, as a matter of fact, never use such an expression, but rather say, "Now there is a good old boy."

Moreover, it is interesting to notice how abstract the language of person is in relation to our first-order moral language through which we live our lives and see the kind of issues I have mentioned above. For example, the reason that we do not use one man for another or society's good is not that we violate his "person," but rather because we have learned that it is destructive of the trust between us to do so. (Which is, in fact, Ramsey's real concern, as his case actually rests much more on his emphasis on the "covenant" between doctor and patient than on the status of the patient as a "person.") For example, it would surely make us hesitant to go to a doctor if we thought he might actually care for us only as means of caring for another. It should be noted, however, that in a different kind of society it might well be intelligible and trustworthy for the doctor rightly to expect that his patient be willing to undergo certain risks for the good of the society itself. I suspect that Ramsey's excessive concern to protect the patient from the demands of society through the agency of the doctor is due to living in an extraordinarily individualistic society where citizens share no good in common.

Even more artificial is the use of "person" to try to determine the moral decision in relation to abortion, death and the care of the defective new-born. For the issues surrounding whether an abortion should or should not be done seldom turn on the question of the status of the fetus. Rather, they involve why the mother does not want the pregnancy to continue, the conditions under which the pregnancy occurred, the social conditions into which the child would be born. The question of whether the fetus is or is not a person is almost a theoretical nicety in relation to the kind of questions that most abortion decisions actually involve.

Or, for example, when people are dying, we seldom decide to treat or not to treat them because they have or have not yet passed some line that makes them a person or non-person. Rather, we care or do not care for them because they are Uncle Charlie, or my father, or a good friend. In the same manner, we do not care or cease to care for a child born defective because it is or is not a person. Rather, whether or how we decide to care for such a child depends on our attitude toward the having and caring for children, our perception of our role as parents, and how medicine is seen as one form of how care is to be given to children.[5] (For it may well be that we will care for such children, but this does not mean that medicine has some kind of overriding claim on being the form that such care should take.)

It might be felt that these examples assume far too easily that our common notions and stories are the primary ones for giving moral guidance in such cases. The introduction of the notion of "person" as regulatory in such matters might be an attempt to find a firmer basis than these more historically and socially contingent notions can provide. But I am suggesting that is just what the notion of "person" cannot do without seriously distorting the practices, institutions and notions that underlay how we have learned morally to display our lives. More technically, what advocates of "personhood" have failed to show is how the notion of person works in a way of life with which we wish to identify.

Yet, we feel inextricably drawn to come up with some account that will give direction to our medical practice exactly, because we sense that our more immediate moral notions never were, or are no longer, sufficient to provide such a guide. Put concretely, we are beginning to understand how much medicine depended on the moral ethos of its society to guide how it should care for children, because we are now in a period when some people no longer think simply because a child is born to them they need regard it as their child. We will not solve this kind of dilemma by trying to say what the doctor can and cannot do in such circumstances in terms of whether the child can be understood to be a "person" or not.

As Paul Ramsey suggests, we may have arrived at a time when we have achieved an unspeakable thing: a medical profession without a moral philosophy in a society without one either. Medicine, of course, still seems to carry the marks of a profession inasmuch as it seems to be a guardian of certain values—that is, the unconditional commitment to preserve life and health; the responsibility for justifying the patient's trust in the physician; and the autonomy of the physician in making judgments on others in the profession. But, as Alasdair MacIntyre has argued, these assumed virtues can quickly be turned to vices when they lack a scheme, or, in my language, a story that depends on further beliefs about the true nature of man and our true end.[6] But such a scheme is exactly what we lack, and it will not be supplied by trying to determine who is and is not a "person."

The language of "person" seems convenient to us, however, because we wish to assume that our medicine still rests on a consensus of moral beliefs. But I am suggesting that is exactly what is not the case and, in the absence of such a consensus, we will be much better off to simply admit that morally there are many different ways to practice medicine. We should, in other words, be willing to have our medicine as fragmented as our moral lives. I take this to be particularly important for Christians and Jews, as we have been under the illusion that we could morally expect medicine to embody our own standards, or, at least, standards that we could sympathize with. I suspect, however, that this may not be the case, for the story that determines how the virtues of medicine are to be displayed for us is quite different from the one claimed by the language of "person."[7] It may be then, if we are to be honest, that we should again think of the possibility of what it might mean to practice medicine befitting our convictions as Christians or Jews. Yet, there is a heavy price to be paid for the development of such a medical practice, as it may well involve training and going to doctors whose technology is less able to cure and sustain us than current medicine provides. But, then, we must decide what is more valuable, our survival or how we choose to survive.

Notes

1. Paul Ramsey, *The Patient as Person* (New Haven: Yale University Press, 1970).

2. For a more extended analysis of this point, see my *Vision and Virtue: Essays in Christian Ethical Reflection* (Notre Dame, Ind.: Fides Press, 1974).

3. Joseph Fletcher, "Indicators of Humanhood," *Hastings Center Report,* November, 1972, pp. 1-3; also see my response in "The Retarded and the Criteria of Human," *Linacre Quarterly,* November, 1973, pp. 217-22.

4. Michael Tooley, "A Defense of Abortion and Infanticide," in Joel Feinberg (ed.), *The Problem of Abortion* (Belmont: Wadsworth Publishing Co., 1973), pp. 51-91.

5. For an extended analysis of these issues, see my "The Demands and Limits of Care: Ethical Reflections on the Moral Dilemma of Neonatal Intensive Care," *American Journal of Medical Science,* March-April, 1975, pp. 269-91.

6. Alasdair MacIntyre, "How Virtues Become Vices: Values, Medicine and Social Context," *Evaluation and Explanation in the Biomedical Sciences* (Dordrecht: Reidel, 1975), pp. 97-111.

7. For I would not deny that advocates of "person," or the regulatory notion of medical care, are right to assume that the notion of person involves the basic libertarian values of our society. It is my claim that such values are not adequate to direct medicine in a humane and/or Christian manner.

46. Man as Patient

ROBERT JENSON

I

Man-as-patient, man as the physician professionally sees him, is an image with at least two sides. One side is determined by the physician's role as a technician of the behavioral sciences, the other by his role as a man dealing with his fellowmen. Let us begin by considering each side separately.

The patient lies—or stands, or sits—before the physician as a complex and malfunctioning system which the physician is called on—perhaps by the patient himself, perhaps not—to repair. In this respect, the physician's situation with respect to the patient is not decisively different from that of a systems engineer working on a rocket's malfunctioning fuel valves; indeed, the parts may well be spread out on a table in very similar fashion. It is important to note here that the physician's recognition of the moral and religious involvement of his patient, as factors which must be dealt with and supported for their health-giving value, does not transcend this picture. The physician is a technician of all the behavioral sciences, which include psychology and sociology. From the therapeutic point of view, recognition of "the whole man" complete with "inner man" is merely recognition of certain subsystems besides the chemical and organic subsystems. These subsystems, too, may need repair, or may be utilized as supporting mechanisms for repair of other subsystems.

As a consequence, the patient, as his title indicates, is notably passive. The understanding on both sides is that the physician will do the thinking and the patient will obey. The good patient is precisely the one who behaves in accordance with this understanding. Indeed, the patient has in all probability "gone to the doctor" on purpose to be relieved of his responsibility: One "calls the doctor" at just those points in life where we formerly "called on the gods." Textbooks on the subject quite properly, therefore, speak of "patient management." The patient has abdicated just that active determination of his affairs which

From *Studies in Man, Medicine and Theology,* vol. 1, *Man, Medicine and Theology.* Division for Mission in North America, Lutheran Church in America, 1967. Used by permission.

might otherwise make "management" an inappropriate word.

Thus man-as-patient is *manipulated* and *manipulable* man. Nor should this be taken too spiritually; the sheer physical and psychological manipulation to which the patient is subjected is of great importance to his situation. Man-as-patient—his guts, his genitalia, his fears, values and convictions, the wax in his ears—is suddenly bereft of all personal mystery. The patient must very really abandon himself to the physician in order to become a patient at all. There is, of course, a certain amount of ritual here which functions to save face for the patient: The physician's decrees are "medical *advice*" and the patient is always free to "call in another man" (as we always were to try another god). Such face-saving is needed because the relation of doctor and patient is also a *personal* relation. We turn next to this other side of the matter.

Despite the depersonalizing tendency of the patient's situation, the physician inescapably sees in the patient a man like himself. Indeed, it is precisely because the doctor sees in the patient a man in need of help that he exercises his technique on him. Their relation is a *human* relation. It may even become the "doctor-patient" relation, which, as the profession is well aware, can be explosively and even magically intimate. Even when the relation is much less than this, it is almost always sufficiently personal that the physician can never see the patient *only* as a reparable, manipulable object. Yesterday the patient was the physician's golf partner; tomorrow—both hope—he will be again. And even if the patient is a total stranger, he could have been a friend and may yet become one.

Is there any conflict between these two sides of the image of man-as-patient? Many physicians seem to believe that a clash does exist. Indeed, the medical profession seems sometimes to have a bad conscience about its inability to reconcile the conflict it feels here (or perhaps it has a bad conscience about *not* feeling any conflict where it supposes that it ought to). Issue after issue of the journals, whose substantive articles discuss the patient solely as a malfunctioning system, include editorials or more philosophical pieces lamenting a felt loss of "the human element" in medical practice and decrying an alleged tendency to practice medicine "merely" as a technology. This literature contrasts "technique" with "medical wisdom;" the "science" with the "art" of medicine. "Humanitarianism," it is said, "is failing to keep pace with the advancement of medical science." Young doctors are exhorted, in slightly despairing tones, to approach the patient as a "person" rather than as a "case." Medicine suffers or—what comes to the same—thinks it suffers from a split in its image of man.

Yet, just as clear as the split is the presence of all the genuine humanity one could wish in actual discussions even of "patient management." In his practice, the physician somehow bridges the chasm which alarms him when he considers it abstractly.

This gives us the direction our further investigation of man-as-patient must take. Further understanding of the image of man-as-patient will be achieved by finding the origin of the apparent incoherence of the image. What *exactly* is there about seeing the patient as a manipulable object to be repaired which may seem to make it hard to see him as a *fellow?*

II

The first side of our preliminary evocation of man-as-patient reflects the physician's role as a technician of the biological and behavioral sciences, applying these sciences to the control of a particular part of nature. It reflects, therefore, the attitude toward nature which is intrinsic to technology, which one adopts in taking up the technological enterprise. It reflects this viewpoint on nature in the form of an image of man because man is the part of nature on which the physician exercises his technique.[1] There are several different ways of getting at the way in which medical technology leads to a particular image of man and in which this image may conflict with at least the traditional form of the image of man as a *fellow* man. We will single out four (A–D following).

A

Medical technique is as old as the human race. But medical technique *as* a part of modern technology is part of something new in human history. Modern technology is new in that the knowledge by which it controls nature is a new kind of knowledge, the kind we call "science."

Scientific knowledge is knowledge wrought in the teeth of observation. Where the observed course of events does not correspond to the predictions made following a particular hypothesis, the hypothesis is altered. This principle may now seem obvious enough, but its consistent application is radically new in human culture and still achieved only by a tiny elite and by them only occasionally.

This radical procedure means that the prescriptions for the control of nature which the technologist draws from science are not like the magician's—the magician is the technologist of pre-scientific culture. The technologist's formulas actually work. If they do not they are withdrawn and replaced by others that will—unlike those of magic, to which success seems ultimately irrelevant.

Scientific technology, therefore, is successful technology. In addition, its success accelerates. Scientific knowledge is continuously self-correcting and so provides an ever-broadening base for its own progress and for the power of the technology based upon it.

Moreover, scientific knowledge is general. It does not suppose that the heavenly bodies are to be approached differently from the rocks on the shore, nor that a man is to be approached differently from an amoeba. This is so because science makes the wager of asserting propositions of the form "*Whenever* A, then B" or "In one hundred cases of A, eighty-five cases of B." Such propositions are overthrown by just one valid instance of A without B, or by one series of tests with a significant deviation from the predicted percentage of B's. Science makes this wager and seems to be winning it.

Thus scientific technology is universal technology. No part of reality is in principle exempt from the control it gives us. No awe holds back the technologist from proposing to establish mines on the moon. No barrier other than the reluctance of the proposed subjects stops us from breeding new varieties of men as we do of dogs.

The result of our technology's practicality and universality is that through it we do acquire vast control over nature. Our technology actually does transform the world and create for its masters a new image of nature. It creates a nature in the image of its informing spirit, in the image of the scientific ideal.

Science sees nature in the pattern "*Whenever* A, then B." Technology produces an image of nature which really conforms to this pattern. The nature transformed by technology is, therefore, a nature *without exceptions,* or with only predictable exceptions, which are thus no exceptions at all. Whatever is true of this nature is true of all of it.

It is precisely by the technological endeavor of the physician that *man* is incorporated into the technological image of nature. By the physician's taking up the technological enterprise with respect to man, man-as-patient becomes a part of that nature which brooks no exceptions. The language here is "In respect of . . . man is just like . . . "

But our traditional understanding of man has based its special regard for him on the conviction of his *exceptionality;* on the conviction that there is inherent in man's nature something which makes him radically different from all other creatures. (The dispute as to what that something might be need not concern us here.) We have believed men worthy of love and hate and fidelity, of all the personal bonds which we do not make with sticks or stones, because we have seen them as a different and "higher" kind of being. But man-as-patient is *defined* as *no exception.*

B

Technology, we have said, creates a version of nature after the pattern of the scientific ideal, after the pattern "Whenever A, then B." Now the practical translation of "Whenever A, then B" is "Whenever I do A, B will also happen." Technologized nature is nature which responds in this way to my orders. It is nature in which if I do A, B will follow; if I do C, D will follow; and in which the choice of doing A or C is my choice or someone else's. Technologized nature is manipulable nature.

Manipulable nature is radically demythologized nature. Pre-technological man lived in a nature whose forces and regularities controlled his destiny and set the pattern of his life. Therefore pre-technological man saw these forces as divine, and regarded those natural events in which they especially impinged on his life as revelations in which deity addressed him in reproach or promise. Water, air, the heavenly bodies—all were gods or demons. For technological man, the gods and demons are gone from nature, because he sees the powers of nature not as controlling him but as actually or potentially controlled by him. Consider, for example, a flood. To pre-technological man it is a revelation of God's wrath. Technological man is, to be sure, as dead as any primitive if the waters close over him, and he may fear them just as intensely. But he does not find a revelation from above in the flood. He finds, rather, proof that the authorities have neglected to perform the "A" which would have prevented it and a reminder to vote for repair of this deficiency if he survives.

In technologized nature there are no divinities, no supernatural beings. The labors of the physician incorporate man into technologized nature. Thereby man is bereft of any claim to divinity. But that is the problem. For our traditional understanding of man has based the possibility of an attitude toward man appropriate only to him on his incipient divinity. "The spark of God in every man" has been the legitimation of our love and honor and fear for each other. Technologized man, here man-as-patient, has no such spark.

C

Traditionally, western man has found God "in the gaps." That is, we have introduced him as the explanation of those events in our experience which we could not otherwise explain, called on him for help in those situations where we could no longer help ourselves, and asked his mercy on the occasions when our morality lapsed. (The utterly unchristian character of this concept of God "in the gaps" is not our present concern.) Our life and world have been conceived of as fundamentally self-contained systems, suffering however from some gaps in the usually smooth series of cause and effect: the inexplicable recovery of an apparently doomed sufferer; the hopeless and undeserved financial crisis of a good man; the sudden failure of my normally good intentions. The traditional God of our society operates in exactly those gaps. He is the watchmaker who made and started the natural and historical processes in the first place and now from time to time intervenes with a miracle to keep the mechanism going on the occasions when it cannot keep going by itself.

The scientific and technological enterprises are inherently an assault upon the "God-in-the-gaps." For the whole point of these enterprises is the attempt to eliminate the gaps: to discover explanations for those events in our experience which we do not yet understand, and to extend our control to those circumstances of our lives not yet subject to our will. Science and technology simply are the labor of walling up God's erstwhile homes in the "gaps." It is, of course, well known that for every mystery which science clears up, it discovers ten others, and for every force of nature which technology tames, others yet more powerful are set loose. There are, and no doubt will be, plenty of gaps in our world. But it is the *attitude toward them* which one adopts in taking up the scientific and technological enterprises that is important. To do science *is* to see an unexplained event not as a mystery to be adored but as a puzzle to be solved. To do technology *is* to see the occurrences before which we are helpless not as fates to be pacified but as challenges to ingenuity. Involvement in these enterprises *is* a declaration of unbelief in the God-in-the-gaps and an installing of ourselves, with our intelligence and strength, in his place.

To the concept of God-in-the-gaps corresponded a concept of nature as inherently *gapped,* as, so to speak, fitted out with receptacles to receive God. As part of such a nature, man was thought of as having certain areas of his existence, such as sickness or moral crisis, where openness to God was built into him. The way one put this was to speak of man's "immortal soul." Moreover, man's openness to *man* was understood as part of his openness to God; man's openness to any other-than-he was conceived of as a function of his openness to *the* Other-than-he. It was thought of as a function of the "soul." Thus it, too, was *located* in man's nature, in, that is, the gaps in his nature.

Since man-as-patient is an image evoked, in part at least, by taking up the scientific and technological enterprises of gap-closing, man-as-patient lacks the built-in openness to God and other men on which we have traditionally relied as the basis of distinctive relations between men. We may say exactly the same thing this way: Traditional esteem for and love of man was esteem for man's supposedly built-in religiosity, his "immortal soul." Man-as-patient, like technologized man generally, lacks this organ.

D

Man-as-patient adopts this role by claiming to be sick, or in danger of becoming sick. The physician is, therefore, compelled to differentiate constantly between sick men and well men; even the physician who dislikes the distinction makes it all the time as he sends one man to the hospital and the other home, tries to inhibit one growth process and promote another. Thus man-as-patient always diverges somehow from what man *ought* to be. For "illness," after all, can only mean "a characteristic of a certain man which that man's physician and he can try to alter and are determined to alter," and "health" can only mean "a characteristic of a certain man which he and his physician are content to leave." The analogy between the way in which a characteristic is determined to be a "fault" and the way in which another characteristic is determined to be an "illness" is obvious and close. Both determinations are *evaluations.* Man-as-patient is, therefore, defined by reference to a partial *ideal* of what man, in certain respects, *should* be like.

As an example, let us consider the case of a man with a stomach-ache which, after all due tests, proves to have "no organic basis." In these psychosomatic days consultations continue. In their course, the patient gives the physician to understand—without of course admitting that he does so—that he needs and wants his stomach-ache. Calling such a stomach-ache "illness" is not a matter of straightforward empirical labelling like calling an artifact in which one can sit a "chair." That it is an *evaluation* is shown by the position in which the physician now finds himself. He may let the patient continue with his stomach-ache, thus accepting that whether this condition is to be alleviated or not lies in the patient's free evaluating choice. Or he may set about to persuade the patient that his symptom is a "crutch" on which he *ought* not rely. Either way we find ourselves in the realm of values. Or to take an example from the other side, no twelfth-century doctor would have *wanted* to cure the ulcerative phenomena of the stigmatics—it would not even have occurred to him that these were the *kind* of thing one might set out to cure or not cure. The diagnostic handbooks are in fact codes of values.

Where does the physician get the standards by which

he makes such evaluations? One can of course say that he uses the standards of his society, that he tries to cure whatever in his society is commonly regarded as illness. But this answer is incomplete. For the physician himself is a major influence in society's decision at this point. It often happens that the medical profession educates the public to regard as illness conditions formerly seen as "natural."

The tests do, of course, seem obvious enough: *Pain* is to be alleviated. *Disablement* is to be prevented or mitigated. Processes which would lead to the *death* of the patient are to be halted or slowed. Yet men in other cultures have sought pain and disablement as virtues and death as the fulfillment of life. That these are characteristics of life to be fought against is apparently not a self-evident universal truth. The comfortable, able and long-lived man is *one particular* ideal of man. Where does it come from? I suggest that it has been drawn from behavioral science's description of organic life: In all sufficiently complex organisms, pain is a stimulus to such activity as will, if successful, effect the cessation of the pain. All organisms seek maximum adaptation to their environments. And all organisms avoid and resist threats to the continuance of life. The picture of what man-as-patient ought to be is given by taking this *description* and making of it a *norm.*

It is inevitable that physicians will use behavioral science's description of man in this normative way. As the enterprise of forming hypotheses subject solely to confirmation or disconfirmation by the facts, science inherently avoids all moral or aesthetic judgment. Insofar, therefore, as medicine is a scientific technology, the physician must refrain in his work from moral or aesthetic evaluation. Yet evaluate he must. Where is he to turn for standards by which to evaluate? It must be remembered that we are not now speaking of the physician's own moral decisions with respect to the patient—here his resources are the same as anyone else's. (Though his problems are not. Bringing resources and problems together is the main task of these studies.) We are speaking of his evaluation of which characteristics of the patient are to be promoted and which inhibited by the exercise of his medical technique. The physician's obvious recourse is to turn to what is said about man by the science on which his technique is based and to treat this description as normative.

Making descriptions into norms is regular procedure in our culture. Wherever it is done, it amounts to a declaration that man as nature provides him is as he ought to be. Such a naturalistic ethos can be and often is noble and fine. But its picture of man excludes any sign of a need for man to become radically different from what he is; it excludes any sign of a need for man to rise above himself, to seek his true self in the future. So here: Man-as-patient rests complete in what he already is. But traditionally we have based our love for man exactly on what we *hoped* for from him.

III

In sum, taking up the technological enterprise with men as the objects, means renouncing the traditional basis for *understanding* why we shall have specifically personal bonds with each other. This is the reason why some feel an incongruity between two sides of the image of man-as-patient. It must be strongly emphasized that adopting the technological attitude toward a man does *not* make it impossible in fact to see and treat him as a fellow—this is proven by many physicians' notable success at doing both. But it does destroy the *image* of man-as-fellow which the tradition of our society provides us. The technological attitude renders implausible the *doctrine* that man, by reason of a reference beyond himself which is part of his very nature, is uniquely related to the divine and so is an exceptional kind of being to whom exceptional attitudes are appropriate—the doctrine by which our tradition has *understood* man as a fellow-man. So long as the image by which we see other men as our fellows is that provided by the tradition of our society, the total image of man-as-patient is incoherent. Whether this is bad or not depends on how important consistency is. Most physicians—like the rest of us—can doubtless continue their humane and concerned relation with their patients whether or not they have a rationale for doing this that is consistent with their other commitments. And yet it seems likely that sooner or later a crisis will occur.

What are the options? How can this incoherence be resolved, or, at least, lived with? An obvious and presumably much practiced option is strict compartmentalization. With one eye, the physician looks at the patient as the object of his technique. With the other eye, he sees in the patient the fellow-man of our traditional doctrines, the fellow-man whom he may serve and by whom he may be morally and spiritually enriched. And he simply refuses to worry about any possible incongruity. Despite the intended derogatory connotation of "compartmentalization," the short-range beneficence of this method should not be denied. Absolute consistency of attitudes is not possible anyway. And sometimes the cost of seeking it may be too high.

One way in which consistency could be purchased would be by denying the fellow-man side of the image of man-as-patient. The disaster here is not that the physician would thereby turn himself into a straight-out engineer—being an engineer is a fine thing. The disaster is that since the physician *cannot* cease to have men as his objects, he can take this option only by directly denying that his patients personally concern him: *i.e.,* by explicitly denying them special human worth. That this nihilist solution is possible, and what its practical consequences might be, has been demonstrated in the concentration camps of Nazi Germany.

The opposite way in which consistency could be purchased would be by ignoring the scientific origin of medical technique, by merely using the material results of scientific investigation without inner participation in the activity by which they are obtained. Just so the magician used poppy-juice to put people to sleep without knowing why it did so. Instead of a structure of testable theory, the magician had a structure of dreaming associations within which he "understood" the efficacy of the poppy. So also the physician could perhaps dissociate himself from the genuine scientific spirit and work within some other, specifically moral and spiritual, framework of ideas, probably that of a political ideology. We can only imagine the pompous mumbo-jumbo which would result—and shudder.

There is another option. The physician may accept all sides of the image of man which his work evokes for him, accept them with their consequences—and *stand up to* the problem they pose. He may work with and for men who show no signs of being exceptions to the principles which describe the actions and relations of things in general, in whom he can find no spark of divinity nor built-in opening to God; yet who *nevertheless* demand to be lived for as would be appropriate to no other beings; who *nevertheless* in challenge and promise open to him the possibility of rising above what they and he are to a final mutual fulfillment of their life and his. What is special *in* man? Nothing, such a courageous physician will tell us—and yet he is to be confronted in an entirely special way. Is man divine? No, he will say—and yet in the commands and beseechings of my brother I am addressed by God. Does man open to a more perfect life beyond him? Not visibly—and yet one must set no limits to one's hopes for him. In sum, that men are unique and directed to some goal beyond themselves is not given in any factor *in their nature*—and yet we are to live with them in the faith that they are so directed.

The physician who from his special confrontation with his fellows, his confrontation with them as *patients,* spoke *so,* would speak an eminently sane and healing word. The great threat to a technological civilization is that men may become increasingly obscured from each other in their uniqueness as men. The cure is *not* retreat from or dilution of the technological enterprise. The cure is absolute clarity about and courage before the image of man evoked by the technological enterprise and before the question the image puts to us. Perhaps the physician, the man-technologist, is called to lead us to this clarity.

The question which our technological civilization calls us to stand up to is: How will you men live humanely *for* each other, without the illusion that in each other you meet semi-divinities or immortal souls? Perhaps the physician is the one specifically called to hear this question and speak it to the rest of us.

The believer is glad to hear this question. For the Christian proclamation shows man as a *creature; i.e.,* as one who in himself, in what he is and has, has no special hope beyond himself. But the Christian proclamation also shows man as one who nevertheless does live by what is beyond himself and by his own future possibility; who does this not by what he is in himself but *because God has addressed and addresses him,* because God has *spoken* to him and called him out of what he is and has in himself. To the question posed by the image of man-as-patient: Wherein is man special, if not in his nature? faith replies: Man is special and the appropriate partner of special, personal, relations not because of anything he is, but because of something that others than he—God and, thereupon, his fellows—have done and do to him, because they speak to him, address him. Because from outside him they call to him to *become* in some way different from what he is; they call him to a future goal beyond himself.

One more specification must be made. The *address* we are speaking of is in no way some sort of wordless or mystic speech. It is what traditional theology has called the "Law" and the "Gospel." The Law is the commands and promises with which our societies fill our ears and call us to be different from what we are (*i.e.,* call us forward into the future); the Gospel is the story which one human tells another about Jesus of Nazareth. And since the address we are speaking of is both the Law and the Gospel, it is by no means only those who hear the specifically Christian story—the Gospel—who are so addressed. By the "Law" we mean *all* the addresses which men make to each other; we call them "Law" because of the way in which all our speech to each other *obligates* us when we hear, and because of Christian faith's conviction that all our obligations are obligations to God. If it is being addressed by God which opens us up to each other, then the possibility and reality of actual humane behavior to each other is not at all limited to believers; for all men are in fact addressed by God.

Indeed, the voice of science itself, the obligating address of the scientific community to each of its members as the work of research goes on, is Law, God's Law, for those who belong to this community. It is not merely that there is no conflict between involvement in the scientific and technological enterprise and being fellow-men to each other; involvement in the scientific enterprise can be itself the address which opens us and makes such personal existence possible. It may well be that a new humane ethos is arising from the very work of science and technology itself, if the humane involvement of those taken up in scientific-technological work can survive the loss of the old doctrines of *why* we should be fellow-men to each other. To these old doctrines—to the traditional image of the fellow-man—scientific technology is indeed fatal. It will be necessary either simply to *be* fellow-men to each other without any image by which to apprehend and understand each other as fellows, or to find that apprehension and understanding in some radically different way than we have traditionally done. I say "radically different" because it would be disastrous if we should simply invent some "scientific" substitute for the traditional doctrine of man. Attempts, for example, to use the uncertainty principle as the basis for a new exaltation of the "subject" are to be viewed with suspicion. For the "observer" with whom the uncertainty principle says we must reckon and the "fellow-men" whom I and my fellows are called to be to each other, are not the same at all, and pretending they are must pervert either the work of science or our human fellowship.

Whether or not, or for how long, it will be possible to live with and for each other as fellows without any doctrine of why we should do so, and without taking to pseudo-scientific ersatz doctrines of man's worth, is a point which it is wiser not to predict. But, to repeat, the believer is glad to hear the question posed by the technological enterprise. For the *knowledge* that—as opposed to the fact that—all men are addressed by God in the Law and that it is this that makes me and my fellow open to each other in a special way, is one of the benefits of that other more particular address of God by which faith lives, the Gospel. The situation of being called to live for my fellows without knowing why is one to which the Gospel can have something to say. And the temptation to cling to the traditional doctrine of man even after we can no longer wholly credit it, or to invent phony substitutes for it, is one from which the knowledge given by the Gospel can save us.

IV

The physician is the technologist who *cannot* be rid of men in all their humanity. Perhaps, therefore, he is the one called to make us fully understand what our technological civilization means for our vision of each other. Understanding this may be just what believers need if we are to see in man what the Gospel wants to point us to—see this clearly and in a way appropriate to our time and culture. The image of man-as-patient may be a hidden pivot of the present epoch in the history of the Gospel and in the history of our culture. If it is, the believing physician will play a decisive role both in his church and in his profession.

Note

1. I use the term "part" because the physician's concern is not delimited by the boundaries of a *discipline.* The physician will use the results of, and if he is a research physician may himself pursue, any of the sciences that offer promise of help to his enterprise. His concern is delimited as concern for a *part* of nature in the most ordinary-language sense of "part."

47. The Basis of Medicine and Religion: Respect for Persons

DAVID C. THOMASMA

On the whole, the present age has lost respect for human life. Literature, music, and art reflect the fact that life is under assault. It is no wonder that mere survival is considered an exalted achievement in these times when human life can be ended before birth by being salinated in the mother's womb or can be born nutritionally brain-damaged and suffer from starvation, food additives, and a polluted environment. Even when human life survives all these assaults, it can be snuffed out in one of a hundred wars which break out all over the earth.

Against this admittedly negative scenario, the medical profession bravely asserts its commitment to respect human persons. Apart from religious organizations, the profession of healing is one of the few effective international forces fostering the dignity and value of individual human beings. But because of its commitment to human life, healing, too, is under assault.

Within the profession, evidence exists of practices for economic gain, destruction of human dignity, and attacks on life. The profession also is under pressure from external sources to fulfill social aims for which it is ill-equipped[1] or to fulfill political purposes, such as the torture of prisoners, for which its commitments demand profound antipathy. Given these anti-life forces, it is all the more important that the healing profession renew its commitment to affirm the value of human life.

A close examination of the role of humanism in patient care reveals not only how current health professionals affirm this value, but also how religious-sponsored health care can develop its goals and values in the future. There is no need to retreat into the past; rather, health care leaders must continue to show courage and wisdom in implementing their convictions. This article will explore three generalizations about humanism in patient care: (1) that respect for persons is a guiding motive of both religion and the healing profession; (2) that ethical norms for the healing profession result from respect for persons; and (3) that religious affirmation can strengthen these ethical norms. This last point will emphasize the Catholic tradition.

The struggle for individual autonomy and recognition has been a long and hard one, and it is not yet completed. Both religion and medicine contain the seeds of that struggle, and both have played a major role in whatever success each has achieved. Religion and the profession of healing share the premise that human life is at once fragile and perfectible. Growth in virtue and health requires awareness of life's finitude and perfectibility and, at the same time, demands an affirmation that happiness and well-being are ideal aims for individuals. Such growth rests upon the altruistic assumption that human beings can help each other to improve. It is significant to note that the earliest priests were also medicine men.

The effects of virtue and health, happiness and well-being were virtually indistinguishable for all but the past 2,000 years, a relatively short part of the human lifespan. Respect for persons is a natural byproduct of the aims of happiness and well-being which are intrinsic to religion and the profession of healing. Respect for persons ascends the ladder of values as both religion and medicine concentrate on the individual.

As long as religion and medicine were both embodied in the person of the medicine man, their social and community aims were indistinguishable. For example, the Babylonians considered illness to be a direct consequence of sin, and healing included a confession of sins and infractions against community mores. But as early as 1500 B.C. Hindu physicians took an oath remarkably like the later Hippocratic Oath in which respect for individual persons was coupled with a real sense of a profession, that is, a public commitment to care for individuals regardless of public mores.[2] Later, in Egypt and Greece the medical profession became sufficiently secure to divorce itself from religious aims. This action led the healing profession to concentrate on its moral commitments to individuals. The Hippocratic Oath clearly reveals this principle of individuation in its solemn promise not to harm the patient to whom one has professional obligations of care, confidentiality, and personal respect.[3]

The growth of respect for persons in religion was also linked to a principle of individuation, although its genesis was different. While anthropologists argue that a common feature of all religions was the respect for the members of one's own tribe, universal respect for persons not in one's tribe or nation was long in coming. The theological movements of greatest import included the rise of universalism, demands for justice,

Reprinted with permission from *Linacre Quarterly,* vol. 47 (May 1984), pp. 142-50. 850 Elm Grove Road, Elm Grove, WI 53122. Subscription rate: $20 per year; $5 per single issue.

and the distinction between creation and redemption concomitant with the emergence of the prophetic movement around 500 B.C.[4]

At the heart of prophetic universalism is the belief that the Creator made all human beings and called all to redemption. Exclusivism and tribal loyalties are not compatible with this conviction, and they were replaced with a belief in the inherent value of individuals which demands respect for all human persons. The growth of Christianity combined this vision with the Roman Empire's stoic view of natural rights.

Thus, professionalism in medicine coupled with the supranatural universalism of religion led to the principle of individuation; the value of respect for persons was firmly intrenched, even though actual behavior often was less than altruistic.

Painting cultural progress in such broad strokes can be dangerous. Nevertheless, the picture painted above is relatively complete. Pedro Lain-Entralgo, in his excellent book *Doctor and Patient,* describes this relationship throughout history.[5] Although the rationale for the obligations in the relationship differs in Greek, Christian, and contemporary times, respect for individual persons underpins the relationship throughout these historical eras.[6] Similarly, respect for persons is at the heart of Judeo-Christian morality, which regards every human being as a child of God called to redemption.

Given this rich religious heritage, it is not surprising that Western political and philosophical thought underscores this same respect for persons. Each individual is regarded as having endowed rights that no individual or government can rescind. In addition to the philosophical movement which emphasized this theory of individual rights, moral philosophers have also highlighted this conviction. Kant held that persons should be treated, not as mere means, but as ends in themselves.[7] John Stuart Mill in *On Liberty* argued that the freedom of persons could not be infringed upon unless they were a danger to others or could not apprehend the negative consequences of their actions on others.[8]

Norms for the Healing Profession

The principle of respect for persons offers norms of moral activity for the healing profession. Such respect is at the root of current guidelines on research and functions as the basis for clinical medicine. Of course, it continues to inform the ethical codes of the healing professions as well. Although this article is limited to an examination of the medical research guidelines and to reflections on clinical medicine, the norms which emerge from these reflections could lead to a rejuvenated code of ethics for the healing profession, a task which is outside the scope of this article.[9]

The Department of Health, Education, and Welfare (HEW) guidelines for human participation in medical research are based on the principle of the rights of subjects as human beings. Basic to the procedures following from this principle is the need for informed consent.[10] The requirement of informed consent is based on the conviction that persons are autonomous beings who, if their autonomy is diminished for some reason, must be protected. Thus respect for persons entails two ethical guidelines: "the requirement to acknowledge autonomy and the requirement to protect those with diminished autonomy."[11]

As the *Belmont Report* of the National Commission for the Protection of Human Subjects points out, respect for persons also entails a medical obligation to promote their well-being.[12] Hence, in addition to obtaining informed consent, medical research must compare risks and benefits to individual participants and must attempt, in scientific design, to maximize the benefit and minimize possible harm. Finally, respect for persons entails a principle of justice that demands that persons be treated fairly, without undue burdens. Thus, to perform all hypertension research only on poor black persons for the benefit of the whole population places an unjust burden on them as a class and diminishes their personal integrity.

Respect for persons leads to moral obligations in the healing profession. The following norms for medical research flow from this principle:

1. *To recognize the autonomy of persons.* This norm rests not only on the principle of liberty proposed by Mill but also on the medical obligation to treat individuals as free agents so that they can be full partners in the research. The relationship of subject and researcher is promoted as a true human relationship.[13]

2. *To protect persons whose autonomy is impaired.* This norm is not simply a sequel to informed consent but follows as a professional obligation. It would be inappropriate to attempt to heal people while simultaneously diminishing their autonomy or taking advantage of their lack of it.

3. *To promote the well-being of persons.* This norm follows directly from the beneficent aim of medicine, i.e., the healing profession's obligation to benefit people exceeds the demands of justice. Caring for whole persons is a real professional obligation.

4. *To treat each person fairly.* This is a minimal norm of medical research. At the very least, healing requires that the person cannot be used for an experiment to benefit others unless the person also derives

some benefit as an individual or as a member of a class.

Norms for Clinical Practice

These norms for medical research can be better understood by comparing them to similar norms for clinical medical practice. Apparently, many persons consent to research—even research that does not benefit them—in which the norms buttressing their individuality are not adequately applied. In studying the practical effects of the HEW guidelines, researchers found that most subjects tolerated lack of information and freedom in consent precisely because they did not want to impair their physician-patient relationship.[14] In other words, this clinical bond is so important and so primary that patients will suffer diminished personal autonomy and respect to maintain it.

Why is this clinical bond so important and what does its existence reveal about respect for persons? The clinical bond between the patient and the healing profession is based on a primary value: health. Persons who are healthy rank other values ahead of health. They see health, as have many philosophers from Aristotle to Dewey, as a condition for freedom and autonomy.[15] When persons become sick, however, they often rate health at the top of their list of values and rate other values, such as freedom and autonomy, secondary to the aim of healing.

Thus, when physicians and staff view persons only as patients, the sick individual suffers from both a diminished state of health and a diminished sense of autonomy. These individuals find themselves in an imbalanced relationship of almost childlike dependency on the healing profession. This feeling of dependency is perhaps the most irksome aspect of admission to a hospital.

The aim of the clinical bond between the patient and the healing profession is to restore health. This value is ranked highest in the patient's priorities and is affirmed by the healing profession. Professional obligations follow from this primary goal.

Clearly, respect for persons would be negated if treatment resulted in harm rather than healing. For this reason, the most ancient norm of medicine, expressed in the Hindu Oath and the Hippocratic Oath, is *primum non nocere* ("first of all, do no harm").[16] This norm is essentially beneficent. The health professional's obligation is primarily to the patient, even though other values of society may impinge on the clinical relationship. The clinical bond is so strong a relationship of obligation that Paul Ramsey calls it a canon or covenant of loyalty to distinguish its human faithfulness from lesser legal, contracted obligations.[17]

Two additional norms for clinical medicine also follow from the nature of the clinical bond.[18] The first of these is to respect the imbalanced relationship itself. The healing profession not only must fulfill its obligation to heal but also must recognize and help to restore those aspects which diminish the patient's personhood in the physician-patient relationship. Since the patient is no longer a fully autonomous and knowledgeable partner in this imbalanced relationship, the patient is in a diminished state as a person. Obligations inherent in such an imbalanced relationship include revealing the truth, supplying sufficient information for free decisions, and respecting the patient's right to refuse treatment.

The third norm of the clinical relationship is to treat each person as a class instance of the human race. This is really an obligation of justice. Since sick persons have an imbalanced relationship with the healing profession, promoting their well-being implies that all persons be treated equitably regardless of social standing and custom. The poor should receive the same care as the rich, blacks the same as whites, the aged the same as the young.

Respect for persons, then, is the guiding principle for the healing profession, in both research and clinical medicine. This respect is tailored to and modified by the healing relationship essential to medicine, from which its professional obligations flow.

Beyond Professionalism: Religion and Medicine

The previous section explained how respect for persons establishes professional obligations. This final section will discuss ways in which religious commitments reinforce professional obligations.

If respect for persons is the guiding motive of the healing profession, then medicine practiced for religious reasons can only strengthen this obligation. What medicine regards as professional obligations, religion views as human obligations. And it is this difference in viewpoints that constitutes any difference between professional and human obligations.

From a religious perspective, the respect due a human being arises from the fact that individuals are created by God and called to His salvation. No human person, regardless of how hopeless his or her life, can be abandoned. All persons are seen as sacramental, that is, extensions of God in human history. Each person is a created presence of God.

Hence the professional requirement to treat each

person as a class instance of the human race means that, from a religious perspective, beyond the professional requirement of justice is a loving requirement of faith. One loves the person, not only as person but as a presence of God. As Jesus said, "Whatever you do for the least of these, you do to me." Thus, to justice is added mercy. From a religious perspective, those who have been ill-treated by society or by national mores deserve even better care than those who have not. St. Augustine's theological definition of justice, "to each according to his need," means that those in greater need of care should have more available.

There is a second point about the class instance norm. Professional obligations of justice and fairness do not address the deeper need of human beings to be loved as individuals. People want to be loved for their singularity, not because they belong to the race. As W. H. Auden says in his poem "Sept. 1, 1939," there is an "error bred in the bones of each woman and each man." What is that error? A craving not to be loved universally "but to be loved alone." Religion does not consider this desire an "error." Persons are to be respected not only through equitable treatment but by individual love for the qualities they portray. Indeed, the well-being of patients is often impeded by a lack of this individualized compassion.[19]

Religious concern for the imbalance inherent in the physician-patient relationship also transcends professional obligations. Seneca explains the role of love in the clinical relationship:

> Why is it that I owe something more to my physician and my teacher, and yet do not complete the payment of what is due to them? Because from being physician and teacher they become friends, and we are under an obligation to them, not because of their skill, which they sell, but because of their kind and friendly goodwill.
>
> If, therefore, a physician does nothing more than feel my pulse and put me on the list of those whom he visits on his rounds, instructing me what to do and what to avoid without any personal feeling, I owe him nothing more than his fee, because he does not see me as a friend but as a client. . . .
>
> Why then are we so much indebted to these men? Not because what they have sold us is worth more than we paid for it, but because they have contributed something to us personally. A physician who gave me more attention than was necessary, because he was afraid for me, not for his professional reputation; who was not content to indicate remedies, but also applied them; who sat at my bedside among my anxious friends and hurried to me at times of crisis; for whom no service was too burdensome, none too distasteful to perform; who was indifferent to my moans; to whom, although a host of others sent for him, I was always his chief concern; who took time for the others only when my illness permitted him.
>
> Such a man has placed me under an obligation, not so much as a physician but as a friend.[20]

Finally, the professional obligation to do no harm can be strengthened by a religious perspective, which goes beyond mere physical health. From a religious perspective, the well-being of patients requires genuine love of the patient as a person. Greater sympathy with the common condition of humankind, attention to family relationships, and the virtues of kindness, mercy, and charity result. Other needs besides just the physical are addressed.

The contrast between professional obligations and their religious affirmation can be understood by comparing the ways in which the prayer of Maimonides, a Jewish physician and philosopher in the Middle Ages, differs from the Oath of Hippocrates. The Oath clearly states professional obligations to individuals. But the Prayer of Maimonides moves beyond this professionalism to a profound sense of common humanity under the Father, to the religious task of healing as a work of God, and to love as the bond with patients:

> I begin once more my daily work. Be Thou with me, Almighty, Father of Mercy, in all my efforts to heal the sick. For without thee, man is but a helpless creature. Grant that I may be filled with love for my art and for my fellow man. May the thirst for gain and the desire for fame be from my heart. For these are the enemies of Pity and the ministers of Hate. Grant that I may be able to devote myself body and soul to the children who suffer from pain.
>
> Preserve my strength, that I may be able to restore the strength of the rich and the poor, the good and the bad, the friend and the foe. Let me see in the sufferer the man alone. When wiser men teach me, let me be humble to learn; for the mind of man is so puny, and the art of healing is so vast. But when fools are ready to advise me or find fault with me, let me not listen to their folly. Let me be intent upon one thing, O Father of Mercy, to be always merciful to thy suffering children.
>
> May there never rise in me the notion that I know enough, but give me strength and leisure and zeal to enlarge my knowledge. Our work is great, and the mind of man presses forward forever.

> Thou hast chosen me in thy grace, to watch over the life and death of thy creatures. I am about to fulfill my duties. Guide me in this immense work so that it may be of avail.

The sacramental character of individual persons, then, reinforces the norms of the healing profession by introducing love as the primary reason for promoting the well-being of human beings.

A close examination of the role of humanism in patient care, particularly the requirements to respect persons, can lead to setting the future goals of religious-sponsored health care institutions. Among the goals and standards already proposed by The Catholic Health Association, several deserve special attention in light of respect for persons.[21] First is that a Catholic healing organization must be committed to healing, especially by respecting each person's autonomy and providing hope to the weary. Second, in light of the imbalanced relationship of healing, the Catholic hospital must place special emphasis on justice for and love of the patient by working for the well-being of whole persons, whatever their religious convictions. Finally, the requirement of treating each person as an embodiment of the human race means that economic and organizational efficiency, however important, must not interfere with providing better care for the disenfranchised.

Because God loves each individual, each person's life is sacred. Catholic health care institutions must take absolute care to affirm and foster this sacredness. For a religious hospital, healing means not only curing but extending God's love to His creatures.

Notes

1. See Ivan Illich, *Medical Nemesis* (New York: Bantam Books, 1977).

2. The oath of Hindu physicians.

3. The Hippocratic Oath.

4. This universalism was especially evident in Zoroastrianism and Judaism. Among Jewish prophets, Second Isaiah is generally regarded as the first to formulate a universalism based upon a theology of creation.

5. Pedro Lain-Entralgo, *Doctor and Patient* (New York: McGraw-Hill, 1969).

6. The Greek relationship was described as one of friendship, the Christian as one of love, and the contemporary as one of comradeship. All of these presuppose respect for persons.

7. Immanuel Kant, *Metaphysical Foundations of Morals,* ed. by C. J. Friedrich (New York: Modern Library Edition, 1965), pp. 140-187; R. S. Downie and Elizabeth Telfer, *Respect for Persons* (New York: Schocken, 1970), pp. 13-37. The authors argue that respect for persons in the Kantian formulation is the basic principle of all ethical theory.

8. John Stuart Mill, *On Liberty,* ed. by C. V. Shields (Indianapolis: Bobbs-Merrill, 1956), pp. 114 ff.

9. Edmund D. Pellegrino, M.D., describes a way in which a new code of morality for the professions may be developed from the norms for clinical practice, both in a book-length manuscript co-authored with me and entitled "A Philosophical Basis of Medical Practice," in preparation at Oxford University Press, and in his "Toward a Reconstruction of Medical Morality," *Journal of Medicine and Philosophy,* March, 1979, pp. 32-56.

10. Dept. of Health, Education and Welfare, "Protection of Human Subjects," *Federal Register,* May 30, 1974, pp. 18914-18920; Rev. Kevin O'Rourke, "Fetal Experimentation: An Evaluation of the New Federal Norms," *Hospital Progress,* Sept., 1975, pp. 60-69.

11. National Commission for the Protection of Human Subjects, *Belmont Report: Ethical Principles and Guidelines for the Protection of Human Subjects of Research,* DHEW Publication No. OS 78-0012 (Washington, D.C.: DHEW, 1978), pp. 4-5.

12. *Ibid.,* p. 6.

13. Alexander Capron, "Informed Consent in Catastrophic Disease Research and Treatment," reprinted in *Ethical Issues in Modern Medicine,* ed. by Hunt and Arras (Palo Alto, Calif.: Mayfield Publishing Co., 1977), pp. 253-264.

14. See, for example, a study on labor induction done by Bradford Gray and reported in his *Human Subjects in Medical Experimentation* (New York: Wiley, 1975), pp. 202-234.

15. Edmund D. Pellegrino, M.D., and I have tried to develop these norms for clinical practice from a philosophy of medical practice, a development differing from the one posed in this article.

16. Kudlein has illustrated how this norm was considered a general guideline for civic behavior during the Greek period. See "Medical Ethics and Popular Ethics in Greece and Rome," *Clio Medica,* 5, 1976, pp. 91-121. However, the use of this norm was part of the general context of *philia,* or friendship, prevailing as the explanation of the bond between physician and patient. See Lain-Entralgo, pp. 17-22.

17. Paul Ramsey, *The Patient as Person* (New Haven: Yale University Press, 1970), pp. 17-32.

18. These norms can also follow from a philosophy of medicine. See footnote 15.

19. To consider respect for persons as an end of human action, it is important to realize that a value is placed on persons for the qualities they portray. See Downie and Telfer, pp. 13-19.

20. Seneca, *De beneficiis,* VI, p. 16.

21. Catholic Health Association, The, *Evaluative Criteria for Catholic Health Care Facilities* (St. Louis: Catholic Health Assoc., 1979).

48.
Agency and an Interactional Model of Society

JAMES M. GUSTAFSON

The practical reasons that one could draw up for adhering to particular views of agency are not sufficient. At their worst they could become useful fictions, rationalizations for the sake of morality and a certain view of humanization. Philosophical or moral beliefs that are defended solely for their utility value deserve no more credence than religious beliefs so defended. The philosophical issues of action theory are the real issues. And one way in which they are distinguished is by looking at action from the agent's perspective on the one hand and the observer's on the other. Intentions as causes are always more persuasive from the agent's perspective. The reduction of intentions and volitions to the end stages of a particular causal sequence is more or less plausible from an observer's perspective; in retrospect, many intentions and actions are susceptible to more refined causal analysis than the agent is conscious of in the moment of choice.

As Midgley says, "Central factors in us *must* be accepted, and the right line of human conduct must lie somewhere within the range they allow."[1] This certainly would have to be admitted by even the most radical libertarians (not political libertarians but theorists of the "will"). Our intentions and choices, whether moral or otherwise, draw upon and give focus to our biological natures. Other factors must be accepted; at least they are not subject to radical revision and alteration in most persons under most circumstances. Cultural and social conditioning, while unpredictable to a degree in their effects, certainly predetermine the range of choices and actions under most circumstances. What we have become as a result of habituations and conscious commitments is a preselective reality that particularizes the limits and possibilities of action at a particular time. Similarly, the specific external location of our activity in both time and space limits and particularizes our human possibilities.

This is not to deny several important things. We can care for and develop our natural capacities so that more possibilities exist for us. This is a matter of choice and discipline. We need not be the prisoners of a given culture or society in the modern pluralistic and mobile world. The relativization of our "natural" cultures and societies occurs not only as a result of unintended exposures to different ones but also by deliberate effort to make contact with alternatives. We appear to have quite natural revulsions against repressive ways of life that have formed us; I take it that much of modern psychotherapy offers explanations of such resentments and individual rebellions. We need not resign ourselves to the limitations and possibilities of action that are prima facie apparent. We can act to alter those conditions so that the range of possibilities is amplified; we can choose to relate ourselves to other circumstances than those that immediately confront us.

In all of these possibilities, however, our agency is exercised to marshall and to direct realities that exist prior to our choices and actions. The scope of our "freedom" is not as vast as it is claimed to be from some points of view. Edwards, in his own eighteenth-century terms, makes a similar point. "[T]he will always follows the last dictate of understanding. But then the understanding must be taken in a large sense, as including the whole faculty of perception or apprehension, and not merely what is called reason or judgment."[2] Our freedom is the exercise of various capacities that are involved in human agency, capacities that earlier were called "faculties." Understanding, motives, desires, will, reason, and judgment are all involved. This view, it seems to me, does not denigrate humanity, and has the merit of more accurately portraying human agency. As Midgley so poignantly asks, "Why should not our excellence involve our whole nature?"[3]

Human accountability is not abolished from this point of view. To be sure, we can rightly indicate that persons have been held accountable in the past for more than they actually should have been. A great deal of misplaced guilt has been evoked by beliefs about the range of human freedom that are not defensible. Persons have been held morally accountable for events and effects for which they were only partially causally accountable. But one might argue that what we are held accountable for can be more complex and more particularized than can be included in a dialectic of freedom and nature, or freedom and destiny, when those are understood as specific and independent roles in the drama of life. We are accountable for the ways in which we bring our "natural" capacities to a focus of choice and action, for the assessment of our interrelations with other persons and other things in determining how we will exercise

---

From James Gustafson, *Ethics from a Theocentric Perspective,* vol. 1, *Theology and Ethics* (Chicago: University of Chicago Press, 1981), pp. 289–93.

our powers, and for the understanding of the circumstances of our action. We are accountable for the ordering of our motives, drives, and desires, as well as for the consequences of our actions that are within our powers to control. We are accountable to ourselves, to the communities of which we are a part, and to those who are affected by our actions.

In contemporary moral philosophy it is almost axiomatic to say that we are to respect the rational autonomy of other agents; that we are to respect their freedom.[4] Certainly it is correct to respect their capacities for agency. But persons are more than their capacities for agency. We must also respect their bodily natures, and we have responsibilities to see that they are not deprived of necessities. We are to respect persons not merely as individuals but as "members one of another" in their communities. What any moralist means when he or she insists on respect for persons depends upon the image or view held of persons. A view can be more or less comprehensive, more or less complex. If persons are viewed as biological entities with an unique capacity for agency, what is respected is amplified beyond "rational autonomy." Indeed, when one sees how restricted is the range in which autonomy is exercised, and when one sees how the exercise of agency is dependent upon and limited by biological, social, cultural, and other conditions, respect only for autonomy can be viewed as denigrating.

It is my conviction that a reader can learn more about human agency from great novels than he or she can from philosophical treatises or scientific accounts of the subject. Novelists such as Jane Austen, George Eliot, and Tolstoy show with poignancy and detail how human agency and particular acts bring to focus many drives, many motives, and require assessments of complex circumstances. In novels that are perspicacious in their development of character and action, we see how choices are made in continuity with what persons had become as a result of their whole natures.

Man is an agent. But agency draws upon all that persons are; it is the capacity to exercise our powers in accordance with purposes and intentions to affect, either by overt action or by restraint, the subsequent course of events.

Our views of the nature of human beings are affected by the selection of a dominant metaphor or analogy for understanding social relations. Social theory in Western culture tends to be divided, in this respect, between an organic analogy and a contractual view of human interrelations. Of course there are combinations of these; the family emerges as a result both of a "contract" of marriage and the natural bonding between the couple and children. As a more or less natural (organic) unit, the family shapes our natural duties; parents do not make contracts with their children that define their obligations to them. In professional life and business transactions the contractual relationship is dominant; we consciously undertake obligations that are specified, and are bound to meet them.

Each of these, when driven to extremes or when used too exclusively, falsifies human experience and misconstrues human nature. The organic metaphor excessively highlights the processes of continuous mutual determination between persons, between groups, and in some instances, as in the extreme sociobiological views, between human beings and the rest of nature. It overcomes the dichotomy between body and "soul" by construing the activities of the intellect and other forms of human agency as necessary and determined outcomes of other processes. Only their ignorance, it would appear, keeps investigators from giving sufficient explanations of human activity, and that is being overcome. The individual is seen primarily as the outcome of the processes of life as a whole, and his or her "autonomy" is underestimated. In morality it is easy to claim, from this perspective, that the good of the whole body is of greater importance than the good of its individual parts. "Surgery," the denial of life and liberty to an individual "organ," is more readily justified.

The contractual model rests strongly on the primacy of individuals. Their being is implicitly if not explicitly judged to be of prior significance to the "whole." The agency of individuals has a more central role; society is seen to be more the result of the actions and choices of individuals, or of contractually bound groups, than as the outcome of "natural" processes. The distinctiveness of man among the animals is stressed more than the similarities and continuities. The autonomy of individuals is highly respected, and with this comes a moral stress on the respect for the autonomy and rights of individuals. In situations of conflict between the rights of individuals and benefits for a social group, the presumption is always in favor of the former. It is more difficult to make a case for restraints and denials of liberty and life for the sake of the well-being of a whole.

An interactional model of society takes into account what is valid in each of the other two models. It can account for the priority of society in the sense that we are the "products" of it to a large extent, and our initiatives are always in response to what exists and to the actions of others upon us. It recognizes that individuals and even most groups do not have the power to create or to recreate their larger societies. Novelty takes place within the developments in social life that are beyond the control of individual and corporate actions. Yet it recognizes the individual and corporate capacities for action. The processes of social change are not mechanically or organically construed; the exercise of powers does alter social orders and the course of historical events; it affects the development of culture. An interactional view provides no simple way of deciding in hard cases whether the individual's autonomy should be curbed for the sake of a larger good any more than it simply sustains the "good of the whole" over against the claims of individuals. Whether the moral weight rests primarily on the individual or particular groups over against the well-being of a larger community—a nation-state or the species—depends on valuations that are not determined by the model itself. Such critical choices, in any case, could not be universally predetermined in the abstract, or in very general terms. They are determined in relation to a particular set of circumstances and events. Societies are developing; their development is governed by a whole complex of processes of which particular events initiated by particular persons and groups are only a part. Multicausality, including human agency, must be taken into account in understanding individual, social, historical, and cultural developments.

Notes

1. Mary Midgley, *Beast and Man: The Roots of Human Nature* (Ithaca: Cornell University Press, 1978), p. 81.
2. Jonathan Edwards, *Freedom of the Will,* ed. Paul Ramsey (New Haven: Yale University Press, 1957), p. 148.
3. Midgley, *Beast and Man,* p. 204.
4. See, for example, Alan Donagan, *The Theory of Morality* (Chicago: University of Chicago Press, 1979), pp. 33-74.

49.

Toward a Human Medicine

HENRY STOB

I am not a physician and am therefore disqualified from speaking in any professional way about the technical, diagnostic, and healing procedures of medical practice. When, as a layman, I nevertheless make an address to the subject of this essay, I do so in the expectation that the reader will place the emphasis, not on the word "medicine," but on the word "human." I shall centrally be asking, "What is man?" That is, what is man that the medical fraternity should "be mindful of him"?

The Judaeo-Christian conception of man is that of a personal being who is first of all an individual. Now an individual, if human, is not a mere atom of existence; he stands within a complex network of relations. But he also stands apart; he is singular. Each man, every man, is distinct, unique. As such he forms an impenetrable boundary to all other existences. Being "separate," he has his own private identity, an identity that may not be ignored, compromised, or invaded, but only respected. Because every man has his individuality, no normal man craves long-run anonymity. To exist means to stand out, and if a man exists he wants to stand out, even when he is not outstanding. He does not want to be lost in the crowd, be absorbed in the mass, or be reduced to a number. He wants to be identified, named, singled out. When in our treatment of someone we fail in any measure to fulfill this need, we to that extent diminish and dehumanize him. This sometimes happens within the medical community.

As an individual, moreover, man is never a mere thing, an object. He is a subject, an active, dynamic center of will and power. He is a focus of energy. The human individual is alive, propulsive, and creative. He is marked not so much by passivity as by activity. He is not so much a patient as an agent. In an engagement with a thing, an object, there is no need to elicit the thing's consent. The thing can be manipulated at will, for it itself has no will, no freedom, no creativity. It is otherwise with man. There is no way, except in extreme emergencies or when a man is in an unconscious state, that one can legitimately bypass

From Henry Stob, *Ethical Reflections: Essays on Moral Themes* (Grand Rapids: Eerdmans, 1978). Used by permission.

his inherent agency and spontaneity. Doctors know this, of course. They know that for healing, not operation, but co-operation is needed, but this is sometimes forgotten, and when it is the medicine is less than human.

Moreover, the human individual is rational. He possesses, is an active embodiment of, reason. Now, to possess reason is to be able to think, and human beings, as we all know, are able to do this. But reason is not exhausted in thinking. Thinking merely as such, is a kind of technical competence. It is not to be despised; it is in fact indispensable to the conduct of human affairs. But it is not uniquely human; the higher animals seem capable of manipulating a simple means-ends calculus. But they are not on that account rational in the true and human sense of the word. Reason, as this is embodied in human beings, extends not only to the cognitive, but also to the affective and evaluational dimensions of existence. Reason in man is not only technical; it is this, but more; it is ontological. Reason in man is an ability to grasp the shape and structure of the universe, and to put himself in touch with that overarching order under which he resides. It is by reason that man is able, not merely to move in prescribed ways from premises to conclusions, but to discern, and if not to discern then to posit, a universal law, and the ends of human striving appropriate thereto. To be rational is not only to know how, but to know what, and to know why. To be humanly rational is, in short, to be constituted not merely narrowly scientific, but metaphysical and moral.

These remarks on rationality are meant in part to remind the physician that the sick man under his care has the gift of intelligence (however great or small) and that account must be taken of this. The so-called patient must be addressed as a hearer and giver of reasons. Proposed procedures, and their actual or possible consequences, should be discussed with him, not simply imposed. And every effort should be made to assure that the consent elicited from him is an *informed* consent. But these remarks bear even more directly on the physician's own grasp of rationality. He is a scientist, and as a scientist he is by training and practice tempted more than most individuals to equate know-how with knowledge and technical mastery with wisdom. Under these circumstances he does well to remind himself that reason or rationality is a much broader and deeper thing than the technological competence that modern philosophy and science have made it out to be.

I have thus far considered man as an individual, in abstraction from the relations he sustains. There is therefore more to be said about him. But I shall pause here to sum up what has been said. I have ventured to declare that in the Judaeo-Christian view man is an individual and as such unique, dynamic, and rational; that he is an individual and as such distinct, creative, and transcendental; that he is an individual and as such inviolable, agential, and valuational; that he is, in short, a centered-self, or person. If this account of man be correct, and I think it is, it sets certain norms for practice, also for medical practice. It means that man is never to be so approached, confronted, or handled as to ignore or violate his unique self-identity, his true agency, and his attachment to and engagement with transcendental norms of being and acting. He is to be treated always and only as a person—never as an anonymous entity, never as a mere patient or object, never as a shallow existent without those dimensions of depth and height by which he sets himself upon ends and is constituted religious and moral.

Man, I suggested, is an individual. But individuality is not atomistic particularity. One *is* an individual, one *becomes* an individual, with all the notes of individuality I have already recorded (identity, agency, and rationality) only in relation. In the Judaeo-Christian view there are three relationships within which the human individual is ineluctably caught up.

The first of these relationships is that between himself and God. The Judaeo-Christian man understands himself to be in an unbreakable ontic (even though a disturbed moral) relation to a transcendent self, who because he is a self cannot be invaded, and who because he is transcendent cannot be comprehended, but who because he is God is an unavoidable presence in man's consciousness. Man, in this view, though estranged from God, is not a stranger to God; and God, though offended by man, is not careless of man. God, in this view, is self-existent, and does not *become* God in and with his relationship to man. Man, on the other hand, is man only as he is related to God. It is because of God's creational activity and his providential ordering that man exists and endures, and that he is *what* he is. Human self-hood is accordingly centrally constituted and perpetually guaranteed by the God-man relation. Man is and becomes a person *coram deo.* It is before the face of God that man attains to self-identity, agency, and rationality—the essential ingredients of responsibility. It is possible, of course, to deny that God exists, and consequently to deny that humanness is basically constituted by an ontic relation to the transcendent, but for theists this does not alter the fact; it only obscures for the denier the depth dimension in every man, and thereby diminishes his dignity. In the Judaeo-Christian view man has dignity, for in his very being he is attached to God, and in his constitution he resembles God. He is *imago dei*—on which account there is a kind of sacredness about him which in each one's dealing with him must be kept inviolate. All this amounts to saying that man is a symbol and mirror of that which transcends the relativities of time and space. On this account we owe each man respect. It means, furthermore, that man's being (and that includes his body) is neither at his own disposal, simply as such, nor at the disposal of a physician or surgeon. We have indeed been made stewards of ourselves, but we are obliged to be responsive and responsible stewards, for we are not our own, but God's, and we are answerable to him for what he has given us in pawn.

What does this entail for the practice of medicine? I hazard the generalization that no procedures should be adopted which tend to horizontalize and secularize, and so de-humanize, the patient. I further opine that the art of the physician is likely to be most effectual when it is exercised in concert with the chaplain, the curator of souls. More importantly, it is to be observed that man being what he is—a being in touch with God—is never to be treated as a means, not even as a means toward increased "scientific" knowledge, but only as an end. The experiments conducted on the cure for syphilis in which a control group of syphilitic patients went untreated for scientific purposes, goes counter to every moral value, and offends humanity. It reduces man to a means, and thus dehumanizes him. As for the matter of dignity, the medical instructor who entered the hospital room trailed by a bevy of interns, and unceremoniously uncovered a sheeted woman and began pointing, was apparently unconscious that it was a person—and not a thing—he was pointing at. The story is that the woman—in defense of her dignity—gathered the sheet about her, and obstructed observation. I must acknowledge that I admire her for that, for she recognized that one may not be undressed before being addressed.

There is a second relation that must now be considered, and it bears with maximum directness on the work of the physician. Man is related not only to God, but also to nature—to the inorganic and organic world about him. Man is, in fact, rooted in this world. It is not only about him; it is in him. Man is physical. Man's kinship with nature in his body is a state of affairs that no amount of idealism or asceticism can manage to obscure, and authentic theism has never wished to deny it. Man in the Judaeo-Christian view is an embodied soul or an ensouled body, a psycho-somatic unity, with the closest of ties to nature. This is why so much can be done for him by natural science and by the arts and techniques of medicine and surgery. But in this view man is not a mere *product* of nature; he is more than a congeries of molecules. Implanted in nature, he yet rises above it. Participating in the vitalities of *bios,* he participates also in the realm of mind, and mind is not matter, not even the most complicated matter. Of course, neither is matter mind. A proper view of man is provided neither by idealism nor by materialism. Man is neither mere *psyche* nor mere *soma,* but the two indefeasibly combined in a psycho-somatic unity. Not in the same way as God, but in analogy to him, man is both immanent in nature and transcendent to it. This is why he can both fall victim to the determinations and ravages of nature, and in freedom rise to superiority and victory over it. In fact, this is why science, and in particular medical science, is possible at all. Were man simply immersed in nature, no rational control of nature would be possible, for nothing rises above its source—and man's source is God.

This state of affairs involves, I judge, entailments for the practice of medicine. Because man is neither (merely) a physical and chemical congeries of atoms, nor a living vegetable, nor a sentient animal, but something which, while akin to these things, supersedes them, the approach to and the treatment of even man's body cannot be simply that which is appropriate to inanimate things, or even to animate things—like animals—which in the hierarchy of beings lie below him. Man, even when contemplated as an organism, must be contemplated as an organism-plus. The *bios* of man's life is not that of even the highest animal. It is attended by psychic, social, and religious relations and dimensions that are transcendent to nature. Man is quantified, chemicalized, physicalized, and vitalized, but he is also spiritualized, and this affects and qualifies all the processes that take place within him. Even the physiology of an animal is different from that of a human, for human physiology is caught up in a matrix foreign to, because transcendent to, that of the animal. It would seem to follow that when a physician treats the body of a man, he does not really treat the body of the man unless he attends to more than the body. The body of a man is palpably not a mere body, but something which has super-bodily dimensions. To treat man only as a body is to treat him abstractly. And this dehumanizes him.

The third relation in which man stands is social. The individual, while being a centered-self, distinct from all others, with his own identity, is nevertheless racial. He is set in the context of other persons, all of whom belong to him, and all of whom in some sense constitute him. A self, if human, is not a self except in the company of what is not *his* self, but that of another. The ego demands the other ego for its very existence. The life of a man is inextricably intertwined with that of other men. No man—not even the most forsaken—is an island; he is part of the main. A man comes into the world through parents—ideally through the loving conjunction of an enduringly wedded man and woman intending a family, but in any case (at least until now) through the conjunction of man and woman. Every man, therefore, has kin, and in the treatment of him this may not be ignored. As an individual a man needs and deserves to be treated as separate and unique, not en masse. As a social creature, however, he needs and deserves to experience belongingness, acceptance, and embracement by his family, the physician, the hospital staff, and everyone else. To the extent such embracement is absent, the man is humanly impoverished.

I fear that with the trend toward scientific-medical specialization, and with the demise of the family doctor, the social side of the healing art has not come into its own. It is good, therefore, to hear that some medical schools have lately introduced special programs to train general practitioners who will make house calls and become once more a friend to the family.

50. The Liberty of the Sick, Theologically Considered

KARL RAHNER

An essay on the liberty of the sick, seen from a theological standpoint, is not just the same thing as an account of the Church's doctrinal statements on the subject. Of course this essay is not intended to go beyond the limits of what the Church's official doctrine says about the liberty of the sick, either directly and expressly, or indirectly and implicitly. But in so far as the teaching of the Church has actually been formulated, it does not come to grips closely enough with what we mean by the phrase 'the liberty of the sick'. Consequently, however carefully the theologian may take the Church's doctrine into consideration, he is bound to try to say something about this subject on his own account and at his own risk, in the light of the theological data and using theological methods.

Here we shall be limiting the subject to those illnesses in which the sick person is confronted, objectively and subjectively, with death as something that is threatening him and that is pressingly close.[1] A cold, an upset stomach, or any illness which does not really force the person affected out of the circle of the people who are actively able to control their lives freely, does not present any theological problem of its own.

In the first section we shall say something about the nature of liberty as the theologian sees it. From the theological standpoint, liberty is something other than a merely psychological freedom of choice in the individual act, and it differs, too, from a purely legal and civic responsibility for one's actions. Of course this first, theological section is bound to be no more than a fragment; and it stresses—and to some degree isolates—those elements of liberty, in its theological essence, which are of particular importance for our question.[2] In the second part we shall ask what the liberty of the sick as such consists of; and we shall finally inquire about the invalid's claim to liberty where this touches on his relationship to his doctor.

From Karl Rahner, *Theological Investigations,* vol. 17, trans. Margaret Kohl (New York: Crossroad, 1981), pp. 100-113. Used by permission.

On the Essence of Liberty

First of all we must mention a number of features of human liberty which are specifically theological and which are of particular importance for our subject. When the word 'liberty' is used in the secular sphere, it is either understood sociologically, as the absence of social compulsions and estrangements; or it is meant psychologically, as the person's freedom of choice in any given act of decision—always provided that we do not adopt the determinist view, which denies the existence of psychological freedom of choice in general, and tries to interpret responsibility, social sanctions and so forth without the concept of free choice. The theological concept of liberty certainly implies the concept of psychological freedom of choice, but it is more comprehensive and more radical.

The theological concept of liberty is theological in the first place because it explicitly or implicitly includes the thesis that whenever there is a radically responsible, true freedom of choice, there is also a definite relation to God. This is so even though in certain circumstances—in fact very often—this relation is not conscious or considered, in any explicit sense. Real, personal freedom of choice is possible only when individual good and individual value are exceeded—even if unconsciously—in man's transcendental self, in anticipation of the Good in general and *per se.* But this means the existence of a theological dimension of liberty—relatedness to God—even if this is not the subject of conscious reflection. And this is inescapable, whether this relatedness is conscious and reduced to terms and terminology or not. It is inescapable, whether liberty accepts this relatedness in true self-affirmation, or whether it rejects it in that ultimate denial of the self to which we theologically give the name of sin.[3]

Liberty in the theological sense, therefore, deeply and fundamentally, is not merely the ability to do one thing rather than another, let alone the possibility of always being able to do the opposite of what one has done before. It is rather the possibility open to the free subject or person of disposing totally and finally of himself and his life, as an individual and a whole. Liberty in the theological sense means, first and last, the one and total subject himself in so far as he is object for himself—in so far as the actor, the act, and what has been performed are one—in so far as the one and total life is set in irrevocable finality through this act of liberty; in so far, that is to say, as what we are accustomed to call the eternal being of man comes into existence. And by eternity we do not mean an endlessly continuing time that succeeds our earthly life. We mean the freely ordered finality of the person and his earthly life before God.

These indications of the theological nature of liberty show that there are two different groups of related problems which we must consider in a little more detail. The first is the problem of the relationship between liberty in the theological sense, and the individual, empirical, single object, which can be objectified and expressed in words. The second is the problem of the relationship between liberty and time.

As far as the first problem is concerned, we must here briefly say that the fulfilment of human liberty (by which we mean the self-determination of the total subject in the direction of finality) is, of course, inevitably mediated through some individual object of an *a posteriori* kind, existing in space, time and history. It is to this that liberty chooses to be related in its act of choice, though of course in order to establish its own real nature, which is the self-fulfilment of the person or subject. But this individual object, which is indispensable if liberty is to be consummated, in itself gives no final and certain information as to what the self-consummation of the subject really is, and whether it is for good or evil. It is possible for a person to align himself with God for his salvation, at least unconsciously, because he lets himself fall into the incomprehensibility of his existence in serene hope; though it may well be that the object on which this saving disposal of the self is exercised is materially not only very unimportant and limited, but even ought not to exist, and ought not to be realised at all, if it is tested against the obligatory norms and circumstances of this world.[4]

It is therefore, fundamentally speaking, quite possible for personal liberty to be fulfilled even when the material for decision which is offered to the actual free subject *a posteriori* can no longer be fitted into the 'normal' contexts of human life and society, with its structures and norms, where the person who is 'served' by his experience only in this way is no longer 'responsible' in the civic and psychiatric sense. It is quite conceivable, basically speaking, for a free and personal self-ordering of the subject to get along with a much smaller amount of mediating material than we have to assume and demand in normal civic life if we are to concede responsibility to someone. It is conceivable that a particular objective material which is presented to a person from outside and is in itself conceptually understood, may not be eligible at all as material for the person's real self-fulfilment, because of the actual structure or make-up of the person himself.

The second problem is the obscure relationship between liberty and time. Theologically, liberty must be understood as the personal self-determination of the subject, through which he completes himself as a whole, together with his whole earthly life, in the direction of its final and ultimate form.[5] But then the conceptual scheme which Christian practice and pastoral care employ is insufficient. For there the assumption is that the final fate of men and women, in the sense of salvation or perdition, is simply determined by the final free act in time, in the history of a given individual. It is decided by an act which stands at the end in temporal isolation, as it were, and this act by itself governs the whole of the person's previous life. On the other hand, the fundamental option of a person over the totality of himself as subject and over a life extending over a period of time, cannot be thought of as simply taking place outside time and history, and as revealing itself from this meta-historical point only in the many temporally distributed acts of the person. Even free acts, in which the person orders himself and his life in its totality, must take place in history, and must have a place in time and space within the history of the person himself. Otherwise history—and salvation-history above all—becomes a semblance without an essence, on to which a liberty which is above time is projected.

Because of the incongruence we have already indicated between the material through which liberty is mediated and the original act of liberty as the self-ordering of the personal subject himself, the place and time at which such an act of liberty takes place in a person's life can never be unequivocally stated. Nor should we maintain that a fundamental option of this kind is possible only once, and that it cannot be revised later by the same existentially radical act of decision in the form of a later choice. It is true that human liberty as self-ordering does not imply the arbitrary revisability of its decisions, as if these decisions could continually be remade indefinitely; it wants these decisions to take the form of final decisions. But as liberty that is finite and materially mediated, it always exposes itself to still current time; and so it arrives at the fulfilment of its own nature only through the fact that time stops, because of an event which is not simply within the power of liberty itself, although by virtue of its own nature it lays itself open to that event.

The Liberty of the Sick Person

Here the liberty of the sick means quite specifically the liberty of the sick person in his confrontation with death. This relationship between liberty, in the theological sense, and death is of a quite particular kind. But it is easily understandable if we remember what we have just said about liberty in the theological sense; and if at the same time we take into account the Christian conviction that in death a person's free history assumes its final form. This means that the final 'Judgement' of the person takes place. It means that the person who in his liberty always has to do consciously or unconsciously with God, finally finds him or loses him.

The situation of approaching death is really an unusual situation for liberty. For death brings to an end the time and space in which a person orders himself in the direction of finality. At all events the free subject cannot be certain that a radical, fundamental choice has already been made in his lifetime in such a way that there is no longer any danger of its being upset again in sickness or dying. This means that the situation of approaching death is really a radical challenge to liberty to decide finally for God on the very basis of the 'material' offered by the process of dying, with its helplessness and loneliness. It should decide for God by accepting serenely and hopefully this 'hopeless' situation of radical helplessness and of being engulfed by the incomprehensibility of what we call God.[6]

This means that a person ought to die 'consciously' as far as possible. He ought not simply to *suffer* death but should also paradoxically *suffer it actively* as an act of liberty. He therefore has the right to know that he is going to die, and when. If and in so far as this knowledge can reach the dying person only by means of a communication made to him by the people round him, this communication must not be withheld. If the moment when this communication is made, and the way in which it is made, are chosen properly, it does not have to come as a frightening shock to the dying person. The very helplessness which the patient experiences inwardly can awake a gently composed awareness of death as the situation confronting him. For unless it is a completely sudden death, biologically speaking, the dying are aware of the situation they are in, even if they suppress their awareness for a while.

Because, and in so far as, death (or the act of dying) is a special situation for liberty in the theological sense, man has a right, and even something of a duty, to mould the situation in such a way that it offers as many opportunities for liberty as possible, even in an empirical sense. An alleviation of suffering which does not simply reduce the sick person to unconsciousness, but leaves him conscious and makes a greater serenity of spirit possible than would be the case if he were overwhelmed by pain in the physiological sense, is therefore not merely a claim made by the vital self-assertion of the patient himself. It is also a demand of liberty in the theological sense, which rightly desires to win for itself as extensive a space as possible and, as far as possible, right up to the frontier of death. The alleviation of pain is not merely important for the patient's physiological and psychological well-being. It is also important in the struggle for the greatest possible area of liberty in the theological sense—an area where a history of salvation may be played out.

What we have just said, however, is not a final answer to the problem of an alleviation of pain which makes the sick person more or less unconscious and incapable of responsible decision. In our present context we need only say that there is no need to dispense with an alleviation of this sort, as long as it does not mean directly killing the patient, and as long as the nature and violence of the pain would in any case permit no more extensive area of liberty.[7]

'Styles of Dying'

In the course of Christian history, the awareness that death (i.e. the act of dying, as distinct from the state of having died) is a special situation for liberty in the theological sense has given rise to what Arthur Jores has called different 'styles of dying'.[8] It is not merely a question of administering the 'sacraments of the dying' (which is not simply and directly obvious). There is not merely a special sacrament for the sick who are near death.[9] Formerly there was also a social and religious ritual for dying, which has largely faded into disuse today. Dying was not merely seen as a biological happening. It was a personal, historical, free event, which quite actively brought life to its final state: eternity. The dying person gathered his family round him, gave them his final blessing, expressed his last wishes, affirmed his faith and hope in a gracious God, prayed the prayers for the dying with those round him and so on. All this can be significant as the completion and proclamation of the task of dying as part of a person's own history of freedom. The sober courage befitting the Christian in the hour of death, and indeed a great deal else in this traditional style of dying, may seem to be the reflection of a genuine kind of liberty in the face of death. All the same, this particular 'style of dying' is, when all is said and done, historically conditioned in many ways, and need not in itself be permanently adopted. (We shall come back later to the sacraments of the dying, which are distinct from the other 'stylistic' elements of dying in its traditional form.)

That is one side of the matter. But it is impossible to maintain that the total and final consummation of liberty on the part of the human subject in the direction of finality—i.e. death as total act of liberty—always takes place in immediate proximity to death in the medical sense. In most cases the doctors will have before them a dying person whose condition in any case makes it difficult to conceive (without arbitrary hypotheses) how he could be capable of any radical personal act in this situation—by which I mean an act through which he freely disposes of himself and the ultimate meaning of his life in a thoroughly radical way. Moreover, there is no cogent theological reason for postulating the opposite of what the medical situation would lead us to suppose. The act in which a person freely orders himself in the direction of finality can, even in the case of a 'responsible' person, take place much earlier and can, for internal or external reasons, be the final act of this kind even though it takes place a considerable time before death in the medical sense. Dying in the medical sense and dying as an act of liberty need not coincide chronologically. What took place and could take place in life as an act of free and final disposal of the self, on the basis of a relatively modest and not at all explicit 'material' for the exercise of liberty, is not necessarily also possible in the case of dying in the medical sense, not even if the 'material' there is more explicitly religious and the situation of the dying person is a 'devout' one.

Human and Religious Help in Dying

There are people who under certain circumstances are called to help the sick person to arrive at a clearly religious death and an explicitly religious act of liberty in dying. (This help does not always have to be an official pastoral duty. It may also be a humane and Christian duty of love on the part of nurses and doctors.) For these people what we have just said has particular consequences. These helpers should draw on the gift of 'testing the spirits', so as to try to help the dying person to the attitude which is open to this particular individual in the light of his life history and his religious knowledge and capabilities. A helper of this kind should not therefore exploit the sick person's weakness in order to clothe his death with the hastily donned garment of a religious act which he is not actually able to perform existentially, and which, therefore, contributes nothing to his eternal salvation. If a dying person rejects the visit of a priest or pastor, or any other religious help, his wish should be respected. There should be no attempt to enlist the indiscreet help of relatives or nurses, in order to influence him to the contrary. These people may perhaps be more concerned about social 'respectability' than about the religious meaning of the anointing of the sick and the viaticum, or the eternal salvation of the sick person. (But this is not intended to lay down rules for a person who is charismatically endowed and who can trust himself to achieve a deeper and more genuine conversion or repentance in the spirit of the sick person.) When a dying person is no longer able to arrive at an obviously religiously articulated acceptance of death, or a free and saving act, the question of his salvation is completely open for the person who is at his side. It is a question he cannot decide. For the dying person the personally decisive hour of salvation may have taken place much earlier, while he was still in the midst of life, and the material for his free act may not have been expressly and verbally religious at all.

When it is possible to help the dying person to find an expressly religious significance in his death, and when this is accepted by the sick person, the most important thing, even for Catholics, is that the dying person should arrive at a religiously existential attitude towards death. Receiving the 'Last Sacraments' is only secondary to this. In the case of a Catholic who has practised his religion with normal zeal, these things normally coincide. But this is not true of people who have hitherto been used to little or no expressly religious observance. With these people it may be possible under certain circumstances—and it is also theologically legitimate—to help them to acquire a right inner attitude to the possibility of death (hopeful resignation to their fate etc.). There is no need to expect them immediately to accept a sacramental act. That would only overtax and shock them. Of course in a situation of this kind an earlier sacramental practice, which the dying person was accustomed to a long time previously, can be revived without any great difficulty, so that the sacramental event, in its tangibility and clarity, may facilitate and confirm the act of hopeful resignation to death as God's decree. But this is not always the case, and where there is any doubt the decision should be in favour of help in the existential acts of the dying person. Nobody should force a sacramental event on him which, quite innocently perhaps, he cannot really endorse, and which for that reason he quite rightly refuses.

Of course a position of this kind also means that the people surrounding the sick person are not simply released from the outset from the duty of giving any kind of religious help, just because the invalid is incapable of receiving the sacraments or rejects them. Explicit contrition for the sins of one's past life is really an essential part of a free and living act at the hour of death—if, and in so far as, this sense of sin is alive in the person or can be awakened out of its suppression. But the hoping act of acceptance of one's own situation can be implicit contrition. A person may sometimes succeed in achieving that more easily than in finding an express relationship to past events, to which he no longer feels related. This must also be remembered in connection with religious help for the sick—for example, with regard to the content of prayers said in the presence of the sick person.

The Free Choice of Doctor

When we come to the claim which the liberty of the sick makes on the physician, we must first of all say something about the free choice of doctor. This is an essential sphere for the liberty of the sick person. If illness were a purely biological event which took place in some realm detached from the actual free person himself, it might be judged an open question whether the sick person must basically have the right to choose his doctor freely, or whether the State could prescribe a health-service functionary, in the same way that it prescribes other functionaries without asking our permission first.

But for the free person as such, a severe illness means a particular and unique situation. In order for him to fulfil his inner liberty, a person must in principle be conceded as wide a sphere of liberty as possible. Consequently the free choice of doctor is one of the essentials for liberty. Institutions and procedures such as the licensing of medical personnel, the appointment of official doctors for particular groups of people, the compulsory medical examinations required by the State—all these things should continually lead us to ask whether they are not reducing the free choice of doctor more than is absolutely necessary. And 'absolutely necessary' means more than is legitimately required by circumstances and by the legitimate pursuit of other benefits for society as a whole.

It is undoubtedly true that the free choice of doctor is often a mere faded ideal, which for social and economic reasons is largely becoming an illusion. Where this is the case, these social and economic conditions must be altered, in order to facilitate, in real terms, as free a choice of doctor as possible. Of course the right to a free choice of doctor must continually be a matter of fresh compromise with other human values and rights. We must not see it in isolation. But we might also ask whether the possibility of choosing one's doctor freely is not restricted by the unjustifiably high fees which doctors themselves charge. We might well ask whether it is right for doctors' fees to be thrown open to free competition, like the prices of other commodities, and whether to do so is not a contradiction of the sick person's right to choose his doctor freely.

The Right to Die

Part of the sick person's liberty with regard to his doctor is the right to die. We need not inquire here whether under certain circumstances the sick person may even have a duty to claim this right. At all events, the patient, as a free person, is not simply the object of the doctor who allows himself to be guided solely by his aim to prolong the biological life of the sick person for as long as possible, without any reference to other points of view held by the patient himself or by society. There are other values and aims which may make the sick person (or, it may be, someone close to him who represents his interests and is also called to defend his other rights too) freely express the wish not to be prevented from dying.

It is true that, according to the general Christian and Catholic view, it is not objectively and morally legitimate to will an action which is aimed directly at causing the death of the sick person. That is to say, no direct control over a person's biological life as a whole can be morally justified. But according to the view of Catholic moral theology, this does not mean that the patient or the doctor has the positive duty to apply every conceivable and actually possible means to prolong biological life. It is the generally accepted view of Catholic moral theology that the application of measures for a positively useful purpose—for example the relief of pain—is permissible even when these measures involve a certain curtailment of the patient's life, if this is an unintentional though known and accepted side-effect. For this is no different from what happens at other times in human life, when a person puts up with something which is harmful from a purely biological point of view if he can thereby arrive at a higher quality of living.

There are theoretical obscurities about these specific rules, which try to distinguish between the legitimate permitting of a person to die, and direct killing. These need further clarification. This clarification might perhaps bring about a considerable re-structuring of the answer to the problems we have touched on here. There are also practical difficulties about the actual application of these rules. But since it is impossible simply to get rid of the problems themselves, we may and must meanwhile work with rules and distinctions of this kind, in order to find a 'middle of the road' between euthanasia on the one hand (by which we mean the direct killing of a sick person at his request) and an absolute, unconditional will to preserve biological life, without taking any other points of view into account. If we reject euthanasia in the sense in which we have defined it, and if we hold the preservation of biological life at all costs (even at the cost of inhumanity) to be wrong, then we shall have to accept the validity of the rule-of-thumb view we have indicated. We must simply see it *as* a pure rule of thumb, and hope that the moral theologians will clarify the problem further in the future.[10]

A more specialised question arises in this context too. Does the sick person's right to be allowed to die merely *permit* the doctor to accept his wishes, or does it actually lay on him the *duty* of allowing the patient to die? In a conflict between the patient's wish for a speedy end, and the doctor's will to preserve life for as long as possible, the doctor will in practice generally have his way and will override the patient's wishes. This will be the case especially if he has the impression that the patient's desire is the expression of his illness and his pain, rather than a genuine, personal decision; and if he is understandably reluctant to do anything except fulfil his primary task as doctor—to defend and preserve life. But this is not a solution to the problem. Does the genuine, personal, carefully considered decision and will of the sick person to accept death, even if it could be postponed for a certain time, correspond on the doctor's side to a real moral duty to carry out his patient's wish? For as doctor he has not merely entered into the service of a physiological defence of life. When he accepts a sick person as patient he accepts the duty to serve a person and his total and entire life history (even if under a particular aspect).

It might be said that a problem of this kind is highly academic and arises only in rare cases, because it can only be a question of the will of a sick person during his illness, not while he is still in good health. A decision of this kind made in health cannot simply be accepted as being valid in the situation of illness. In illness itself a truly personal will of this kind seldom exists, and the doctor is seldom able to discern unequivocally that it exists. But we cannot view such cases as impossible, and that means that the problem exists. In addition there is the problem of whether the relatives of an unconscious and dying person can on his behalf express the will to allow him to die, and can express it in such a way that the doctor has the duty to carry out their wish.

The question seems an obscure one. For in general a person's wish, even though it may be morally legitimate, does not imply another's duty to enable him to carry out his intention. Also—unless there is an express agreement between patient and doctor—it is impossible to prove that the acceptance of medical duties towards a particular patient necessarily implies the readiness to carry out the patient's wishes in this particular respect. Admittedly the opposite cannot be proved either, in view of the doctor's role towards the patient as a total person. We must also consider whether a doctor can opt out of a doctor-patient relationship which was freely entered into on both sides, if he is clearly confronted with the sick person's will to be allowed to die. This question is hard to answer too; for on the one hand a relationship that has been freely entered into can equally freely be terminated; on the other hand, a sick person in the cases we are assuming here will find it hard to find another doctor.

Basically speaking, I incline to the view that the doctor does have the duty we have been discussing. This is the only way in which an inhumane and undignified prolongation of life can be prevented. And a doctor who recognises this duty will more easily get over his understandable reluctance to let a person die, even though he could have preserved his life for a while longer. But in these questions even Christian ethics no longer succeed in formulating rules which are factually unambiguous, directly applicable and generally comprehensible.

Liberty is a mystery. In its fundamental character, it is the necessity imposed on man to decide freely for or against the Incomprehensibility which we call God. It is the possibility of letting oneself fall in hope and in unconditional trust into this Incomprehensibility as goal, bliss and human fulfilment. The highest power which liberty has is consummated in the helplessness of death. The doctor, too, is drawn into this individual history of liberty and death. He can really fulfil his very own, specific task (as distinct from other human acts) only if he is more than a physician—if, in the fulfilment of his medical task, he is truly man and even (anonymously[11] or expressly) a Christian. For that reason the liberty of the sick person, which arrives at its final frontier and its completion in the process of dying, cannot be a matter of indifference to him. He, too, is fighting for the space for, and the right to, this same ultimate liberty. He—as well as the sick person—should resign himself in silent and serene hope to the mystery of death, after he has fought for this earthly life to the last possible moment. The doctor is a servant of liberty.

Notes

1. The original text of this essay was published in *StdZ* 193 (1975), pp. 31-40, but notes and cross-references have been supplied for the present version. Some points considered here have already been dealt with by the present author in *Zur Theologie des Todes* (Quaestiones Disputatae 2), 4th edn (Freiburg 1963); ET *On the Theology of Death* (Edinburgh and London 1961). The new angle from which the subject is treated here may, however, open up some fresh aspects.

2. On the problem of liberty, cf. especially *Gnade als Freiheit,* Herder Bücherei 322 (Freiburg 1968), with the second group of essays: 'Ermächtigung zur wahren Freiheit', pp. 31-89.

3. For additional material which may give added depth to our view of the subject, cf. what has been said about 'choice' in the following essays in *Theological Investigations* XVI (London 1979): 'Experience of the Spirit and Existential Commitment', pp. 24-34; 'Modern Piety and the Experience of Retreats', pp. 135-55; and 'Reflections on a New Task for Fundamental Theology', pp. 156-66.

4. For the idea of decision as fundamental option, the author is indebted to Ignatius Loyola's *Spiritual Exercises.* His theological work has been continually influenced by the desire to work out the theological implications of the spiritual stimulus he has found there, and to make that stimulus fruitful theologically; cf. the essays quoted in n. 3.

5. On the question of time, seen theologically, cf. the essays on the subject which have been gathered together from the different volumes of *Theological Investigations* and printed in paperback form in K. Rahner, *Zur Theologie der Zukunft* (dtv 4076) (Munich 1971).

6. In view of the process of dying, the present author does not share the familiar 'hypothesis of a final decision' which is supported by L. Boros in *The Movement of Truth: Mysterium Mortis* (London 1965).

7. On the problem of illness and the sick person, cf. especially 'The Saving Force and Healing Power of Faith', *Theological Investigations* V (London 1966), pp. 460-7; 'Proving Oneself in Time of Sickness', *Theological Investigations* VII (London 1971), pp. 275-84.

8. Cf. A. Jores, *Menschsein als Auftrag* (Bern 1964), especially pp. 114-17 and 121-34.

9. On the sacrament of the anointing of the sick, cf. K. Rahner, *Kirche und Sakramente* (Quaestiones Disputatae 10) (Freiburg 1960), especially pp. 100-4; 'Bergend und heilend—Über das Sakrament der Kranken' in K. Rahner, *Die siebenfältige Gabe—Über die Sakramente der Kirche* (Munich 1974), pp. 115-37.

10. For moral theology's view of euthanasia, cf. the articles by W. Schöllgen in *LThK* III, 2nd edn (Freiburg 1959), 1207-8, and H. Vorgrimler in *LThK* IX, 2nd edn (Freiburg 1964), 1053-4; also the bibliographies.

11. For 'anonymous' in this sense, cf. 'Anonymous and Explicit Faith', *Theological Investigations* XVI (London 1979), pp. 52-9.

Part III
ISSUES IN MEDICAL ETHICS

Chapter Ten
CONTRACEPTION

Introduction

The simple narrative of the first birth (Genesis 4:1) seems almost quaint today: "Now Adam knew Eve his wife, and she conceived and bore Cain, saying 'I have gotten a man by the help of the Lord.' " Since Genesis we humans have developed a wide variety of interventions into the natural processes of procreation. Already in Exodus we hear of the midwife, and more and more we have subdued the natural process of human begetting and have brought it more and more under our control, until today it is possible to intervene at a number of different points of the reproductive process, in a number of different ways, and for a number of different reasons.

The next few chapters provide a sampling of the theological reflection prompted by these new powers and also an invitation to engage in such reflection. This chapter deals specifically with the power to prevent conception.

Public discussion has focused on two principles in the consideration of contraceptive techniques, freedom and utility. This is not hard to demonstrate. The decision whether to use contraceptives or not is basically considered a private matter and protected from interference by one's right to privacy, by the right to do as one pleases as long as it doesn't impinge on another's equal freedom. When one's freedom is restricted or when there is publicly sanctioned advice about what to decide, the justification usually involves some calculation of risks and benefits, whether to the mother or the embryo or society.

It is not surprising that freedom and utility are the principles which are publicly appealed to. The options in contemporary moral philosophy are often seen to be either formalism, with its Kantian heritage and its emphasis on freedom and autonomy, or utilitarianism, with its pedigree in Mill and Bentham and its principle of the greatest good for the greatest number. The philosophers have not convinced us which principle is the right impartial principle, but they have evidently succeeded in convincing us that public moral discourse, including discourse about reproduction, must be limited and governed by principles we can and must hold on the basis of reason alone, specifically, freedom and utility.

The strength of such an impartial perspective should not be neglected, especially in a pluralistic society; and a theological ethic need not disown impartial rationality. But for all the importance of freedom and utility when we deal with strangers, they provide little help in understanding the moral significance of the family or of being and becoming a parent (or not). The impartial principle of freedom tends to reduce such role relationships to contractual relationships between independent individuals; and utility tends to reduce them to instrumental relationships designed to achieve some extrinsic good. These impartial principles may need to be qualified by Christian convictions about freedom and about the good to be sought and done as well as supplemented by reflection about the significance of human sexuality and parenting—at least if we are to live with Christian integrity as well as with impartial rationality. Our new powers over reproduction, including our power to prevent conception, demand theological reflection if we are to preserve Christian integrity in our exercise of human powers. That theological reflection involves a number of issues, many of them introduced before.

One issue is the relation of theological ethics to "natural" moral wisdom. One may contrast the claim of the pope that the church only defends "natural" morality with the candidly Christian perspective of Karl Barth *post Christum natum* (after the birth of Christ). Of course it is also important to identify the "natural" morality to which one relates Christian reflection. Charles Curran differs from the pope in part in terms of their reading of "natural law," and one may ask whether some Protestants and Catholics have simply identified theological ethics with a Kantian emphasis on autonomy and/or a utilitarian assessment of the consequences.

Another issue is the meaning of respect for persons and their agency. Barth's essay makes significant appeals to "freedom," but it is hardly the conventional understanding of freedom as autonomy, as the capacity of a neutral agent to will what he will, unconstrained and uncoerced. Rather, it is the freedom given by God which recognizes that the Christian is not a law to himself (autonomous) but stands in and under the command of God. How should Christians think of freedom and of the respect due persons? Certainly it is theologically warranted to require respect for the capacities for agency, but is respect for persons identical to respect for their capacities for agency? Or are persons more than their capacities for agency? Does respect for persons also require respect for their bodily natures (for example, does it require that we not unjustly deprive them of necessities)? Again, does respect for persons entail respect for them not only as autonomous individuals but also as "members of one another," as members of communities some of which at least are not of their own choosing? The burden of proof may shift, depending on how one answers these questions, either to those who would limit the autonomy of individuals, asserting the moral significance of our bodily natures and the natural, indeed biological, communities by which we are members one of another, or to those who deny or ignore all that, seeing humans as merely autonomous individuals.

Still another issue which has been examined earlier and now bears concretely on this question is the issue of nature and its mastery. Is the normatively human to be found in nature or in mastery over nature? Is the natural process of procreation normative, or is it distinctively human procreation when it is controlled and planned, when the natural processes are brought under human control? Perhaps we are human precisely in being both children of nature and children of spirit,[1] but what are the implications of that for reflection about birth control? Is the human sexual act ever simply "natural" or always "unnatural" insofar as it is formed by human intentions? Even the appeal to the "natural" is a form of human intentionality, and it is worth pondering *Humanae Vitae* as an attempt to protect not the "nature" of the act but the human and Christian significance of the act. Then, of course, it will be very important to state and defend the convictions that determine the significance of the sexual act and the institution of marriage and the practice of having children.

These questions are critically important not only to guide and direct the use or nonuse of birth control and other powers over procreative processes but also because unthinking use of contraceptives jeopardizes the quality of the sexual act by trivializing it, making it facile and insignificant. Theological reflection is necessary not only to limit our powers but also to preserve our capacities for expressing and gesturing our gratitude to God and our confidence in God with our sexuality. "It is," as Paul Ricoeur said, "probable that a rational use of contraception can only succeed where men are spiritually aroused to the need for maintaining the quality of sexual language."[2]

Notes

1. See Reinhold Niebuhr, *The Nature and Destiny of Man,* vol. I, *Human Nature* (New York: Charles Scribner's Sons, 1964), p. 270.

2. Paul Ricoeur, quoted in "Sexuality and the Modern World: A Symposium," *Cross Currents* 14 (Spring 1964): 247.

Suggestions for Further Reading

Cerling, C. E., Jr. "Abortion and Contraception in Scripture." *Christian Scholars Review* 2 (Fall 1971): 42-58.

Curran, Charles E., ed. *Contraception: Authority and Dissent.* New York: Herder and Herder, 1969.

Dyck, Arthur J. "Ethics, Policy, and Population Debates." Chapter in *On Human Care,* 32-51. Nashville: Abingdon Press, 1977.

"The Family in Contemporary Society" (an Anglican report). In *Christian Ethics and Contemporary Philosophy,* edited by Ian T. Ramsey. New York: Macmillan, 1966.

Noonan, John T. *Contraception: A History of Its Treatment by the Catholic Theologians and Canonists.* Cambridge, Mass.: Belknap, 1965.

Potter, Ralph. "Religion, Politics, and Population: A Time for Change." *Harvard Medical Alumni Bulletin* 41 (1967): 14-21.

Spitzer, W. O., and C. L. Saylor. *Birth Control and the Christian: A Protestant Symposium on the Control of Human Reproduction.* Wheaton, Ill.: Tyndale, 1964.

Thielicke, Helmut. *The Ethics of Sex.* Translated by John W. Doberstein. New York: Harper & Row, 1964. See pp. 200-225.

Veatch, Robert M., ed. *Population Policy and Ethics: The American Tradition.* New York: Irvington, 1977.

51.
Of Human Life (Humanae Vitae)

Encyclical Letter of His Holiness on the Regulation of Birth

PAUL VI

To the venerable Patriarchs, Archbishops and Bishops and other local ordinaries in peace and communion with the Apostolic See, to priests, the faithful and to all men of good will.

Venerable brothers and beloved sons:

The Transmission of Life

The most serious duty of transmitting human life, for which married persons are the free and responsible collaborators of God the Creator, has always been a source of great joys to them, even if sometimes accompanied by not a few difficulties and by distress.

At all times the fulfillment of this duty has posed grave problems to the conscience of married persons, but, with the recent evolution of society, changes have taken place that give rise to new questions which the Church could not ignore, having to do with a matter which so closely touches upon the life and happiness of men. . . .

Doctrinal Principles

A Total Vision of Man

The problem of birth, like every other problem regarding human life, is to be considered, beyond partial perspectives—whether of the biological or psychological, demographic or sociological orders—in the light of an integral vision of man and of his vocation, not only his natural and earthly, but also his supernatural and eternal vocation. And since, in the attempt to justify artificial methods of birth control, many have appealed to the demands both of conjugal love and of "responsible parenthood" it is good to state very precisely the true concept of these two great realities of married life, referring principally to what was recently set forth in this regard, and in a highly authoritative form, by the Second Vatican Council in its pastoral constitution Gaudium et Spes (Constitution on the Church in the Modern World).

Conjugal love reveals its true nature and nobility when it is considered in its supreme origin, God, who is love,[1] "the Father, from whom every family in heaven and on earth is named."[2]

Marriage is not, then, the effect of chance or the product of evolution of unconscious natural forces; it is the wise institution of the Creator to realize in mankind His design of love. By means of the reciprocal personal gift of self, proper and exclusive to them, husband and wife tend towards the communion of their beings in view of mutual personal perfection, to collaborate with God in the generation and education of new lives.

For baptized persons, moreover, marriage invests the dignity of a sacramental sign of grace, inasmuch as it represents the union of Christ and of the Church.

Its Characteristics

Under this light, there clearly appear the characteristic marks and demands of conjugal love, and it is of supreme importance to have an exact idea of these.

This love is first of all fully human, that is to say, of the senses and of the spirit at the same time. It is not, then, a simple transport of instinct and sentiment, but also, and principally, an act of the free will, intended to endure and to grow by means of the joys and sorrows of daily life, in such a way that husband and wife become one only heart and one only soul, and together attain their human perfection.

Then, this love is total, that is to say, it is a very special form of personal friendship, in which husband and wife generously share everything, without undue reservations or selfish calculations. Whoever truly loves his marriage partner loves not only for what he receives, but for the partner's self, rejoicing that he can enrich his partner with the gift of himself.

Again, this love is faithful and exclusive until death. Thus in fact do bride and groom conceive it to be on the day when they freely and in full awareness assume the duty of the marriage bond. A fidelity, this, which can sometimes be difficult, but is always possible, always noble and meritorious, as no one can deny. The example of so many married persons down through the centuries shows, not only that fidelity is according to the nature of marriage, but also that it is a source of profound and lasting happiness and finally, this love is fecund for it is not exhausted by the communion between husband and wife, but is destined to continue, raising up new lives. "Marriage and conjugal love are by their nature ordained toward the begetting and educating of children. Children are

From the St. Paul Editions, 1968. Used courtesy of the Daughters of St. Paul, 50 St. Paul's Ave., Boston, MA 02130.

really the supreme gift of marriage and contribute very substantially to the welfare of their parents."[3]

Responsible Parenthood

Hence conjugal love requires in husband and wife an awareness of their mission of "responsible parenthood," which today is rightly much insisted upon, and which also must be exactly understood. Consequently it is to be considered under different aspects which are legitimate and connected with one another.

In relation to the biological processes, responsible parenthood means the knowledge and respect of their functions; human intellect discovers in the power of giving life biological laws which are part of the human person.[4]

In relation to the tendencies of instinct or passion, responsible parenthood means that necessary dominion which reason and will must exercise over them.

In relation to physical, economic, psychological and social conditions, responsible parenthood is exercised, either by the deliberate and generous decision to raise a numerous family, or by the decision, made for grave motives and with due respect for the moral law, to avoid for the time being, or even for an indeterminate period, a new birth.

Responsible parenthood also and above all implies a more profound relationship to the objective moral order established by God, of which a right conscience is the faithful interpreter. The responsible exercise of parenthood implies, therefore, that husband and wife recognize fully their own duties towards God, towards themselves, towards the family and towards society, in a correct hierarchy of values.

In the task of transmitting life, therefore, they are not free to proceed completely at will, as if they could determine in a wholly autonomous way the honest path to follow; but they must conform their activity to the creative intention of God, expressed in the very nature of marriage and of its acts, and manifested by the constant teaching of the Church.[5]

Respect for the Nature and Purpose of the Marriage Act

These acts, by which husband and wife are united in chaste intimacy, and by means of which human life is transmitted, are, as the council recalled, "noble and worthy,"[6] and they do not cease to be lawful if, for causes independent of the will of husband and wife, they are foreseen to be infecund, since they always remain ordained towards expressing and consolidating their union. In fact, as experience bears witness, not every conjugal act is followed by a new life. God has wisely disposed natural laws and rhythms of fecundity which, of themselves, cause a separation in the succession of births. Nonetheless the Church, calling men back to the observance of the norms of the natural law, as interpreted by its constant doctrine, teaches that each and every marriage act (quilibet matrimonii usus) must remain open to the transmission of life.[7]

Two Inseparable Aspects: Union and Procreation

That teaching, often set forth by the magisterium, is founded upon the inseparable connection, willed by God and unable to be broken by man on his own initiative, between the two meanings of the conjugal act: the unitive meaning and the procreative meaning. Indeed, by its intimate structure, the conjugal act, while most closely uniting husband and wife, capacitates them for the generation of new lives, according to laws inscribed in the very being of man and of woman. By safeguarding both these essential aspects, the unitive and the procreative, the conjugal act preserves in its fullness the sense of true mutual love and its ordination towards man's most high calling to parenthood. We believe that the men of our day are particularly capable of seizing the deeply reasonable and human character of this fundamental principle.

Faithfulness to God's Design

It is in fact justly observed that a conjugal act imposed upon one's partner without regard for his or her condition and lawful desires is not a true act of love, and therefore denies an exigency of right moral order in the relationships between husband and wife. Hence, one who reflects well must also recognize that a reciprocal act of love, which jeopardizes the responsibility to transmit life which God the Creator, according to particular laws, inserted therein, is in contradiction with the design constitutive of marriage, and with the will of the Author of life. To use this divine gift destroying, even if only partially, its meaning and its purpose is to contradict the nature both of man and of woman and of their most intimate relationship, and therefore it is to contradict also the plan of God and His will. On the other hand, to make use of the gift of conjugal love while respecting the laws of the generative process means to acknowledge oneself not to be the arbiter of the sources of human life, but rather the minister of the design established by the Creator. In fact, just as man does not have unlimited dominion over his body in general, so also, with particular reason, he has no such dominion over his generative faculties as such, because of their intrinsic ordination towards raising up life, of which God is the principle. "Human life is sacred," Pope John XXIII recalled;

"from its very inception it reveals the creating hand of God."[8]

Illicit Ways of Regulating Birth

In conformity with these landmarks in the human and Christian vision of marriage, we must once again declare that the direct interruption of the generative process already begun, and, above all, directly willed and procured abortion, even if for therapeutic reasons, are to be absolutely excluded as licit means of regulating birth.[9]

Equally to be excluded, as the teaching authority of the Church has frequently declared, is direct sterilization, whether perpetual or temporary, whether of the man or of the woman.[10] Similarly excluded is every action which, either in anticipation of the conjugal act, or in its accomplishment, or in the development of its natural consequences, proposes, whether as an end or as a means, to render procreation impossible.[11]

To justify conjugal acts made intentionally infecund, one cannot invoke as valid reasons the lesser evil, or the fact that such acts would constitute a whole together with the fecund acts already performed or to follow later, and hence would share in one and the same moral goodness. In truth, if it is sometimes licit to tolerate a lesser evil in order to avoid a greater evil or to promote a greater good,[12] it is not licit, even for the gravest reasons, to do evil so that good may follow therefrom,[13] that is, to make into the object of a positive act of the will something which is intrinsically disorder, and hence unworthy of the human person, even when the intention is to safeguard or promote individual, family or social well-being. Consequently it is an error to think that a conjugal act which is deliberately made infecund and so is intrinsically dishonest could be made honest and right by the ensemble of a fecund conjugal life.

Licitness of Therapeutic Means

The Church, on the contrary, does not at all consider illicit the use of those therapeutic means truly necessary to cure diseases of the organism, even if an impediment to procreation, which may be foreseen, should result therefrom, provided such impediment is not, for whatever motive, directly willed.[14]

Licitness of Recourse to Infecund Periods

To this teaching of the Church on conjugal morals, the objection is made today, as we have elsewhere observed, that it is the prerogative of the human intellect to dominate the energies offered by irrational nature and to orientate them towards an end conformable to the good of man. Now, some may ask: in the present case, is it not reasonable in many circumstances to have recourse to artificial birth control if, thereby, we secure the harmony and peace of the family, and better conditions for the education of the children already born? To this question it is necessary to reply with clarity: the Church is the first to praise and recommend the intervention of intelligence in a function which so closely associates the rational creature with his Creator; but she affirms that this must be done with respect for the order established by God.

If, then, there are serious motives to space out births, which derive from the physical or psychological conditions of husband and wife, or from external conditions, the Church teaches that it is then licit to take into account the natural rhythms immanent in the generative functions, for the use of marriage in the infecund periods only, and in this way to regulate birth without offending the moral principles which have been recalled earlier.[15]

The Church is coherent with herself when she considers recourse to the infecund periods to be licit, while at the same time condemning, as being always illicit, the use of means directly contrary to fecundation, even if such use is inspired by reasons which may appear honest and serious. In reality, there are essential differences between the two cases; in the former, the married couple make legitimate use of a natural disposition; in the latter, they impede the development of natural processes. It is true that, in the one and the other case, the married couple are concordant in the positive will of avoiding children for plausible reasons, seeking the certainty that offspring will not arrive; but it is also true that only in the former case are they able to renounce the use of marriage in the fecund periods when, for just motives, procreation is not desirable, while making use of it during infecund periods to manifest their affection and to safeguard their mutual fidelity. By so doing, they give proof of a truly and integrally honest love.

Grave Consequences of Methods of Artificial Birth Control

Upright men can even better convince themselves of the solid grounds on which the teaching of the Church in this field is based, if they care to reflect upon the consequences of methods of artificial birth control. Let them consider, first of all, how wide and easy a road would thus be opened up towards conjugal infidelity and the general lowering of morality. Not much experience is needed in order to know human weakness, and to understand that men—especially the young, who are so vulnerable on this point—have need of encouragement to be faithful to the moral law, so that they must not be offered some easy means of eluding its observance. It is also to be feared that the man, growing used to the employment of anticonceptive practices, may finally lose respect for the woman and, no longer caring for her physical and psychological equilibrium, may come to the point of considering her as a mere instrument of selfish enjoyment, and no longer as his respected and beloved companion.

Let it be considered also that a dangerous weapon would thus be placed in the hands of those public authorities who take no heed of moral exigencies. Who could blame a government for applying to the solution of the problems of the community those means acknowledged to be licit for married couples in the solution of a family problem? Who will stop rulers from favoring, from even imposing upon their peoples, if they were to consider it necessary, the method of contraception which they judge to be most efficacious? In such a way men, wishing to avoid individual, family, or social difficulties encountered in the observance of the divine law, would reach the point of placing at the mercy of the intervention of public authorities the most personal and most reserved sector of conjugal intimacy.

Consequently, if the mission of generating life is not to be exposed to the arbitrary will of men, one must necessarily recognize insurmountable limits to the possibility of man's domination over his own body and its functions; limits which no man, whether a private individual or one invested with authority, may licitly surpass. And such limits cannot be determined otherwise than by the respect due to the integrity of the human organism and its functions, according to the principles recalled earlier, and also according to the correct understanding of the "principle of totality" illustrated by our predecessor Pope Pius XII.[16]

The Church, Guarantor of True Human Values

It can be foreseen that this teaching will perhaps not be easily received by all: Too numerous are those voices—amplified by the modern means of propaganda—which are contrary to the voice of the Church. To tell the truth, the Church is not surprised to be made, like her divine founder, a "sign of contradiction,"[17] yet she does not because of this cease to proclaim with humble firmness the entire moral law, both natural and evangelical. Of such laws the Church was not the author, nor consequently can she be their arbiter; she is only their depositary and their interpreter, without ever being able to declare to be licit that which is not so by reason of its intimate and unchangeable opposition to the true good of man.

In defending conjugal morals in their integral wholeness, the Church knows that she contributes towards the establishment of a truly human civilization; she engages man not to abdicate from his own responsibility in order to rely on technical means; by that very fact she defends the dignity of man and wife. Faithful to both the teaching and the example of the Savior, she shows herself to be the sincere and disinterested friend of men, whom she wishes to help, even during their earthly sojourn, "to share as sons in the life of the living God, the Father of all men."[18]

Notes

1. Cf. I John 4:8.
2. Cf. Eph. 3:15.
3. Cf. Second Vatican Council, Pastoral constitution Gaudium et Spes, no. 50.
4. Cf. St. Thomas, Summa Theologica, I-II, q. 94, art. 2.
5. Cf. Pastoral constitution Gaudium et Spes, nos. 50, 51.
6. Ibid., no. 49.
7. Cf. Pius XI, encyc. Casti Connubii, in *Acta Apostolicae Sedis* XXII (1930), p. 560; Pius XII, in AAS XLIII (1951), p. 843.
8. Cf. John XXIII, encyc. Mater et Magistra, in AAS LIII (1961), p. 447.
9. Cf. Catechismus Romanus Concilii Tridentini, part. II, Ch. VIII; Pius XI, encyc. Casti Connubii, in AAS XXII (1930), pp. 562-564; Pius XII, discorsi e Radiomessaggi, VI (1944), pp. 191-192; AAS XLIII (1951), pp. 842-843; pp. 857-859; John XXIII, encyc. Pacem in Terris, Apr. 11, 1963, in AAS LV (1963), pp. 259-260; Gaudium et Spes, no. 51.
10. Cf. Pius XI, encyc. Casti Connubii, in AAS XXII (1930), p. 565; decree on the Holy Office, Feb. 22, 1940, in AAS L. (1958), pp. 734-735.
11. Cf. Catechismus Romanus Concilii Tridentini, part. II, Ch. VIII; Pius XI, encyc. Casti Connubii, in AAS XXII (1930), pp. 559-561; Pius XII, AAS XLIII (1951), p. 843; AAS L (1958), pp. 734-735; John XXIII, encyc. Mater et Magistra, in AAS LIII (1961), p. 447.
12. Cf. Pius XII, alloc. to the National Congress of the Union of Catholic Jurists, Dec. 6, 1953, in AAS XLV (1953), pp. 798-799.
13. Cf. Rom. 3:8.
14. Cf. Pius XII, alloc. to Congress of the Italian Association of Urology, Oct. 8, 1953, in AAS XLV (1953), pp. 674-675; AAS L (1958), pp. 734-735.
15. Cf. Pius XII, AAS XLIII (1951), p. 846.
16. Cf. AAS XLV (1953), pp. 674-675; AAS XLVIII (1956), pp. 461-462.
17. Cf. Luke 2:34.
18. Cf. Paul VI, encyc. Populorum Progressio, March 26, 1967, no. 21.

52. The Contraceptive Revolution and the Human Condition

CHARLES E. CURRAN

The Council of the Society for Health and Human Values has determined that the most significant and far-reaching advance produced by the new biology is contraception. The purpose of this paper is to study from the perspective of moral theology or Christian ethics the phenomenon of contraception—the great revolution of the new biology—and to see what this tells us about new images of the human condition.[1]

I. The Contraception Revolution

The fact of the contraception revolution must be admitted by all. In 1976 only 7.7 percent of American married women were classified as fertile, not wanting to become pregnant, and nonusers of contraception in their marriage.[2] The changes brought about by contraception have been enormous. At the family level in all parts of the world the procreation of offspring can now be controlled by the marriage partners. No longer are sexual relationships necessarily connected with procreation. Family planning has replaced biological necessity as the way in which parents bring children into the world. Such family planning has above all freed the woman from the biological necessity of spending most of her life as a bearer and nurturer of children. The ability to plan, to limit the number of children, or even to have no children at all has already contributed much to the changing role of women in contemporary society. However, in parts of the world there is still some resistance to family planning and the use of contraception.

Effective contraceptive methods have made it possible at least in theory for the population of countries and of the world to be controlled. According to the "World Population Plan of Action" adopted by the World Population Congress meeting in Bucharest in 1974 under the auspices of the United Nations, if the world population growth continues at the rate of 2 percent, which has been occurring since 1950, there would be a doubling of the world population every thirty-five years.[3] There are different theories about the meaning and extent of the population problem, but at the very minimum all recognize the need for population control in some countries of the world. Effective and cheap contraceptive devices make the control of population much easier.

For individuals engaging in sexual relations contraception does away with the fear of pregnancy. It is difficult to correlate the exact relationship between sexual activity among young nonmarrieds and contraception, but the general wisdom maintains that contraception has definitely contributed to the fact that more unmarried people are sexually active today than ever before. A recent study shows a remarkable upsurge in premarital intercourse by unmarried teen-aged women living in metropolitan areas. A survey taken in 1971 indicated that 30 percent of these young unmarried women had sexual intercourse by age nineteen. In 1976 the percentage rose to 43 percent. The latest survey puts the figure at 50 percent.[4]

The term "revolution" is often abused in our media conscious age, but perhaps the word is justified in referring to the use of contraception and the resultant change brought about for individuals, for families, and for nations in dealing with the problem of human control over births. Effective contraceptive devices have given human beings control over the procreative aspect of sexual relationships and have contributed greatly to significant societal changes. However, the contraceptive revolution has not been without its problems. There have been a number of significant debates in the area of contraception that can help us to evaluate better the whole question of contraception as an illustration of the ethical and human possibilities and dilemmas brought about by the new biology. The debates have centered on a number of issues—the morality of using contraception; the safety and side effects of contraceptive devices, especially the pill; the problems connected with population control; and the uses and abuses of the power of contraceptive technology.

The Morality of Contraception

The morality of using contraception as a means of family planning has been attacked primarily by the Roman Catholic Church. In 1968 Pope Paul VI reiterated the condemnation of artificial contraception in his encyclical *Humanae vitae.* The Catholic Church, however, believes in responsible parenthood. Couples should bring into the world only those children that they can care for and educate properly. As early as 1951 Pope Pius XII acknowledged that medical, eugenic, economic, and social conditions can justify the desire to limit the size of one's family. But the

From *American Journal of Philosophy and Theology* 3 (May 1982): 42-59. Used by permission of the publisher and the author.

official hierarchical Catholic teaching does not allow the use of any means that interfere with the natural act of sexual intercourse or with the sexual faculty. The God-given purpose of the sexual faculty is for the procreation and education of offspring and for the love union of the spouses. Every act of sexual intercourse must be open to this twofold finality. Human beings cannot directly interfere with the faculty or with the act so that the natural finality is frustrated.[5]

There are both practical and theoretical objections to this official teaching within Roman Catholicism. Archbishop John Quinn of San Francisco, president of the National Conference of Catholic Bishops, has recognized the serious pastoral problems existing in the American church on this issue. Quinn recently quoted statistics showing that 76.5 percent of American Catholic married women of child-bearing age use some form of contraception, and 94 percent of these were employing means condemned by the pope. Many theologians have disagreed with the conclusion and the reasoning proposed by the pope. Human beings do have the power and responsibility to interfere with the sexual faculty and act. The official Catholic teaching is often accused of a physicalism or biologism because the biological or physical structure of the act is made normative and cannot be interfered with.[6] I take this dissenting position.

Some Catholics and others have been advocating natural family planning whereby a couple determines the time of ovulation by an examination of the woman's cervical mucus and limits conjugal relations to the sterile time. Promoters of natural family planning (NFP) support this approach with many reasons—often using arguments proposed against other forms of contraception. Natural family planning capitalizes on the contemporary appreciation of the natural, which seeks to avoid additives and pills. NFP appeals to the highest aspect of the human—the love and discipline of the spouses—and is not merely a scientific technique. The method is totally safe and avoids many of the dangers often associated with the pill. NFP requires the joint cooperation of both spouses and does not put the burden of contraception on one—especially the woman.[7] There do seem to be many attractive aspects about NFP, but I personally see no moral problem in using other forms of contraception as a means of exercising responsible parenthood. Unfortunately, NFP does not appear to be effective where discipline, training, and high motivation are not present, so that its effectiveness with regard to population control is questionable.[8]

A related but different moral problem concerns the use of contraception by unmarried people. Although a surprising number of sexually active teenagers do not use contraception, still there can be no doubt that the availability of contraception has contributed to the growing frequency of extra and premarital sexual relations. In general the Judaeo-Christian tradition has historically condemned sexual relations outside the context of marriage. The vast majority of philosophical and theological ethicists seem to agree in insisting that sexual relations must be seen in the context of person relations. Casual and impersonal sex violates the human meaning of sexuality. Many, myself included, understand the full meaning of human sexuality in terms of the total commitment of one person to another in marriage. On the other hand, while maintaining that casual and impersonal sex and sex without full personal commitment are morally wrong, I and many others would urge people engaging in such sexual intercourse to use contraception as a way of avoiding conception. Such people obviously are not prepared to bring children into the world and educate them.

Safety and Side Effects

The most discussed question in the area of oral contraception has been the safety and side effects of the pill. In a period of twenty years the pill has become the most widely used form of artificial contraception. Recent estimates (1978) from the World Health Organization indicate that somewhere between 50 and 80 million women in the world are using the pill. Not only is the pill effective, but it is now comparatively inexpensive. The cost of oral contraceptives in large government projects has been reduced to about fifteen cents per woman per month.[9] Effectiveness and availability are two very important characteristics significantly influencing the importance of the pill as a form of contraception. In the United States about half of all married women practicing contraception (as distinguished from sterilization) use the pill. However, there is a significant change in women aged 35 to 44. In this category over 50 percent of the married couples are sterile, and 28.9 of the total number of married couples are sterile because of contraceptive sterilization—either tubal ligation for the women or vasectomy for the males. Of the 49.9 percent of women in fertile marriages in this age bracket, 72 percent use contraceptives in their marriage. But only one out of five of these contraceptors uses the pill. These figures show the diminishing percentage of women over 35 years who use the pill apparently because of the health risk involved.[10]

The question of safety and risk has been a constant worry for women and also a matter for frequent discussion in both the scientific and popular literature. An article in the *New York Times Magazine* in 1976 accepted the conclusion proposed by Professor Martin Vessey of Oxford, whose study group based their findings on the medical histories of seventeen thousand users of the pill. The benefits of the pill outweigh its disadvantages, but there are some qualifications. Pill users should be kept under general supervision by their doctors. They should limit the length of time they stay on the pill. After 35 years, since the adverse effects tend to increase, for example, the risk of a thromboembolic event, other methods of contraception are suggested.[11]

A 1978 study by Mishell in the *American Journal of Diseased Children* listed the following absolute contraindications for the pill: estrogen dependent neoplasia; cancer of the breast; active, acute, or marked chronic liver disease with abnormal function; a history of thrombophlebitis, thromboembolism, or thrombotic disease, including cerebral, vascular, and coronary artery disease; undiagnosed abnormal uterine bleeding; pregnancy; congenital hyperlipidemia; diabetes mellitus; history of gestational diabetes; hypertension. Relative contraindications include: depression, migraine headache, leiomyomata of the uterus, epilepsy, oligomenorrhea, amenorrhea. Note that in addition to the problems of safety and risk there also are the unwanted side effects such as possible weight gain, headaches, and menstrual irregularities. The study concludes that women over 35 years should discontinue oral contraceptives; women under 35 years with hypertension, diabetes, and hyperlipidemia and those who are heavy smokers should not use the steroid pills.[12]

The most intense study in the United States, conducted by the Kaiser-Permanente Medical Center at Walnut Creek, California, has involved more than sixteen thousand pill users over a period of ten years. The final report of this study, which will now cease because of its high cost (4.3 million dollars), is being readied for publication. Newspaper accounts report the findings that in a population of young, adult, white, middle-class women the risks of oral contraception use appear to be negligible. But the final word is not in, and women must weigh the pros and cons among the uncertainties. Smoking, long sun exposure, and having multiple sex partners increase the risks.[13]

However, there has been a continuing opposition to the use of the contraceptive pill, especially from some feminist groups who view the risks connected with the pill as unacceptable and unnecessary. There are other forms of safe contraception which do not put such a burden on the woman.[14]

One can conclude there will probably never be a form of contraception which is absolutely safe with no negative side effects and no inconveniences. The woman using the pill now must make a prudential judgment based on the available information. However, one should remember that there are also risks in childbearing itself.

The possible dangers and side effects connected with the pill have made the public and regulatory agencies, particularly the Food and Drug Administration (FDA), more conscious of the need for safety in the use of drugs in general and in the area of contraception especially. There is some dispute about whether the United States is too stringent in its requirements of testing before allowing new drugs and especially new forms of contraception to go on the market. Some even claim that under the present directives the original contraceptive pill would never have appeared. In the future it will be very difficult to come up with newer contraceptive pills and devices precisely because of the large cost involved in research and in the necessary testing before the pill could be approved.[15]

One very significant, continuing debate concerns the contraceptive Depo-Provera, which is injected intramuscularly in women and is effective for three months. Depo-Provera has not been approved by the FDA in the United States for contraceptive use, although it has been approved for use in treating advanced endometrial cancer. In the United States groups such as the National Women's Health Network have opposed the drug.[16] However, the medical board of the International Planned Parenthood Federation has endorsed the widespread use of Depo-Provera as a contraceptive.[17]

In general I support the strict testing standards and regulations which are now in effect. The danger is great that researchers and drug companies with their primary interest of marketing drugs as quickly as possible will tend not to recognize the need for adequate safeguards and testing before such drugs are put on the market. Government regulations with strict and fair procedures are absolutely necessary even though such testing will inevitably cause delays before drugs are used and will raise the cost of marketing new drugs.

There is one other "side effect" of the pill that should be mentioned, but with side effects understood in a broader way. This is the great rise in the rate of VD. In the mid-1950s there was a general feeling that VD was no longer a real problem in the United States. Federal appropriations for VD fell from a high of 17 million dollars to 3 million dollars in 1955. But in the late 1950s after the introduction of the pill the reported cases of infectious syphilis and gonorrhea began to rise. By the 1970s gonorrhea had become the number one of all the reportable communicable diseases in the United States. Similar growth in VD has been reported in other countries of the first world such as England, Canada, Australia, and Denmark.[18] One can legitimately presume that the use of the pill is causally related in some manner to the increase in VD because the pill (unlike the condom) does nothing to prevent the spread of VD. The linkage between the use of the pill and the rise of VD is another indication that there is no such thing as a contraceptive which is perfect from every perspective.

Population Control

The macro aspects of the contraception revolution involve especially the question of population control. Here, too, there has been much discussion in the last decades. Of primary importance is the very definition and understanding of the problem itself. I agree with the approach of Philip Hauser, who insists on a complex understanding of the problem, including four elements or even four crises. The population explosion refers to the growing number of people. The population implosion indicates the increasing concentration of people on relatively small portions of the earth's surface. The population displosion means the increasing heterogeneity of people who share the same geographical state as well as the same social, political, and economic conditions, as exemplified by current problems in Northern Ireland, in many African countries, and even in Canada. Finally, the technoplosion refers to the accelerated pace of technological innovation which has characterized our present era. Hauser maintains that the problems created or exacerbated by implosion and displosion will create more human misery during the remainder of this century than the problems produced by excessive fertility and growth.[19] However, we must not forget the long-range problems.

A fundamental ethical problem concerns the means used by governments to control the growth of population. The moral values involved here are the freedom of the individual, justice, and the general welfare of the nation, including security and survival.[20] On a scale of government interference in a continuum from freedom to coercive policies, the following general approaches can be identified: education, motivation, and propaganda for population control together with provision of acceptable means to control fertility to all who want them; change of structures which affect demography; incentives offered to control population; coercive methods.[21]

In general I am opposed to coercive measures except as an absolutely last resort, but it is necessary to evaluate properly the role and meaning of freedom in these discussions about contraception and population control. Too often freedom in these matters can be poorly understood in an overly individualistic sense. Insistence on reproductive autonomy can forget the social dimensions of human sexuality and procreation. Sexuality and procreation involve a relationship to the human species. Precisely because of the social aspects of procreation the individual couple must give consideration to the broader question of overpopulation. The possibility of accepting coercion as a last resort, at least from a theoretical position, is based on this more social understanding of freedom and responsibility in the matter of marriage. However, in practice, the complexity of the population problem and the dangers of abuse argue against the acceptance of coercion.

The reasoning behind the official Catholic Church's teaching on procreation and its condemnation of artificial contraception is most instructive in this matter of freedom. The Catholic condemnation of artificial contraception rests on the assumption that the sexual faculty has a purpose and finality related to the species and including more than merely the individual or the couple. Freedom of the spouses is not the only ethical concern; the species must also be considered. The official Catholic approach is insightful in recognizing the need to consider more than the freedom of the spouses. Apart from the question of the means employed, the official Catholic position can and does support the need to control population if this is truly necessary for the human good. Catholic teaching in this and other related matters has never absolutized the freedom of the individual person but has constantly stressed the social nature of human existence. As mentioned above, I disagree with the aspect of official Catholic teaching which maintains that every single act must be open to procreation so that one cannot directly interfere with artificial means.

Contraception as Power

In the last few decades there has been a growing skepticism and criticism of science and technology. Much of the recent ferment surfaced again at the Conference on Faith, Science, and the Future sponsored by the World Council of Churches at the Massachusetts Institute of Technology in July 1979. One of the most significant divergencies in the conference, in the preparatory papers, and in meetings concerns the very meaning of science itself. Note that we are not talking about technology as applied science but rather about pure science itself. The one perspective, which has been typical of traditional Western understanding, sees science as an objective search for knowledge and a method for solving problems. The objectivity of science calls for the scientist to abandon all subjective prejudices and presuppositions and enter into give-and-take with fellow scientists in the objective and disinterested search for truth. The method of test and experiment facilitates this objective search. Yet there is no doubt that science itself can and has been abused. The tremendous cost of scientific research today means that pure science is subject to the industries and governments which support it. Likewise, the results of science and the technology it produces have been abused and put to wrong purposes. In this connection one can mention the question of atomic and nuclear weapons.[22]

A second view, often connected with a more radical perspective, sees science not so much as knowledge but as power. The sociology of knowledge reminds us that knowledge is always a function of practical interests. Science is power over nature and over people wielded by the strong against the weak. Science is what scientists do in the social situations in which they work. Science objectively exists only as a social reality and is closely related to economic and political interests. The objectivity and disinterestedness of science are a myth.[23]

Both positions seem to have some truth, but it is not necessary for us to become involved in a long discussion of the problem, since we are dealing with contraceptive technology, or applied science. All must recognize the connection between power and contraceptive technology. An examination of some of the debates in the matter of contraception shows that contraceptive technologies have constituted a power which has been used against the weak and the disadvantaged. Aspects of contraception as power have arisen vis-à-vis individual poor in this country, against women in general, and against the developing nations of the world.

First of all, contraception as power has been used against the poor in this country. Perhaps the best illustration has been the sterilization of people against their will. Headlines were created with the revelation that people in Virginia public institutions had been sterilized without their consent. Questions have also been raised about the free consent given by poor women to sterilizations when they did not truly understand the nature of the operation.[24] The dangers here are very real, and there have been many illustrations of such abuses of power without the truly informed consent of the persons involved.

Second, some feminists have maintained that women have been victimized by the pill. Men have used their dominant power to make sure that it is the woman who puts up with the risks of using the pill. While many look upon the pill as something which has brought about greater freedom for women, these feminists see the pill as another form of male oppression forcing the woman to take all the risks involved in contraception. Feminists and others also resent the importance given to the psychological fears often mentioned as deterring the male from sterilization, even though male sterilization (vasectomy) is a much simpler medical procedure than female sterilization (tubal ligation). Contraception can become another form of male dominance.[25]

A third aspect of contraception as power is seen in the attitudes of many of the countries of the first world to the population problems in the developing nations. Too often official United States policy and the opinions of many Americans, especially before the 1974 United Nations Conference in Bucharest adopted its World Population Plan of Action, saw the solution of the overpopulation problem only in terms of a reduction of the birth rate through efficient, inexpensive, and readily available contraception. Population growth was seen as the cause of many other problems such as retarded economic growth, shortage of food resources, pollution of the environment. One can readily recognize the temptation of employing a technological fix without realizing the complexity of the reality involved and above all without acknowledging the many problems created by the United States and other nations of the first world.

The complexity of the population problem is such that merely providing the means for individuals to control fertility is not enough. Other population factors are involved such as population distribution and structure, migration, mortality rates, and the role of women in society. Above all, the position of Americans with their unilateral approach to the population problem was suspect precisely because they failed to recognize the underlying problems to which the first world is contributing so much. Overconsumption by the first world creates just as many, if not more, problems than overpopulation by others. Above all the population question cannot be viewed apart from its interdependence with social phenomena such as economic change, environmental factors, and technological developments.[26]

There is some evidence to support the position that programs aimed at lowering fertility will not be successful unless they are accompanied by social and economic changes. To poverty-striken mothers in American ghettos a child is a source of joy, hope, and contentment which cannot be had in any other ways.[27] India's programs for population control based on massive contraception and sterilization have been failures apparently because they did not recognize the interrelatedness of the population problem with other factors, especially the economic.[28] One can understand how the poorer nations of the world saw in the

American insistence on contraception and sterilization as the solution to the population problem another instance of the strong trying to hold on to their power and oppress the weak.

II. The Human Condition

What do this analysis of the contraceptive revolution and the ethical questions raised by it tell us about our image of the human condition? Our understanding of the human condition obviously influences our evaluation of contraceptive technology, but an analysis of the contraceptive revolution and its human and ethical ramifications also sheds some light on our appreciation of the human condition. Three different aspects of the human condition will be discussed—anthropology in general, human progress, and technological progress.

Anthropology

As might be expected, there have been and are different approaches to anthropology in the Christian tradition, and these differences continue to exist today. In general, one can distinguish more optimistic anthropologies and more pessimistic anthropologies. Harvey Cox with his emphasis on the secular city represented a more optimistic anthropology in his writings in the 1960s.[29] Cox did not deny the reality of sin, which in Christian theology has usually been the grounding for more pessimistic anthropology, but Cox attempted to reinterpret the very meaning of sin. The Christian tradition sees the primary sin of human beings as pride—the unwillingness to accept the limitations and dependency of our human condition. The good Christian thus becomes the individual who does not expect too much of oneself and is content to live within limitations. But today we need a doctrine of sin that will not encourage defense and dependency. We need an anthropology that will accentuate the responsibility that human beings must take for the cosmos and its future. An emphasis on guilt and forgiveness has made Christians look backward, but the gospel is a call to leave what is behind and open ourselves to the promises of the future. The primary sin is not pride but sloth—*acedia*—an abdication of our power and a failure to take responsibility for the world in which we live. Today the gospel calls the Christian to an adult stewardship, originality, inventiveness, and the control of the world. Even the sin of Adam and Eve was not pride but sloth. Self-doubt, hesitant activity, and dependency preceded that fatal nibble.[30]

Paul Ramsey, especially in his writings on the new biology, takes a more pessimistic view of anthropology and stresses that *hubris,* or pride, is the primary sin of human beings. Ramsey sees many ethical violations on the horizontal plane of human existence brought about by the new biology—coercive breeding or nonbreeding, injustices done to individuals or mishaps, the violation of the nature of human parenthood. All these ethical violations on the horizontal plane point to a fundamental flaw in the vertical dimension—*hubris,* or playing God. In attempts of the new biology to fabricate human beings, to prevent aging, to make cyborgs, to control intimate human moods and powers, Ramsey perceives the human desire to have limitless dominion over our lives—the fatal flaw of *hubris,* or the denial of our own creatureliness. Ramsey insists on the limitations of human wisdom as a guide for the rosy future portrayed by the messianic positivists. If our genetic planning policy is no better than our foreign policy or our urban policy, then we will truly be in trouble. Human beings must be willing to accept our finitude and our limitations, to say nothing of our sinfulness.[31]

My understanding of Christian anthropology is greatly influenced by what is logically the first step in any theological ethics—what has been called the stance, perspective, posture, or horizon of Christian ethics. The stance is the logically first step broad enough to encompass the entire matter of Christian ethics but also able to provide a perspective within which the field of moral theology can be viewed. As a stance for Christian ethics I proposed in *Personal Ethics* the need to see all human reality in terms of the fivefold Christian mysteries of creation, sin, incarnation, redemption, and resurrection destiny. In the light of this stance anthropology tends to find a balance between the extremes of Cox and Ramsey as mentioned above. Creation, incarnation, and redemption all point to human goodness and the power which is ours as God's gracious gift. However, creation also reminds us of our finitude and limitations; sin affects us without ever destroying our basic goodness and without totally escaping the reality of redemption; resurrection destiny as the fullness of the kingdom always lies beyond our attainment in this world.

Such a theoretical framework for anthropology, which recognizes the positive aspects of human existence but also cautions about continuing limitation, sinfulness, and incompleteness, is confirmed by our consideration of contraceptive technology and by developments in the new biology. Human beings through technology have a greater power and corresponding responsibility than we ever had before. With the new medical technology human beings are called upon to make decisions about life and death itself, e.g., pulling the plug on the respirator or deciding who will receive lifesaving technologies. But, on the other hand, finitude and sinfulness will always affect our human existence. Contraception has enhanced human responsibility and freed us from a determinism by the forces of nature, but biological or any other kind of technology cannot overcome our basic creatureliness. Likewise, the proclivity to abuse based on our continuing sinfulness must always be recognized. Contraception, despite its many contributions to human development, has also contributed somewhat to a depersonalization of human sexuality in some areas of human behavior. Technological contraceptive power has been used by the strong at the expense of the weak. A series of checks and balances on researchers, drug companies, and contraception programs of governments is an absolute necessity.

The recognition of the greater power and responsibility that human beings have achieved because of science, technology, and other developments has led some to describe the human being as a self-creator. In one sense the concept of the human person as a self-creator is not all that new. Thomas Aquinas grounded his anthropology in a similar concept. In the prologue to the second part of the *Summa theologiae* which describes the ethical life, Aquinas briefly explains that he will now consider the human being who is an image of God precisely because the human being is endowed with intellect, free will, and the power of self-determination.[32] In contemporary theology Karl Rahner has emphasized the concept of the person as a self-creator. Such assertions must be properly understood. Rahner does not mean to deny all creaturely limitation, but he emphasizes that the human person truly creates and determines one's own self and subjectivity by one's free action. The German theologian stresses that the new aspect in this concept today is the fact that our transcendental self-manipulation can take on new historical and categorical forms because of our science and technology, especially in the biological area.[33] Rahner's emphasis on the subject is part of his transcendental approach, which can be criticized for not giving enough importance to the physical, social, political, and cosmic dimensions of human existence. However, Rahner would agree that we cannot speak of the human person as a self-creator understood in terms of one who makes something out of nothing. Human beings today, thanks to science and technology, have great power over our world, our environment, and even our bodies, but we can never deny our creaturely existence and limitations.

Intimately connected with the improper notion of the person as a self-creator is the ethical reductionism of seeing the human being only in terms of freedom. A proper human anthropology must recognize both our freedom and our limits. We are embodied spirits living in multiple relationships with others. As already pointed out in our discussion of contraceptive technology, a stress on individual freedom and autonomy has often failed to recognize that procreation involves us in a broader web of human relationships. Procreation can never be adequately considered only under the rubric of the freedom of the individual person or couple.

We do not exist in the world apart from our bodies, and to a certain extent we are limited by the givenness of our bodies. The official Catholic teaching condemns contraception as an unwarranted interference in the bodily structures of human existence. I do not agree with such a position, but I also do not agree with those who fail to recognize both the importance and the limitations of the bodily. Joseph Fletcher, for example, maintains that laboratory reproduction is more human than sexual reproduction precisely because it is more rational.[34] However, the bodily is a part of the human, and there are limitations connected with our body that we cannot forget. Fatigue and pain are two readily experienced limitations with which we constantly live. In the discussion of contraceptive technologies the best illustration of bodily limitations is the problem with the safety and side effects of the pill. The complex hormonal systems of the human body cannot be interferred with at will. There are intricate relationships and connections that must be taken into account. The chemicals that prevent ovulation can and do have deleterious effects on other bodily organs and functions. These limitations of the complex bodily system are analogous to the limitations of the "eco-systems" in our cosmos. The ecological crisis has made us aware of these continuing material limitations of the cosmic world that we inhabit. By overstressing our dominion, our power, and our freedom to intervene in our natural world, we fail to give due importance to the limitations inherent in our bodies and in our cosmos. Yes, human beings have great power and responsibility, but we also have limits, and true responsibility calls for us to recognize these limits.

Human Progress

The question of human progress is ultimately connected with anthropology. What about human progress, especially in the light of the contraceptive revolution? Christian theology has taken a number of different approaches to human progress. In the early part of the twentieth century liberal Protestantism in general and the social gospel in particular emphasized human progress. Influenced by the theory of evolution and recent technological developments, these theologians accepted an evolutionary human progress, some even going so far as to accept the inevitability of such progress.[35]

Protestant liberalism was severely challenged by Karl Barth in Germany and by Reinhold Niebuhr in the United States. It was no coincidence that Barth's commentary on the Epistle to the Romans appeared in 1919,[36] and Niebuhr's *Moral Man and Immoral Society* was published in 1932.[37] The horror of the First World War burst the bubble of an optimistic progress which, according to the caricature, proclaimed that every day and in every way we were becoming better and better. The brutal reality of war contradicted the bland slogans of the social gospel—the fatherhood of God and the brotherhood of men. It is a sad commentary that the sharpest attack in the United States against the progressivism of liberal Protestantism was occasioned by the economic problems of the depression rather than by the war! But, whatever the occasion, the progressive and optimistic theology of the early part of the century was no longer acceptable in the light of the brutality of war and the harshness of the industrial revolution with its ever-widening gulf between the rich and the poor. The neoorthodoxy of Barth and the Christian realism of Niebuhr stressed the transcendence of God rather than immanence, placed heavy emphasis on human sinfulness, and insisted that the fullness of the kingdom lies beyond the world, or "beyond tragedy" as Niebuhr entitled one of his books of sermons.[38] The Second World War reinforced the mood of realism with its denial of dramatic human progress within history.

In the 1960s a change occurred which can be seen in the theology of secularity and the death of God theology.[39] Secularity was no longer something opposed to the gospel, but the gospel according to the theologians of secularity calls for us to accept secularity with all its hopes and promises. The older pessimistic theology no longer attracted universal support, especially in the light of the power and the responsibilities that were in the hands of human beings to shape their own future and the destiny of the world. There are those who said that the secular city theology was just a warmed-over version of the social gospel, but it captured the attention of many in the middle 1960s.[40]

Once again, however, human experience shifted. The great hopes of the early 1960s, as expressed for example in the inaugural addresses of John F. Kennedy in 1960 and Lyndon Johnson in 1964, were dashed against the stark realities of discrimination, war, and poverty. Many thought that the school desegregation decision of 1954 and the march on Selma marked the beginning of a new era in race relations, but the urban riots of the late 1960s reminded Americans of how deeply racism and poverty were engrained in our society. The 1960s began with great hopes of peace throughout the world, but the involvement in Vietnam disillusioned many Americans. On a worldwide basis the poverty problem indicated the structural problems of economic neocolonialism, because of which the first world was systematically keeping the developing world in the shackles of poverty. In the light of many of these developments the overly optimistic theology of the early 1960s was no longer convincing.

Changing attitudes to human progress from the 1960s to the present can be seen in the work of many theologians. Take, for example, Johannes Metz. In the early 1960s Metz put heavy emphasis on secularity and the world as history. This incarnational approach with its stress on history rather than on nature emphasized human freedom and responsibility in the world in which we live.[41] By the middle 1960s Metz's understanding of the problematic shifted from secularity to futurity, from an incarnational to an eschatological approach. Eschatology, futurity, and hope characterized the work of many theologians in this period. In this eschatology there was some continuity between the present and the future.[42] In the early 1970s a change emerged in Metz's development. The tone becomes more pessimistic as the aspect of suffering is added. The relationship of human beings to history now occurs through suffering, which is seen in the light of the dangerous memory of Jesus.[43] Finally in the later 1970s the eschatological element in Metz now emphasizes not the continuity but the discontinuity between the present and the future. Apocalyptic becomes a central theme in Metz, who strongly opposes an evolutionary and teleological view of eschatology which is often associated with the Western technological perspective.[44]

Thus we are confronted with the question: Is there truly human progress in history and how does it occur? Again, my theoretical approach is based on the stance or perspective. The goodness of creation, the incarnation, and the fact that redemption has already occurred argue for some continuity between the present and the future of the kingdom. However, human finitude, sinfulness, and resurrection destiny as future call for some discontinuity between the present and the future. The fullness of the kingdom is always beyond our grasp. Such a perspective has room for some truly human progress in history, but the negative aspects of finitude, sin, and eschatological incompleteness are limits against a naive, evolutionary, and too optimistic view of human progress. Such a perspective, especially when looking at history in the long view, does not expect to see any great or dramatic breakthroughs in human progress. Yes, there can and will be some limited progress over time, but there will be no utopias existing in this world. My approach thus differs from both evolutionary progressivism and contemporary apocalypticism.

How does this theoretical view of human progress stand up in the light of experience in history? The interpretation of history is always risky. One can point to great deformations that have occurred in the development of history. Modern war with its nuclear weapons has become infinitely more destructive than earlier wars. However, I think there has been limited but significant historical advance in terms of truly human progress. A very basic ethical reality concerns the rights, dignity, and equality of human beings. Here one can note some true historical progress. Slavery is nowhere near as prevalent as it was at one time. Our society today is much more aware of the equal rights of women. Contemporary human beings have a greater area in which to exercise their freedom and responsibility in many aspects of human life. Democratic government has given individuals a greater participation in their government. The Declaration of Human Rights of the United Nations points to an ever-growing awareness on the international level of basic human rights. Without claiming any utopian or dramatic breakthroughs one can make an argument for some true but limited human progress in history.

It seems as if theology has somewhat flip-flopped in its approach to human progress and has been too easily influenced by the immediate situations of the times. There will always be more optimistic and more pessimistic periods in human history, but a theological worldview must be supple enough to recognize these ups and downs without losing sight of the overall perspective which in my judgment recognizes some true but limited progress in the course of history. Struggle, with penultimate victories somewhat outweighing penultimate defeats, will characterize our historical existence.

Technological Progress

What is the relationship between technological progress and truly human progress? One significant factor contributing to the optimistic understanding of human progress in the 1960s was technological progress. There can be no doubt that technology has made great progress. Human beings have come from the discovery of the wheel to the animal drawn cart, to the steam engine, the automobile, the airplane, and the rocket ships that landed human beings on the moon. Technological developments seem to be ever progressive in the sense that new developments build on older discoveries and constantly move forward as illustrated in the case of transportation. However, the experience of the late 1960s and the 1970s caused many to take a quite critical look at technological progress.

First, technological progress is not the same as human progress. The apparently steadily progressive thrust of technological progress is not true of human progress. Newer technology always builds on the old and improves on it, but look at other areas of human existence. Why do we still read Shakespeare, listen to Bach and Beethoven, admire the sculpture of ancient Greece and Rome, and recognize the artistry of Michelangelo or Raphael? Literature, art, drama, and music do not show this always-advancing progress which is true of science and technology. Human progress and technological progress are not the same precisely because the technological is only one small part of the human. Technology is never going to solve the great human problems of life and death, love and sharing, hope and endurance. Yet technology is not something evil or necessarily opposed to the human, but rather science and technology are the result of human creativity and therefore good. However, science and technology are also quite limited in terms of the truly and fully human. Since the human encompasses much more than the technological the human at times must say no to the possibilities of technology.

Second, technological progress is not as unilaterally progressive and developmental as was supposed. Technological progress itself is ambiguous. Developments in transportation were used to illustrate the presumably always progressive nature of technological development, but later experience and reflection recall some negative aspects of such development. Think, for example, of the problem of air pollution or the flight from the cities occasioned by the mass use of automobiles. Technological advances, even apart from their relationship to the wider aspect of the human, are not without ambiguous side effects.

III. Conclusion

This paper has studied the contraceptive revolution and has analyzed the understanding of anthropology and of human and technological progress from the perspective of theological ethics. In light of all these considerations, some conclusions can now be drawn with regard to contraceptive technology and its relationship to the human.

First, contraceptive technology in general has been good for human beings. The effects of contraception in the matter of family planning and population control have been very beneficial. To free human beings from physical necessity and to give them greater control and responsibility enhances the reality of the human. The very term "responsible parenthood," accepted by about all people today, calls attention to the human good which has been brought into being by contraceptive technology.

Second, contraceptive technology is a limited human good. Technology itself can never solve or even touch the deeper human questions and problems of life and death, loving concern, or egoism. Contraception can contribute to the well-being of spouses and of families. Population control can help nations and the whole world. However, the human problems and possibilities facing individuals, spouses, nations, and the world transcend the level of biological technologies or of all technologies combined. Recall the dangerously unilateral approach which viewed the problems of limiting population in the narrow terms of providing safe, cheap, and effective contraceptives and failed to recognize the many other aspects of the problem.

Third, this limited human good remains somewhat ambiguous. The best example of the ambiguity in contraceptive advances had been the dangers and side effects associated with the pill. There will undoubtedly never be a perfect contraceptive in the sense of something that is perfect from every single perspective—the hygienic, the eugenic, the aesthetic, etc. At the very minimum all existing contraceptive technologies seem to have some limitations and imperfections about them.

Fourth, contraception is a limited good which can be abused. While contraception has made it possible for people to practice responsible parenthood, it has also made it somewhat easier for others to engage in impersonal and irresponsible sexuality. Limited human goods are always subject to such abuse.

Fifth, contraceptive technology is susceptible to takeover by the strong at the expense of the weak. The poor in our country, women in general, and the poor nations of the world have all been victims of the contraceptive technology of the powerful. Thus contraceptive technology has been a good for human beings but a good that is somewhat limited, ambiguous, and vulnerable to takeover by the powerful at the expense of the weak. This assessment and understanding of contraceptive technology should provide us with a framework for judging the newer biological technologies that will come our way in the future.

Notes

1. This article was originally presented at the annual meeting of the Society for Health and Human Values in October 1980. Throughout the article contraception will be used in the strict sense to include both contraception and sterilization but *not* abortion.

2. Kathleen Ford, "Contraceptive Use in the United States, 1973-1976," *Family Planning Perspectives* 10 (1978), 264-269.

3. United Nations Economic and Social Council, "World Population Plan of Action," *World Population Conference* (October 2, 1974), E/5585, par. n. 3.

4. Melvin Zelnik and John F. Kantner, "Sexual Activity, Contraceptive Use and Pregnancy among Metropolitan Area Teenagers: 1971-1979," *Family Planning Perspectives* 12 (1980), 230-237.

5. For a summary of this hierarchical Catholic teaching, see Thomas J. O'Donnell, *Medicine and Christian Morality* (Staten Island, New York: Alba House, 1976), pp. 238-257.

6. Archbishop John R. Quinn, "New Context for Contraception Teaching," *Origins: N.C. Documentary Service* 10 (October 9, 1980), 263-267. For an overview of the discussion within Catholicism on the occasion of the encyclical *Humanae vitae,* see William H. Shannon, *The Lively Debate: Response to Humanae Vitae* (New York: Sheed and Ward, 1970); Joseph A. Selling, "The Reaction to *Humanae Vitae:* A Study in Special and Fundamental Theology" (S.T.D. diss., Catholic University of Louvain, 1977).

7. Mary Shivanandan, *Natural Sex* (New York: Rawson, Wade Publishers, 1979).

8. World Health Organization, *Special Programme of Research, Development and Research Training in Human Reproduction,* 7th Annual Report, Geneva, November 1978. This report is quoted in Carl Djerassi, *The Politics of Contraception* (New York: W.W. Norton, 1980), pp. 9-10. For a defense of the effectiveness of NFP, see Shivanandan, *Natural Sex.*

9. Djerassi, *The Politics of Contraception,* p. 33.

10. Ford, *Family Planning Perspectives* 10 (1978), 264-369; Djerassi, *The Politics of Contraception,* pp. 33ff.

11. Paul Vaughan, "The Pill Turns Twenty," *The New York Times Magazine,* June 13, 1976, pp. 9ff. The scientific source for *The New York Times Magazine* article is M.P. Vessey and R. Doll, "Is the Pill Safe Enough to Continue Using?" *Proceedings of the Royal Society of London,* vol. B.195 (1976), 69-80.

12. David R. Mishell, "Contraception," *American Journal of Diseases of Children* 132 (September 1978), 912-921.

13. *The Washington Post,* Tuesday, October 21, 1980, p. A7.

14. Barbara Seaman, *The Doctor's Case against the Pill* (New York: Doubleday, 1980).

15. Djerassi, *The Politics of Contraception,* pp. 67-167.

16. Carol Levine, "Depro-Provera and Contraceptive Risk: A Case Study of Values in Conflict," *The Hastings Center Report* 9, 4 (August 1979), 8-11.

17. *The New York Times,* October 19, 1980, section 1, p. 56.

18. Louis Lasagna, *The VD Epidemic* (Philadelphia: Temple University Press, 1975), pp. 1-11.

19. Philip M. Hauser, "Population Criteria in Foreign Aid Programs," in *The Population Crisis and Moral Responsibility,* ed. J. Philip Wogaman (Washington: Public Affairs Press, 1973), pp. 233-239.

20. This is the conclusion of the Population Research Group of the Institute of Society, Ethics and the Life Sciences, which was charged by the Commission on Population Growth and the American Future to examine the relevant ethical values and principles. See *Population Policy and Ethics: The American Experience,* ed. Robert M. Veatch (New York: Irvington Publishers, 1977), especially pp. 477-484.

21. Robert M. Veatch, "An Ethical Analysis of Population Policy Proposals," in *Population Policy and Ethics,* pp. 445-475.

22. Robert Hanbury Brown, "The Nature of Science," in *Faith and Science in an Unjust World: Report of the World Council of Churches' Conference on Faith, Science and the Future,* vol. I, *Plenary Sessions,* ed. Roger L. Shinn (Philadelphia: Fortress Press, 1980), pp. 31-40.

23. Rubem Alves, "On the Eating Habits of Science," in *Faith and Science in an Unjust World,* pp. 41-43.

24. *The Washington Post,* February 23, 1980, p. A1. Patricia Donovan, "Sterilizing the Poor and Incompetent," *The Hastings Center Report* 6, 5 (October 1976), 7, 8; see also the symposium "Sterilization of the Retarded: In Whose Interest?" *The Hastings Center Report* 8, 3 (June 1978), 28-41.

25. See Seaman, *The Doctor's Case against the Pill.*

26. United Nations Economic and Social Council, "World Population Plan of Action," *World Population Conference* (October 2, 1974), E/5585, par. nn. 20-67. For other authors who stressed the multidimensional aspects of the problem, see Donald P. Warwick, "Ethics and Population Control in Developing Countries," *The Hastings Center Report* 4, 3 (June 1974), 1-4; Peter J. Henriot, "Global Population in Perspective: Implications for U.S. Policy Response," *Theological Studies* 35 (1974), 48-70.

27. Arthur J. Dyck, "American Global Population Policy: An Ethical Analysis," *Linacre Quarterly* 42 (1975), 60.

28. John F.X. Harriott, "Bucharest and Beyond," *The Month* 7 (1974), 630.

29. Harvey Cox, *The Secular City: Secularization and Urbanization in Theological Perspective* (New York: Macmillan, 1965).

30. Harvey Cox, *On Not Leaving It to the Snake* (New York: Macmillan, 1967), pp. ix-xix.

31. Paul Ramsey, *Fabricated Man: The Ethics of Genetic Control* (New Haven: Yale University Press, 1970), especially pp. 90-96, 150-160.

32. Thomas Aquinas, *Summa theologiae,* Ia-IIae, Prologue.

33. Karl Rahner, *Theological Investigations,* vol. IX, *Writings of 1965-1967,* I (New York: Herder and Herder, 1972), pp. 205-252.

34. Joseph Fletcher, "Ethical Aspects of Genetic Controls: Designed Genetic Changes in Man," *New England Journal of Medicine* 285 (September 30, 1971), 780, 781; see also Fletcher, *The Ethics of Genetic Control: Ending Reproductive Roulette* (Garden City, New York: Doubleday Anchor Books, 1974).

35. For an overview of this period in Protestantism, see John Dillenberger and Claude Welch, *Protestant Christianity: Interpreted through Its Development* (New York: Charles Scribner's Sons, 1954), pp. 160-254.

36. Karl Barth, *The Epistle to the Romans,* tr. from the 6th ed. by Edwyn C. Hoskyns (New York: Oxford University Press, 1968). For a study of Barth's ethics, see Robert E. Willis, *The Ethics of Karl Barth* (Leiden: E. J. Brill, 1971).

37. Reinhold Niebuhr, *Moral Man and Immoral Society* (New York: Charles Scribner's Sons, 1932; republished in 1960). For a recent evaluation of Niebuhr, see Ronald H. Stone, *Reinhold Niebuhr: Prophet to Politicians* (New York: Abingdon Press, 1972).

38. Reinhold Niebuhr, *Beyond Tragedy: Essays on the Christian Interpretation of History* (New York: Charles Scribner's Sons, 1937; republished in 1965).

39. As illustrations of this approach, see Harvey Cox, *The Secular City,* and Thomas J.J. Altizer and William Hamilton, *Radical Theology and the Death of God* (Indianapolis: Bobbs-Merrill Company, 1966).

40. *The Secular City Debate,* ed. Daniel Callahan (New York: Macmillan Company, 1966).

41. Johannes B. Metz, *Theology of the World* (New York: Seabury Press, 1973), part one, pp. 13-77. In the preface Metz indicates that the essays in this book were written between 1961 and 1967. Although Metz does not explicitly acknowledge any development in the preface, the reader can readily see the development in the book, with part one representing the incarnational stage. See Francis Fiorenza, "The Thought of J. B. Metz," *Philosophy Today* 10 (1966), 247-252.

42. Metz, "Chapter Three: An Eschatological View of the Church and the World," *Theology of the World,* pp. 81-97.

43. Johannes B. Metz, "The Future in the Memory of Suffering," *New Concilium* 76 (1972), 9-25; Metz, "The Future *Ex Memoria Passionis,*" in *Hope and the Future of Man,* ed. Ewert Cousins (Philadelphia: Fortress Press, 1972), pp. 117-131.

44. Johannes B. Metz, "For a Renewed Church before a Renewed Council: A Concept in Four Theses," in *Towards Vatican III: The Work That Needs to Be Done,* ed. David Tracy with Hans Küng and Johannes B. Metz (New York: Seabury, 1978), pp. 137-145. The suffering and apocalyptic themes are also found in his latest book containing articles published in the 1970s—Johannes Baptist Metz, *Faith in History and Society: Toward a Practical Fundamental Theology* (New York: Seabury, 1980).

53.
Parents and Children

KARL BARTH

Man can be father or mother. A husband and a wife can together become parents. Their relationship to their children in the light of the divine command must now occupy our attention. But first we must answer two unavoidable preliminary questions.

The first is posed by the fact that there are men who do not become parents. We are thinking of all those who broadly speaking might do so, and perhaps would like to do so, but either as bachelors or in childless marriage do not actually fulfil this possibility. What attitude are they to adopt to this lack? What has the divine command to say to them concerning it? In some degree they will all feel their childlessness to be a lack, a gap in the circle of what nature obviously intends for man, the absence of an important, desirable and hoped for good. And those who have children and know what they owe to them will not try to dissuade them. The more grateful they are for the gift of children, so much the more intimately they will feel this lack with them. Parenthood is one of the most palpable illuminations and joys of life, and those to whom it is denied for different reasons have undoubtedly to bear the pain of loss. But we must not say more. If we can use the rather doubtful expression "happy parents," we must not infer that childlessness is a misfortune. And we must certainly not speak of an unfruitful marriage, for the fruitfulness of a marriage does not depend on whether it is fruitful in the physical sense. In the sphere of the New Testament message there is no necessity, no general command, to continue the human race as such and therefore to procreate children. That this may happen, that the joy of parenthood should still have a place, that new generations may constantly follow those which precede, is all that can be said in the light of the fact which we must always take into fresh consideration, namely, that the kingdom of God comes and this world is passing away. *Post Christum natum* there can be no question of a divine law in virtue of which all these things must necessarily take place. On the contrary, it is one of the consolations of the coming kingdom and expiring time that this anxiety about posterity, that the burden of the postulate that we should and must bear children, heirs of our blood and name and honour and wealth, that the pressure and bitterness and tension of this question, if not the question itself, is removed from us all by the fact that the Son on whose birth alone everything seriously and ultimately depended has now been born and has now become our Brother. No one now has to be conceived and born. We need not expect any other than the One of whose coming we are certain because He is already come. Parenthood is now only to be understood as a free and in some sense optional gift of the goodness of God. It certainly cannot be a fault to be without children. . . .

The first point to be inferred as God's command to the childless is thus that they do not let themselves be misled about the matter. They must set their hope on God and therefore be comforted and cheerful. Their lack cannot be a true or final lack, for the Child who alone matters has been born for them too. And we must then continue that they may and must interpret their childlessness as something which specifically frees them for other tasks and cares and joys. To bring up children is a beautiful and promising thing, but the end and purpose of human life cannot and must not be sought in this, as all too happy parents would often have it, since the meaning of this activity is only earthly and temporal. One may and can and must live for God and one's fellows in a very different way. May not childlessness be an indication to those who are troubled by it that they should look all the more seriously to other and perhaps very obvious fields which might have lain fallow had there not been men and women without the desire or worry of bringing up children? And childless married couples in particular should feel the persuasion that as such they are all the more called and empowered to build up their life-companionship with particular care both outwardly and inwardly. Parenthood may be a consequence of marriage which is both joyful and rich in duties, but from a Christian point of view the true meaning and the primary aim of marriage is not to be an institution for the upbringing of children. On the contrary, children may be at least a serious threat to what man and wife should together mean in marriage for the surrounding world. From this point of view, childlessness can be a release and therefore a chance which those concerned ought to seize and exploit instead of merely grieving about it. And finally, should we not ask whether a man and his wife, and even those who are single, are any the less called to be elders, to fatherliness and motherliness, because they are not parents in the physical sense—elders who in regard to all young people have the same task as physical par-

---

From Karl Barth, *Church Dogmatics,* III/4, trans. A. T. Mackay et al. (Edinburgh: T&T Clark, 1961), pp. 265–76. Used by permission.

ents have towards their physical offspring? May there not be young persons in their locality whose physical parents may be dead, or for some reason do not fulfil their duty, so that they can help both them (and themselves) if they are willing directly or indirectly to fill the gap? Where the great message of divine comfort is not known and believed, such suggestions will be scorned as an offering of stones for bread. But where it is perceived and accepted, it is hard to see why the childless should not act upon one or other of these suggestions. The divine command, which is only the practical form of this comfort, will certainly draw them out of their grief and warn them to take some such action.

The second preliminary question to be considered is posed by the fact that, while it does not depend on the wishes of a man and woman if their sexual intercourse leads to the birth of a child and therefore to parenthood, they do have the technical possibility of so guiding their sexual activity that it does not have this consequence. Hence in regard to the prolongation of their existence in that of children they have at least this negative power of control. We allude to the problem of what is called birth control. From a Christian point of view, is the exercise of this control permissible, and if so may it sometimes be obligatory? . . .

Our starting point is again the fact that *post Christum natum* the propagation of the race ("Be fruitful, and multiply," Gen. I[28]) has ceased to be an unconditional command. It happens under God's longsuffering and patience, and is due to His mercy, that in these last days it may still take place. And it does actually do so with or without gratitude to the One who permits it. There may even be times and situations in which it will be the duty of the Christian community to awaken either a people or section of a people which has grown tired of life, and despairs of the future, to the conscientious realisation that to avoid arbitrary decay they should make use of this merciful divine permission and seriously try to maintain the race. But a general necessity in this regard cannot be maintained on a Christian basis. . . .

From this standpoint, then, there can be no valid objection to birth control.

The matter is rather different, however, when we consider the problem of marital fellowship.

We must first insist that this life-fellowship as such, whether or not it includes parenthood, is a relationship which is sanctified by the command of God. We do not refer to sexual intercourse in itself and as such. Sexual intercourse performed for its own sake, whether within marriage or without, whether with or without birth control, is a nonhuman practice forbidden by the divine command. We say deliberately, however, that according to the command this life-fellowship as such, including its physical basis in sexual intercourse, has its own dignity and right irrespective of whether or not it includes parenthood. It was always crude to define marriage as an institution for the production of legitimate posterity. Even sexual intercourse may have a first essential meaning simply in the fact that it is integral to the completion of marital fellowship. From the standpoint of this fellowship, then, it may not be generally and necessarily required that it should be linked with the desire for or readiness for children. It may rather be that from the standpoint of this fellowship sexual intercourse should be performed in a way which implies that its meaning is simply the love relationship of the two partners and excludes the conception and birth of children.

At this point there does, of course, arise a question which in my judgment is the only one which weighs against the acceptability of birth control. Sexual intercourse as the physical completion of life-partnership in marriage can always be, not merely human action, but an offer of divine goodness made by the One who even in this last time does not will that it should be all up with us. Hence every act of intercourse which is technically obstructed or interrupted, or undertaken with no desire for children, or even refrained from on this ground, is a refusal of this divine offer, a renunciation of the widening and enriching of married fellowship which is divinely made possible by the fact that under the command of God this fellowship includes sexual intercourse. Can we really do this? Should we do so? Do we realise what it means? Does not a real unwillingness at this point involve an imperilling of marital fellowship, slight perhaps but possibly more serious, to the extent that the latter includes the possibility of this broadening? Can even sexual intercourse as the physical complement of marriage be perfect within its limits if it is thus burdened by reluctance in face of this possibility, or even its deliberate refusal? Or can it be neglected through such reluctance without intimately threatening the whole structure of marriage? Those who basically affirm freedom for birth control cannot too severely put to themselves this practical question. The exercise of this freedom must have valid reasons if the gravity of this renunciation and the seriousness of this threat are to be dispelled, and what one does is therefore to be done with a clear conscience. By this question all frivolity and expediency are excluded. If married life includes sexual intercourse it means that the possibility of parenthood is a natural consequence. To be sure, the attempt to evade this consequence is not always the result of arbitrariness or sloth. Yet those who exclude this possibility and deliberately avoid this consequence must be asked whether they do so under the divine command and with a sense of responsibility to God, and not out of caprice. From this standpoint, therefore, a strong warning must be inserted which we must always consider. In the light of what marital fellowship demands, the use of this freedom may be something which the divine law strictly forbids. The fact remains, however, that even from this standpoint there can be no absolute denial of this freedom.

In favour of this essential freedom, we have to consider that not only the physical consummation of marriage in sexual intercourse as such, but within this the phenomena of procreation and conception, if they are not to elude the imperative of God's command, must be understood as a responsible action on the part of both those concerned. If marital fellowship, including sexual intercourse, has its own right and dignity, the same is true of the act of generation and conception. Just as the former is not merely an arrangement for the continuance of the species, so the latter are not to be regarded as merely the inevitable consequence of the physical intercourse which forms the climax of the fellowship. This means, however, that generation and conception are the effects of an action which is in its own particular way responsible. And as a responsible action it must and will be a choice and decision between Yes and No. Why should we not ask at this point concerning the divine command as though it were already known in this respect? Why should there not have to be a choice and decision at this point? With what right may it be said that these are not necessary here, but it is better to leave things to pot luck, i.e., to chance? It might be objected that they should be left to the rule of divine providence. Man should not interfere with this and therefore with the course of nature. With this, and therefore with "the course of nature"—this is the flaw in the reasoning. For surely the providence of God and the course of nature are not identical or even on the same level. Surely the former cannot be inferred from the latter! Surely the providence and will of God in the course of nature has in each case to be freshly discovered by the believer who hears and obeys His word, and apprehended and put into operation by him in personal responsibility, in the freedom of choice and decision. Surely the specific question: May I try to have a child? has in each case to be given a specific answer as he sets himself in the hands of the living God. Surely he is not allowed to dispense with rational reflection or to renounce an intelligent attitude at this point. The very opposite is the case. At this point especially intelligent reflection may and must constantly and particularly prevail, and nothing must be done except in responsible decision.

I gladly quote what Ernst Michel (*Ehe,* p. 189 f.) says on this point: "Believing trust (in the government of providence) vouches also for the potential blessing given in the gift of children and adopts a responsible attitude with regard to the question of generation and conception, not a religiously masked naturalism.... To reveal its full potentiality as blessing, the blessing of children demands the responsible Yes of parents, just as every good gift of God is meant for the acceptance of the human being for whom it is intended, and only then is able to unfold its character as a gift and blessing.... We thus affirm birth control as a matter for responsible consideration. For it is part of the dignity of man that in responsibility he moulds nature intelligently to his purposes. It is hard to see why in the domain of sex he should simply accept the course of nature or even make it an ethical norm for himself."

The danger of such reflection and decision is obvious. We have already mentioned one of its forms. Broadly speaking, it may happen that in consequence of mistaken reflection an actual divine gift may be refused and a child who might have been the light and joy of its parents is not generated and conceived and does not come into existence. On the other hand, something may be affirmed which was not offered by God. Again in consequence of mistaken reflection, a child may be generated of whom it might well be said from the parents' standpoint that they would have been better without it. Thus the possibility of error exists on both sides. And both errors may mean an imperilling of marital and even sexual fellowship. Both may entail a divine judgment in some form. The danger of thus failing to do the will and command of God is no smaller, but also no greater, at this point than everywhere where responsible action and the venture of faith and obedience are required. The venture, however, is required at this point too. Hence it would be false to say that in view of the risk an unthinking *laissez faire* is better in this matter than action in free responsibility and decision.

It may be that in a given case the faith of a man and a woman will assume the form and character of a homely and courageous confidence in life. Thus the husband thinks that he is entitled to expect of his wife the ordeal of giving birth to children, and the wife believes that she may understand and accept this prospect not merely as a threat but also as a promise. Both of them believe that they are equal to the task imposed upon them with the possibility of generation and conception and therefore with that of the birth and existence of a child. When both together and each individually can believe this, then they ought to believe it, and therefore in all seriousness they should seek to have a child in the name of God, and what happens, even if they are mistaken, will at least happen in responsibility and therefore in a right relation to the divine command.

The idea of birth control can and should also and especially have this positive connotation. Birth control can also be the conscious and resolute refusal in faith of the possibility of refusing, i.e., the joyful willingness to have children and therefore to become parents. Undoubtedly it rests upon false ideas of the good old days to try to maintain that people were then so much more reckless with regard to procreation because they all had this confidence in life rooted in faith. Prudence, and a practice determined by it, were no less characteristic then than they are now. Yet in relation to the modern increase of carefulness in this direction, and the corresponding prevalence of birth control in the negative sense, the question arises why it is that to-day so many people obviously do not seem able to command this confidence in life. Changed social conditions are partly but not wholly responsible, for it was not among small farmers and workers that the modern habit arose and spread, but among the propertied middle and upper classes. It was, for example, an accompaniment of the high standard of living in modern America. A certain degeneration and impoverishment of faith rather than outward circumstances undoubtedly plays some part. And there can be no doubt that a positive choice and decision ought to be made far more often than they are to-day on the basis of this confidence in life grounded in faith.

Yet it is certainly not a Christian but a very heathen or even Jewish type of thought to try to make it an invariable rule that faith should self-evidently produce and exercise in all cases and circumstances this cheerful confidence in life. The fact may be that in certain circumstances a man cannot believe himself justified in expecting this of his wife. Indeed, various considerations regarding her physical and psychological health may forbid him to do so. There must be room for such considerations. Failure to take them into account was and is always to be described as male brutality. But the wife may also be forbidden to understand conception as a promise and therefore to desire it. And both may be prevented from believing that they can rightly assume responsibility for the birth and existence of a child. For both of them it may be impossible for one reason or another really to desire a child in the name of God and therefore in faith. It might also involve an imperilling of their marital fellowship if either or both were to do so in spite of these serious considerations. They must examine their consciences to be sure that these reasons are not merely pretexts of expediency and frivolity. But if their reasons stand this test, they ought not to desire a child (again at the risk of being mistaken), and what happens will happen in responsibility and therefore in a true relation to God's law.

Up to this point there is agreement to-day among all serious Christian moralists, whether doctors, theologians or ecclesiastics. It is accepted that, although the choice for or against generation and conception is not a matter for human caprice, it should not be left to chance and therefore lack the character of true decision, but must always be a matter of free obedience and therefore free consideration and decision. The disagreement that remains and cannot easily be overcome, especially between the Evangelical and Roman Catholic view, concerns the question how the negative decision, when taken in obedience to the divine command, is to be put into effect in harmony with this command and therefore in responsibility.

What is to happen when a man and woman actually believe they cannot accept the responsibility of generation and conception? Four possibilities arise: 1. the practice of complete sexual restraint; 2. sexual intercourse at periods when the woman cannot conceive; 3. *coitus interruptus;* and 4. the use of contraceptives. It must be said of all four, even of the first, let alone the second, (1) that in relation to the course of nature as such they have the character of human arrangement and control. To be consistent, those who on principle decline such a possibility must refuse all these possible courses of action. But if we cannot on principle refuse this possibility, we cannot basically and absolutely give one of these alternatives preference over another. Again, it must be said of all of them (2) that in each there is something painful, troublesome and we may say unnatural or artificial. Since it is a question of controlling the course of nature, and in this case its biological rhythm, this is not surprising. It is obvious that the negative decision in this matter must be paid for no less than the positive, and that the cost cannot be small either way, whichever possibility we choose on the negative side. The costliness is not in itself an argument against any of these four possibilities. If something preventive has to be done, then one of these four possibilities will have to be chosen in spite of their technical and therefore unnatural or artificial character and the painfulness inherent in each of them.

Sexual restraint or connubial asceticism, which was once the only possible course for Christians in the case of a negative decision, has been described in our times as at least the higher path and therefore to be recommended. The fact that it seems to be the most difficult and sometimes heroic makes it most impressive. It would be wrong to say that its practice is always impossible, and that it may not be obligatory for certain men in certain situations. Hence I do not think that it should be generally described as a terrible *tour de force* (so E. Brunner, *The Divine Imperative,* p. 369). But we must be clear that even this method is a matter of technique and therefore unnatural, artificial and painful. Where it is adopted we do not usually have to reckon seriously with injuries to the health of the two partners, but rather with undesirable psychological repressions which might have fatal consequences for the marital fellowship, which as such includes sexual intercourse. And what Paul says to married people in 1 Cor. $7^{3f.}$, and especially in v. 5: "Defraud ye not one the other, except it be with consent for a time, that ye may give yourself to fasting and prayer; and come together again, that Satan tempt you not for your incontinency," hardly seems to point in this direction, although the reference is not, of course, to the problem of birth control. To strict but careful thinking this course cannot therefore claim to be the only possible solution to the problem.

In the second possibility, i.e., sexual intercourse at periods when there is no danger of conception, we have the great and so far the only concession which the Papacy can allow apart from complete continency. The relevant clause in the Encyclical *Casti connubii* is put very guardedly and cautiously, but it is quite unmistakeable: *Neque contra naturae ordinem agere ii dicendi sunt coniuges, qui iure suo recta et naturali ratione utuntur, etsi ob naturales sive temporis sive quorundam defectuum causas nova inde vita oriri non possit.* Apart from the main purpose of marriage (the procreation of children, as the Encyclical firmly maintains), there are also certain *secundarii fines* such as the *mutuum adiutorium* and *mutuus amor* of the married partners, which they may freely cultivate, so long as the *intrinseca natura* of the sexual act remains intact, its centrality is preserved and it takes place normally. T. Bovet (*Die Ehe,* p. 162) recommends his Roman Catholic readers to keep strictly to this injunction, "for it is especially important that they should be in harmony with their Church." They may thus adopt this course, and others with them who see in it a right and happy *via media.* It is certainly feasible. Indeed, since it is distinct from the way of absolute asceticism on the one side, and obviously does less violence to the *intrinseca natura* of the sexual act on the other, it might well seem to be relatively the most feasible course of all. But we cannot take it too blithely. Why did not the papal pastor say expressly that the whole burden of the question whether we may exclude the possibility of procreation on our own judgment cannot be evaded even if we take this course, and that this question is really more serious than that with which he is clearly preoccupied, namely the normality or abnormality of the sexual act as such? And is not this, too, a painful course with its complicated technique and all the statistics and calculations which it involves? Indeed, does the *natura intrinseca* of the sexual act really remain unaffected when its performance, although quite normal, is cramped by so much calculation which seems open to objection even from the medical standpoint, and by all the anxious considerations and obvious fears of the participants? What becomes of its spontaneity if it necessarily involves a constant glancing at the calendar of conception? And what becomes of its character as the joyful consummation of marital fellowship if its spontaneity is threatened in this way?

The simplest and perhaps the oldest and most popular method of preventing conception is that of *coitus interruptus* (*copula diminuata*). In a decree of the Holy Office, 22 Nov. 1922, Denz. 2240 note) the Roman Catholic Church forbids confessors spontaneously (*sponte sua*) and indiscriminately (*promiscue omnibus*) to advise this course, but according to the same text it does not seem to exclude it absolutely in individual cases, provided certain reservations are made by confessors. One cannot allege in objection to it the story of Onan the son of Judah (Gen. 38^{7-10}), because what is described as a sin worthy of death in that story does not consist in the substance of the act and therefore in what normally goes under this name to-day, but in his refusal to give adequate satisfaction to the Levirate law of marriage. We need not waste words, however, on the particularly unsatisfactory nature of this course. And there also seem to be medical objections to it on account of its psychological and physiological dangers. T. Bovet (*op. cit.,* p. 167) declares that for these reasons he must issue an emphatic warning against it, and that it can be harmlessly practised only for a time and by less sensitive married couples. In any event, we have always to reckon with the fact that it constitutes a special threat to marital fellowship.

It is obvious that with the fourth possibility, the use by man or woman of mechanical or chemical means of contraception, the technical and therefore unnatural or artificial character of the whole business is more immediately apparent than in the case of the previous alternatives. At this point, then, Roman Catholic moral and pastoral theology issues what is for the moment, at any rate in theory, an inflexible veto. The difficulty of the whole problem is again revealed in miniature by the fact that none of these means—

assuming this fourth possibility is chosen—seems to be free from objection or even reliable, and that each of them is in some way suspect or even repellent. Some of them are even dangerous, so that they should not be used except on medical advice. And it is perfectly natural that even some who do not disallow birth control as such should feel a kind of instinctive or aesthetic repugnance to all the means suggested. The only thing is that they must not make their repugnance a law for others. Nor must it be supposed and asserted that at this point, where the artificiality is so apparent, we enter the sphere of what is evil and illegitimate. The use of these means is not evil just because they are so manifestly artificial. It is evil when it takes place for reasons of self-seeking, pleasure-seeking or expediency (cf. the statement of the Lambeth Conference 1930). The earlier courses are no less evil when they are adopted for these reasons. And the same holds good not only of these courses, or of birth control as a whole in its negative sense, but of the failure to exercise it if this is grounded in self-seeking, pleasure-seeking or expediency.

Among the various possibilities of negative birth control there is thus none to which, all things considered, an absolute and exclusive preference can be given, but there is also none which can be flatly rejected. Hence it is impossible to formulate any general rule facilitating choice among the four possibilities indicated. Does this mean that we can only conclude that in this matter each individual must choose and decide for himself in the freedom which faith confers? This is true enough. Yet we may still mention and seriously insist upon certain universal principles which must govern the choice made.

1. The choice will be correctly made if it is made, not without difficulty of course, yet with a clear and not an uneasy conscience, with the realisation that in the special responsibility in which one finds oneself it must take the form it does and may therefore do so. Whatever the outcome of the choice may be, if it is to be right it must be made in this freedom of obedience, i.e., it must be made and executed in faith, not in fear, doubt or dismay. As a human act it may, of course, be mistaken. And in any case it will be made only in transition through a more or less difficult set of problems. Hence it can be made—otherwise how could it be related to the freedom of faith?—in reliance upon God's forgiving grace and therefore upon the fifth petition of the Lord's Prayer. But this does not mean that here any more than elsewhere we may desire to sin with a view to forgiveness, and therefore act with a bad conscience. What we can desire only as conscious sin, and can therefore do only with a bad conscience, we ought not to desire and do at all either here or elsewhere.

2. If it is to be correct, the choice must in any case be made only in joint consideration and decision by the two partners. There must be no dictation, overreaching or deceit on either side, but they must both act in full freedom, i.e., they must both take the decision in the free responsibility of their faith and in such a way that they can be open with each other both before and after. Their resolve and its execution must be a communal task, a product of their whole life of fellowship in marriage, so that they can rejoice together in spite of all difficulties, and their solidarity can remain unbroken even though later they may have cause to regard the step as an error and therefore have to repent of it together. What the two partners will and do together will be well willed and done for all the unavoidable problems and the possibility of better information later.

3. The choice must be made with due regard to the fact that so far as possible the inevitable painfulness of each available course must be the burden of the husband and not of the wife. In this whole question of positive and negative birth control, and in all the various possibilities mentioned, it is the wife who is directly and primarily affected and concerned. Here if anywhere there is an opportunity intelligently to respect the order of the relationship of man and woman, and therefore to express the priority and demonstrate the masculinity of the man in such a manner that in every possible choice he takes into decisive account, first individually and then in common discussion and decision with his wife, the fact that biologically she is always in greater danger than he is, and that she must therefore bear the lighter burden, he himself the heavier. It is on this assumption that the decision must then be made which of the alternatives is to be adopted and which rejected. This does not mean that the wife may not be ready for sacrifice as her love requires. But if the husband does not take the initiative in surrendering his own wishes and shouldering the dangerous burden, there can be no genuine achievement in concert, the conscience of the two parties cannot be free, and the decision to adopt a particular course cannot be a good one. No doubt the problem of birth control is not immediately envisaged in 1 Pet. 3[7], but this text is a valid criterion for genuine answers to the problem: "Ye husbands, dwell with them according to knowledge, giving honour unto the wife, as unto the weaker vessel, and as being heirs together of the grace of life; that your prayers be not hindered."

54.
The Ethics of Conception and Contraception

CARL BRAATEN

In dealing with the morality of contraceptive means and with a specific series of "borderline situations" [in the book *The Ethics of Conception and Contraception*], I proceeded from a Christian understanding of the meaning of sex and love in the marriage relation. I stressed that the sexual function of man and woman is not primarily to propagate the race but to serve each other. A married couple does not and ought not marry to have children, but to have each other. Sexual intercourse in marriage has a profound personal value in reflecting a human dimension of love which Christians have interpreted as an earthly analogy of the love of God. Because this is so, it is necessary for the church to make absolutely clear that it now rejects the teaching of some previous theologians who held that the only excuse for coitus in marriage was either to procreate or, if necessary, to satisfy irrepressible lust. Love and sexuality are primarily in the service of the two persons whom God has joined together in a one-flesh union.

A possible, and now controllable, result of this union is that husband and wife may become father and mother. This possibility may be chosen as a vocation; it need not be viewed any longer as a fateful duty or burden which nature foists upon us. Protestant Christians may consider themselves free to use any means of contraception which do not violate the integrity of the love relationship in marriage and which are medically sound. Therefore, in an evangelical ethic love cooperates with reason to determine the specific course of action in a given situation. Yet, if a couple should choose to practice birth control, the ethical question has not been answered. For whether they do or don't, the question remains whether they are following this course in order better to exercise their parental responsibility. Many who earnestly reject birth control measures are only swimming with the stream of nature's instincts, equating that with the will of God. We have found that a Christian ethic may not equate the two, since the nature we know and experience is the world under the conditions of sin. Others who with equal sincerity advocate contraceptive aids in family planning may fail to realize that these can be used as alibis for their egoistic existence. The refusal to have children merely for reasons of personal convenience should not be dignified as a virtue. An evangelical ethic must be sensitive to the subtleties of sin that manage to creep into every solution to every human problem.

A couple planning a family should not consult merely their own convenience. To bring a child into the world is to become involved in a long-term covenant with a new person whom parents are to love and nurture into physical, moral, and spiritual maturity. Love will cause the couple to fix the number of children primarily in the interest of their children. Our essay on the conception of life deals with a very important but certainly fragmentary part of the parents' role. When the child is born, then the vocation of the parents is still barely beginning. Whether they are parents not only in the biological but also in the spiritual sense will, from a Christian point of view, be determined by whether they represent God to their children; whether they hand down the tradition of salvation and teach them the language of faith. For the lives they conceive need to be reconceived by a new act of the Holy Spirit working through the word which Christian parents speak to their children.

From Carl Braaten, *The Ethics of Conception and Contraception,* pp. 39–40. Division for Mission in North America, Lutheran Church in America, 1967. Used by permission.

Chapter Eleven
TECHNOLOGICAL REPRODUCTION

Introduction

It is possible to intervene in the natural processes of procreation not only to prevent conception but also to accomplish it. Artificial insemination, for example, is a relatively simple procedure using a syringe to deposit sperm into a woman's uterus during her time of ovulation. It can use the sperm of either the husband or another donor and can deposit it in either the wife or a surrogate mother. In vitro fertilization is a more complex procedure involving the surgical removal of ova, their fertilization in vitro, and their implantation into the wall of the uterus. It could use an egg from either the wife or another donor and could fertilize it with sperm provided by either the husband or some other donor, implanting it finally in either the wife or a surrogate mother.

These techniques—and others like them—can be used for a variety of ends. The reasons for developing and using these forms of technological reproduction include enabling an infertile couple to circumvent their infertility and to have a child conceived of their seed, enabling a childless couple simply to have a child, enabling a couple to have a particular sort of child—say, a "normal" child or a "gifted" child—or enabling society to influence the genetic endowment of the next generations. The next chapter will focus specifically on the human capacity to influence the genetic endowment of our children and the coming generations. This chapter focuses on technological reproduction itself—and especially on in vitro fertilization.

Several years and several hundred babies after the birth of Louise Brown, the first "test tube" baby, in vitro fertilization procedures are becoming a clinical commonplace, taking their place alongside hormone therapy and artificial insemination as a clinically accepted remedy for infertility. And little wonder, for there are hundreds of thousands of women whose infertility can be traced to problems in their fallopian tubes, which ordinarily carry the eggs released by the ovaries to the womb. For these women in vitro fertilization and embryo transfer provide a way to remedy their infertility. Moreover, the success of these procedures has been remarkable. The outcome is a viable pregnancy nearly 20 percent of the time. That approaches the "success rate" of normal intercourse during the fertile period of the menstrual cycle. And there appears to be no increase in the incidence of abnormalities. The success of in vitro fertilization and the difficulty—not to mention the inhumanity—of indifference to the desperate longing of some childless couples for a baby of their own have almost silenced the voices (like some of those included here) once raised in cautionary cries of alarm and prohibition.

The issues of in vitro fertilization and technological reproduction in general remain worth considering, however, if we are to guide and limit their use, and worth considering theologically if we are to preserve Christian integrity in the exercise of human powers. But what are the issues?

Public discussion of technological reproduction, like public discussion of contraception, focuses on the issues of freedom and utility. "Freedom" comes up again and again: proponents of the research leading to such powers defended it in terms of "freedom of inquiry"; couples defend reproductive technologies in terms of their freedom to have a child (or the child of their choosing); single people have begun to insist on an equal freedom to have children. The only issue that has come up more frequently is the calculation of risks and benefits, whether to the embryo, the mother, or society. Freedom and utility, however, and the impartial perspective which sponsors these principles, still provide only a minimal account of what is morally at stake in these new powers. They are morally appropriate to our relationships with strangers, but can they sustain or nurture any moral significance in being part of a marriage or a family? To understand becoming a parent in terms of freedom or utility is surely a minimal account and may be a real distortion if it is not recognized as such.

A fuller account may still consider freedom and risks and benefits, as do many of the essays below, but it is worth asking whether the concern for consequences is supplemented by a concern about other features of the act or practice and also whether the vision of the goods to be sought and the limits to be imposed on our seeking them is illumined and qualified by a larger vision of human life than that supplied by either the quest for happiness or the assertion of autonomy. All of the essays finally move to a consideration of nature and its mastery, the moral significance of the sexual act, and the role of becoming and being a parent. The application of impartial principles like freedom and utility finally depends on more profound convictions about our appropriate relations and dispositions toward nature, toward our capacities for procreation, and toward our children. Public discourse in a pluralistic society would be well served by candor about these convictions. Christians, too, must participate in the discussion as they formulate their own convictions in ways appropriate to their relation to God, not simply to contribute to public discourse but also to live (and beget) with Christian integrity.

While we are seizing technological control of reproduction, we had better pause to consider technology, sexuality, and parenting. Without some sense of the significance of these, we will never develop the wisdom to guide or limit our new powers.

Few of us would accept the position that every technological intervention into natural processes is wrong ("It's not nice to fool Mother Nature") or the position that any technological intervention is morally licit ("If we can, we may"), but how shall we think about technology and moral responsibility concerning it? Is it simply a function of existing values, a way of getting what we already want—a child, say—or is that view of technology naive? Does it stimulate our wants rather than satisfying them? Does it shape our values as much as it is a function of them? Might in vitro fertilization shape and form our views of becoming and being parents as much as it is a function of our desire to be parents?

The new powers of reproduction, therefore, raise questions about how we understand the moral significance of becoming and being a parent. May we, for example, sharply distinguish the sexual act as a gesture of the covenant fellowship of marriage from the process of generating human life—lovemaking from babymaking, as Joseph Fletcher put it?[1] Or is there a relationship between sexual love and the generation of human life by which God has creatively and providentially ordered the beginnings of human life in an act which also can (and should) express the commitments between a woman and a man? Again, is parenting to be understood primarily and essentially in terms of a vocation to nurture rather than in terms of acts of begetting? Or are acts of begetting essentially parental, conferring responsibilities for nurturing the life generated? Does the desire of a couple for their own biological child itself suggest that parenting not be understood in terms that are altogether abiological? But if so, can the means to achieve the couple's desire be justified by sundering the relationship of biology to parenting?

As long as the Christian church thinks of children as gifts of God and thinks of having children as a gesture of our confidence in God's future, may we do anything but welcome a ministry of physicians to infertile couples? But if the technology to circumvent infertility tempts us to see our children as a human achievement rather than as God's gift, may it still celebrate such a ministry? If the technology commended as a way of becoming parents when we could not before also shapes our way of understanding what it means to be a parent (as a responsibility, for example, to make perfect children and to make children perfect), then may the Christian church still be hospitable to the new powers of procreation? At least such questions can remind us all that the new powers to intervene in reproduction require wise people, not just clever ones.

Notes

1. Joseph Fletcher, "Ethical Aspects of Genetic Control," *The New England Journal of Medicine* 285 (1971): 781.

Suggestions for Further Reading

Curran, Charles. *Issues in Sexual and Medical Ethics.* Notre Dame, Ind.: University of Notre Dame Press, 1978.

Haring, Bernard. *The Ethics of Manipulation.* New York: Seabury Press, 1975.

Holmes, Helen, Betty Hoskins, and Michael Gross, *The Custom-Made Child? Woman-Centered Perspectives.* Clifton, N.J.: Humana, 1981.

Kass, Leon. "Making Babies Revisited." *The Public Interest* 54 (Winter 1979).

Lebacqz, Karen. "Reproductive Research and the Image of Woman." In *Women in a Strange Land,* edited by Claire B. Fischer, et al. Philadelphia: Fortress, 1975.

———. *Genetics, Ethics, and Parenthood.* New York: Pilgrim Press, 1983.

McCormick, Richard A. "Ethics and Reproductive Interventions." Chapter in *How Brave a New World?* 306–35. Washington, D.C.: Georgetown University Press, 1981.

Ramsey, Paul. *Fabricated Man.* New Haven: Yale University Press, 1970.

"Symposium on the Warnock Report," *Ethics & Medicine* 1, no. 2 (1985).

Thielicke, Helmut. *The Ethics of Sex.* Translated by John W. Doberstein. New York: Harper & Row, 1964. See pp. 248–68.

Walters, LeRoy. "Human *In Vitro* Fertilization: A Review of the Ethical Literature," *Hastings Center Report* 9 (August 1979).

55. In Vitro Fertilization

RICHARD A. MCCORMICK

The Ethics Advisory Board, an interdisciplinary board of which I was a member, was established at the behest of the National Commission for the Protection of Human Subjects. It included physicians, geneticists, lawyers, lay people, and two of us in the field of ethics. We chose to begin by considering this question: Is in vitro fertilization (IVF) with embryo transfer ethically acceptable? We defined ethically *acceptable* as ethically *defensible,* although not necessarily ethically *right.* Some 14 months later, we concluded that IVF was ethically defensible even though controversial, because the heart of it involves an evaluation that can't be proved.

The response to our conclusions was overwhelmingly negative. We received some 15,000 letters criticizing us severely, some of them pointing out that the Catholic moral theologian was no longer a Catholic.

I'd like to summarize some of our reflections, touching on the basic issues. Four points were of concern to the public: the naturalness or unnaturalness of the procedure; the question of zygote loss; the possibility of danger to the prospective child; and the problem of containment.

Is IVF Natural?

It might be helpful to review quickly the history of the Catholic community's attitude. In 1897, the Congregation of the Inquisition was asked: May artificial insemination be applied to a woman? The answer, given with the approval of Pope Leo XIII, was no. This despite the fact that the procreation and rearing of children was regarded by the Roman Catholic community as the primary end of marriage.

Here is what Pope Pius XII said in 1949: "The simple fact that the desired result is attained by this means does not justify the use of the means, nor is the desire to have a child sufficient to prove the permissibility of artificial insemination to achieve this end." In 1951, he returned to the subject again, arguing that, for the good of the child and the family, the child ought to be born from an action which is of itself the expression of personal love between a man and a woman. Human sexual expression has two dimensions, the procreative and the unitive, and we ought not to separate those dimensions. We ought not to procreate apart from intimate sexual lovemaking and we should not have intimate sexual lovemaking apart from a context of responsibility for procreation. The Holy Father saw that sexual intercourse had what he called a "divine design," and we shouldn't tamper with it. Therefore, no contraception, and no artificial insemination, and, *a fortiori,* no in vitro fertilization.

In the past 25 years, a lively discussion within the Catholic community and elsewhere has centered on whether the Pope's interdict might not absolutely prohibit artificial procreative procedures. Perhaps it should be looked upon as a general admonition to be careful in the way we proceed. Some would say the child ought to be born of an act of love, but sexual intercourse is not the only act of love in marriage. If artificial procedures began to replace sexual intimacy as a way of childbearing, that would be an attack on marriage because it would deprive the typical marital act of its grandest achievement. But many of us are convinced that the urge to merge is not likely to disappear from our midst, and therefore artificial procedures are not likely to become substitutes for sexual lovemaking.

The strongest presentations made to the Ethics Advisory Board were from people concerned about tampering with nature. Are we justified in doing that? I believe that the mere artificiality of IVF cannot be a decisive reason for rejecting it, just as I believe that the mere artificiality of measures that are used to prevent birth cannot be the reason for condemning them.

Does Embryo Loss Constitute Abortion?

Originally, the procedure did involve embryo loss. Some 3 or 4 years ago, Steptoe and Edwards estimated that they had lost between 200 and 300 fertilized ova before they got a uterine fix. Hyperovulation is still used, so obviously there are failures to implant.

Objections to these losses are raised vociferously and continuously by those in our community who identify themselves as pro-life. Are these losses mini-abortions? Dr. Robert Edwards stated that such protests appear almost irrelevant, when 4-month fetuses, or older, are being aborted for social reasons. That is not a good argument. The problem of embryo loss raises the evaluative question of how we are to assess human life at the embryo stage. Ethically, this is the

From *Contemporary OB/GYN* 20 (November 1982): 227-32.

most difficult problem. How are we to evaluate embryonic life before implantation? Physicians on the Board insisted that before human IVF could be attempted, a certain amount of experimentation was necessary.

There are three possible positions on human life at that stage. At one extreme are those who say it is simply disposable maternal tissue. At the other are those who insist that this is a human being, who merits the protections given to all humans. In the middle are those who hold that there is a human, living being, demanding respect but not yet meriting the full panoply of personal rights.

In moral matters, you can't prove evaluations. Here's a gold coin weighing an ounce; that's a scientific fact. What is it worth? That's a matter of evaluation. That's why the abortion discussion is so intractable. I believe that there are serious reasons, of a physiologic nature, for evaluating the embryo before implantation differently from the embryo that has implanted, or from the newborn. At least 50% of fertilized ova never implant. As Dr. Mishell has pointed out (see page 223 of *Contemporary OB/GYN* 20), many of those that do, abort naturally. The loss of an embryo at this stage is not as critical an issue as many people think.

Those who argue the thesis of the continuity of human life along a spectrum will quote Dr. Edwards [*Science Digest,* October 1978, p. 9]. He says of Louise Brown: "The last time I saw her she was eight cells in a test tube. She was beautiful then and she is beautiful now." Along with the members of the Board, I feel there is reason to conclude that as long as artificial procedures do not result in many more lost embryos than the large numbers lost in the natural processes, this is not a key argument against IVF.

What Are the Risks to the Child?

Some ethicists, such as Paul Ramsey at Princeton, maintain that embryo transfer necessarily means producing at least some severely defective infants. To Ramsey, this is immoral because it exposes some individuals to unknown but very serious risks, without their consent, for the benefit of others. In his opinion, we may not choose for others the risks that they undergo.

Other ethicists—Mark Lapee and Charles Curran—have responded by calling for an examination of the natural processes of procreation. There's some risk of producing a deformed baby when any couple undertakes procreation. The risk is measurably higher when one or both partners are over 35. Does that mean they can't have sexual intercourse any more? Are they running risks for a prospective child if they do? Again, if the risks of the artificial procedures are no greater than those of natural procreation, perhaps even lower, then clearly the heart is taken out of this argument. By January 1983 there will be about 100 children born through IVF, and the experience so far is that this is a safe procedure; there is little evidence that we're dealing with a process remarkably more dangerous than natural procreation.

In taking testimony before the Ethics Advisory Board, we discovered disagreement within the research community. Some felt there had been enough prior animal research, especially in nonhuman primates; others that there hadn't been enough.

Can It Be Contained?

There are those who fear that IVF will lead to donor sperm and surrogate wombs. These would raise basic questions about our values: lineage, the identity of the child, the nature of parenting, and the biologic structure of the family. At some point we might ask: Who gets the Mother's Day card?

Further, there is the matter of moral justification. Some argue that the principle used to justify IVF will eventually justify more than we intend. It seems to me that this depends on the principle applied. Here are two to consider: Principle 1: Husband and wife, using their own gametes, may use artificial means. Principle 2: Couples are permitted to overcome their sterility by artificial procedures such as AID. Principle 1 has a built-in exception stopper. Principle 2 is a wedge.

In summary, the Ethics Advisory Board concluded unanimously that this procedure is ethically acceptable—under certain conditions. We wrote into our recommendation that the gametes of the husband and wife must be used; that embryonic loss must be containable and not much greater than it is in normal processes; that dangers to the prospective child must be no greater than they are in the natural processes; and that sufficient animal research must precede implementation in human beings. Finally, I believe—although I know many of you won't agree and certainly some of the members of the Board did not—abortion should not be part of the contract. Those philosophers, theologians, and physicians who feel that approach is justified would take a different position.

Purely Social Concerns

Now, let's turn to the purely social concerns. Contemporary medicine has often depersonalized the dying process. The danger is that we will overtechnologize the procreative process. What sometimes happens in the NICU is an example of what I fear—maintenance of low-birthweight preemies way beyond where it can do them any good. The other side of that coin is the problem of positive eugenics—preferential breeding of superior genotypes. Researchers and ethicists run from this as if it were a plague. You hear questions like: Is more intelligent necessarily better? Who decides? Isn't diversity part of survivability? I don't think we should be doing these things for positive eugenics. We should be involved only insofar as we are overcoming infertility.

Then there is the matter of priorities. Our health care delivery system is not meeting the needs of the poor. In 1978, there were 135 US counties without a single physician and many more without a hospital. When primary care requisites are not met for so many, to what extent can the government get involved in funding research and clinical implementation of highly sophisticated technologies that benefit relatively few people? Anyone seriously concerned with the ethics of IVF must face questions similar to the ones I have raised.

56. Ethical Implications of In Vitro Fertilization

JANET DICKEY McDOWELL

On December 28, 1981, Elizabeth Carr made headlines as the first child born in the United States as the result of in vitro fertilization (IVF). Worldwide, the IVF total is more than 120 births. Clinics currently exist in 11 countries, and new facilities willing to offer IVF are springing up rapidly, especially in the U.S. IVF is a technique in which a woman's ovum is surgically removed, fertilized with sperm in a petri dish, incubated until successful cell division is observed, and then inserted into the woman's uterus. With luck, the tiny cluster of eight to 16 cells will implant in the uterine wall and mark the beginning of an otherwise uneventful pregnancy.

In the U.S. at present the procedure is available only to stable married couples otherwise unable to conceive and give birth to their own children, often because of the woman's blocked fallopian tubes. However, such new applications of IVF as ova banks and embryo banks have been proposed in England and implemented in Australia. These and other potential uses of IVF should prompt serious reflection within the Christian community. What should be the Christian response to IVF and associated techniques?

Some Christians believe that the response ought to be uniformly negative. The earliest and strongest objections to even limited employment of IVF came from within Christian traditions committed to the indivisibility of sexual union and reproduction. Those who oppose artificial forms of birth control (notably the Roman Catholic Church in its official statements) most often do so on the grounds that these forms deliberately sever a natural—that is, biological—link between intercourse and procreation, a connection which ought not to be broken simply because to do so is unnatural. Their objection to IVF rests on the same premises. They contend that because IVF removes conception from its natural context, intercourse, it is impermissible. If sex without the potential for conception is wrong, then so, they say, is conception without sex.

These opponents to artificial birth control and IVF

may be faulted at several points. Initially, one must question whether artificiality per se is reason enough to oppose a procedure like IVF. Kidney dialysis, respirators, even blood transfusions are also unnatural medical interventions, yet they are not opposed with the vigor of the Vatican's response to IVF. One may choose to distinguish between artificial birth control and a technique such as dialysis by pointing out that dialysis *supports* or *mimics* natural physiological function, whereas artificial birth control *thwarts* natural function. However, such a distinction would work against those who oppose IVF on grounds of its artificiality, for in fact it is far more analogous to dialysis, in that it also attempts to replace (by admittedly complex technological means) a deficient physiological function. Thus the Roman Catholic response to IVF appears inconsistent with its acceptance of other medical technologies.

A second difficulty with this most conservative rejection of IVF is that it presumes an absolute indivisibility of reproductive potential and the sexual expression of love in every single act of intercourse. The majority of Protestants (and a great many Roman Catholics who stand in tension with their tradition's stand on artificial birth control), while perceiving an important connection between reproduction and sexual love, do not assert that the reproductive purpose of sexuality needs to be served at all times. Instead, the unitive purpose of sexuality—its capacity to express love—is claimed as fundamental. Procreation will often be an outgrowth of a mature sexual relationship, but the temporary postponement of reproduction, or even a decision not to conceive children at all, is acceptable within this less naturalistic perspective.

This understanding of the values associated with intercourse would hold that love (as expressed in sexual activity) is preconditional to reproduction, and in that sense the two purposes remain linked. But because this view is less act-oriented, more concerned with the total relationship than with every instance of intercourse, there would be no reason to object to IVF. The fact that conception does not take place as the *direct* result of love made concrete through intercourse is less significant; provided that both love and the desire to procreate are elements of the couple's total relationship, IVF would not be problematic.

Other critics raise quite a different objection. They fear that IVF will encourage (by providing a means) an obsessive concern with having one's own child, a child genetically related to its parents. It is thought that those who choose to accept the discomfort, expense and inconvenience of IVF, rather than opting for adoption, may perceive parenthood too biologically. These critics are concerned that IVF candidates will fail to keep in mind that Christian parenthood is above all a moral commitment to nurture a child, not the contribution of ova or sperm.

It would seem, however, that this danger is not substantially greater for couples using IVF than for other couples. All parents are potentially prey to this sort of idolatry: a veiled worship of self and the continuation of self in future generations. Christian churches rightly ought to discourage all of its manifestations, whether in candidates for IVF or prospective parents who anticipate ordinary conception.

At the same time, it is important to remember that genetic inheritance is not incidental. A sense of lineage—connectedness to parents and grandparents and great-grandparents—while far from vital to successful family relationships, ought not to be discounted entirely. If only for very practical reasons, such as medical records, children often need to identify their genetic parents. Many contemporary adoptees testify to the psychological value of learning about those to whom one is bound by genetic ties. Additionally, a child resulting from the unique combination of the parents' reproductive cells—in a very real sense, their selves—may be a significant sign of their life together.

Kept in proper perspective, genetic parenthood is valuable. It would be unreasonable to deny couples unable to conceive without IVF the chance to experience such parenthood merely because the potential for misunderstanding exists. It is highly unlikely that Christians will ever totally disregard genetic parenthood. (Random child-swapping at birth or mandatory communal child care from very early ages would seem to be ways a community could curb a fixation on genetic parenthood. These have not, to my knowledge, been endorsed by any major Christian group.) Unless and until such a state of affairs comes about, it would be cruel to denounce as selfish or idolatrous those who desire to establish a genetically based family, even when a procedure like IVF is required.

Other objections to IVF have focused more narrowly on the technique itself. Some fear that fertilized ova created by the procedure may be destroyed or used for experimentation, rather than transferred to the uterus of the woman from whom they were obtained. Recovering and fertilizing several ova during IVF is very common; hormonal stimulation of the ovaries is a standard element of the procedure and frequently results in the production of more than one mature ovum.

Objections to possible destruction of or experimentation with fertilized ova stem from a contention that human life is worthy of moral respect (and even legal protection) from its origins in the fertilized ovum. To use fertilized ova for experimental purposes or to discard them would be, according to these critics, tantamount to abortion or human experimentation without consent.

This potentially serious reservation about IVF, however, is overcome by the particular procedure in use at the Eastern Virginia Medical School in Norfolk (the most "prolific" clinic in the U.S.). Where more than one ovum is recovered by the laparoscopy, all are exposed to sperm. Any which manifest successful cell division (and thus are "alive") are inserted into the woman's uterus and thus given an opportunity for implantation. None is used for experimental purposes or destroyed.

However, if a clinic chose to deviate from this procedure and retain some fertilized ova, the objection would be properly focused on the morality of destroying or experimenting with fertilized human ova, not on IVF itself. Setting aside the question of whether discarding a fertilized ovum *would* constitute abortion (and further, whether such abortion ought to be prohibited or discouraged), it is clear that this objection does not necessarily apply to present procedures, especially those used in U.S. clinics. Respect for human life at its very earliest stages is not inherently incompatible with in vitro fertilization and thus need not be the basis for opposing the technique.

It seems, then, that IVF is not inherently immoral. When employed to facilitate conception by loving couples, it is no more problematic than an artificial fallopian tube would be. The abuse of fertilized ova is not necessarily an element of the procedure, and those who would object on grounds of unnaturalness must be prepared to reject other medical interventions that bypass pathological conditions. Conceptions via IVF ought not simply to be tolerated; they should be celebrated, for they enable otherwise infertile couples to join in passing along the gift of life.

Nevertheless, future procedures relying in part on the IVF technique may pose moral dilemmas. Two in particular, embryo transfer (the insertion of a fertilized ovum into the uterus of a woman who did not provide the ovum) and ova and embryo banking (stockpiling frozen ova and fertilized ova), are being quietly attempted in Australia and perhaps elsewhere. Whereas IVF as currently practiced aids in the establishment of genetically connected families, these new applications run significant risks of confusing lineage, distorting traditional family structures, and/or depersonalizing human reproduction.

Defenders of ova and embryo banking argue that it need not be used in tandem with embryo transfer to a nondonor woman. They contend that frozen ova, fertilized or not, would merely be stored until such time as the donor chose to use them. Theoretically this would reduce the need for multiple surgeries to recover ova when implantation does not take place and the procedure must be repeated. This use of ova/embryo banks raises no objections not already discussed herein with regard to the basic IVF technique.

However, embryo transfer in combination with ova banking or embryo banking could be used in a variety of circumstances. For example, in the case of a woman with healthy ovaries but uterine disease (or the absence of a uterus) such that she could not carry a child, embryo transfer would make it possible for her to have her ovum removed, fertilized, then transferred to the uterus of another woman. This "genuine surrogate" would experience pregnancy and birth, and after birth the child would be surrendered to its genetic parents.

For another example, a woman with a healthy uterus who did not wish to have her own ovum fertilized (perhaps for eugenic reasons) could elect to have an ovum provided by an anonymous donor fertilized with her partner's sperm and then transferred to her uterus. Or she could choose to have an already fertilized ovum inserted. Using a donated unfertilized ovum would be strongly analogous to artificial insemination by an anonymous donor; employing the services of an embryo bank has been likened to very early adoption.

What objections might be raised to the genuine surrogate application of IVF and embryo transfer? Primarily, one must be concerned with the attitude such a practice would engender toward the surrogate. Would she view herself merely as an incubator-for-hire, or be viewed in that light by those who employ her? Probably—perhaps even certainly. It would, in fact, be almost imperative for the surrogate to see herself in this way in order to maintain an emotional distance during pregnancy and thus be able to surrender the child at birth. She would have to guard zealously against viewing herself as a "mother," as more than a temporary "repository" for someone else's child. Do Christians wish to encourage women to perceive procreative capacities as mere services available for hire?

Further, an impersonal, businesslike attitude toward the surrogate on the part of the genetic parents seems crucial to a successful surrogate arrangement, unless the couple genuinely welcomes ongoing third-party involvement in their family life. The couple would seem to have only two choices: viewing the surrogate simply as a means to their reproductive end, or creating a new form of extended family. While the latter choice is not unthinkable (and perhaps not undesirable), the former is more likely. One must ask whether Christians wish to be the sort of people who treat one another in this way; the answer seems clearly negative. The kind of interactions among the primary parties necessary to make the genuine surrogate situation work are not those fostered by Christian values. It would be difficult (though not impossible) to structure a surrogate situation in such a way that people are fully respected as persons.

Ova banking is, as was suggested earlier, analogous to artificial insemination by donor (AID). Therefore qualms about AID—such as concern about psychological damage to the noncontributing partner, pseudo-adultery, confusion of the child's genetic inheritance, and devaluation of the anonymous donor—apply also to ova banking. Large numbers of people, many of them Christian, believe that the potential pitfalls of AID can be avoided through sensitive counseling and maximum participation by the male partner during the insemination process. The fact that embryo transfer would enable a woman to experience pregnancy and the birth of the child (conceived with an ovum not her own) would ensure in this case an even greater sense of full contribution to procreation by the partner whose genes are absent. Those who permit AID should welcome ova banking; those who find AID troublesome will view ova banking in a similar light.

In contrast to ova banking, embryo banking has some genuinely novel features—features which could well rule out its use. Fundamentally, objections to embryo banking stem from its deliberate creation of nascent life not desired by either genetic parent. While unintended conceptions do occur with some frequency as a result of intercourse, such conceptions are accidental—perhaps even tragic—and not normative. And many couples who conceive unintentionally do, upon reflection, welcome the child. But the anonymous contributors to a bank will never have such a change of heart. Presumably they will not even know whether their genetic offspring exist.

The analogy to adoption employed to defend the practice of anonymous embryo banking (and subsequent transfer) breaks down when one considers that it induces genetically broken families. The child will never have a chance to know biological kin. Adoption, in contrast, *copes with* broken biological relations; it does not create them. Such deliberate scrambling of lineage seems to serve only the purpose of allowing a couple to experience pregnancy and birth—a purpose that does not seem sufficiently important to warrant the possible confusion.

In summary, I have argued that IVF per se is not morally troublesome. It seems, in fact, to be a positive good in overcoming medical conditions that preclude procreation by some couples. However, other procedures relying on the IVF technique are less acceptable. Ova banking ought to be employed only with the same caution as AID. Genuine surrogate situations seem acceptable only under very rare circumstances that preserve respect for the surrogate. And the transfer of embryos provided by anonymous donors ought virtually to be prohibited altogether.

57. On In Vitro Fertilization*

PAUL RAMSEY

To state my considered judgment in advance of the reasons for it: *in vitro* fertilization and embryo transfer should not be allowed by medical policy or public policy in the United States—not now, not ever. I venture no comment on whether sufficient "animal work" has been done, by *scientific* standards, for this technology safely to be applied within general practice or in trials on human beings. That question and such like questions you will explore with scientific experts. I limit myself to basic ethical and policy considerations that any knowledgeable citizen can understand; and it is in this capacity that I submit this written testimony.

It is my conviction that the Ethics Advisory Board, the Department of Health, Education and Welfare, the National Institutes of Health and the Congress of the United States—and, in absence of action from these Federal sources, the medical profession itself if it has any remaining power to enforce standards or the legislatures of the several States—should take appropriate action to the extent of their jurisdictions to stop embryo manipulation as a form of human genesis.

I am not unmindful of the gift of a child this procedure promises to women with oviduct blockage. Still there are, I judge, *conclusive* reasons for not continuing these experimental trials and for not allowing the procedure to become standard practice in the United States.

I offer four reasons in support of this verdict: (1) the need to avoid bringing further trauma upon this nation that is already deeply divided on the matter of the morality of abortion, and about when the killing of a human being (at tax expense) can occur; (2) the *irremovable* possibility that this manner of human genesis may produce a damaged human being; (3) the *immediate* and not unintended assault this procedure brings against marriage and the family, the *immediate* possibility of the exploitation of women as surrogate mothers with wombs-for-hire, and the *immediate* and not unintended prospect of beginning right now to "design" our descendants; and (4) the remote—but still very near—prospect of substituting laboratory generation from first to last for human procreation. We ought not to choose—step by step—a world in which extracorporal gestation is a possibility. Since I wish to testify to things *distinctively* characteristic of embryo manipulation, reasons (2), (3), and (4) are more significant, in my opinion.

I

Nevertheless, the abortion issue cannot simply be passed by. Millions of U.S. citizens who oppose abortion will bring the same moral objection against *in vitro* fertilization because of the numerous "discards" the procedure requires.

Let me be clear about this first point. I am not speaking of traditional Roman Catholics only. I refer also to the growing number of "evangelical" Protestants whose voice in Washington is the Christian Action Council. I also have in mind the hundreds of thousands of our fellow citizens in the "mainline" Protestant churches who conscientiously oppose abortion despite their leaders. I also have in mind Orthodox Jews and many Conservative Jews and all Mormons, and for all I know many humanists as well, who agree in this common opposition. We are a pluralistic society, like none other in the world.

I do not here open the question of the morality of abortion. Instead, I mean only to call attention to the additional trauma that will be brought upon a nation morally divided on this issue if *any* Federal funding by the Department of Health, Education and Welfare or the National Institutes of Health goes to support *in vitro* fertilization as a form of human genesis, or to support any research tending in that direction. Millions and millions of our fellow citizens do not want their pockets picked by the Internal Revenue Service if any portion of their income taxes goes to support what they sincerely believe to be repeated abortions.

The Supreme Court has declared that public policy in regard to funding abortion is not a question of constitutional right, but rather a matter to be determined by the democratic processes of Federal, State, and even municipal legislation.[1] The Ethics Advisory Board will play a crucial role in determining public policy by "administrative law," not by legislation. Your hearings on *in vitro* fertilization may eventuate, or may not eventuate, in a policy that uses citizens' taxes for purposes to which vast millions are conscientiously opposed. I urge you to consider that constitutionally,

From Paul Ramsey, "On In Vitro Fertilization," Studies in Law and Medicine, no. 3 (Chicago: Americans United for Life, 1978). Used by permission.

*Testimony on In Vitro Fertilization before the Ethics Advisory Board, Department of Health, Education and Welfare, by Paul Ramsey.

on this point alone, you have the legal authority to make whatever "value judgment" or public policy judgment you wish to make. It is within your power of recommendation to encourage or discourage, to allow or to prohibit, the funding of the number of "discards" that are required in the course of *in vitro* fertilization as a new form of human genesis.

To this first point I add the following. To me, at least, it would be significant to find out—if Dr. Robert G. Edwards or Dr. Patrick C. Steptoe could be called to testify—how many, if any, of their monitored trials (from 60 to 200 "failures" have been estimated) have required abortion after the embryo had become, technically, a fetus; and how many, if any, monitored trials required abortion at a stage after viability, which the Supreme Court in *Wade* declared the States could go so far as to prohibit.

Whatever policy the EAB-DHEW (or the Congress) promulgates, it is clear that the several States can constitutionally prohibit *in vitro* fertilization in their jurisdictions, as many have done in the case of fetal research. I would prefer a *national* solution flowing from the recommendation of the Ethics Advisory Board or by Congressional legislation. My plea is that the consciences of millions of our fellow citizens ought not to be additionally burdened by forced cooperation, through funding, in believed evil. You would not want any one of these millions of people to be your friends or neighbors if they thought it right to kill 60 or 200 human lives in order to give birth to one. You would want them to resist, instead of tacitly consenting to, such a spectacular increase of "elective abortions." So my first point is that a prudent medical and public policy on this matter should not, for the sake of so few for whom there are other alternatives including improved oviduct reconstruction, further exacerbate our "civil war" over the morality of abortion.

As a matter of national public policy, I ask you to consider the result of allowing embryo manipulation to become first a trial and then standard medical practice. Already it is the case that Federal and State "conscience clauses" allowing freedom from participation in elective abortions for individuals and medical institutions are not working. For them to be effective would require "affirmative action" such as is now devoted to racial and women's rights.[2] So I ask: if the Ethics Advisory Board and DHEW approves, and if then the Congress negligently approves (or lets research continue on) embryo manipulation and discard, what obstacles will this raise against the adoption of a national health plan in which these procedures could become standard medical practice?

A judicious approach would surely be to exclude such procedures from among the medical procedures claiming public support or general approval. If any American supports a comprehensive national health plan, he or she should exclude *in vitro* fertilization, and other deeply divisive proposals, from such a plan. For the same reasons, we ought not to ask our conscientiously-opposed fellow citizens to support elective abortions with their taxes. I see no other practical compromise that will not increase the polarization and tear further asunder the fragile moral fabric of our nation.

II

My final three points do not touch upon the issue of the morality of abortion, or Federal funding of it. The *distinctive* arguments I submit to you are, first, the *irremovable* possibility that this manner of human genesis may produce a damaged child and that this constitutes a *conclusive* argument against allowing such attempts to be made in the human community, in the United States or any other society.

One "successful" case does not settle the issue I am raising. Besides, who now knows that Louise Brown was a scientific accomplishment? Physical characteristics are not enough to show this.

Here I detour beyond my depth to invoke an analogy with amniocentesis. This procedure has been judged by medical authorities to be safe, no longer experimental. That verdict seems to be concentrated on the mother's safety, and on the unlikelihood that the procedure would induce spontaneous abortion. Incidentally, one percent chance of "false positive" diagnosis for the unborn child, i.e., one in one hundred, does not seem to one to be a negligible risk for the child. My point here, however, goes beyond the physical destruction of normal unborns instead of physically defective fetuses because of mistaken diagnosis. The point is rather whether the procedure of amniocentesis does or does not induce unknown and unknowable *psychological* damage to the children who are saved from genetic abortion. Henry Nadler, M.D., wrote that, while amniocentesis detects gross anomalies, "There is no way, with present studies, our own included, of establishing, ten or fifteen years from now, if these children [the children saved from genetic abortion] lose 5 or 10 I.Q. points"; "The risks of 'induced' congenital malformations are difficult to determine and the subtle damage in terms of loss of intelligence is almost impossible to evaluate."[3]

The comparison with human genesis by embryo manipulation should be clear. No one knows the future of these children. We ought not to try to discover these truths by human experimentation upon them.

But there is no other way to find out. The argument is *conclusive,* unless as a people we mean to make technical medical advance by creating our progeny at risk of unknown and unknowable damage from the procedure itself.

This would violate the primary principle of medical ethics, "Do no harm." To understand that this is the case, we have to distinguish clearly between the procedure in question and medical treatments given the "maternal-fetal unit" when both mother and fetus are actual patients. Sometimes procedures are necessary that are hazardous to the fetus (e.g., intrauterine blood transfusions), but the life that is exposed to hazard stands also to be benefited. In such treatments, possible harm may be risked. Embryo manipulation is quite different: here the mother seeks a benefit; this benefit can be delivered only at some risk of grave injury to the future possible child. Oviduct reconstruction (now a much improved art) is by contrast a treatment that can be undertaken at no risk to another life than the one who elects the operation—since no other life has yet been conceived or will be manipulated.

In his series of articles in *The New York Times,* [4] Walter Sullivan brought up another possibly deleterious outcome that is impossible to remove. Notably, he was quoting the British scientists. The eggs taken after superovulation of the female may not be those that would mature normally. The sperm that in natural reproduction reach their goal are "a highly selective sample," Dr. Edwards noted, "relatively free from genetic defects." There is no such "screening" in *in vitro* fertilization. The "screen" may be the opposite. Such subtle effects, Sullivan correctly concluded, "may not be evident until babies born by the Steptoe-Edwards method reach maturity." No woman should have wanted a baby under these stated conditions, nor should a (tax exempt) American Foundation have funded the Steptoe-Edwards trials, nor should any such thing ever be approved by the Ethics Advisory Board. Only an unexamined preference for *human design* over nature can support any other conclusion.

No answer to the foregoing objection can be found in more time for trying *in vitro* fertilization in the sub-human primates, or the proposal that medical and public policy be to *delay* permission for applying this procedure to human beings until more "animal work" has been done. In other connections—when scientists need normal volunteers to place *themselves* at risk—the stress is always correctly placed on the unknown risk involved in moving from animals to the human.

In a 1974 scientific article one member of the winning team, Dr. Robert G. Edwards[5] of Cambridge University, asserted, "If there is no *undue* risk of deformity additional to those of natural conception, and *publicity is avoided,* the children should grow up and develop normally and be no more misfits than other children born today after some form of medical help." Here Edwards raised two points: how we are to estimate "undue" additional risks of deformity (whether *any* such risks should be imposed) and the psychological damage that may result because publicity was not avoided in the case of Louise Brown.

On the first point, Dr. Edwards argues for 15 pages that there is no risk of deformity from the procedure. I understand why the risks are very low. The developing life (the blastocyst, not yet called an embryo) that is manipulated is a cluster of cleaving cells. These cells have "toti-potency." None is as yet on its way to becoming, say, blood, or has "clicked-off" its potency for becoming, say, a liver cell or a bone. At this point in human development the individual can renew itself even if momentarily injured (like an earthworm). After differentiation into various tissues and organs, the embryo and fetus are more vulnerable to irreversible damage. For example, by thalidomide taken by the mother during pregnancy.

Still there is risk of procedurally induced injury, however small. The question of "undue" additional risk remains at the heart of the moral question whether human genesis should ever be attempted in this way. Having carefully built the case for no undue risk, Dr. Edwards—to my amazement—then spends four pages warning all participants in this procedure that they are liable to "wrongful life" suits for tort compensation. As defendants, all the participants would have to prove that any manifest damage did not result from manipulating the blastocyst.

I was stunned by this contradiction in a single article by an eminent scientist because I heretofore supposed that only theologians were reputed to "fudge" in their arguments. In any case, knowing that one may induce injury, though not foreseen injury, cannot be excluded. This seems to me to be significant in a *conclusive* moral argument against the experiments that have gone on for more than a decade. Moreover, even if longitudinal studies of *in vitro* children for the next five or ten years determine that they are in every respect normal, this will prove only that this kind of human genesis is at that point in time and for the future not to be condemned for *this* reason. Such success will *not* show that all the past trials at irremovable *possible* risk (including Louise Brown's) were for that period of time excusable. Two decades of morally unacceptable human experimentation, by rough reckoning: one decade to perfect the technology; another to prove it *was* safe.

I once expressed the "macabre 'hope' " that the first

child by laboratory fertilization would prove to be a bad result—and that it be well advertised, not hidden from view. That might halt the practice! Dr. Edwards missed my irony, failing to note what else I said: "I do not actually believe that the good to come from public revulsion in such an event would justify the impairment of that child. But then for the same reasons, neither is the manipulation of embryos a procedure that can possibly be morally justified"—even if the result happens to be a Mahalia Jackson.[6] A small risk of grave induced injury is still a morally unacceptable risk.

Concerning the second source of possible grave damage—publicity—I do not know whether or why Dr. Edwards changed his mind. Perhaps there was only a breakdown of communication between him and Dr. Steptoe, the gynecologist who advised that the next Brown be capitalized from birth. "Checkbook publicity," the British press calls it. One can speculate, however, as follows concerning the dilemma the winning team faced. They needed to prove their accomplishment to the scientific community and to the world at large. Already a British doctor had announced that there were one or more babies already born in Europe by this procedure. He offered no proof, and was *disbelieved.* Nobody wins a Nobel prize for science that way.

If the Steptoe-Edwards team wanted *both* to advance science and/or their scientific reputations *and* to protect the next Brown from damaging publicity, they should have tried to create a new "institution" for doing both. The British Medical Association could have been asked to appoint a monitor who could now certify the team's achievement while at the same time avoiding publicity focused upon the subjects (the Browns) with whom the scientist-physician team have achieved their success.

In the absence of this anticipatory solution, there was no other recourse than to try to control the publicity and to enable Louise Brown to garner the revenues. She will be hailed or stigmatized all her life as the first laboratory fertilized progeny to be birthed in all human history. Think of the enormity of that reputation! "Brown" is an ordinary name; the father is a railway worker. Louise Brown can in no way have a natural human life. If she is not psychologically damaged from her beginning, socio-psychological ruin seems invited. If she is Britain's best tennis player at Wimbledon or if she becomes a juvenile delinquent, the outcome will be explained or excused by the child's unique genesis. Mahalia Jackson had a more obscure and normal passage into maturity. So also did the parents of Brown, and Drs. Steptoe and Edwards. What now have they visited upon this child?

Perhaps Dr. Edwards' warnings about "wrongful life" suits could be taken up, and used to advantage. Such suits (for having been born illegitimate, or in poverty) have not succeeded in American courts. Judges have reasoned that the plaintiff would not be there to sue if he or she had never been born. The plaintiff can have no legal standing to sue, because that depends upon the wrongful life he complains of. This seems to me to be the sound legal decision.[7]

In vitro fertilization and embryo manipulation, however, introduce quite different considerations. This form of human genesis *reaches back* to before the beginning. If tort damage results, there were human agents who did it—knowing the possibility could not be excluded. They should be liable. I do not say liable to punishment or to pay damages; but liable to suits that will determine their accountability. It can, therefore, be recommended that our several State legislatures create a special category of "wrongful life" cases limited to torts occurring in this, and coming, new forms of human genesis. Then perhaps the practice can be stopped while there is still time.

III

Among the parties liable and warned by Dr. Edwards in his 1974 article[8] was the "semen donor," not only the husband. This demonstrates that one member of the winning team does not intend the procedure to be used only to the good end of overcoming a married woman's oviduct blockage.[9] This brings me to my third point, which brings against marriage and the family, the *immediate* (not remote) possibility of the exploitation of women as surrogate mothers with wombs-for-hire, and the *immediate* (not remote and not unintended) spectre that we are going right now to begin to "design" our descendants up to the limit that is scientifically possible.

We are told that this sort of "assisted pregnancy" is a "far cry" from Aldous Huxley's *Brave New World.* This is true for the moment. Women with fallopian tube blockage now will be able with their husbands to have children. That is all.

Still there is more to be said about medical and public policy than that a woman's infertility can be "cured." This medical technology is another "long step for mankind" (to quote from the moon landing) toward Aldous Huxley's womb-free paradise. Host "mothers" with wombs-for-hire are immediately possible. Nothing technically limits the fertilization to the husband's sperm. We already have sperm banks. Egg banks will be next. People will go to either to select. No loved-woman need bear the child. This can be arranged by contract, and financial payment. The consequences to come from the opening of the human uterus to medical technological control are not likely to contribute to the emancipation of women.[10]

There is still more. We are not limited to human progeny growing with their own natural genetic endowments. We are not limited to the child the Browns wanted. Gene splicing soon can be done before the blastocyst or embryo is transferred to the womb of the woman—*any* woman. "The procedures leading to replacement and implantation," Edwards and D.J. Sharpe wrote in a 1971 scientific article,[11] "*open the way* to further work on human embryos in the laboratory." The authors do not mean only benign attempts to correct genetic defects. They also mention cloning and the creation of "chimeras" by importing cells from other blastocysts (perhaps from other species). These creations also now need women to carry them through pregnancy. Noting that the first principle of medical ethics, "Do no harm," permits the alleviation of infertility, and that this "*has been stretched* to cover destruction of fetuses with hereditary defects," Edwards and Sharpe ask rhetorically whether the first principle of medical ethics can be stretched to justify "the more remote techniques of modifying embryos?"

Even more ominous is the announced claim that scientists have the "right" to "exercise their professional activities *to the limit that is tolerable by society* . . . as lay attitudes *struggle to catch up* with what scientists can do." Publics must be "helped to keep pace." In short, science does not operate within the ethics of a wider human community. It is a scientific ethics, or whatever *can* be done, that should shape our public philosophy. Let laggards beware.

True, in his 1974 article,[12] Dr. Edwards stated that there is "hardly any point in making chimeras until some clinical advantage can be shown to accrue from the method." But he also speaks of "*sexing* blastocysts" before transfer. His remedy for the problems this will lead to is: "Imbalance of the sexes could probably be prevented by recording the sex of newborn children, and adjusting the choice open to parents." Scientist-kings will manage everything. Concerning the use of "surrogate mothers," his only reservation is that this should be avoided *at the present time* until more is known about the interlocking psychological relationships among the parties. Edwards does not say how we can acquire such knowledge without (on his own terms) doing unethical experimentation now in order to find out whether we ought to do it or not.

IV

I have not yet mentioned the *remote*—but still very near—prospect of substituting laboratory generation from first to last for human procreation.

Pope Pius XII once warned against reducing the cohabitation of married persons to the transmission of germ life. This would, he said, "convert the domestic hearth, sanctuary of the family, into nothing more than a biological laboratory."[13] That quaint language was spoken about artificial insemination. The Pontiff feared the nemesis of humanity under the fluorescent light of laboratories. He warned of this in 1951—ages ago in technological time. To the fluorescent light of the laboratory has been added the glare of media protection and copyrighted publicity.

The first book to be printed entitled *Test Tube Babies* was published in 1934[14]—again ages ago in technological time. Its subject matter was not at all what we mean by this expression. The book's subtitle was "A History of the Artificial Impregnation of Human Beings, Including a Detailed Account of its Technique, together with Personal Experiences, Clinical Cases, A Review of its Literature, and the Medical and Legal Aspects Involved."

Clearly ours is an age of galloping biomedical technology. Aldous Huxley and C.S. Lewis had the prescience to see already the future that comes ever closer. Not the abuse of political power by Hitler nor of nuclear power but the unchecked employment of powers the biological revolution places in human hands was for these authors the final threat of the "abolition of man."

The human womb is a half-way technology. It is replaceable by more "perfect" artifices.[15] Human life has been maintained in petri dishes for two weeks; and our National Commission for the Protection of Human Subjects used 20-24 weeks as its definition of a "possibly viable" infant. Only about 18 to 22 weeks remain to be conquered in which the human female must necessarily participate in procreation, except as the source of the ovum. Then "reproduction" can replace procreation, and we will come to Huxley's Hatcheries. His was a vision of society in which everyone was quite happy. The way there is also a happy one, and we go along that way always motivated by good ends, such as the relief of women's infertility and salvaging "premies" earlier and earlier.

For all the motherhood intended at present, the truth is that (as C.S. Lewis once wrote[16]): "We should not do to minerals and vegetables what modern science threatens to do to man himself."

Members of the Ethics Advisory Board may wish to perform the following experiment on themselves.

Turn off the tube. Don't pick up the newspaper for two days. Instead, read the third of C.S. Lewis' space-science trilogy, *That Hideous Strength.* The final assault upon humanity is gathering in Edgestow, a fictional British college town. The forces of technology, limited no more by the Christian ages, are trying to combine with pre-Christian forces, represented by Merlin the Magician whose body is buried on the Bracton College grounds. Only the philologist Ransom can save humankind from the powers of the present age concentrated in the National Institute for Coordinated Experimentation (acronym NICE).

It is NICE that the Browns have a wonderful baby girl; her middle name is Joy. Lewis need not have thought of his fictional college, Bracton. Cambridge University is NICE too. So is Vanderbilt. To give couples a baby sexed to their desires will be NICE. Every other step taken will certainly be NICE. Finally, *Brave New World* is entirely NICE. For everyone is happy in Huxley's pharmacological, genetic and womb-free paradise. Only there is no poetry there. Nor does a baby have the right to be a *surprise.*

Notes

1. *Beal v. Doe,* no. 75-554, 45 LW, pp. 4781-87; *Maher v. Roe,* no. 75-1440, 45 LW, pp. 4787-94; *Poelker v. Doe,* no. 75-442, 45 LW, pp. 4794-97 (the three decisions handed down June 21, 1977).

2. See my *Ethics at the Edges of Life* (New Haven: Yale University Press, 1978), Chapter Two.

3. Henry Nadler, M.D. in Maureen Harris, ed.: *Early Diagnosis of Human Genetic Defects.* Washington, D.C.: U.S. Government Printing Office, 1972, pp. 315, 230.

4. Walter Sullivan, "Successful Laboratory Conception Intensifies Debate over Procedures," *The New York Times,* July 27, 1978.

5. R.G. Edwards, "Fertilization of Human Eggs in Vitro: Morals, Ethics and the Law." *The Quarterly Review of Biology,* 49:1 (March 1974), pp. 3-26. (Stoney Brook Foundation, Inc.) Italics added.

6. Paul Ramsey, "Shall We Reproduce?", *Journal of the American Medical Association,* 220:11 (June 12, 1972), p. 1482. My suggestion paraphrased and reversed a statement by Dr. Joshua Lederberg concerning whether "cloning" human beings will be socially acceptable. This depends, he wrote, on the first clonant's batting average; and on his good looks, success and being well advertised. Joshua Lederberg, "Experimental Genetics and Human Evolution," *The American Naturalist,* Vol. 100 (Sept.-Oct., 1966), pp. 519-31; slightly revised and reprinted. *Bulletin of Atomic Scientists,* Oct., 1966, pp. 4-11. See also my *Fabricated Man* (New Haven: Yale University Press, 1970), Chapter Two.

7. A convenient reference for those decisions, with commentary, is Joel Feinberg, ed., *The Problem of Abortion.* Belmont, California: Wadsworth Publishing Company, 1973.

8. See note 5 above.

9. Testifying before the Sub-Committee on Health and the Environment, U.S. House of Representatives, on August 4, 1978, Dr. James C. Gaither, Chairman of the Ethics Advisory Board, offered the opinion not only that implantation of human fertilized ova should not be done until the safety of the procedure is demonstrated *as far as possible* in subhuman primates. He also testified that it was the opinion of some 20 experts in ethics and the life sciences convened by DHEW that such a procedure should await definition of the responsibilities of the *donor,* recipient "parents," and of the research institution. Walter J. Wadlington, professor of law at the University of Virginia Law School, urged that Congress propose model legislation for use by the States in coping with such problems as *legitimacy* and parental responsibility if *in vitro* fertilization becomes widespread. *The New York Times,* August 5, 1978.

10. Here I quote from a striking letter to *The New York Times* (August 6, 1978) by Judith Lorber, Department of Sociology, Brooklyn College:

"I am thankful that the first child born from laboratory fertilization is a girl. At least now there are *two* female principals in the drama, instead of one lonely woman surrounded by powerful and prestigious male doctors, male scientists, male legal, ethical and religious experts, male newspapermen, and so on and on.

"Men now have the ability to freeze their sperm, fertilize eggs *in vitro* and deliver the children surgically, and the potential ability for freezing embryos and transplanting them in women other than the egg producers. Fortunately, a woman's body is still needed to carry the fetus to term.

"But women of the future had better get more than a toehold in the bastions of power. Otherwise, when male-dominated technological reproduction develops artificial wombs, too, women, except for a select few egg producers, may end up totally superfluous."

11. R.G. Edwards and D.J. Sharpe, "Social Values and Research in Human Embryology." *Nature* 231:87-91 (1971). Italics added.

12. See note 5 above.

13. *Acta Apostolicae Sedis* 43:850 (1951).

14. Dr. Herman Rohleder, *Test Tube Babies.* New York: The Panurge Press, 1934. Can we use "panurge" as a symbol for the basic problem of modern times, since Bacon unfurled the flag for "the relief of the human estate" of disease, suffering, death, and any other deficit?

15. If I were a reproductive biologist in need of funds and reputation, and anyway a sincere believer in progress by science, I would begin now to search for an animal species whose gestation is close enough to the human for it to be not impossible to use its females as hosts for human embryos. After all, "herds" of prime cattle in embryo have been flown across the Atlantic within rabbits, thereafter to be transferred again to scrub cows to bear them. So my idea is not a fanciful one (if we ought to treat the human embryo like cattle). If I can secure funds for my trials I may gain Senator Proxmire's "golden fleece" award,

even if I do not gain an honored place in the moral history of mankind.

16. C.S. Lewis, *The Abolition of Man.* New York: Macmillan Co., 1947.

58. Biotechnical Parenting

PAUL SIMMONS

Biotechnical parenting has a symbolic value that brings together several biblical principles. First, it points to the goodness and rightness of sexual intercourse on its own. Coitus is not primarily for procreation but for the expression of intimate love in the context of marital commitments. Secondly, the love of the couple may be served by their deliberate choice to become parents. Choice, not chance, governs this pregnancy. The child is assured of caring love from the very first. God's intention for every child is thus symbolized. Finally, parenthood is related to calling, not to accident or mere biological capacity. Emotional and spiritual commitments to the tasks of parenthood are far more important than the relatively simple process of giving birth. Those who confront the frustration of childlessness, who weigh the commitments that may and will be required and are willing to invest time, energy, devotion, and considerable financial outlay to become a parent, symbolize the consideration and commitments that are integral to the biblical sense of calling. These are parents by design, intention, and purpose. They will recognize their child as the extraordinary gift it truly is. They will not resent the pregnancy as an untimely accident or reject the child as an unwelcome intruder. Every child should be as fortunate. To such commitments every parent is called.

Chapter Twelve
GENETIC CONTROL

Introduction

Advances in medical science and technology have provided a remarkable control not only over whether to have a child but also over the sort of children we will have. The rapidly expanding knowledge of human genetics has made contraception and technological reproduction serviceable to eugenic ends, and both parents and society have a new capacity to affect the genetic endowment of their own children and the coming generations.

Some uses of the new knowledge of genetics, it must be observed, serve the more traditional ends of medicine. A number of genetic diseases can be diagnosed by means of genetic tests, and appropriate therapy can be prescribed to at least forestall or limit the effects of the disease, even if it cannot be cured. PKU (or phenylketonuria), a genetically based metabolic disease, for example, can be detected in newborns by a simple test and, if detected, can be controlled by a special diet, forestalling and limiting the serious brain damage which would otherwise surely result. Indeed, the test for PKU is not simply made available to parents in consultation with their physician; it is routinely done in the PKU screening programs mandated by law. The value of genetic testing for diagnosis may one day be matched by genetic therapy, but the prospect of genetic cures for genetic diseases remains on the distant horizon.

The use of genetic information for eugenic purposes is already a reality. It is possible, for example, to identify the carriers of a number of genetic diseases and so to calculate some of the genetic risks a particular couple would undertake for the sake of having a child. Such information can be used by prospective parents to make an informed decision about whether to take the known genetic risks for the sake of having a child. They might choose not to have a child and might choose either contraception or sterilization. Or they might choose to circumvent the known risks by using artificial insemination with sperm from a donor or in vitro fertilization with ova from a donor. But when donor sperm or ova are used, what genetic characteristics of the donor should be considered relevant—race? health? intelligence? Should the purpose be to prevent the genetic risk to the child or to give the parents the sort of child they want or to improve the general gene pool? If we can improve the genetic endowment of our children or of the next generation by using donor seed, should that be the preferred model of reproduction? Many years ago the Nobel Prize-winning geneticist H. J. Muller made precisely that recommendation, suggesting freezing and banking sperm from distinguished men in order to improve the genetic characteristics of the race. Given now in vitro fertilization, it would be only equitable to bank ova from distinguished women as well.

The ability to detect the carriers of certain genetic diseases requires decisions not only by parents but by society as well. Society might decide to fund mass screening programs to identify the carriers of certain genetic diseases. The programs could be voluntary or mandatory (as a 1971 Massachusetts law—Chapter 491 of Acts and Resolves—"requiring the testing of blood for sickle trait or anemia as a prerequisite for school attendance"). The information could be provided to the individual or to prospective mates or could be used publicly to discourage or prohibit certain marriages or procreation by certain partners.

It is also possible to diagnose certain genetic diseases prenatally. In amniocentesis, a procedure done after the fourteenth week, a small sample of amniotic fluid is removed from the sac which surrounds the fetus and then analyzed for genetic and chromosomal characteristics. Other procedures have been and are being developed to enable the diagnosis to be made much earlier in a woman's pregnancy. Chorionic villi sampling, for example, can be done as early as the fifth week. In this procedure a physician suctions up a sample of the chorionic villi, the branching extensions of the outer membrane of the developing egg, through a long thin tube inserted through the vagina. A number of disorders can be detected in these ways, including Down's syndrome, and the number continues to grow. The information provided by such a test can then be used by parents to make an informed decision about therapy for the fetus (if there is such available) or abortion or simply to ready themselves for the demands of being parents to the child. Some sex-linked diseases like kinky hair disease (Menkes' syndrome), a metabolic disorder which affects the absorption of copper and which is usually fatal before three years, cannot be diagnosed, but any male child of a carrier mother has a fifty-fifty chance of being affected. In such a case, the prenatal test can at least tell whether the child is male or female, and the parents can then make a decision on the basis of those risks. Indeed, these procedures have already been used to support aborting fetuses diagnosed to be the "wrong" sex.

Prenatal diagnosis calls for decisions from physicians and society as well as from parents. May or should physicians say no to the clients who would use amniocentesis to determine the sex of the fetus? May or should health insurance programs refuse to pay for the care of a Down's infant whose condition could have been predicted and whose birth could have been prevented? May or should government entitlement programs divert funds from the care of the genetically retarded and diseased to the education of "normal" and "gifted" children to encourage "genetic responsibility" and advance the interests of society? Such recommendations are not only plausible but real.

The new powers have prompted new questions but these new questions, in turn, demand attention to some very old questions among reflective people.

One set of questions has to do with the mode of ethical reflection. How shall we decide what we ought to do or leave undone—on the basis of consequences? But then what is the good to be sought and the evil to be avoided? Or are other aspects of the act relevant—the means as well as the end, the values expressed as well as achieved by the act? And how does theological reflection warrant or qualify answers to these questions? The articles included below provide clearly contrasting models for ethical reflection and an invitation to think clearly and carefully and Christianly about this issue.

Another set of questions has to do with the image of man. Is there an image of the "normatively human" which we can and should use to warrant and guide and limit our powers, including our power to intervene in genetics? The judgment, for example, that rational control of our own life and environment is the "normatively human" will have quite different implications from the judgment that our embodiment and dependency on communities not of our own choosing are essential to the "normatively human." Again, is the "normative human" an independent individual or an interdependent individual? How can such judgments be made and defended; and how does the Christian vision of humanity affect them? What, according to a Christian vision, are people meant to be and to become, and how does Christian eschatology bear on their becoming it? These questions are quite clearly at issue in the articles included below, and it is fascinating to compare the perspectives and to see the implications drawn out and qualified. But fascination aside, it is important for members of believing communities to form and defend their own theological account of what human persons are meant to be and to become, not only in order to contribute to public discussion but to live, to exercise their powers, in ways that have religious integrity.

There are other questions posed by these new powers. Is there a professional ethic relevant to their use? How does a theological ethic relate to it? What is the meaning of "health," specifically, in this context, "genetic health"? What is the moral significance of being a parent? Does genetic technology simply enable parents to get the child they want or does it affect our view of being a parent by introducing a calculating nurture in place of an uncalculating nurture? What are the rights and responsibilities of people with respect to marriage and procreation? What are the rights and responsibilities of society? May a society with a history of sexism be open to the sex selection of fetuses? May a society with a history of racism run a screening program for the sickle-cell trait? And what about the abortion of "defective" fetuses? That last question, however, invites you too quickly to the subject of the next chapter, abortion.

Suggestions for Further Reading

Birch, Charles, and Paul Albrecht. *Genetics and the Quality of Life.* Elmsford, N.Y.: Pergamon, 1975.

Fletcher, John. *Coping with Genetic Disorders.* San Francisco: Harper & Row, 1982.

Glover, Jonathan. *What Sort of People Should There Be?* New York: Penguin, 1984.

Gustafson, James M. "Genetic Engineering and the Normative View of the Human." In *Ethical Issues in Biology and Medicine,* edited by Preston N. Williams, 46-58. Cambridge, Mass.: Schenkman, 1973.

Hamilton, Michael, ed. *The New Genetics and the Future of Man.* Grand Rapids: Eerdmans, 1972.

Lebacqz, Karen, ed. *Genetics, Ethics, and Parenthood.* New York: Pilgrim Press, 1983.

McCormick, Richard. "Genetic Medicine: Notes on the Moral Literature." Chapter in *How Brave a New World?* 281-305. Washington, D.C.: Georgetown University Press, 1981.

Ramsey, Paul. "Screening: An Ethicists' View." In *Ethical Issues in Human Genetics: Genetic Counseling and the Use of Genetic Knowledge,* edited by Bruce Hilton, et al. New York: Plenum Press, 1973.

Simmons, Paul D. *Birth and Death: Bioethical Decision-Making.* Philadelphia: Westminster, 1983. See pp. 193-246.

Verhey, Allen D. "The Morality of Genetic Engineering." *Christian Scholars Review* 14, no. 2 (1985): 124-139.

59. The Ethics of Genetic Control: Some Answers

JOSEPH FLETCHER

When we discuss issues calling for more than a merely technical solution the effect can be much like a centrifuge. We whirl the things we wonder about around and around and the answers finally take shape. They make their appearance by their own weight. Here, then, are a couple of dozen such answers to questions; questions about what is good and what is evil in the new biology and medicine, or what has been called bioengineering.

As we have seen, these answers are based upon a humane concern for the well-being of people, according to actual needs in actual situations. They do not rest on religious doctrines or metaphysical ideas, nor on the prejudicial notion that we ought to follow moral rules regardless of cases or consequences. The "God Squad" approach is too inflexible to fit the variety of real-life situations. In other words, we do not suppose that what is right or wrong can be settled dogmatically in advance of the facts.

Sometimes abortion would be right, sometimes wrong; sometimes egg transfers would be a good thing, sometimes not. The same thing holds true with test tube conceptions, sterilizations, artificial gestations, preselection of sex, cloning, insemination and enovulation from storage banks, and so on. This is the "clinical" approach typical of biomedical ethics.

The main guidelines we have established are these six: compassion, consideration of consequences, proportionate good, the priority of actual needs over the ideal or the potential, a desire to enlarge choice and cut down on chance, and a courageous acceptance of our responsibility to make decisions. With these principles we can arrive at some reasonable conclusions about the morality of human reproduction and genetics.

For convenience's sake the answers are laid out by title in alphabetical order; it will be obvious that a good deal of cross-reference and blending ("interface") develops between many of them—a kind of moral fabric.

From Joseph Fletcher, *The Ethics of Genetic Control* (Garden City, N.Y.: Anchor, 1974), pp. 147-87. Used by permission of the author.

Adultery

The traditional literary sense of "adultery," as an interpersonal and intergenital affair, is the correct one. Properly understood, adultery is *only* a personal and genital act. No longer can we say that a monogamous marriage agreement means exclusive access to any or all of the wife's or husband's "generative" faculties. It might exclude third-party genitalia but not third-party sperm and ova, nor graft gonads which can overcome childlessness and barren marriages. It is morally absurd if the law allows, even only by implication, that a donor of seeds could be named a correspondent in a divorce action.

The law will slowly catch up with humanitarian medicine. Donors of sperm and ova, as such, are *not* adulterers in any ethical sense; they are far less adulterers than the Old Testament "levirate" men who impregnated their dead brothers' childless widows for the sake of their brothers' posterity. Their good deeds were intimately intergenital—which is not true of donors. Adultery cannot apply any longer to the donation of the powers of our "loins" to persons in need just because they are not one's spouse.

Artificial Germination

Inseminating and enovulating artificially stand together, ethically. They are ways of conceiving when other and more familiar methods cannot work. The opinion that these procedures are wrong, promulgated officially by the Catholics and backed by a few Protestants and Jews, rests on two assertions: one is that conception by artificial means is immoral because to be ethical conception "must" be accomplished by intercourse, and the other is that donating and accepting sperm and ova between the unmarried is adultery. It is this dogmatic objection which we are rejecting.

Some people find artificial insemination distasteful or esthetically objectionable, but they do not brand it as unethical. They do not try to stigmatize the assisting physician as an accessory to a crime or a "sin." It is simply ridiculous to argue that a consenting husband in "AID" [Artificial Insemination from a Donor] makes himself a party to an immoral and criminal conspiracy. Oklahoma's law giving it legal status and protecting children so conceived is a precedent for similar laws elsewhere. To say, however, that the practice is not wrong in and of itself does not mean it is *always* the right thing to do. There are still problems of when and how it should be done. If the benefits are too meager or the foreseeable consequences too onerous for parents, donors, or children, it is wrong in those particular cases.

Artificial insemination from a donor is often in order when the husband is azoospermic or has a low sperm count. Premature ejaculation, malformation, and psychological hang-ups are other reasons. It is both silly and sad when people are mired down in a physical rather than a moral notion of true family relationship. Out of this error comes the practice of mixing the husband's ineffective semen with the donor's, so that the husband can be regarded as the "putative" father—a pathetic legal fiction. Most happily of all, we can see in artificial insemination and enovulation from donors a means at last whereby we can have children and still avoid crippling or killing them with our known inheritable defects or diseases.

The glaring fault in our practice of assisted conception, up to the present, has been its secrecy. It is wrong to keep the truth not only from the public but also from the child. This used to be done in adoptions until experience began to discourage it. Deception undermines family relationships psychologically, as well as courting the shock of disclosure or discovery. A brother and sister innocently married some years ago in England, having been adopted when they were infants by different families and renamed; only then did they learn the truth, by a fluke. Insemination and enovulation from donors should be matters of agreement with the husband, and a formal record made.

To receive an egg or sperm without the spouse's knowledge and consent would be an odd business, hard to justify. It should be recorded officially by the physician along with his notes of serological tests (e.g., venereal disease and the Rh factor), with proper dates, just as in any other medical service. A child could be wrecked emotionally if he found it out without any preparation; an angry spouse or confidant could disclose it for revenge; "rich uncles" could claim criminal conspiracy if they settled money on such children in ignorance of the truth.

In states where the law does not yet protect the rights of "AID" children it should be revealed in order to adopt them, thus securing their status. (What an irony it is that a child who is at least one-half the biological descendant of his parents has less standing in most states than an adopted child who is altogether unrelated biologically.)

Birth Control

As we have seen, birth control covers a great many things besides contraception. Contraconception, a wider category, includes sterilization, whether by chemical, biological, or surgical means. And literally, the control of *birth* as distinct from conception prevention lies in genetic and fetological interventions. The key to the morality of control is that it should be consistent and complete, not half-baked.

Our moral obligation is to control the quality as well as the quantity of the children we bring into the world. We owe it to a prospective child, to ourselves as parents of integrity, to our families which have only so much in the way of human and economic resources, and to society. Ethically it is in the discretion of a woman to prevent or end any pregnancy she does not want, unless she has promised the child to a husband or lover who justifiably insists on it, or unless a clear case can be made that society has a supervening interest in its birth. (Rarely indeed would either of these limitations cut into her personal freedom.)

Morally this biological self-determination extends as much to legally minor females as to an adult; hence the rapid increase of Minor Consent laws which protect their rights to obstetrical care in spite of obstruction by parents or others.

The looming moral issue has to do with *compulsory* birth control. Up to the present we have relied upon a voluntary policy, and everything else being equal it is better to be responsible for our reproduction of our own free will than to be compelled to. But the two control goals, quality and quantity, cannot rightly be ignored by individuals to the common hurt. Birth control is not merely a private matter. We may have to face compulsory controls of fertility and dysgenic inheritances, however regrettably, as we have had to face compulsory vaccination for communicable diseases.

A contemporary and morally responsible ethics of reproduction calls for whatever policy works. An English clergyman, typifying a not uncommon and truly nihilistic irresponsibility, said recently that without a free private option to reproduce we lose our humanity, and that if therefore population reaches disastrous proportions, "well, then we die."[1]

Laissez-faire has not proved to be altogether a just policy in the production of economic goods and services, Adam Smith to the contrary notwithstanding, and the same can be said of human reproduction. Fortunately, birth control is spreading through all the world, including Asia and Africa, in spite of various religions and customs. We ought not to forget that the original Latin for population, *populare,* meant to devastate or lay waste; it can come exactly to that.

Birth Defects

Children born with defects become at once objects of loving concern. We must do what we can for them, and in some cases *much* can be done. Sometimes, however, voluntary societies seeking help for the mentally "handicapped" or retarded, for the victims of muscular dystrophy, cystic fibrosis, even spina bifida, are—to say the least—sentimental. As much as possible such misery should be *prevented,* not ameliorated. Morally, honest concern for such unfortunate creatures should be based as much on an effort to prevent their birth as to help them when they are born anyway.

Many people plead loud and long for the means to help them, yet they oppose preventive measures such as genetic screening, therapeutic abortion (or embryotomy), gene engineering, artificial germination, sterilization, and most if not all of the reproductive technology which could avoid these tragedies. This is a strange and contradictory species of compassion; it shows up as absurd or phony.

For example, a few die-hard extremists say, "We may not abort defective fetuses; we should work instead on finding cures for genetic and congenital disorders." This is a false either-or, a red herring. Study of abortuses is what gives us the knowledge to eliminate and alleviate these ills. There are those who denounce even embryological studies of blastocysts and primitive embryos; this is a particularly bizarre instance of false compassion.

As it is, obstetricians and pediatricians are put unnecessarily and often in an intolerable quandary. They have to stretch the truth, telling a woman her baby was "stillborn" when it wasn't, after having simply not respirated the delivered fetus—out of mercy for her and her family. If such creatures manage to be born anyway (start breathing) physicians may then resort to high-risk surgery with the unspoken hope that it will be fatal, or they may hold back on antibiotics, a lethal tactic. When these maneuvers fail they then advise putting seriously defective infants in institutions which are nothing more than "warehouses." This is more nearly immoral than moral; it could be escaped as a quandary if our reproductive ethics was honestly based on compassion.

Cloning

Good reasons in general for cloning are that it avoids genetic diseases, bypasses sterility, predetermines an individual's gender, and preserves family likenesses. It wastes time to argue over whether we should do it or not; the real moral question is when and why.

By cloning from the same source, perhaps to preserve biological qualities, clonants would be able to be lifesaving donors to each other of paired or cadaver organs with no risk of failure due to the rejection of alien tissue; this is true already in the case of monozygotic or identical twins. (When an immunosuppressive is found, for what Rostand calls "biological xenophobia," this particular reason for cloning will have lost its weight.) Clonants could always marry nonclonants if they chose to (at the price of thinning out the clone's qualities) but staying strictly within the clone's genotype would be necessary to be sure of nonrejection in transplant operations.

Robert Sinsheimer has remarked that cloning will "permit the preservation and perpetuation of the finest genotypes that arise in our species—just as the invention of writing has enabled us to preserve the fruits of their life work."[2] There could be many other personal and clinical reasons for it in particular cases.

There could also be reasons of the social good. Individuals might need to be selectively reproduced by cloning because of their special resistance to radiation, their small body size and weight, because they are impervious to high-decibel sound waves; these things could be invaluable for professional flights at high altitudes and space travel, for example. In a stretch of imagination, a biologist could solve the weight problem by going alone to a distant planet with a supply of different somatic cells, and colonize it from a cloning start. Even without any need to specialize people we might some day have to turn to either cloning or genetic engineering to correct for the loss of quality we suffer as our recessive defects get spread around in our common gene pool. Dangerous roles within society or on its frontiers might justify cloning, to safeguard those who take risks in the social interest.

What cloning's constructive uses will be cannot, of course, be wholly predicted or even anticipated. Some things can be ruled out. For example, it would be wrong of lesbian or male homophile extremists to want to use cloning to reproduce a general population of their own sex (the males would need at least a few captive ovulators); the fault with it, obviously, would be the loss of genetic variety due to asexual reproduction on such a wide scale, and its undermining effect on the survival of the species.

Inhumane, inordinate suggestions have been made to use cloning to produce legless people, dwarfs, individuals distorted functionally in various ways—for example, to man spaceships to Jupiter. But this seems impossible to justify, given our present knowledge, and would accordingly be morally wrong. Similar is a proposal to solve the fruit picking problem in a future leisure society by using a genetically "designed" and then cloned submental people with prehensile tails to do the work. It can be countered immediately with, "Why not monkeys?" (which are already being considered for some orchards).

There is no ethical objection to cloning when it is *morally* (that is, humanely) employed. Artificial virgin births and cloned "multiplets" promise real benefits not only to human beings but to the "green revolution" also. Whole orange groves are sometimes copied tree by tree, from a single high yield tree. Herds of meat and coat animals cloned from a champion Kenya or Kazakhstan sheep could increase our meat supply two or three times in just a couple of years. Fish farming in controlled waters is another option; we need not rely altogether on delicate eco-balances. What men can do by cloning with their plants and animals they could and sometimes should do for themselves. There is no moral reason why we must follow biological heterogeneity in all human beings, whenever homogeneity can serve a constructive purpose.

Control for Quality

An editorial by Dr. Malcolm Watts in the journal of the California Medical Association in 1970 remarked that "man exercises ever more certain and effective control" over the quality of human life. "It will become necessary and acceptable to place relative rather than absolute values on such things as human lives, the use of scarce resources, and the various elements which are to make up the quality of life or of living which is to be sought."[3] All of this, he said, requires "a new ethic" in "a rational development" of "what is almost certain to be a biologically oriented world society."

Physicians in the past, the editorial points out, have tried "to preserve, protect, repair, prolong, and enhance every human life which comes under their surveillance." This was the old vitalistic, undiscriminating sanctity-or-quantity-of-life ethics, now giving way to a responsible, decisional quality-of-life ethics. To repair and prolong lives, indiscriminately, may be a kind of technical virtuosity but it is not *control.* To control means to choose, and therefore any absolute morality about always keeping life going, before or after birth, regardless of quality considerations, is the very opposite of control and a denial of quality.

If we choose family size we should choose family health. This is what the controls of reproductive medicine make possible. Public health and sanitation have greatly reduced human ills; now the major ills have become genetic and congenital. They can be reduced by medical controls. We ought to protect our families from the emotional and material burden of such diseased individuals, and from the misery of their simply "existing" (not *living*) in a nearby "warehouse" or public institution.

We have an example in hemophilia. If a man has a recessive gene for it, even though he himself is all right, he passes it on—not to his sons but to his daughters. They won't have the disease (it is sex-linked) but they will pass it on to their children. By controlling his reproduction through sex selection or pre-emptive abortion, keeping only male embryos, this man would stop the scourge once and for all in his family line. That is his moral responsibility.

If the State is morally justified in repelling an unwelcome invader, why should not a woman do so when burdened or invaded by an unwelcome pregnancy? And why shouldn't the family be protected from an idiot or terribly diseased sibling? Control is human and rational; submission, the opposite of control, is subhuman. Suffering and misfortune cannot be utterly escaped, it is true, and human beings can grow tremendously in pain and disappointment. But a basic ethical principle of medicine and health care is nonetheless the minimization of human suffering, by deliberate control.

Producing our children by "sexual roulette" without preconceptive and uterine control, simply taking "pot luck" from random sexual combinations, is irresponsible—now that we can be genetically selective and know how to monitor against congenital infirmities. As we learn to direct mutations medically we should do so. Not to control when we can is immoral. This way it will be much easier to assure our children that they really are here because they were *wanted,* that they were born "on purpose."

Controlling the quality of life is not negative; it just rejects what fails to come up to a positive standard. The new biology equips us to save and improve the defective, as well as to maintain a sensible standard. For example, it was once prohibitively expensive to correct dwarfism when HGH (human growth hormone) had to be extracted from human pituitaries at autopsy, but biochemistry has synthesized HGH and one day soon it will be available economically. (Such achievements are undesirable only if we allow the dwarfs we treat to pass their genetic defect along to innocent progeny.)

We began our human history by learning to control the physical environment (and still make serious mistakes). We have made some progress in controlling our social life, and we are learning to control our behavior. It is time, then, that we accepted control of our heredity.

Costs and Benefits

The essence of tragedy is the conflict of one good with another. The conflict of good with evil is only melodrama. We often have to calculate the relative desirability of things. We pay for what we get, always. Choosing high quality fetuses and rejecting low quality ones is not tragedy; sad, but not agonizing.

A heavier trial of the spirit and a real test of responsible judgment, if we want to exert serious control, would be a problem like deciding whether to induce abortion when only one of a pair of nonidentical twins has an untreatable metabolic disorder. It would mean losing a good baby to prevent a bad one. But even here compassionate control should not hesitate: the good one is still only potential, and pregnancy could—at least ordinarily—be restarted. It is far more callous not to prevent the fate of a foreseeably diseased baby than it is disappointing to postpone a good one for a matter of only months.

To be responsible, to take control and reject low quality life, only seems cruel or callous to the morally superficial. Actually, it is practical compassion. Robert Louis Stevenson was shocked at first when he found the Polynesians practicing "infanticide." Their ignorance of contraception and obstetrics meant they had to resort to "abortion at birth" when a newborn turned out to be defective, or when the small atolls they lived on simply could not yield food and shelter for any more people. It was loving concern for *actual* children in their radically finite world which led them to abortion and population control; a matter of costs and benefits.

Stevenson said, somewhat bemused, that never had he seen people anywhere who loved their children as much as those coral reef dwellers did. Of course. The world's finiteness is harder to hide on a Pacific coral reef.

Not to control, and not to weigh one thing against another, would be subhuman. A mature ethics is social, not egocentric. Call it what you will—mathematical morality, ethical arithmetic, moral calculus—we are obliged in conscience to think of benefits relative to costs.

Trying to be responsible we have to calculate. We issue drivers' licenses, for example, even though the cars of some will become lethal weapons; it is the price we pay for motor transport. If we could tell which applicants for a license will be killers we would not license them. It used to be that we had no way of knowing which couples were carrying a common gene defect or which pregnancies were positive for it. But now we *can* know; we have lost that excuse for taking genetic risks. To go right ahead with coital reproduction in many couples' cases is like walking down a line of children blindfolded and deliberately maiming every fourth child. It is cruel and insane to deprive normal but disadvantaged children of the care we could give them with the $1,500,000,000 we spend in public costs for preventable retardates.

Ethics is not loftily independent of economics and utilitarian or distributive justice. Economics deals with preferences among competing choices, and utility aims at spreading expectable benefits. What we need morally is a telescope, not just a microscope.

Cryogenics

There is no ethical reason, at least in principle, not to keep vital human tissue "on ice." The use of cryogens (low temperature agents) is practical or applied physics, bioengineering, put to work in the freeze-storage of sperm—and eventually of ova and even embryos. (Its workability and value for *whole* human bodies is still very speculative.)

In particular cases cryogenics is easily justifiable for treatment reasons. Because a married man has oligospermia his sperm might be collected over a period of time, to aggregate it for fertilization. In another situation he might bank it for a future marriage because he faces a sterilizing operation, either for therapeutic reasons or as a method of voluntary birth control. A wife may be ill and temporarily unable to "carry" a conceptus at just the time when the husband learns of the need for the operation. Stored semen could be used for several inseminations at the ovulation period, thus increasing the chances of a hoped-for conception. As laboratory fertilization develops, the relevance and utility of banked germ plasm is obvious. It will also be a helpful adjunct to cloning.

Cryogenics could be simple fertility insurance for those who are going to war or other dangerous enterprises, and for those who work near nuclear power piles or who risk irradiation on a nuclear submarine or commercial freighter. Telegenesis (baby making from germ cells stored in order to conceive when a partner is far away) is one class of its uses, and paleogenesis (for those separated by time—even by death) is another. Sterilization, the most reliable method of contraception, need no longer entail inevitable childlessness, now that we have cryogenics; a combination of both sterilization *and* fertility is possible now.

The voluntary choice of germ plasm, that is, of one's children's biological quality, is a great boon. It buttresses quality control and, like genetic mutations, helps heredity to be rational and responsible.[4] Storage banks will carry descriptions, even the names of the donors of sperm, eggs, and embryos. "Celebrity Seed for Sale," one wag has suggested for the display signs.[5] Since it is done through these organized banks, involving physicians and nurses, conceptions from storage will have to give up the secrecy and anonymity of some of the past practice of artificial insemination. Too many people will have to be "in the know." Candor is better than deception.

Sensible regulatory laws and policies will need to be worked out, to set guidelines. Should corporations as well as individuals be allowed to get germs or embryos, to artificially produce children? Could a "fictitious person" be a proper parent? Should we allow a business or any other such entity to produce its own labor force, bypassing the "labor market"? Should we encourage monetary payment to donors of bank-distributed germ cells and embryos—it is done already in some clinical procedures? Would clients ever have any right to return, reject, or pass on to others what they receive from a bank? Must they only be the reproducers? These are some of the legal and prudential questions at stake; there are others, of course—but apart from contingent questions like these there is no ethical objection to cryogenics as such.

Donating—Giving—Sharing

"It is more blessed to give than to receive," said Jesus. This is a moral sentiment that certainly needs no defense. Artificial insemination, egg transfers, gonad transplants, substitute gestation, and the like, now make it possible to put our generosities very close to home—in one's very own person. How "blessed" it was, to get down to cases, of the forty-five-year-old mother in Greece in 1973 who gave up her vagina for transplant to her twenty-one-year-old daughter, a victim of vaginal atresia, whose marriage was saved by the graft.[6]

Narcissism, egoism, and selfishness have heretofore had at least one last refuge that could never be threatened—one's own private and exclusive reproductivity. Every one of us either had it all to himself or herself, or lacked it altogether and were without hope. Now we can and will be asked to share our reproductivity with others, if they should lack fertility or have the wrong kind. The old alibis for the old selfishness are shot down, gone for good.

Unless there are foreseeably undesirable consequences in a particular case, we *ought* upon occasion to be donors of germ cells, gonads, or, in the case of women, of hostess gestation. It would be selfish to be sterilized by a simple tubal section, for example, if excision and transplant of the gonads could help a sterile neighbor to have a child. If we have a chance to donate one of our paired organs, should we not? Generosity and human community now have a richer range and depth. Whether or not we ourselves choose to be reproducers—by whatever method—we can and should help our friends and neighbors if they need to share our reproductivity. This is the meaning of the Roman nuns' donation of urine to facilitate the preparation of FSH. If we have acceptable help to give—no matter if we are married or not, celibate or not, parents or not—our obligation is to give it.

Ectogenesis: Outside the Womb

Nonvivaporous birds and animals lay their eggs and tend them until they hatch (are born)—it is all done outside the parents' bodies. Humans can do this too, for humane reasons and for quality's sake. If a wetnurse can supply another woman's child with her milk, and if we can give our blood to others, then how could there be any moral barrier to donating even more basic gifts, such as germ cells and placental sustenance, in hostess gestation?

No doubt trivial reasons will be given for extrauterine gestation sometimes ("I'd like to keep my figure"), but there will be more substantial reasons, too. Yet surely it is not necessary to have a solemn or highly exigent reason. Mothers are entitled to decide against using their own wombs even though the great majority will probably always opt for gestation as an important part of becoming a mother. Besides physical conditions that call for ectogenesis—serious genetic disorders, incorrigible infertility, hysterectomy, chronic heart disease, blocked tubes—there are personal vocational reasons as well.

Transcending these difficulties does *not* make mothers "obsolescent," as some have suggested. In Huxley's *Brave New World* normal birth with its physiological pain was never openly mentioned. Is such pain desirable for any real reason, other than a masochistic urge and "because the Bible says it's so" (Genesis 3:16)? As the Peking newspaper *Jenmin Jin Pao* put it, "Nine months of pregnancy is no light or easy burden and such diseases as poisoning due to pregnancy are detrimental to health. If children can be had without being borne, working mothers need not be affected by childbirth. This is happy news for women."[7]

Plastic, glass, or steel wombs, as an alternative for substitute (hostess) human carrywomen, will soon become "operational"—once we compound artificial placentas. Biochemistry has yet to work through the problem of the placenta, to figure out the chemistry of "nature." It is easy, alas, to underestimate the problem. J. B. S. Haldane wildly predicted in his little book *Daedalus* (1923) that by 1968 France would have sixty thousand babies by ectogenesis.

The glass womb is after all nothing more than an extension of the "extracorporeal membrane oxygenator," the incubator which already feeds "preemies" and babies with hyaline membrane disease. An artificial placenta, like a heart-lung machine, is a substitute for a natural function; it provides amniotic fluid chemically. Glass wombs are a radical version of early Caesarean sections. With artificial placentas we could save a fetus which might otherwise have to be lost in a medical abortion; both the patient *and the baby* could be saved. If we can save people with kidney failure by putting them on machines (artificial kidneys), and people with heart disease by putting machines in them (artificial hearts), why not do the same for *potential* people? When cloning becomes fully operational for humans, ectogenesis would in some situations eliminate the reimplantation stage, to advantage.

As in cryogenics, there will be regulatory questions. Is the genetic mother of a baby gestated by a hostess the "real" mother in the eyes of the law, or is the gestator? For example, should hostess gestators be married or single; would their husbands have veto powers; what, if any, would be the legal rights of the surrogates? These are all matters of social policy, and yet to be carefully thought through.

Egg Transfers

Egg grafts or artificial enovulations from a donor would be perfectly ethical if a person is, for example, without ovaries or has a hopeless infection of her tubes, or if she fears to pass on a genetic disease. A transfer is psychologically happier than AID because the husband is the genetic father and the wife can at least "carry" her own baby if she wants. But the *method* is more complicated—for example, getting her and the donor's ovulation periods together. Furthermore, the donor's time and discomfort is markedly greater than in AID.

Present feasibilities favor *in vitro* fertilization before the implantation of borrowed ova, rather than *in vivo* fertilization in coitus. In February 1970 a couple went to Edwards and Steptoe in England for an *in vitro* fertilization and implantation, even though the procedure is still tentative. The patient's tubes were blocked and her own ova, not a donor's, were to be used. Somehow it was aired on the BBC and a great "debate" arose. Reactionaries and sensationalists used put-down language, such as "Guinea Pig Mother of Test Tube Baby." It was said that they should be refused the investigative treatment they wanted because it is unethical, irreligious, and an unnatural medical service.

A leading Methodist ethicist countered that it was morally all right if no harm was done to the zygote. That condition is of course impossible to meet. The clinicians can be confident only that whenever their procedure results in a defective conceptus they should do what nature does when the *natural* process produces a defective conceptus—abort it, and try again.

To the warning that this artificial reproduction is playing God and is irreverent, an Anglican bishop quite wisely said, "The church would not want any restrictions imposed upon research into the beginning of life and it is certain that the outcome will never undermine belief in God as the creator."

Family and Marriage

Women who had never copulated will have children, and women who have often copulated will never have children. Babies without sex, sex without babies. Some children will have only one parent—a parent who may be either a man or a woman. Bachelor mothers and fathers will become more common. Single parents are already having children. Marriages will be contracted less often than in the past. Families, at least nuclear families, are sure to be smaller in size or frequency.

How far do we want to depart from the conventional and familiar marriage syndrome—monogamous, permanent, exclusive, heterosexual? With the separation of love making from baby making, plus the reduction of progeny numbers and the escape of women from the baby-machine role, the family is losing some of its pragmatic importance. Historically marriage and the family, which "began as a physical union and then became a legal one—to give men property rights in women and their offspring—has now reached the threshold of a moral union: a free one, elective to start, and elective to stop."[8]

The family functions primarily for the sake of the children, and rightly so; they create it. A childless couple is a "hominid pair bond," not a family. Under the influences of the new biology and social change the family's shape will change too. (Recall, for example, Alvin Toffler's futuristic option of pro-parents or professional child-rearers, in relation to bio-parents or those who generate the child.[9])

Nostalgic critics see these emerging patterns as a moral decline, a weakening of the family. One such critic even thinks we are disastrously "creating a new conception of what it means to be human." But the essence of the family—adults giving loving personal care to children—will be basically unchanged by new modes of reproduction. Children will still have ancestors, parents, siblings. The new biology only enlarges the family and deepens what it means to be human. We cannot repeat it too often; new and refined modes of reproduction are still thoroughly biological and natural—and because they are highly rational and purposive, not just sexual roulette or marital lottery, *they are more fully human,* as well as more humane.

With artificial insemination and egg transfer, children are truly chosen, definitely wanted. No happenstance about it. By comparison, "normal" parents are far more apt to be casual or flighty. It has been found, for example, that there is only one divorce in 800 AID couples compared to one divorce in every four couples of the general population.[10]

What an extraordinary *volte face* it is for Christians to have turned and twisted along a line from St. Paul's legalistic claim that the only reason for marriage is that it legitimates sex ("better to marry than to burn") to St. Augustine's insistence that the only excuse for sex is that babies are made by means of it (a very antisexual posture indeed) to the present-day reactionary view of typical objectors to noncoital asexual reproduction—the reverse opinion, now, that the only justification for babies is that they come from sex.

Genetic Engineering

Of all phases of the new molecular biology and reproductive medicine, what we call "genetic engineering" is furthest from being "operational" or in practical use. Genetic intervention in humans to eliminate inborn physical and mental defects is not here yet. But it looms ahead. Since Crick and Watson deciphered DNA's three dimension double-helix base-pair structure more than twenty years ago we have already seen the nucleic acid code broken, then an active viral gene synthesized, and at the practical level the green revolution's genetic production of supercereals and miracle rice in the "hungry Third World."

Morally, genetic engineering is good when it serves human needs, both health and happiness. If genetic manipulation were not possible in agriculture and plant physiology we would be back where Stalin and Lysenko stalled Soviet biology. If we were unable to do it in animal husbandry we would have to say good-bye to the rational reproduction of meat, work and hide animals, livestock improvement, and so on. These farming and herding techniques are for human benefit, and there is no ethical cut-off point at which to clamp an arbitrary stop on the use of genetic controls for the health and quality of human beings themselves.

Two different uses are up for approval: therapeutic or medical treatment, and the *design* of genotypes preconceptively. While some people object to all genetic intervention, others only object to genetically designing human beings—not to repairing genetic faults *after* they are conceived or born. In short, they justify it for treatment but not for prevention.

This is somewhat more humane than the blanket condemnations but hardly any more rational. It is absurd to be willing to cure human ills or lacks but unwilling to avoid or supply them before they afflict us. Such a strange posture is ethical nonsense. For example, in the relatively benign area of cosmetic surgery for disfiguring physical traits, who would prefer to have it done over and over again from generation to generation when it could be obviated once and for all by genetic intervention?

Still others would condemn any use of genetic controls to produce a "strain" of men with long arms to fit them to be orchard workers, or to produce a family of people with oversize lungs for sponge fishing or pearl diving.

Ethical questions are raised about using genetic control to choose the phenotypes of *future* individuals. (Gerald Feinberg has put it neatly. Much as we dislike making plans which restrict the freedom of future generations, we cannot escape doing so. "An inescapable result of the one-way flow of time is that we are born into a world we never made." He adds, "I do not think that any new moral principle is established" when we exercise our honest judgment about what is best for our descendants.)[11] But this is after all only another version of the ethical questions we are already facing when we reproduce with known traits. We have always had to weigh the cost of our choices and purposes against our needs, and we always will. The only change would be for the good, because we would have more control with which to do what we think is right.

A sensible policy is to breed animals for special purposes instead of humans, where possible, if the specialization delimits human capacities. Dolphins, fish, pigeons, primates are even now being used to do dull or dangerous work for us. We could even design species from scratch. There is no need to drag humans down genetically to do special or menial jobs; we can bring animals *up,* to do them. As Sir George Thompson sees it, "Very large modifications in the wild species can no doubt be made."[12] For example, animal brains can be markedly improved by doses of the twenty-first human chromosome. And rather than providing people with low I.Q.s to do dull work we might take Shaw's advice (*The Intelligent Woman's Guide to Socialism*) and pay normal people extra-high wages to do what most of us don't want to do.

Human Beings, Being Human

Human beings, in order to qualify as human, have to be something more than just biologically classifiable as organisms of the species *homo sapiens.* They have to have individual or separate existence ("viability") and they have to be actually "sapient"—that is, possessed of a functioning cerebral cortex—some minimal level of intelligence.

Therefore an individual of the species who is not yet human, a fetus, and one who has ceased to be, a "brain dead" patient, is without the status of being human or of human being. The sadness of abortion is that it means letting a potential go—but it is only a potential, not a reality; the sadness of "pulling the plug" on an irreversibly comatose patient is that it means accepting the bitter fact of a loss—acknowledging that a human being is now no more. But the point is that abortion and "brain death" terminations are *biocide,* not homicide. All talk of "killing a human being" in such cases is therefore ethically off the track.

Incidentally, the nearest thing to a specifiable "moment" for *becoming* human is when a fetus is respirated after birth—that reflexive and explosive gulp of air starting the lungs to work. This is what Plato contended. Only on his terms can it make sense to speak of the "moment" of becoming human. The "moment" of death, of *ceasing* to be human, is quite commonly unspecifiable. In any case, being human is two things essentially—intelligence and "going it alone" as an individual on one's own lungs.

Hybrids

But hold on. What if an ape had the intelligence and sensibilities of a human, and a human had only the capabilities of an ape? Which would be the human being? The answer is plain; the ape would be the human being.

This is no mere play on words. All mammals, man among them, are remarkably close biologically. Modern biology can devise "chimeras" or combinations of humans and animals, and also "cyborgs" or combinations of humans and machines. Gerald Leach warns us against the Minotaur, a mythical creature half man and half bull who was hidden away because it was too horrible to look upon.[13] The basic fact is that the body cells of all species will cross-fuse, and the germ cells of many—though not all—will unite sexually.

If a prosthetic device, perhaps an intricate mechanical hand or leg, supplies a person with 50 per cent or more of the function lost in an amputation, that is morally good. An artificial kidney or hemodialysis machine is morally good. This applies equally to heart pacemakers, dacron arteries, metal bones, ceramic hip-joints. All such technical contrivances are cyborgs or man-machine "hybrids."

Man-animal combinations are in the same ethical class. If a cow's kidney is "grown" into a patient's thigh to help cleanse his blood, after his own kidney function is gone, that is morally good. If an animal's organ or tissue is used to replace something lost by a human (an interspecific transplant) that is good. These are examples of man-animal combinations for medical purposes. And the day may come when replacement medicine will be keeping herds of animals on hand, to supply physicians with what they need. It would mean more "live" rather than transshipped cadaver transplants, and it would relieve human beings of the risks or inconveniences of the donor role.

But what of hybridization for nonmedical reasons? Chimeras or parahumans might legitimately be fashioned to do dangerous or demeaning jobs. As it is now, low grade work is shoved off on moronic and retarded individuals, the victims of uncontrolled reproduction. Should we not "program" such workers thoughtfully instead of accidentally, by means of hybridization? Cell fusion and putting human cell nuclei into animal tissue is possible (such hybrid tissue exists already as a matter of fact).

Hybrids could also be designed by sexual reproduction, as between apes and humans. If interspecific coitus is too distasteful, then laboratory fertilization and implant could do it. If women are unwilling to gestate hybrids animal females could. Actually, the artificial womb would bypass all such repugnances. In some cases even the sterility of hybrids might be overcome. (Euphenic changes, such as cell fusion tissues would be, are not transmissible genetically.)

Contrived in order to protect human beings from danger, a social reason, or from disease, a medical reason, chimeras and cyborgs would be morally justified. What counts is human need and well-being.

Incest

The prohibition of incest among humans is a fictive

(in the sense of a nonbiological) rule. It exists for socially pragmatic reasons. On the whole it has been a good rule. It has enforced a healthy "exogamy" or marriage outside the group or family, with a consequent variation of human genotypes—resulting from the input of different strains. Also it has the effect of distributing wealth and spreading power.

Other animals have no aversion to incest, and breeders often reinforce their livestock's natural incestuousness for quality purposes. The so-called "instinct" against incest is a matter of cultural conditioning, not a biologically based aversion. Religious claims that it is against "nature" or the "laws of nature" are groundless. Brother-sister reproduction goes on on a wide scale all of the time, occasionally even among human beings. Exogamy or outbreeding is a sound policy for distributing bad genes and avoiding the locked-in concentration of faults which has ruined famous families such as the Jukes and Kallikaks and some royal family lines. In the same way endogamy or inbreeding is a sound policy for holding good genes together and preserving superior genotypes—provided, of course, that the "strain" does not include too many subfaults which might aggregate and subvert the good qualities.

Warnings that artificial insemination might end up in incest have no biological force. As a matter of fact, the statistics are that there would be only one occurrence in fifty to a hundred years, at the rate of two thousand AIDs performed per year, if each donor contributed only five times. And clonants, having the same sex as the parent cell, could not possibly engage in incest with a fellow clonant—unless it was homosexual incest.

We have here a case of conduct in which there is nothing inherently or absolutely wrong, yet the greatest good of the greatest number might best be served by disapproving it. Having said as much, however, we may then hold that in particular cases it could be right to practice incest. It would depend on the situation, presumably an odd and highly unusual situation. The only argument against meeting human needs in such cases, other than the *a priori* "law of nature," would have to be the slippery slope or wedge argument—that *any* exceptions at all to the rule would lead to abandoning its wisdom as a general policy. This would be hard to make stick, just as it is in surgery in spite of "do the patient no harm" or executive clemency in spite of "criminals should pay for their crimes."

Trying to imagine situations where incest would be desirable, even if tolerable, is exceedingly difficult. But there is an important difference ethically; incest is tolerable because it is not in and of itself an evil, even though it would only rarely be possible to show that it is positively desirable. The main point is: Instead of twisting biology to fit an ethical system, let's build our ethics to fit biology and human well-being.

Love Making

Love as an interpersonal sentiment is of course wider and deeper than sexual intercourse, just as "sexuality" is. But in the restricted sense of intercourse "love making," like other human acts, is not inherently either right or wrong. Our moral judgments on sex acts are determined by many extrinsic and contextual variables—such factors as the intentions and attitudes of the parties, their marital status or lack of it, their health, their age and competence, and so on.

If we keep two crucial realities in mind—the separation biologically of love making from baby making, and the critical need socially and ecologically to arrest or even reverse population growth—we will see that our moral scheme must have a place for sex freedom and variety. Love making has a two-dimensional nature, "procreation and recreation." On its procreative side, sex should be well controlled, a discipline of careful calculation, whether it is carried out naturally or artificially. On its recreative side, spontaneity and personal feeling should reign.

Women are not baby machines, men are not baby machine operators, and homes are not human manufacturing plants. Women are persons first of all, not wives or spinsters. Fathers-in-law no longer require a bride price from husbands, nor do they lose it if the bride is not a virgin. Virginity (a condition) as distinguished from chastity (a virtue) is not so much valued any more. Spouses (especially wives) are no longer private property; husbands no longer bury two or three wives in a lifetime. Legalistic language like "the marital debt" does not fit authentic love making.

Terms which tie love making so closely to marriage—we speak of premarital, comarital and extramarital sex—are archaic. They reflect an outmoded inflexibility of sexual role, too stereotyped to fit our deepening sense of personal freedom and responsibility. (Francoeur lists as many as twenty telltale variants in patterned sexual behavior.[14]) More and more people remain single, and extramarital sex or "adultery" increases, as among the retired elderly who often have very practical reasons for not marrying—and aren't really expected to. The blackmailing business, to put it another way, is in decline.

Heterosexual, monogamous, permanent, and sexually exclusive marriage still remains an ideal and a reality for many and possibly even for most people. At the same time, divorce figures indicate a general acceptance of serial polygamy—as being more humane than a relentless maintenance of one-shot monogamy, regardless of the unhappiness of the partners.

Reproduction will be moving away to some extent from sexual intercourse and marriage is losing its old simplistic foundation. We must either find new moral guidelines for old values—or change our values.

Parenthood

Mothers and fathers are of several different kinds now. Take mothers: Some are genetic (they provide the egg), some are natal (they carry the fetus), some are social (they rear or "bring up" the child). All of them can play a part in a child's creation—yet no one of them needs to fill more than one of these roles. All of them, or any combination, would be ethical as far as the functions themselves are concerned.

Parental (and kin) relationships need to be reconceptualized. They cannot any more be based on blood or wombs or even genes. Parenthood will have to be understood nonbiologically or, to be specific, *morally.* Its own achievements have forced biology out of court in validating parental relations. The mere fact of conceiving a child or donating the elements of its conception or gestating it does not establish anybody as a father or a mother. Parental love has by this time become truly interpersonal; no longer can it be merely germinal, somatic, or physiological—and certainly not merely genital. An authentic parental bond is established morally, by care and concern, not by some simple physicalist doctrine.

Uterine and ovarian transplants, like egg and embryo transfers, further extend the legalistic questions about paternal rights raised nearly fifty years ago when AID was started. Maternity now is in question too, as paternity used to be. The old rule that only paternity is not self-evident (*"Mater semper certa est, pater est quem nuptiae demonstrat"*) is overthrown by reproductive medicine.

Morally, donors of seed or ova ought to have no claims of any kind on recipient or child, nor recipient or child on a donor, nor recipient or child on the spouses of either a donor or a recipient. What counts morally is the commitment of the participants, not what they contribute. All of this complexity forces us to embrace a moral rather than physical definition of parenthood.

Research and Ignorance

The geneticist Joshua Lederberg said in his paper at the Nobel symposium in Stockholm in September 1969 ("Orthobiosis, the Perfection of Man"), "The suppression of knowledge appears to me unthinkable, not only on ideological but on merely logical grounds. How can the ignorant know what they should not know?"[15]

Dr. Lederberg's remark is aimed at those who want to suppress research because they are afraid of "dangerous" knowledge, especially in the field of human reproduction. It may be conceded that we ought not to embark on irreversible innovations if we are sure we know them to be both irreversible and imprudently dangerous—such things (presumably) as immortality pills, untraceable poisons, or a hydrogen bomb that could be made in private bedrooms. The new biology, however, is not of that caliber or character.

"The answer to dangerous knowledge," as Van Rensselaer Potter has noted, "continues to be more knowledge."[16] Deliberately to choose ignorance is unethical, immoral. It is comforting, therefore, to recall that the risks of damage to *in vitro* conceptions and implanted embryos is no greater than the errors in natural or *in vivo* pregnancies; neither is risk free.

A related moral issue is raised around the research use of live fetuses obtained from either medically prescribed or personally elected abortions. "Right to life" or "pro-life" agitators in 1973 actually intimidated the U.S. National Institutes of Health into (at least temporarily) suspending their approval of many programs of research into the causes of genetic and fetal disorders. On the other hand, a conference of Britain's leading obstetricians, chaired by Sir John Peel, settled in 1972 on a fairly sensible policy, ethically regarded—although at some points it shows more compromise than logic.[17] An inviable fetus (less than five months) and fetal material at any stage (placenta, fluids, membranes) may be used. Nothing is said in their policy statement, incidentally, about any "rights" of the fetus. A good deal is quite properly said about the patient's rights of consent or objection.

It is contended that an abortee's permission should be given before any use is made of her fetus or fetal material and this would seem ordinarily to be the right principle. But surely this limiting principle could be disregarded in some situations—for example, when a woman stubbornly refuses consent even though her fetus holds a promising clue to an epidemic or, equally hypothetical, if it were discovered that the abortus contains an agent that will cure or control cancer. The antiabortionists, of course, object to postabortional fetal research even if the patient's permission is given, and no matter what the excuse.

Rights and Regulation

All alleged human rights cease to be right, become unjust, when their exercise would victimize innocent third parties and bystanders. All rights are "imperfect," not absolute or uncontingent. We might say this particularly of the so-called "right to privacy" as it bears on propagating at will and inordinately. The social welfare and protection of third parties has a prior claim. The "right" to reproduce, like all others, is—morally weighed—really only a privilege.

A worrisome side to the practice of control is whether it should ever be imposed or must always be voluntary. If people could be relied upon to be compassionate we would have no reason to even consider mandatory controls. But there are too many who do not control their lives out of moral concern; they are self-centered about what they do or neglect to do, even though they may be "cagey" about it. Large families and a pious disregard of genetic counseling, like refusing to undergo vaccinations until it is made a matter of police enforcement, show how the common welfare often has to be safeguarded by compulsory control or what Garrett Hardin calls "mutual coercion mutually agreed upon."[18]

Coercion is a dirty word to liberals, but all social controls—e.g., the government's tax powers—are really what the majority agree upon, however reluctantly, out of enlightened self-interest and a *quid pro quo* willingness to give up something to get something better. It might be protection from overpopulation, for instance. Ideally it is better to do the moral thing freely, but sometimes it is more compassionate to force it to be done than to sacrifice the well-being of the many to the egocentric "rights" of the few. This obviously is the ethics of a sane society. Compulsory controls on reproduction would not, of course, fit present interpretations of due process in the fifth and fourteenth amendments to the Constitution.[19] Here, as in so many other ways, the law lags behind the ethics of modern medicine and public health knowledge.

Screening

A good illustration of the tension between rights and regulation takes shape in trying to control hereditary disease. Each of us carries from five to ten genetic faults. If they match up in sexual roulette, tragedy results. How can we avoid or curtail the danger? Denmark prohibits marriages of certain couples unless they are sterilized. But if this method of control and prevention is used, or any other, how do we find out *who* are the ones who should not marry or, if they do, should not have babies by the natural or coital mode? Screening by one means or another is the obvious way to fulfill our obligation to potential children, as well as to the community which has to suffer when defectives are born.

The law in most countries is far behind our emerging medical information. People are not required to make their bad genes known to their mates nor are physicians required to reveal the facts. A man with polycystic kidney disease is not required to let it be known—even though it is highly immoral (unjust) to keep knowledge of such a hereditary disaster (renal failure in middle age) from his children and those they marry. Medical genetics will continue to isolate more and more such diseases, so that as our ability to prevent disease and tragedy increases so does the moral guilt of secrecy, indifference to the consequences for others, and fatalistic inaction.

Conquering infectious diseases reduces the cause of the trouble, but to conquer genetic diseases *increases* the cause or source of the trouble. This dysgenic effect is the first big-scale moral dilemma for medicine—truly a dilemma. Infections come from the environment around us but genetic faults come from within us, and therefore any line of genetic sufferers allowed to propagate will spread their disease through more and more carriers. As we cut down on the infectious diseases we are threatened with a relative rise in deaths and debility due to genetic disorders. We are now approaching a situation in which genetic causes account for as many *or more* deaths than "disease" in the popular sense.

Our moral obligation to undergo voluntary screening, if it is indicated, is too obvious to underline. The squeeze here, ethically, is that the social good often requires *mass* screening. When it is voluntary it is "nicer," as we see in the popular acceptance of tests for cervical cancer. But let it be compulsory if need be, for the common good—Hardin's "mutual coercion mutually agreed upon." Francis Crick has said that "if we can get across to people the idea that their children are not entirely their own business and that it is not a private matter, it would be an enormous step forward."[20] The biophysicist Leroy Augenstein estimated in 1972 that a total of 6 per cent of births or one out of seventeen, are defective. Of these, he said, forty thousand to fifty thousand children every year "are so defective that they don't know that they are human beings."[21] His figures are more impressive than his formulation, however; if an individual cannot "know" he is a human being he is not a human being.

Parents of adopted children and donors of AID are much more carefully screened and selected than "natural" parents—which is logically ridiculous even though we can understand how it came about. A socially conscientious system would be a national registry; blood and skin tests done routinely at birth and fed into a computer-gene scanner would pick up all anomalies, and they would be printed out on data cards and filed; then when marriage licenses are applied for, the cards would be read in comparison machines to find incompatibilities and homozygous conditions.

The objection is, predictably, that it would "violate" a "right"—the right to privacy. It is even said, in a brazen attack on reason itself, that we have a "right to *not* know." Which is more important, the alleged "privacy" or the good of the couple as well as of their progeny and society? (The couple could unite anyway, of course, but on the condition Denmark makes—that sterilization is done for one or both of them. And they could even still have children by medical and donor assistance, bypassing their own faulty fertility.)

Screening is no more an invasion of privacy than "contact tracing" in the treatment of venereal disease, or income tax and public health records, or compulsory fluoridation of the water, or the age-old codes of consanguinity (which were only based on nonsense). A good education for those who balk would be a week's stay in the wards of a state institution for the "retarded"—a term used to cover a host of terrible distortions of humanity. Just let them *see* the nature and extent of it; that would convince them.

Sex Selection

The ethical issues raised about preselection of children's sex are mainly two: whether it is wrong to exercise that much control over our progeny, and whether it is right to throw the sex ratio out of balance. The second "issue" is based on an assumption that most people would prefer boys to girls.

By way of answering, we would say that control as such is good, not evil, and the more the better, but that it should not be used for immoral purposes. Throwing the sex ratio out of near balance might be undesirable if it denied some people their aliquot share of sexual partnership. This could be the case in a strictly monogamous culture, even though single persons and celibates (to say nothing of group-marriage members) could have children asexually. With fewer progeny needed or wanted, and sexual intercourse freer in part because of that fact, there is now much less need for a near balance of the sexes. And in the last resort, reproduction no longer will have to depend on marital-coital-gestational reproduction.

The assumption that the male gender is better and more desirable is a bare-faced piece of male chauvinism and androcentric psychology. To suppose that fetal sex choice and freedom of abortion would mean throwing out "worthless females" is both hilarious and foolish. If men were stupid enough to do it (they aren't) the women would soon set things straight.

There is also the related issue, the assertion that embryos are human beings and that superfetation and selection is "mass murder." This strident protest is not ethically tenable. Even its metaphysical validity is dubious, to say nothing of its unethical and antimedical consequences if it were followed out logically.

Sterilization

In May 1973 the Supreme Court upheld a lower court's decision that it was unconstitutional when the Worcester (Massachusetts) City Hospital denied a patient's request for a voluntary sterilization. That settled the legal side of it.

On the ethical side sterilization is plainly a matter of personal freedom and responsibility. It is as moral a means to the end as any other form of birth control. In fact, its reliability makes it more responsible. Sterilization is not absolutely ethical, of course. Nothing is. But unless it either violates a promise or denies some real obligation to propagate (which would be rare situations indeed) it is morally right.

As a matter of fact, even after a woman has had a sterilization she could still have children. Once we worried about the irreversibility of sterilization. But now a woman can have the tubes finally closed off, yet aspirate the eggs by laparascope, fertilize them *in vitro,* and then have one egg implanted in her own womb for nurture. We could drop vasectomies and the pill, and practically eliminate any abortions except those done for therapeutic and genetic reasons.

Value, Values

Human acts and things are both like poker chips, they have whatever value or worth we—human beings—choose to assign to them. A red one is worth so much, a blue one so much, a white one so much. Put negatively, nothing has intrinsic value—things have no value apart from how human beings feel about them. As in games where chips are used, so in real affairs we agree about the relative values of what we do and what we want in terms of humanly desirable and exchangeable needs and aspirations.

For example, would we on principle "bump" a suicide from an intensive care unit (ICU) to save an auto accident victim, if it had to be one or the other? The answer, surely, is No. We cannot say that all suicides want to die, nor that all auto accident casualties want to live. It depends. Every case has to be looked at on its own merits.

How we judge or weigh our decisions in real life situations will depend on what we know or suppose we know about the alternatives. One thing we can be sure of; it is immoral in the extreme to say, as one member of the British Parliament did in the debate on the Abortion Act of 1967, "We are not here to listen to professional opinion, we are here to legislate." That posture, Don't Bother Me With the Facts, My Mind Is Made Up, is the last word in irresponsibility.

As we have seen in nearly all of our ethical problems, the pressure comes when the social interest fails to phase with the personal. The conviction throughout my *Ethics of Genetic Control,* perhaps because we believe that without survival of the species all talk about ethics is academic, is that the general welfare comes first. Look at Robert Louis Stevenson's turnaround experience. He went to Polynesia *sure* that "infanticide" is wrong. What happened to him?

Stevenson already knew "in the back of his mind" that we exist in a finite world inescapably. But he never really understood what he "knew" until he stood on a small atoll in the vast surrounding sea, trying to identify with the outlook of the inhabitants. Then he could grasp the fact that these tiny atolls are true paradigms of the finite "spaceship Earth." When too many babies were born (because the atoll dwellers did not yet know how to prevent it) they accepted the moral responsibility of "aborting at birth" *because they loved their children* and knew that there is a point of too much. He finally saw the ethical error of his simplistic prohibition of infanticide.

This may appear to be a remote example or *ultima ratio* of the relativity of values. But before we dismiss it too lightly we should hold it long enough in mind to test the ethical validity of the concepts of species survival and social conscience.

Wrongful Life

We have already reached the conclusion that sometimes it is wrong to procreate a life, but let it be nailed down again. In the law they speak of wrongful death—deaths due, for example, to criminal negligence. Now the new biology and reproductive medicine are confronting us ethically with the reality of wrongful *life,* too.

A wrongful death is one which results from a "tort" or injurious, blameworthy act for which the victim or his agents and beneficiaries should be indemnified or somehow compensated. In any case, the tort is by definition blameworthy, wrong. People who know a child will be defective, or could have known if they had cared but nonetheless allowed it to be born, are as guilty of wrongdoing as those who culpably contribute to a wrongful death.

The ethical principle, as distinct from (but not unrelated to) the legal category of wrongful death, is that there is indeed such a thing as wrongful life. Already the courts have accepted two or three suits by the victims of misconception and misgestation, or by others involved; the principle is taking form, inevitably. We are as morally responsible for what we do at the start of a life as we are for what we do at the end of it. And the test, at both the alpha and the omega on the continuum, is loving concern.

Notes

1. G. Dunstan, *Morals and Medicine,* ed., Archie Clow, p. 67.
2. "Genetic Engineering," *Engineering and Science,* 35 (June 1972), 7.
3. "A New Ethic for Medicine and Society," *California Medicine,* 113 (September 1970), 67-68.
4. See H. Muller, "Human Evolution by Voluntary Choice of Germ Plasm," *Science,* 134 (September 8, 1961), 643-49 for a suggestive exposition.
5. In a play by J. Costigan, *Baby Want a Kiss?*
6. *Hospital Tribune,* 7:14 (April 9, 1973), 1, 24.
7. Quoted by E. Grossman, "The Obsolescent Mother," *Atlantic Monthly,* 227 (May 1971), 39-50.
8. Joseph Fletcher, in *Marriage: For and Against,* intro. by H. Hart. New York: Hart Publishing Co., 1972, p. 205.
9. *Future Shock.* New York: Random House, 1970, p. 208.
10. S. Behrman, in Behrman and Kistner, *Progress in Infertility.* Boston: Little, Brown and Company, 1967.
11. *The Promethean Project.* Garden City, N.Y.: Doubleday & Company, 1969, pp. 203-5.
12. *The Foreseeable Future.* New York: The Viking Press, 1960, p. 98.
13. *The Biocrats.* New York: McGraw-Hill Book Co., 1970, p. 98.
14. R. Francoeur, *Adam's New Rib,* op. cit., pp. 221-24.
15. In *The Place of Value in a World of Facts,* ed., A. Tiselius and S. Nilsson. New York and London: John Wiley & Sons, 1971.
16. *Bioethics: Bridge to the Future.* Englewood Cliffs, N.J.: Prentice-Hall, 1971, p. 70.

17. *The Use of Fetuses and Fetal Material for Research.* London: Her Majesty's Stationery Office, 1972.
18. *Exploring New Ethics for Survival.* New York: The Viking Press, 1972, pp. 260-62.
19. F. Grad, "Legislative Responses to the New Biology: Limits and Possibilities," *U.C.L.A. Law Review,* 15 (February 1968), 486.
20. Quoted by A. Rosenfeld, op. cit., p. 161.
21. "Birth Defects," *Humanistic Perspectives in Medical Ethics,* ed., M. Visscher. London: Pemberton Publishing Co., 1972, p. 207.

60.
Moral and Religious Implications of Genetic Control

PAUL RAMSEY

The Genetic Apocalypse and the End of Man

In order to analyze the moral implications of genetic control for western religions, it is necessary to lift up to view certain aspects of what it means to intend the world as a Christian or as a Jew. These also are modes of being human, and of how values are "otherwise known" in this world and ethical judgments made. On the assumption that it is a Christian *subject* who has come into the possession of all this genetic knowledge and who faces our genetic dilemma, what will be the attitude he takes toward eugenic proposals? Two ingredients are of chief importance. First, we have to contrast biblical or Christian eschatology with genetic eschatology, and observe how these practical proposals may change their hue when shifted from one ultimate philosophy of history to the other. This will be the matter of the present section of this chapter. Then, secondly (in the following section), we have to explore the bearing which the Christian understanding of the union between the personally unitive purpose and the procreative purpose of human sexual relations (sex as at once an act of love and an act of procreation) may have upon the question of the means to be used in genetic control.

The writings of H. J. Muller give the most vivid portrayal of the genetic cul-de-sac into which the human race is heading. He describes, in fact, a genetic apocalypse. His fellow geneticists can correct, if they must, the extremism of this vision. For the purpose of making clear, however, how one intends the world as a Christian, even in the face of such an apocalyptic account of the end toward which we are proceeding, or which is coming upon us, it is better to leave the vision unaltered and assume it to be a true account of the scientific facts.

Within a period of a few million years, according to Muller, provided that during this period our medical men have been able to continue to work with the kind of perfection they desire, "the then existing germ cells of what were once human beings would be a lot of hopeless, utterly diverse genetic monstrosities." Long before that, "the job of ministering to infirmities would come to consume all the energy that society could muster," leaving no surplus for general or higher cultural purposes.[1] People's time and energy would be mainly spent in an effort "to live carefully, to spare and prop up their own feebleness, to soothe their inner disharmonies and, in general, to doctor themselves as effectively as possible." Everyone will be an invalid, and everyone's accumulated internal disability would amount to lethality if he had to live under primitive conditions.[2] If any breakdown occurs in the complex hospital system that civilization will have become, mankind will be thrown back into a wretchedness with which his primitive beginnings cannot be compared.

> Our descendants' natural biological organization would in fact have disintegrated and have been replaced by complete disorder. Their only connection with mankind would then be the historical one that we ourselves had after all been their ancestors and sponsors, and the fact that their once-human material was still used for the purpose of converting it, artificially, into some semblance of man. However, it would in the end be far easier and more sensible to manufacture a complete man *de novo,* out of appropriately chosen raw materials, than to try to refashion into human form those pitiful relics which remained. For all of them would differ inordinately from one another, and each would present a whole series of most intricate research problems, before the treatments suitable for its own unique set of vagaries could be decided upon.[3]

It is unreasonable to expect medicine to keep up with the problem (especially because medical men themselves in that near, or distant, future will be subject to the same genetic decomposition); "at long last even the most sophisticated techniques available could no longer suffice to save men from their biological corruptions"[4] (and, again, I add to Muller's assumptions, medicine in that future could not be all that sophisticated, because of the genetic deterioration of the medical men who would be alive in the generation before the genetic *eschaton*).

Stripped of rhetoric, this means that, according to the genetic apocalypse, there shall come a time when *there will be none like us to come after us.* There have been other such scientific visions of the future. Whether this results from the pollution of our atmosphere and water by industrial refuse, or of the atmosphere by strontium 90, or from a collision of planets, the burning up of the earth, or the entropy of energy until our planet enters the eternal night of a universe run down, these scientific predictions—without exception—portray a planet no longer fit for human habitation, or a race of men no longer fit to live humanly. Because these are science-based apocalypses, the gruesome details of the "last days" can be filled in, and our imagination heightened in its apprehension of the truth concerning physical nature and the prospects of human history in the one dimension that is scientifically known to us. All these visions quite realistically teach that there will come a time when there will be none like us to come after us. It is as obvious as the ages are long that it is an infirm philosophy which teaches that "man can be courageous only so long as he knows he is survived by those who are like him, that [in *this* sense] he fulfils a role in something more permanent than himself."[5] Every scientific eschatology (with the single exception of the view that human history is eternal) places in jeopardy courage and all other values that are grounded in the future of the human generations. It does not matter whether the end comes early or late. Nor do the gruesome details do more than heighten the imagination. They do not add to the ultimate meaninglessness to which all human affairs were reduced when meaning came to rest in the temporal future (unless that future is foreknown to be eternal—and, if one thinks this through, it too is a melancholy prospect). All that can be said to the credit of the genetic apocalypse, or to the credit of any science-based eschatology, is that it makes *impressive* the truth that was already contained in the thought that men live in "one world."

Anyone who intends or perceives the world as a Christian will have to reply that he knew this all along, and that he has already taken into his system the idea that one day there will be none like us to come after us. Even gruesome details about what will happen in the "last days" are not missing from the Christian's Apocalypse, even though admittedly these are not extrapolations from scientific facts or laws. The Revelation of St. John is still in the Bible; and even the so-called little apocalypse (Mark 13 and parallels) had this to say: "In those days shall be affliction, such as was not from the beginning of the creation which God created unto this time, neither shall be.... But in those days, after that tribulation, the sun shall be darkened, and the moon shall not give her light, and the stars of heaven shall fall, and the powers that are in heaven shall be shaken" (Mark 13:19, 24-25). Again, stripped of rhetoric, there will be none like us to come after us on this planet.

This means that Christian hope into, and through, the future depends not at all on denying the number or seriousness of the accumulating lethal mutations which Muller finds to be the case (let his fellow geneticists argue with him however they will).

Where genetics teaches that we are made out of genes and unto genes return, Genesis teaches that we are made out of the dust of the ground and unto dust we and all our seed return. Never has biblical faith and hope depended on denying or refusing to face any facts—either of history, or of physical or biological nature. No natural or historical "theodicy" was ever required to establish the providence of God, for this providence was not confined to the one dimension within which modern thought finds its limits.

It is as easy (and as difficult) to believe in God after Auschwitz, as it was after Sennacherib came down like a wolf on the fold to besiege and destroy the people of God. The Jews who chanted as they went to meet their cremation, "*Ani Ma'amin . . .* "—"I believe with unswerving faith in the coming of the Messiah"—uttered words appropriate to that earlier occasion, and to all temporal occasions. It is as easy (and as difficult) to believe in God after Mendel and Muller, as it was after Darwin or the dust of Genesis. Religious people have never denied, indeed they affirm, that God means to kill us all in the end, and in the end He is going to succeed. Anyone who intends the world as a Jew or as a Christian—to the measure in which this is his mode of being in the world—goes forth to meet the collision of planets or the running down of suns, and he exists toward a future that may contain a genetic apocalypse with his eye fixed on another *eschaton: "Ani Ma'amin . . .* " He may take these words literally, or they may imaginatively express his conviction that men live in "two cities" and not in one only. In no case need he deny whatever account science may give him of this city, this history, or this world, so long as science does not presume to turn itself into a theology by blitzing him into believing that it knows the one and only apocalypse.[6]

This does not mean a policy of inaction, or mere negative acceptance, of trends in history or in biology on the part of anyone who is a Christian knowing-*subject* of all that he knows about the world. Divine determination, properly understood, imposes no iron law of necessity, no more than does genetic determination. Only the ultimate *interpretation* of all the action that is going on is different, and significantly different. We shall have to ask what practical difference this makes as one man goes about responding (in all the action that comes upon him) to the action of the laws of genetics, while another goes about responding (in all the action coming upon mankind) to the action of God; or, as one gives answers to the ultimate untrustworthiness of the force behind genetic trends, while another answers with his life and choices to a trustworthiness beyond all real or seeming untrustworthy things.[7]

The differences are two—one pervasive and the other precise. In the first instance, one must notice the tone of assertive or declaratory optimism based on the ultimate and unrelieved pessimism that pervades the thought of some proponents of eugenics. The writings of H. J. Muller cannot be accounted for simply by the science of genetics, or even by the fact that his ethics is that of a man who intends the world as a scientist and who finds the whole dignity of man to consist in thought. As such, and in themselves, these things might be productive of more serenity, or serenity in action. But it is the whole creation, as it is known in genetics to be effectively present today and into the future, that Muller is fighting. No philosophy since Bertrand Russell's youthful essay[8] has been so self-consciously built upon the firm foundations of an unyielding despair. Mankind is doomed unless positive steps are taken to regulate our genetic endowment; and so horrendous is the genetic load that it often seems that Muller means to say that mankind is doomed no matter what steps are taken. Yet his optimism concerning the solutions he proposes is no less evident throughout; and all the more so, the more it is clear that his solutions (dependent as they are upon voluntary adoption) are unequal to the task. The author's language soars, he aspires higher, he challenges his contemporaries to nobler acts of genetic self-formation and improvement, all the more because of the abyss below. The abyss sets up such powerful wind currents that mankind seems destined to be drawn into it no matter how high we fly. These are some of the consequences of the fact that when all hope is gone, Muller hopes on *in despair.* An Abraham of genetic science, if one should arise, would be one who, when all hope is gone, hopes on *in faith,* and who therefore need neither fear the problem nor trust the solution of it too much.

The more precisely identifiable difference is the greater room there will be for an "ethics of means" in the outlook of anyone who is oriented upon the Christian *eschaton* and not upon the genetic cul-de-sac alone. Anyone who intends the world as a Christian or as a Jew knows along his pulses that he is not bound *to succeed* in preventing genetic deterioration, any more than he would be bound to retard entropy, or prevent planets from colliding with this earth or the sun from cooling. He is not under the necessity of *ensuring* that those who come after us will be like us, any more than he is bound to *ensure* that there will be those like us to come after us. He knows no such *absolute* command of nature or of nature's God. This does not mean that he will do nothing. But it does mean that as he goes about the urgent business of doing his duty in regard to future generations, he will not begin with the desired *end* and deduce his obligation exclusively from this end. He will not define *right* merely in terms of conduciveness to the good end; nor will he decide what *ought to be done* simply by calculating what actions are most likely to succeed in achieving the *absolutely imperative end* of genetic control or improvement.

The Christian knows no such absolutely imperative end that would justify any means. Therefore, as he goes about the urgent business of bringing his duty to people now alive more into line with his genetic duty to future generations, he will always have in mind the premise that there may be a number of things that might succeed better but would be intrinsically wrong means for him to adopt. Therefore, he has a larger place for an ethics of means that is not wholly dependent on the ends of action. He knows that there may be a great many actions that would be wrong to put forth in this world, no matter what good consequences are expected to follow from them—especially if these consequences are thought of simply along the line of temporal history where, according to the Christian, success is not promised mankind by either Scripture or sound reason. He will approach the question of genetic control with a category of "cruel and unusual means" that he is prohibited to employ, just as he knows there are "cruel and unusual punishments" that are not to be employed in the penal code. He will ask, What are right means? no less than he asks, What are the proper objectives? And he will know in advance that any person, or any society or age, expecting ultimate success where ultimate success is not to be reached, is peculiarly apt to devise extreme and morally illegitimate means for getting there. This, he will know, can easily be the case if men go about making themselves the lords and creators of the future race of men. He will say, of course, of any historical and future-facing action in which he is morally obliged to engage: "Only the end can justify the means" (as Dean Acheson once said of foreign policy). However, because he is not wholly engaged in future-facing action or oriented upon the future consequences with the entirety of his being, he will immediately add (as Acheson did): "This is not to say that the end justifies any means, or that some ends can justify anything."[9] An ethics of means not derived from, or dependent upon, the objectives of action is the immediate fruit of knowing that men have another end than the receding future contains.

The ethics which, as we have seen, governs genetic proposals says as much. A fruit of intending the world as a geneticist is an ethics whose means are determined by the values of free will and thought. This puts a considerable limit upon the actions which can be proposed for the prevention of the genetic apocalypse (which, if a correct prediction, belongs only to the *contents* of the science of genetics). Still, this is not a sufficient substance for the morality of action, or at least not all the substance a Christian will find to be valid. One who intends the world as a Christian will know man's dignity consists not only in thought or in his freedom, and he will find more elements in the nature of man which are deserving of respect and should be withheld from human handling or trespass. Specifically in connection with genetic proposals, he will know that there are more ways to violate man-womanhood than to violate the *freedom* of the parties; and that something voluntarily adopted can still be wrong. He will pay attention to this as he goes about using indifferent, permitted, or not immoral means to secure the *relatively* imperative ends of genetic control or improvement. To this ethics of means we turn in the next section.

The Covenant of Marriage and Right Means

In relation to genetic proposals, the most important element of Christian morality—and the most important ingredient that the Christian acknowledges to be deserving of respect in the nature of man—which needs to be brought into view is the teaching concerning *the union between* the two goods of human sexuality.

An act of sexual intercourse is at the same time an act of love and a procreative act. This does not mean that sexual intercourse always in fact nourishes love between the parties or always engenders a child. It simply means that it *tends,* of its own nature, toward the strengthening of love (the unitive or the communicative good), and toward the engendering of children (the procreative good). This will be the nature of human sexual relations, provided there is no obstruction to the realization of these natural ends (for example, infertility preventing procreation, or an infirm, infertile, or incurving heart that prevents the strengthening of the bonds of love).

Now, there has been much debate between Protestants and Roman Catholics concerning whether the unitive or the procreative good is primary, and concerning the hierarchial order or value-rank to be assigned these goods. I have shown elsewhere[10] that, contrary to popular belief, there is in the present day little or no essential difference between Roman Catholic and Protestant teachings on this point. The crucial question that remains is whether sexual intercourse as an act of love should ever be separated from sexual intercourse as a procreative act. This question remains to be decided, even if the unitive and procreative goods are equal in primacy, and even if it be said that the unitive end is the higher one. It still must be asked, Ought men and women ever to put entirely asunder what God joined together in the covenant of the generating generations of mankind? Assign the supreme importance to sexual intercourse as an act of personal love, and there still remains the question whether, in what sense, and in what manner, intercourse as an act of love should ever be divorced from sexual intercourse as in and of itself procreative.

Now, I will state as a premise of the following discussion that an ethics (whether proposed by nominal Christians or not) that *in principle* sunders these two goods—regarding procreation as an aspect of biological nature to be subjected merely to the requirements of *technical* control while saying that the unitive purpose is the free, human, personal end of the matter—pays disrespect to the nature of human parenthood. *Human* parenthood is not the same as that of the animals God gave Adam complete dominion over. Such a viewpoint falls out of the bounds which limit the variety of Christian positions that may be taken up by, and debated among, people who undertake to intend the world as Christians.

It is important that these outer limits be carefully defined so that we see clearly the requirements of respect for the created nature of man-womanhood, and so that we do not rule out certain actions that have traditionally been excluded. Most Protestants, and nowadays a great many Catholics, endorse contraceptive devices which separate the sex *act* as an act of love from whatever tendency there may be in the act (at the time of the act, and in the sexual powers of the parties) toward the engendering of a child. But they do *not* separate the sphere or realm of their personal love from the sphere or realm of their procreation, nor do they distinguish between *the person* with whom the bond of love is nourished and *the person* with whom procreation may be brought into exercise. One has only to distinguish what is done in particular *acts* from what is intended, and done, in a whole series of acts of conjugal intercourse in order to see clearly that contraception need not be a radical attack upon what God joined together in the creation of man-womanhood. Where planned parenthood is not planned *un*parenthood, the husband and wife clearly do not tear their own one-flesh unity completely away from all positive response and obedience to the mystery of procreation—a power by which at a later time their own union originates the one flesh of a child.

Moreover, the fact that God joined together love and progeny (or the unitive and procreative purposes of sex and marriage) is held in honor, and not torn asunder, even when a couple for grave, or for what in their case is to them sufficient, reason adopt a lifelong policy of planned *un*parenthood. This possibility can no more be excluded by Protestant ethics than it is by Roman Catholic ethics, which teaches that under certain circumstances a couple may adopt a systematic and possibly lifelong policy of restricting their use of the unitive good to only such times as, it is believed, there is no tendency in the woman's sexual nature toward conception. The "grave reasons" permitting, or obliging this, have been extended in recent years (the original "reason" being extreme danger to a woman's life in childbirth) to include grave family financial difficulties (because the end is the procreation *and education* of the child). These "grave reasons" have been extended even to the point of allowing that the economy of the environing society and world overpopulation may be taken into account, by even the healthy and the wealthy, as sufficient reason for having fewer children or for having no more at all.[11] Once mankind's genetic dilemma is called to the attention of the Church and its moral theologians, I see no intrinsic reason why these categories of analysis may not be applied to allow ample room for voluntary eugenic decisions, either to have no children or to have fewer children, for the sake of future generations.

After all, Christian teachings have always held that by procreation one must perform his duty to the future generations of men; procreation has not been a matter of the selfish gratification of would-be parents. If the fact-situation disclosed by the science of genetics can prove that a given person cannot be the progenitor of healthy individuals (or at least not unduly defective individuals) in the next generations, then such a person's "right to have children" becomes his duty not to do so, or to have fewer children than he might want (since he never had any right to have children simply for his own sake). Protestant and Roman Catholic couples in practicing eugenic control over their own reproduction may (unless the latter's church changes its teaching about contraception in the wake of the Vatican Council) continue to say to one another: you in your way, and I in God's! In the turmoil over Pope Paul VI's encyclical *Humanae Vitae,* one Catholic couple says, in effect, to another: you in your way, I in the Church's or at least the Pope's. Still, it is clear that the Roman Catholic no less than the Protestant Christian could adopt a policy of lifelong nonparenthood, or less parentage, for eugenic reasons. Such married partners would still be saying by their actions that if either has a child, or if either has more children, this will be from their own one-flesh unity and not apart from it. Their response to what God joined together, and to the claim He placed upon human life when He ordained that procreation come from sexual love, would be expressed by their resolve to hold acts of procreation (even the procreation they have not, or have no more) within the sphere of acts of conjugal love, within the covenant of marriage. . . .

Let us continue our examination of the various methods that have been proposed for the control or improvement of man's genetic inheritance, evaluating these in the light of the requirement that there be no complete, or radical, or "in principle" separation between the personally unitive and the procreative aspects of human sexual life. By this standard there would seem to be no objection to eugenically motivated birth control, if the facts are sufficient to show that genetic defects belong among those grave reasons that may warrant the systematic, even lifelong, prevention of conception. A husband and wife who decide to practice birth control for eugenic reasons are still resolved to hold acts of procreation (even the procreation they have not, or have no more) within the sphere of conjugal love.

This understanding of the moral limits upon methods that may properly be adopted in voluntary genetic control leads, I would argue, to the permissibility of artificial conception control (no less than to the permissibility of the so-called rhythm method) and to the endorsement of voluntary sterilization for eugenic reasons. I know that many of my fellow Christians do not agree with these conclusions. Yet it seems clear that both are open for choice as means (if the ends are important enough)—provided Christian ethics is no longer restricted to the analysis of individual *acts* and is concerned instead with the coincidence of the *spheres* of personal sexual love and of procreation (the spheres to which particular actions belong). Neither the husband (or wife) who practices artificial birth control nor the husband who decides to have a vasectomy is saying by the total course of his life anything other than that *if* either marriage partner has a child, or more children, it will be within their marriage-covenant, from their own one-flesh unity and not apart from it. In principle, they hold together, they do not put completely asunder, what God joined together—the sphere of procreation, even the procreation they have not or have no more, and the sphere in which they exchange acts that nurture their unity of life with one another. They honor the union between love and creation at the heart of God's act toward the world of his creatures, and they honor the image of this union in the union of love with procreativity in their own man-womanhood. Their morality is not oriented upon only the genetic consequences which are believed to justify any voluntary means; nor is it only an ethic of inner intention which is believed to make any sort of conduct right. They *do* something, and are constantly engaged in doing it. This gives their behavior a character that is derived neither wholly from the desired results nor from subjective intention. Through a whole course of life they actually unite their loving and their procreativity (which, incidental to this, they have not). So they do not do wrong. They do no wrong that good may come of it. They do right that good may come of it. (In this moral reasoning, the present writer can see no difference between the case for contraception and the case for voluntary contraceptive sterilization, except in not unimportant differences in the findings of fact that may warrant the one form of birth control or the other—and except for the fact that as yet sterilization is ordinarily irreversible. Even in terms of the more static formulations of the past, it should certainly be said that a vasectomy may be a far less serious invasion of nature than massive assault upon the woman's generative organism by means of contraceptive pills.) . . .

The notation to be made concerning genetic surgery, or the introduction of some anti-mutagent chemical intermediary, which will eliminate a genetic defect before it can be passed on through reproduction, is simple. Should the practice of such medical genetics become feasible at some time in the future, it will raise no moral questions at all—or at least none that are not already present in the practice of medicine generally. Morally, genetic medicine enabling a man and a woman to engender a child without some defective gene they carry would seem to be as permissible as treatment to cure infertility when one of the partners bears this defect. Any significant difference arises from the vastly greater complexity of the practice of genetic surgery and the seriousness of the consequences if, because of insufficient knowledge, an error is made. The cautionary word to be applied here is simply the moral warning against culpable ignorance. The science of genetics (and medical practice based on it) would be obliged both to be fully informed of the facts and to have a reasonable and well-examined expectation of doing more good than harm by eliminating the genetic defect in question. The seriousness of this consideration arises from the serious matter with which genetic surgery will be dealing. Still, the culpability of actions performed in unjustifiable ignorance cannot be invoked as a caution without allowing, at the same time, that in the practice of genetic medicine there doubtless will be errors made in inculpable ignorance. But genetic injuries of this order would be *tragic,* like birth injuries under certain circumstances. They would not entail *wrong*-doing; nor should applications of genetic science be stopped until all such eventualities are impossible. That would be an impossible demand, which no morality imposes.

The paradox is that the most unquestionably moral means of genetic control (direct medical action for the sake of the genotype by some "surgical" or chemical anti-mutagent before the genotype is produced) is technically the most difficult and distant in the future,[12] while a number of the means presently available (phenotypic breeding in or breeding out) are of quite questionable morality, and questionable for reasons that the voluntariness of the practice would not remove. . . .

H. J. Muller, of course, respects man's quality as a thinking animal; he would not violate his freedom, and he challenges men to noble action. This ethics, we have pointed out, is not to be found among the contents of the science of genetics, but is rather the necessary presupposition of man the geneticist and the fruit of intending the world with a scientific mind. Or, perhaps, Muller's humanism is a fruit of intending the world as a man within the community of men. Christian ethics, too, is not found among the contents of any natural science, nor can it be disproven by any of the facts that such sciences know. It is a fruit of intending the world as a Christian. (There is no conflict here between religion and science, but a conflict between two philosophies.) The Christian understands the *humanum* of man to include the body of his soul no less than the soul (mind) of his body. In particular, he holds in honor the union of the realm of personal love with the realm of procreativity in man-womanhood, which is the image of God's creation in the midst of His love. Since artificial insemination by means of semen from a nonhusband donor (AID) puts completely asunder what God joined together, this proposed method of genetic control or genetic improvement must be defined as an exercise of illicit dominion over man no less than the forcing of his free will would be. Not all dominion over man's own physical nature, of course, is wrong, but *this* would be—for the reasons stated above.

In outline, Muller proposes that "germinal choice" be secured by giving eugenic direction to AID (Julian Huxley called this technique "pre-adoption"—it has already become a minority "institution" in our society). Muller also proposes that comparable techniques be developed and employed: "foster pregnancy" (artificial inovulation) and parthenogenesis (or stimulated asexual reproduction). The enormous difficulties in the way of perfecting punctiform genetic surgery or mutational direction by chemical intermediaries impel Muller to concentrate on presently available techniques of parental selection. Similarly, the apparently small gains for the race that can be secured by negative eugenics (because the genes will continue in great numbers as recessives in heterozygotes) impel him to advocate positive or progressive eugenics.[13] In positive genetics, one does not have to identify the genetic defects, or know that they do not add vigor in hybrids. One has only to identify the desired genotype (no small problem in itself!) and breed for it.

Muller rejects the following practices: choosing a donor who is likely to engender a child resembling the "adopting" father, using medical students (notoriously not of the highest intelligence) or barhops, using AID only when the husband is infertile or the carrier of grave genetic defect, and keeping the matter secret. Instead he proposes the selection of donors of the highest proven physical, mental, emotional, and moral traits, and he suggests that publicity be given to the practice so that more and more people may follow our genetic leaders by voluntarily deciding to bestow upon their "children" the very best genetic inheritance instead of their own precious genes.

In order for this practice to be most effective, Muller proposes that a system of deep-frozen semen banks be established and that records of phenotypes be kept and evaluated. At least twenty years should be allowed to elapse before the frozen semen is used, so that a sound judgment can be made upon the donor's capacities. The men who earn enduring esteem can thus be "manifolded" and "called upon to reappear age after age until the population in general has caught up with them."[14] It is an insufficient answer to this proposal to point out that in his 1935 book, *Out of the Night,* Muller stated that no intelligent and morally sensitive woman would refuse to bear a child of Lenin, while in later versions Lenin is omitted and Einstein, Pasteur, Descartes, Leonardo, and Lincoln are nominated.[15] Muller might well reply either by defending Lenin or by saying that not enough time had elapsed for a sound judgment to be made on him.

To his fellow geneticists can be left the task of stating and demonstrating scientific and other socio-psychological objections, some of which follow: (1) the genes of a supposedly superior male may contain injurious recessives which by artificial insemination would become widespread throughout the population instead of remaining in small proportion, as they now do;[16] (2) the validity of this proposal is not demonstrated by the present-day children of geniuses; (3) "it might turn out that parents who looked forward eagerly to having a Horowitz in the family would discover later that it was not so fine as they expected because he might have a temperament incompatible with that of a normal family," and "it is bad enough if we take responsibility only for the environment of our children; if we take responsibility for their genetic make-up, too, the guilt may become unbearable;"[17] (4) we know nothing about the mutation rate that would continue in the frozen germ cells; (5) the IQ's of criminals would be raised,[18] (6) we could not have a "healthy society" because not many men would be "emotionally satisfied by children not their own."[19] Without debating these issues, my verdict upon the eugenic use of semen banks has been negative, in terms of the morality of means which Christian ethics must use as its standard of judgment.[20] . . .

Ends in View

Finally, we need to bring under scrutiny the ends or objectives of genetic control, and the choice to be made between negative eugenics (by breeding-out or by back-mutation) and progressive eugenics (by breeding-in or by the positive direction of mutation).

H. J. Muller had supreme confidence that those pioneering spirits who lead the way in this generation in the employment of germinal selection can be trusted to choose, from a variety of choice-worthy genotypes (described to them by the keepers of the semen banks), the types that will be good for mankind to produce in greater numbers. "Can these critics," he asks, "really believe that the persons of unusual moral courage, progressive spirit, and eagerness to serve mankind, who will pioneer in germinal choice, and likewise those who in a more enlightened age will follow in the path thus laid down, will fail to recognize the fundamental human values?"[21] Muller expresses the guiding aims of particular eugenic decisions in quite general terms: "practically all peoples," he writes, "venerate creativity, wisdom, brotherliness, loving-kindness, perceptivity, expressivity, joy of life, fortitude, vigor, longevity."[22] Or again: "What is meant by superior is whatever is conducive to greater wisdom, cooperativeness, happiness, harmony of nature, or richness of potentialities."[23] This understanding of the goals of eugenic decisions may be open to the objection that, in animal husbandry, one has to have very narrowly defined criteria governing the selection to be made. It is less open to the objection stated by Theodosius Dobzhansky: "Muller's implied assumption that there is, or can be, *the* ideal human genotype which it is desirable to bestow upon everybody is not only unappealing but almost certainly wrong—it is human diversity that acted as a leaven of creative effort in the past and will so act in the future."[24] There is range enough, it would seem, in Muller's description of ideal man to permit a great variety of specific genotypes. The fact is that within these very general value assumptions, Muller counts on individual couples to pick the specific genotype they want to bestow on their "preadoptive" children.[25] "Couples so enlightened as to resort in this and the next generation to germinal choice will not require a corps of axiologists or sociologists to tell them what are the most crying genetic needs of the man of today."[26] Thus, Muller is confident that a host of particular choices, made by people who have concrete options, can be laid, as it were, end to end with similar choices made by people in succeeding generations. The choices of the latter people will doubtless improve as their genetic inheritance improves, thus producing a continuity of choices in the ascending direction of genetic improvement (which was formerly the work of natural selection). This hope is only exceeded by Muller's certainty that, unless man assumes the direction of his genetic goals, the descent of the species is the sole alternative expectation.

Place beside this the objection, raised by Donald M. Mackay, based on the fact that the generation that first initiates genetic control cannot determine the goals that will be set by future generations—or establish any directional continuity. No one can prevent "the 'goal-setting' from drifting and oscillating as time goes on, under the influence of external or even internal factors." Suppose genotype X is chosen in a majority of instances in the first generation. No one can know "what kind of changes these men of type X would think desirable in their successors—and so on, into the future." If we cannot answer this question and establish a continuity from the beginning, then "to initiate such a process might show the reverse of responsibility, on any explication of the term." (Moreover, unless this question is answered and unless future answers to it are assured, then the process would be quite unlike animal husbandry.) "In short, to navigate by a landmark tied to your own ship's head is ultimately impossible."[27]

Now, how does one adjudicate between these opposing views? It is obvious that these judgments fall far outside the science of genetics itself. There may even be operative here a kind of ultimate determination of one man's individual mode of being in the world toward making man the creator and determiner of his own evolution, and, on the part of the other scientist, a personal determination away from that dizzy prospect. The present writer would say that in order to refuse to concede some degree of truth to Muller's opinion, one has to be a rather thoroughgoing relativist who denies to man any fundamental competence to make moral judgments. This is why, in addition to supporting genetically motivated conception control and voluntary sterilization, I have conceded that, if AID is not to be prohibited by law, it might morally be a better wrong to use AID with the intention of bestowing a better genetic inheritance upon a child than if it is used with complete anonymity in regard to the donor's genotypic qualities and only for the sake of securing a child as much like the putative parents as possible. In any case, the voluntariness of the genetic decisions made in any one generation, and through the generations, insures the *usus* of Muller's proposal against such *abusus* as would forbid it *from the point of view of the ends only,* and would seem to render somewhat inconsequential such oscillation in goal-setting as might take place. Such oscillation in genetic decisions would be roughly comparable to oscillations in cultural decisions (taking place under the guidance of Muller's *jus gentium*) that may occur over the sweep of centuries; and the one would be no more and no less consequential than the other, while reciprocating strength to the other.

On the other side of this question, it must be acknowledged that this way of characterizing the goals to be set for positive human betterment does, despite its generality, describe the characteristics of a good geneticist, or the virtues of a good community of scientists, or at least the special values of man in the contemporary period. This is a science-based age, and an age of rapid social change in which men dream of inhabiting other planets after despoiling this one. It is an age in which "progressives" are in the saddle and ride mankind—ahead if not forward. In such an age it is natural enough that most of man's problems are defined in terms of "social lag" of one sort or another, and in terms of the laggard type of characters our genes continue to produce. Still, in the long view, mankind might be in the greatest peril if it succeeded in finding a way to increase its own momentum by selecting on a large scale for the special values of this present culture. In the long view, the race may have need of laggard types and traditional societies, who could take up the history of humanity again after the breakdown of the more momentous civilizations. If positive genetics gained its way, even under the aegis of a quite unexceptionable *jus gentium* setting the goals, would this not unavoidably take the form of genetically instituting some parochial *jus civilis?*

Partly because of the difficulties concerning goal-setting and because the negative goals would seem to be clearer, the present writer leans in the direction of approving preventive eugenics only. I do so also because the means to the ends of preventive genetics—whether these be the voluntary control of conception, or anti-mutagent surgery or chemicals—seem, at our present state of knowledge, to have the good effect of eliminating bad effects without as much danger of also producing an overflow of incalculable, unintended bad consequences. We may say with Hampton L. Carlson, "let us recommend preventive eugenics but proceed very cautiously in progressive eugenics. A firm scientific basis for the latter does not now exist."[28]

It must be admitted that the results on the total population of negative genetics may not be very effective in bringing about large-scale prevention of the deterioration of the gene pool. Nevertheless, faced by such pessimistic predictions, "it is well to remember that every defective individual that can be avoided represents a positive gain."[29] Also, if genetics can identify the *carriers* of genetic defects and thus we no longer need restrict preventive genetics to persons who are identifiably unfit themselves—if a qualitative control of reproduction can wisely be adopted by, and at some time in the future back-mutation can be performed helpfully upon, a larger proportion of the population—then the results of preventive eugenics need not be so limited as it has been in the past. To sterilize *forcibly* all persons suffering from serious genetic defect would have hardly any influence on the proportion of that particular recessive gene in the population. But if carriers can be identified, and if each heterozygous carrier has only half as many children as he would otherwise have, we would reduce the abnormal-gene frequency by fifty percent. This alone would greatly reduce the incidence of the defect in the next generation, and prevent untold future human misery.[30]

To make preventive eugenics more effective will require the development and widespread adoption of an "ethics of genetic duty." It is shocking to learn from the heredity clinics that have been established in recent years in more than a dozen cities in the United States, how many parents will accept grave risk of having defective children rather than remain childless. "When a husband and wife each carry a recessive deleterious gene similar to the one carried by the other, the chances of their having a defective child are one in four, with two children carriers of a single gene, but themselves without defect, and [only] the fourth child being neither a carrier nor defective. Couples in such a position, knowing that they have one chance in four of having a seriously defective child, and that two out of four of their children are likely to be carriers, still frequently take a chance that things will turn out all right."[31] This can only be called genetic imprudence, with the further notation that imprudence is gravely immoral.

In making genetic decisions to be effected by morally acceptable means, the benefits expected from a given course of action must be weighed against any risk (or loss of good) incurred. This is exactly the mode of moral reasoning used in deciding whether or not to use X rays in medical diagnosis, or radiation therapy in medical treatments. Should patients with cancerous growths, for whom (because of age and/or condition of health) the expectation of parenthood is quite small, be subjected to massive radiation therapy? The answer here is obviously affirmative. But how does one compare the detection of a case of tuberculosis by X-ray survey with the genetic harm that will befall someone in generations to come? How compelling should the indication be before an unborn child is subjected to damage by a fluoroscopic examination of its mother?[32] Moral reasoning that applies the principle of prudence, or the principle of proportion between effects both of which arise from a single action, is notoriously inexact. Still, it is certain that it is *immoral* to be imprudent, and it is a dereliction of duty not to make this sort of appraisal as best one can, and to act upon the best knowledge one can secure.

It is hardly utopian to hope that with the dissemination of genetic knowledge there will arise increased concern about this problem, and among an increasing number of people a far greater moral sensitivity to their responsibilities to the future generations of mankind. Such an "ethics of genetic duty" was well stated by H. J. Muller: "Although it is a human right for people to have their infirmities cared for by every means that society can muster, they do not have the right knowingly to pass on to posterity such a load of infirmities of genetic or partly genetic origin as to cause an increase in the burden already being carried by the population."[33]

There is ample and well-established ground in Christian ethics for enlarging upon the theme of man's genetic responsibility. Having children was never regarded as a selfish prerogative. Instead, Christian teachings have always held that procreation is an act by which men and women are to perform their duty to future generations of men. If a given couple cannot be the progenitors of healthy individuals—at least not unduly defective individuals—or, if they are the carriers of serious defect, then such a couple's "right to have children" becomes their duty not to do so, or to have fewer children. The science of genetics may be able to inform them with certain knowledge of the fact-situation. That would be sufficient to place eugenic reasons among those serious causes justifying the systematic practice of lifelong *un*parenthood, or of less parentage.

What is lacking is not the moral argument but a moral movement. The Christian churches have in the past been able to promote celibacy to the glory of God—men and women who for the supreme end of human existence "deny themselves" (if that is the term for it) both of the goods of marriage. These same Christian churches should be able to promote voluntary or "vocational" childlessness, or policies of restricted reproduction, for the sake of the children of generations to come. In place of Muller's "foster pregnancy," the churches could set before such couples alternatives that might be termed "foster parentage"—all the many ways in which human parental instincts may be fulfilled in couples who for mercy's sake have no children of their own. These persons would be called upon to "deny themselves" (if that is the term for it) one of the goods of marriage for the sake of that end itself. And they would honor the Creator of all human love and procreation, in that they would hold in incorruptible union the love that they have and the procreation they never have, or have no more.

Notes

1. H. J. Muller, "The Guidance of Human Evolution," in *Perspectives in Biology and Medicine* (Chicago: University of Chicago Press, 1959) 3 (Autumn 1959): 11.

2. H. J. Muller, "Our Load of Mutations," in *The American Journal of Human Genetics* 2 (June 1950): 146, 171.

3. Ibid., p. 146. Cf. also Muller, "Should We Strengthen or Weaken our Genetic Heritage?" in Hudson Hoagland and Ralph W. Burhoe, eds., *Evolution and Man's Progress* (New York: Columbia University Press, 1962), p. 27. It does not seem a sufficient answer to all this to reply: "Norway rats . . . have been kept in laboratories since some time before 1840 and 1850. . . . But it does not follow that laboratory rats are decadent and unfit; nor does it follow that the 'welfare state' is making man decadent and unfit—to live in a welfare state!" (Theodosius Dobzhansky, *Mankind Evolving* [New Haven: Yale University Press, 1962], p. 326).

4. Muller, "Better Genes for Tomorrow," in Stuart Mudd, ed., *The Population Crisis and the Use of World Resources* (The Hague: Dr. W. Junk Publishers, 1964), p. 315.

5. Hannah Arendt, quoted in a *Worldview* editorial, Sept. 1958, p. 1.

6. In an article entitled "Sex and People: A Critical Review" (*Religion and Life* 30 [Winter 1960-61]: 53-70), I sought to apply the edification found in Christian eschatology in refutation of certain genial viewpoints sometimes propounded by Christians on the basis of a doctrine of creation. These Christians hold that religious people *must* believe that God intends an abundant *earthly* life for every baby born, and that we would deny His providence if we doubt that world population control, combined with economic growthmanship, can finally succeed in fulfilling God's direction of human life to this end. Such a belief is secular progressivism with religious overtones. Taken seriously enough, it can lead, as easily as any other utopianism can, to the adoption of any means to that end, the control of the world's population. In essence, an independent morality of means, or righteousness

in conduct, is collapsed into utilitarianism when the *eschaton* or man's supernatural end is replaced by any future *telos.*

7. The language of this paragraph reflects that of H. Richard Niebuhr, *The Responsible Self* (New York: Harper and Row, 1963).

8. "A Free Man's Worship." There is less posturing in Muller's despair, more in the optimism that floats over this despair, than in Russell.

9. "Ethics in International Relations Today," an address delivered at Amherst College, Dec. 9, 1964; quoted from *The New York Times,* Dec. 10, 1964.

10. "A Christian Approach to the Question of Sexual Relations Outside Marriage," in *The Journal of Religion* 45 (Apr. 1965): 100–18.

11. Gerald Kelley and John C. Ford, "Periodic Continence," in *Theological Studies* 23 (Dec. 1962): 590–624.

12. H. J. Muller, who favors phenotypic selection, describes the enormous difficulties in the way of perfecting methods of genotypic change in "Means and Aims in Human Genetic Betterment," in *The Control of Human Heredity and Evolution* (New York: The Macmillan Co., 1965). In the advancement of science toward direction or change of the germ cells themselves, Muller believes "there may be in time a race between genetic surgery and robotics, and we may find that 'this old house will do no longer' " (p. 109). I take him to mean that a new type of man may be as easily made as present man can be remade by direct action on his genes. Neither, for Muller, is "utterly visionary." Since both robotics and the direction of mutation are visionary, however, Muller wants to proceed with parental selection by all the voluntary means presently available.

13. "As in most defensive operations, it is dreary, frustrating business to have to run as fast as one can merely to stay in the same place. Nature did better for us. Why can we not do better for ourselves?" ("Guidance," p. 17). Thus, only progressive eugenics would be the equivalent of natural selection, which was phenotypic and preserved the genes of the strongest types.

14. "Guidance," p. 35.

15. Dobzhansky, p. 328; and Klein's comment in the discussion in *Man and His Future,* a Ciba Foundation Volume (London: J. and A. Churchill, 1963), p. 280.

16. J. Paul Scott in the discussion in *Evolution and Man's Progress,* p. 48.

17. R. S. Morison in ibid., p. 64.

18. Donald M. MacKay in the discussion in *Man and His Future,* p. 298.

19. John F. Brock in ibid., p. 287. Or that, in view of the incredible diversity of opinions expressed by the scientists, it is impossible to know what we should try to educate people to do in making genetic choices (Medawar in *Man and His Future,* p. 382).

20. There is an exceedingly profound and open-minded discussion of artificial insemination, from the point of view of a Lutheran ethics, in Helmut Thielicke's *The Ethics of Sex,* trans. John W. Doberstein (New York: Harper and Row, 1964), pp. 248–68.

21. "Better Genes for Tomorrow," p. 336.

22. "Genetic Progress by Voluntarily Conducted Germinal Choice," in *Man and His Future,* p. 260.

23. *The World View of Moderns,* University of Illinois 50th Anniversary Lecture Series (Urbana, Ill.: University of Illinois Press, 1958), p. 26. Without some consensus on the ultimate question of values, he points out elsewhere, all man's cultural activities, no less than his germinal choices, would be at cross-purposes ("Guidance," p. 19).

24. Bruce Wallace and Theodosius Dobzhansky, *Radiation, Genes, and Man* (New York: Henry Holt, 1959), p. 330.

25. "Couples desiring to have in their own families one or more children who are especially likely to embody their own ideals of worth will be afforded a wide range of choice. They will be assisted by records of the lives and characteristics of the donors and of their relatives, and by counsel from diverse specialists, but the final choice will be their own and their participation will be entirely voluntary" ("Means and Aims," p. 122).

26. Ibid., p. 118.

27. Donald M. MacKay in the discussion in *Man and His Future,* p. 286.

28. Hampton L. Carson, *Heredity and Human Life* (New York: Columbia University Press, 1963), p. 189.

29. Ibid., p. 188.

30. See James F. Crow, "Mechanisms and Trends in Human Evolution," in *Evolution and Man's Progress,* p. 18.

31. Frederick Osborn, "The Protection and Improvement of Man's Genetic Inheritance," in *The Population Crisis and the Use of World Resources,* pp. 308–09.

32. See Wallace and Dobzhansky, *Radiation,* pp. 184–85. Since these authors had just cogently stated (perhaps without knowing it) the "rule of double effect," I frankly do not understand their meaning in the following paragraph: "The importance one places on genetic damage depends, really, on the value one places on human life. If the importance of human life is absolute, if human life is infinitely precious, then the exact number of additional victims of genetic damage is not crucial. One death is as inadmissible as 100, 1,000, or 1,000,000. Infinity multiplied by any finite number is still infinity. Whoever claims that the number of genetic deaths is an important consideration in this problem claims that human life is of limited value" (p. 188). To the contrary, it is precisely because each human life has such value that it becomes important to take the numbers into account as one element in the proportion in situations where *not all can be saved.* Prudence is a matter of estimating the cost-benefit where infinite values (the lives of persons) are in conflict, where, e.g., persons in the present generation must be saved at the expense of persons in a future generation, or vice versa; and there is *no other alternative.*

33. H. J. Muller, *Man's Future Birthright* (University of New Hampshire, Feb., 1958), p. 18. See also Muller's "Guidance," p. 8.

61. Moral Theology and Genetics

CHARLES E. CURRAN

Through technology and science man has been able to improve his lot in this world. In the last decade science has acquired an almost undreamed of knowledge about genetics and man's genetic development. There is the definite possibility that in the future, and to some extent even now, man can eliminate deleterious genes from the human gene pool and add desirable genes which will improve human individuals and the human species. We are thus faced with ethical problems concerned with man's interference in his own evolutionary development to better the individual and the human species. In addition, man may very well have to interfere in his evolutionary future to prevent a gradual and perhaps even apocalyptic deterioration of the future of the human race. This is because conditions in modern civilization (e.g., exposure to radiation) bring about deleterious changes in man's genetic makeup, while advances in medical science now make it possible for many genetically deficient people—who in earlier times would not have survived—to live and reproduce; as a result, there are more and more deleterious genes present in the human gene pool.

From the outset, one must realize that the relationship between the scientist and the ethician is not one of opposition or exclusion. The scientist in his own field and in his daily life is constantly making ethical decisions. Many conscientious scientists, perhaps influenced by the horrible use of nuclear power, believe they have a duty to make all of us cognizant of the possibilities that lie ahead in the area of human genetics. Man should be prepared for such possible developments so that all the people in our society can have a part in determining how man will handle the genetic powers that he has now and might have in the future. The ethician or moral theologian, on the other hand, does not claim to be a more moral person than any other in society. He tries to study the way in which men make their decisions and to point out those choices he believes to be right, good, or fitting. (It is difficult to choose a particular word, for different ethical systems would look at it differently.) The Christian ethician looks at a particular problem in the light of the Christian understanding of man, his life, and his world. Everyone, of course, is required constantly to make ethical judgments; the professional ethician tries to criticize and analyze human decisions. In any case, although the ethicist and the scientists have different roles, their functions should be complementary and not antagonistic.

To discuss the problems raised by the possible genetic patterning of man, one must know the facts—the possibilities and the needs. First, the actual situation. Is the genetic future of the human species in danger because of a deleterious gene load in its own population? Scientific opinion is divided on this point. Hermann J. Muller, the late Nobel Prize winner, was quite pessimistic: "It is evident that under modern conditions, so long as the dying out is seriously interfered with, human populations must become ever more defective in their genetic constitution, until at long last even the most sophisticated techniques available could no longer suffice to save men from their biological corruptions."[1]

Muller's appears to be a minority opinion. Theodosius Dobzhansky is more optimistic about the human future, though he does admit the problem created by deleterious gene mutations coupled with the fact that modern medicine allows genetically deficient people to live and reproduce. The majority opinion is that more positive factors will outbalance those negative considerations. "Man is a product of his cultural development as well as of his biological nature. The preponderance of cultural over biological evolution will continue or increase in the forseeable future."[2] The theologian is not capable of deciding which viewpoint is correct.[3]

Even if there is no need to interfere in human evolution to divert a genetic apocalypse, the ethical problems raised by the fact that man can better the human species still remain. Let me briefly summarize the ways in which modern science is now, or will in the future, be able to control and direct human evolution through genetics. Although various authors employ diverse terminology, we will speak of three generic types of approach: eugenics, genetic engineering, and euphenics.

Eugenics is simply described as good breeding. More technically, it is described as the selection and recombination of genes already existing in the human gene pool. Negative eugenics aims at removing the deleterious genes; positive or progressive eugenics tries to improve the existing genes.

The biologists quite generally admit that negative eugenics will have little or no effect in reducing the load of genetic defects in the human species. Recessive genetic defects are generally carried in heterozy-

From *Crosscurrents* 20 (Winter 1970): 64–82.

gotes and thus escape detection. Even if one could detect such recessive genetic defects in heterozygotes, the very fact that most people have some such recessive genetic defects would make it practically impossible to eliminate them from the human population. Negative eugenics is a matter of real concern on a more personal basis in considering problems of the immediate family. Through genetic counselling, a couple may be provided with information which at times should convince them not to marry, or at least not to have children. If a couple knows that the chances are one out of four that their child will be mentally retarded and two out of four that the child will be a carrier of such retardation, there seems to be a strong moral argument not to have children. In addition to voluntary decisions, there could also be laws forbidding such people to marry or laws requiring the sterilization of some genetically defective people. The compulsory aspect and the interference by the government in the reproductive lives of human beings, however, raise moral questions about such solutions.

Positive eugenics embraces a much more ambitious program for the betterment of the human species. Hermann J. Muller and Julian Huxley think that in the future there may be other means available, but man must now use those means for improving and saving the human species that are already available. Muller proposes that sperm banks be established to store the frozen sperm of men of outstanding characteristics. A panel would decide, preferably after a waiting period of twenty years, which sperm should be used. Women would then be artificially inseminated with this sperm, and the whole genetic future of man would improve. Muller even looks forward to a veritable utopia of never-ending progress in the development of the human species, but in his later writing talks more of the small number who would voluntarily accept such practice in the beginning. This small group would then serve as an experiment for future development.[4]

A more radical approach, which is not yet possible in men, has been suggested by Joshua Lederberg and others. Lederberg speaks of clonal reproduction, which like Muller's suggestion would begin with the genetic types now known to be strong and make sure these types would be reproduced in great numbers in the future. Clonal reproduction would replicate in an a-sexual way already existing genotypes. Science can now remove the nucleus from a fertilized frog's egg and replace it with a nucleus from one of the cells of a developing embryo (part of the problem is that the genes must not be already differentiated, as is the case in most cells). The fertilized egg thus develops into a frog which is the genetic twin of the frog from which the nucleus of the cell was taken. Cloning would thus be an even surer way than artificial insemination of insuring that genetically gifted people continue to exist and multiply in the future.[5]

A second generic type of approach has been called genetic engineering, genetic surgery, algeny, or transformationist eugenics as distinguished from selectionist eugenics.

The aim of genetic engineering is to change the genes in such a way as to eliminate a certain deleterious type (negative) or to improve the genotype (positive). Genetic engineering aims at changing a particular molecule in the complex structure of the gene. At the present time, science does not have the finesse necessary to change a very specific molecule in the complex structure without affecting other molecules. In the future, however, man may be able to direct genetic mutations. Genetic engineering also embraces the phenomena of transformation and transduction. In transformation scientists are now able to take a strain of bacteria not containing a certain genetic property and introduce this property with the DNA extracted from another strain. Transduction tries to transfer such properties through a virus. Such experiments have already been successful with bacteria. However, there are tremendous problems of specificity, directivity, and efficiency which must be overcome before genetic engineering could be a possibility on human beings. Also, the fact that human traits have a polygenic base greatly complicates the problem. The individual diversity of every human being tends to make some scientists quite pessimistic about the future possibilities of genetic engineering. Others, however, think it remains a real possibility, though still many years away.

A third generic type of improving human species has been called euphenics. Euphenics is somewhere between eugenics and euthenics or environmental engineering. In the past, and probably even more so in the future, human development occurs primarily because of man's intervention in and control over his environment. Lederberg has proposed euphenics as that part of euthenics concerned with human environment. Euphenics aims at the control and regulation of the phenotype rather than the genotype. This would involve all efforts at controlling gene expression in man without changing the genotype, and thus would not involve hereditary changes. Eyeglasses to correct poor vision is one example; insulin for diabetes sufferers is another. Lederberg believes there are a number of areas in which medical science should proceed: accelerated engineering in the development of artificial organs; development of industrial methodology for synthesis of specific proteins; eugenic experiments with animals to produce genetically homogeneous materials for spare parts in man. Lederberg was arguing in 1962 that priority should now be given to euphenics and then later to long-range eugenic concerns of the human genotype.[6] Also, there is the future possibility that science will know how to switch on and off different genes at specific periods of development and greatly change the individual.

In general, these are the various ways in which it might be scientifically possible for man to interfere in and direct his own human development. At the present time, however, the only available positive means that might be efficacious is the positive eugenics proposed by Muller, and many scientists would agree with Paul Ramsey that this means raises more moral problems than the forms of genetic engineering possible in the future.[7] Indeed, the majority of scientists writing on the subject are unwilling at the present time to accept the proposals of Muller on both scientific and moral grounds. They are raising these questions for discussion today so that man will not suddenly be confronted with these problems in the future without having thought of any way to cope with them.[8] In this paper we are primarily concerned with the various elements in the discussion that not only involve problems about the ethical use of this scientific power, but also raise methodological questions for moral theology itself.

At first it might seem strange that possible advances in man's control over his heredity should raise questions for moral theology. History, however, reminds us of the dangers of a totally a priori theological approach to newer developments in science. Theology is not totally settled once and for all, but is itself in a continual process of growth and change. As the study of Christian man and his actions, moral theology is constantly in dialogue with the empirical and social sciences in order better to understand its own subject.

There would appear to be three emphases that must be present in any theological approach to the problems raised by man's possible power over his own future development. The first is a greater appreciation of historicity and historical consciousness. Catholic theology, in many ways following the lead of Protestant theology, first adopted an historical perspective through the renewal of the study of Scripture. As the Word of God in the words of men, the books of the Bible are historically and culturally limited documents. Theology has also learned from the mistakes of nineteenth and twentieth century liberal Protestantism in assuming a simple identity between the historical experience of the contemporary interpreter and the first century biblical witness.[9]

The notion of historicity or historical development has been employed by some theologians to show that the teachings of Gregory XVI and Pius IX in the area of religious liberty were not contradicted by the later teachings of Vatican II. In the light of the historical contexts of the times, both teachings could be correct in their own circumstances.[10] John Courtney Murray saw the primary reason for the different approaches to religious liberty in the different understanding of the role and function of the state in the nineteenth and twentieth centuries. Perhaps those theologians who have been defending the teaching of the nineteenth century Popes on religious liberty have been somewhat too facile in explaining differences in terms of historicity.[11] But at least Catholic theology has come to see the need for an historical understanding in its approach.

The growth and progress of modern civilization in all areas, not just science and technology, have made contemporary theology more aware of historical growth and change. Changes in politics, science, economics and sociology cannot remain unreflected in approaches to moral theology. Philosophy today illustrates the greater emphasis on historicity in many of its contemporary trends such as process philosophy. According to Rahner, theology's possibility of error is ultimately rooted in its historical character.[12] The very fact that contemporary advances in the science of genetics present dangers for moral theology is another indication of the historicity of theology itself.

A more historically conscious theology will tend to have a different concept of man—one that is more open than closed. Man is not totally determined by a fixed nature existing within him. The genius of modern man is his ability for self-creation and self-direction. Man is constantly open to a tremendous variety of actions and options. Any theological position based on a closed concept of human nature, something already within man to which he must conform himself and his actions, will be an inaccurate understanding of the human reality and tend to result in unacceptable moral conclusions. Thus the predominate concept can no longer be an immutable and unchangeable nature, but rather the concept of historicity. Notice that historicity provides both for continuity and discontinuity, thus avoiding the extreme of an immobile classicism or the complete discontinuity of sheer existentialism.

In the area of questions raised by the possible drastic developments in genetics, the theologian must be ever mindful of the need for an historical approach; but he must also avoid the danger of uncritically accepting every new scientific possibility as something necessarily human and good.

The progressive eugenics proposed by Muller would call for the separation of procreation and the love-union aspect of sexuality. Christian ethics has generally maintained that these two aspects are joined by the design of the Creator, and man cannot separate what God has joined together. However, there is a methodological problem in proving this simply by citing the first chapters of Genesis in which the unitive and procreative nature of human sexuality is taught. Obviously, the teaching of Genesis is itself historically conditioned. Can the theologian merely extrapolate from the circumstances of Genesis and make an absolute and universal norm for the understanding of human sexuality?

Ramsey argues against Muller's plan just because it breaks the bond between the procreative and unitive aspects of sexuality. Ramsey does not base his case primarily on Genesis, or creation, or nature. Ramsey argues primarily from the "Second Article of the Creed," which specifies the Christian concept of creation and conjugal love in the Prologue of John's gospel and the fifth chapter of Ephesians.[13] Just as the creative and redeeming act of God is a life-giving act of love, so human sexuality is both procreative and loving. Nevertheless, the teaching that Ramsey finds in Ephesians might itself be historically conditioned.

I believe that in our circumstances at the present time sexuality has its proper expression, value and meaning in the marital realm, within which the procreative and love union aspects of sexuality are joined together. However, one can envision a possibility in which greater values might be at stake and call for some alteration of the way in which Christian marriage now tries to preserve these important values. For example, if the dire predictions of Muller were universally accepted and mankind faced a genetic apocalypse in the near future, the entire situation might be changed. Even the Scriptures provide cases in which the understanding of marriage had to be changed because of the conditions of the times (e.g., polygamy). Ramsey himself admits some possible relativity in his teaching by saying that there might be some redeeming features in Muller's proposals, but this is not "sufficient to place the practice in the class of morally permitted actions."[14] I agree with Ramsey's understanding of things as they are at present, but this argumentation and his projection for the future do not seem to give enough place to historicity.

A second danger in the approach of moral theology to genetics is that of an individualistic methodology, a logical result of the failure to emphasize the communitarian and societal dimensions of reality. Christian thinking deserves much credit for upholding the dignity of the individual, in many ways the foundation of our modern society, although at times Christian practice has not always lived up to theory. Today, however, man is much more conscious of his communitarian nature and his relationships with all other people and the world. The approach of moral theology will have to balance more adroitly the proper claims of the individual and of society. The Christian notions of *agape, koinonia,* and the reign of God all seem to be more open to communitarian and social understandings. Problems facing contemporary men in politics, sociology and economics all show a greater role being given to the communitarian, the social and the cosmic. Moral theology cannot employ models that are exclusively individualistic or narrowly interpersonal.[15]

In the past, moral theology has been somewhat ambivalent about the tension between the individual and the community. In many areas the approach has been too individualistic, but there were other instances in which too much stress was placed on the power of the community over the rights of the individual. For example, theologians affirmed the obligation of the defendant to admit his guilt publicly, which would deny the right of the individual not to incriminate himself.[16] The long-standing failure to accept religious liberty fully is another indication of an unwillingness to accept the total freedom and dignity of the individual. The area of social ethics furnishes examples where Catholic theology was too individualistic in its approach. Such an emphasis can be partly explained in the light of reaction to communism and socialism. More recently, some Catholics have become upset at the papal call for "socialization," which they look upon as an invasion of the rights of the individual. Pope John's encyclicals emphasized the social dimension of man, while still preserving the legitimate claims of the individual, by basing his social ethics on the two principles of subsidiarity and socialization.[17] The danger of individualism can also be seen in the overemphasis on private property in some Catholic teaching. Leo XIII acknowledged the social aspect of property, but it was not emphasized. Contemporary Catholic theology, along with Pope Paul's *Progressio Populorum,*[18] stresses the social aspect of property because the goods of creation exist primarily for all mankind.

Too individualistic a concept of man has also affected Catholic understandings of medical morality, especially as this was influenced by the principle of totality, developed by Pius XII in many of his discourses on medical matters. According to the principle of totality, the individual may dispose of the members or functions of his body for the good of the whole, but a part may be sacrificed "only when there is the subordination of part to whole that exists in the natural body."[19] Pius XII wrote in the context of totalitarian governments, and was very careful to deny that by virtue of the principle of totality the government had power over the life of the individual, for the individual is not merely a part of the totality which is the state. At times, Pius XII limited the application of totality to physical organisms with their physical unity or totality.[20] Thus the principle of totality cannot be used to justify the transplantation of organs or experimentation for the good of others, since in this case the strict relationship of part to physical whole does not exist. Some Catholic theologians went further and denied that organic transplantation or experimentation for the good of others was morally permitted.[21] Others, however, justified such practices, either by introducing other principles (e.g., charity) or by attempting to expand the principle of totality itself.[22] Thus the principle of totality, at least in its narrower understanding and application, apart from other considerations, can overly emphasize the individual at the expense of other aspects of reality.

Perhaps the area of greatest disagreement in the past between the medical ethics proposed by Catholics and other ethical theories concerns the generative organs. In accord with the understanding of the generative organs and functions of man as existing for the good of the species, as well as for the good of the individual, the principle of totality would not justify the direct suppression of the generative organs or functions for the good of the individual. This results in the condemnation, among other things, of direct sterilization. However, if the totality of the person is somewhat enlarged to consider "his relationship to his family, community and the larger society," one would at times find a justification for direct sterilization.[23] Or one could justify direct sterilization by talking about the marital union and relationship itself as a whole or a totality. Again, notice the dangers of applying too individualistically the principle of totality without taking into account other important aspects.

The present historical situation calls for a greater understanding of man as existing in community with other persons intertwined with many different relationships. The task for moral theology is to develop a methodology which does justice to the communitarian, social and cosmic needs of the present without falling into a collectivism. The ever-growing consciousness of the one world in which we all share has tended to underline the need for such a communitarian approach. The economic problems of England and the United States affect the whole world; the political decisions in Moscow and Washington have immediate repercussions everywhere. Scientific advances in controlling our environment are affecting more and more people in all parts of the globe.

Precisely in the area of genetics and heredity the individual realizes the existence of other responsibilities which limit his own options and freedom. Traditional Catholic theology also recognized some limitations in this area. The older manuals of theology spoke of the primary end of marriage, which included the procreation and education of offspring. Responsible parenthood is a moral imperative for couples, and responsible parenthood entails some responsibility for the children who will be born and to the race itself. As we have seen, genetic reasons at times should compel a couple not to bring children into the world, but what if the community should positively intervene to prevent and prohibit marriages in which there is a serious possibility that children born of them would be retarded? In the past, Catholic theology has been willing to accept somewhat similar practices. The impediments to marriage in the Code of Canon Law include consanguinity, which may have been based on some eugenic reasoning. Another question arises in regard to compulsory sterilization of certain classes of people. I do not believe that such interference with the individual person is called for today, especially without a first attempt to employ genetic counselling on a wide scale. Most scientists are also somewhat unwilling to propose such compulsory measures; they are aware of the abuses of power to which such practices would be susceptible.

The very complexity of the overall problem will in the long run call for some community control. In other areas of human life the more power that an individual has and the more complex things become, the greater is the need for community intervention and control. Such things as the right of people to fly their own airplanes, or to hunt and fish, to say nothing of questions of economics, politics and education, have required some type of community control. The very power which science and genetics can bring into existence must be under some greater control than the individual can provide. In the not-too-distant future, there may well be need for some type of community control in the area of genetics and heredity. What if man acquires the power to determine the sex of his children? Tremendous problems could very easily result for society if the proportion between the sexes was greatly affected. What could be done? Society could forbid its members to use such means of determining the sex of their children, or it could set up an elaborate control system. Obviously, there will be many problems no matter which choice is made, but the point is that society may very well have to make such a choice. Nor can one avoid the problem by merely condemning the research that might lead to such power. I am not euphoric at the prospect of such power, but it is man's creative challenge to use it for his betterment despite all the inherent human limitations. My contention is that the complexity and interrelatedness of human existence, plus the tremendous power that science may put into the hands of men, are going to call for a more communitarian and social approach to the moral decisions facing our society.

A third required emphasis in the approach of moral theology to questions raised by man's control over his own hereditary future concerns the power which man has over his own life. Christian thought has constantly emphasized that man does not have complete dominion over his own life; he is the steward of the gift of life he has received from the Creator; his final destiny lies outside and beyond this world. On the other hand, a man is the glory of creation and the greatest sign of God's handiwork in this world.

Today more than ever in the past man is conscious of the power that he has over his own life and his own future. Catholic theologians do not hesitate to say that man today is his own self-creator, for in a sense man is unfinished and capable now of creating himself. The power of self-creation has always been rooted in the spiritual power of man himself—a truth recognized by Thomas Aquinas. Thomas does not hesitate to see man as an image of God precisely because he is "endowed with intelligence, free will, and a power of his actions which is proper to him . . . having dominion over his own activities."[24] Thanks to the marvels of science, man is now able to extend this dominion into many other facets of his own existence.

The Christian attitude toward man tries to balance or even hold in dialectical tension these two aspects of man—his greatness precisely because he is free and the guide of his own development, and also his creatureliness and sinfulness. Corresponding to these two aspects of human existence are what the older theological tradition called the two capital sins of sloth and pride. Harvey Cox has pointed out that too frequently we forget that the great sin of man is sloth or the failure to take responsibility for the world which is his to make.[25] Although it is true that sloth has been an often neglected aspect of Christian life, we should not forget the terrible evils connected with pride through which men have used all kinds of power—social, economic, political, military, and even religious—to pursue their own particular ends and gain advantage over others.[26] Just as Cox has at times overemphasized sloth, Paul Ramsey, especially in his writing on genetics, seems to overemphasize *hubris* or pride. "In fact it may be said that the ethical violations we have noted on the *horizontal* plane (coercive breeding or non-breeding, injustice done to individuals or to mishaps, the violation of the nature of human parenthood) are a function of a more fundamental happening in the *vertical* dimension, namely *hubris,* and playing God."[27] Certainly Ramsey is correct in seeing that some genetic proposals fail to take account of the limitations and sinfulness of man; but one cannot deny that since man does have a greater dominion over his life and future today, there is also the danger of man's not using responsibly the dominion or power he either has now or may possess in the future.

Although I agree with most of Ramsey's conclusions on the questions of genetics at the present time, I believe he does not give enough importance to the aspects of historicity and the greater dominion that man has today. Both of these differences stem from a basic theological stance in terms of which I would attribute greater importance to man's own efforts in cooperating with the building of the new heaven and the new earth. This difference raises the fundamental question of ethics and eschatology. Ramsey views eschatology primarily, and sometimes exclusively, in terms of apocalypse: "Religious people have never denied, indeed they affirm, that God means to kill us all in the end, and in the end He is going to succeed. Anyone who intends the world as a Jew or as a Christian—to the measure in which this is his mode of being in the world—goes forth to meet the collision of planets or the running down of suns, and he exists toward a future that may contain a genetic Apocalypse with his eyes fixed on another *eschaton*. . . . "[28]

Ramsey rightly emphasizes the aspect of apocalypse or discontinuity between this world and the next, as against the naive progressivists who see the future age in perfect continuity with the present. However, Christian eschatology includes three aspects, all of which have to be retained if one is going to have a proper understanding of the relationship between this world and the next: the teleological, the apocalyptic, and the prophetic.[29] By stressing just the apocalyptic, Ramsey fails to give due, even if limited, importance to man's efforts in cooperating with God in bringing about the new heaven and the new earth. Ramsey emphasizes exclusively the apocalyptic aspect of eschatology because of his polemic with those who see man as bringing about the blessed future through his own efforts and technology, but this leads him to see Christian ethics on the model of deontological ethics rather than of teleology or responsibility.[30]

Man does have more dominion over his life today than he had in the past—a fact that has already had a great impact on Catholic moral theology. The dissatisfaction with some explanations of natural law theory, especially as illustrated by arguments against artificial contraception, stems from the fact that man now has the power and ability to interfere with the physical and biological laws of nature. Scientific and technological progress have given man a greater power over both his life and death so that today Catholic theologians even acknowledge "the right to die."[31] Obviously this raises questions about those arguments against euthanasia that are based on the lack of dominion man has over his own life and death. All these indications point out the need for theologians to be very precise and cautious in applying the notion of man's limited dominion over his life to the theological questions raised by advances in genetics.

This paper will now criticize from a viewpoint of Catholic moral theology some of the attitudes seen in various scientific approaches. Especially in the proposals of Muller, there is a utopian outlook on the future, although in his later writings his proposals were scaled down somewhat to an experimental nucleus. His overall goal, however, remained the same: "By these means the way can be opened up for unlimited progress in the genetic constitution of man to match and reinforce his cultural progress, and reciprocally to be reinforced by it, in a perhaps never-ending succession."[32] Muller advocates the use of sperm banks and artificial insemination of women with this superior semen because there are no other means available at present. He does not think other techniques of genetic surgery will be available until the twenty-first century, if then; but such genetic surgery may very well "do much better than nature has done."[33]

Muller does recognize an element of the tragic in man, but he believes many of the problems could be overcome by progressive eugenics. "Thus, men grievously need the Golden Rule, but the Golden Rule grievously needs men in whose very nature it is more deeply rooted than in ours. These men would not require the wills of saints, for their way of life would be normal to them. They would take it for granted, and could live full wholesome lives, joyously carrying out the ever greater enterprises made possible for their strengthened individual initiative, working hand in hand in free alliance with their enhanced cooperative functionings. At the same time their personal relationships would be warmer and more genuine, so that they could enjoy more of the love that gives itself away. Along with this, less forcing would be required of them in extending their feelings of kinship to those remote from their contacts."[34]

The Christian vision of man and his world cannot accept any utopian schemes. Modern life and science give man much greater dominion than he had before, but he remains a creature and a sinner. The final stage of the reign of God is in the future and not totally continuous with man's present existence. Although, in the past, many Christians may have been guilty of what has been called "eschatological irresponsibility," since they forgot about the possibility of bringing about a relative justice here and now, contemporary Christians can never forget the transcendent aspect of the reign of God which is his gracious gift to us. Science and technology can do much to help man, but they cannot overcome the creatureliness and sinfulness which mark man in the Christian perspective.

Christian theology has also learned from its own history the dangers of utopian thinking and the temptations of a naively optimistic outlook on human growth and progress. Not so long ago some Roman Catholics naively looked to the past and saw a romantic utopia in "the thirteenth, greatest of centuries." Liberal Protestantism less than a century ago made the mistake of thinking that man could bring about the kingdom of God in this world by his own work and effort. Christian theologians are chastened by the well-known statement (in my judgment too negative and critical) of H. Richard Niebuhr: "In this one-sided view of progress, which saw the growth of the wheat, but not that of the tares, the gathering of the grain, but not the burning of the chaff, this liberalism was indeed naively optimistic. A God without wrath brought men without sin into a kingdom without judgment through the ministrations of a Christ without a cross."[35]

The ambitious genetic proposals of Muller (sperm banks) and Lederberg (cloning) would call for large-scale changes in our contemporary society if they were to be successful even from a biological viewpoint. Lederberg points out that a system of tempered clonality would be necessary to provide for the variety and adaptability necessary if the human gene pool is to progress. Thus some people would reproduce clonally and some sexually.[36] Among the many problems that would arise for both Muller and Lederberg would be the selection of the ideal types. Who is to decide? What criteria are to be employed? How do we know if a person will do as well in a different type of environment? Why is it that many children of geniuses have not made contributions themselves? Even Muller agrees that men would have a difficult time selecting the ideal person and what characteristics he should have. Commentators occasionally note that Muller himself changed his opinion about who would be ideal types. In 1935 he claimed no woman would refuse to have a child by Lenin, but a later list leaves Lenin out of the acceptable "fathers."[37] These problems are raised to illustrate the complexities that are often not given sufficient attention by the proponents of such approaches.

Human history seems to confirm the Christian understanding of human limitation and sinfulness.

Even if man does acquire such tremendous power over genetics and his heredity, there is every indication that such power will not always be used for the good of all mankind. History shows that man uses his power for evil as well as for good: the horrible use of eugenics by totalitarian regimes still is a clear and horrendous memory in the minds of many people. Industrialization has brought about a tremendous increase in economic power, but such power probably has been used more often to exploit people than to help them. And can one claim that dominance and self-interest have not played the greatest role in the shaping of the foreign policy of our own nation? Does the priority of certain domestic programs indicate a true willingness to share the goods of our society with others, or rather an attempt to make sure that the gulf widens between the "haves" and the "have nots" in society? The very thought that our genetic planners would be of the same type as our domestic, economic, political, and foreign policy planners does not augur for a utopia on the way.

Catholic theologians generally admit the axiom that abuse does not take away the use. Preliminary discussion and planning might help to eliminate some possible abuses, but history indicates that as more solutions are found, further questions and problems will also arise. It is also important to note that the vast majority of scientists writing on these issues disavow the utopian proposals that have been put forth—e.g., those of Muller. Also, in fairness to Lederberg, he has not to my knowledge advocated the proposal of clonal reproduction, although he presents it as a very likely possibility, if and when it is biologically possible.

A second danger found in the writings of some scientists is the identification of the scientific with the human, but the human—and *a fortiori* the Christian—includes much more than just science and technology. The scientific and the human do not necessarily coincide; there exists a potential source of conflict, as was pointed out by Pope Pius XII in an address to the First International Symposium on Genetics in 1953.[38] The very fact that man is scientifically capable of doing something does not mean that it should be done, for man must control the evolution and development of science. Too often one has the impression that it is science and technology that are going to control man. Men today are somewhat more aware of the need to give human direction and guidance to technology. Just because our nation has the ability and knowledge to send a man to the moon does not mean that such projects should have priority over more pressing human needs. Just because science can keep a dying man alive for a few more hours, does not mean that such means should be employed. At times there are important human values involved which should not be sacrificed for the good of any science.

Such a narrowness of view does seem to color some of the writings of Muller. Muller argues that man should adopt a progressive eugenic program through sperm banks and A.I.D. rather than wait for the genetic surgery which might be available in the next century. His argumentation is most revealing: "The obstacles to carrying out such an improvement by selection are psychological ones, based on antiquated traditions from which we can emancipate ourselves, but the obstacles to doing so by treatment of the genetic materials are substantive ones rooted in the inherent difficulties of the physico-chemical situation."[39] Notice that the only substantive obstacles are those rooted in the biological order.

Muller dismisses the obstacles in the way of his progressive eugenics program as merely "psychological ones based on antiquated traditions." Thus the only things that stand in the way of scientific development are those to which science has not as yet found a suitable answer. However, it does seem that there can be, and are, important human values which would stand in the way of the geneticist on some occasions. Not even Muller would allow the scientist to experiment on man the same way in which he experiments on bacteria. Elsewhere Muller refers to the primary obstacle standing in the way of the adoption of his eugenic program as the attitude of "individual, genetic proprietorship, or pride of so-called blood."[40] But many people see in these obstacles very important human and moral values, since parenthood and family bonds are more than antiquated traditions. For the Christian, the bond between procreation and love union is more than a mere arbitrary arrangement even if one can envision certain historical situations in which it might be sacrificed for greater values.

The narrowness of vision of one who sees all reality through the eyes of an individual science can be illustrated by the consequences that such a program might have on many other facets of human existence. A sociologist, for example, would have some very significant things to say about how marriage and family serve important functions and roles in our contemporary society. If sexual behavior is completely separated from reproduction, why should there be any regulation of sexual behavior at all? Muller's plan would raise grave problems for the psychologist who would then have to try to find some substitute for the stability and deep personal relationships now provided for in marriage and the family. For the ethician, of course, these things also constitute important moral values.

The third danger follows from what has been said

about the difference between the scientific and the ultimate human horizon. The scientific and technical worlds are success oriented and look at reality primarily in terms of effects and performances. Thus there arise several sources of conflict with the human and the Christian horizon. The first concerns the ultimate reason for the dignity of the human person which, from the Christian perspective, cannot be measured in terms of utility or performance. The greatness of human life stems from the free gift of the loving God of creation and redemption. The Christian notion of love, modeled on the love of Yahweh for his people and Christ for his Church, indicates that the ultimate reason for the lovability of a person does not depend on his qualities or deeds or successes or failures; in fact, the covenant commitment of God to his chosen people appears as a sheer gift, especially in the light of the constant infidelities of his people. The Christian view of man does not see his value primarily in terms of what he does or can do for himself or others, but in terms of what God has first done for him.

On the level of ethical theory, an overemphasis on the importance of effects leads to a theory of consequentialism. In such a theory there remains the difficulty of judging the hierarchy of the different consequences and also the difficulty in that man can never know all the consequences of his actions. But even more fundamental is the danger of seeing all moral values in terms of consequences so that the model of the means-end relationship becomes centrally normative. Our basic human intuitions reject the manipulative spirit that tries to use everything as a means for a further end—e.g., we react against people "using friends" or "using other human lives," etc. Thus, especially in the area of genetics Ramsey has pointed out the need for an ethic of means as well as an ethic of ends, since there are certain values that cannot be sacrificed as means for certain other ends.[41] Pius XII, in his 1953 address, likewise pointed out the danger of making a good end justify any means.[42] However, in Catholic moral theology there has been a tendency to view the means-end relationship in too physical a manner and to forget that on occasion the end truly specifies the means.[43]

Most scientists are aware of the possible collision of values and other problems arising from the difference between the human and the scientific horizons. In many cases, for example, they see no problem in performing certain experiments on plants or animals which they would not employ on man. Lederberg himself has brought up the problem of the first experiment in genetic surgery and especially the first attempts to clone a man.[44] This question of experimentation will become even more acute in the future, and will be faced long before the problems created by the use of techniques for directing the human evolutionary process.

The scientists I have read readily admit the dignity of man, and constantly emphasize that nothing should be done to man without his consent. Nevertheless, I would agree with Ramsey in pointing out that man is the body of his soul just as much as he is the soul of his body.[45] In more modern terms, man is not merely his freedom but also his corporality. One can offend against man not only by violating his spirituality, but also his corporality. There is the danger of a neo-dualism that sees man only as spirit. The very fact that a man consents to something does not mean that the act is necessarily right. Such a principle is rejected in our jurisprudence which holds that a man cannot give up his inalienable rights even if he gives his consent. Too often today in many ethical problems one hears that there is nothing wrong with a particular act, provided that everybody agrees and consents. The Catholic tradition has unfortunately tended to make the biological normative, but the opposite extreme of paying no attention to man's corporality also goes against human dignity precisely insofar as it is human.

This paper has tried, from the viewpoint of both theology and biology, to raise some of the dangers implicit in man's control of his evolution. Since the scientists themselves, and especially Ramsey, have given extensive ethical criticisms of some of the genetic proposals, I have concentrated more on the problems such genetic questions raise for moral theology or Christian ethics. I agree with the scientists that now is the time to begin discussing these important issues. In the meantime, it seems that voluntary negative eugenics should be encouraged through a more widespread use of genetic counselling. As for Muller's program, the majority of the scientists themselves who have written in this area do not believe that it should be put into practice even from the limited viewpoint of biology. From the moral viewpoint, I agree that such a program should not be adopted now. In my view, whatever the future brings, it will not be a utopia. Scientific advances will also bring problems and difficulties especially in the control of such great power that man will have. However, these problems are not sufficient reason to stop all experimentation and work toward acquiring a greater power over man's heredity and genes. In the experimentation and continual probing, it will be necessary to respect human dignity and not totally subordinate the individual to the goals of scientific advancement. Since man may have such power within a century, it is not too early to continue in a more structured way the dialogue that has already been initiated.

Notes

1. Herman J. Muller, "Better Genes for Tomorrow," *The Population Crisis and the Use of World Resources,* ed. Stuart Mudd (The Hague: Dr. W. Junk Publishers, 1964), 315. For most of Muller's articles and addresses in the field of genetics before 1961, see *Studies in Genetics: The Selected Papers of H. J. Muller* (Bloomington, Ind.: Indiana University Press, 1962).

2. Theodosius Dobzhansky, "Changing Man," *Science* 155 (1967), 409. Dobzhansky (411) maintains that we do not have enough knowledge to be sure of the value, even from the biological perspective, of mankind freed from all genetic loads. For a fuller explanation of his thought, see Dobzhansky, *Mankind Evolving* (New Haven: Yale University Press, 1962). Others who are not as pessimistic as Muller and maintain the need to wait for more knowledge include: S. E. Lurie, "Directed Genetic Change: Perspectives from Molecular Genetics," *The Control of Human Heredity and Evolution,* ed. T. M. Sonneborn (New York: Macmillan, 1965); John Maynard Smith, "Eugenics and Utopia," *Daedalus* 94 (1965), 487-505; Curt Stern, "Genes and People," *Perspectives in Biology and Medicine* 10 (1966-67), 500-523; and many others.

3. In the preparation of this paper, in addition to the bibliography already mentioned, the following studies from the scientific viewpoint were helpful: E. Shils, et al., *Life or Death: Ethics and Options* (Seattle: University of Washington Press, 1968); Frederick Osborne, *The Future of Human Heredity* (New York: Weybright and Talley, 1968); John D. Roslansky, ed., *Genetics and the Future of Man* (New York: Appleton-Century-Crofts, 1966); T. M. Sonneborn, ed., *The Control of Human Heredity and Evolution* (New York: Macmillan, 1965); Gordon Wolstenhomme, ed., *Man and His Future* (Boston: Little, Brown, and Co., 1963); also Leonard Ornstein, "The Population Explosion, Conservative Eugenics, and Human Evolution," *Bulletin of the Atomic Scientists* 23 (June 1967), 57-60; Joshua Lederberg, "Experimental Genetics and Human Evolution," *Bulletin of the Atomic Scientists* 22 (Oct. 1966), 4-11; James F. Crowe, "The Quality of People: Human Evolutionary Changes," *Bioscience* 16 (1966), 863-867; N. H. Horowitz, *Perspectives in Biology and Medicine* 9 (1965-66), 349-357; Roland D. Hotchkiss, "Portents for a Genetic Engineering," *Journal of Heredity* 56 (1965), 197-202; T. M. Sonneborn, "Genetics and Man's Vision," *Proceedings of the American Philosophical Society* 109 (August 1965), 237-241; Sonneborn, "Implications of the New Genetics for Biology and Man," *A.I.B.S. Bulletin* 13 (April 1963), 22-26 (A.I.B.S. is the American Institute of Biological Sciences).

4. Later articles by Muller include: "Genetic Progress by Voluntary Conducted Germinal Choice," *Man and His Future,* 247-262; "Means and Aims in Human Genetic Betterment," *The Control of Human Heredity and Evolution,* 100-123; Julian Huxley, *The Humanist Frame* (London: Allen and Unwin, 1961); *Eugenics in Evolutionary Perspective* (London: Eugenics Society, 1962); *Essays of a Humanist* (New York: Harper and Row, 1964).

5. Lederberg, *Bulletin of the Atomic Scientists* 22 (Oct. 1966), 4-11.

6. Joshua Lederberg, "Biological Future of Man," *Man and His Future,* 263-273.

7. Paul Ramsey, "Moral and Religious Implications in Genetic Control," *Genetics and the Future of Man,* 153.

8. This conclusion is based on the works cited above and is the same conclusion reached by James M. Gustafson in reviewing *Life or Death: Ethics and Options* in *Commonweal* 89 (4 Oct. 1968), 28.

9. Lloyd J. Averill, *American Theology in the Liberal Tradition* (Philadelphia: Westminster Press, 1967), 125-127.

10. Roger Aubert, "La liberté religieuse du Syllabus de 1864 à nos jours," *Recherches et Débats* 50 (1965), 13-25. Among Murray's many writings, see especially for this aspect, John Courtney Murray, S.J., *The Problem of Religious Freedom* (Westminster, Md.: Newman Press, 1965).

11. Étienne Borne, "Le problème majeur du Syllabus: vérité et liberté," *Recherches et Débats* 50 (1965), 26-42.

12. Karl Rahner, S.J., "The Historical Dimension in Theology," *Theology Digest,* Sesquicentennial Issue (1968), 30-42.

13. Ramsey, *Genetics and the Future of Man,* 145-147.

14. *Ibid.,* 159.

15. Johannes B. Metz, "Relationship of Church and World in the Light of a Political Theology," *Theology of Renewal* II, ed. L. K. Shook, C.S.B. (New York: Herder and Herder, 1968), 255-270; Metz, "The Church's Social Function in the Light of a Political Theology," *Concilium* 36 (June 1968), 2-18.

16. Patrick Granfield, O.S.B., "The Right to Silence," *Theological Studies* 26 (1965), 280-298; 27 (1966), 401-420.

17. John F. Cronin, S.S., *The Social Teaching of Pope John XXIII* (Milwaukee: Bruce Publishing Co., 1963).

18. For a fine summary of this changing emphasis, see Edward Duff, S.J., "Property, Private," *New Catholic Encyclopedia* 11, 849-855.

19. Gerald Kelly, S.J., *Medico-Moral Problems* (St. Louis: Catholic Hospital Association, 1958), pp. 8-11.

20. *Acta Apostolicae Sedis* 44 (1952), 786; 48 (1956), 461.

21. Gerald Kelly, S.J., "Pope Pius XII and the Principle of Totality," *Theological Studies* 16 (1955), 373-396. A summary and applications of the principle of totality are found in Kelly, *Medico-Moral Problems,* 8-11; 245-269. Kelly on the basis of other moral principles would allow organic transplants and experimentation for the good of others. Note that Kelly wrote before the address of Pius XII in 1958 in which Pius developed and extended the principle of totality: "To the subordination, however, of the particular organs to the organism and its own finality, one must add the subordination of the organism to the spiritual finality of the person himself." *A.A.S.* 50 (1958), 693, 694.

22. For an interpretation which broadens the notion of

totality in the light of Pius' 1958 discourse, see Martin Nolan, O.S.A., *The Principle of Totality in the Writings of Pope Pius XII* (Rome: Pontifical Gregorian University, 1960).

23. Martin Nolan, O.S.A., "The Principle of Totality in Moral Theology," *Absolutes in Moral Theology?*, ed. Charles E. Curran (Washington: Corpus Books, 1968), 244.

24. *Summa Theologiae,* IaIIae, Prologue.

25. Harvey G. Cox, *On Not Leaving It to the Snake* (New York: Macmillan, 1967), "Introduction: Faith and Decision," and throughout the book.

26. E.g., Reinhold Niebuhr, *Moral Man and Immoral Society* (New York: Charles Scribner's Sons, 1933 and 1960); *Love and Justice: Selections from the Shorter Writings of Reinhold Niebuhr,* ed. D. B. Robertson (Cleveland: Meridian Books, 1967), especially 46-54.

27. Paul Ramsey, "Shall We Clone a Man?" an address given at a conference on "Ethics in Medicine and Technology" sponsored by the Institute of Religion at the Texas Medical Center and by Rice University, Houston, Texas, March 25-28, 1968. Professor Ramsey kindly sent me a copy of his address. This problem of the greater dominion possessed by modern man, who still remains a sinful creature, is recognized by Leroy Augenstein, *Come, Let Us Play God* (New York: Harper and Row, 1969).

28. Ramsey, *Genetics and the Future of Man,* 136.

29. Harvey Cox, "Evolutionary Progress and Christian Promise," *Concilium* 26 (June 1967), 35-47; M. C. Vanhengal, O.P., and J. Peters, "Death and Afterlife," *Concilium* 26 (June 1967), 161-181.

30. Paul Ramsey, *Deeds and Rules in Christian Ethics* (New York: Charles Scribner's Sons, 1967), 108-109.

31. John R. Cavanagh, "Bene Mori: The Right of the Patient to Die with Dignity," *Linacre Quarterly* 30 (May 1963), 60-68. This right follows from the traditionally accepted principle that man does not have to use extraordinary means to preserve his life.

32. Muller, *Studies in Genetics,* 590.

33. Muller, *The Control of Human Heredity and Evolution,* 109.

34. Muller, *The Population Crisis and the Use of World Resources,* 332.

35. H. Richard Niebuhr, *The Kingdom of God in America* (New York: Harper and Row, 1937; Torchback, 1959), 193.

36. Lederberg, *Bulletin of the Atomic Scientists* 22 (Oct. 1966), 9-10.

37. E.g., M. Klein, *Man and His Future,* 280.

38. *A.A.S.* 45 (1953), 602, 603.

39. Muller, *The Control of Human Heredity and Evolution,* 100.

40. Muller, *The Population Crisis and the Use of World Resources,* 323.

41. Most of the points briefly mentioned in this third danger have been developed at greater length by Ramsey in various articles and books, although I would again disagree with the eschatology sometimes expressed in these contexts. On consequentialism in general, see *Deeds and Rules in Christian Ethics,* especially 176-225. His two essays on genetics develop the need for an ethic of means.

42. *A.A.S.* 45 (1953), 605, 606.

43. William H. Van der Marck, O.P., *Toward a Christian Ethic* (Westminster, Md.: Newman Press, 1967), 48-69.

44. Lederberg, *Bulletin of the Atomic Scientists* 22 (Oct. 1966), 10. Ramsey develops the point at great length in his paper on cloning.

45. Ramsey, *Genetics and the Future of Man,* 155-157.

62. The Problem of Genetic Manipulation

KARL RAHNER

Man's finite nature implies that, however much he may conceivably (and even legitimately) submit his own self to planning, he is no less a being whose essence has been predetermined. He must accept this particular *existentiale* as well as the task of self-determination. We must now relate this fundamental anthropological and ethical insight to the concrete problem under discussion, and then draw the appropriate and necessary conclusions.

1. Man must freely accept his nature as being predetermined. For he has not called *himself* into existence. He has been projected into a particular world, and although this world is presented to him for his free acceptance or rejection, he has not *chosen* it himself. It is rather that the world confronts him as something which has been determined from another quarter, *before* he embarks on his own history as a free being. Consequently the world can never be 'worked over' to such an extent that man is eventually dealing only with material *he* has chosen and created. Even if it were exhaustively calculated and planned in advance by the parents, the very stuff which is the precondition of the test-tube baby's freedom is (as far as the baby *itself* is concerned—and this 'self' is what is decisive) something already decided by someone else, something alien, like the genes one receives according to natural conception at the present time. It is part of the test-tube child's freedom to ask why he is obliged to shape his whole lifelong history out of the particular material which his parents have so wisely and thoughtfully selected for him by means of technology and planning. The question still remains as to whether, having had one's 'good fortune' planned and predetermined, one really considers oneself to be 'fortunate'. Accepting this necessarily alien determination of one's own being *is* and *remains,* therefore, a fundamental task of man in his free moral existence. All this can be understood, by 'transcendental deduction', as a necessarily given factor of man's nature. Wherever the *amor fati—fatum* in the sense of what is uniquely committed to the individual—is no longer achieved, and wherever this *fatum* is no longer accepted confidently in patience and humility as the gift of an *incomprehensible* love, man is subject to total neurosis, to a basic fear concerning his destiny which weighs more heavily on him than all the things which, as a result of this fear, he tries to escape from. Man's fundamental guilt is the consequence of his freely refusing to accept this gift.

2. However, although this *existentiale* and what it implies (the task of free decision) exercises its sovereign influence in the ultimate ground of man's being, it must also take on a corresponding 'categorial', tangible form in time and space, lest, banished from man's existence, it should be forgotten and ultimately freely denied by him.

Now man is in a certain respect most free when he is not dealing with a 'thing' but calling into being another, freely responsible person. If he is not to conceal or fall short of his nature, man must be presented clearly with the dialectically opposite position of his freedom as a man. And in concrete terms that means that the freedom to determine another person must remain a clear-cut and radical destiny, which one has *not chosen* but *accepted.* Procreation in particular must not become an act of neurotic anxiety in the face of fate. The other person must remain the one who is both *made* and *accepted;* both an elevating influence, because he has been chosen, and a burden to be accepted and carried. If man, when confronted with his child, saw only what he had himself planned, he would not be looking at his own nature, nor would he experience his true self which is both free *and* the object of external determination. Genetic manipulation is the embodiment of the fear of oneself, the fear of accepting one's self as the unknown quantity it is.

Someone might say that even genetic manipulation cannot really get rid of every indeterminate element in procreation and that therefore genetic manipulation does not run counter to what we have said. (In any case, surely certain 'eugenic precautions' are not really reprehensible?) In this case we must answer with another question: What, in actual fact, is the driving force behind genetic manipulation? What sort of person is driven to it? And the answer would be, in the first place, the *hate* of one's destiny; and secondly, it is the man who, at his innermost level, is in despair because he cannot *dispose* of existence. In genetic manipulation such a man clearly and unequivocally oversteps the boundary between legitimate eugenic precautions and the realm tyrannised by the desperate fear of destiny. Even in those cases where no precise boundary can be set, one can see that a particular action undoubtedly exceeds it. This is plain in the

From Karl Rahner, *Theological Investigations,* vol. 9, trans. Graham Harrison (New York: Crossroad, 1972), pp. 244-52. Used by permission.

case in hand, since the concrete genetic manipulation is governed by the desire to banish the *fatum* from existence, at a particular point. To the extent that this intention does not quite succeed, it is contrary to the original desire, for this desire hates destiny and can only love—as the product of its own free action—what it has calculated and planned. It no longer desires to say 'I have gotten a man from the Lord'—from *God,* who cannot be manipulated and who must be concretely present in man's existence. The essence of this rather more theological conclusion can be seen just as clearly in the dimensions of concrete anthropology: *Does* man in the concrete—who is not a mere abstract concept—really wish, in accepting genetic manipulation, to accept what *cannot* be predetermined? Has he actually the courage to take a decision, the results of which are unforeseeable? Does he really want to enter into a future of open possibilities, full of both threatening and promising surprises? And if his will fails at this point, will he ever find it again in any other area of his existence? Or is he like a man who only wants to perform a particular function of his nature when it is too late for him to do otherwise, and who will thus not be really able to carry it out even then? These are the decisive questions.

3. Man has his own sphere of intimacy. Historically and sociologically its concrete form can vary considerably. But whether it is technologically possible to abolish it is not the point, for this sphere of intimacy *should* exist, and ought to be resolutely safeguarded. It forms the innermost region of freedom which man needs in order to be really self-determining. At whatever point anyone else is able and is permitted arbitrarily to invade another person's private area of free decision, freedom itself ceases to exist.

Man is right to designate the ultimate achievement of sexual union as belonging to this area of intimacy. For human sexuality, as a free activity, both is and ought to be more than a merely biological function; namely, an activity of the whole human being: the appearance and realisation of personal love.[1] Now this personal love which is consummated sexually has within it an essential inner relation to the child, for the child is an embodiment of the abiding unity of the marriage-partners which is expressed in marital union. Genetic manipulation, however, does two things: it fundamentally separates the marital union from the procreation of a new person as this permanent embodiment of the unity of married love; and it transfers procreation, isolated and torn from its human matrix, to an area outside man's sphere of intimacy. It is this sphere of intimacy which is the proper context for sexual union, which itself implies the fundamental readiness of the marriage-partners to let their unity take the form of a child.

The fact that it is technologically *possible* to effect the changes involved in genetic manipulation while at the same time producing a new *human being* is no argument against the essential connectedness of the factors we have just referred to (the sphere of intimacy—the union of marital love—the child as the permanent form of this union). For the child produced by such a method is, in this sense, the child of the mother *and* of the donor. The latter refuses, however, to acknowledge his fatherhood in an act of personal love: he remains anonymous or at least does not wish to be the donor in respect of this particular mother; precisely through his anonymity he robs the child of the right and ability to fulfil the obligation of his existence, namely to accept himself as the child of these particular parents. Genetic manipulation of this sort is no more 'human', merely because it produces a human being, than a case of rape. The fact that a biological chain of cause-and-effect is not broken, even when the moral/human unity and the whole of really human meaningfulness receives a mortal blow (for the 'biological' side is intended to be an expression of this total meaningfulness), does nothing, in itself, to justify its own occurrence.

4. What we have just said is directed against the *desire* (which is at least implicit in genetic manipulation) to plan man totally; it runs counter to the nature of man in the sense we have outlined. Consequently saying 'No' to this desire is not dependent on the question of its feasibility, and it is both possible and permissible to ask the further question, whether this desire *could* be totally realised, and what would be the moral implication of a failure in the execution of these plans.[2]

Initially we should have to answer the first part of the question in the negative. It can confidently be said that it would be impossible, from the technological point of view, to implement a genetic manipulation involving *all* future human beings, because, however much apparatus and 'automation' one had at one's disposal, the fact that one would have to deal with each human being as an individual[3] would imply such a vast quantity of active 'manipulators' that it would take up, *per absurdum,* the whole of mankind's attention and energy. But what would be the moral significance of the impossibility of producing the *whole* of future mankind by genetic manipulation?

In the first place it does *not* mean—as we shall show more clearly *a posteriori*—that a *partial* genetic manipulation is morally admissible, i.e. on the grounds that in any case 'not much' will happen. The practical impossibility of overstepping a particular quantitative limit is by no means a reason for morally justifying any action within that limit. If everyone told lies, for instance, the telling of lies would have no effect, because no-one would believe a liar any more. But that does not make a limited dose of lies a morally justifiable thing. Furthermore, if a *partial* genetic manipulation became normal practice, consciously recognised by society, it would create two new 'races' in mankind: the technologically manipulated, super-bred test-tube men who inevitably would have a special status in society, and the 'ordinary', unselected, mass-produced humans, procreated in the old way. But what new social tensions would arise from this, and at a time when racial discrimination and racial conflicts are laboriously being dismantled so that a gigantic, tightly-packed humanity can exist peacefully! Or is one to believe that this group of test-tube men, whose intelligence quotients would be clearly considerably higher from birth, would not aspire to such a unique position in society, and that the remaining herd of humanity (*without* 'pedigree') would obey them? But would the rest of mankind, remaining at least as intelligent, revolutionary and violent as *we* are, readily accept the leadership of pedigree test-tube men? All this would probably not happen provided that the number of genetically manipulated men were *very* small, and that for that very reason they could not lay claim to be the exclusive leaders of society. But in such a case the spokesmen of manipulation would not have achieved the very results they want, namely, to create mankind's elite of leaders, able to claim the right of leadership on account of their genetic qualifications. However, it must be declared immoral to plan to produce such conflict-laden material with its unforeseeable consequences. It constitutes a threat to man and to mankind.

5. Nowadays we are trying to extend and secure the individual's area of freedom. It is one of mankind's moral commissions. To pursue the practical possibility of genetically manipulating man is to threaten and encroach upon this free area. For it offers incalculable opportunities of man's manipulation—reaching to the very roots of his existence—*by organised society,* i.e. the state. This in turn subjects the state to the strong temptation of itself manipulating the genetic manipulation. And unless one adopts the radically false view (which is untenable from both the philosophical and the Christian standpoints) that what the state wants is automatically good and just, it must be acknowledged that, over and above the essential inner perversity of genetic manipulation, this gives the state the power of further immoral action in using it for its own purposes, to create men who suit its own predilections.

Let no-one say that *every* new and legitimate possibility always involves the temptation for man to misuse it, and that it is not thereby immoral, but must just be protected against abuse. The danger of misusing a newly created possibility may be taken into account *if* this new possibility is in itself justifiable and seems to be inevitable and required by man. But is this the case in genetic manipulation? What compelling aims does it have in view? That men should be able to grow a little older? But is that really desirable with the present size of world population, etc.? In any case, is this the right way—it is not the *only* way—to set about it? Or is the main aim that man should be genetically more intelligent and cultured? But is it true that higher intelligence is clearly correlated with a more highly developed humane sensitivity? Is the kind of intelligence which can be 'bred' in this way the kind we need today, i.e. the intelligence of wisdom, moral responsibility and selflessness? (For the other kind, the 'technical' kind of intelligence can be adequately increased by means of computers and cybernetics.) What is the point of genetic manipulation if not to extend the state's area of control and thus to diminish, instead of to increase, man's sphere of freedom? It would be wiser not to put weapons into the hands of one's aggressors.

6. In future man must develop a critical attitude towards the fascination exercised by every new possibility. Here, in general terms, we have a new moral commission.

Essentially it has always been possible to see that not everything which *can* be done, *ought* to be done.[4] The possibilities available to man in earlier days were, however, very stable, and as a result they had been tested countless times. The possibilities for evil (and they were relatively simple and clear-cut) were recognised promptly as such, since they were of a common and general nature, e.g. that 'cheats never prosper', tyranny is eventually self-destructive, excessive indulgence destroys the ability to enjoy, etc. The situation was simple: one knew what one ought not to do because one had already experienced the fact that such things were not really lasting possibilities in the long run, although one could 'get away with it' for a time. But the past did teach a sound doctrine: one should *not* do everything one is *able* to do; there are times when the attraction of the possible must be resisted.

Nowadays the situation is different. New and practical possibilities are set before us in relatively rapid succession, and they have vast and far-reaching effects. It is a strange factor of the dialectic of the accelerating movement of our history that these new possibilities can be discovered more quickly than their ultimate effects can be ascertained by practical tests. This is why it is so vital for humanity to develop a resistance to the fascination of novel possibilities. Of course there are 'feedback' effects in the field of social morality too, and they put a brake on the lure of novelty: the latest attraction in the form of the mini-skirt becomes monotonous when everyone is wearing it; and if almost everyone adopts the policy of limiting the size of the family because of the demands it makes, a large family will suddenly become an 'attractive' possibility and even gain a new social prestige. But there is no guarantee that such feedback effects can be relied upon in social morality in every case. The irreparable catastrophe can already have taken place before any feedback has had time to take effect. In certain cases to create immunity from moral diseases requires more time than the disease itself allows.

Nowadays there are things with which one cannot have a preliminary run through, in order to gain experience for the next occasion and become wiser through trial and error. Or should one first of all arrange a 'trial run' for a total atomic war, for instance, before deciding to avoid a second one? Today we must be aware that a thing may have irreversible consequences. This is a fundamental conviction of Christianity's theology of history; in spite of the multifarious possible recombinations Christianity sees the course of history as being ultimately a one-way street. At all events, if the new humanity of the future is to survive, it must cultivate a sober and critical resistance to the fascination of novel possibilities.

Genetic manipulation seems to be, initially, a case in point. Are there any reasons against such a view? There could only be objections if there were considerable reasons *in favour* of genetic manipulation from other quarters. Like what, for instance? That we must bring the decline of intelligence and bodily health under control? But has anyone proved such a decline to be a fact? Or if it *is* partially the case, has it been shown that it could not be brought under control in another way? No such proofs are forthcoming.

7. There is another side to the fascination of novelty. The suggestion is that new possibilities will become actualities *all the same;* that nothing can resist them and that to offer any resistance is to be backing a loser; that one is being old-fashioned and stick-in-the-mud by not joining forces with the heralds of the 'new age'. On the contrary, it is one of the fundamental duties of a genuinely moral and Christian man to endeavour to do precisely this: to be *absolutely* faithful to a thing in a situation where it seems hopelessly doomed to failure. The biological end of an individual is not the only death of which one must not be afraid. There are other kinds of apparent death which one must not fear. History is not made by those who try to foresee what is 'inevitable' so that they can jump on the cart of fate in good time, but by those who are prepared to take the ultimate risk of defeat. No-one can say that genetic manipulation *inevitably* will come. The only person who 'knows' such a thing is the man who secretly *wishes* it to be so.

Is that kind of man a trustworthy prophet? Why should not mankind as a whole have to learn the lessons every individual has to learn in his own life if he is to survive, namely, the lessons of sacrifice and renunciation? After all we have said, the issue of sacrifice and renunciation is in this sense a 'rational' one and not the unreal fantasy of masochistic minds perversely obstructing their own progress. It is by no means certain that mankind will always be able to remain at the juvenile stage where it can only do the sort of 'mischief' which does not matter very much. That is surely another most valuable insight of our time. So then, if mankind as a whole must seek to learn the renunciation characteristic of maturity, it cannot be said that a rejection of genetic manipulation has 'no prospects' from the very beginning.

In conclusion let us recapitulate in order to understand the whole in the proper light. We do not claim that these observations against genetic manipulation are complete; rather they constitute an appeal to, and the inadequate objectifying of, a humane and Christian 'instinct' which can be discovered in the moral field. A moral awareness of this kind (which both is and does more than we have mentioned here) forms the context in which man has the courage to make decisions; thus a decision is also more than its rationale, because the act is always more than its theoretical foundation. This 'instinct' justifiably has the courage to say *Stat pro ratione voluntas* because such a confession need not necessarily be overcautious about making a decision. On the contrary it can claim to be the first really to make room for the possibility of genuine criticism and to bring to light the justification, implications and limitations of a real theoretical foundation. All theoretical reasoning always says (among other things), 'We do not *want* to manipulate man genetically'; but this will is meaningful in spite of the fact that it neither claims nor is obliged to be exhaustively analysable by theoretical reason; measured against the opposite will, *this* will is more deeply meaningful and more genuinely human. It must accept the risks involved in history and the unpredictable, in order to find out whether it is stronger than its converse, and whether it can endow its theoretical meaningfulness with the particular radiance which is the exclusive characteristic of *performed* reality. Modern man is faced with making this decision.

Of course, in saying this we have raised yet another problem. Right from the beginning, rejecting man's genetic manipulation is not a merely theoretical declaration but a deliberate act. Consequently this theoretical discussion cannot be supported conclusively by the general, formal authority of the Christian churches alone. And so, as in many other cases in moral theology, we are faced today with a new, additional question of great importance: How, in concrete terms, can such a rejection (of genetic manipulation) be established in modern society as society's *own* maxim, its own inner attitude and 'instinct', in the face of society's 'pluralism'? However, this particular problem of moral and pastoral theology is part of a wider issue[5] which cannot be pursued further within the limits of the present discussion.

Notes

1. Cf. the Pastoral Constitution of the Second Vatican Council, *Gaudium et spes,* Nos. 47-52.

2. We need not go into the first part of the question in so far as the concrete details are concerned; that belongs to the field of natural science.

3. Here we can pass over the question as to whether it is possible or impossible to synthesise the hereditary material itself in large quantities.

4. Of course, in a real and most profound sense one cannot 'do' something which is really immoral, for evil, measured against the *whole* of reality (including man in all his dimensions and God as well), is always impotent and ineffectual. Cf. also B. Welte, *Über das Böse* (Freiburg, 1959).

5. Some pointers are given in K. Rahner, 'Reflections on Dialogue within a pluralistic society', *Theological Investigations* VI (London and Baltimore, 1969), pp. 31-42.

Chapter Thirteen
ABORTION

Introduction

On January 22, 1973, the Supreme Court of the United States ruled in *Roe v. Wade* that state laws prohibiting abortion before a fetus is viable were unconstitutional. The court held that decisions about abortion were fundamentally private decisions, to be made in the context of conversations between a woman and her physician.

The public controversy about abortion did not begin with *Roe v. Wade,* and of course it did not end there either. But in the years since the ruling, the debate has become increasingly intractable. The arguments by both partisans in the debate, the advocates of a woman's right to control her own powers of reproduction and the advocates of a fetus's right to life, are familiar—and remain unpersuasive to the other side.

The argument has sometimes seemed deceptively simple, the questions at least readily identifiable if not readily answerable. The one most important question has frequently been identified as the question of the status of the fetus. On the answer to that question all the law and the prophets with respect to abortion are sometimes presumed to hang. It is indeed an important question, and answers to it have important implications for abortion. On the one side are those who claim that the genetic uniqueness and completeness of a fertilized ovum should be enough to identify it as an individual member of the human species and so worthy of all the respect due any other human individual. On the other side are those who claim that the fetus does not have the necessary or sufficient attributes of human persons and so need be neither ascribed nor granted in practice the full rights of human persons, including the right to life. In between these two poles are developmental views of the fetus which regard some stage or stages of fetal development as morally significant and as demanding increasing respect and restraint. The question "Who counts as a person?" is relevant quite concretely to the discussion of abortion, and the earlier essays of Joseph Fletcher and Stanley Hauerwas should be read alongside the essays by Albert Outler, Karl Barth, David Smith, Margaret Farley, and Beverly Harrison in this section.

The question is easily identified—but not easily answered. *Roe v. Wade,* for example, recognized that the moral status of the fetus was the point of controversy, but the court stood back and did not pretend to be wise enough to decide this issue. A frequent criticism of the reasoning of the court, however, is that although it acknowledged its inability to decide this "difficult" question, for all practical purposes it did decide it, ruling that before viability the fetus is simply not protectable by law. The court held that the *legal status* of the fetus may be distinguished from the moral status and that there was no precedent for holding that its legal status entitles it to the same protection extended to persons. The point is not that the legal ruling of the court was right or wrong, but that it clearly distinguished legal from moral questions. That its legal holding was taken as moral license may provide an occasion to judge our society rather than the courts.

At any rate, the issue of the relation of law to morality, of public policy to the moral passions and projects that give one moral identity, is an issue which also demands attention. Christians may have reasons for ascribing a certain moral status to the fetus which can hardly be articulated in the courts or legislatures. Though Christians may sign and seal their trust in God's future by having and loving children, by resisting the "solution" of consigning even nascent life to the realm and powers of darkness, the convictions which evoke and sustain such behavior are not legally enforceable. David Smith pays special attention to the relation of public policy and personal moral discernment, but many of the essays included make certain assumptions about it. It is related (but not identical) to questions about the relation of an impartial moral perspective and a candidly Christian perspective. Whatever one thinks about the relation of social policy and Christian morality, Christians should not permit their attention to be monopolized by the legal issues. They should not hesitate to articulate their fundamental convictions about human life, even though they may not be legally enforceable. If they do, they may lose the capacity to act with integrity themselves and may abandon society to a minimal account of morality in terms of legality.

One of the reasons the question of the status of the fetus has loomed so large is the public focus on autonomy as the relevant impartial principle. Public discussion has tended to make abortion an issue of the "rights" of individuals; then the only important questions are whether the fetus is an individual person or not and, if it is, what its rights are. A woman contemplating an abortion is sometimes considered as though she were simply exercising ownership rights over her own body, like a landlady with an undesirable tenant or pest. Partisans on both sides of the debate have relied heavily on the logic and language of individual autonomy and rights, but we should ask whether a focus on autonomy can do justice to the interdependence of people, whether it can attend both to the values which people freely choose and to the values of social relations and embodied existence which are not matters of choice, and whether it can appreciate the limitations on choice imposed by social arrangements and conditions.[1] Perhaps a religious perspective would qualify or challenge the focus on the autonomy of individuals with attention to human relatedness and vulnerability.

Some feminist perspectives have relied on the logic and language of autonomy and rights, but others have called attention to human relatedness and vulnerability and to the limited choices some women contemplating an abortion have. The perspective on the situation changes not only in terms of how we see the fetus, but also in terms of how we see the woman. Is she an autonomous individual exercising ownership rights over her body? Or is she a character in a tragedy—a story in which evils have gathered and cannot all be avoided, a story in which goods have collided and cannot all be sought, a story wrought in part by a social context pervasively oppressive to women? Such a woman might understand abortion as violence, as a desperate violence inflicted not only upon an embryo but upon herself, but also as a tragic necessity. If such a challenge to a focus on autonomy is accepted, and if one sees the woman contemplating an abortion in this way, then opposition to abortion may perhaps be softened but surely must be joined by an effective support system—financial, social, psychological, moral, and spiritual—for women and their children. If tragedy is acknowledged this side of the eschaton, then Christians may acknowledge that sometimes abortion may mournfully, repentantly, tearfully be indicated. But does tragedy fit with the Christian story? Do principles or values conflict genuinely or only apparently? If tragedy is acknowledged, then Christians are obliged to say what goods can weigh against the good of life and what indications there may be for abortion as a tragic choice.

Finally, it may be observed that in *Roe v. Wade* the court presumed that the question of abortion would be a "medical decision" and that the professional integrity of physicians would restrict what the law could not prohibit. "Basic responsibility for [the decision to abort] must rest with the physician," it said.[2] That the court's legal ruling was taken as an entrepreneurial opportunity by some physicians may be reason to judge the profession rather than the ruling. At any rate, it raises again the question of a professional ethic and its relation to a Christian ethic. Is the profession simply the body of skills learned by training and accessible to consumers, or are there goods intrinsic to medicine as a practice and a profession, goods which can be violated when the skills are used for alien ends? And can those goods, if there are such, be nurtured or qualified by a Christian vision?

The issues identified for the reader's theological reflection include the relation of social policy recommendations to personal moral decisions; the relation of a professional ethic and a Christian ethic; the appropriate perspective on the situation involving the fetus, the woman, and their wider social context; and the relevance and meaning and possible conflict of a number of principles, including autonomy, the sanctity of life, the protection of the vulnerable, and the liberation of the oppressed.

Notes

1. For a perceptive analysis and critique of the focus on autonomy see Helen John, SND, "Reflection on Autonomy and Abortion," in *Respect and Care in Medical Ethics,* ed. David Smith (Lanham, Md.: University Press of America, 1984).

2. *Roe v. Wade,* 410 U.S. 113 (1973). See also *Biomedical-Ethical Issues: A Digest of Law and Policy Development* (United Ministries in Education, 1983), p. 16.

Suggestions for Further Reading

Batchelor, Edward, Jr., ed. *Abortion: The Moral Issues.* New York: Pilgrim Press, 1982.

Burtchaell, James Tunstead, C.S.C. *Rachel Weeping and Other Essays on Abortion.* New York: Andrews and McMeel, 1982.

Callahan, Daniel. *Abortion: Law, Choice and Morality.* London: Macmillan, 1970.

Callahan, Sidney, and Daniel Callahan, eds. *Abortion: Understanding Differences.* New York: Plenum Press, 1984.

Grisez, Germain. *Abortion: The Myths, The Realities, and the Arguments.* New York: Corpus Books, 1970.

Hartshorne, Charles. "Scientific and Religious Aspects of Bioethics." In *Theology and Bioethics: Exploring the Foundations and Frontiers,* edited by Earl E. Shelp. Dordrecht: Reidel, 1985.

John, Helen. "Reflections on Autonomy and Abortion." In *Respect and Care in Medical Ethics,* edited by David H. Smith. Lanham, Md.: University Press of America, 1984.

Meilaender, Gilbert. "Against Abortion: A Protestant Proposal." *Linacre Quarterly* 45 (May 1978): 165-78.

Noonan, John T., Jr., ed. *The Morality of Abortion.* Cambridge: Harvard University Press, 1970.

Ramsey, Paul. *Ethics at the Edges of Life.* New Haven: Yale University Press, 1978. See pp. 1-142.

Schaeffer, Francis, and C. Everett Koop. *Whatever Happened to the Human Race?* Old Tappan, N.J.: Revell, 1979.

Simmons, Paul D. *Birth and Death: Bioethical Decision-Making.* Philadelphia: Westminster, 1983. See pp. 65-107.

Sojourners, November 1982.

Wennberg, Robert N. *Life in the Balance: Exploring the Abortion Controversy.* Grand Rapids: Eerdmans, 1985.

63. The Beginnings of Personhood: Theological Considerations

ALBERT C. OUTLER

There are two fairly obvious constants in the abortion debate thus far.[1] The first is a general agreement, by all but the hard-line abortionists, that abortion is a genuine *moral* dilemma—not least because all its crucial terms are actually question begging. This might suggest the prudence of a suspended judgment, but we have no such option. Abortion is a stark dilemma confronting us now—with far-reaching decisions that have already been made about it on presumptions about human existence that run far past verified knowledge. The resulting crisis has generated more heat than light and many of us are more eager to defend our prejudices than to reach for a new consensus. Hence, our adversary proceedings in a problem-area that is as baffling as life itself, since it clearly *may*—as some of us believe it clearly *does*—involve just that: life, death and destiny.

A second constant in the debate is its reflection of the mercurial shifts in popular opinion in recent years—shifts that are functions of the cataclysmic collapse of the moral-demand systems that have guided Western society (more or less!) for two millennia.[2] Twenty years ago, there were not two sides in the debate, really. Ten years ago, our findings would have been practically foreclosed by the then prevailing sentiments.[3] Now, there is a *real* debate in which many pro-abortionists, flushed with victory, are confident that the future is theirs.

In all such upheavals of customary morality, familiar terms become newly ambiguous and value-judgments, long distilled into ordinary language, require new analyses and transvaluations. In the abortion debate, such transvaluations confront us at every turn, all of them buttressed by self-assured rationalizations. Is fetal life already human or still sub-human, personal or non-personal? The answer here, obviously, depends on the biases of one's notions about "human" and "personal." Then there is that poignant phrase, "unwanted life"—which naturally prompts such questions as "unwanted by *whom?*" and "why?" Again, there is the notion of "privacy," whose connotation has been so dramatically extended by the Supreme Court. But just how

From *Perkins Journal* 27 (Fall 1973): 28-34. Used by permission.

private an affair is pregnancy, after all—since, from time immemorial, it has been the primal *social* event in most human communities? If feticide is innocuous, why then should medical research on aborted fetuses be disallowed?[4] Every answer to all such questions (and many others like them) is rooted in our intuitions as to what human fetal life amounts to and these intuitions rest, in turn, on our prior convictions as to what makes human life human, in the first place.

This, then, is the focal question of all our common concerns: what is the truly *human,* what are its real origins and grounds, what are its valid ends? If the human person is understood as a divine intention, with a transcendental ground and context, this will surely guide our analysis of its origins. If abortion is a matter of life and death—*human* life and *human* death—then all decisions about it should reflect this awe-full supposition. If, on the other hand, a fetus is mere tissue—and never more than sub-human till birth—then abortion is an elective, minor surgery and we may cast aside our scruples and disregard all outcries against this kind of "slaughter of the innocents."[5] But this either/or (*either* human life *or* mere tissue) is just precisely the issue that still remains undecided—except on arbitrary grounds—and cannot finally be resolved by any of the arguments that I have yet heard, or have been able to conceive.

The deepest confusion in the debate stems from the confusions generated by the tradition of body-soul dualism which has lasted so long, from its origins in Persia and Greece, through Western philosophy and theology, down to our own times.[6] And it is confusing, since all its versions involve *some* kind of invidious comparison between "lower" and "higher" levels in the *humanum,* and it commits one to *some* sort of "magic moment theory" as to when and how animal tissue becomes "ensouled" or "animated"—and hence to some "magic moment" along the human lifeline when the defenseless finally deserves to be defended. Now the difficulty here is that every decision about such a moment is *arbitrary,* despite all the arguments for or against it.[7] For instance, in a recent (very interesting!) lecture at Rice University, Dr. Engelhardt concluded that, "though the fetus is obviously an example of *human life,* it is in *no way* suggestive of *personal* life."[8] It's a wry comfort for a theologian to catch a scientist in such a hyperbole, since we, too, have the same bad habit of saying "none at all" when we mean "not much." Thus, at the very least, it would seem to be simply a fact that *some* fetuses do, in *some* ways, suggest "personal life" to *some* people! But the real point at issue here is the thesis that something (a fetus) which is *totally* devoid of *any* sign of "personal life" should then regularly develop into "personal life" and to nothing else except a "personal life"—unless accidentally thwarted in its normal development. This is at once a commonplace and a profound ambiguity.

The same "magic moment theory" has been carried further, with less sophistication, by the Supreme Court. Mr. Justice Blackmun began with what, apparently, is a *fait accompli* in constitutional law: viz. that "the term 'person' does not include the unborn."[9] But then he found it possible (arbitrarily, of course) to divide pregnancy into progressive trimesters, with disparate values arbitrarily assigned to each successive trimester—from none, to some, to a good deal.

This is less helpful than it was meant to be, for *birth* is not *the* "magic moment," either. Even "normal" neonates (as well as the premature ones) are not yet decisively human, in their neurological or social maturations. And a discouragingly large fraction of the population never attain to Dr. Engelhardt's norm of "rationality" as the sign of "personhood."[10] Most neurologists agree, or so I am told, that an infant is not yet distinctively "human" until its frontal granular cortex is integrated into the rest of the brain—about the third month *after* birth.[11] Pediatricians and sociologists largely agree that social differentiations take longer than that![12] Professor Lederberg specifies "the acquisition of language" as the *transitus* when an infant "enters the cultural tradition which has been the special attribute of man."[13] Dr. Engelhardt disjoins "the human-biological process" (devoid of "intrinsic value") from "the human-personal process" which climaxes (if it ever does) in "rationality, consciousness, and self-consciousness."[14] As a distinction, this is illuminating. As a radical disjunction, it excludes a very large number of human beings (the very young, the sub-normal, the senescent) from "personhood"—from whence it would follow that they are devoid of intrinsic personal value, or any morally assured human status!

It would follow, further, that human status may validly be decided by dominant codes of social evaluation. When human life is "socially appreciated" its value is thereby assured. By the same token, "unwanted life" would have no such value and no such assurance. This principle might then, with equal consistency, cover not only unappreciated fetuses but also defectives in variety, and the unwanted old as well. I know that such extensions of this principle of social validation are often denied, and I do not propose to belabor all its consequences. What I am suggesting, however, is that the "magic moment" approach entails unmanageable ambiguities and that all conceptions of "personhood" that presume to resolve the dilemma of abortion—as innocuous on the one hand, or absolutely proscribed, on the other—are too crude to correspond to the nuances of personal existence, as we know it in ourselves, and intuit it in others.

Thus, it would seem that the strength of the pro-abortion cause lies in its sentimental appeal: positively, to current approved social values (e.g. population control); negatively, to the personal values of the anguished mother of her rights. These are certainly not negligible considerations, either, for an over-populated planet, with underdeveloped technologies of contraception, and a newly promiscuous society, there is bound to be a plethora of unwanted pregnancies and anguished mothers. What is more, the world is already overburdened with lives that might very well be adjudged "unwanted" on any calculus of *social utility.*

But here the ways part again. When the case for contraception is linked too closely with the case for or against abortion, nothing but confusion follows, since most of the analogies are misleading. The prevention of conception, or nidification—at one end of the spectrum—and adoption, on the other, represent a common view of human life and personhood that is very different from the notion that the human life process, once stabilized, may be terminated without moral scruple. For in the decision for or against abortion, what is being weighed is the *life* of the fetus against the *anguish* of the mother, and these incommensurables create a profound moral dilemma.

This may serve to bring the issue between utilitarian and theological views of life into focus (and to give the phrase in my title, "theological considerations," some specificity). If with the utilitarians and secularists, you are confident that human life is autonomous, in this world, and that human values are created and validated by social consensus, then, obviously, there are no "theological considerations" pertinent to this question (or any other)—and the rest of what I shall be saying is bound to sound a mite uncouth. For I am prepared to affirm, openly and without much embarrassment—except for my awareness of how unfashionable it may appear to some of you—that the primal origins, the continuing ground and final ends of human life are truly transcendental. In the Christian tradition, at least, to be human and personal is to be God's own special creation. Our lives and potentials are ours on trust from God. They are, therefore, never at our own selfish disposal. All our truly human experiences (identity, freedom, insight, hope, love) are also self-transcending—despite their being bracketed in space and time. The *humanum* is a genuine oddity, differing from its animal congeners not only in kind but in degree as well.[15] And, in the Christian tradition, this self-transcendence has been valued as a sign of life's *sacredness*—a way of pointing to God's involvement in, and concern for, the human enterprise. Thus, the notion of life's sacral quality places it over against all merely utilitarian codes.

Terms like "person," "personality," "personhood," "self" are all code-words for a trans-empirical reality. Whatever it is that they denote, it does not "exist" in space and time or in the causal nexus; all our efforts at introspection are infinitely regressive.[16] "Personhood" is not a *part* of the human organism, nor is it inserted into a process of organic development at some magic moment. It *is* the human organism oriented toward its transcendental matrix, in which it lives and moves and has its human being.[17] The self is "there" long before self-consciousness or any self-conscious acceptance or rejection of the primal intention which it represents. Thus, its lifeline stretches from an aboriginal God-knows-when to an eschatological God-knows-whenever—and all our efforts to draw precise lines between sub-human and truly human are dangerously parallel to our other efforts to distinguish between "inferior" and "superior" human beings.

In this theological perspective, therefore, "personhood" is a divine intention operating in a life-long process that runs from nidification till death.[18] It is never perfectly achieved and it is all too often thwarted in ways too tragic for glib rationalizations or even bitter tears. Our personhood is our identity, and this is always experienced as prevenient. *Homo est et qui est in futurus* (as Tertullian put it): "He who is ever going to be a man already is one."[19] Dr. Engelhardt has rightly observed that "stepping on a pile of acorns is not the same as destroying a forest of oaks."[20] But abortion is rather more like clipping off a sprouted *sapling,* and that's a categorically different business.

There is a human-biological continuum that is life-long, and there is also a human-personal continuum equally life-long—always in the making and always reaching out beyond. Both processes, unsurprisingly, have somatic substrates that are also life-long and concurrent. Our DNA codings are primal and perduring. The "hard-wired receptors" that make possible our earliest experiences are correlated with "the soft-wired receptors" that are malleable to culture—and they are active from birth to death.[21] Human thought and feeling are functions of cranial and blood-chemical processes and yet the brain does not secrete thought and blood-chemical explanations of consciousness are significantly inadequate. Instead of searching for magic moments when the subpersonal becomes personal, we would do better to envisage each individual human process as a unique slice of being, in which "personhood" is its "longitudinal axis"—each with its own divine intention and destiny.

One of Christianity's oldest traditions is the sacredness of human life, as implications of the Christian convictions about God and the good life. If all persons are equally the creatures of the one God, then none of these creatures is authorized to play god toward any other. And if all persons are cherished by God, regardless of merit, we ought also to cherish each other in the same spirit. This was the ground on which the early Christians rejected the prevalent Graeco-Roman codes of sexuality in which abortion and infanticide were commonplace.[22] It was not that these codes were not socially useful—as population controls, etc. —and they help cut down the welfare rolls! But the Christian moralists found them profoundly irreligious and proposed instead an ethic of compassion (adopted from their Jewish matrix) that proscribed abortion and encouraged "adoption."[23]

The theological ground for such an ethic was God's hallowing of life through sex and pregnancy, in the familial matrix. The value of this human life or that is not, in the first instance, "intrinsic." It comes, instead, from God's special and costing love. This impulse of compassion for the defenseless has always been the glory of the Christian ethic at its best. And despite our shameful record in practice (or malpractice!) its influence has been strong enough through the centuries to call down Nietzsche's scorn upon it as an ethic of weakness—unfit for any race of Supermen.

The essence of the tradition is that no human life has a right to its own *self*-enhancement at the cost of other human life. And it is all of human life that is sacred, from its mysterious origins to its equally mysterious ends. In the sex-procreation-fetus-infant-family syndrome we see a paradigm of human obligation at every level: freedom of choice issuing in consequences that are then accepted as personal and collective responsibilities. Care for the unborn is a mutuality between weaker and stronger. It is the essence of every relationship of unselfish love.

Always, therefore, we are driven back to this bedrock perplexity about the human status of the fetus and the neonate—and any warrants we may allege for their disposability. Obviously, the right to life is in no way absolute—death itself is sufficient evidence of *this!* There is, therefore, an undeniable case for some kinds of "therapeutic" abortions, and I would be greatly interested in the exploration of this category with a view to its possible enlargement—if such explorations could start from some higher view of fetal life than mere tissue.

My own conviction is that we not only lack *proof* that a fetus is mere tissue but that all the probabilities look the other way. And if it is only *probable* that a fetus is a human being—and thus personal, in the sense of being a divine intention—then we would do better to recognize abortion as a moral evil in every case and thus, even when chosen, a tragic option of what has been judged to be the lesser of two real evils. And if it is this serious, then every decision, for or against it, is a momentous crisis demanding the solemn involvement of *all* the parties concerned—and with all feasible alternatives conscientiously canvassed.[24]

The issue comes down to this: whether or not human-personal life is a real continuum[25] and whether or not it is truly sacred. For if it is, then fetal life, infant life, senescent life—even when "unwanted"—deserve humane care and compassion, even when pitted against the personal values of youthful or adult lives. And I believe that our continuing scruples against infanticide and euthanasia are the residues of an older conscience that where human *life* is at stake, life outweighs *utility.* Once *that* conscience goes, the only barriers between us and Auschwitz will be societal moods that, on their record, can give us very little real security.

Abortion is now *legal* (up to "viability")—and this leaves us with the agonizing *moral* issue as to whether, or whenever, it is "right" (still, I would insist, in the sense of the lesser of two evils). This shift from legal to moral grounds might very well be an advance—*if* the value-shaping agencies in our society were agreed that abortion *is* a life-and-death choice; *if* there were legal and social supports for conscientious doctors in their newly appointed role as killers as well as healers; *if* we had a general will in our society to extend our collective commitments to the unborn and the newly born; and *if,* above all, there were any prospects in our time for higher standards of responsible sexuality. What has actually happened, however, is that in our liberation from abortion as a "crime," many of us have also rejected any assessment of it as a *moral evil*—and this will further hasten the disintegration of our communal morality.

It has occasionally been explained to me somewhat impatiently, that an aging, WASP, male, theologian cannot possibly understand human realities and the human damage of unacceptable pregnancies—and, therefore, that all my notions about abortion are "academic." My response to this is also *ad hominem,* and it comes in two parts: the one frankly sentimental; the other, grimly prophetic. My personal sentiments in this matter root in the fact that we are adoptive parents and that none of our adopted children would have seen the light of day in these new times. To tell me *now* that the social values that might have accrued to their three anguished mothers (had they aborted) would have outweighed the human and personal worth of these three persons is, I'm afraid, moral nonsense.

And as for my prophetic forebodings, it seems certain that in America alone, over the next few years, millions of fetal lives will be snuffed out—*with little moral outcry!* There are ways of arguing that this is not comparable to the Nazi holocaust, or to the tragedy in Indo-China, or the widening stains of child abuse here at home. But it will be comparable statistically—and morally it will be even more ominous, for it will be sponsored by many whose professional ordinations are to healing and compassion. Moreover, it will have, for its rationalization, theories of fetal life that define it as a chattel to a mother's private value-judgments. Who then will be surprised if our human sensitivities are still further calloused, if sex becomes yet more promiscuous—with our scruples against euthanasia crumbling and the moral cements of our society dissolving?

I began by stressing how little we really can ever *know* about the mystery of human origins and, therefore, about the final grounds for human compassion.[26] And I'm still unable to *prove* the thesis that I have been urging: that human life is sacred and, therefore, precious at every point along the entire human lifeline. But, obviously, the alternative theories—which fix a point before which a fetus has no human standing—are equally *unproved* and unproveable. This leaves us at a dialogical impasse.

Our best recourse, in such a situation, is to look to the *practical* consequences of the two contrary perspectives, each taken in turn *as if* it were true. If fetal life is regarded *as if* it were human and sacred and potentially personal in some truly important sense—*as if* its values were rooted in its transcendental origins and ends—then it must not readily be violated by others on grounds of disparate self-interests. If, on the contrary, fetal life is viewed *as if* it were sub-human, *as if* its values were conferred on it, or denied it, by other human beings, in terms of self-interest or social sentiment, then abortion is a legitimate failsafe against defective births and beyond that, euthanasia an acceptable failsafe against lives no longer useful. By then, of course, abortion would have ceased to be the central issue, but rather human life itself. But that, precisely, is what this debate has been all about, all along!

Notes

1. Cf., e.g., Robert E. Cooke, ed., *The Terrible Choice: The Abortion Dilemma* (New York, 1968)—the proceedings of "An International Conference on Abortion," sponsored by Harvard Divinity School; or Kenneth Vaux, ed., *Who Shall Live?,* "The Houston Conference on Ethics in Medicine and Technology" (Philadelphia, 1970); or the even more recent *Symposium on the Beginnings of Personhood* at The Institute of Religion and Human Development (Houston, 1973) under the chairmanship of Dr. Albert Moracewski, O.P. See also *The Hastings Center Report,* Vol. 2, No. 5 (November, 1972).

2. Cf. Philip Rieff, *The Triumph of the Therapeutic* (London, 1966), p. xi and ch. I.

3. Cf. the Report of the decennial of the Lambeth Conference of Anglican Bishops (1960) and the special statement of the National Council of Churches (1961): "*All* Christians are agreed in condemning abortions [on demand]. . . . The destruction of life already begun cannot be condoned as a method of family limitation." Karl Barth (*Church Dogmatics* III-IV, 1961, pp. 415–16) called abortion "a monstrous thing"; Dietrich Bonhoeffer (*Ethics,* 1955, pp. 175–76) denounced it as "nothing but murder." Helmut Thielicke (*The Ethics of Sex,* 1964, p. 227) says that "in abortion, the order of creation is infringed upon. . . . " Cf. Robert F. Drinan, "Contemporary Protestant Thinking on Abortion" in *America,* #117 (December 9, 1967), pp. 713ff. By this time, though, Joseph Fletcher had joined the pro-abortionist ranks; cf. *Situation Ethics* (Westminster, 1966). Since then, the switch to official church support for abortion on demand has almost been pell-mell. Cf. *The Book of Discipline of the United Methodist Church,* Part III, §72-D.

4. Cf. *The New York Times,* April 18, 1973, for a report on the action to this effect by the *National Institutes of Health.*

5. Cf. the almost startling shift from his former position by an eminent black theologian, in C. Eric Lincoln's "Why I Reversed My Stand on Laissez-Faire Abortion," *The Christian Century,* Vol. XC, No. 17 (April 25, 1973), pp. 477–79.

6. Cf. D. R. G. Owen, *Body and Soul: A Study on the Christian View of Man* (Westminster, 1956).

7. From a one-sided interpretation of Descartes' dualism—the passivity of "body" (*res extensa*)—has come the mechanistic tradition of "Man, the Machine" that runs unbroken from Holbach and La Mettrie down to B. F. Skinner's *Beyond Freedom and Dignity* (Knopf, 1971).

8. "The Ontology of Abortion," February 16, 1973, p. 27. Cf. the lecture "The Beginnings of Personhood," May 15, 1973, p. 21: "There is *nothing* 'personal' about the fetus."

9. Roe *vs.* Wade, in *Supreme Court Reporter,* February 15, 1973.

10. Cf. Engelhardt's article in *Perkins Journal* 27 (Fall 1973): 20.

11. Cf. James Skinner, M. D., "Neurological Considerations Relevant to the Beginnings of Personhood," in the transcript of The Houston Symposium (1973), *op. cit.,* pp. 11-12; 76–78.

12. Cf. Robert Zeller, M.D., in The Houston Symposium, *op. cit.,* pp. 12–13.

13. Joshua Lederberg, "A Geneticist Looks at Contraception and Abortion," in *Annals of Internal Medicine,* Vol. 67, No. 3, Part 2 (September, 1967), pp. 26–27.

14. Engelhardt, in *Perkins Journal,* p. 20.

15. This is the central issue in Mortimer Adler, *The Difference of Man and the Difference It Makes* (New York:

Holt, Rinehart and Winston, 1967), and this is Adler's "conclusion," although he is very much aware of its problematic character. What is clear is that *if* men are to act and be treated as moral agents, a difference in kind is presupposed thereby (pp. 292-94).

16. Cf. a similar comment about "intelligence" in Carl Eisdorfer, M.D., "Intellectual and Cognitive Changes in the Aged," in Busse and Pfeiffer (eds.), *Behavior and Adaptation in Later Life* (Boston, 1969), p. 238.

17. Cf. St. Paul's reported allocution on Mars' Hill in Acts 17:24-28.

18. Cf. Karl Rahner, *Hominisation; The Evolutionary Origin of Man as a Theological Problem* (Herder & Herder, 1965).

19. Tertullian, *Apology,* IX: . . . *etiam fructus omnis iam in semine est* ("because the fruit is already in the seed").

20. Engelhardt, in *Perkins Journal,* p. 21.

21. An hypothesis of Dr. Skinner's, *op. cit.,* pp. 9-10.

22. Cf. W. E. H. Lecky, *History of European Morals, From Augustus to Charlemagne* (London, 1894), I, 45, 92, and II, 20-24. For example, "the general opinion among the ancients seems to have been that the foetus was but a part of the mother and that she had the same right to destroy it as to cauterise a tumour upon her body" (I, 92).

23. Cf. Lecky, *ibid.,* II, 20-24 on abortion; and then pp. 24-39 for a summary of Christianity's crusade against infanticide. See also David M. Feldman, *Birth Control in Jewish Law* (New York, 1968), Part 5, pp. 251-96, and Immanuel Jakobovitz, *Jewish Medical Ethics* (New York, 1959), especially pp. 190-91. Typical Christian condemnations of abortion and infanticide may be seen in Tertullian, *Apology,* IX, in Minucius Felix, *Octavius,* 30, and *The Epistle to Diognetus,* 5 ("Like everyone else, Christians marry and have children but they do not 'expose' their infants").

24. It is worth noting how casually, in a pro-abortion article in the April *Reader's Digest* (1973), p. 280, Dr. William Sweeney speaks of "killing the baby."

25. Cf. Louis Dupré, "A New Approach to the Abortion Problem," in The Houston Symposium (1973), p. 6. "If personhood is irreducible to its functions alone, its origins cannot be an acquired reality. This leaves us no choice but to place that origin at the beginning of human life. All human life then is personal at least in a minimal way, though by no means to an equal degree."

26. Cf. B. A. Brody, "Abortion and the Law" in *The Journal of Philosophy,* Vol. 68 (June, 1971), pp. 357-69 and especially p. 357: "The status of the fetus and of whether destroying the fetus constitutes the taking of a human life . . . seem difficult, if not impossible, to resolve on rational grounds [alone]." Brody concludes against abortion on demand because of the *possibility* of its involving the destruction of human life.

64.

Respect for Life in the Womb

Address to the Medical Association of Western Flanders (April 23, 1977)

PAUL VI

Modern medicine is becoming more and more remote from the uninitiated because both its techniques and its language have become so complicated. At the same time, however, the high scientific level every physician should attain must not be allowed to overshadow or lessen that sense of the human reality and that attention to persons which have always characterized the medical profession and been the source of its greatness.

In the matter of medical ethics, We wish to insist once again on the foundation of everything else, namely, an unconditional respect for life from its very beginnings. It is important to understand why this principle, so essential to every civilization worthy of the name, is today being challenged and why we must firmly oppose what is being improperly termed a "liberalization."

The Catholic Church has always regarded abortion as an abominable crime because unqualified respect for even the very beginnings of life is a logical consequence of the mysteries of creation and redemption. In our Lord Jesus Christ every human being, even one whose physical life is utterly wretched, is called to the dignity of a child of God. That is what our faith teaches us.

Every Christian must draw the necessary conclusions from this premise and not let himself be blinded by what are claimed to be social or political necessities.

Still less may he excuse himself on the ground that he must respect the opinions of those who do not share his convictions for, in this area, the Christian faith simply casts a further, supernatural light on a moral attitude which is a universal and basic demand imposed by every rightly formed conscience and which is, therefore, legitimately regarded as a requirement of humanness itself, that is, of human nature in the philosophical sense of the term.

Every Christian must attribute the proper importance to this higher morality, this unwritten law which exists in the very heart of man and alone can provide

From *The Pope Speaks* 22 (Fall 1977): 281-82. Used courtesy of Our Sunday Visitor, Inc.

a basis for an authentic social consensus and a legislation worthy of the name.

As doctors, moreover, as men and women who know the scientific and ethical norms of your profession, you have a special and very important role to play in informing and forming others, each of you according to your special competence, and in pointing out the serious errors on which propaganda for abortion is based. Who more than you are frequently in a position to denounce the manipulation of statistics, the overhasty claims in the area of biology and the disastrous physiological and psychological repercussions of abortion?

In encouraging you to fight on behalf of life, We do not forget—as We are sure you realize—the serious problems you face in the exercise of your profession. You need an enlightened conscience if you are to find practical solutions, often painful to implement, which will not sacrifice any of the values at stake. Is it not in this way that the role of physician, which is based on but involves more than technical competence, takes on its full dimensions: the role, We mean, of being a person to whom nothing human is alien?

In your researches may you advance equally in knowledge and in awareness of your responsibilities! You can be sure that We lift up your intentions to the Lord, asking him to bless you, your families and all who come to seek your help.

65. The Protection of Life

KARL BARTH

What makes a man an arbitrary killer is that, even though he knows he should not kill, after long or very short deliberation he thinks that he himself can decide that in his own particular case the killing of a man is not murder but a justifiable, necessary and even incontestable action, the co-existence of this fellow-man with himself and the world at large being so intolerable that he is under obligation to extinguish it. The arbitrary killer thus has his own morality. He is an arbitrary killer, and therefore a murderer, to the degree that this morality is exclusively his private morality, whether carefully weighed or discovered in a lightning flash of intuition. "Private" is derived from *privare.* He has constructed the exception out of his own sovereign opinion and in accordance with the *desiderata* of his situation. Ignoring the doubtful and arbitrary nature of his motives, he has appropriated to himself the right in a single person to act towards his fellow-man the roles of law-giver, judge and executioner. In so doing, he has allowed the wolf to break out. Setting up his private code of morality, independently deciding that the exception has arrived, and thus trying to put himself in the right, he commits a crime, falls under the corresponding guilt, and becomes what even he never meant to be, namely, a murderer.

We speak of him because his existence intensifies the warning under which alone we may approach the problems now calling for attention. We have not only to consider that, in virtue of the dark factor latently operative in all men, we are all a little too close to the murderer and are thus inclined to take these problems too lightly. We have also to realise that on every occasion on which even for what seem to be the best of reasons we count on the presence of the exceptional case, we move in the vicinity of the murderer and therefore in a very dangerous neighbourhood. Whenever we dare even think that the killing of men by men is not only not forbidden but even necessary in certain circumstances, there is always the possibility of the same *privare,* of the same independent construction of the exceptional case on the ground of very dubious and quite arbitrary desires, of the same

From Karl Barth, *Church Dogmatics,* III/4, trans. A. T. Mackay et al. (Edinburgh: T&T Clark, 1961), pp. 414-23. Used by permission.

attempted self-justification by moral sophistry. In such cases we are always in danger of approving that which the civil law with more or less assurance and consistency condemns as a crime and the command of God as a sin. The line which keeps us from falling under this condemnation will always be razor sharp, and how near we shall sometimes be to crossing it! But if this is a warning to be most circumspect, it must not deter us from being prepared point by point even in this dangerous neighbourhood to stand by the truth that at some time or other, perhaps on the far frontier of all other possibilities, it may have to happen in obedience to the commandment that men must be killed by men.

We mention first the problem of the deliberate interruption of pregnancy usually called abortion (*abortus,* the suppression of the fruit of the body). This question arises where conception has taken place but for varying reasons the birth and existence of the child are not desired and are perhaps even feared. The persons concerned are the mother who either carries out the act or desires or permits it, the more or less informed amateurs who assist her, perhaps the scientifically and technically trained physician, the father, relatives or other third parties who allow, promote, assist or favour the execution of the act and therefore share responsibility, and in a wider but no less strict sense the society whose conditions and mentality directly or indirectly call for such acts and whose laws may even permit them. The means employed vary from the most primitive to relatively sophisticated, but these need not concern us in the first instance. Our first contention must be that no pretext can alter the fact that the whole circle of those concerned is in the strict sense engaged in the killing of human life. For the unborn child is from the very first a child. It is still developing and has no independent life. But it is a man and not a thing, nor a mere part of the mother's body.

The embryo has its own autonomy, its own brain, its own nervous system, its own blood circulation. If its life is affected by that of the mother, it also affects hers. It can have its own illnesses in which the mother has no part. Conversely, it may be quite healthy even though the mother is seriously ill. It may die while the mother continues to live. It may also continue to live after its mother's death, and be eventually saved by a timely operation on her dead body. In short, it is a human being in its own right. . . .

Before proceeding, we must underline the fact that he who destroys germinating life kills a man and thus ventures the monstrous thing of decreeing concerning the life and death of a fellow-man whose life is given by God and therefore, like his own, belongs to Him. He desires to discharge a divine office, or, even if not, he accepts responsibility for such discharge, by daring to have the last word on at least the temporal form of the life of his fellow-man. Those directly or indirectly involved cannot escape this responsibility.

At this point again we have first and supremely to hear the great summons to halt issued by the command. Can we accept this responsibility? May this thing be? Must it be? Whatever arguments may be brought against the birth and existence of the child, is it his fault that he is here? What has he done to his mother or any of the others that they wish to deprive him of his germinating life and punish him with death? Does not his utter defencelessness and helplessness, or the question whom they are destroying, to whom they are denying a future even before he has breathed and seen the light of the world, wrest the weapon from the hand of his mother first, and then from all the others, thwarting their will to use it? Moreover, this child is a man for whose life the Son of God has died, for whose unavoidable part in the guilt of all humanity and future individual guilt He has already paid the price. The true light of the world shines already in the darkness of the mother's womb. And yet they want to kill him deliberately because certain reasons which have nothing to do with the child himself favour the view that he had better not be born! Is there any emergency which can justify this? It must surely be clear to us that until the question is put in all its gravity a serious discussion of the problem cannot even begin, let alone lead to serious results.

The mediaeval period, which in this case extended right up to the end of the 18th century, was therefore quite right in its presuppositions when it regarded and punished abortion as murder. It is indeed an action which in innumerable cases obviously has the character of murder, of an irresponsible killing which is both callous and wicked, and in which one or more or perhaps all the participants play more or less consciously an objectively horrible game. If only the rigour with which the past judged and acted in this matter, as in child murder strictly speaking, had been itself more just and not directed against the relatively least guilty instead of the relatively most guilty! If only its draconian attitude had at least made an impression on the consciousness of the people and formed even in later recollection an effective dyke against this crime! But it obviously failed to do this. For no sooner had this attitude decayed externally than its inner strength also collapsed, and transgression swept in full flood over the land.

In the circumstances there is something almost horribly respectable in the attitude of the Roman Church. Never sparing in its extreme demands on women, it has to this day remained inveterate and never changed its course an inch in this matter. In the encyclical *Casti connubii* of 1930 (Enc. 2242 f.), deliberate abortion is absolutely forbidden on any grounds, so that even Roman Catholic nuns raped when the Russians invaded Germany in 1945 were not allowed to free themselves from the consequences in this way.

This attitude of the Roman Church is undoubtedly impressive in contrast to the terrible deterioration, to what one might almost call the secret and open mass murder, which is the modern vogue and custom in this respect among so-called civilised peoples. This can be partly explained by the social and psychological conditions in which modern man finds himself, and by the estrangement from the Church and palpable paganism of the modern masses, the age of the *corpus Christianum* being now, as it seems, quite definitely a thing of the past. But there is more to it than this. It concerns both the rich and the poor, both those who suffer and are physically in danger and innumerable others who are in full or at least adequate possession of their spiritual balance. Nor is it restricted to the so-called world; it continues to penetrate deeply into the Christian community. It is a simple fact that the automatic restraint of the recognition that every deliberate interruption of pregnancy, whatever the circumstances, is a taking of human life, seems to have been strangely set aside in the widest circles in spite of our increasing biological appreciation of the facts. Even worse, the possibility of deliberate killing is sometimes treated as if it were just a ready expedient and remedy in a moment of embarrassment, nothing more being at issue than an unfortunate operation like so many others. In short, it can be and is done. Even official statistics tell us in a striking way how it can be and is done; and we may well suspect that these figures fall far short of the reality. It remains to be seen how legal regulation will finally work out where it is introduced, but the first result always seems to be a violent campaign for the widest possible interpretation.

Who is to say where the error and wickedness operative in this matter have their ultimate origin? Are they to be traced to the morality or immorality of the women and girls who are obviously for some reason troubled or distressed at their condition? Do they lie in the brutality or thoughtlessness of the men concerned? Are they to be sought in the offer of the sinister gentleman who makes use of both? Are we to look to the involved lack of conscientiousness in some medical circles? Do they originate in a general increase of self-pity in face of the injustices of life, which were surely just as great in the past as they are to-day? Or do they arise from a general decline in the individual and collective sense of responsibility?

We certainly cannot close our eyes to these happenings. Nor can we possibly concur in this development. Nevertheless, there can be no doubt that the abstract prohibition which was pronounced in the past, and which is still the only contribution of Roman Catholicism in this matter, is far too forbidding and sterile to promise any effective help.

The fact that a definite No must be the presupposition of all further discussion cannot be contested, least of all to-day. The question arises, however, how this No is to be established and stated if it is to be a truly effective No. In face of the wicked violation of the sanctity of human life which is always seriously at issue in abortion, and which is always present when it is carried out thoughtlessly and callously, the only thing which can help is the power of a wholly new and radical feeling of awe at the mystery of all human life as this is commanded by God as its Creator, Giver and Lord. Legal prohibitions and restrictions of a civil, moral and supposedly spiritual kind are obviously inadequate to instil this awe into man. Nor does mere churchmanship, whether Romanist or Protestant, provide the atmosphere in which this awe can thrive. The command of God is based on His grace. He summons man to the freedom in which he may live instead of having to live. At root, the man who thinks he must live cannot and will not respect life, whether his own or that of others, far less the life of an unborn child. If it is for him a case of "must" rather than "may," he lacks perspective and understanding in relation to what life is. He is already burdened and afflicted with his own life. He will only too readily explore and exploit all the supposed possibilities by which to shield himself from life which is basically hostile. He will also fall into the mistake of thinking that the life of the unborn child is not really human life at all, and thus draw the inference that he has been given a free hand to maintain or destroy it. Mothers, fathers, advisers, doctors, lawgivers, judges and others whom it may concern to desire, permit, execute or approve this action, will act and think in true understanding of the meaning of human life, and therefore with serious reluctance to take such a step, only if they themselves realise that human life is not something enforced but permitted, i.e., that it is freedom and grace. In these circumstances they will not be at odds with life, whether their own or that of their fellows. They will not always desire to be as comfortable as possible in relation to it. They will not simply take the line of least resistance in what they think and do concerning it. Those who live by mercy will always be disposed to practise mercy, especially to a human being which is so dependent on the mercy of others as the unborn child.

This brings us back to the point at which we cannot evade the question where was and is the witness of the Protestant Church in face of this rising flood of disaster. This Church knows and has the Word of the free mercy of God which also ascribes and grants freedom to man. It could and can tell and show a humanity which is tormented by life because it thinks it must live it, that it may do so. It could and can give it this testimony of freedom, and thus appeal effectively for the protection of life, inscribing upon its heart and conscience a salutary and resolute No to all and therefore to this particular destruction of human life. Hence it neither could nor can range itself with the Roman Catholic Church and its hard preaching of the Law. It must proclaim its own message in this matter, namely, the Gospel. In so doing, however, it must not underbid the severity of the Roman Catholic No. It must overbid its abstract and negative: "Thou shalt not," by the force of its positive: "Thou mayest," in which, of course, the corresponding: "Thou mayest not," is included, the No having the force not merely of the word of man but of the Word of God. The Protestant Church had and has this Word of God for man but against his depravity in so far as its task was and is to bear witness to it. For this reason it cannot have clean hands in face of the disastrous development. It need not enquire whether or not it has restrained this development, or may still do so. The truth is plain that it has not been faithful to its own commission in the past, but that its attitude has resembled far too closely that of the Roman Church, i.e., that it has been primarily a teacher of the Law. The truth is also plain that only now is it beginning to understand its commission, and that it has not yet grasped it with a firm hand. It is still almost with joy that we hear perspicacious doctors, perhaps of very different beliefs (cf. Lk. 16^8), express a view which the Protestant Church, if it had listened and borne witness to the Word of God, ought to have stated and championed long since, namely, the kindly and understanding No which will prevail as such.

At this point it may be interjected that, when this No is established as a divine No, namely, when it is in virtue of the liberating grace of God that deliberate abortion is irrefutably seen to be sin, murder and transgression, it cannot possibly be maintained that there is no forgiveness for this sin. However dangerous it might sound in relation to all that has been said thus far, it must also be said that in faith, and in a vicariously intercessory faith for others too, there is a forgiveness which can be appropriated even for this sin, even for the great modern sin of abortion. God the Creator, who by His grace acquits and liberates man that he may live and let live in the most serious sense, who in and by this liberation claims man incontestably as the great protector of life, who inexorably reveals the true character of man's transgression as sin—this God is our Father in Jesus Christ, in whom He has not rejected sinful man but chosen him for Himself and reconciled him to Himself, in whom He Himself has intervened for sinful man who has violated His command, in order that the latter may not be lost to him even in and by reason of this terrible transgression. God sees and understands and loves even modern man in and in spite of all the dreadful confusions and entanglements of his collective and individual existence, including this one. Those who see themselves placed by the Gospel in the light of the relevant command, and are thus forced to admit that they, too, are in some degree entangled in this particular transgression, and are willing, therefore, to accept solidarity with more blatant transgressors, cannot and will not let go the fact, nor withhold it from others, that the same Gospel which reveals this with such dreadful clarity is the Gospel which, proclaiming the kingdom of God to all, summons all to repentance and promises and offers forgiveness to all. Nor does it weaken the command and its unconditional requirement that the one free grace, which in its one dimension unmasks sin as such, implies in the other that God has loved this sinful world in such a way that He has given His Son, and in Him Himself, on its behalf, that it should not perish. Without this second dimension we cannot really understand the first. Indeed, only those who really grasp the promise of divine forgiveness will necessarily realise that sin as such is inexorably opposed by the divine No, and will never be able to keep this either from themselves or others.

If the No is securely grounded as seen from this angle, it inevitably raises here, too, the problem of the exception. Human life, and therefore the life of the unborn child, is not an absolute, so that, while it can be protected by the commandment, it can be so only within the limits of the will of Him who issues it. It cannot claim to be preserved in all circumstances, whether in relation to God or to other men, i.e., in this case to the mother, father, doctor and others involved. In His grace God can will to preserve the life which He has given, and in His grace He can will to take it again. Either way, it is not lost before Him. Men cannot exercise the same sovereignty in relation to it. It does not really lie in their power even to preserve it. And only by an abuse of their power, by a sinister act of overweening arrogance, can they wilfully take it. But they do have the power, and are thus commissioned, to do in the service of God and for the preservation of life that which is humanly possible if not finally decisive. Trained in the freedom which derives from the grace of God, they can choose and will only the one thing. In the case of the unborn, the mother, father, doctor (whose very vocation is to serve the preservation and development of life) and all concerned, can desire only its life and healthy birth. How can they possibly will the opposite? They can do so only on the presupposition of their own blindness towards life, in bondage to the opinion that they must live rather than that they may live, and therefore out of anxiety, i.e., out of gracelessness and therefore godlessness.

On the other hand, they cannot set their will absolutely upon the preservation of this life, or rather upon the service of its preservation. They all stand in the service of God. He orders them to serve its preservation and therefore the future birth of the child. There is an almost infinite number of objections to the possibility of willing anything else in obedience to Him. But it is not quite infinite. If a man knows that he is in God's service and wills to be obedient to Him, can he really swear that he will never on any occasion will anything else as God may require? What grounds have we for the absolute thesis that in no circumstances can God will anything but the preservation of a germinating life, or make any other demand from the mother, father, doctor or others involved? If He can will that this germinating life should die in some other way, might He not occasionally do so in such a way as to involve the active participation of these other men? How can we deny absolutely that He might have commissioned them to serve Him in this way, and that their action has thus been performed, and had to be performed, in this service? How, then, can we indict them in these circumstances?

This is the exceptional case which calls for discussion. In squarely facing it, we are not opening a side-door to the crime which is so rampant in this sphere. We refer to God's possibility and His specific command. We cannot try to exclude this. Otherwise the No which has to be pronounced in every other case is robbed of its force. For, as we have seen, it is truly effective only as the divine No. Hence no human No can or should be given the last word. The human No must let itself be limited. God can limit this human No, and, if He does so, it is simply human obstinacy and obduracy and transgression to be absolutely logical and to try to execute the No unconditionally. Let us be quite frank and say that there are situations in which the killing of germinating life does not constitute murder but is in fact commanded.

We hasten to lay down some decisive qualifications. For these will be situations in which all the arguments for preservation have been carefully considered and properly weighed, and yet abortion remains as *ultima ratio.* If all the possibilities of avoiding this have not been taken into account in this decision, then murder is done. Genuine exceptions will thus be rare. If they occur too often, and thus become a kind of second rule, we have good reason to suspect that collective and individual transgression and guilt are entailed. Again, they will be situations in which all those concerned must answer before God in great loneliness and secrecy, and make their decision accordingly. If the decision has any other source; if it is only the result of their subjective reflection and agreement, this fact alone is enough to show that we are not dealing with the genuine exception in which this action is permitted and commanded. With these qualifications, there are undoubtedly situations of this kind.

And we can and must add that, even if only in general terms and in the sense of a guiding line, these situations may always be known by the concrete fact that in them a choice must be made for the protection of life, one life being balanced against another, i.e., the life of the unborn child against the life or health of the mother, the sacrifice of either the one or the other being unavoidable. It is hard to see why in such cases the life of the child should always be given absolute preference, as maintained in Roman Catholic ethics. To be sure, we cannot and must not maintain, on the basis of the commandment, that the life and health of the mother must always be saved at the expense of the life of the child. There may well be mothers who for their part are ready to take any risk for their unborn children, and how can we forbid them to do so? On the basis of the command, however, we can learn that when a choice has to be made between the life or health of the mother and that of the child, the destruction of the child in the mother's womb might be permitted and commanded, and with the qualifications already mentioned a human decision might thus be taken to this effect. It goes without saying that the greatest possible care must be exercised in its practical execution. That is to say, it cannot be left to the mother herself or to quacks, but is a matter for the experienced and trained physician. More detailed consideration would take us rather beyond the sphere of ethics. The question obviously arises in what particular circumstances and from what standpoint the life of the mother might be regarded as in peril, and therefore this alternative indicated. To try to answer this question, however, is to expose oneself to the risk of making assertions which inevitably prove to be either too broad or too narrow from the standpoint of ethics, especially theological ethics. We must be content, therefore, simply to make our general point.

Physicians and lawyers speak in terms of the "indication" of abortion, a distinction being made between medical (whether somatic or psychiatric) on the one side and social on the other. The Swiss Penal Code regards it as nonindictable in an emergency, generally defined as a danger to life, body, freedom, honour or capacity, which cannot be averted in any other way (§ 34). In practice, however, it allows it only where there exists an immediate danger which cannot otherwise be warded off, or the risk of severe and permanent injury to the health of the pregnant woman. It also insists that it be undertaken by a certified doctor who is under obligation to report it to the responsible cantonal authorities (§ 120). It will be seen that this is in line with what we have just said. It must be remembered, however, that by no means every action allowed and exempted from punishment even on a strict, let alone a laxer, interpretation of these rules is for this reason permitted and enjoined ethically, i.e., by the command of God, as if those involved did not have to keep to a much narrower restriction of "indication" than that of the law. On the other hand, while Swiss legislation finds valid reason for abortion in an emergency affecting the life or body of the pregnant woman, the same does not hold good of an emergency affecting her freedom, honour or capacity. This means that, whereas medical "indication" is fully accepted, sound reasons are seen for not including social, and therefore for its implicit rejection. It does not follow, however, that a doctor is generally and radically guilty of transgressing the command of God, though he may expose himself to legal penalty, if he thinks he should urge a socio-medical "indication," i.e., in terms of a threat presented to the physical or mental life of the mother, or of economic or environmental conditions. For occasionally the command of God may impose a judgment and action which go beyond what is sanctioned by the law, and this may sometimes serve as a summons to all of us to consider that a sound social policy might well be a most powerful weapon in the struggle against criminal abortion. The legal rules are obviously useful, and even have an indirect ethical value as general directions to those involved, particularly doctors and judges. On the other hand, they are not adapted to serve as ethical criteria, since obedience to the command of God must have the freedom to move within limits which may sometimes be narrower and sometimes broader than even the best civil law. The exceptional case in the ethical sense is in general something very different from an extension of the permissible and valid possibilities established by human law.

The required calculation and venture in the decision between life and death obviously cannot be subject to any human law, because no such law can grasp the fulness of healthy or sick, happy or unhappy, preserved or neglected human life, let alone the freedom of the divine command and the obedience which we owe to it. Hence we shall have to be content with the following observations. 1. For all concerned what must be at stake must be life against life, nothing other nor less, if the decision is not to be a wrong decision and the resultant action murder either of the child or the mother. 2. There is always required the most scrupulous calculation and yet also a resolute venture with a conscience which is bound and therefore free. Where such thought as is given is only careless or clouded, and the decision weak and hesitant, sin couches at the door. 3. The calculation and venture must take place before God and in responsibility to Him. Otherwise, how can there possibly be obedience, and how can the content be good and right, even though apparently good human reasons and justification might be found in one direction or another? 4. Since the calculation and venture, the conviction that we are dealing with the exception, are always so dangerous, they surely cannot be executed with the necessary assurance and joy except in faith that God will forgive the elements of human sin involved.

66.
A Protestant Ethical Approach

JAMES M. GUSTAFSON

In the ethics of abortion, the differences of opinion surface not only on the substantial moral question of whether it is permissible but also on the question of what is the proper method of moral reflection. The two questions are not entirely independent of each other, as this essay demonstrates. Catholics and Protestants have been divided on the question of method, as well as on the substantial moral judgment.

I. Salient Aspects of Traditional Catholic Arguments

Any Protestant moralist writing about abortion is necessarily indebted to the work of his Roman Catholic colleagues. Their work on this subject shows historical learning that is often absent among Protestants; it shows philosophical acumen exercised with great finesse once their starting principles are accepted; it shows command of the medical aspects of abortion beyond what one finds in cursory Protestant discussions; and it shows extraordinary seriousness about particular moral actions. Debt must also be acknowledged to the contemporary Protestant moralist who has learned most profoundly from the Catholics, namely Paul Ramsey, for his voluminous writing about problems of war and of medical ethics have introduced a note of intellectual rigor into Protestant ethics that was too often absent.

Every moral argument, no matter who makes it and what is the issue at hand, must limit the factors that are brought into consideration. No one can handle all possible relevant bits of data, ranges of value, sources of insight, and pertinent principles in a manageable bit of discourse. What one admits to the statement of the moral issue in turn is crucial to the solutions given to it. The determination of which factors or principles are primary, or at least of greater importance than others, in the way one argues is also fairly decisive for the outcome of the argument. The traditional Catholic arguments about abortion can be characterized in part by the following delineations of the perspective from which they are made.[1]

First, the arguments are made by an *external judge.* They are written from the perspective of persons who claim the right to judge the past actions of others as morally right or wrong, or to tell others what future actions are morally right or wrong. To make the point differently, moral responsibility is ascribed to others for their actions, or it is prescribed or proscribed.

The perspective of the external judge can be distinguished from those of the persons who are more immediately involved in an abortion situation. It is clear, of course, that those involved, for example, physicians or mothers, might interpret their situations in terms that they have been taught by the external judges. Even if they do, however, the *position of personal responsibility* that physicians, mothers, and others have is different from that of the writer of a manual of moral theology, or of the priest who judges the moral rectitude of others and determines the penance that is to be required. To assume responsibility for an action is quite a different order of experience from ascribing responsibility to others for an action.[2] Physicians, mothers, and others are initiators of action, they are agents in the process of life who determine to a great extent what actually occurs. Their relationship to a situation involves their senses of accountability for consequences, their awareness of particular antecedents (for example, the conditions under which a pregnancy occurred), their sensibilities and emotions, their private past experiences and their private aspirations for the future, their personal commitments and loyalties.

Second, the arguments are made on a basically *juridical model.* The action is right or wrong depending on whether it conforms to or is contrary to a rule, a law, and the outcome of a moral argument. The rules or laws, of course, are defended on theological and philosophical grounds; they are not arbitrary fiats imposed by an authoritarian institution. Traditional authorities are cited; theological and philosophical principles are given to support the rules; the consequences of different possible courses of action are considered. The argument's principal terms and its logic, however, are directed toward the possibility of defining a morally right act and a morally wrong act. As with the civil law, there is a low tolerance for moral ambiguity. The advantages of this for the person whose behavior conforms to the outcome of the authoritative argument is that he probably can act with a "clear conscience," and he can justify his actions on the basis of authorities other than himself. His own responsibility for his actions, including its

---

Reprinted by permission of the publishers from *The Morality of Abortion: Legal and Historical Perspectives,* edited by John T. Noonan, Jr., Cambridge, Mass.: Harvard University Press,

consequences, is decisively limited, for with reference to the juridical model of morality he has done what is determined by those whose authority he accepts to be correct. If the primary agents of action, mothers and physicians, for example, do not judge themselves only in the light of the rules, if they exercise the virtue of prudence, and the virtue of *epikeia,* or equity in interpreting the law in a particular case, they are in a slightly different situation. Their own degree of responsibility is increased, and yet they have the advantage of the clarity of reflection that is given in the moral prescription.

The juridical model can be distinguished from others that view the justification for the moral rectitude of actions in different ways or that have different views of how moral judgments are to be made. Some persons have sought virtually to quantify the good and ill effects of courses of action, and as a result of this have suggested that action which assures the greatest good for the greatest number is right. Others have relied heavily on "moral sentiment" to be sensitive to the moral issues in a situation, and relied upon compassion, the sense of altruism, or the sense of moral indignation to determine the act. Some have relied upon insight and rational intuition to size up what is going on in a time and place and to discern what the proper human response ought to be. Or "love" has been asserted to have sufficient perspicacity and motivating power to enable one to perceive what is right in a situation. It has been cogently argued that morality develops out of experience, and that when laws become abstracted from experience, their informing and persuasive powers begin to evaporate.

Third, the traditional Catholic arguments largely confine the relevant data to *the physical.* The concern is with physical life, its sanctity and its preservation. Obviously, other aspects of human life depend upon the biological basis of the human body, and thus the primacy of this concern is valid. But on the whole, the arguments have not been extended to include concern for the emotional and spiritual well-being of the mother or the infant. The concern has been largely for the physical consequences of abortion.

Fourth, the arguments are limited by concerning themselves almost *exclusively with the physician and the patient* at the time of a particular pregnancy, isolating these two from the multiple relationships and responsibilities each has to and for others over long periods of time. The obvious basis for this is that the physician has to decide about abortions with individual patients as these patients come to him. But he also has responsibilities for the well-being of the whole of his society, and for the spiritual and moral well-being of the patient's family. It could be argued that there is no dissonance between what would be decided in a particular relationship between two people and what is good for society, but that is not self-evident. The focus on the mother's physical condition, and on her as a statistical instance of a general and uniform category of mothers, makes it difficult to consider this particular mother, her particular relationships, and her past spiritual as well as physical history. For example, arguments pertaining to "saving the life of the mother" do not admit as important evidence such factors as whether she is the mother of six other children dependent upon her, or no other children. In some other ways of discussing abortion such information might make a difference in the argument. I am suggesting that the time and space limits one uses to isolate what is "the case" have a considerable effect on the way one argues.

Fifth, the traditional Catholic arguments are *rationalistic.* Obviously to make an argument one has to be rational, and to counter an argument one deems to be rationalistic he has to show what would be better reasons for arguing differently. What I refer to as rationalistic can be seen in the structure of many of the sections of the manuals of moral theology that deal with questions such as abortion, or the structure of manuals of medical ethics. One often finds brief assertions of "fundamental truths" which include definitions of terms used in these truths or in subsequent arguments. This might be followed by "basic principles" which will include distinctions between the kinds of law, principles pertaining to conscience, principles of action, a definition of the principle of double effect, and others. The principle of the sanctity or inviolability of human life is discussed at great length since its application is primary to particular cases.

One must recognize that any argument about abortion will use principles. But the rationalistic character of the arguments seems to reduce spiritual and personal individuality to abstract cases. The learning from historical experiences with their personal nuances seems to be squeezed out of the timeless abstractions. The sense of human compassion for suffering and the profound tragedy which is built into any situation in which the taking of life is morally plausible are gone. Individual instances must be typified in order to find what rubric they come under in the manual. While it is eminently clear that any discussion must abstract facts and principles from the vitality and complexity of lived-experience, the degree of abstraction and the deductive reasoning of the traditional Catholic arguments remove the issues far from life. The alternative is not to wallow in feeling and visceral responses, nor is it to assume that one's deep involvement with the persons in a situation and one's awareness of the inexorable concreteness of their lives are sufficient to resolve the issues. But an approach which is more personal and experientially oriented is another possibility.

Sixth, the traditional perspective seeks to develop arguments that are based on *natural law,* and thus ought to be persuasive and binding on all men. Intentionally the particular historical standpoint and substance of the Christian message are subordinated to the natural law in the arguments. To be sure, arguments can be given for the consistency between the natural law and particular Christian affirmation; also any one who would begin with particular Christian affirmations would have to show their viability on moral questions to those who did not share his religious outlook and convictions. To indicate that arguments from natural law can be distinguished from arguments that place particular historical aspects of Christian thought at a different point in the discussion is not to assert that the answer to questions about abortion can be found in "revelation," or that the use of human reason is less necessary. It is to suggest, however, that one's basic perspective toward life might be altered, and one's ordering of values might be different if the first-order affirmations dealt with God's will not only to preserve his creation, but to redeem it. One's attitude toward the persons involved might well be more tolerant, patient, loving, and forgiving, rather than judgmental. One might look for consistency between one's principles and the great themes of the Christian faith at a more central place in the discussion than the traditional Catholic arguments do. To predict that the outcome of the argument would be greatly different in every case would be folly, though it might very well be in some cases. Since theologically based moral arguments, like all others, are arguments made by human beings, many other factors than commonly held convictions enter into them.

These six points are meant to provide a descriptive delineation of salient aspects of traditional Catholic arguments. I have sought to indicate that alternative ways of working are possible with regard to each of them. To claim them to be insufficient or invalid without providing an alternative would be presumptuous. As a way of suggesting and exploring an alternative, I shall describe a situation, and indicate how I would go about making and justifying my moral judgment pertaining to it. In its basic structure it is in accord with the situations of persons who have sought me out for counsel, although for various reasons I have made a composite description.

II. A Discussion of a Human Choice

The pregnant woman is in her early twenties. She is a lapsed Catholic, with no significant religious affiliation at the present time, although she expresses some need for a "church." Her marriage was terminated by divorce; her husband was given custody of three children by that marriage. She had an affair with a man who "befriended" her, but there were no serious prospects for a marriage with him, and the affair has ended. Her family life was as disrupted and as tragic as that which is dramatically presented in Eugene O'Neill's *Long Day's Journey into Night.* Her alcoholic mother mistreated her children, coerced them into deceptive activity for her ends, and was given to periods of violence. Her father has been addicted to drugs, but has managed to continue in business, avoid incarceration, and provide a decent income for his family. The pregnant woman fled from home after high school to reside in a distant state, and has no significant contact with her parents or siblings. She has two or three friends.

Her pregnancy occurred when she was raped by her former husband and three other men after she had agreed to meet him to talk about their children. The rapes can only be described as acts of sadistic vengeance. She is unwilling to prefer charges against the men, since she believes it would be a further detriment to her children. She has no steady job, partially because of periodic gastro-intestinal illnesses, and has no other income. There are no known physiological difficulties which would jeopardize her life or that of the child. She is unusually intelligent and very articulate, and is not hysterical about her situation. Termination of the pregnancy is a live option for her as a way to cope with one of the many difficulties she faces.

The Christian Moralist's Responsible Relationship

In indicating that the position of writers of moral argument about abortion in traditional Catholicism is that of an external judge, I did not wish to suggest that priests are not compassionate, understanding, and loving in their relationships to physicians and to mothers, nor did I intend to suggest that they overrule the liberty of conscience of others through authoritarian ecclesiastical sanctions. No doubt some have acted more like rigorous judges than loving pastors, but many have been patient, tolerant, loving, and aware of the limitations of any human authority. (This is not the place to raise the difficult problem of the magisterial authority of the Church, which logically could be raised here, an authority still used to threaten, coerce, and suspend dissident voices.) I do wish to suggest, however, that I believe the responsible relation of a Christian moralist to other persons precludes the primacy of the judgmental posture, either in the way we write or in the way we converse with others.

The moralist responding to this woman can establish one of a number of ways of relating to her in his conversations. The two extremes are obvious. On the one hand, he could determine that no physiological difficulties seem to be present in the pregnancy, and thus seek to enforce her compliance with the standard rule against abortions. The manuals would decide what right conduct is; her predicament would be defined so that factors that are important for others who respond to her are not pertinent to the decision about abortion. Both the moralist and the woman could defer further moral responsibility to the textbooks. On the other hand, he could take a highly permissive approach to the conversation. In reliance on a theory of morality that would minimize the objective moral considerations, and affirm that what a person feels is best is morally right, he could affirm consistently what her own dominant disposition seemed to be, and let that determine the decision.

Somewhere between these is what I would delineate as a more responsible relationship than either of the two extremes. It would recognize that the moralist and the woman are in an interpersonal relationship; this is to say that as human beings they need to be open to each other, to have a high measure of confidence in each other, to have empathy for each other. Obviously the moralist, like any other counsellor, is in a position to have more disclosed to him than he discloses of himself to the other, and he has professional competence that enables him to be relatively objective within the intersubjectivity of the relationship. But as a Christian moralist his obligation is first to be open and to understand the other, not to judge and to prescribe. He will recognize that his judgement, and that of others who have informed him, while learned, mature, and hopefully sound, remains the judgment of a finite being with all the limitations of his perspective. He will, in a situation like this, acknowledge the liberty of her conscience, and will not immediately offer an authoritative answer to her question; indeed, the context of her question, and its nuances might make it a subtly different question than the one the textbooks answer. All this is not to say that he has nothing to contribute to the conversation. As a moralist he is to help her to objectify her situation, to see it from other perspectives than the one she comes with. He is to call to her attention not only alternative courses of action with some of the potential consequences of each (including the violation of civil law), but also the value of life and those values which would have to be higher in order to warrant the taking of life. He is to help her to understand her past, not as a way of excusing anything in the present, but as a way of gaining some objectivity toward the present. He is to find what constitutes her moral integrity and convictions, her desires and ends. He may find himself bringing these into the light of other ends which he deems to be important, or he may find himself inquiring whether potential courses of action are more or less in accord with the values and convictions she has. It is his obligation as a Christian moralist to bring the predicament into the light of as many subjective and objective considerations as his competence permits, including concerns for the wider moral order of the human community of which she is a part as this is sustained in civil laws.

Salient Facts in One Christian Moralist's Interpretation

The relationship of a moralist to a person who seeks conversation with him is by no means simple. Thus it is not easy to isolate what the salient facts of the predicament are, and to give a ready valence to each of them. Efforts at this analytical task are incumbent upon him, but he also *perceives* the person and the situation in some patterns or in a single whole pattern which already establish in his perception some of the relationships between the factors. He never confronts the salient facts as isolates, or as discrete entities that can be added arithmetically into a sum. The person confronts him not as isolable elements, and her experiences are not detached moments only chronologically related to each other. He does not respond to her any more than he responds to a portrait first of all as a series of colors, or a series of lines. He can in reflection discriminate between the colors and talk about the lines, but even then these are in particular relationships to each other in the portrait, and in his perception of it. He does not perceive the woman in pure objectivity, nor as she perceives her own predicament, though obviously he seeks to have his own perception informed by the actual predicament insofar as possible. Even in this, however, his perspective conditions how he "sees" and "feels" the relationships between factors that can be abstracted and isolated. This preface to a statement of salient facts is important, for it precludes both oversimplification and dogmatic analytical authority. He can never say to another person, "In comparable situations find out the answers to the following factual questions, and you will have an accurate picture of the predicament."

In the personal situation under discussion, it is clear that if medical factors alone were to be considered grounds for an abortion, none would be morally permissible. The woman had three pregnancies that came to full term, and the children were healthy. To the best of her knowledge there are no medical problems at the present time. Periodic gastro-intestinal illnesses, which might be relieved with better medical care, would not be sufficient medical grounds. Although the present pregnancy is disturbing for many reasons, including both the occasion on which the pregnancy occurred and the future social prospects for the woman and the child, in the judgment of the moralist the woman is able to cope with her situation without serious threat to her mental health. The medical factors, insofar as the moralist can grasp them, would not warrant a therapeutic abortion.

Legal factors potentially involved in this situation are serious. First, and most obvious, the woman resides in a state where abortion of pregnancies due to sexual crimes is not at present legally permissible. Since there are not sufficient grounds for a therapeutic abortion, a request to a physician would put him in legal jeopardy. Even if abortion was permissible because of the rapes, this woman was unwilling to report the rapes to the police since it involved her former husband and had potential implications for the care of her children. To report the rapes would involve the woman in court procedures which seem also to require time and energy that she needs to support herself financially. To seek an abortion on conscientious moral grounds would be to violate the law, and to implicate others in the violation. Not to press charges against the rapists is to protect them from prosecution. Disclosure of the rapes would make the abortion morally justifiable in the eyes of many, but it might lead to implications for her children. The legal factors are snarled and are complicated by social factors.

The moralist has to reckon with the financial plight of the woman. She is self-supporting, but her income is irregular. There are no savings. Application for welfare support might lead to the disclosure of matters she wishes to keep in confidence. If a legal abortion was possible, the physician would receive little or no remuneration from the patient. There are no funds in sight to finance an illegal abortion, and the medical risks involved in securing a quack rule that out as a viable prospect. The child, if not aborted, could be let out for adoption, and means might be found to give minimum support for the mother during pregnancy. If she should choose to keep the child, which is her moral right to do, there are no prospects for sufficient financial support, although with the recovery of her health the woman could join the work force and probably with her intelligence earn a modest income.

The spiritual and emotional factors involved are more difficult to assess. While the moralist is impressed with the relative calm with which the woman converses about her predicament, he is aware that this ability is probably the result of learning to cope with previous inhumane treatment and with events that led to no happy ending. Socially, she is sustained only by two or three friends, and these friendships could readily be disrupted by geographical mobility. She has no significant, explicit religious faith, and as a lapsed Catholic who views the Church and its priests as harsh taskmasters, she is unwilling to turn to it for spiritual and moral sustenance. She has a profound desire not merely to achieve a situation of equanimity, of absence of suffering and conflict, but also to achieve positive goals. Her mind is active, and she has read fairly widely; she expresses the aspiration to go to college, to become a teacher, or to engage in some other professional work, both for the sake of her self-fulfillment and for the contribution she can make to others. She has not been defeated by her past. She can articulate the possibility of keeping the child, and see the child as part of the world in which there would be some realization of goals, especially since she has been deprived of her other children. She has confidence, she has hope, and she seems to be able to love, though she wonders what else could happen to make her life any more difficult than it is. She carries something of a guilt load; the courts gave custody of her three children to the husband because of adultery charges against her. Yet, her interpretation of that marriage in her youth was that it freed her from her parental home, but that the marriage itself was a "prison." She responds to the rapes more in horror than in hatred, but is too close to that experience to know its long-range impact on her.

The more readily identifiable moral factors are three, though in the ethical perspective of this paper, this constitutes an oversimple limitation of the "moral" and of the nature of moral responsibility. One is the inviolability of life, the sanctity of life. My opinion is that since the genotype is formed at conception, all the genetic potentialities of personal existence are there. Thus it is to be preserved unless reasons can be given that make an exception morally justifiable. A second is rape—not only a crime, but a morally evil deed. The sexual relations from which the pregnancy came were not only engaged in against the woman's will, but were in her judgment acts of retaliation and vengeance. The third is the relation of morality to the civil law. If abortion were considered to be morally justifiable, to have it done would be to break the civil law. It would be an act of conscientious objection to existing laws, and is susceptible to scrutiny by the moral arguments that pertain to that subject in itself.

All of these factors in isolated listing, and others that could be enumerated, do not add up to a moral decision. They are related to each other in particular ways, and the woman is related to her own ends, values, and to other beings. And the moralist's relationship is not that of a systems analyst sorting out and computing. His relationship is one of respect and concern for the person; it is colored by his perspective. It is necessary, then, to state what seem to be the factors that are present in the perspective of the moralist that influence his interpretation and judgment.

Salient Aspects of the Moralist's Perspective

The perception and the interpretation of the moralist are not a simple matter to discuss. It would be simpler if the author could reduce his perspective to: (a) theological and philosophical principles; (b) moral inferences drawn from these; and (c) rational application of these principles to a narrowly defined case. But more than belief, principles, and logic are involved in the moral decision. A basic perspective toward life accents certain values and shadows others. Attitudes, affections, and feelings of indignation against evil, compassion for suffering, and desire for restoration of wholeness color one's interpretation and judgment. Imagination, sensitivity, and empathy are all involved. For Christians, and many others presumably, love is at work, not merely as a word to be defined, and as a subject of propositions so that inferences can be drawn from it, but love as a human relationship, which can both move and inform the other virtues, including prudence and equity (to make a reference to St. Thomas). All of this does not mean that a moral judgment is a total mystery, it does not mean that it is without objectivity.

The perspective of the Christian moralist is informed and directed by his fundamental trust that the forces of life seek the human good, that God is good, is love. This is a matter of trust and confidence, and not merely a matter of believing certain propositions to be true. (I believe certain statements about my wife to be true, including the statement that she wills and seeks my good, but the reasons for my trust in her cannot be described simply by such a statement.) Yet the way in which I state my convictions about this trust defines in part my moral perspective and my fundamental intentionality. (What I know *about* my wife sustains my trust in her, and in part sets the direction of our marriage.) Life, and particularly human life, is given to men by God's love: physical being dependent upon genetic continuity; the capacity of the human spirit for self-awareness, responsiveness, knowledge, and creativity; life together in human communities, in which we live and care for others and others live and care for us.

God wills the creation, preservation, reconciliation, and redemption of human life. Thus, one can infer, it is better to give and preserve life than to take it away; it is better to prevent its coming into being than to destroy it when it has come into being. But the purposes of God for life pertain to more than physical existence: there are conditions for human life that need delineation: physical health, possibilities for future good and meaning that engender and sustain hope, relationships of trust and love, freedom to respond and initiate and achieve, and many others. The love of God, and in response to it, the loves of men, are particularly sensitive to "the widow, the orphan, and the stranger in your midst," to the oppressed and the weak.

These brief and cryptic statements are the grounds for moral biases: life is to be preserved, the weak and the helpless are to be cared for especially, the moral requisite of trust, hope, love, freedom, justice, and others are to be met so that human life can be meaningful. The bias gives a direction, a fundamental intention that does not in itself resolve the darknesses beyond the reach of its light, the ambiguities of particular cases. It begins to order what preferences one would have under ideal conditions and under real conditions. One would prefer not to induce an abortion in this instance. There is consistency between this preference and the Christian moralist's faith and convictions. But one would prefer for conception to arise within love rather than hate, and one would prefer that there would be indications that the unknowable future were more favorably disposed to the human well-being of the mother and the child.

The perspective of the Christian moralist is informed and directed by his understanding of the nature of human life, as well as his convictions about God. Abbreviated statements of some convictions are sufficient here. These would be first, that moral life is a life of action, in which intentions, judgments, the exercise of bodily power and other forms of power and influence give direction to our responses to past events, and direction to future events themselves. Persons are active, responsive, creative, reflective, self-aware, initiating. The second would be that we can discern something of the order of relationships and activity that sustains, preserves, and develops our humanity. The child conceived in love, within a marriage (an order of love), within an order of society that maintains justice, is more likely to have a higher quality of life than one who is conceived in other conditions. The decision to seek an abortion is human, the act of abortion would be human, the relationships before, during, and after the abortion are human. The consequences are not fully predictable beyond the physical, and yet the human is more than perpetuation of the body. A moral order was violated in rape; are the human conditions present that would sustain and heal the humanity of the child and the mother in the future? The answer to that question is a finite, human answer, and how it will be answered by the mother and others deeply affects a most decisive act.

A third pertinent affirmation about human life is important: to be a creature is to be limited, and the good and the right are found within the conditions of limitation. Present acts respond to the conditions of past actions, conditions which are usually irrevocable, unalterable. Their consequences will be projected into the future and quickly become part of other actions and responses so that the actors in the present cannot fully know or determine the future. The limitations of knowledge, both of potentially verifiable facts and of good and evil, while no excuse for not knowing what can be known, nonetheless are present. Thus not only physical risk, but moral risk is fundamental to human action, and this risk in the life of this woman involves potential tragedy, suffering, and anguish. But her condition itself is the fruit both of events beyond her control (for example, the rapes) and events that have occurred because of choices (for example, earlier adultery). What many men find out about the dark side of existence through novels and dramas, she has experienced. Action is required within the limits; the good or the evil that is involved will be concrete, actual. Thus there is no abstract standard of conduct that can predetermine without moral ambiguity what the right action is in this predicament. Since predicaments like this have emerged before, however, one's conscientious moral interpretation can use those generalizations that have emerged out of the past for illumination, and for direction. They may present values or principles so universally valid that the present decision, if contrary to them, must be justified as a clear exception. Since action is specific, either the following of established rules, or the finding exceptions to them, refers to specifics. Specificity of good and evil is the human condition (I never know either in the abstract); choices are agonizingly specific. The moralist has the obligation conscientiously to assess the specific in the light of principles and arguments that pertain to it; the woman is entitled to see her predicament and potential courses of action in the light of as much distilled wisdom and experience as she can handle. Indeed, the principle of double effect (preferably multiple effects none of which are totally evil, and none of which are totally good) might assist in the reflection. But the choice remains in the realm of the finite, the limited, and the potentially wrong as well as right.

Pertinent Principles That Can Be Stipulated for Reflection

Neither the moralist nor the woman comes to a situation without some convictions and beliefs that begin to dissolve some of the complexity of the particularities into manageable terms. Perhaps the traditional Catholic arguments simply assume that one can begin with these convictions and principles, and need not immerse one's self in the tragic concreteness. The pertinent ones in this case have already been alluded to, but here they can be reduced to a simpler scheme.

1. Life is to be preserved rather than destroyed.
2. Those who cannot assert their own rights to life are especially to be protected.
3. There are exceptions to these rules.

Possible exceptions are:

a. "medical indications" that make therapeutic abortion morally viable. Condition not present here.

b. the pregnancy has occurred as a result of sexual crime. (I would grant this as a viable possible exception in every instance for reasons imbedded in the above discussion, if the woman herself were convinced that it was right. In other than detached academic discussions I would never dispatch an inquiry with a ready granting of the exception. If the woman sees the exception as valid, she has a right to more than a potentially legal justification for her decision; as a person she has the right to understand why it is an exception in her dreadful plight.)

c. the social and emotional conditions do not appear to be beneficial for the well-being of the mother and the child. (In particular circumstances, this may appear to be a justification, but I would not resort to it until possibilities for financial, social, and spiritual help have been explored.)

In the short-hand of principles this can be reduced to an inconsistency between on the one hand the first and second, and on the other hand 3.b. and perhaps 3.c. While I am called upon to give as many reasons for a decision between these two as I can, the choice can never be fully rationalized.

The Decision of the Moralist

My own decision is: (a) if I were in the woman's human predicament I believe I could morally justify an abortion, and thus: (b) I would affirm its moral propriety in this instance. Clearly logic alone is not the process by which a defense of this particular judgment can be given; clearly, the facts of the matter do not add up to a justification of abortion so that one can say "the situation determines everything." Nor is it a matter of some inspiration of the Spirit. It is a human decision, made in freedom, informed and governed by beliefs and values, as well as by attitudes and a fundamental perspective. It is a discernment of compassion for the woman, as well as of objective moral reflection. It may not be morally "right" in the eyes of others, and although we could indicate where the matters of dispute between us are in discourse, and perhaps even close the gap between opinions to some extent, argument about it would probably not be persuasive. The judgment is made with a sense of its limitations, which include the limitations of the one who decides (which might well result from his lack of courage, his pride, his slothfulness in thinking, and other perversities).[3]

Continuing Responsibilities of the Moralist

The responsibilities of the moralist, like the consequences for the woman, do not end at the moment a decision might be made in favor of an abortion. Some of them can be briefly indicated, since they have already been alluded to in the discussion. Since the moralist concurs in the decision, and since the decision was made in a relationship in which he accepts limited but real responsibility for the woman, he is obligated to continue his responsible relationship to her in ways consistent with the decision, and with her well-being. He cannot dismiss her to engage in subsequent implications of the decision on her own and to accept the consequences of such implications on her own. First, he is obligated to assist, if necessary, in finding competent medical care. In such a situation as the one described, with abortion laws as they now stand in most states, this is not necessarily an easy matter and not a trivial one. Second, financial resources are needed. To put her on her own in this regard would be to resign responsibility prematurely for a course of action in which the moralist concurred, and might jeopardize the woman's health and welfare. Third, the woman needs continuing social and moral support in her efforts to achieve her aspirations for relief from anguish and for a better human future. To deny continued support in this case is comparable to denying continued care and concern for the well-being of those who have large families as a result of a moral doctrine prohibiting contraception, or for children born out of wedlock, both reprehensible limitations of responsibility in my judgment. Fourth, the moralist is under obligation, if he is convinced of the propriety in this human situation of an abortion, to seek reform of abortion legislation which would remove the unjust legal barrier to what he believes to be morally appropriate. Other considerations must be brought to bear on the discussion of legal reform, such as the crucial matter of the legal and moral rights of the defenseless unborn persons, but it is consistent with the moral judgment in this case that the laws permit an action which is deemed to be morally approvable. To judge an action to be morally appropriate, and not to seek the alteration of legislation which would make such an action possible without penalties would be a serious inconsistency in the moralist's thinking and action. It would be comparable to approving conscientious objection to specific wars on moral grounds and not seeking to make such objection a legal possibility.

These points are made to indicate that the time and space limits of a moral issue extend beyond the focal point of a particular act. Indeed, the focal point has not been the abortion, but the well-being of the woman over a long range of time. If such a delineation of the situation is made, the responsibility of the moralist must be consonant in its dimensions with that. These points are made to reiterate an earlier one, then, namely that the delimitation which a moral issue receives from its discussants is a crucial factor in determining what data are significant and what the extent of responsibilities is.

III. The Location of This Discussion on the Current Map of Moral Theology

This essay began with a description of salient aspects of the traditional Catholic arguments. With reference to each of these, I have emphasized a different way of working. The discussion of this paper does not provide a totally different way of thinking about the matter; indeed, the concerns of traditional moral theology are brought into it.

In place of the external judge, the position of the persons who must assume responsibility for the decision has been stressed. This requires empathy with the woman and the physician who might become involved. But the moralist himself is responsible for his decision: if he offers recommendations he is responsible to all who accept and act upon them. If an abortion is induced, he shares moral responsibility for it. Moral decisions, however, are not made wallowing in sympathy and empathy. The element of disinterested objectivity is a necessity, something of the stance of the external judge or observer is involved. In a process of conversation with one who has the serious moral choice, however, the interpersonal relationship not only establishes the possibilities of open communication, but provides insight and understanding, and sensitizes the affections.

In place of the determination of an action as right or wrong by its conformity to a rule and its application, I have stressed the primacy of the person and human relationships and the concreteness of the choice within limited possibilities. There can be no guarantee of an objectively right action in the situation I have discussed, since there are several values which are objectively important, but which do not resolve themselves into a harmonious relation to each other. Since there is not a single overriding determination of what constitutes a right action, there can be no unambiguously right act.

Whereas the moral theology manuals generally limit discussion to the physical aspects of the human situation, I have set those in a wider context of human values, responsibilities, and aspirations. While this does not make the physical less serious, it sets it in relation to other matters of a morally serious nature, and thus qualifies the way one decides by complicating the values and factors to be taken into account.

I find it difficult in discussing possible abortions to limit the personal relationships as exclusively to the physician and the patient as do the manual discussions, and to limit the time span of experience to the fact of pregnancy and action pertaining to it alone. Most significantly in the instance discussed, the conditions under which the pregnancy occurred modify the discussion of the abortion.

The role of compassion and indignation, of attitudes and affections in the process of making a decision is affirmed in my discussion to a degree not admitted in traditional moral theology. Indeed, I indicated the importance of one's basic perspective, and the way in which one's perception of a situation is conditioned by this perspective. Situations cannot be reduced to discrete facts; one's response to them is determined in part by one's faith, basic intentions, and dispositions, as well as by analysis and the rational application of principles.

Although I have only sketched most briefly the theological convictions that inform the perspective, they perhaps have a more central place in the ways in which I proceed than is the case in traditional moral theology. I wish not to suggest that there is a deposit of revelation, supernaturally given, which I accept on authority as a basis of moral perspective; such a position is not the alternative to natural law. Ampler elaboration of this, however, is beyond the bounds of this paper.

Although the structure I have used as a model differs from that model used by the Roman Catholic manuals of moral theology, in a specific instance a Catholic moralist might reach a conclusion not strikingly dissimilar from my own in counselling the woman. He could do so by means of the classic Catholic doctrine of "good faith." As expounded by Alphonsus Liguori, a confessor is not to disturb the good faith of the penitent if he believes that telling the penitent he is committing a sin will not deter him from his course of action, but will merely put him in "bad faith," that is, in a state of mind where he is aware that what he is doing is opposed to the will of God. There are exceptions to this doctrine where the penitent must be informed of what is necessary to salvation, or where the common good is endangered by the proposed actions. These exceptions, however, do not seem applicable to the special kind of case I have outlined. Consequently, a Catholic moralist faced with a woman who believes she is doing what is right in seeking an abortion, and who in all probability would not be deterred by advice to the contrary, might well conclude that his responsibility was not to put the woman in bad faith.[4]

This Catholic approach to a particular case accords with mine in recognizing a principle of personal responsibility which the moralist must honor. He cannot coerce the person; in some sense each person must decide for himself. This approach differs from mine, however, in the analysis of the act of abortion, which is treated in a special sense as a sin. Elucidation of this difference would require extensive discussion of the relation of religion and morality in the two approaches, in the uses of the concept of sin, and other matters too large to be developed here. This Catholic approach also differs from mine in the limits it would impose on cooperation with the act by the counsellor.

A Catholic moral theologian, if he approved of the outcome of the discussion presented here, might compliment it by indicating that it is an example of prudence informed by charity at work, or that it is an exercise in the virtue of *epikeia,* applying principles to particular cases. If such generosity were shown, I would not be adverse to being pleased, for it would indicate that some of the polarizations of contemporary moral theology between ethics of law and situational ethics are excessively drawn. I would also suggest, however, that there is a different valence given to prudence and equity, indeed, to the moral virtues, in the order of ethical analysis here than is the case in the treatises on medical ethics. There is a sense in which the present discussion subordinates law to virtue as points of reliance in making moral decisions.

Since there is no fixed position called "situation ethics," it would be futile to distinguish the approach taken here from what cannot be readily defined. I would say in general that in comparison with Paul Lehmann's ethics of the theonomous conscience,[5] with its confidence in a renewed sensitivity and imagination to perceive what God is doing in the world to make and keep human life human, the approach of this paper is more complex, and ultimately less certain about its answer. Further, the weight of responsibility for reflection and for action rests heavily upon the actor, since no perceptive powers I have enable me to overcome the distance between God and the action that I respond to. I cannot claim to perceive what *God* is doing. The polemical force with which Lehmann attacks "absolutist ethics" is foreign to this approach;[6] while I clearly believe that abstract principles and logic alone do not contain the dynamics of suffering and evil, or of love and good, their utility in bringing clarity to discussion is much treasured.

As the morally conscientious soldier fighting in a particular war is convinced that life can and ought to be taken, "justly" but also "mournfully,"[7] so the moralist can be convinced that the life of the defenseless fetus can be taken, less justly, but more mournfully.

Notes

1. The generalizations do not do injustice to the treatment of abortion in at least the following books: Thomas J. O'Donnell, S.J., *Morals in Medicine,* 2nd ed. (Westminster, Md.: Newman Press, 1960); Charles J. McFadden, O.S.A., *Medical Ethics,* 5th ed. (Philadelphia: F. A. Davis Co., 1961); John P. Kenny, O.P., *Principles of Medical Ethics,* 2nd ed. (Westminster, Md.: Newman Press, 1962); Gerald Kelly, S.J., *Medico-Moral Problems* (St. Louis: The Catholic Hospital Association, 1958); Allan Keenan, O.F.M. and John Ryan, F.R.C.S.E., *Marriage: A Medical and Sacramental Study* (New York: Sheed and Ward, 1955). They apply also to manuals of moral theology that are more comprehensive than these which focus on medical care.

2. Albert Jonsen, S.J., in *Responsibility in Modern Religious Ethics* (Washington, D.C.: Corpus Books, 1968), demonstrates the importance of the distinction made here. See pp. 36ff.

3. This procedure can be applied to cases other than pregnancy due to rape, obviously, and *might* lead to similar conclusions in instances of unwed girls, or older married women with large families, etc.

4. See Bernard Häring, "A Theological Evaluation," in *The Morality of Abortion: Legal and Historical Perspectives,* ed. John T. Noonan, Jr. (Cambridge: Harvard University Press, 1970).

5. Paul Lehmann, *Ethics in a Christian Context* (New York: Harper & Row, 1964).

6. *Ibid.,* pp. 124-132.

7. See Roland H. Bainton's discussions of the mournful mood of the just war theorists, in *Christian Attitudes toward War and Peace* (New York: Abingdon Press, 1960), pp. 98, 112, 139, 145, and 221-222.

67.
The Abortion of Defective Fetuses: Some Moral Considerations

DAVID H. SMITH

I

The dinosaur Stegosaurus did not have much of a brain. To compensate for this deficiency it had bony plates sticking up along the crest of its back and, more to the point, two large ganglia in its spinal chord. These knots of nerve cells, located over the legs, were many times larger than the animal's brain. This seeming duplication of "brains" led someone to write of Stegosaurus:

> As he thought twice before he spoke,
> He had no judgments to revoke,
> For he could think without congestion
> Upon both sides of every question.[1]

As this paper proceeds, it will become clear that so far as I am concerned evolution has not progressed very far. I want to say two things about the abortion of defective fetuses: First, parents should have the liberty to decide for those abortions; second, at least within the context of the Christian community, it will usually (but not always) be wrong for them to have abortions for the sake of the fetus.

At the core of my argument is a distinction that I find myself unable to make with sufficient precision. It is a distinction among kinds of moral discourse, reasoning and evaluation; very loosely: a distinction in points of view. One way of making this distinction is to stress the difference between discussions of our duties or obligations to other persons, and our assessment of the character of individual persons. The latter theories of virtue find themselves especially concerned with character traits such as honesty, loyalty or courage. The discussion rests on a philosophical description of human nature and its "excellence" or "flourishing." Thus considerable use can be made of the writings of some psychologists and problems of philosophical psychology are central.[2] In any case on the normative level one's primary concern is with the discernment of the congruity between a particular choice, act or habit and the person's vision or perception of moral ideals. Integrity of conscience is presumed to be a value.

In contrast we may concentrate on the duties owed to one person by another. These obligations may be based on commitments made, the rationality of a greatest happiness principle, or roles assumed. The obligations of one person are correlative to the rights of another; thus it is essential that the form of reasoning used be one that is intelligible to all persons and not involve private or sectarian categories. The preoccupation is with actual performance, enactment or forebearance in accordance with social agreements and expectations. Motive for action is reduced to secondary importance.[3]

This way of distinguishing among kinds of moral discourse provides me with my starting point, but it leaves me very uneasy. The causes of this disquiet are several. To start with, it is unclear that discussions of virtue or character can be excluded from our second or "public" realm. While it may not be fundamental, there is a kind of "civic virtue" required in a populace, if social life is to go on. This will involve a disposition to obey the law, to treat people fairly, and to honor commitments made. Character is not simply a private or confessional matter. At the same time, as various writers have suggested,[4] a concern for integrity or virtue will very likely lead to specification of general obligations.

Most important, use of this virtue-obligation contrast may lead to an over-strong assertion about the canons of reasonableness to be employed on one side or another. Specifically, one might be tempted to say that discussions of obligations must work on analogy with scientific method—using quantifiable goods and cost-benefit analyses as sufficient components in social debate. In contrast, the implication would be that assessments of character and conscience are irrational and arbitrary. That there is a difference of emphasis here I would concede. The general intelligibility requirement of public discourse will tend to require the development of a common normative political language. That leads to a dilution of the traditional symbolic content of any categories of moral obligation. Assessments of character, however, necessarily refer to the history, the accidents, the significant mythology in an individual's biography. Nevertheless, a strictly a-historical and value neutral framework for discussions of social obligation has yet to be designed, and there are sensible requirements of coherence, stability and order incumbent on individual persons. We describe as insane or fanatical someone who has lost sight of those requirements.

For these reasons, I am less than satisfied with the

From David H. Smith and Linda M. Bernstein, eds., *No Rush to Judgment* (Bloomington: The Poynter Center, 1978), pp. 126-51.

virtue-obligation distinction. Yet something like it is of great importance and too-often lacking in discussions of normative issues such as abortion. There is a set of duties essential to social life, duties that we can define and expect everyone to follow. However, moral life and character require much more than this minimum, in particular the embodiment of diverse moral ideals.[5] Neither component can be dropped out of the analysis without seriously impoverishing the discussion.

Nothing reveals this impoverishment better than the essays on abortion written by two of the religious moralists to whom I owe the greatest debts. Paul Ramsey has wrestled repeatedly with the complexity of the issue[6] and the question he forces, over and over again, is the straightforward one of which abortions are compatible with the obligation of fidelity (agape, or covenant-love). While he defends a decision to allow some defective premature infants to die,[7] his major claim is that it is only faithful to bring about fetal death to protect the life of the mother. There have been changes in his formulations, but the general idea has always been that abortions are moral, if "we are not turning directly against the basic value of the child's (i.e., fetus's) life . . . (but) the target is that child's fatal function (active or passive)." Specifically this implies that " 'removal' (i.e., justified abortion) is what *is done* and is justified in all cases where 'necessity' foredooms that only one life can be saved. . . . "[8] He criticizes Germain Grisez for adopting a broader definition of what constitutes legitimate protective killing because such reasoning "is subjectivism gone riot in scrutinizing intention."[9]

As I hope will emerge, I think there is an important place for an argument like this one in a discussion of the morality of abortion. Yet its striking limitation seems to me to be the kinds of factors it excludes or—by omission—makes trivial. The difference in the abortion choices of promiscuous young middle-class adults and illiterate female heads of households in the ghetto becomes "subjectivism gone riot." The circumstances of conception are explicitly made of secondary relevance.[10]

Speaking very generally, I suggest that the basic reason for these limitations lies in Ramsey's attempt simultaneously to state a plausible set of public obligations and to spin out the *full* requirements of the Christian conscience.[11] General obligations do require formulae that abstract from the variability or fluctuations of what Ramsey calls motive: my students have a right to a coherent lecture no matter why I give it. But the understanding of sexuality, parenthood and fetal personhood that Ramsey presupposes is not plausible apart from a background in Christian theology. These ideas only make sense within the context of a particular theological tradition (although there, they are profound). The result of using them outside (or presupposing) that context is to discredit the idea that there are any plausible and nonarbitrary general obligations referring to the morality of abortion. In effect, Ramsey's overly-vigorous *way* of rejecting moral relativism tends to undercut itself. At the same time, if less conspicuously, the preoccupation with the formulation of public standards means that Ramsey can allow characteristically theological categories like grace and forgiveness to drop into the background. Both parties—theology and general discourse, obligation and virtue—lose in a symbiotic marriage.

If Ramsey loses sight of the need for an independent discussion of the requirements of conscience, Stanley Hauerwas talks of nothing else. He writes with great power of the forms of self-deception and subjectivism often associated with analyses of abortion, "from the agents' perspective."[12] Then he discusses fetal personhood and the intentionality of abortion decisions in ways that I find very instructive, as what follows will make clear. But Hauerwas gives us no indication of what moral bases there should be for a *general* social policy on abortion. He (rightly) rejects "the assumption that a personal moral decision such as abortion should be determined in terms of some vague criteria such as the 'needs' of society." Instead such decisions should be honest reflections of an individual's perception of the truth. "If society does not provide the context in which the individual can do the good, the conclusion to be reached is that the society should be changed and not the individual's decision."[13] Thus, "the good of society must be determined not by what is possible, but by what men should be."[14]

And what should men be? This is determined by their perceptions, and perceptions are a product of one's life-story. Ethics begins with the "specificity" of a particular set of beliefs. These beliefs may be religious; for some (including Hauerwas) they will be Christian. "It cannot be assumed that moral behavior for Christians is the same as for other persons, though there may be great areas of agreement."[15] Hauerwas does not draw the conclusion that there is *no* "realm of morality accessible to all men,"[16] but so far as I can tell he makes no attempt, beyond his concession of a universalizability principle,[17] to indicate what the *content* of such a morality might be in our society.

Not only does this limit the relevance of his normative discussions to those who "tell the same story," it tends—at least by omission—to suggest a privileged place for the Christian story. This is ironical in a writer as clearly aware of pluralism as Hauerwas. Furthermore, he glosses over the loyalty of tellers of a

Christian story to those whose experience differs,[18] for that loyalty would seem to require the development of a shared moral language, a set of categories with which to criticize the general social ethos. Finally, great stress on truth and Christian vision means that Hauerwas insufficiently grasps the extent to which the Christian story itself can become a vehicle of self-deception.[19] There may be times and situations in which action perceived to be truly Christian is immoral because not congruent with general social obligations. Thus some abortion choices may be right (or wrong) despite their irreconcilability with a Christian conscience. Correction from "outside" is possible. There seems to be something true in the old poem:

> "That ain't my style," said Casey.
> "Strike one," the umpire said.

II

Before any analysis of abortion can go very far something must be said about the question of fetal personhood.[20] On a practical level, our concern with fetuses known to be defective minimizes this problem somewhat, for most ante-natal diagnoses are not done early in pregnancy. Thus it is only in the very rare case that the technique involved will be a D and C operation done within the first month of pregnancy. We are dealing with second trimester, or later, abortions. Is personal life taken in these abortions? Some conservative writers suggest that all abortions involve the taking of human personal life;[21] other liberal spokesmen imply that none do.[22] The conservative view runs into difficulty because of the phenomenon of twinning; it seems to ignore the role of interaction (including interaction in utero) and phenotype in the formation of personhood; and it presupposes difficult theses about potentiality.[23] The liberal, in contrast, tends to be excessively rationalistic and anti-physical. "The hard question put to those who regard the fetus as (merely) tissue is not the factual one, but rather what view of life have they accepted by doing so."[24]

Some of these difficulties can be avoided if we realize that our moral term, *abortion,* is too broad. We use it to denote and often evaluate any termination of life within the uterus, but not all such life is the same. Suppose we consider four different actions: (1) contraception using a diaphragm, (2) a D and C done seventy-two hours after intercourse, (3) a saline abortion in the twenty-eighth week of pregnancy, and (4) a potassium injection into an infant forty-eight hours after birth. Let us ask which pairs of actions show the greatest similarities? Which non-moral consequences—losses of life in three cases—are most similar? If we begin our debate over this question by asking which procedures are *abortions,* we will be forced to the conclusion that procedures two and three are most alike. Yet I think this contravenes the sensibility of almost all of us. Set aside the question of the morality of these actions, we feel that there has been a much greater loss, something more significant has died, in three and four than in two. In fact, we may well feel that (2) is more like (1) than it is like (3).

The implication, of course, is that late abortions are a much more serious matter than early ones, and it may not be possible or necessary to go beyond this differentiation. It is easy to cause problems for this minimal distinction, as "conceptionalists"[25] are eager to do, by inquiry about the seriousness of abortions in the fifteenth to twentieth weeks. Are those more like my category two or three? The question is unanswerable, but not much is gained. The fact of continuity of process in embryonic and/or fetal development does not prove that no real change occurs in the course of that process. Inability to identify the moment of twilight does not mean there is no difference between day and night. Thus, one may be very hard pressed to specify exactly what dies in many abortions. Quite literally, there may be occasions when we do not know *what* we are doing. Yet this ambiguity should not lead us to be more vacillating on early and late abortions than we would otherwise be. Each may be right or wrong in a certain situation, but they differ and resemble other non-abortive processes (contraception and infanticide) more than they resemble each other.

With these considerations in mind, I shall assume that a decision to abort because of known fetal defect is significantly similar to—if it is not always in fact—a decision to terminate the life of a defective newborn. We are, at least, dealing with a case of doubt, and doubt about the personhood of a being ought to be resolved in that being's favor.[26]

III

How should Christian parents decide when faced with a diagnosis of fetal defect? Is a decision for such an abortion congruent with the basic affirmations of Christian conscience? Answers to this question range all the way from Joseph Fletcher's approval of any freely chosen abortion decision to the total exclusion of this particular possibility by traditional Roman Catholic moralists. These answers seem to me to distort the complex ingredients in Christian literature and experience as well as to oversimplify the practical problem. There are various lines of analysis that must be made and somehow woven together. These will include something like the following ingredients, formed by a Christian perception of the world.

1. The fundamental Christian affirmation is that through Jesus Christ human beings are related to the greatest power and the most profound truth that are to be found. This power and truth is called God. Obviously this is no place to attempt to develop a full theology, but it is essential to notice that Christian conscience is always relational. Persons do not, ultimately, live by themselves: they live, according to Christian confession, with God through Christ.

The first relevant implication of this fact for reasoning about abortion is that it suggests that God, rather than persons, is sovereign over the world. This is an idea captured in the creation stories, in the recurrent metaphor of the "kingdom" of God—so central in ancient Israel and the proclamation of Jesus—and of course in the Lord's Prayer—"Thy kingdom come. . . . " Probably I do not need to go on. The point to stress at this stage is the negative one: God's sovereignty implies the less-than-ultimate sovereignty of human persons. We are men and not God.[27] Thus we should not make absolutes of our fears, hopes, or purposes.

The implication for reasoning about the abortion of defective fetuses is that disruption of established and gratifying life-patterns, forced changes of plans, the necessity completely to rethink and rework personal and family expectations—all these, and many more, challenges that a prospective defective child implies are not really challenges to something unquestionably right. If God is sovereign people must learn to sit loose to comfortable habits and dreams. The necessity to rethink a present set of values, and the future, should come as no surprise to the Christian. Thus one ingredient in the conscientious consideration of abortion of defective fetuses should be a willingness to put one's prior plans and values at least temporarily into the realm of the provisional. The Christian does not pray, "*my* kingdom come."

On the other hand, Christians claim that the fundamental use God has made of his sovereignty has been to involve himself with, to relate himself to, the world. The same creation stories that imply God's transcendence suggest the goodness of nature as his product. And human nature, in particular, takes on value from its relation to God.[28] Thus persons are made "in the image of God" with dominion over the creation; the Christian claim is that God disclosed himself in a person; indeed a vigorous recent critique of traditional Western Christianity is that it is excessively "anthropocentric."[29] Christianity implies that because of God's special relation to human persons, human life is a much more significant value than anything non-human.

This claim does not settle the basic question of when embryos or fetuses become human persons,[30] but it does suggest that insofar as they are persons they have the same kinds of value that the rest of us have. The consequence is that fetuses perceived by us as persons have personal rights. They do not cease to make claims because they are young, dependent, not fully developed, or invisible. Of course many, although not all, fetuses aborted because of fetal defect are perceived as persons. The parents understand themselves to have an obligation *to that fetal person* to prevent his existence.[31] If such an obligation exists, then the fetus has been included as a person, and one can not consistently reason about his death except as one would about the deaths of other persons.

2. Life before God, moreover, has certain definite characteristics. The Christian has an understanding of human nature and social life that is rooted in his perception of his relationship to God in Christ. Three ingredients of this perception are of some relevance here.

(i) To start with, our individual lives are involved in relationships with several other human beings. We can not help but be bound to or concerned with more than one other person. Thus, supposing us to have obligations to others, these obligations are diverse and may well conflict. There is always more than one person, more than one relationship, to be taken into account. Consequently, reasoning about a possible abortion of a defective fetus can not bracket off consequences for spouse, siblings or fellow workers any more than it can discount a sense of obligation to the fetus. Effects on all others, and on the self, are relevant to any abortion decision.

(ii) Furthermore, the created world in which we live has natural characteristics that must be related to this decision. The old traditional notion of *proles* as a *justification* for sexuality did presuppose that sex was in some way bad and in need of justification; it should therefore be junked. But a modified notion of the reproductive character of ideal sexuality may be an interesting normative claim: the "best" sex leads beyond itself to personal novelty and growth, and nothing is more novel than a human child.

However that may be, the most basic point remains that human sexual acts of love may have procreative consequences undesired by lovers. Sometimes those are consequences for which couples are responsible. Responsibility for pregnancy resulting from an ill-fitting diaphragm is different from responsibility for pregnancy caused by failure to take any contraceptive precautions. An attempt to deny responsibility for the latter pregnancy, on the basis of an appeal to desires or "intentions," only shows an inability accurately to perceive the nature of the world in which we live. In reality sexuality is procreative.

Consequently, in reasoning about the abortion of a defective fetus the circumstances of conception are of considerable relevance. Most men, it seems, regard all pregnancies as occurrences "caused" by women, as the result of female *actions.* Women, in contrast, often think of pregnancy as something that *happens* to them. In the final portion of this paper, I will stress the truth in the second (female) interpretation. For now, I merely mean to note that there are some times when the "male" view is correct—when unwanted pregnancy is a woman's, or her lover's, responsibility. Insofar as someone is responsible for the pregnancy, a justification of abortion for fetal defect becomes more problematical.[32]

(iii) Finally under the heading of the structured nature of life before God, we should note the very general implication of individual human finitude of knowledge and discernment. There is always the possibility that one's perceptions are wrong, that one can learn from the individual and collective judgments of others. Moreover, there is the constant tendency for self-deception. As a result the standards of one's society become of considerable relevance. Such standards may, of course, be perverse. Legalization of abortion does not make it right. But nevertheless, legal prohibitions, regulations and/or permissions are morally relevant facts.

3. Christians understand themselves to have an ideal character in their life before God. Most generally this can be described as a life of passion for God and compassion for others.[33] The New Testament portraits of Jesus are the basis for the sketch of this ideal. They show a man faithful to the needs of his fellow men.[34] The needs of the weak and helpless are stressed.[35]

Given all we have said, is a life of fidelity compatible with a decision for the death of a defective fetus? The major justification for taking life in Christian tradition has been protection. Human life as the highest value under God could be destroyed only to protect other human life. Defective fetuses may threaten lives and so can be reasoned about in this way. Then the hard questions arise—what is the exact extent and kind of the harms done to others by the fetus's life? Are the psychological strain, social and economic dislocation, equivalent to the price the fetus will pay? Is the fact that the fetus is caught in this situation anyone's responsibility? Are there alternatives which would allow the fetus to live, yet save the endangered other persons? In conscience it may be that these questions can be answered in a way that abortion for fetal defect is justified, but that justification will not be the usual result.

Going beyond this, however, it may be that some fetuses have a need to die that finite persons in fidelity should respect or even work to meet. Fetal defect is a very broad term. The fact that a faithful decision to abort because of Down's syndrome will be rare, should not blind one to the possibility that a life may be very likely to be nasty, brutish and short. If there are no possibilities of happiness or flourishing, if the only value a person is likely to receive is disvalue, then it would make sense to abort for the sake of the fetus.[36] I have in mind an ante-natal diagnosis of Tay-Sach's disease, or other more rare and terrible anomalies.

The danger in this possibility, of course, is that it will be abused. On the level of individual conscience, however, it seems to me that the way to avoid abuse is not to foreclose a possibility on principle, but to insist that the decision-maker focus, for the moment, on the needs and prospects of the specific defective fetus. Comparisons with the prospects of "healthy" fetuses should be ruled out. Is the disorder so severe that the only good we can bring to the fetus is a ministry and fidelity to his death? If so, we should act accordingly.

In sum, Christian conscience will tend to be conservative about the decision to abort defective fetuses. Arguments from protection of others and from fidelity to the fetus are both admissible on principle, but neither will in fact often lead to the conclusion that a decision for abortion is compatible with Christian life.

IV

Social duties must be defined in terms that are widely understood. I will here assume that those duties include fundamental principles of fidelity and equality.[37] Moreover, though this is not the place to argue the claim, I suggest that Christian character requires a commitment to both these general principles as a product of a compassionate and faithful stance towards others.[38] Various derivative principles will follow from these basic ones—these will include a prohibition on killing and a requirement to respect the liberty of conscience and action of other persons. *Ceteris paribus,* people have equal needs to exist, to act and to choose for themselves.

It follows from this that parents and society have important obligations to the life and health of infants. These include more than prohibitions on harm. We understand ourselves to be obliged positively to act to feed, clothe, medicate and educate. On the other hand, our commitment to equality means that we cannot provide any one individual, of any age, with everything he may need. Our liabilities to other individuals must be limited by the fact that we must consider the needs of several people. There are times when we must say, in effect, "although he needs it, I (we) cannot give it." Such a decision follows plausibly from a commitment to equality, although it could also be derived from a theory of personal rights.

What then are the obligations or duties of women to the defective fetuses they carry? It is hard for me to see how these obligations can be seen as an exception to the general rule on limited liability. Pregnant women can not be *obliged* to make unlimited sacrifices for the sake of their unborn children. Professor Judith Thomson makes this point in a justly well-known essay.[39] She creates the hypothetical situation of a person who awakens to discover that all his vital systems have been connected to those of the world's greatest violinist. The violinist is suffering from a serious disease and can only survive the next nine months if his "host" remains in bed and connected to him. Could one say he is "obliged" to spend the next months so constrained? "No," Professor Thomson argues. Such a self-sacrificial decision would be noble, but it can not be required of anyone; it is not part of our basic, common moral obligations.

Attacks that I have heard on this argument from analogy usually stress the disanalogy of cause.[40] The critics argue that waking up pregnant is not a surprise like that experienced by the person with the violinist hook-up. People become pregnant because they made love, and love-making is procreative. Thus, so the criticism seems to run, women are always responsible for being pregnant.

My partial sympathy for this point of view has, I hope, already come out, but it is important to observe that this objection to Professor Thomson glosses over the frequent occurrence of *responsible accidental* pregnancy. Pregnancy following rape or incest is the obvious, but by no means the only, case of this. Generally, many pregnancies in stable relationships following contraceptive failure must fall under this heading. In such cases it is Draconian to refer to the pregnancy as something *caused* by the woman. Rather, as most women perceive, those pregnancies are things that happen to women. In this sense the wide availability of effective contraceptives is a very significant moral fact; if they did not exist, it would be impossible to intend non-procreative love-making. Since contraceptives are available, however, we must see that although not every unwanted pregnancy is "responsibly accidental," some are.

The implication, of course, is that women can not be understood to be obliged to carry "accidental" pregnancies, with or without fetal defect, to term. We may often praise them for a willingness to make sacrifices—and those who operate from a Christian sense of virtue will do so. But they can not be *obliged* to pay the price, to be Good Samaritans.

Abortions that follow pregnancies for which couples are responsible (non-accidental) are not justified by this line of reasoning, however. If a couple either meant to get pregnant or failed to take reasonable contraceptive precautions, they can not then claim that the pregnancy, the perilous situation of the fetus, is one for which they have no responsibility. Sissela Bok has considered the distinction involved with some rigor. She writes that "ceasing bodily life support *of a fetus or of anyone else* cannot be looked at as a breach of duty except where such a duty has been assumed in the first place. Such a duty is closer to existing when the pregnancy has been voluntarily begun. And it does not exist at all in cases of rape."[41] She goes on to concede that "there are many cases where these distinctions cannot be so clearly made. It may be difficult to know whether there was an intention to have a baby, or to risk becoming pregnant."[42] Yet, she rightly suggests, some difficult problems of line-drawing do not invalidate the importance of the distinction at issue.

In fact, the only problem with Professor Bok's discussion involves her reluctance to press the distinction involved as far as it will go. Unfortunately, she does not explicitly say that some *unwanted* pregnancies are, nevertheless, pregnancies for which lovers are responsible. Thus she implies that absence of the *desire* to have a child is the crucial moral fact. According to Professor Bok, omission of contraceptive measures is not immoral but "insensitive"[43] when abortion is used as a check.

The degree of responsibility for conception affects the morality of an abortion decision. Bok suggests three different degrees of responsibility through use of an analogy with death by drowning. We can schematize this as follows.[44]

Drowning

1. X drowns, and a passerby, Y, does not attempt to save him.
2. X drowns after swimming where/when Y assured him it was safe.
3. X drowns after Y pushes him into the water.

Pregnancy

1. The abortion of a fetus conceived against a woman's wishes.
2. The abortion of a fetus which was conceived despite certainty of being "protected against pregnancy."
3. The abortion of an intentionally conceived pregnancy.

The basic point is that responsibility (on the part of Y or the pregnant woman) for death in #3 is much greater than it is at #1. My difficulty is that there is a wide range of cases[45] that fall under #2, so that the category should be subdivided as follows:

2a. X drowns after swimming on the advice of a well-informed and reasonable friend, Y.
2b. X drowns when a friend, Y, urges him to water ski at night immediately after a banquet.

2a. The abortion of a fetus conceived despite reasonable contraceptive precautions.
2b. The abortion of a fetus conceived when no or inadequate (e.g., rhythm, foam) contraceptive precautions are taken.

The friend of the drowned person (Y) and the parents of the fetus have, I suggest, responsibilities in 2b that their counterparts do not have in 2a. Although they did not consciously plan for (or cause) a death to occur (and thus are different from case #3), they do have responsibility for the situation in virtue of their negligence and prior actions. If this is so, then failure to use adequate contraceptives is not "insensitive" but, like drunken driving, immoral and potentially murderous. In neither case should an appeal to wishes absolve from moral responsibility.

The number of responsible accidental pregnancies (1, 2a), then, is not as great as might be supposed. Certainly it is smaller than the number of "unwanted" pregnancies. Supposing, now, that in this instance social policy should follow moral guidelines, which abortions are to be allowed? Who is to decide if a particular pregnancy is one for which people are responsible—or an accident that occurred? One logical possibility would be a public board to inquire into the circumstances of conception as well as a range of other matters, but such inquisitorial agencies have everywhere proven themselves inconsistent, arbitrary and discriminatory.[46] Others suggest that fathers should have a veto power, forgetting that many fathers take no responsibility for their children. The only legitimate final decision-maker is the pregnant woman herself who may, of course, make a moral mistake, one way or the other. It is incumbent on lover and society to provide her support of all kinds.

The social implication of this is that women should have the right to bring their pregnancies to an end whenever they choose. Women should have a right to "unplug from the violinist," to their liberty, to avoid being forced to remain pregnant. But that is all women should have. This reasoning does not give women the right to kill a fetus whom the rest of us could save. Although she does not stress it, Professor Thomson makes this point very well.[47] To paraphrase her jargon: the right to unplug does not imply a right to kill a violinist plugged in to someone else. The fact that I am not obliged to save a drowning man I happen to see does not suggest that I have a justification for keeping *you* from saving him. Thus this argument does not establish a right to kill a viable fetus—i.e., one that others could save. There is a distinction between choosing liberty for oneself and choosing death for another. Society should honor the first but not the second choice.

If this is correct, it follows that some abortion techniques, and late abortions generally, become very problematical. Late fetuses are not only like persons in certain significant respects, they are (or soon will be) viable,[48] i.e., savable by someone besides the mother. Abortion techniques like saline injection and hysterotomy are, in effect, ways of doing something besides liberating the mother. They are ways of insuring that no one else will save, nurture and care for the fetus. Except in the very most rare instance they are, therefore, immoral. This is a consideration that should regulate medical policy and perhaps our laws; such regulation would be constitutional under recent Supreme Court rulings.[49]

Abortions before viability, in contrast, do not create quite the same problem for society, since they do not involve society in destroying a life it morally can save. The only way a public group could insure the safety of non-viable fetuses is by denying to women rights that, I contend, they should have. It is not exactly that society must condone and/or approve of all early abortions, any more than we condone thousands of daily deaths from automobile accidents. Rather, our commitment to other values, generally liberty, means that society must tolerate a certain amount of unjustified sacrifice of fetal life.

Moreover, this restriction on late abortions should not be absolute. There may be late fetuses for whom the life prospects are so bleak that they are better off dead. My point has been that the mother's right to be free does not settle all questions about the fetus's fate, not that no fetuses should be allowed to die. But a decision for the death of a viable fetus should be made solely with reference to its prospects; it is indistinguishable from parallel choices about defective newborns. Thus the number of such decisions for death that is morally legitimate will be small. It will matter how, as well as whether, the fetus's death comes about.[50]

V

I conclude, therefore, that two factors, often not stressed, are of considerable importance in deciding about the abortion of a defective fetus: 1) The stage of fetal development is a relevant moral fact, but not because some clear line distinguishing fetal persons from fetal non-persons can be drawn. From the perspective of social duties, the crucial point in development is viability extra-utero, for that viability makes possible sustaining care by others besides the mother. From the perspective of Christian parents, stage of development has less relevance, but early enactment of an otherwise conscientious abortion decision would seem preferable as involving less suffering for mother/fetus/embryo, or others. 2) Also relevant are the circumstances of conception. Because pregnancy may not be a situation for which women are responsible they should have the liberty to terminate pregnancy (if not to feticide). Because of their perception of themselves and the world, Christians must accept responsibility for some unwanted pregnancies—whether a handicapped child is expected or not.

In summary, our social duties require the honoring of a female right to terminate pregnancy. Before viability this is equivalent to a right to decide to destroy the fetus; after viability it is not. A faithful and just society can morally *require* no less—and no more. In contrast, a Christian perception of the world does not lead parents to think in terms of rights. Instead, the questions Christian parents put to themselves concern responsibility: for other persons, for nascent life, for the limitations of their preconceptions and projects, for cowardice and self-deception. These considerations may lead to a choice for abortion because of fetal defect, but only when the choice is an act of fidelity. Integrity, not liberty, is the fundamental concern. There is, in other words, a "natural" logic of social duties that leads to certain liberties and restrictions on abortion practices (i.e., no abortions of viable fetuses); there is a contrasting theological analysis that should inform and control Christian behavior. The two lines of reasoning are equally important; each should be pursued independently.

Of course, many people find a self-consciously Christian theological perspective uncongenial. Some prefer an alternative theological structure; others may assess character in "humanistic" terms. My overriding point, however, is to suggest the difficulty that occurs for writers on the morality of abortion who do not distinguish questions of social duty from those of character. Indeed, it is incumbent on us not only to distinguish the issues but to address them both. The alternatives are confusion, parochialism, or moral impoverishment. Single track analyses leave too much out of account. Our ongoing problem is maintaining balances—between protection and liberty, virtue and duty, beliefs and public life. I hope I have suggested the importance of relating differing kinds of analyses of the problem, and I imagine it is now clear why I began with a poem about Stegosaurus, a dinosaur with two *small* brains!

Notes

1. Quoted in Alice Fitch Martin and Bertha Morris Parker, *Dinosaurs* (Racine, Wis.: Western Publishing Company, 1973), p. 29.

2. A landmark in the contemporary discussion with this emphasis is G. E. M. Anscombe's "Modern Moral Philosophy," *Philosophy* 33 (1958): 1-19. For a very suggestive appropriation of virtue-theory by a theologian see Stanley Hauerwas, *Vision & Virtue* (Notre Dame: Fides, 1974), especially Part I; and "Obligation and Virtue Once More," *Journal of Religious Ethics* 3 (Spring 1975): 27-44. Erich Fromm's *Man for Himself* (New York: Fawcett, 1947) is a very potent critique of theistic theories of ideal character.

3. As one illustration of this consider John Stuart Mill in *Utilitarianism:* "It is the business of ethics to tell us what are our duties, or by what test we may know them: but no system of ethics requires that the sole motive for all we do shall be a feeling of duty: on the contrary, ninety-nine hundredths of all our actions are done from other motives, and rightly so done if the rule of duty does not condemn them. . . . Utilitarian moralists have gone beyond almost all others in affirming that the motive has nothing to do with the morality of the action, though much with the worth of the agent. He who saves a fellow creature from drowning does what is morally right, whether his motive be duty, or the hope of being paid for his trouble. . . . " Quoted in Max Lerner, ed., *The Essential Works of John Stuart Mill* (New York: Bantam Books, 1961), p. 205.

4. Cf. Frederick S. Carney, "The Virtue-Obligation Controversy," *Journal of Religious Ethics* 1 (Fall 1973): 5-19; William Frankena, *Ethics,* 2nd ed. (Englewood Cliffs, N.J.: Prentice-Hall, 1973); "The Ethics of Love Conceived as an Ethics of Virtue," *Journal of Religious Ethics* 1 (Fall 1973): 21-36; and "Conversations with Carney and Hauerwas," *Journal of Religious Ethics* 3 (Spring 1975): 45-62.

5. Cf. J. O. Urmson, "Saints and Heroes," in A. I. Melden,

ed., *Essays in Moral Philosophy* (Seattle: University of Washington Press, 1958); and P. F. Strawson, "Social Morality and Individual Ideal," in Ian Ramsey, ed., *Christian Ethics and Contemporary Philosophy* (London: SCM Press, 1966), pp. 280-98.

6. His first discussion is found in *War and the Christian Conscience,* pp. 34-59, but other important treatments are "The Morality of Abortion," in Daniel H. Labby, ed., *Life or Death: Ethics and Options* (Seattle: University of Washington Press, 1968), pp. 60-93; "Reference Points in Deciding About Abortion," in John T. Noonan, ed., *The Morality of Abortion* (Cambridge, Mass.: Harvard University Press, 1970), pp. 60-100; and "Abortion: A Review Article," *The Thomist* 37 (January 1973): 174-226.

7. "Reference Points in Deciding About Abortion" (cited in note 6), pp. 87-100.

8. "Abortion: A Review Article" (cited in note 6), pp. 222f.

9. *Op. cit.,* p. 223.

10. *Ibid.,* p. 224. Professor Ramsey concedes that a threat to the psychological health of the mother may, on principle, be equivalent to a threat to her life. He seems to feel this will be a very small number of cases in fact. See his additions to "The Morality of Abortion," in James Rachels, ed., *Moral Problems* (New York: Harper & Row, 1971), pp. 17f.

11. I tried to get at some of the general problems in Ramsey's discussion of this and similar topics in "Paul Ramsey, Love and Killing," in James T. Johnson and David H. Smith, eds., *Love and Society* (Missoula, Mt.: Scholar's Press, 1974), pp. 3-18.

12. "Abortion: The Agent's Perspective," in *Vision & Virtue* (cited in note 2), pp. 147-65.

13. *Ibid.,* p. 164.

14. *Ibid.,* p. 165.

15. *Ibid.,* p. 75.

16. *Ibid.,* p. 87.

17. *Ibid.,* pp. 82-89.

18. There is New Testament precedent for the idea that the Christian should acknowledge a plurality of legitimate standards. Paul tells the Corinthians, who know that they can eat meat offered to idols, to *avoid* doing so if the eating would offend the conscience of another (I Corinthians 10:14-30; cf. Romans 14:13-23). Far from stressing the importance of discovering *the* true Christian style, Paul stresses mutual "upbuilding" (Romans 14:19) and keeping the consciences of others intact. On the level of constructive theology, Hauerwas's refreshing stress on honesty as a core virtue has meant that he allows it to displace fidelity (or love) as the central determinant of Christian character. Yet for Paul and other New Testament writers telling truth has value insofar as it relates to *being* true.

19. This problem seems to be the obvious omission in David Burrell and Stanley Hauerwas, "Self-Deception and Autobiography: Theological and Ethical Reflections on Speer's *Inside the Third Reich,*" *Journal of Religious Ethics* 2 (Spring 1974): 99-117. Do the authors mean to imply that a teller of the Christian story could not do things as wicked as those done by Speer?

20. An interesting and well-intentioned attempt to circumvent this issue is Ronald Green, "Conferred Rights and the Fetus," *Journal of Religious Ethics* 2 (Spring 1974): 55-76. See, however, James Childress, "A Response to Ronald Green 'Conferred Rights and the Fetus,'" *Journal of Religious Ethics* 2 (Spring 1974): 77-83.

21. E.g., John T. Noonan, "An Almost Absolute Value in History," in Noonan, ed., *The Morality of Abortion* (cited in note 6), pp. 1-59. Paul Ramsey's view (see "Reference Points in Deciding About Abortion") is not far from this.

22. Joseph Fletcher has defended this view in many contexts, but it is clear as early as *Morals and Medicine* (Boston: Beacon Press, 1960), pp. 141-71. A more philosophically sophisticated statement is Michael Tooley, "A Defense of Abortion and Infanticide," in Joel Feinberg, ed., *The Problem of Abortion* (Belmont, Cal.: Wadsworth Publishing Co., 1973), pp. 51-91. See also the responses to Tooley in *Philosophy and Public Affairs* 2 (Summer 1973): 407-32.

23. On potentiality see Tooley, "A Defense of Abortion" (see note 22); and Richard B. Brandt, "The Morality of Abortion," *The Monist* 56:503-26.

24. Hauerwas, *Vision & Virtue,* p. 153.

25. I take the term "conceptionalist" from Paul Camenisch, "Abortion, Analysis and the Emergence of Value," *Journal of Religious Ethics* 4 (Spring 1976): 131-58.

26. This view was held in *Abortion: An Ethical Discussion* (Westminster, Eng.: Church Information Office, 1965). Exactly how to respond to this question of uncertainty is the final problem faced in Roger Wertheimer, "Understanding the Abortion Agreement," in Feinberg, *The Problem of Abortion* (see note 22), pp. 33-51.

27. The stress on the sovereignty of a transcendent God was the major theme of the later work of H. R. Niebuhr. See *The Responsible Self* (New York: Harper & Row, 1963) and *Radical Monotheism and Western Culture* (New York: Harper & Row, 1960). To my knowledge, the best working out of the implications of this general theological style for abortion choices is James M. Gustafson, "A Protestant Ethical Approach," in Noonan, ed., *The Morality of Abortion,* pp. 101-22.

28. Ramsey makes this point very effectively in "The Morality of Abortion" (previously cited), pp. 72-78.

29. Lynn White, Jr., "The Historical Roots of Our Ecological Crisis," in Ian Barbour, ed., *Western Man and Environmental Ethics* (Reading, Mass.: Addison-Wesley, 1973), pp. 18-31.

30. As may be clear, I do not think it sensible to speak of a particular religious resolution to this question.

31. Although he pushes his argument in a more conservative direction than I follow here, Paul Camenisch is very acute on this. He writes: "If aborting the diagnosed malformed fetus is to be considered a moral duty or obligation . . . and if . . . no person has yet emerged, to whom do we have that duty or obligation?" See "Abortion: For the Fetus's Own Sake?" *Hastings Center Report* 6 (April 1976): 40.

32. See section IV below.

33. H. R. Niebuhr, *Christ and Culture* (New York: Harper & Row, 1951), p. 19.

34. This theme is the core of Paul Ramsey's Christian ethics. See his *Basic Christian Ethics* (New York: Charles

Scribner's Sons, 1950) and Paul Camenisch, "Paul Ramsey's Task: Some Methodological Clarifications and Questions," in Johnson and Smith, eds., *Love and Society,* pp. 67-90.

35. For a very different interpretation of this idea see John C. Bennett, *The Radical Imperative* (Philadelphia: The Westminster Press, 1975).

36. Obviously there would be a fuller specification of the factors to be taken into account in such a decision. At the moment my only point is to avoid foreclosing the moral possibility of abortion choices for the fetus's sake. Self-deception is certainly a possibility, but so is a "life not worth living." Thus, if he means to refer to *all* abortions for the fetus's sake I can not agree with Camenisch: " . . . describing such an abortion as being done for the sake of the fetus is at least inadequate and at most deceptive not only to the observer but to the participants as well." See "Abortion: For the Fetus's Own Sake?" p. 41.

37. See William Frankena, *Ethics;* and Paul Ramsey, *Basic Christian Ethics* (previously cited).

38. Fidelity, however, is a more fundamental Christian principle than equality.

39. "A Defense of Abortion," in Feinberg, ed., *The Problem of Abortion,* pp. 121-39.

40. See Paul Camenisch, "Abortion, Analysis and Value," pp. 136-38.

41. "Ethical Problems of Abortion," *The Hastings Center Studies* 2 (January 1974): 33-52.

42. *Op. cit.,* p. 46.

43. *Ibid.*

44. Adapted from *ibid.,* p. 35.

45. As Professor Bok concedes on *ibid.,* p. 35, n. 5.

46. See Daniel Callahan's discussion of the situation in the United Kingdom in *Abortion: Law, Choice and Morality* (New York: Macmillan, 1970), pp. 142-48, 284-304, 486-92.

47. "A Defense of Abortion," p. 139.

48. I assume that the development of medical technology will move the point of extra-uterine viability earlier and earlier into pregnancy. As this occurs there will be fewer and fewer moral abortion decisions that result in fetal death. Even presuming her own rationale for life-saving, I do not understand why Professor Bok stipulates that for moral purposes the moment of viability must remain where it is. "Ethical Problems of Abortion," p. 45.

49. Cf. Roe *v.* Wade, 93 Supreme Court 705 (1973).

50. I have tried to develop these points, first, in my essay "On Letting Some Babies Die," *Hastings Center Studies* (May 1974); second and more happily, in "Death, Ethics and Social Control," at the symposium "Medical Wisdom and Ethics in the Treatment of Severely Defective Newborn and Young Children," Center for Bioethics of the Clinical Research Institute of Montreal (November 1976).

68.

Theology and Morality of Procreative Choice

BEVERLY WILDUNG HARRISON

Much discussion of abortion betrays the heavy hand of misogyny, the hatred of women. We all have a responsibility to recognize this bias—sometimes subtle—when ancient negative attitudes toward women intrude into the abortion debate. It is morally incumbent on us to convert the Christian position to a teaching more respectful of women's concrete history and experience.

My professional peers who are my opponents on this question feel they own the Christian tradition in this matter and recognize no need to rethink their positions in the light of this claim. As a feminist, I cannot sit in silence when women's right to shape the use of our own procreative power is denied. Women's competence as moral decision makers is once again challenged by the state even before the moral basis of women's right to procreative choice has been fully elaborated and recognized. Those who deny women control of procreative power claim that they do so in defense of moral sensibility, in the name of the sanctity of human life. We have a long way to go before the sanctity of human life will include genuine regard and concern for every female already born, and no social policy discussion that obscures this fact deserves to be called moral. We hope the day will come when it will not be called "Christian" either, for the Christian ethos is the generating source of the current moral crusade to prevent women from gaining control over the most life-shaping power we possess.

Although I am a Protestant, my own "moral theology"[1] has more in common with a Catholic approach than with much neoorthodox ethics of my own tradition. I want to stress this at the outset because in what follows I am highly critical of the reigning Roman Catholic social teaching on procreation and abortion. I believe that on most other issues of social justice, the Catholic tradition is often more substantive, morally serious, and less imbued with the dominant economic ideology than the brand of Protestant theo-

From Beverly Wildung Harrison, *Making the Connections: Essays in Feminist Social Ethics* (Boston: Beacon Press, 1985). Revised from an earlier version with the collaboration of Shirley Cloyes.

logical ethics that claims biblical warrants for its moral norms. I am no biblicist; I believe that the human wisdom that informs our ethics derives not from using the Bible alone but from reflecting in a manner that earlier Catholic moral theologians referred to as consonant with "natural law."[2] Unfortunately, however, all major strands of natural law reflection have been every bit as awful as Protestant biblicism on any matter involving human sexuality, including discussion of women's nature and women's divine vocation in relation to procreative power. And it is precisely because I recognize Catholic natural law tradition as having produced the most sophisticated type of moral reflection among Christians that I believe it must be challenged where it intersects negatively with women's lives.

Given the depth of my dissatisfaction with Protestant moral tradition, I take no pleasure in singling out Roman Catholic moral theology and the activity of the Catholic hierarchy on the abortion issue. The problem nevertheless remains that there is really only one set of moral claims involved in the Christian antiabortion argument. Protestants who oppose procreative choice[3] either tend to follow official Catholic moral theology on these matters or ground their positions in biblicist anti-intellectualism, claiming that God's "word" requires no justification other than their attestation that divine utterance says what it says. Against such irrationalism, no rational objections have a chance. When, however, Protestant fundamentalists actually specify the reasons why they believe abortion is evil, they invariably revert to traditional natural law assumptions about women, sexuality, and procreation. Hence, direct objection must be registered to the traditional natural law framework if we are serious about transforming Christian moral teaching on abortion.

To do a methodologically adequate analysis of any moral problem in religious social ethics it is necessary to (1) situate the problem in the context of various religious communities' theologies or "generative" stories, (2) do a critical historical review of the problem as it appears in our religious traditions and in the concrete lives of human agents (so that we do not confuse the past and the present), (3) scrutinize the problem from the standpoint of various moral theories, and (4) analyze existing social policy and potential alternatives to determine our "normative moral sense" or best judgment of what ought to be done in contemporary society. Although these methodological basepoints must be addressed in any socioethical analysis, their treatment is crucial when abortion is under discussion because unexamined theological presumptions and misrepresentations of Christian history figure heavily in the current public policy debate. Given the brevity of this essay, I will address the theological, Christian historical, and moral theoretical problematics first and analyze the social policy dimensions of the abortion issue only at the end, even though optimum ethical methodology would reverse this procedure.

Abortion in Theological Context

In the history of Christian theology, a central metaphor for understanding life, including human life, is as a gift of God. Creation itself has been interpreted primarily under this metaphor. It follows that in this creational context procreation itself took on special significance as the central image for the divine blessing of human life. The elevation of procreation as the central symbol of divine benevolence happened over time, however. It did not, for instance, typify the very early, primitive Christian community. The synoptic gospels provide ample evidence that procreation played no such metaphorical role in early Christianity.[4] In later Christian history, an emergent powerful antisexual bias within Christianity made asceticism the primary spiritual ideal, although this ideal usually stood in tension with procreative power as a second sacred expression of divine blessing. But by the time of the Protestant Reformation, there was clear reaffirmation of the early Israelite theme of procreative blessing, and procreation has since become all but synonymous among Christians with the theological theme of creation as divine gift. It is important to observe that Roman Catholic theology actually followed on and adapted to Protestant teaching on this point.[5] Only in the last century, with the recognition of the danger of dramatic population growth in a world of finite resources, has any question been raised about the appropriateness of this unqualified theological sacralization of procreation.

The elevation of procreation as the central image for divine blessing is intimately connected to the rise of patriarchy. In patriarchal societies it is the male's power that is enhanced by the gift of new life. Throughout history, women's power of procreation has stood in definite tension with this male social control. In fact, what we feminists call patriarchy—that is, patterned or institutionalized legitimations of male superiority—derives from the need of men, through male-dominated political institutions such as tribes, states, and religious systems, to control women's power to procreate the species. We must assume, then, that many of these efforts at social control of procreation, including some church teaching on contraception and abortion, were part of this institutional system. The perpetuation of patriarchal control itself depended on wresting the power of procreation from women and shaping women's lives accordingly.

In the past four centuries, the entire Christian story has had to undergo dramatic accommodation to new and emergent world conditions and to the scientific revolution. As the older theological metaphors for creation encountered the rising power of science, a new self-understanding including our human capacity to affect nature had to be incorporated into Christian theology or its central theological story would have become obscurantist. Human agency had to be introjected into a dialectical understanding of creation.

The range of human freedom to shape and enhance creation is now celebrated theologically, but only up to the point of changes in our understanding of what is natural for women. Here a barrier has been drawn that declares No Radical Freedom! The only difference between mainstream Protestant and Roman Catholic theologians on these matters is at the point of contraception, which Protestants more readily accept. However, Protestants like Karl Barth and Helmut Thielicke exhibit a subtle shift of mood when they turn to discussing issues regarding women. They follow the typical Protestant pattern: They have accepted contraception or family planning as part of the new freedom, granted by God, but both draw back from the idea that abortion could be morally acceptable. In *The Ethics of Sex,* Thielicke offers a romantic, ecstatic celebration of family planning on one page and then elaborates a total denunciation of abortion as unthinkable on the next.[6] Most Christian theological opinion draws the line between contraception and abortion, whereas the *official* Catholic teaching still anathematizes contraception.

The problem, then, is that Christian theology celebrates the power of human freedom to shape and determine the quality of human life except when the issue of procreative choice arises. Abortion is anathema, while widespread sterilization abuse goes unnoticed. The power of man to shape creation radically is never rejected. When one stops to consider the awesome power over nature that males take for granted and celebrate, including the power to alter the conditions of human life in myriad ways, the suspicion dawns that the near hysteria that prevails about the immorality of women's right to choose abortion derives its force from the ancient power of misogyny rather than from any passion for the sacredness of human life. An index of the continuing misogyny in Christian tradition is male theologians' refusal to recognize the full range of human power to shape creation in those matters that pertain to women's power to affect the quality of our lives.

In contrast, a feminist theological approach recognizes that nothing is more urgent, in light of the changing circumstances of human beings on planet Earth, than to recognize that the entire natural-historical context of human procreative power has shifted.[7] We desperately need a desacralization of our biological power to reproduce[8] and at the same time a real concern for human dignity and the social conditions for personhood and the values of human relationship.[9] And note that desacralization does not mean complete devaluation of the worth of procreation. It means we must shift away from the notion that the central metaphors for divine blessing are expressed at the biological level to the recognition that our social relations bear the image of what is most holy. An excellent expression of this point comes from Marie Augusta Neal, a Roman Catholic feminist and a distinguished sociologist of religion:

> As long as the central human need called for was continued motivation to propagate the race, it was essential that religious symbols idealize that process above all others. Given the vicissitudes of life in a hostile environment, women had to be encouraged to bear children and men to support them: childbearing was central to the struggle for existence. Today, however, the size of the base population, together with knowledge already accumulated about artificial insemination, sperm banking, cloning, make more certain a peopled world.
>
> The more serious human problems now are who will live, who will die and who will decide.[10]

A Critical Historical Review of Abortion: An Alternative Perspective

Between persons who oppose all abortions on moral grounds and those who believe abortion is sometimes or frequently morally justifiable, there is no difference of moral principle. Pro-choice advocates and anti-abortion advocates share the ethical principle of respect for human life, which is probably why the debate is so acrimonious. I have already indicated that one major source of disagreement is the way in which the theological story is appropriated in relation to the changing circumstances of history. In addition, we should recognize that whenever strong moral disagreement is encountered, we simultaneously confront different readings of the history of a moral issue. The way we interpret the past is already laden with and shaped by our present sense of what the moral problem is.

For example, professional male Christian ethicists tend to assume that Christianity has an unbroken history of "all but absolute" prohibition of abortion and that the history of morality of abortion can best be traced by studying the teaching of the now best-remembered theologians. Looking at the matter this way, one can find numerous proof-texts to show that some of the "church fathers" condemned abortion and equated abortion with either homicide or murder. Whenever a "leading" churchman equated abortion with homicide or murder, he also *and simultaneously* equated *contraception* with homicide or murder. This reflects not only male chauvinist biology but also the then almost phobic antisexual bias of the Christian tradition. Claims that one can separate abortion teaching into an ethic of killing separate from an antisexual and antifemale ethic in the history of Christianity do not withstand critical scrutiny.[11]

The history of Christian natural law ethics is totally conditioned by the equation of any effort to control procreation with homicide. However, this antisexual, antiabortion tradition is not universal, even among theologians and canon lawyers. On the subject of sexuality and its abuse, many well-known theologians had nothing to say; abortion was not even mentioned in most moral theology. An important, untold chapter in Christian history is the great struggle that took place in the medieval period when clerical celibacy came to be imposed and the rules of sexual behavior rigidified.

My thesis is that there is a relative disinterest in the question of abortion overall in Christian history. Occasionally, Christian theologians picked up the issue, especially when these theologians were state-related, that is, were articulating policy not only for the church but for political authority. Demographer Jean Meyer, himself a Catholic, insists that the Christian tradition took over "expansion by population growth" from the Roman Empire.[12] Christians opposed abortion strongly only when Christianity was closely identified with imperial state policy or when theologians were inveighing against women and any sexuality except that expressed in the reluctant service of procreation.

The Holy Crusade quality of present teaching on abortion is quite new in Christianity and is related to cultural shifts that are requiring the Christian tradition to choose sides in the present ideological struggle under pressure to rethink its entire attitude toward women and sexuality. My research has led me to the tentative conclusion that, in Protestant cultures, except where Protestantism is the "established religion," merging church and state, one does not find a strong antiabortion theological-ethical teaching at all. At least in the United States, this is beyond historical debate.[13] No Protestant clergy or theologian gave early support for proposed nineteenth-century laws banning abortion in the United States. It is my impression that Protestant clergy, usually married and often poor, were aware that romanticizing nature's bounty with respect to procreation resulted in a great deal of human suffering. The Protestant clergy who finally did join the antiabortion crusade were racist, classist white clergy, who feared America's strength was being threatened because white, middle-class, respectable women had a lower birth rate than black and ethnic women. Such arguments are still with us.

One other historical point must be stressed. Until the late nineteenth century the natural law tradition, and biblicism following it, tended to define the act of abortion as interruption of pregnancy after ensoulment, which was understood to be the point at which the breath of God entered the fetus. The point at which ensoulment was said to occur varied, but most typically it was marked by quickening, when fetal movement began. Knowledge about embryology was primitive until the past half-century, so this commonsense understanding prevailed. As a result, when abortion was condemned in earlier Christian teaching it was understood to refer to the termination of a pregnancy well into the process of the pregnancy, after ensoulment. Until the late nineteenth century, when Pope Pius IX, intrigued with the new embryonic discoveries, brought the natural law tradition into consonance with "modern science," abortion in ecclesiastical teaching often applied only to termination of prenatal life in more advanced stages of pregnancy.

Another distortion in the male-generated history of this issue derives from failure to note that, until the development of safe, surgical, elective abortion, the act of abortion commonly referred to something done to the woman, with or without her consent (see Exodus 22), either as a wrong done a husband or for the better moral reasons that abortion was an act of violence against both a pregnant woman and fetal life. In recent discussion it is the woman who does the wrongful act. No one would deny that abortion, if it terminates a pregnancy against the woman's wishes, is morally wrong. And until recent decades, abortion endangered the woman's life as much as it did the prenatal life in her womb. Hence, one premodern moral reason for opposing abortion was that it threatened the life and well-being of the mother more than did carrying the pregnancy to term. Today abortion is statistically safer than childbearing. Consequently, no one has a right to discuss the morality of abortion today without recognizing that one of the traditional and appropriate moral reasons for objecting to abortion—concern for women's well-being—now inheres in the pro-choice side of the debate. Anti-abortion proponents who accord the fetus full human standing without also assigning positive value to women's lives and well-being are not really pressing the full sense of Christian moral tradition in the abortion debate.

Beyond all this, the deepest moral flaw in the "pro-life" position's historical view is that none of its proponents has attempted to reconstruct the concrete, lived-world context in which the abortion discussion belongs: the all but desperate struggle by sexually active women to gain some proximate control over nature's profligacy in conception. Under the most adverse conditions, women have had to try to control our fertility—everywhere, always. Women's relation to procreation irrevocably marks and shapes our lives. Even those of us who do not have sexual contact with males, because we are celibate or lesbian, have been potential, even probable, victims of male sexual violence or have had to bear heavy social stigma for refusing the centrality of dependence on men and of procreation in our lives. The lives of infertile women, too, are shaped by our failure to meet procreative expectations. Women's lack of social power, in all recorded history, has made this struggle to control procreation a life-bending, often life-destroying one for a large percentage of females.

So most women have had to do whatever we could to prevent too-numerous pregnancies. In societies and cultures, except the most patriarchal, the processes of procreation have been transmitted through women's culture. Birth control techniques have been widely practiced, and some primitive ones have proved effective. Increasingly, anthropologists are gaining hints of how procreative control occurred in some premodern societies. Frequently women have had to choose to risk their lives in order not to have that extra child that would destroy the family's ability to cope or bring about an unmanageable crisis.

We have to concede that modern medicine, for all its misogyny, has replaced some dangerous contraceptive practices still widely used where surgical abortion is unavailable. In light of these gains, more privileged western women must not lose the ability to imagine the real-life pressures that lead women in other cultures to resort to ground-glass douches, reeds inserted in the uterus, and so on, to induce labor. The radical nature of methods women use bespeaks the desperation involved in unwanted pregnancy and reveals the real character of our struggle.

Nor should we suppress the fact that a major means of birth control now is, as it was in earlier times, infanticide. And let no one imagine that women have made decisions to expose or kill newborn infants casually. Women understand what many men cannot seem to grasp—that the birth of a child requires that some person must be prepared to care, without interruption, for this infant, provide material resources and energy-draining amounts of time and attention for it. The human infant is the most needy and dependent of all newborn creatures. It seems to me that men, especially celibate men, romanticize this total and uncompromising dependency of the infant on the already existing human community. Women bear the brunt of this reality and know its full implications. And this dependency is even greater in a fragmented, centralized urban-industrial modern culture than in a rural culture, where another pair of hands often increased an extended family unit's productive power. No historical interpretation of abortion as a moral issue that ignores these matters deserves moral standing in the present debate.

A treatment of any moral problem is inadequate if it fails to analyze the morality of a given act in a way that represents the concrete experience of the agent who faces a decision with respect to that act. Misogyny in Christian discussions of abortion is evidenced clearly in that the abortion decision is never treated in the way it arises as part of the female agent's life process. The decision at issue when the dilemma of choice arises for women is whether or not to be pregnant. In most discussions of the morality of abortion it is treated as an abstract act[14] rather than as a possible way to deal with a pregnancy that frequently is the result of circumstances beyond the woman's control. John Noonan, for instance, evades this fact by referring to the pregnant woman almost exclusively as "the gravida" (a Latin term meaning "pregnant one") or "the carrier" in his *A Private Choice: Abortion in America in the Seventies.*[15] In any pregnancy a woman's life is deeply, irrevocably affected. Those such as Noonan who uphold the unexceptional immorality of abortion are probably wise to obscure the fact that an unwanted pregnancy always involves a life-shaping consequence for a woman, because suppressing the identity of the moral agent and the reality of her dilemma greatly reduces the ability to recognize the moral complexity of abortion. When the question of abortion arises it is usually because a woman finds herself facing an unwanted pregnancy. Consider the actual circumstances that may precipitate this. One is the situation in which a woman did not intend to be sexually active or did not enter into a sexual act voluntarily. Since women are frequently victims of sexual violence, numerous cases of this type arise because of rape, incest, or forced marital coitus. Many morally sensitive opponents of abortion concede that in such cases abortion may be morally justifiable. I insist that in such cases it is a moral good because it is not rational to treat a newly fertilized ovum as though it had the same value as the existent, pregnant female person and because it is morally wrong to make the victim of sexual violence suffer the further agonies of unwanted pregnancy and childbearing against her will. Enforced pregnancy would be viewed as a morally reprehensible violation of bodily integrity if women were recognized as fully human moral agents.

Another more frequent case results when a woman—or usually a young girl—participates in heterosexual activity without clear knowledge of how pregnancy occurs and without intention to conceive a child. A girl who became pregnant in this manner would, by traditional natural law morality, be held in a state of invincible ignorance and therefore not morally culpable. One scholarly Roman Catholic nun I met argued—quite appropriately, I believe—that her church should not consider the abortions of young Catholic girls as morally culpable because the Church overprotected them, which contributed to their lack of understanding of procreation and to their inability to cope with the sexual pressures girls experience in contemporary society. A social policy that pressures the sexually ill-informed child or young woman into unintended or unaware motherhood would be morally dubious indeed.

A related type of pregnancy happens when a woman runs risks by not using contraceptives, perhaps because taking precaution in romantic affairs is not perceived as ladylike or requires her to be too unspontaneous about sex. Our society resents women's sexuality unless it is "innocent" and male-mediated, so many women, lest they be censured as "loose" and "promiscuous," are slow to assume adult responsibility for contraception. However, when pregnancies occur because women are skirting the edges of responsibility and running risks out of immaturity, is enforced motherhood a desirable solution? Such pregnancies could be minimized only by challenging precisely those childish myths of female socialization embedded in natural law teaching about female sexuality.

It is likely that most decisions about abortion arise because mature women who are sexually active with men and who understand the risk of pregnancy nevertheless experience contraceptive failure. Our moral schizophrenia in this matter is exhibited in that many people believe women have more responsibility than men to practice contraception and that family planning is always a moral good, but even so rule out abortion altogether. Such a split consciousness ignores the fact that no inexorable biological line exists between prevention of conception and abortion.[16] More important, such reasoning ignores the genuine risks involved in female contraceptive methods. Some women are at higher risk than others in using the most reliable means of birth control. Furthermore, the reason we do not have more concern for safer contraceptive methods for men and women is that matters relating to women's health and well-being are never urgent in this society. Moreover, many contraceptive failures are due to the irresponsibility of the producers of contraceptives rather than to bad luck.[17] Given these facts, should a woman who actively attempts to avoid pregnancy be punished for contraceptive failure when it occurs?

In concluding this historical section, I must stress that if present efforts to criminalize abortion succeed, we will need a state apparatus of massive proportions to enforce compulsory childbearing. In addition, withdrawal of legal abortion will create one more massively profitable underworld economy in which the Mafia and other sections of quasi-legal capitalism may and will profitably invest. The radical right promises to get the state out of regulation of people's lives, but what they really mean is that they will let economic activity go unrestrained. What their agenda signifies for the personal lives of women is quite another matter.

An adequate historical perspective on abortion recognizes the long struggle women have waged for some degree of control over fertility and their efforts to regain control of procreative power from patriarchal and state-imperial culture and institutions. Such a perspective also takes into account that more nearly adequate contraceptive methods and the existence of safe, surgical, elective abortion represent positive historic steps toward full human freedom and dignity for women. While the same gains in medical knowledge also open the way to new forms of sterilization abuse and to social pressures against some women's use of their power of procreation, I know of no women who would choose to return to a state of lesser knowledge about these matters.

There has been an objective gain in the quality of women's lives for those fortunate enough to have access to procreative choice. That millions upon millions of women as yet do not possess even the rudimentary conditions—moral or physical—for such choice is obvious. Our moral goal should be to struggle against those real barriers—poverty, racism, and antifemale cultural oppression—that prevent authentic choice from being a reality for every woman. In this process we will be able to minimize the need for abortions only insofar as we place the abortion debate in the real lived-world context of women's lives.

Abortion and Moral Theory

The greatest strategic problem of pro-choice advocates is the widespread assumption that pro-lifers have a monopoly on the moral factors that ought to enter into decisions about abortion. *Moral* here is defined as that which makes for the self-respect and well-being of human persons and their environment. Moral legitimacy seems to adhere to their position in part because traditionalists have an array of religiomoral terminology at their command that the sometimes more secular proponents of choice lack. But those who would displace women's power of choice by the power of the state and/or the medical profession do not deserve the aura of moral sanctity. We must do our homework if we are to dispel this myth of moral superiority. A major way in which Christian moral theologians and moral philosophers contribute to this monopoly of moral sanctity is by equating fetal or prenatal life with human personhood in a simplistic way and by failing to acknowledge changes regarding this issue in the history of Christianity.

We need to remember that even in Roman Catholic natural law ethics, the definition of the status of fetal life has shifted over time and in all cases the status of prenatal life involves a moral judgment, not a scientific one. The question is properly posed this way: What status are we morally wise to predicate to prenatal human life, given that the fetus is not yet a fully existent human being? Those constrained under Catholic teaching have been required for the past ninety years to believe a human being exists from conception, when the ovum and sperm merge.[18] This answer from one tradition has had far wider impact on our culture than most people recognize. Other Christians come from traditions that do not offer (and could not offer, given their conception of the structure of the church as moral community) a definitive answer to this question.

Even so, some contemporary Protestant medical ethicists, fascinated by recent genetic discoveries and experiments with deoxyribonucleic acid (DNA), have all but sacralized the moment in which the genetic code is implanted as the moment of humanization, which leaves them close to the traditional Roman Catholic position. Protestant male theologians have long let their enthrallment with science lead to a sacralization of specific scientific discoveries, usually to the detriment of theological and moral clarity. In any case, there are two responses that must be made to the claim that the fetus in early stages of development is a human life or, more dubiously, a human person.

First, the historical struggle for women's personhood is far from won, owing chiefly to the opposition of organized religious groups to full equality for women. Those who proclaim that a zygote at the moment of conception is a person worthy of citizenship continue to deny full social and political rights to women. Whatever one's judgment about the moral status of the fetus, it cannot be argued that that assessment deserves greater moral standing in analysis than does the position of the pregnant woman. This matter of evaluating the meaning of prenatal life is where morally sensitive people's judgments diverge. I cannot believe that anyone, if truly morally sensitive, would value the woman's full, existent life less than they value early fetal life. Most women can become pregnant and carry fetal life to term many, many times in their lifetimes. The distinctly human power is not our biologic capacity to bear children, but our power to actively love, nurture, care for one another and shape one another's existence in cultural and social interaction.[19] To equate a biologic process with full normative humanity is crass biologic reductionism, and such reductionism is never practiced in religious ethics except where women's lives and well-being are involved.

Second, even though prenatal life, as it moves toward biologic individuation of human form, has value, the equation of abortion with murder is dubious. And the equation of abortion with homicide—the taking of human life—should be carefully weighed. We should also remember that we live in a world where men extend other men wide moral range in relation to justifiable homicide. For example, the just-war tradition has legitimated widespread forms of killing in war, and Christian ethicists have often extended great latitude to rulers and those in power in making choices about killing human beings.[20] Would that such moralists extended equal benefit of a doubt to women facing life-crushing psychological and politicoeconomic pressures in the face of childbearing! Men, daily, make life-determining decisions concerning nuclear power or chemical use in the environment, for example, that affect the well-being of fetuses, and our society expresses no significant opposition, even when such decisions do widespread genetic damage. When we argue for the appropriateness of legal abortion, moral outrage rises.

The so-called pro-life position also gains support by invoking the general principle of respect for human life as foundational to its morality in a way that suggests that the pro-choice advocates are unprincipled. I have already noted that pro-choice advocates have every right to claim the same moral principle, and that this debate, like most debates that are morally acrimonious, is in no sense about basic moral principles.

I do not believe there is any clear-cut conflict of principle in this very deep, very bitter controversy.

It needs to be stressed that we all have an absolute obligation to honor any moral principle that seems, after rational deliberation, to be sound. This is the one absolutism appropriate to ethics. There are often several moral principles relevant to a decision and many ways to relate a given principle to a decisional context. For most right-to-lifers only one principle has moral standing in this argument. Admitting only one principle to one's process of moral reasoning means that a range of other moral values is slighted. Right-to-lifers are also moral absolutists in the sense that they admit only one possible meaning or application of the principle they invoke. Both these types of absolutism obscure moral debate and lead to less, not more, rational deliberation. The principle of respect for human life is one we should all honor, but we must also recognize that this principle often comes into conflict with other valid moral principles in the process of making real, lived-world decisions. Understood in an adequate way, this principle can be restated to mean that we should treat what falls under a reasonable definition of human life as having sanctity or intrinsic moral value. But even when this is clear, other principles are needed to help us choose between two intrinsic values, in this case between the prenatal life and the pregnant woman's life.

Another general moral principle from which we cannot exempt our actions is the principle of justice, or right relations between persons and between groups of persons and communities. Another relevant principle is respect for all that supports human life, namely, the natural environment. As any person knows who thinks deeply about morality, genuine moral conflicts, as often as not, are due not to ignoring moral principles but to the fact that different principles lead to conflicting implications for action or are selectively related to decisions. For example, we live in a time when the principle of justice for women, aimed at transforming the social relations that damage women's lives, is historically urgent. For many of us this principle has greater moral urgency than the extension of the principle of respect for human life to include early fetal life, even though respect for fetal life is also a positive moral good. We should resist approaches to ethics that claim that one overriding principle always deserves to control morality. Clarification of principle, for that matter, is only a small part of moral reasoning. When we weigh moral principles and their potential application, we must also consider the implications of a given act for our present historical context and envision its long-term consequences.

One further proviso on this issue of principles in moral reasoning: There are several distinct theories among religious ethicists and moral philosophers as to what the function of principles ought to be. One group believes moral principles are for the purpose of terminating the process of moral reasoning. Hence, if this sort of moralist tells you always to honor the principle of respect for human life, what he or she means is for you to stop reflection and act in a certain way—in this case to accept one's pregnancy regardless of consequences. Others believe that it is better to refer to principles (broad, generalized moral criteria) than to apply rules (narrower, specific moral prescriptions) because principles function to open up processes of reasoning rather than close them off. The principle of respect for life, on this reading, is not invoked to prescribe action but to help locate and weigh values, to illuminate a range of values that always inhere in significant human decisions. A major difference in the moral debate on abortion, then, is that some believe that to invoke the principle of respect for human life settles the matter, stops debate, and precludes the single, simple act of abortion. By contrast, many of us believe the breadth of the principle opens up to reconsideration the question of what the essential moral quality of human life is all about and to increase moral seriousness about choosing whether or when to bear children.

Two other concerns related to our efforts to make a strong moral case for women's right to procreative choice need to be touched on. The first has to do with the problems our Christian tradition creates for any attempt to make clear why women's right to control our bodies is an urgent and substantive moral claim. One of Christianity's greatest weaknesses is its spiritualizing neglect of respect for the physical body and physical well-being. Tragically, women, more than men, are expected in Christian teaching never to honor their own well-being as a moral consideration. I want to stress, then, that we have no moral tradition in Christianity that starts with body-space, or body-right, as a basic condition of moral relations. (Judaism is far better in this regard, for it acknowledges that we all have a moral right to be concerned for our life and our survival.) Hence, many Christian ethicists simply do not get the point when we speak of women's right to bodily integrity. They blithely denounce such reasons as women's disguised self-indulgence or hysterical rhetoric.[21]

We must articulate our view that body-right is a basic moral claim and also remind our hearers that there is no unchallengeable analogy among other human activities to women's procreative power. Pregnancy is a distinctive human experience. In any social relation, body-space must be respected or nothing deeply human or moral can be created. The social institutions most similar to compulsory pregnancy in their moral violations of body-space are chattel slavery and peonage. These institutions distort the moral relations of a community and deform a community over time. (Witness racism in the United States.) Coercion of women, through enforced sterilization or enforced pregnancy, legitimates unjust power in intimate human relationships and cuts to the heart of our capacity for moral social relations. As we should recognize, given our violence-prone society, people learn violence at home and at an early age when women's lives are violated!

Even so, we must be careful, when we make the case for our right to bodily integrity, not to confuse moral rights with mere liberties.[22] To claim that we have a moral right to procreative choice does not mean we believe women can exercise this right free of all moral claims from the community. For example, we need to teach female children that childbearing is not a purely capricious, individualistic matter, and we need to challenge the assumption that a woman who enjoys motherhood should have as many children as she and her mate wish, regardless of its effects on others. Population self-control is a moral issue, although more so in high-consuming, affluent societies like our own than in nations where a modest, simple, and less wasteful lifestyle obtains.

A second point is the need, as we work politically for a pro-choice social policy, to avoid the use of morally objectionable arguments to mobilize support for our side of the issue. One can get a lot of political mileage in U.S. society by using covert racist and classist appeals ("abortion lowers the cost of welfare rolls or reduces illegitimacy" or "paying for abortions saves the taxpayers money in the long run"). Sometimes it is argued that good politics is more important than good morality and that one should use whatever arguments work to gain political support. I do not believe that these crassly utilitarian[23] arguments turn out, in the long run, to be good politics for they are costly to our sense of polis and of community. But even if they were effective in the short run, I am doubly sure that on the issue of the right to choose abortion, good morality doth a good political struggle make. I believe, deeply, that moral right is on the side of the struggle for the freedom and self-respect of women, especially poor and non-white women, and on the side of developing social policy that ensures that every child born can be certain to be a wanted child. Issues of justice are those that deserve the deepest moral caretaking as we develop a political strategy.

Only when people see that they cannot prohibit safe, legal, elective surgical abortion without violating the conditions of well-being for the vast majority of women—especially those most socially vulnerable because of historic patterns of oppression—will the effort to impose a selective, abstract morality of the sanctity of human life on all of us cease. This is a moral battle par excellence, and whenever we forget that we make it harder to reach the group most important to the cause of procreative choice—those women who have never suffered from childbearing pressures, who have not yet put this issue into a larger historical context, and who reverence women's historical commitment to childbearing. We will surely not reach them with pragmatic appeals to the taxpayer's wallet! To be sure, we cannot let such women go unchallenged as they support ruling-class ideology that the state should control procreation. But they will not change their politics until they see that pro-choice is grounded in a deeper, tougher, more caring moral vision than the political option they now endorse.

The Social Policy Dimensions of the Debate

Most people fail to understand that in ethics we need, provisionally, to separate our reflection on the morality of specific acts from questions about how we express our moral values within our social institutions and systems (that is, social policy). When we do this, the morality of abortion appears in a different light. Focusing attention away from the single act of abortion to the larger historical context thrusts into relief what "respect for human life" means in the pro-choice position. It also illuminates the common core of moral concern that unites pro-choice advocates to pro-lifers who have genuine concern for expanding the circle of who really counts as human in this society. Finally, placing abortion in a larger historical context enables proponents of pro-choice to clarify where we most differ from the pro-lifers, that is, in our total skepticism that a state-enforced anti-abortion policy could ever have the intended "pro-life" consequences they claim.

We must always insist that the objective social conditions that make women and children already born highly vulnerable can only be worsened by a social policy of compulsory pregnancy. However one judges the moral quality of the individual act of abortion (and here, differences among us do exist that are morally justifiable), it is still necessary to distinguish between how one judges the act of abortion morally and what one believes a societywide policy on abortion should be. We must not let those who have moral scruples against the personal act ignore the fact that a just social policy must also include active concern for enhancement of women's well-being and, for that, policies that would in fact make abortions less necessary. To anathematize abortion when the social and material conditions for control of procreation do not exist is to blame the victim, not to address the deep dilemmas of female existence in this society.

Even so, there is no reason for those of us who celebrate procreative choice as a great moral good to pretend that resort to abortion is ever a desirable means of expressing this choice. I know of no one on the pro-choice side who has confused the desirability of the availability of abortion with the celebration of the act itself. We all have every reason to hope that safer, more reliable means of contraception may be found and that violence against women will be reduced. Furthermore, we should be emphatic that our social policy demands include opposition to sterilization abuse, insistence on higher standards of health care for women and children, better prenatal care, reduction of unnecessary surgery on women's reproductive systems, increased research to improve contraception, and so on. Nor should we draw back from criticizing a health care delivery system that exploits women. An abortion industry thrives on the profitability of abortion, but women are not to blame for this.

A feminist position demands social conditions that support women's full, self-respecting right to procreative choice, including the right not to be sterilized against our wills, the right to choose abortion as a birth control means of last resort, and the right to a prenatal and postnatal health care system that will also reduce the now widespread trauma of having to deliver babies in rigid, impersonal health care settings. Prolifers do best politically when we allow them to keep the discussion narrowly focused on the morality of the act of abortion and on the moral value of the fetus. We do best politically when we make the deep connections between the full context of this issue in women's lives, including this society's systemic or patterned injustice toward women.

It is well to remember that it has been traditional Catholic natural law ethics that most clarified and stressed this distinction between the morality of an individual act on the one hand and the policies that produce the optional social morality on the other. The strength of this tradition is probably reflected in the fact that even now most polls show that slightly more Catholics than Protestants believe it unwise for the state to attempt to regulate abortion. In the past, Catholics, more than Protestants, have been wary of using the state as an instrument of moral crusade. Tragically, by taking their present approach to abortion, the Roman Catholic hierarchy may be risking the loss of the deepest wisdom of its own ethical tradition. By failing to acknowledge a distinction between the church's moral teaching on the act of abortion and the question of what is a desirable social policy to minimize abortion, as well as overemphasizing it to the neglect of other social justice concerns, the Roman Catholic church may well be dissipating the best of its moral tradition.[24]

The frenzy of the current pope and many Roman Catholic bishops in the United States on this issue has reached startling proportions. The United States bishops have equated nuclear war and the social practice of abortion as the most heinous social evils of our time.[25] While this appallingly misguided analogy has gained credibility because of the welcome if modest opposition of the bishops to nuclear escalation, I predict that the long-term result will be to further discredit Roman Catholic moral wisdom in the culture.

If we are to be a society genuinely concerned with enhancing women's well-being and minimizing the necessity of abortions, thereby avoiding the danger over time of becoming an abortion culture,[26] what kind of society must we become? It is here that the moral clarity of the feminist analysis becomes most obvious. How can we reduce the number of abortions due to contraceptive failure? By placing greater emphasis on medical research in this area, by requiring producers of contraceptives to behave more responsibly, and by developing patterns of institutional life that place as much emphasis on male responsibility for procreation and long-term care and nurturance of children as on female responsibility.

How can we reduce the number of abortions due to childish ignorance about sexuality among female children or adult women and our mates? By adopting a widespread program of sex education and by supporting institutional policies that teach male and female children alike that a girl is as fully capable as a boy of enjoying sex and that both must share moral responsibility for preventing pregnancy except when they have decided, as a deliberative moral act, to have a child.

How would we reduce the necessity of abortion due to sexual violence against women in and out of marriage? By challenging vicious male-generated myths that women exist primarily to meet the sexual needs of men, that women are, by nature, those who are really fulfilled only through our procreative powers. We would teach feminist history as the truthful history of the race, stressing that historic patterns of patriarchy were morally wrong and that a humane or moral society would be a fully nonsexist society.

Technological developments that may reduce the need for abortions are not entirely within our control, but the sociomoral ethos that makes abortion common is within our power to change. And we would begin to create such conditions by adopting a thoroughgoing feminist program for society. Nothing less, I submit, expresses genuine respect for all human life.

Notes

1. I use the traditional Roman Catholic term intentionally because my ethical method has greater affinity with the Roman Catholic model.

2. The Christian natural law tradition developed because many Christians understood that the power of moral reason inhered in human beings qua human beings, not merely in the understanding that comes from being Christian. Those who follow natural law methods address moral issues from the consideration of what options appear rationally compelling, given present reflection rather than from theological claims alone. My own moral theological method is congenial to certain of these natural law assumptions. Roman Catholic natural law teaching, however, has become internally incoherent by its insistence that in some matters of morality the teaching authority of the hierarchy must be taken as the proper definition of what is rational. This replacement of reasoned reflection by ecclesiastical authority seems to me to offend against what we must mean by moral reasoning on best understanding. I would argue that a moral theology cannot forfeit final judgment or even penultimate judgment on moral matters to anything except fully deliberated communal consensus. On the abortion issue, this of course would mean women would be consulted in a degree that reflects their numbers in the Catholic church. No a priori claims to authoritative moral reason are ever possible, and if those affected are not consulted, the teaching cannot claim rationality.

3. For a critique of these positions, see Paul D. Simmons, "A Theological Response to Fundamentalism on the Abortion Issue," in *Abortion: The Moral Issues,* ed. Edward Batchelor, Jr. (New York: Pilgrim Press, 1982), pp. 175-187.

4. Most biblical scholars agree that either the early Christians expected an imminent end to history and therefore had only an "interim ethic," or that Jesus' teaching, in its radical support for "the outcasts" of his society, did not aim to justify existing social institutions. See, for example, Luke 4 and 12; Mark 7, 9, 13, and 14; Matthew 25. See also Elişabeth Schüssler Fiorenza, "You Are Not to be Called Father," *Cross Currents* (Fall 1979), pp. 301-323. See also her *Bread Not Stone: The Challenge of Feminist Biblical Interpretation* (Boston: Beacon Press, 1985).

5. Few Roman Catholic theologians seem to appreciate how much the recent enthusiastic endorsement of traditional family values implicates Catholicism in Protestant Reformational spirituality. Rosemary Ruether is an exception; she has stressed this point in her writings.

6. Helmut Thielicke, *The Ethics of Sex* (New York: Harper and Row, 1964), pp. 199-247. Compare pp. 210 and 226ff. Barth's position on abortion is a bit more complicated than I can elaborate here, which is why one will find him quoted on both sides of the debate. Barth's method allows him to argue that any given radical human act could turn out to be "the will of God" in a given context or setting. We may at any time be given "permission" by God's radical freedom to do what was not before permissible. My point here is that Barth exposits this possible exception in such a traditional prohibitory context that I do not believe it appropriate to cite him on the pro-choice side of the debate. In my opinion, no woman could ever accept the convoluted way in which Barth's biblical exegesis opens the door (a slight crack) to woman's full humanity. His reasoning on these questions simply demonstrates what deep difficulty the Christian tradition's exegetical tradition is in with respect to the full humanity and moral agency of women. See Karl Barth, "The Protection of Life," in *Church Dogmatics,* part 3, vol. 4 (Edinburgh: T. and T. Clark, 1961), pp. 415-22.

7. Compare Beverly Wildung Harrison, "When Fruitfulness and Blessedness Diverge," *Religion and Life* (1972), vol. 41, no. 4, pp. 480-496. My views on the seriousness of misogyny as a historical force have deepened since I wrote this essay.

8. Marie Augusta Neal, "Sociology and Sexuality: A Feminist Perspective," *Christianity and Crisis* 39, no. 8 (14 May 1979), pp. 118-122.

9. For a feminist theology of relationship, see Carter Heyward, *Toward the Redemption of God: A Theology of Mutual Relation* (Washington, D.C.: University Press of America, 1982).

10. Neal, "Sociology and Sexuality." This article is of critical importance in discussions of the theology and morality of abortion.

11. Susan Teft Nicholson, *Abortion and the Roman Catholic Church,* JRE Studies in Religious Ethics II (Knoxville: Religious Ethics Inc., University of Tennessee, 1978). This carefully crafted study assumes that there has been a clear "antikilling" ethic separable from any antisexual ethic in Christian abortion teaching. This is an assumption that my historical research does not sustain.

12. Jean Meyer, "Toward a Non-Malthusian Population Policy," in *The American Population Debate,* ed. Daniel Callahan (Garden City, N.Y.: Doubleday, 1971).

13. See James C. Mohr, *Abortion in America* (New York: Oxford University Press, 1978), and James Nelson, "Abortion: Protestant Perspectives," in *Encyclopedia of Bioethics,* vol. 1, ed. Warren T. Reich (New York: Free Press, 1978), pp. 13-17.

14. H. Richard Niebuhr often warned his theological compatriots about abstracting acts from the life project in which they are embedded, but this warning is much neglected in the writings of Christian moralists. See "The Christian Church in the World Crises," *Christianity and Society* 6 (1941).

15. John T. Noonan, Jr., *A Private Choice: Abortion in America in the Seventies* (New York: Free Press, 1979). Noonan denies that the history of abortion is related to the history of male oppression of women.

16. We know now that the birth control pill does not always work by preventing fertilization of the ovum by the sperm. Frequently, the pill causes the wall of the uterus to

expel the newly fertilized ovum. From a biological point of view, there is no point in the procreative process that can be taken as a clear dividing line on which to pin neat moral distinctions.

17. The most conspicuous example of corporate involvement in contraceptive failure was the famous Dalkan Shield scandal. Note also that the manufacturer of the Dalkan Shield dumped its dangerous and ineffective product on family planning programs of third world (overexploited) countries.

18. Catholic moral theology opens up several ways for faithful Catholics to challenge the teaching office of the church on moral questions. However, I remain unsatisfied that these qualifications of inerrancy in moral matters stand up in situations of moral controversy. If freedom of conscience does not function *de jure,* should it be claimed as existent in principle?

19. I elaborate this point in greater detail in "The Power of Anger in the Work of Love" in my *Making the Connections.*

20. For example, Paul Ramsey gave unqualified support to U.S. military involvement in Southeast Asia in light of just-war considerations but finds abortion to be an unexceptional moral wrong.

21. See Richard A. McCormick, S.J., "Rules for Abortion Debate," in Batchelor, Abortion: The Moral Issues, pp. 27-37.

22. One of the reasons why abortion-on-demand rhetoric—even when it is politically effective in the immediate moment—has had a backlash effect is that it seems to many to imply a lack of reciprocity between women's needs and society's needs. While I would not deny, in principle, a possible conflict of interest between women's well-being and the community's needs for reproduction, there is little or no historical evidence that suggests women are less responsible to the well-being of the community than are men. We need not fall into a liberal, individualistic trap in arguing the central importance of procreative choice to issues of women's well-being in society. The right in question is body-right, or freedom from coercion in childbearing. It is careless to say that the right in question is the right to an abortion. Morally, the right is bodily self-determination, a fundamental condition of personhood and a foundational moral right. See Beverly Wildung Harrison, *Our Right to Choose: Toward a New Ethic of Abortion* (Boston: Beacon Press, 1983).

23. A theory is crassly utilitarian only if it fails to grant equal moral worth to all persons in the calculation of social consequences—as, for example, when some people's financial well-being is weighted more than someone else's basic physical existence. I do not mean to criticize any type of utilitarian moral theory that weighs the actual consequences of actions. In fact, I believe no moral theory is adequate if it does not have a strong utilitarian component.

24. For a perceptive discussion of this danger by a distinguished Catholic priest, read George C. Higgins, "The Prolife Movement and the New Right," *America,* 13 Sept. 1980, pp. 107-110.

25. Philip J. Murnion, ed., *Catholics and Nuclear War: A Commentary on the Challenge of the U.S. Catholic Bishops' Pastoral Letter on War and Peace* (New York: Crossroads, 1983), p. 326.

26. I believe the single most valid concern raised by opponents of abortion is that the frequent practice of abortion, over time, may contribute to a cultural ethos of insensitivity to the value of human life, not because fetuses are being "murdered" but because surgical termination of pregnancy may further "technologize" our sensibilities about procreation. I trust that all of the foregoing makes clear my adamant objection to allowing this insight to justify yet more violence against women. However, I do believe we should be very clear that we stand ready to support—emphatically—any social policies that would lessen the need for abortion *without* jeopardizing women's right to control our own procreative power.

69. Liberation, Abortion and Responsibility

MARGARET A. FARLEY

The Present Impasse

When I was asked to write this article, it was suggested that I might want to assess the Roman Catholic Church's position on abortion from my standpoint as a woman. It might also have been suggested that I evaluate the Women's Liberation position on abortion from my standpoint as a Roman Catholic. I have found it impossible to do either without falling into a recitation of concerns which anti-abortionists and pro-abortionists have presented to one another almost to the point of tedium. It occurred to me that it might be interesting, but on the whole unenlightening, to discuss rather the blurring of stereotypical positions when they are seen coming from concrete individuals who nonetheless stand in identifiable groups. I came finally to the conclusion that my own central concern now with the state of the abortion debate focuses on the present impasse between strong anti-abortionists (though clearly not equated with Roman Catholics, at least well represented by them) and strong pro-abortionists (though surely not equated with feminists, yet most significantly represented by them). It is an impasse not only in moral discourse, or in struggles between wants and beliefs, or in political battles for different sorts of laws (the battles are for the time being largely over on the legal front, and where they continue, they cannot be described as being at an impasse).[1] It is, rather, an impasse in efforts either to mediate or to join issue between what are fundamentally opposing conscience claims, profoundly different experiences of moral obligation. If such an impasse remains unresolved for long, it seems to me that it can only contribute to a deepening moral anguish or a growing moral apathy, and to an overall societal fragmentation or self-deception.[2] One need not, perhaps, paint the picture so dramatically in order to recognize in it a cause for moral concern.

It is to be expected that in a genuinely pluralistic society there will at times emerge between different groups of persons contradictory experiences of moral obligation. Not only diversity but conflict will appear in regard to moral values. Intellectual convictions regarding moral action will produce opposing ethical arguments, but more than this, different and opposing experiences of obligation to action may bring persons in the practical order to painful cross purposes and attempts at mutually exclusive patterns of behavior.

Sophisticated forms of pluralism eliminate conflict by allowing diverse beliefs, ways of action, modes of decision, in so far as these do not seriously interfere with one another. One may (within some limits) worship as one wills, drink as one wills, speak as one wills, marry as one wills, beget children as one wills, because all of these are possible without preventing other persons from doing these and more things in other ways. Peaceful coexistence, in terms of responding to diverse experiences of moral obligation, is a highly developed pattern of social living. Conflict that would arise from infringement upon selves, property or action, is avoided by a society's acceptance of protective laws whose effectiveness depends in part on their ability to allow each member of society at least to follow his or her conscience (if not to pursue his or her every desire).

Some conscience calls (or experiences of moral obligation), however, are not so easily harmonized into patterns of coexistence. This is the case when moral obligations are perceived so differently that they demand of different persons actions that cannot be neatly relegated to a carefully apportioned private sphere. Thus, for example, opposing perceptions of obligations in relation to innocent third parties can constitute acute and seemingly unresolvable points of public conflict between private experiences of moral obligation. I take it that such a situation obtains relative to the issue of abortion. On the one hand, some persons experience a profound and compelling obligation to alleviate situations which are oppressive and harmful to women. On the other hand, some persons experience an equally profound and compelling obligation to protect the lives of human fetuses.[3] In terms of their perceptions of the ways to respond to these obligations, these two groups of persons are led inevitably into public conflict. The goal of the one cannot be had if the goal of the other is to be achieved.

Given the nature of the experience of moral obligation (that is, its experience as an unconditional claim addressed to one's freedom), neither party to a dispute such as the one I have been describing (that is, one which involves concretely opposing courses of action) can simply retire to the sidelines. It would be a strange notion of conscience which would allow for passive acceptance of what is perceived as inherently harmful and unjust to third parties. Thus, those who under-

From *Reflection* 71 (May 1974): 9-13. Used by permission.

stood restrictive abortion laws to be part of the overwhelming structures of oppression for women experienced themselves as obligated to work for liberalization of those laws. But those who understood abortion to be the taking of human life experienced no less an obligation to try to withstand the efforts of the others. And now, too, each of these groups of persons experiences a continuing obligation to secure the rights and welfare of either women or fetuses. The current legal status of the question does not settle the moral struggle which must continue between these groups. It is this struggle, however, which seems to me to be at an impasse—unresolved and, without some advance in moral discourse, unresolvable. It can simply remain unresolved, of course (as long as in the realm of action there is at least no fighting in the streets—or in the hospitals and clinics), but the price of leaving a conflict which has been so large a concern for such large portions of society in a state of limbo may be, as I have suggested above, greater than it immediately appears to be. The conflict may never be resolved, but it seems to me crucial that we attempt to resolve the present impasse in which the conflict is caught. The only way open to such a resolution is precisely some advance in the moral discourse which engages the parties to the conflict.

The nature of the stalemate in moral discourse about abortion is suggested in the frequent observations that the opposing sides never really join issue. There is sometimes the implication given that this failure to come to terms with the opposite position is the result of malice, culpable insensitivity, or stupidity. On the contrary, it seems to me quite possible that it is a consequence of the very intensity of the experience of moral obligation which characterizes those on both sides of the question. The difficulty is that the objects which give rise to these experiences of obligation are not the same, and hence the focus of attention for anti-abortionists and for pro-abortionists is different. The issue is not, in fact, perceived by them as being for or against the same thing. Thus, anti-abortionists do not perceive themselves as against women, but rather for fetuses. Similarly, pro-abortionists do not understand themselves as against fetuses, but rather for women. The possibility that what each is for does indeed oppose what the other is for is perceived only in a defensive way. The strength of the concern which each side has for one object rather than the other does in fact, however, prevent each side from sharing the moral awareness of the other, and does in fact, also, make each the opponent of the other's concern.[4] Hence, there arise the mutual accusations that one side refuses to attend to the reality of the object with which the other side is concerned. The impasse is, indeed, a "passing in the night."

Conflicting experiences of moral obligation may be resolved by one person's being convinced by another that there is, after all, no justification for what was perceived as an obligation. It is not likely that either side in the abortion debate will soon be convinced in this way. Nor, I would argue, ought they to be. But past efforts have also persuaded me that there is little to be gained in simply calling on one side or the other to take into account the reality of the object with which the other is concerned. What might begin to break the impasse, however, is a decision by each to consider seriously the experience of the other precisely as a genuine experience of moral obligation. This would not entail a legitimizing of the experience of the other (for we can clearly have experiences of moral obligation which turn out to have been objectively unfounded, or consciences which turn out to have been mistaken), but only a recognition of it in the other as a moral experience which includes—at least for the other—a perceived obligation and hence a perceived responsibility. Such a recognition may in itself expand the possibilities for sharing the moral awareness of an object hitherto seen only as a marginal concern in relation to the focal concern with which each side begins.

Areas of "Bad Faith"

The breaking of the impasse in the abortion debate may require yet another kind of dislodging, however. The "passing in the night" by the two groups in this debate has to some extent been maintained by the suspicion which each has harbored of the other's fundamental "bad faith"—"bad faith" in the Sartrean sense of self-deception, pretentiousness, hypocrisy, perhaps self-righteousness, and final non-involvement. It may not be enough merely to recognize the "good faith" of the opponent's reported concern and experienced claim. It may be essential that each group take serious account of the opponent's charge against it of "bad faith." That is, it may be necessary that each consider in a self-critical way the possibility that it may itself be partially, and importantly, in "bad faith." The most immediate consequence of "bad faith" is not that one fails to understand an opponent's position; it is that one fails to understand and to disclose one's own position. It may be obvious, then, how self-recognition of areas of "bad faith" can help to clarify issues, discern points of convergence as well as divergence, work out morally acceptable compromises, or sustain energy to continue a prophetic stance. Let me show what I think might emerge and/or be left behind in the advancing debate were both sides to take such a recommendation seriously.

There are, it seems to me, at least three areas in the abortion debate where it is possible that both sides are to some extent in "bad faith." That is to say, there are three areas in which arguments are put forth which represent logical inconsistencies, abstractions from qualifying contexts, misapplication of principles, or rejection of verifiable counterevidence. These arguments at least appear to arise not from a failure of intellect, nor from malicious intent to deceive or confuse, but from some form of unwillingness to reflect fully on the data or reasoning at hand. The deficiencies in the arguments are in some way the result of irresponsibility, however slight or grave, however explicitly or implicitly conscious.[5]

The first of these areas is located within the debate regarding *the nature of the fetus.* On the one hand, it is difficult not to wonder about "bad faith" in a pro-abortion position which, in contradiction to persistent empirical evidence, rests its arguments wholly on the claim that the fetus is simply a part of the pregnant woman, a piece of tissue no more unique than an appendix. What is effective rhetorically is defective logically, however little weight one may wish to give to purely biological data. Arguments for total dependency in spite of some kind of autonomy of the fetus in relation to its mother seem in the long run more fruitful as well as more honest.[6] On the other hand, one must also wonder about "bad faith" in anti-abortion positions which admit no ambiguity, no uncertainty whatsoever, regarding the nature of the fetus, and thus argue for an absolute proscription of abortion. Such arguments belie the traditions to which they appeal and hide the important options which are able to be maintained within a position which unequivocally affirms the existence of human life from the time of conception.[7] They are all the more questionable as they seem to admit inconsistencies such as the simultaneous proscription of all direct abortion and the allowance of curettage after rape.[8] It seems clear that the conflict regarding abortion will neither be sustained in discourse nor ever advanced in thought or policy by opponents whose positions take the grounds of their own arguments with so little seriousness. On the contrary, a sober meeting of opponents in areas of recognized certainty and uncertainty may yet yield clarity, though disagreement, in moral appeal, and may yet yield helpful guidelines for a context of legal compromise.

The second area in which some amount of "bad faith" must at least be allowed as a possibility is the area in which consideration is given to *the needs and claims of women, of pregnant mothers, in regard to abortion.* The credibility of anti-abortionists is stretched considerably in this area, and that on several counts. (1) Present interpreters of the anti-abortion position allude very little to the anti-woman aspects of the long tradition of anti-abortion arguments. Surely it could only help contemporary debate were they to point up the obscurities in a tradition where abortion appears almost always juxtaposed to largely inadequate views of human sexuality and marriage. Conditions conducive to abortion, if not arguments justifying it, have derived in some ways from these views. (2) While some proponents of the anti-abortion position have begun to see the need for alternate ways of dealing with problem pregnancies,[9] and have indeed made efforts to fill gaps in societal structures designed to care for women and children, few have sensed the kind of overall nature of the problem. One cannot help wondering about the increased credibility of anti-abortionists were their voices to be heard leading the challenge against cultural and societal frameworks which still give to women almost total responsibility for the rearing of children. (3) In their understandable concern to safeguard the independent reality of the fetus, anti-abortionists have too easily overlooked the nonetheless intimate relationship of mother and fetus. In order to understand anti-abortion principles one need not abstract from the experience of a mother who finds herself possessed by as well as possessing new life within her. "She feels it as at once an enrichment and an injury. . . . A new life is going to manifest itself and justify its own separate existence, she is proud of it; but she also feels herself tossed and driven, the plaything of obscure forces. It is especially noteworthy that the pregnant woman feels the immanence of her body at just the time when it is in transcendence: it turns upon itself in nausea and discomfort; it has ceased to exist for itself and thereupon becomes more sizable than ever before."[10] The recognition of the complexity as well as intimacy of this relationship may indeed not lead to the justification of abortion, but it is surely not irrelevant to the concrete moral context, and it surely must be taken into account when anti-abortionists consider the implications of a return to abortion laws which would depend upon coercion rather than moral suasion.

But pro-abortionists, too, must not consider themselves innocent of all possibility of "bad faith" in this area. In their very cry for attention to the plight of the mother, for consideration of her as subject and not only as object, they all too often objectify her by removing the relations of mutuality which are constitutive of subjectivity. Experiences of disrelation need not be denied in the recognition of possible experiences of mutuality between mother and fetus, or between mother and father. Tragedies of aloneness are not remedied by rigidifying them into paradigms for the understanding of womanhood and motherhood. When calls for liberation from oppressive situations and repressive laws turn to ideological claims which abstract from the fullness of human experience, their credibility must inevitably suffer. When distortive claims for self-sacrificial love are rightly rejected, but are replaced by counterclaims which recognize no covenant opportunities or responsibilities, the cause of women is not well served. One heavy burden gives way to another.

The third area for self-reflection regarding "bad faith" is the area in which *valuations are made of human life—whether of mother or fetus,* and in which *moral terms are assigned to the act of abortion.* Anti-abortionists appear at times to give absolute value to human life, to make absolute the prescription to preserve life. They have, then, frequently been faulted for the inconsistency of this position with other positions they may take regarding war and capital punishment, and with positions they fail to take regarding the desperate claims for life and human welfare by oppressed and forgotten peoples. Their credibility is further stretched by a reading of the history which has broadened then narrowed the possibilities for justified therapeutic abortion, and by a reading of the agonized casuistry which at times allows greater evils for the sake of purer consciences.[11] Finally, assignment of abortion to the category of murder may prove politically effective, but it does not accurately represent the carefully nuanced history of the anti-abortion tradition.[12]

Pro-abortionists, on the other hand, appear at times to consider human life so relative a value as to make response to it almost morally neutral. The more careful of feminist positions, however, find significance in the need to weigh values, to discern gradations of evil, and to regret the need for abortions at all.[13] "If it is not true that abortion is murder, it still cannot be considered in the same light as a mere contraceptive technique; an event has taken place that is a definite beginning, the progress of which is to be stopped."[14] Pro-abortion slogans, no less than anti-abortion ones, can benefit from carefulness of description vis-a-vis abortion and the methods of abortion.

New Levels of Moral Concern

We return, finally, to the obverse side of self-criticism. Recognition of the possibility of one's own "bad faith" enhances the possible recognition of genuine moral experience in the other. We need not fear that this will relativize all moral principles important to either side, or that it will dull the edges of a conflict which must grow more acute before it can begin to be resolved. If it succeeds in breaking the impasse in the moral debate, then new lines will need to be drawn, and new arguments will need to be given, and new obligations to action may need to be assumed. The line can no longer be, for example (at least in the moral realm, if not in the legal), between abortion on demand on the one side and absolute proscription of abortion on the other. Pro-abortionists must take seriously the recommendations now being offered for line-drawing in terms of the time of abortion, the method, the justifying reasons, possible alternatives, and shared decision-making.[15] Arguments for abortion can no longer give the impression that the highest form of feminine consciousness and the most comprehensive form of feminine liberty are to be found in the choice for abortion. And pro-abortionists must reflect soberly on the kind of moral leadership needed to avoid promoting alienation and spiritual as well as physical sterility. But so, too, must anti-abortionists consider seriously the need for new lines when the situation is one of violent disrelation or two-fold danger of death or truly intolerable burden to the spirit or the body.[16] And so, too, must anti-abortionists take seriously their natural law position (if such is their source of appeal) and respect conscience wherever it appears, addressing it with reasons and not accusations. And so, finally, must anti-abortionists translate what has been a pastoral sensitivity for the individual person into the broader sphere of concern for change in centuries-laden structures of oppression. They, too, must ask what kind of moral leadership is needed to change abortion-conducive societies and abortion-producing relationships.

Each side in the abortion debate must continue to submit its position to the structures whereby a pluralistic society attempts to mediate conflict through law or through a judicial system. Yet each must continue to make moral appeals to the other. In so far as impasses in conflict are transcended, there may emerge greater clarity and modesty of claim along with stronger and more prophetic voices. There may also emerge the gradual recognition that the moral concerns in both the pro-abortion and anti-abortion positions lead finally to a kind of shared position that argues for a social context in which abortion becomes unnecessary. There is, after all, a "beyond abortion" position which must argue for values and structures that will liberate women, and men, and that will conduce to mutuality in child-rearing. Only through such a position can human life finally be valued, from its beginning to its end, wherever it is to be found.

Notes

1. They do, of course, continue. In fact, 200 abortion bills were introduced in state legislatures in 1973. Some of these aimed at regulating abortions in the second and third trimesters. Others attempted to clarify issues such as the place for consent of the husband, consent for a minor, conscientious objection for medical personnel and hospitals, etc. There is federal legislation pending regarding experimentation on fetuses, etc., as well as continuing efforts at the federal level to bring about a constitutional amendment.

2. There is evidence of this, for example, in the efforts of society to carry on "business as usual" in deciding questions regarding human genetics. The issue of abortion continues to sit in the middle of such decisions, but there is almost an agreed-upon silence about it, as if none were aware of the continuing diversion in its regard.

3. It would be inaccurate to insist that the only participants in the abortion debate are feminists and pro-life partisans, or that the only issues in the debate are ones which pit women against fetuses. Clearly, for example, the population issue has been an important one in the ongoing debate. Nonetheless, I would maintain that the impetus of the pro-abortion movement gained immeasurably with the growth of the Women's Liberation Movement, and that the poles of the debate have gradually come to mirror the issues raised by that movement.

4. Needless to say, not all partisans in the debate abstract thus from one another's position. The overall image which each side presents, however, is, I think, accurately described in these terms.

5. This does not contradict my assertion that the failure of one side to take account of the moral concern of the other can arise from the very intensity of the moral experience of each. "Bad faith" can be found in even the strongest and most sincere of moral positions. It does not vitiate moral concern, but it does in some way blind it.

6. See, for example, Jean MacRae, "A Feminist View of Abortion," *Proceedings of the Working Group on Women and Religion, American Academy of Religion* (1973), p. 113.

7. Noonan reads the history of Christianity's rejection of abortion as a gradual achievement of clarity and certainty. Nonetheless, the recurring "agnosticism on ensoulment" seems not yet transcended. Noonan, for example, cites the important role of the writings of Bernard Häring in settling the question. But Häring, a few years later, acknowledged a continuing degree of uncertainty. See John T. Noonan, "An Almost Absolute Value in History," in *The Mortality of Abortion: Legal and Historical Perspectives* (Harvard, 1970), pp. 1–59. See also Bernard Häring, "A Theological Evaluation," in *The Mortality of Abortion: Legal and Historical Perspectives,* p. 132. Paul Ramsey, too, admits a certain unclarity in this regard: "While my statement of the argument from genotype was a stronger one than Noonan's . . . my adherence to it was never full or certain." See Paul Ramsey, "Abortion: A Review Article," *The Thomist,* XXXVII (January, 1973), 188. Ramsey finally opts for the time of segmentation, or "the time at or after which it is settled whether there will be one or two or more distinct individuals," as the point at which human life begins.

It is never in question for anti-abortionists whether or not abortion is justified (it is not), but it is in question for some anti-abortionists whether justification is needed from the moment of conception or the time of implantation, segmentation, the development of brain impulses, etc.

8. Roman Catholic moral theologians still teach that for a time after rape, a woman may receive a D and C. This may have been founded originally on the belief that conception never takes place immediately after intercourse. The teaching has not been changed, however, even though such a belief is by no means always verifiable.

9. The important position and concern of Birthright is a case in point.

10. Simone de Beauvoir, *The Second Sex* (Bantam, 1953), pp. 466–67.

11. This is the case when, in justifying abortion of an ectopic pregnancy, a tube must be removed in order to indirectly remove the fetus.

12. See Noonan, pp. 15, 23, 32, 35. It would be misleading to imply that in spite of different terminology, even different assessment of guilt entailed, the anti-abortion tradition within Christianity ever considered the obligation to prevent the killing of the fetus as anything other than an obligation of the highest order of seriousness.

13. See, for example, Sissela Bok, "Ethical Problems of Abortion," *The Hastings Center Studies,* II (January, 1974), 33–52.

14. S. de Beauvoir, p. 462.

15. See Bok, p. 52.

16. It seems necessary for anti-abortionists to admit such lines at least in the legal order. Even morally, however, serious grounds can be found, within an anti-abortion position, for such line-drawing.

Chapter Fourteen
CHOOSING DEATH AND LETTING DIE

Introduction

There are few times more personally wrenching than when someone close to us is dying. That time can be made still more difficult when the dying person is or appears to be suffering uncontrollably. What may we do to and for those who suffer in dying? Are we obligated to continue all forms of medical intervention in order to preserve their life? May we discontinue medical interventions aimed at preserving life while we continue those to relieve pain? May we relieve their pain by choosing their death? Must we? It is usually in this context that the discussion of killing and letting die first appears.

By now we know that medicine has at least two goals, the preservation of life and the relief of suffering. Medical personnel face directly the limitations on what they can do for patients. Although they may be able to hold off death for a time, eventually all born of human flesh die. Thus medical personnel know that at some point they can no longer cure but can still continue to care for patients and attempt to relieve their suffering.

The justifications for this behavior are contested in our society. There seems to be little disagreement over the legitimacy of withdrawing medical interventions in some cases, but other cases are vigorously contested. What is at stake are the reasons we can give to one another for either letting die or choosing death.

The impartial perspective suggests two answers. One school suggests that everyone has a right to die. If patients or their duly appointed guardians decide that medical interventions should be withdrawn, then we must respect their wishes. Indeed, this point is sometimes applied to nonterminal as well as to terminal cases. Another group asks us to consider the costs and benefits of continuing such treatment. The patients' wishes are not primary but an assessment of the costs and benefits of withdrawing care is in order. These assessments must take into account society as a whole in addition to the family and the patient.

Traditionally, Christian thinkers have argued that not everything that could be done for a patient necessarily had to be done. This has been justified on a number of grounds. Some have argued that people are not obligated to submit to extraordinary treatments, treatments which would impose a grave burden upon them. Other thinkers have argued that care need not be continued if it is useless. As Lisa Cahill points out below, a therapy which has no hope of curing a terminal illness is not obligatory.

Christian thinkers did not think of death as the greatest evil. Life indeed may be sanctified by God and death is a great evil, to be sure, but there are greater. Thus a Christian may choose a course of action, witnessing to Christ, knowing that it will result in death. The martyr did not seek death but saw unfaithfulness as the greater evil.

For better or for worse, the solutions of the past have given rise to new questions today. First, the meaning of medical care for the dying is contested. Most people agree that medical care may utilize antibiotics and respirators. These are forms of medical care that may, in certain circumstances, when they are no longer necessary for care, be withdrawn. But what of liquids and nourishment that are given to a person intravenously or through a nasogastric tube? Are these forms of medical care that may be withdrawn, or are they a form of service, a giving of drink to the thirsty and food to the hungry, a service that we owe to all human beings, even and especially the dying? If we withdraw them, must we see our action as aiming at or choosing the death of the person, or may we understand it in a different way?

When persons withdraw some forms of medical intervention from a patient, they often know that the patient will die. This is justified, say some, if the intention in withdrawing the medical intervention is the relief of suffering. But, say others, if withdrawing care results in death, is this really different from more actively aiming at the death of the patient? In many cases it would be kinder to the patients, so it is claimed, to kill them and relieve them of their suffering. Thus begins the discussion of euthanasia.

The original meaning of euthanasia was "good death." Today, the term is used in different ways. Some thinkers use it to refer to taking active, direct steps to kill someone for his or her own sake. Others make a distinction, calling these acts of killing "active euthanasia" and calling the withholding of care for the sake of the (eventual) victim "passive euthanasia." Some people believe that if passive euthanasia is permitted in order to relieve suffering, active euthanasia should be permitted as well.

Clearly the most difficult case is the one in which a

dying person is suffering from uncontrollable pain. What if that person requests death? For those who are convinced that the patient's wishes are the central value, this request is a powerful reason for killing him or her. Though the case of the terminally ill person suffering in uncontrollable pain is not as common as it once was, it does provide us with a clear example with which we might more easily sort out the relevant issues. Is it justifiable to kill in such circumstances? If it is, on what grounds?

In all of this, the mode of analysis is critical. Does one look to the positive consequences of actions and then measure them against the evils of death? Or does one assert throughout that life is sacred and that we may never intentionally and directly end the life of an innocent person, even though the consequences might appear to be better, not only for us, but for that person.

The discussion of autonomy is important here. Is special weight to be given to the decision of a terminally ill patient to be allowed to die? If we honor that decision, do we do so simply because it was freely arrived at by an autonomous person, because it is coherent with the integrity of the one making the request? That is, may we honor the request against our own wishes, respecting the autonomy of the other, or may we do so only if we, too, freely arrive at the same decision? What other values might be at stake? What if the patient requests not only to die but to be killed? What questions does this raise for those of us who hear the request? Is our cooperation, or lack of it, to be respected because of *our* autonomy, because it is an expression of *our* integrity? What obligations, if any, do we have toward the person making the request? Does a request by a patient on these matters prove to be a special difficulty for medical professionals? In what way is their integrity involved in requests by patients to be allowed to die or to be killed? Is it possible to honor one of these requests and not the other? Why or why not?

The issues here relate in part to the earlier chapter on care and suffering. How is suffering to be understood? One approach in this context would be to argue that both suffering and death are great evils, and where possible, are both to be avoided. But what do we do when we can avoid neither? When suffering makes it impossible for people to continue in relatedness to others, are we permitted to choose death for them or to kill them at their request? Death cannot be chosen in preference to some lesser evil; but if suffering has destroyed meaningful relatedness to others, there is a tragic conflict in which not all the significant evils can be avoided and one must choose between them.

In our society, even that question has not been the final one. What about those who are permanently vegetative but not terminally ill: Is it wrong to withhold food and water from them? Is it wrong to kill them? Note that here the issue is not the terminal condition of the patient or her wishes or even her suffering. The issue concerns what kind of people we wish to be, what we think true personhood is. That may turn out to be the critical issue we must confront here, as elsewhere in medicine.

Suggestions for Further Reading

Lord Amultree, et al. *On Dying Well: An Anglican Contribution to the Debate on Euthanasia.* London: Church Information Service, 1975.

Childress, James. *Priorities in Medical Ethics.* Philadelphia: Westminster, 1981.

Foot, Phillippe. "Euthanasia." Chapter in *Virtues and Vices.* Oxford: Basil Blackwell, 1978.

Glover, Jonathan. *Causing Death and Saving Lives.* London: Penguin, 1977.

Hare, R. M. "Euthanasia: A Christian View." *Philosophical Exchange* 2 (Summer 1975).

Maguire, Dan. *Death by Choice.* New York: Schocken, 1975.

McCormick, Richard A. *How Brave a New World?* Washington, D.C.: Georgetown University Press, 1981. See pp. 339-430.

Ramsey, Paul. *Ethics at the Edges of Life.* New Haven: Yale University Press, 1978. See pp. 143-335.

Simmons, Paul. *Birth and Death: Bioethical Decision-Making.* Philadelphia: Westminster, 1983.

Oden, Thomas C. *Should Treatment Be Terminated?* New York: Harper & Row, 1976.

Vaux, Kenneth. *Will to Live—Will to Die: Ethics and the Search for a Good Death.* Minneapolis: Augsburg, 1978.

Veatch, Robert M. *Death, Dying and the Biological Revolution: Our Last Quest for Responsibility.* New Haven: Yale University Press, 1976.

Verhey, Allen D. "Christian Community and Identity: What Difference Do They Make to Physicians and Patients Finally?" *Linacre Quarterly,* May 1985.

70.
Euthanasia

Declaration of the Sacred Congregation for the Doctrine of the Faith (May 5, 1980)

JOHN PAUL II

The inherent rights and values of the human person hold an important place among the questions preoccupying the people of our day. Against this background the Second Vatican Council solemnly reaffirmed the eminent dignity of the human person and, especially, the person's right to life.

In keeping with this restatement the council denounced crimes against life, including "murder, genocide, abortion, euthanasia or willfull self-destruction."[1]

More recently, the Sacred Congregation for the Doctrine of the Faith has reminded all followers of Christ of the Church's teaching on deliberate abortion.[2]

The same congregation now deems it opportune to set forth the Church's teaching on euthanasia.

It is true that on this point of doctrine recent popes have expounded principles which remain fully valid.[3]

On the other hand, recent medical advances have focused attention on new aspects of euthanasia which call for further explanation of the ethical norms.

In modern society, in which even the fundamental values of human life are frequently threatened, cultural changes influence the way people view death and suffering.

Another point to be noted is the increasing ability of medical science to heal and to prolong life under certain conditions which, at times, raise questions of morality. Consequently, people living in these new circumstances ask anxious questions about the meaning of extreme old age and death.

They ask themselves, not unreasonably, whether or not they have the right to secure for themselves or their loved ones an "easy death" which shortens suffering and seems to them more in keeping with human dignity.

From *The Pope Speaks* 25 (Winter 1980): 289-96. Used courtesy of Our Sunday Visitor, Inc.

Purpose of the Document

On this subject a number of episcopal conferences have sent questions to the Sacred Congregation for the Doctrine of the Faith. The congregation has sought the views of experts on the various aspects of euthanasia and now intends this declaration as a reply to the inquiries of the bishops.

The statement will make it easier for them to present correct doctrine to the faithful committed to their care and will supply them with principles which they can communicate to civil authorities for their consideration in connection with this extremely serious problem.

The themes presented in this document are meant primarily for those who place their faith and hope in Jesus Christ, whose life, death and resurrection have given new meaning to the life and, especially, the death of Christians. As St. Paul says, "while we live we are responsible to the Lord, and when we die we die as His servants. Both in life and in death we are the Lord's."[4]

Among those who profess other religions, many are in agreement with us that faith in God as provident Creator and Lord of life—if indeed they share this faith—gives all human persons an eminent dignity and is their guarantee of respect.

Our hope is that this declaration will also win the assent of persons of good will who, though following divergent philosophies or ideologies, nevertheless have a keen awareness of the rights of the human person. In fact, these same rights have in recent years been the subject of declarations issued by international congresses.[5]

Since we are dealing here with fundamental rights inherent in every human person, it is evidently wrong to argue from religious pluralism or freedom of religion in order to deny the universal validity of these rights.

I The Value of Human Life

Human life is the basis of all values; it is the source and indispensable condition for every human activity and all society. While the majority of human beings regard life as sacred and maintain that no one can dispose of it at will, the followers of Christ see it as being something even more excellent: a loving gift from God, which they must preserve and render fruitful. This further consideration entails certain consequences:

1. No one may attack the life of an innocent person without thereby resisting the love of God for that

person; without violating a fundamental right which can be neither lost nor alienated and, therefore, without committing an extremely serious crime.[6]

2. All human beings must live their lives in accordance with God's plan. Life is given to them as a possession which must bear fruit here on earth but which must wait for eternal life to achieve its full and absolute perfection.

3. Intentional death or suicide is just as wrong as is homicide. Such an action by a human being must be regarded as a rejection of God's supreme authority and loving plan.

In addition, suicide is often a rejection of love for oneself, a denial of the natural instinct to live and a flight from the duties of justice and charity one owes one's neighbors or various communities or human society as a whole.

At times, however, as everyone realizes, psychological factors may lessen or even completely eliminate responsibility.

Suicide must be carefully distinguished from the sacrifice of life in which men and women give their lives or endanger them for some noble cause such as the honor of God, the salvation of souls or the service of the brethren.[7]

II Euthanasia

If we are to deal properly with the question of euthanasia, we must first explain carefully the meaning of our terms.

Etymologically, euthanasia meant, in antiquity, an *easy death,* that is, one free of severe pain. Nowadays, it is no longer this original meaning that comes to mind. Euthanasia refers, instead, to a medical intervention that lessens the suffering of illness or of the final agony, an intervention that at times carries with it the danger of terminating life prematurely.

Finally, the word euthanasia may also be used in a more limited sense to mean mercy killing, the purpose being to put a complete end to extreme suffering or to keep defective children, the incurably ill or the mentally subnormal from living out a wretched and, perhaps, lengthy life that might impose an excessive burden on families or society.

We must make quite clear which of these meanings euthanasia is to have in the present document.

Euthanasia here means an action or omission that by its nature or by intention causes death with the purpose of putting an end to all suffering. Euthanasia is, therefore, a matter of intention and method.

We must firmly state once again that no one and nothing can, in any way, authorize the killing of an innocent human being, whether the latter be a fetus or embryo, or a child or an adult or an elderly person, or someone incurably ill or someone who is dying.

In addition, no one may ask for such a death-dealing action for oneself or for another for whom one is responsible, nor may one explicitly or implicitly consent to such an action. Nor may any authority legitimately command or permit it. For such an action is a violation of divine law, an offense against the dignity of the human person, a crime against life and an attack on the human race.

Always Objectively Wrong

It may be that long drawn out and almost unbearable pain, or some emotional or other reason, may convince individuals that they may legitimately ask for death for themselves or others. Although in these cases guilt may be diminished or completely lacking, such an error or judgment into which conscience may fall, perhaps in good faith, does not change the nature of the death-dealing action, which will always be impermissible.

The pleas of the very seriously ill as they beg at times to be put to death are hardly to be understood as conveying a real desire for euthanasia. They are almost always anguished pleas for help and love. What the sick need, in addition to medical care, is love: the warm human and supernatural affection in which all those around—parents and children, doctors and nurses— can and should enfold them.

III Meaning of Suffering

Death does not always come in wretched conditions and after almost intolerable suffering. Nor should we always be focusing our attention on very unusual cases. Many concordant testimonies persuade us to believe that nature itself has taken steps to ease separations at the moment of death, which would be extremely bitter if they involved a person in good health.

The length of an illness, advanced age, a state of loneliness and abandonment create psychological conditions in which it becomes easier to accept death.

We must admit, nonetheless, that death, often preceded or accompanied by severe and prolonged suffering, is an event that naturally causes anguish.

Bodily suffering is certainly an unavoidable part of the human condition. Viewed biologically, pain acts as an undeniably useful warning. But pain also affects the psychological life of the person, where its severity often outweighs its biological value and can become so intense that the person longs for its termination at any cost.

Suffering in the Plan of Salvation

According to Christian teaching, however, suffering, especially in the final moments of life, has a special place in God's plan of salvation. It is a sharing in the passion of Christ and unites the person with the redemptive sacrifice which Christ offered in obedience to the Father's will.

It is not surprising, then, that some Christians desire to use painkillers only in moderation so that they can deliberately accept at least a part of their suffering and thus consciously unite themselves with the crucified Christ.[8]

It would be imprudent, nonetheless, to impose this heroic response as a general norm. On the contrary, in the case of many sick people, human and Christian prudence urges the use of such medications as may alleviate or eliminate suffering, even though they cause secondary effects such as lethargy and diminished awareness.

In the case of persons who are unable to express themselves, it may legitimately be presumed that they want to take painkillers and have them administered according to the advice of the doctors.

Problems in the Use of Painkillers

The concentrated and protracted use of painkillers is not, however, without its difficulties, since habituation usually requires that the dosage be increased in order to maintain effectiveness. It is worth recalling here a statement of Pius XII that is still valid. A group of physicians had asked: "Is the removal of pain and consciousness by means of narcotics . . . permitted by religion and morality to both doctor and patient even at the approach of death and if one foresees that the use of narcotics will shorten life?" The pope answered: "Yes—provided that no other means exist and if, in the given circumstances, the action does not prevent the carrying out of other moral and religious duties."[9]

In this case, as is clear, death is by no means intended or sought, although the risk of it is being incurred for a good reason; the only intention is to diminish pain effectively by use of the painkillers available to medical science.

Painkillers which cause the sick to lose consciousness call for special attention for it is important that people be able not only to satisfy moral obligations and family duties but also and especially to dispose themselves with full awareness for their meeting with Christ. Pius XII therefore warns: "The sick person should not, without serious reason, be deprived of consciousness."[10]

IV The Proportionate Use of Therapeutic Agents

In our day it is very important at the moment of death to safeguard the dignity of the person and the Christian meaning of life, in the face of a technological approach to death that can easily be abused. Some even speak of a "right to die." By this they mean, however, not a right of persons to inflict death on themselves at will by their own or another's hand, but rather a right to die peacefully and in a manner worthy of a human being and a Christian.

In this context the application of the healing art can sometimes raise questions.

In many cases the situation may be so complicated as to raise doubts about how to apply moral principles. In the last analysis, the decision rests with the conscience of the sick person or of those who have a right to act in the sick person's name or of the doctors, who must bear in mind the principles of morality and the several aspects of the case.

All have an obligation to care for their health or to seek such care from others. Those in charge of the sick must perform their task with care and apply the remedies that seem necessary or useful.

Does this mean that all possible remedies must be applied in every circumstance?

The Basis of Judgment

In the not too distant past moralists would have replied that the use of "extraordinary" means can never be obligatory. This reply is still valid in principle but it is, perhaps, less evident today because of its vagueness or because of rapid advances in the treatment of illness. For this reason some prefer to speak of "proportionate" and "disproportionate" means.

In any case, a correct judgment can be made regarding means, if the type of treatment, its degree of difficulty and danger, its expense, and the possibility of applying it are weighed against the results that can be expected, all this in the light of the sick person's condition and resources of body and spirit.

The following clarifications will facilitate the application of these general principles:

—If other remedies are lacking, it is permissible, with the consent of the sick person, to use the most recent medical techniques, even if these are not yet fully tested and are not free of risk. The sick person who agrees to them can even give an example, thereby, of generous service to the human race.

—It is also licit to discontinue the use of these means as soon as results disappoint the hopes placed in them but, in making this decision, account should be taken of the legitimate desire of the sick person and his or her family as well as of the opinion of truly expert physicians. The latter are better placed than anyone else for judging whether the expense of machinery and personnel is disproportionate to the foreseeable results and whether the medical techniques used will cause the sick person suffering or inconvenience greater than the benefits that may be derived from them.

Use Only of Ordinary Means

—It is always licit to be content with the ordinary remedies which medical science can supply. Therefore, no one may be obliged to submit to a type of cure which, though already in use, is not without risks or is excessively burdensome.

This rejection of a remedy is not to be compared to suicide; it is more justly to be regarded as a simple acceptance of the human condition or a desire to avoid the application of medical techniques that are disproportionate to the value of the anticipated results or, finally, a desire not to put a heavy burden on the family or the community.

—When death is imminent and cannot be prevented by the remedies used, it is licit in conscience to decide to renounce treatments that can only yield a precarious and painful prolongation of life.

At the same time, however, ordinary treatment that is due to the sick in such cases may not be interrupted. There is no reason for the doctor to feel anxious in such cases as though he had not come to the aid of a person in danger.

The norms contained in this declaration are motivated by an intense desire to help human beings in a way that accords with the plan of the Creator. While life is to be regarded as God's gift, it also is true that death is unavoidable. We must be able, therefore, without in any way hastening the hour of death, to accept it with full consciousness of our responsibility and with full dignity for death, indeed, puts an end to this earthly life but in doing so it opens the way to undying life.

All human beings, therefore, must properly dispose themselves for this event in the light of human values and Christians even more in the light of their faith.

Health Care Personnel and Death

Those engaged in health care should certainly omit no effort in applying the full skills of their art to the advantage of the sick and dying. They should also bear in mind, however, that there is another consolation such people need and need even more urgently: unlimited kindness and devoted charity. When service of this kind is rendered to human beings, it is also rendered to Christ himself, who said: "As often as you did it for one of my least brothers, you did it for me."[11]

Notes

1. *Pastoral Constitution on the Church in the World of Today,* no. 27 [*TPS* XI, 276].

2. Declaration on Abortion, November 18, 1874: AAS 66 (1974) 730-47; translated in *TPS* XIX, 250-62.

3. Pius XII, Address to the International Union of Societies of Catholic Women, September 11, 1947: *AAS* 39 (1947) 483; Address to the Italian Union of Catholic Midwives, October 29, 1951: *AAS* 43 (1951) 835-54; Address to the International Commission of Inquiry into Military Medicine, October 9, 1953: *AAS* (1953) 744-54; Address to the 11th Congress of the Italian Society of Anesthesiology, February 24, 1957: *AAS* (1957) 146. See also Pius XII, Address on the Question of Reanimation, November 24, 1957: *AAS* 49 (1957) 1027-33. Paul VI, Address to the Special United Nations Committee on Apartheid, May 22, 1974: *AAS* 66 (1974) 346. John Paul II, Address to the Bishops of the United States of America, October 5, 1979: *AAS* 71 (1979) 1225.

4. *Rom* 14, 8; see *Phil* 1, 20.

5. See, in particular, Recommendation 779 (1976) on the rights of the sick and dying, which was adopted by the Assembly of Deputies of the Council of Europe at its 27th regular meeting. See *SIPECA,* no. 1 (March, 1977), pp. 14-15.

6. We leave completely aside here the questions of the death penalty and of war. These involve special considerations which fall outside the scope of this declaration.

7. See *Jn* 15, 14.

8. See *Mt* 27, 34.

9. Address to the 11th Congress of the Italian Society of Anesthesiology, February 24, 1967: *AAS* 49 (1957) 147 [*TPS* b IV, 48].

10. Ibid.: *AAS* 49 (1957) 145 [*TPS* IV, 47]. See the same pope's address of September 9, 1958: *AAS* 50 (1958) 694.

11. *Mt* 25, 40.

71.
A "Natural Law" Reconsideration of Euthanasia

LISA SOWLE CAHILL

Respect for the value of human life and care for its preservation in a state of physical well-being have traditionally motivated the practice of medicine in Western societies. Because of the relatively recent but very rapid advancement of medical technology, it has become commonplace to observe that the proper affirmation of that respect and the adequate fulfillment of that care are perplexing ethical issues. It is often no easy matter for the physician to determine how best to honor his obligation "to render service to humanity with full respect for the dignity of man."[1]

Some of the moral uncertainty which surrounds our current perceptions of the relation of the sick to the healthy (especially to members of the health care professions) and to alternative courses of treatment, might be alleviated by careful reflection upon the meaning of "the sanctity of life" and its implications for action. Difficult questions about life and death ought to be considered in light of the totality of the human person to whom this principle has reference. Biological life is said to be "sacred" because it is a fundamental condition of human meaning. But physical existence is not an *absolute* value for the human person. What are some conflict situations in which other values are foremost? What kinds of acts are compatible both with respect for life and with the recognition that it is not an absolute? Ought direct euthanasia or "mercy-killing" always to be excluded from such acts, even in cases of severe terminal suffering or permanent unconsciousness?

The conviction that human life has a value and commands respect not comparable to that of lower forms of life can be expressed variously and rests upon a broad base of support from diverse ethical traditions. The Judaeo-Christian communities have endorsed the principle of the sanctity of life because it is consistent with a religious belief in a God Who creates and preserves human life, and Who imposes a moral obligation of life to life, consisting in its preservation and protection. The Roman Catholic tradition of Christianity in particular has attempted in the realm of medical ethics to supply this rather abstract principle with appropriate moral content. Only God has full "dominion" or right of control over human life; man's dominion over his own life is limited. "God is the creator and master of human life and no one may take it without His authorization."[2] Although religious belief in a Divine Maker Who loves and sustains personal life provides a strong warrant for respect, the principle of the sanctity of life can also be defended on philosophical grounds, by an appeal to common human experience. Many an atheistic or agnostic humanist would agree that since life is the fundamental and irreplaceable condition of the experience of all human values, it is a basic, or *the* basic, value and must not be destroyed without grave cause.[3]

In Catholic medical-moral theology, the principle of the sanctity of life has been affirmed not only because it is compatible with biblical anthropologies, but because it is part of the natural moral law. As such, it indicates a universal ethical obligation, known to all men and women, not to Christians only. In the natural law moral theology of Catholicism, the principle has been given two primary expressions, one negative and one positive. First, we may consider the negative prohibition of the violation or destruction of life, patterned on Thomas Aquinas's arguments against murder.[4] It is often formulated as, "It is always wrong directly to kill an innocent human being."[5] This has been the basis for the Church's stance against abortion (as murder) and euthanasia (as suicide or murder or both).[6] Second, we have the positive affirmation of respect for the integrity of human personhood, also rooted in Aquinas.[7] It is called "the principle of totality," the standard medical formulation of which proclaims the proper subordination of an organ to the good of the body as part to whole. This affirmation of the value of life has provided a framework within which to justify surgical mutilation of the body (e.g., excision of a diseased organ) in order to further its total well-being.[8] The intention of the principle of totality is to respect and safeguard the integrity and welfare of the whole human being.

The referent of the principle of totality has usually been the life of the human individual considered as a physical organism. However, it can be argued that the fullest meaning of this principle, as it is actually used by Catholic theologians writing on medical ethics, includes the subordination of the physical aspect of man to the whole "person" which also includes his spiritual aspect.

During his pontificate, Pius XII addressed himself repeatedly to contemporary problems of ethics confronting the medical professions. These teachings are

Reprinted with permission from *Linacre Quarterly,* Vol. 44 (February 1977), pp. 47-63. 850 Elm Grove Road, Elm Grove, WI 53122. Subscription rate: $20 per year; $5 per single issue.

significant both because they are expressions of "natural law" thinking about medical morality and because they were promulgated as authoritative (although not infallible) for members of the Catholic Church. The principle of totality is frequently used in Pius's analyses of the medical-moral issue of which he speaks, and it is his formulations of that principle which are most often invoked by Catholic theologians. Pius XII delivered a now well-known speech on medical research to the First International Congress of the Histopathology of the Nervous System convened in Rome on September 13, 1952. Therein he declared that since "the parts exist for the whole," it is true of any physical entity that "the whole is a determining factor for the part and can dispose of it in its own interest."[9] Therefore, "the patient can allow the individual parts to be destroyed or mutilated when and to the extent necessary for the good of his being as a whole."[10]

Consideration of the principle of totality in its abstract version leads us to ask whether the "totality" of a person's "being as a whole" can be adequately defined in terms of the "physical organism" here mentioned by Pope Pius XII. On the contrary, Catholic teaching does in fact provide a strong basis for describing human personhood as a totality which is essentially constituted by the integration of both physical and *spiritual* aspects. The Pope himself states in his encyclical *The Mystical Body of Christ* that "the whole of man" is not "encompassed within the organism of our mortal body."[11] Perhaps his most forthright statement on the matter is given in an address to the International College of Psychoneuropharmacology on September 9, 1958. Speaking of medical experimentation, the Pope affirmed that "there must be added to the subordination of the individual organs to the organism and its end the subordination of the organism itself to the spiritual end of the person."[12]

An expanded and perhaps more technical version of the Pope's view of human personhood is given in a 1958 address to a Congress of the International Association of Applied Psychology. The self is explicitly described as a "totality" having "parts." Says Pius, "We define personality as 'the psychosomatic unity of man in so far as it is determined and governed by the soul'. . . . "[13] Thus in an address to the International Union Against Cancer, in 1956, the Pope feels constrained to warn that "before anything else, the doctor should consider the whole man, in the unity of his person, that is to say, not merely his physical condition but his psychological state as well as his spiritual and moral ideals and his place in society."[14] The question to be asked is whether Pius's strong concern for the "whole man" is consistent with his absolute prohibition of euthanasia.[15] If the body is a "part" of the total person, are there any circumstances in which it may, through a direct act, be sacrificed for the good of the whole? This problem will bear reflection which goes beyond the past prohibitions of such acts.

Considering Life and Death

It is certainly essential to a Thomistic version of Roman Catholic moral theology to consider human life and death in view of the final end of the human person. Consequently, it would seem most inconsistent for any theologian who ostensibly stands within that tradition to interpret moral dilemmas according to a principle of human "totality" which neglects not only man's supernatural goal, but his natural goal of mature integration of body and spirit. It is this total human nature which contemporary Catholic theologians want to give its proper due in considerations of medical ethics. This concern is related specifically to the practice of medicine in the current *Ethical and Religious Directives for Catholic Health Facilities,* which maintains that a Catholic hospital has a "responsibility to seek and protect the total good of its patients." This good is not just a physical one. "The total good of the patient, which includes his higher spiritual as well as his bodily welfare, is the primary concern of those entrusted with the management of a Catholic health facility."[16] Kieran Nolan, a priest and theologian involved in pastoral care of the sick, reminds us that if euthanasia is to be morally acceptable, it must be a sign of "the deep Christian respect for the integrity of the individual."[17] According to the positive sense of the sanctity of life principle, the good of the totality of an individual's human personhood must be foremost in all deliberations about his welfare and the obligations of others to him in his living and his dying. As Nolan significantly puts it, "The Christian concern must be to provide for human survival and not for mere biological preservation."[18]

Why is it that the protection of biological life is usually considered to be an essential factor in respect for the whole human person? Both the negative and the positive versions of the sanctity of life principle express an insight into the human "right" to life and the concomitant human "duty" to protect it. An individual is not to be unjustly deprived of his life, and, furthermore, his total personal well-being is to be promoted. These insights are based on the judgment that life is the fundamental condition of all other human values and is therefore to be preserved itself insofar as it can ground those values. The foremost human value is the love of God achieved at least in part through love of other persons. This Christian view of the meaning of life as the condition of personal love has been given consistent expression in the context of Catholic medical ethics. Pius XII, in "The Prolongation of Life," mentions the ultimacy of a "higher, more important good," the good of love for God, over bodily life.[19] Thomas J. O'Donnell, S.J., observes that life as a "relative good" is valuable because it is a context for other values which contribute to the "absolute good," man's pursuit in charity of his supernatural end, God.[20] Recently, Richard A. McCormick, S.J., has employed a very similar line of argument in discussing the life prospects of defective newborn children. He states that life is to be preserved only insofar as it can ground the highest human good of loving relationships with other persons. A meaningful life is one in which the individual has relational consciousness and is free from physical pain or suffering so severe that the sheer effort to survive distracts the person from the primary human good, love.[21]

Because the Christian affirms the transcendence of full human personhood over sheer biological existence, life is for him never an *absolute* value, a value to be salvaged at all costs. Sometimes continued life does not constitute a good for a certain individual because it cannot offer him the conditions of meaningful personal existence. Sometimes the continued life of an individual is incompatible with the preservation of other values which also claim protection. In such instances, the Christian does not deny that human life is a value to be respected. However, he realizes that under the finite and sinful conditions of historical moral choice, he is called upon responsibly to mediate between conflicting values and the rights and duties which are devolved from them. Occasions of moral choice do not always involve clear-cut issues and alternatives neatly organized into a hierarchy of ethical preferability.[22] While this does not remove from us the obligation to choose, it does forestall false confidence in the finality of particular moral judgments and in the ability of the moral agent to avoid responsibility for the undesirable consequences of a difficult moral choice. At times, decisions about life and death necessitate arbitration among competing values which cannot all be actualized in a given instance.

Classical examples of ethical dilemmas in which this reality must be acknowledged are war, self-defense, and capital punishment. In these three cases, the "right to life" of one individual conflicts with the right of another individual, or even of the community, to life itself, or to the pursuit of goods still more valuable than life, for which life may be sacrificed. If we recall the standard prohibition of killing, we will observe that each instance can be exempted from the range of the prohibition because the object of the act of direct killing can be said in some sense not to be "innocent."[23]

Even the lives of the innocent, however, are not absolutely inviolable goods. In consistence with its concern for the "total good" of the person, the Catholic moral tradition affirms that preservation of the life of even the just man is sometimes not the highest value to be maintained in a situation of conflict. It is clear, however, that in the past only indirect killing of the innocent has been considered to be justifiable. For instance, the martyr may allow his physical welfare to be negated in order to testify to the highest good of love for God in Christ. Here the individual permits (but does not directly cause) his own death in order to protect a greater value. The frequent distinction in medical ethics between "ordinary" means of life support (as mandatory) and "extraordinary" means (as elective) is given similar warrants. Death may be permitted (or "indirectly caused") by withholding treatments which do not serve the best interests of the patient. According to the current definition, a means is not obligatory if it is difficult to maintain or use, *or* if it will probably not offer much benefit to the patient in terms of either quality or duration of life. A treatment need not be used if it will not restore an individual's life to a state in which it can support the development of life's highest (spiritual) goods or which will prevent it from furnishing such support in the future.[24] On the other hand, a human life is indeed worth prolonging if it can provide an opportunity to enjoy forgetfulness of self in love of others. Personal relations are that for the sake of which life is to be sustained.

Direct/Indirect Causes of Death

When an innocent person is involved, an act of killing falls outside the sphere of efficacy of the sanctity of life prohibition if it may be described as "indirect."[25] The martyr neither wills nor directly causes his own death; it is an undesired consequence of his steadfast faith commitment. Similarly, to omit to provide extraordinary life support to a patient is not to directly cause his death, but to permit it to occur as a result of disease. The decision is made in light of the judgment that the active pursuit of life's continuation is not consistent with concern for and protection of the total welfare of that person. His right to life and the physician's concomitant duty to preserve it must, in this particular instance of conflict, be subordinated to his "right to die." Life for him no longer provides the sufficient conditions for the fruitful development of loving relationships, both with other humans, and through them, with God. When extraordinary or ultimately useless treatments are not used, recognition is given to the patient's right to be freed from physical and spiritual deterioration and suffering and to the physician's duty to care for his patient's physical well-being within the larger context of human personhood. This is not to say that the patient no longer has a right to life or that he may be deprived of his life against his will or for the good of any other person or of society. Both the right to life and the right to death must be subsumed under the promotion of the welfare of the whole human person himself. In situations where the values of life and of death conflict, the patient or his proxy may prefer to exercise voluntarily the right to die as most appropriate to the patient's own total well-being.

"Respect" may be shown to a person both by acting in ways which express esteem for his or her dignity and by not acting in ways which express contempt for or indifference to his or her dignity. What does "respect for life" as an ethical principle now mean, demand, require in choices about death in medical practice? There is consensus in theological ethics (though perhaps not always in medicine) that respect for life does not always entail its indefinite prolongation. Sometimes respect is most adequately conveyed by a refusal to intervene or to continue intervention in the progress of the human organism toward biological death. This is the main argument of Pius XII in "The Prolongation of Life"; it is not a new one in Christian or philosophical ethics.

The "hard question" remains and at this juncture unrelentingly confronts us: Can respect ever mean *direct* intervention to end the life of a patient? (We now move from the consideration of the morality of an act of omission to that of one of commission, to use the technical language of moral theology.) It is clear that the magisterial Roman Catholic rejoinder to this specific question has been negative.[26] Life-sustaining treatments may be omitted, but death may not be hastened directly. It must now be asked whether this position in fact meets the test of consistency with other values explicitly upheld and protected by the Church, such as the value of the dignity and welfare of the whole human person.

It will be recalled that the sanctity of life principle in Catholic theology has been given two ethically normative expressions. Its prohibitive form supplies warrants for condemning voluntary euthanasia. Its affirmative form supplies warrants for respecting and promoting the integrity of the individual. But can both of these conclusions from the more generally valid principle of respect for life be observed together in every particular situation? Can the obligation not to cause death directly and the obligation to respect the goods and proper goals of human personhood ever be in conflict? If a conflict should arise in medical practice, which obligation should be given preference on the basis that it best fulfills the grounding principle of life's sanctity?

Let us consider a possible case, one which is very frequently mentioned in discussion of euthanasia because it appropriately frames decision-making about causing death in a context of personal agony, both for the performer and the recipient of the act. A patient with terminal cancer is in "the dying process."[27] The best medical judgment offers a prognosis of only a few days' life. He is undergoing extreme personal suffering, involving both physical and "spiritual" aspects. Bodily pain is intimately related to mental stress, to one's total outlook on life and to one's ability to make the most of biological existence as the condition for fully human meaning, centered on personal relationships. The physical pain of our patient cannot be effectively alleviated by the use of analgesics (this may be either because of the nature of his particular disease, or because of the state of medical practice in the locale in which he is receiving treatment). The integrity and maturity of personality which he has acquired as the goal of his lifetime thus far is slipping rapidly away as he endures the demoralizing experience of physical and mental deterioration. He acknowledges that the life which was once a good to him is now approaching its conclusion. He is reconciled to death and perhaps hopes for peace or joy in an existence beyond death. He requests that his physician hasten his progress toward death and out of his unbearable suffering. He asks that this be done not only out of mercy, but out of respect for his claim to freedom from severe threats to his personal integrity and to the achievement without undue delay of the appropriate goal of this now dying life.

The first objections which will be raised against a physician's compliance with this request will be directed at the very possibility of describing a case in these terms. Some will argue that there is always chance of a wrong diagnosis; examples are recounted of "miracle recoveries" in which an unexplained remission ensued upon the diagnosis of a "hopeless case" of cancer. Anyone who reflects upon human moral experience must grant the fallibility of all creaturely decision-making. Human persons must act, nonetheless, on the basis of strong probabilities, acknowledging that while outside possibilities do exist, they do not provide a reasonable basis for action in the face of far more persuasive evidence.

Other Objections

Others may object that no human being ever has a true desire to die and, with the assistance of a supportive medical team and family, will cherish even the last few hours of his or her existence. Elisabeth Kübler-Ross, M.D., has offered plentiful evidence on the basis of clinical experience that terminal patients are able to achieve acceptance of and readiness for death.[28] When this information is combined with an appreciation of the fact that critical suffering cannot in all circumstances be alleviated, one is able to envision more readily a patient who desires death after he has realistically assessed his prospects for human fulfillment during the short span left to him. Although most patients may be able to live meaningfully even during terminal illness, this does not negate the responsibility to consider the situation of the one who is not able to do so.

The moral character of such a case, admittedly exceptional in medical practice, may be examined in terms of the two expressions of the sanctity of life principle. The first furnishes the traditional prohibition, which describes voluntary euthanasia as a direct act to kill a man (oneself or another) who is "innocent."[29] If one views the moral act through the lens of this principle, the only legitimate killing is that in which either the term "direct" does not apply to the act, or the term "innocent" does not apply to the object of euthanasia.[30] This is certainly not to say that a dying patient is "guilty." The real question to be considered is whether the context of innocence and guilt is an appropriate one within which to ponder the moral character of voluntary euthanasia.

How ought we to interpret the negative phrasing of the natural law command to protect the individual's right to life? In Thomas, the adjective "innocent" refers primarily to the man who is "righteous" in the sense that he has *not forfeited* his right to life so that he may be deprived of it by lawful authority. To have lost one's innocence means to have injured the common good.[31] Thus the command not to kill the innocent seems fundamentally to be a prohibition against the deprivation of another's life against his will, unless that other has somehow forfeited his right to protection. The phrasing of this prohibition envisions correlative exceptions such as war, capital punishment and self-defense. The terms of the prohibition make an awkward context within which to approach suicide and euthanasia, where the "innocent" person is willing.[32]

More importantly, since in the latter cases the argument is made that death is in the better interests of the person, the language of "innocence" vs. guilt, forfeiture, and deprivation is not really applicable. The "innocent" man is one whose rights, among them the "right to life," must be respected. What about another right also belonging to the "righteous man" leading a God-oriented moral life, the "right to death"? Sometimes this right contravenes the importance of the first right. When this is so, it makes little sense to apply the word "innocent" out of its original context of forfeiture and punishment. The individual may be "innocent" in the sense of "legally or morally blameless," but what is the moral relevance of this fact?

It can be granted that the dying individual is innocent. However, it is the duty of those who care for and about him to consider that with which he has a right to be provided, as well as that of which he has a right not to be deprived. There may exist a positive duty to support his desire to die, *if* no conflict exists with other overriding rights and duties. The central problems are deciding, first, whether the duty to sustain life or the duty to end life is in the concrete case more important, and second, what are the morally legitimate means of upholding the predominant right. In care of the sick, the obligation to prolong life is foremost *until* that point at which an individual's life no longer offers to him or her the opportunity to nurture relationships as life's central endeavor. It has traditionally been granted that "hopeless cases" have, in such circumstances, a right to die which it may be the duty of others to support by withholding or withdrawing extraordinary means of treatment. Can the right to die ever justify direct killing? Does a terminal patient have a right to death which in some cases entails a duty on the part of those entrusted with his care to hasten positively its arrival?

Principle of Life's Sanctity

This brings the discussion to the affirmative expression of the principle of life's sanctity. What does it mean to respect and protect the life of a dying person? First, Kieran Nolan has remarked that a patient in the last phases of a terminal illness may be said to be oriented toward death as the appropriate goal of his existence, just as the healthy are appropriately oriented toward continued life.[33] Death is also the natural end of the biological organism. Although the death of a human as a personal being is not a good in itself, it still may be understood as a mediate and necessary goal of the Christian in his hope for eternal life in God. Secondly, the terminal patient who may be a candidate for euthanasia is one who is suffering both physically and spiritually or even "morally" in the sense of proximity to sin. In the first place, personal integration is threatened with degeneration. Physical pain, accompanied by mental exhaustion or sedation, often makes it difficult to sustain a vital concern for the needs of loved family members and friends. Furthermore, as Pius XII has stated, "suffering can also furnish occasion for new faults."[34] Nolan concurs that prolonged physical and mental torment can conduce to rebellion against God or despair.

Death for the Christian is never an unambiguous good, but it is sometimes a lesser evil than the evil of suffering, and is for the Christian a good in a limited but positive sense.[35] If in the light of these considerations, it is agreed that death is a good for a particular suffering and dying patient here and now, and if death will not follow quickly if treatment is ended, then can voluntary euthanasia ever constitute a legitimate moral option? From the evidence thus far (evidence which must be verified in every case from consideration of the situation of a particular individual), it would seem so. Life is not a value to be preserved absolutely. Sometimes it must yield to greater values. If death is for this person the better alternative, there exists sufficient reason for causing it.[36] Deliberately-caused death is not so great an evil that it can never be outweighed by greater goods.

The usual and most well-founded argument against voluntary euthanasia in even exceptional cases is made in terms of social consequences. It is not based on the alleged immorality of the individual act. The act itself may be conceded to result in desirable consequences for the patient, consequences which it would, in fact, be the responsibility of others to hasten directly, were it not for the evil long-range effects of such an act. However, it is argued that it is wrong to commit any act which, while good in itself, would lead to eventual consequences whose evil character would be disproportionate to the initial good. This venerable rejoinder is called the "wedge argument," a contemporary proponent of which is Richard McCormick.[37]

McCormick agrees with those who are convinced that "the direct causing of death involves dangers, especially for the living, not associated with conservative procedures. . . . "[38] Thus he gives a "prudential validity" to a rule against euthanasia of a "virtually exceptionless" sort. Direct killing as a premoral evil would be justified were there sufficient reason, but the reasons in favor of euthanasia in concrete cases are outbalanced by the reasons against instituting euthanasia as a general practice. McCormick believes that an immediate act, perhaps morally justifiable "in itself," is to be refrained from because of consequences such as an attitudinal decrease in mercy and sensitivity on the part of the hospital staff, or the ambiguities inherent in the procedures of ascertaining consent, etc.

This argument is a forceful one, but it need not signal the end of the discussion. Although McCormick has enumerated real dangers, he has not eradicated the problem with which any proposed wedge argument must deal, i.e., whether the long-term effects of an act ought to have the same moral importance as the immediate effects of an act. In cases where the latter are very certain and unavoidable, the former may be relatively uncertain because further moral choices (by others who share responsibility) will have to intervene in order either to actualize or to prevent the anticipated danger.

Traditional Catholic morals have held that it is always wrong to cause a moral evil in order to achieve a moral good or to prevent another moral evil even if it is greater. We also have a responsibility to try to avoid even that moral evil for which we are not directly responsible. Some ethicists have suggested that, at least in some cases, to refuse to hasten the death of a grossly suffering terminal patient is to permit, if not cause, in extreme cases, a moral evil—the despair of the dying man or woman.[39] Even in less severe cases, there is frequently present the clear spiritual, or personal, evil of mental enervation and distress, and of inability to escape the circle of suffering which encloses and limits all efforts to transcend oneself in concern for others. This is not moral evil in the sense of sin, but it is a clear disvalue for the whole human person as composed of both body and "spirit." It is a violation of the purpose and meaning of human existence.

Aquinas distinguishes between a certain and an uncertain moral evil; there exists a greater responsibility to avoid the former than the latter.[40] In the case of euthanasia, there are two possible dangers of moral evil, that to the patient if the act is not performed, and that to future generations if it is performed. In addition, there is the more realistic threat to personality, or fully personal spirit, not to mention the physical evil of bodily degeneration. Does the avoidance of an uncertain future evil actually constitute a proportionate reason for permitting a present evil, which, while of much narrower scope, is of much greater certainty? Is the failure to avoid an immediate moral evil, such as a loss of faith in the ultimate meaning of life, *or even* excruciating and prolonged spiritual and physical evil, such as conscious suffering or unconscious degeneration, sufficiently justified by the "proportionate reason" of avoidance of the danger (not the certainty) of future moral evil? In fact, this future evil seems more than the present one to be described most accurately as "permitted" rather than "caused." This is to say that our moral responsibility for the attitudes toward death of future physicians, etc., is more indirect than is our responsibility for the total personal distress (moral, mental, and physical) of our neighbor suffering here and now and immediately dependent upon our care.

I believe the usual criticism of the wedge argument has force against its use in the condemnation of euthanasia. The opposing contention is that each act must be judged right or wrong primarily *in itself* and only secondarily in its relation to other acts. "In itself" does indeed include effects, and it is admittedly difficult to draw a line around the more "immediate" ones. But the range of effects of an act cannot be extended indefinitely or the very meaning of a discrete "occasion of moral choice" is dissipated to the point of disappearance.

In addition, the social effects of the wedge will more likely be cut short where there is a standard by which to differentiate the first case from other similar but morally distinct cases.[41] The stipulation that a candidate for euthanasia be "in the dying process" is such a standard, and a relatively clear one, though its application is not in every case entirely unambiguous. There is a marked difference between euthanasia for those dying and in pain and euthanasia for the sick but not dying, for the socially useless, for the insane, etc., which can be judged by a relatively objective standard. Where such a criterion is available we must at least say that the "future danger" becomes more "uncertain." Another standard is the one McCormick offers as a justification for permitting death to occur, that of relational consciousness. Such a standard might apply also to the patient with a grossly damaged neocortex, whose vital functions are still maintained spontaneously by the brainstem. The prolonged and meaningless physical deterioration of a permanently comatose individual can be construed as an insult to his or her total personhood. In such a case, as well as that of the dying person, euthanasia may present a viable moral option. Once a patient is in the terminal stage of a fatal illness or is permanently comatose, it may become evident that his or her life is past the point of possible restoration to a quality which would support significant pursuit of the highest human values.

Christian Respect for Life

This discussion of moral responsibilities of and toward the dying does not represent a comprehensive grasp of the problem but rather an indication of appropriate ways to think about it. Through a consideration of Christian respect for the sanctity of human life, which is ultimately a concern for the good of the total person, I have tried to indicate that some relatively limited number of cases may constitute an arena of moral choice about euthanasia.[42] Life can fail to constitute a sufficient condition for the fulfillment of human value in either the presence of gross suffering or the absence of consciousness. These circumstances are predictably permanent if one is in the dying process or is irretrievably brain-damaged. It is at this point that the prospect of a choice about euthanasia arises. Such choices would involve only terminal or comatose patients for whom it is impossible to continue to pursue those human values for which the Creator intended life to serve as the condition. Every such choice must be informed by an authoritative respect for the dignity of human life as God's image and by the intent to protect that dignity. It is essential to remember that no such choices can be free from ambiguity, since death is never an unambiguous good. In particular, it is necessary to repudiate any attempt to define circumstances in which there always exists a moral obligation to perform an act of euthanasia. There is no definable "class" of patients for whom euthanasia is the only morally responsible alternative.

Most importantly, it must be made clear that there weighs on the community of fellow human beings, of which the dying patient is a member, the obligation to exhaust every resource in an effort to make the last phase of that patient's life positively meaningful. This obligation especially impinges upon the Christian, if love is in any sense to be taken as normative for conduct. At least it must be conceded that euthanasia ought always to be a final resort, not an option to be considered before all others have been explored. It goes without saying that such a stipulation ensures that authentic candidates for euthanasia will be few. We may say with confidence that euthanasia would be morally wrong where it is an act which deprives an individual of a real opportunity to live within self-offering relationships to others. In such a case, euthanasia would not be in the best interest of the patient, since life could be of further value *to him* or *her.*

In general, euthanasia is to be avoided or rejected on the basis of what is commonly termed "the sanctity of life principle." Human life has an inherent claim to respect. In certain circumstances, however, other considerations come into play which may influence persons to manifest respect by causing death. Life may cease, in some sense, to be a "good." It may inhibit or prevent the pursuit of human values instead of providing conditions conducive to their fulfillment. In addition, the continuation and development of a personal life history may lose considerable weight as a real alternative among others if terminal illness promises to critically abbreviate the life in question. A positive "choice" to end life in such a case is not a choice of significant continuation of life or of death but a choice of immediate death or of a wait for impending death. In such situations, the positive value of death may gain the ascendancy over the negative value, although both are always co-present. It must be said that euthanasia may not be justified because death is ever a value, right, or goal which can clearly cancel out the value of life. It must be said that euthanasia is never justified because the obligation of the living to the dying, or of the individual to attempt to live meaningfully, is ever ended.

In the resolution of these conflicts of value, the overriding concern must be the good of the patient himself or herself, who is the primary subject concerned. When conditions preclude the patient's voluntary selection of an option, that selection must be made on the basis of his or her own benefit and inferred interests. If these interests are assessed on the basis of a Christian anthropology which views the human being as a body-soul entity, then the primary consideration in life and death decisions in medical practice will be the good of the whole human person, not simply the perpetuation of physical existence.[43] Since the distinctive and controlling element of human nature is the personal self or spirit, then according to the principle of totality, the body which is a "part" may in some cases be sacrificed for the good of the "whole" body-soul entity. Even direct intervention as a final option will not necessarily entail diminishing communal protectiveness toward human life's sanctity, if death is encompassed reluctantly and with a profound (and Christian) reverence for the personal existence within which it is an event.

Notes

1. A.M.A., "Principles of Medical Ethics," *Journal of the American Medical Association,* 226 (1973), 137.
2. Kelly, Gerald, S.J., *Medico-Moral Problems* (St. Louis, 1958), p. 62.
3. For an extended discussion of the sanctity of life principle as a basis of consensus in matters of life and death, see Daniel Callahan, "The Sanctity of Life," *Updating Life and Death,* ed. Donald R. Cutler (Boston, 1968), pp. 181-250.
4. Aquinas, Thomas, *Summa Theologica,* II-II. Q 64, especially article 6.
5. *Cf.,* Kelly, pp. 62, 117.
6. *Cf., Ethical and Religious Directives for Catholic Health Facilities* (St. Louis, 1971), Directives 10, 11, 28, 29.
7. Aquinas, *Summa,* I. Q 61, a5; II-II. Q 64. a 2, 5, 6, Q 65; I-II. Q 17. a 4, Q 2. a 8; and *Summa Contra Gentiles,* Book 3, Chapter 112.
8. Kelly, "The Morality of Mutilation," *Theological Studies,* 17 (1956), 322-344; *Medico-Moral Problems,* pp. 8-11, 246-248; "Pope Pius XII and the Principle of Totality," *Theological Studies,* 16 (1955), 373-396. *Cf., Ethical and Religious Directives for Catholic Health Facilities,* Directives 4, 5, 6, 33.
9. Pope Pius XII, "Moral Limits of Medical Research," *The Major Addresses of Pope Pius XII,* ed. Vincent A. Yzermans (St. Paul, 1961), I, 233.
10. *Ibid.,* p. 228.
11. Pope Pius XII, *The Mystical Body of Christ* (New York, 1943), p. 36.
12. Pope Pius XII, "Tranquilizers and Christian Morals," *The Pope Speaks,* 5 (1958), 8-9.
13. Pope Pius XII, "Applied Psychology," *The Pope Speaks,* 5 (1958), 10.
14. Pope Pius XII, "Cancer: A Medical and Social Problem," *The Pope Speaks,* 3 (1957), 48.
15. Pope Pius XII, *The Mystical Body of Christ,* p. 55; and "Anesthesia: Three Moral Questions," Address to a Symposium of the Italian Society of Anesthesiologists (1957), *The Pope Speaks,* 4 (1957), 48.
16. *Ethical and Religious Directives for Catholic Health Facilities,* pp. 3, 1.
17. Nolan, Kieran, O.S.B., "The Problem of Care for the Dying," *Absolutes in Moral Theology?,* ed. Charles Curran (Washington, D.C., 1968), p. 249.
18. *Ibid.,* p. 249.
19. Pope Pius XII, "The Prolongation of Life," An Address to an International Congress of Anesthesiologists (1957), *The Pope Speaks,* 4 (1958), 396.
20. O'Donnell, Thomas J., S.J., *Morals in Medicine* (Westminster, Maryland, 1959), pp. 71-72.
21. McCormick, Richard A., S.J., "To Save or Let Die," *America,* 30 (1975), 6-10.
22. *Cf.,* Karl Rahner, *The Christian of the Future* (West Germany, 1967), pp. 42-44, 62-63; McCormick, *Ambiguity in Moral Choice,* The 1973 Pere Marquette Theology Lecture (Milwaukee, 1973), p. 106.
23. *Cf.,* Aquinas, *Summa,* II-II. Q 40, Q 64. An individual may be killed who presents a grave *material* danger, even if he is not *morally* guilty of an intended offense against the rights of another. Examples are the killing of enemy soldiers in war and the killing of an insane person who threatens one's life.
24. Kelly, "The Duty of Using Artificial Means of Preserving Life," *Theological Studies,* 11 (1950), 204; Pope Pius XII, "The Prolongation of Life," p. 396; McCormick, "To Save or Let Die," p. 9. Such would be the theological justification for refusing or withdrawing treatments such as a respirator from patients whom responsible medical prognosis designates as "hopeless." The well-publicized case of Karen Ann Quinlan recently decided before the New Jersey Supreme Court is a case in point. Legal ramifications aside, Pius's address provides more than ample ethical justification for allowing death to occur by removing life-sustaining equipment. In general, "ordinary" means of life support (obligatory) are those which can be obtained and used without excessive expense, inconvenience, or difficulty or repugnance for the patient, and which offer a reasonable hope of benefit to his or her total condition.

25. Thomistic natural law morality uses the language of direct and indirect acts to define the degree of responsibility which the agent has for a particular moral act. Since a fully human act is one performed in the use of reason and free will, the agent is not fully responsible for any act to which he does not fully consent. For a standard definition of "indirect effect," see Kelly, *Medico-Moral Problems,* pp. 13-14.

26. *Cf.,* the prohibition of euthanasia by the Congregation of the Holy Office, December, 1940, cited in full by Kelly, *Medico-Moral Problems,* pp. 116-117.

27. Cavanagh, John R., M.D., describes the "dying process" as "the time in the course of an irreversible illness when treatment will no longer influence it. Death is inevitable." "Bene Mori: The Right of the Patient to Die with Dignity," *Linacre Quarterly,* 30 (1963), 65.

28. Kübler-Ross, Elisabeth, *On Death and Dying* (New York, 1969), *Questions about Death and Dying* (New York, 1974), and ed., *Death: the Final Stage of Growth* (Englewood Cliffs, New Jersey, 1975).

29. *Cf.,* Kelly, *Medico-Moral Problems,* pp. 117-118.

30. A case can also be made for the inapplicability of the word "direct." Space does not allow me to pursue that argument at length here. I will mention only that Aquinas defends killing in self-defense because, even though the act is directly willed and performed, the intention of the agent does not terminate in the death for its own sake, but in self-protection. Similarly, an act of euthanasia is "indirectly" intended (although directly performed) in that its final object is not the death of the patient for itself but for the sake of his protection from suffering.

31. Aquinas, *Summa,* II-II. Q 64. a 2, 6.

32. Direct voluntary euthanasia for the terminal patient is a subclass of suicide, but differs from suicide in general in that the end of the person's lifespan is imminent because of reasons beyond human control.

33. Nolan, p. 256.

34. Pope Pius XII, "Anesthesia: Three Moral Questions," p. 46.

35. Thomas Aquinas prohibits suicide in order to avoid suffering because he sees death as "the ultimate and most fearsome evil of this life" (II-II. Q 64, a 5. r. obj. 3). I cannot agree with this and do not think it is consistent with Thomas's own anthropology. St. Thomas states many times that a properly ordered view of human nature places the good of the spiritual aspect of man over that of the physical. Spiritual evils far outweigh bodily ones, even when the latter include death. (*Cf., Summa,* II-II. Q 25. a 7, 12, Q 26. a 4; *Summa Contra Gentiles,* Chapter 121.)

36. Aquinas has stated that "evil must not be done that good may come" (II-II. Q 64. a 5. r. obj. 3). But this is only true when the good violated by the "evil" act is equal to or greater than the good pursued. In *Ambiguity in Moral Choice* (p. 55), Richard McCormick has suggested that death may be caused directly for sufficient reason, since death is a physical and therefore a "premoral" evil. Life may be overriden by other goods. The only sort of evil which may never be directly caused is the spiritual and moral evil of sin. (McCormick himself does not find "proportionate reason" to justify euthanasia, not because causing death is an evil which outweighs all goods, but because he envisions disastrous social consequences of a policy of euthanasia.)

37. McCormick, "The New Medicine and Morality," *Theology Digest,* 21 (1973), 308-321. For a classical use of the "wedge argument" against euthanasia, see Joseph V. Sullivan, S.J., *The Morality of Mercy Killing* (Westminster, Maryland, 1950), pp. 54-55.

38. McCormick, "The New Medicine and Morality," p. 319.

39. Nolan, p. 257; Antony Flew, "The Principle of Euthanasia," *Euthanasia and the Right to Death,* ed. A. B. Downing (Los Angeles, 1970), p. 33; Joseph Fletcher, *Morals and Medicine* (Boston, 1954), p. 175; *cf.,* Daniel Maguire, *Death by Choice* (New York, 1974), p. 155; Pope Pius XII, "Anesthesia: Three Moral Questions," p. 46.

40. Aquinas, *Summa,* II-II. Q 64. a 5.

41. This is important, since the telling point in arguments for and against euthanasia (e.g., the present author in contrast to McCormick) is whether one believes that the future danger is so probable and so serious that it outweighs harm done or permitted in the present instance, or whether it in fact represents the "lesser evil." Such an estimation is more a product of moral insight into human nature and moral responsibility than of rational deduction with probative force. We can only hope to persuade the opposition, not dismantle it!

42. Of course, the practical medical and legal circumstances of such choices remain to be specified, an important task not easily to be accomplished.

43. Religious faith is not a necessary precondition for arguing that the total human person is more than physical existence. An atheist or agnostic might agree that human life has a spiritual dimension which transcends the body. Even if the spirit is believed to die with the body, it may be the key element in one's concept of human dignity. Thus, when living becomes destructive to personal integrity, one may have a right to die.

72.
Euthanasia & Christian Vision

GILBERT MEILAENDER

Every teacher has probably experienced, along with countless frustrations, moments in the classroom when something was said with perfect lucidity. I still recall one such moment three years ago when I was teaching a seminar dealing with ethical issues in death and dying. Knowing how difficult it can be to get students to consider these problems from within religious perspectives, I decided to force the issue at the outset by assigning as the first reading parts of those magnificent sections from Volume III/4 of Karl Barth's *Church Dogmatics* in which he discusses "Respect for Life" and "The Protection of Life." I gave the students little warning in advance, preferring to let the vigor and bombast of Barth's style have whatever effect it might.

The students, I must say in retrospect, probably thought more kindly of Barth (who had, after all, only written these sections) than of their teacher (who had assigned them to be read). But they good-naturedly went about doing the assignment, and our seminar had a worthwhile discussion—with students criticizing Barth and, even, sometimes defending him. However, neither criticism nor defense was really my goal. It was understanding—understanding of death and dying within a perspective steeped in centuries of Christian life and thought—that I was seeking. And at one moment, even in a moment of criticism, we achieved that understanding.

One young woman in the class, seeking to explain why Barth puzzled her so, put it quite simply: "What I really don't like about him is that he seems to think our lives are not our own." To which, after a moment of awed silence, I could only respond: "If you begin to see that about Barth, even if it gets under your skin and offends you deeply, then indeed you have begun to understand what he is saying."

In his discussion of "The Protection of Life," and, in fact, within his specific discussion of euthanasia, Barth notes many of the difficult questions we might raise which seem to nudge us in the direction of approving euthanasia in certain tormenting cases. And then, rejecting these "tempting questions," he responds with his own typical flair. "All honour to the well-meaning humanitarianism of underlying motive! But the derivation is obviously from another book than that which we have thus far consulted."[1] In this brief essay I want to think about euthanasia not from the perspective of any "well-meaning humanitarianism" but from within the parameters of Christian belief—though, as we will see, one of the most important things to note is that, within those parameters, only what is consonant with Christian belief can be truly humane.[2]

The Paradigm Case

Determining what really qualifies as euthanasia is no easy matter. Need the person "euthanatized" be suffering terribly? Or, at least, be near death? Suppose the person simply feels life is no longer worth living in a particular condition which may be deeply dissatisfying though not filled with suffering? Suppose the person's life is filled with suffering or seemingly devoid of meaning but he is unable to request euthanasia (because of a comatose condition, senility, etc.)? Or suppose the person is suffering greatly but steadfastly says he does not want to die? Suppose the "euthanatizer's motive is not mercy but despair at the continued burden of caring for the person—will that qualify?

The list of questions needing clarification is endless once we start down this path. But I intend to get off the path at once by taking as our focus of attention a kind of paradigm case of what must surely count as euthanasia. If we can understand why *this* is morally wrong, much else will fall into place. James Rachels has suggested that "the clearest possible case of euthanasia" would be one having the following five features:[3]

(1) The person is deliberately killed.
(2) The person would have died soon anyway.
(3) The person was suffering terrible pain.
(4) The person asked to be killed.
(5) The motive of the killing was mercy—to provide the person with as good a death as possible under the circumstances.

Such a case is not simply "assisted suicide," since the case requires the presence of great suffering, the imminence of death in any case, and a motive of mercy. Furthermore, considering this sort of case sets aside arguments about nonvoluntary and involuntary euthanasia and gives focus to our discussion.[4] If this case of voluntary euthanasia is permissible, other cases may also be (or may not). If this case is itself morally wrong, we are less likely to be able to

Reprinted by permission of the publisher from "Euthanasia and Christian Vision," *Thought* 57, December 1982 (New York: Fordham University Press, 1982).

argue for euthanasia in nonvoluntary and involuntary circumstances.

Aim and Result

One way of arguing that the paradigm case of euthanasia is morally permissible (perhaps even obligatory) is to claim that it does not differ in morally relevant ways from other acts which most of us approve. Consider a patient whose death is imminent, who is suffering terribly, and who may suddenly stop breathing and require resuscitation. We may think it best not to resuscitate such a person but simply to let him die. What could be the morally significant difference between such a "letting die" and simply giving this person a lethal injection which would have ended his life (and suffering) just as quickly? If it is morally right not to prolong his dying when he ceases breathing for a few moments, why is it morally wrong to kill him quickly and painlessly? Each act responds to the fact that death is imminent and recognizes that terrible suffering calls for relief. And the result in each case is the same: death.

In order to appreciate the important difference between these possibilities we must distinguish what we *aim* at in our action from the *result* of the action. Or, to paraphrase Charles Fried, we must distinguish between those actions which we invest with the personal involvement of purpose and those which merely "run through" our person.[5] This is a distinction which moral reflection can scarcely get along without. For example, if we fail to distinguish between aim and result we will be unable to see any difference between the self-sacrifice of a martyr and the suicide of a person weary of life. The result is the same for each: death. But the aim or purpose is quite different. Whereas the suicide aims at his death, the martyr aims at faithfulness to God (or loyalty of some other sort). Both martyr and suicide recognize in advance that the result of their choice and act will be death. But the martyr does not aim at death.

This distinction between aim and result is also helpful in explaining the moral difference between euthanatizing a suffering person near death and simply letting such a person die. Suppose this patient were to stop breathing, we were to reject the possibility of resuscitation, and then the person were suddenly to begin breathing again. Would we, simply because we had been willing to let this patient die, now proceed to smother him so that he would indeed die? Hardly. And the fact that we would not indicates that we did not *aim* at his death (in rejecting resuscitation), though his death could have been one *result* of what we did aim at (namely, proper care for him in his dying). By contrast, if we euthanatized such a person by giving him a lethal injection, we would indeed aim at his death; we would invest the act of aiming at his death with the personal involvement of our purpose.

A rejoinder: It is possible to grant the distinction between aim and result while still claiming that euthanasia in our paradigm case would be permissible (or obligatory). It may be true that there is a difference between allowing a patient to die and aiming at someone's death. But if the suffering of the dying person is truly intense and the person requests death, on what grounds could we refuse to assist him? If we refuse on the grounds that it would be wrong for us to aim at his death (which will certainly result soon anyway after more terrible suffering), are we not saying that we are unwilling to do him a great good if doing it requires that we dirty our hands in any way? To put the matter this way makes it seem that our real concern is with our own moral rectitude, not with the needs of the sufferer. It seems that we are so concerned about ourselves that in our eagerness to narrow the scope of our moral responsibility we have lost sight of the need and imperative to offer care.

This is, it should be obvious, what ethicists call a *consequentialist* rejoinder. It suggests that the good results (relieving the suffering) are sufficiently weighty to make the aim (of killing) morally permissible or obligatory. And, as far as I can tell, this rejoinder has become increasingly persuasive to large numbers of people.

Consequentialism may be described as that moral theory which holds that from the fact that some state of affairs *ought to be* it follows that we *ought to do* whatever is necessary to bring about that state of affairs. And, although teleological theories of morality are very ancient, consequentialism as a full-blown moral theory is traceable largely to Bentham and Mill in the late 18th and early 19th centuries. To remember this is instructive, since it is not implausible to suggest that such a moral theory would be most persuasive when Christendom had, in large measure, ceased to be Christian. Those who know themselves as creatures—not Creator—will recognize limits even upon their obligation to do good. As creatures we are to do all the good we can, but this means all the good we "morally can"—all the good we can within certain limits. It may be that the Creator *ought to do* whatever is necessary to bring about states of affairs which *ought to be,* but we stand under no such godlike imperative.[6]

One of the best ways to understand the remarkable appeal today of consequentialism as a moral theory is to see it as an ethic for those who (a) remain morally serious, but (b) have ceased to believe in a God whose providential care will ultimately bring about whatever ought to be the case. If God is not there to accomplish what ought to be the case, we are the most likely candidates to shoulder the burden of that responsibility.[7] Conversely, it may be that we can make sense of distinguishing between two acts whose *result* is the same but whose *aim* is different only if we believe that our responsibilities (as creatures) are limited—that the responsibility for achieving certain results has been taken out of our hands (or, better, never given us in the first place). It ought to be the case that dying people not suffer terribly (indeed, that they not die). But, at least for Christians, it does not follow from that "ought to be" that we "ought to do" whatever is necessary—even euthanasia—to relieve them of that suffering.[8]

We are now in a position to see something important about the argument which claims that euthanasia (in the paradigm case) is permissible because it does not differ morally from cases of "letting die" which most of us approve. This argument often begins in a failure to distinguish aim and result; however, it is, as we have seen, difficult for moral theory to get along without this distinction. Seeing this, we recognize that the argument really becomes a claim that if the results are sufficiently good, any aim necessary to achieve them is permissible. And precisely at this turn in the argument it may be difficult to keep "religion" and "morality" in those neat and separate compartments we have fashioned for them. At this point one steeped in Christian thought and committed to Christian life may wish to say with Barth: All honor to the well-meaning humanitarianism—and it is well-meaning. But the derivation—fit only for those who would, even if reluctantly, be "like God"—is obviously "derived from another book" than that which Christians are wont to consult.

Aim and Motive

If the distinction between aim and result makes it difficult to justify euthanasia in the paradigm case, another distinction may be more useful. We might suggest that the act of euthanatizing be redescribed in terms of the motive of mercy. We could describe the act not as killing but as relieving suffering. Or, rather than engaging in such wholesale redescription of the act, we might simply argue that our moral evaluation of the act cannot depend solely on its *aim* but must also consider its *motive.*

Consider the following illustration.[9] A condemned prisoner is in his cell only minutes before his scheduled execution. As he sits in fear and anguish, certain of his doom, another man who has managed to sneak into the prison shoots and kills him. This man is either (a) the father of children murdered by the prisoner, or (b) a close friend of the prisoner. In case (a) he shoots because he will not be satisfied simply to have the man executed. He desires that his own hand should bring about the prisoner's death. In case (b) the friend shoots because he wishes to spare his friend the terror and anguish of those last minutes, to deliver him from the indignity of the sheer animal fright he is undergoing.

Would it be proper to describe the father's act in (a) as an act of killing and the friend's in (b) as an act of relieving suffering? Although many people may be tempted to do so, it muddies rather than clarifies our analysis. If anything is clear in these cases, it is that both the vengeful father and the compassionate friend *aim* to kill though their *motives* are very different. Only by refusing to redescribe the aim of the act in terms of its motive do we keep the moral issue clearly before us. That issue is whether our moral evaluation of the act should depend solely on the agent's *aim* or whether that evaluation must also include the *motive.*

That the motive makes *some* difference almost everyone would agree. Few of us would be content to analyze the two cases simply as instances of "aiming to kill" without considering the quite different motives. The important question, however, is whether the praiseworthy motive of relieving suffering should so dominate our moral reflection that it leads us to term the act 'right.' I want to suggest that it should not, at least not within the parameters of Christian belief.

One might think that Christian emphasis on the overriding importance of love as a motive would suggest that whatever was done out of love was right. And, to be sure, Christians will often talk this way. Such talk, however, must be done against the background assumptions of Christian anthropology. Apart from that background of meaning we may doubt whether we have really understood the motive of love correctly. We need therefore to sketch in the background against which we can properly understand what loving care for a suffering person should be.[10]

Barth writes that human life "must always be regarded as a divine act of trust."[11] This means that all human life is "surrounded by a particular solemnity," which, if recognized, will lead us to "treat it with respect." At the same time, however, "life is no second God, and therefore the respect due to it cannot rival the reverence owed to God." One who knows this will seek to live life "within its appointed limits." Recognizing our life as a trust, we will be moved not by an "absolute will to live" but a will to live within these limits. Hence, when we understand ourselves as creatures, we will both value God's gift of life and recognize that the Giver himself constitutes the limit beyond which we ought not value the gift. "Temporal life is certainly not the highest of all goods. Just because it belongs to God, man may be forbidden to will its continuation at all costs." And at the same time, "if life is not the highest possession, then it is at least the highest and all-inclusive price" which human beings can pay. In short, life is a great good, but not the greatest (which is fidelity to God).

Death, the final enemy of life, must also be understood dialectically. The human mind can take and has quite naturally taken two equally plausible attitudes toward death.[12] We can regard death as of no consequence, heeding the Epicurean maxim that while we are alive death is not yet here, and when death is here we are no more. Thus the human being, in a majestic transcendence of the limits of earthly life, might seek to soar beyond the limits of finitude and find his good elsewhere. If death is of no consequence, we may seek it in exchange for some important good. Equally natural to the human mind is a seemingly opposite view—that death is the *summum malum,* the greatest evil to be avoided at all costs. Such a view, finding good only in earthly life, can find none in suffering and death.

The Christian mind, however, transcending what is "natural" and correcting it in light of the book it is accustomed to consult, has refused to take either of these quite plausible directions. Understood within the biblical narrative, death is an ambivalent phenomenon— too ambivalent to be seen only as the greatest of all evils, or as indifferent. Since the world narrated by the Bible begins in God and moves toward God, earthly life is his trust to be sustained faithfully and his gift to be valued and cared for. When life is seen from this perspective, we cannot say that death and suffering are of no consequence; on the contrary, we can even say with Barth that the human task in the face of suffering and death is not to accept but to offer "final resistance."[13] It is just as true, however, that death could never be the greatest evil. That title must be reserved for disobedience to and disbelief in God—a refusal to live within our appointed limits. So we can also repeat with Barth that "life is no second God."[14] We remember, after all, that Jesus goes to the cross in the name of obedience to his Father. We need not glorify or seek suffering, but we must be struck by the fact that a human being who is a willing sufferer stands squarely in the center of Christian piety. Jesus bears his suffering not because it is desirable but because the Father allots it to him within the limits of his earthly life. Death is—there is no way to put the matter simply—a great evil which God can turn to his good purposes. It is an evil which must ordinarily be resisted but which must also at some point be acknowledged. We can and ought to acknowledge what we do not and ought not seek. George Orwell, himself an "outsider," nicely summarized these background assumptions of Christian anthropology:

> The Christian attitude towards death is not that it is something to be welcomed, or that it is something to be met with stoical indifference, or that it is something to be avoided as long as possible; but that it is something profoundly tragic which has to be gone through with. A Christian, I suppose, if he were offered the chance of everlasting life on this earth would refuse it, but he would still feel that death is profoundly sad.[15]

This vision of the world, and of the meaning of life and death, has within Christendom given guidance to those reflecting on human suffering and dying. That moral guidance has amounted to the twofold proposition that, though we might properly cease to oppose death while aiming at other choiceworthy goods in life (hence, the possibility of martyrdom), we ought never aim at death as either our end or our means.

Against this background of belief we can better understand what *love* and *care* must be within a world construed in Christian terms. In *this* world no action which deliberately hastens death can be called 'love.' Not because the euthanatizer need have any evil motive. Indeed, as the case of the compassionate friend makes clear, the one who hastens death may seem to have a praiseworthy motive. Rather, such action cannot be loving because it cannot be part of the meaning of commitment to the well-being of another human being within the appointed limits of earthly life. The benevolence of the euthanatizer is enough like love to give us pause, to tempt us to call it love. And *perhaps* it may even be the closest those who feel themselves to bear full responsibility for relief of suffering and production of good in our world can come to love. But it is not the creaturely love which Christians praise, a love which can sometimes do no more than suffer as best we can with the sufferer.

Christian Love Enacted and Inculcated

Against this background—a background which pours meaning into words like 'love' and 'care'—we can contemplate the kind of case often considered in discussions of euthanasia.[16] A person may be in severe pain, certain to die within only a few days. Most of us would agree that further "lifesaving" treatments were not in order for such a person, that they would do no more than prolong his dying. Why, one may ask, do we not subject such a patient to useless treatments? Because, we reply, he is in agony and it would be wrong to prolong that agony needlessly. But now, if we face the facts honestly, we will admit that it takes this patient longer to die—and prolongs his suffering—if we simply withhold treatment than if we euthanatize him. Hence, there seems to be a contradiction within our reasoning. The motive for withholding treatment was a humanitarian one: relief of suffering. But in refusing to take the next step and euthanatize the patient we prolong his suffering and, thereby, belie our original motive. Hence the conclusion follows, quite contrary to the moral guidance embedded in the Christian vision of the world: Either we should keep this person alive as long as possible (and not pretend that our motive is the relief of suffering), or we should be willing to euthanatize him.

The argument gets much of its force from the seeming simplicity of the dilemma, but that simplicity is misleading. For, at least for Christian vision, the fundamental imperative is not "minimize suffering" but "maximize love and care." In that Christian world, in which death and suffering are great evils but not the greatest evil, love can never include in its meaning hastening a fellow human being toward (the evil of) death, nor can it mean a refusal to acknowledge death when it comes (as an evil but not the greatest evil). We can only know what the imperative "maximize love" means if we understand it against the background assumptions which make intelligible for Christians words like 'love' and 'care.' The Christian mind has certainly not recommended that we seek suffering or call it an unqualified good, but it is an evil which, when endured faithfully, can be redemptive. William May has noted how parents in our time think that love for their children means, above all else, protecting those children from suffering. "As conscientious parents, they operate as though the powers that are decisive in the universe could not possibly do anything in and through the suffering of their children. . . . They take upon themselves the responsibilities of a savior-figure. . . . "[17] May sees clearly that "minimize suffering" and "maximize love" are not identical imperatives and do not offer the same direction for human action. Perhaps the direction they give may often be the same, but at times—especially when we consider what it is proper to do for the irretrievably dying—we will discover how sharply they may differ.

I suggested above that we should not redescribe the *aim* of an act in terms of its *motive.* (We should not say that an act of killing a suffering person was simply an act of relieving suffering. We should say rather that we aimed at the death of the person in order to relieve his suffering. This keeps the moral issue more clearly before us.) But by now it will be evident that I have in fact gone some way toward redescribing the *motive* of the act in terms of its *aim.* (If the act is aimed at hastening the death of the suffering person, we should not see it as motivated by love.) Is this any better? The answer, I think, is "it depends."

It would not be better, it might even be worse, if my purpose were to deny any humanitarian motive to the person tempted to euthanatize a sufferer. Few people would find such a denial persuasive, and because we would not we are tempted to turn in the opposite direction and describe the act's aim in terms of its motive. We *do* recognize a difference between the vengeful father and the compassionate friend even though both aim to kill the condemned prisoner, and we want our moral judgments to be sufficiently nuanced to take account of these differences. The simple truth is that our evaluation of the act (described in terms of aim) and our evaluation of the act (described in terms of motive) often fall apart. In a world broken by sin and its consequences this should perhaps come as no surprise. Christians believe that we sinners—all of us—are not whole, and many of the stubborn problems of systematic ethical reflection testify to the truth of that belief. It is our lack of wholeness which is displayed in our inability to arrive at one judgment (or even one description) "whole and entire" of a single act. We find ourselves in a world in which people may sometimes seem to aim at doing evil from the best of motives (and think they must do so). And then we are tempted to elide aim and motive and call that evil at which they aim 'good.'

No amount of ethical reflection can heal this rift in our nature. From that predicament we will have to look for a deliverance greater than ethics can offer. However, here and now, in our broken world, we do better to take the aim of an act as our guiding light in describing and evaluating the act—and then evaluate the motive in light of this aim. This is better because moral reflection is not primarily a tool for fixing guilt and responsibility (in which case motive comes to the fore). It is, first and foremost, one of the ways in which we train ourselves and others to see the world rightly. We would be wrong to assert that no euthanatizer has or can have a humanitarian motive. But if we want not so much to fix praise or blame but to teach the meaning of the word 'love,' we are not wrong to say that love could never euthanatize. In the Christian world this is true. And in that world we know the right name for our own tendency to call those other, seemingly humanitarian, motives 'love.' The name for that tendency is *temptation.* We are being tempted to be "like God" when we toy with the possibility of defining our love—and the meaning of humanity—apart from the appointed limits of human life.

To redescribe the motive in terms of the act's aim, to attempt to *inculcate* a vision of the world in which love could never euthanatize, is therefore not only permissible but necessary for Christians. It is the only proper way to respond to the supposed dilemmas we are confronted with by reasoning which brackets Christian background assumptions from the outset. The Christian moral stance which emerges here is not a club with which to beat over the head those who disagree. It does not provide a superior vantage point from which to deny them any humanitarian motive in the ordinary sense. But it *is* a vision of what 'humanity' and 'humanitarian motives' should be. We may therefore say of those who disagree: "All honour to the well-meaning humanitarianism of underlying motive! But the derivation is obviously from another book than that which we have thus far consulted."

Notes

1. Karl Barth, *Church Dogmatics,* Vol. III/4, ed. G. W. Bromiley and T. F. Torrance (Edinburgh: T. & T. Clark, 1961), p. 425.

2. I will be exploring some of the *moral* issues involved in euthanasia without taking up *legal* problems which also arise. I do not assume any answer to the question, Should what is morally wrong be legally prohibited?

3. James Rachels, "Euthanasia," *Matters of Life and Death: New Introductory Essays in Moral Philosophy,* ed. Tom Regan (New York: Random House, 1980), p. 29.

4. Nonvoluntary euthanasia occurs when the person euthanatized is in a condition which makes it impossible for him to express a wish (e.g., senile, comatose). Involuntary euthanasia occurs when the person euthanatized expresses a desire *not* to be killed but is nevertheless euthanatized.

5. Charles Fried, *Right and Wrong* (Cambridge: Harvard University Press, 1978), p. 27.

6. Cf. Joseph Butler, Dissertation "On the Nature of Virtue," appended to *The Analogy of Religion Natural and Revealed.* Morley's Universal Library edition (London: George Routledge & Sons, 1884), p. 301: "The fact then appears to be, that we are constituted so as to condemn falsehood, unprovoked violence, injustice, and to approve of benevolence to some preferably to others abstracted from all consideration, which conduct is likely to produce an overbalance of happiness or misery; and therefore, were the Author of Nature to propose nothing to Himself as an end but the production of happiness, were His moral character merely that of benevolence; yet ours is not so." In other words, though the Creator may be a consequentialist, creatures are not! For a contrary view, see Peter Geach, *The Virtues* (Cambridge University Press, 1977), pp. 95ff.

7. Whether this enlargement of the scope of our responsibility really works is another matter. Being responsible for everything may, for human beings, come quite close to being responsible for nothing. Charles Fried comments: "If, as consequentialism holds, we were indeed equally morally responsible for an infinite radiation of concentric circles originating from the center point of some action, then while it might look as if we were enlarging the scope of human responsibility and thus the significance of personality, the enlargement would be greater than we could support. . . . Total undifferentiated responsibility is the correlative of the morally overwhelming, undifferentiated plasma of happiness or pleasure" (*Right and Wrong,* pp. 34f.).

8. It is a hard, perhaps unanswerable, question whether there might ever be exceptions to this general standard for Christian conduct which I have enunciated. There might be a circumstance in which the pain of the sufferer was so terrible and unconquerable that one would want to consider an exception. To grant this possibility is not really to undermine the principle since, as Charles Fried has noted, the "catastrophic" is a distinct moral concept, identifying an extreme situation in which the usual rules of morality do not apply (*Right and Wrong,* p. 10). We would be quite mistaken to build the whole of our morality on the basis of the catastrophic; in fact, it would then become the norm rather than the exception. One possible way to deal with such extreme circumstances without simply lapsing into consequentialism is to reason in a way analogous to Michael Walzer's reasoning about the rules of war in *Just and Unjust Wars* (New York: Basic Books, Inc., 1977). Walzer maintains that the rules of war are binding even when they put us at a disadvantage, even when they may cost us victory. But he grants that there might be "extreme emergencies" in which we could break the rules; namely, when doing so was (a) morally necessary (i.e., the opponent was so evil—a Hitler—that it was morally imperative to defeat him) and (b) strategically necessary (no other way than violating the rules of war was available for defeating this opponent). Reasoning in an analogous way we might wonder whether the rule prohibiting euthanasia could be violated if (a) the suffering was so unbearable that the sufferer lost all capacity to bear that suffering with any sense of moral purpose or faithfulness to God; and (b) the pain was truly unconquerable. Whether such extreme circumstances ever occur is a question whose answer I cannot give. And even if such circumstances are possible, I remain uncertain about the force of this "thought experiment," which is offered tentatively.

9. This illustration is "inspired" by a different set of hypothetical cases offered by Paul Ramsey in "Some Rejoinders," *The Journal of Religious Ethics,* 4 (Fall, 1976), p. 204.

10. In what follows I draw upon my own formulations in two previous articles: "The Distinction Between Killing and Allowing to Die," *Theological Studies,* 37 (September, 1976), 467-470 and "Lutheran Theology and Bioethics: A Juxtaposition," *SPC Journal,* 3 (1980), 25-30.

11. The passages cited in this paragraph may be found

scattered throughout pages 336-342 and pages 401-402 of Vol. III/4 of *Church Dogmatics.*

12. For what follows cf. C.S. Lewis, *Miracles* (New York: Macmillan, 1947), pp. 129ff., and Paul Ramsey, *The Patient as Person* (New Haven and London: Yale University Press, 1970), pp. 144ff.

13. *Church Dogmatics,* III/4, p. 368.

14. *Ibid.,* p. 342.

15. George Orwell, "The Meaning of a Poem," *My Country Right or Left, 1940-1943.* Volume II of *The Collected Essays, Journalism and Letters of George Orwell,* ed. Sonia Orwell & Ian Angus (New York: Harcourt Brace Jovanovich, 1968), p. 133.

16. For a strong statement of such a case see James Rachels, "Active and Passive Euthanasia," *New England Journal of Medicine,* 292 (1975), pp. 78-80.

17. William May, "The Metaphysical Plight of the Family," *Death Inside Out,* ed. Peter Steinfels and Robert M. Veatch (Harper & Row, 1974), p. 51.

73.
Rational Suicide and Reasons for Living

STANLEY HAUERWAS

1. Suicide and the Ethics of Autonomy

There is a peculiar ambiguity concerning the morality of suicide in our society. Our commitment to the autonomy of the individual at least implies that suicide may not only be rational, but a "right."[1] Yet many continue to believe that anyone attempting suicide must be sick and therefore prevented from killing themselves. This ambiguity makes us hesitant even to analyze the morality of suicide because we fear we may discover that our society lacks any coherent moral policy or basis for preventing suicide.

Therefore the very idea of "rational suicide" is a bit threatening. We must all feel a slight twinge of concern about the book soon to be published by the British Voluntary Euthanasia Society that describes the various painless and foolproof methods of suicide. But it is by no means clear why we feel uncomfortable about having this kind of book widely distributed. As Nicholas Reed, the general secretary of the Society, suggests: suicide is "more and more seen as an acceptable way for a life to end, vastly preferable to some long, slow, painful death. We're simply helping in the fight for another human right—the right to die."[2]

We think there must be something wrong with this, but we are not sure what. I suspect our unease about these matters is part of the reason we wish to deny the existence of rational or autonomous suicide. If all potential suicides can be declared ill by definition then we can prevent them ironically because the agent lacks autonomy. Therefore we intervene to prevent suicides in the name of autonomy which, if we were consistent, should require us to consider suicide a permissible moral act.

Once I was a participant in a seminar in medical ethics at one of our most prestigious medical schools. I was there to speak about suicide, but the week before the seminar had considered abortion. At that time I was told by these beginning medical students they decided it was their responsibility to perform an abortion if a woman requested it because a woman has the

From *Rights and Responsibilities in Modern Medicine,* ed. Marc D. Basson (New York: Alan R. Liss, 1981). Used by permission.

right to determine what she should do with her body—a ethical conclusion that they felt clearly justified on grounds of protecting the autonomy of the patient. Moreover this position, they argued, was appropriate if the professional dominance and paternalism of the medical profession was to be broken.

However, I asked them what they would do if they were attending in the Emergency Room and someone was brought in with slashed wrists with a suicide note pinned to their shirt front. First of all would they take the time to read the note to discover the state of the patient? Secondly would they say this is clearly not a medical matter and refuse to accept the patient? Or would they immediately begin to save the person's life? With the same unanimity concerning their responsibility to perform abortion they felt they must immediately begin trying to save the person's life.

The reason they gave to justify their intervention was that anyone taking their life must surely be sick. But it was not clear what kind of "sickness" was under consideration unless we define life itself as some kind of syndrome. Failing to make the case that all suicides must be sick they then suggested they must act to save such a person's life because it was their responsibility as doctors. But again I pressed them on what right they had to impose their role-related responsibilities on those who did not seek their services and, in fact, had clearly tried to avoid coming in contact with them. They then appealed to experience, citing cases when people have recovered from suicide attempts only to be thankful they had been helped. But again such appeals are not convincing since we can also point to the many who are not happy about being saved and soon make another attempt.

Our discussion began to be more and more frustrating for all involved, so a compromise was suggested. These future physicians felt the only solution was that when a suicide came to the Emergency Room the first time, the doctor's responsibility must always be to save their life. However if they came in a second time they could be allowed to die. That kind of solution, however, is not only morally unsatisfactory, but pragmatically difficult to institutionalize. What happens if each time the person is brought to the hospital they get a different physician?

I have told this story because I think it nicely illustrates the kind of difficulties we feel when we try to get a moral handle on suicide. We feel that Beauchamp and Childress are right that if a suicide is genuinely autonomous and there are no powerful utilitarian reasons for "reasons of human worth and dignity standing in the way, then we ought to allow the person to commit suicide, because we would otherwise be violating the person's autonomy."[3]

However, I want to suggest that this way of putting the matter, while completely consistent with an ethics of autonomy, is also deeply misleading. It is misleading not only because it reveals the insufficiency of autonomy either as a basis or ideal for the moral life[4] but also it simply fails to provide an appropriate account of why any of us decides or should decide to stay alive. Indeed it is odd even to think of our willingness to live as a decision. For example Beauchamp and Childress do not explain how anyone could take account of *all* relevant variables and future possibilities in considering suicide. Indeed that seems an odd condition for if we required it of even our most important decisions it would stop us from acting at all.

Yet by challenging this account I want clearly to distinguish my position from those who are intent to deny the possibility of rational suicide. I think that suicide can be and often is a rational decision of an "autonomous" agent, but I do not therefore think it is justified. It is extremely interesting, for example, that Augustine did not claim that suicide was irrational in criticizing the Stoic acceptance and even recommendation of suicide. Rather he pointed out that their acceptance of suicide belied their own understanding of the relation between evil and happiness and how a wise man thus should deal with adversity. Though the quote is long I think it worth providing the full text. Augustine says,

> There is a mighty force in the evils which compel a man, and, according to those philosophers, even a wise man, to rob himself of his existence as a man; although they say, and say with truth, that the first and greatest utterance of nature, as we may call it, is that a man should be reconciled to himself and for that reason should naturally shun death—that he should be his own friend, in that he should emphatically desire to continue as a living being and to remain alive in this combination of body and soul, and that this should be his aim. There is a mighty force in those evils which overpower this natural feeling which makes us employ all our strength in our endeavor to avoid death—which defeat this feeling so utterly that what was shunned is now wished and longed for, and, if it cannot come to him from some other source, is inflicted on a man by himself. There is a mighty force in those evils which make Fortitude a murderer—if indeed she is still to be called fortitude when she is so utterly vanquished by those evils that she not only cannot by her endurance keep guard over the man she has undertaken to govern and protect,

but is herself compelled to go so far as to kill him. The wise man ought, indeed, to endure even death with a steadfastness, but a death that comes to him from outside himself. Whereas if he is compelled, as those philosophers say, to inflict it on himself, they must surely admit that these are not only evils, but intolerable evils, when they compel him to commit this crime.

It follows from this that the life weighed down by such great and grievous ills, or at the mercy of such chances, would never be called happy, if the men who so term it, and who, when overcome by the growing weights of ills, surrender to adversity encompassing their own death—if these people would bring themselves to surrender to the truth, when overcome by sound reasoning, in their quest for the happy life, and would give up supposing that the ultimate, Supreme God is something to be enjoyed by them in this condition of mortality.[5]

The question is not, therefore, the question of whether suicide is "rational." Augustine knew well that the Stoics could provide outstanding examples of cool, unemotional, and rational suicide. He rather asks what kind of blessedness we should expect out of life. For Augustine the Stoic approval of suicide was an indication of the insufficient account they provided about what human existence should be about—namely they failed to see that the only happiness worth desiring is that which came from friendship with the true God. "Yet," he says, "these philosophers refuse to believe in this blessedness because they do not see it; and so they attempt to fabricate for themselves an utterly delusive happiness by means of a virtue whose falsity is in proportion to its arrogance."[6] So the issue, if Augustine is right as I believe him to be, is how suicide is understood within a conception of life we think good and worthy.

2. The Grammar of Suicide

Before developing this line of reasoning, however, it should be pointed out that the discussion to this point has been trading on the assumption that we know what suicide is. Yet that is simply not the case. For as Beauchamp and Childress suggest, definitions of suicide such as "an intentionally caused self-destruction not forced by the action of another person" are not nearly as unambiguous as they may at first seem. For example they point out when persons suffering from a terminal illness or mortal injury allow their death to occur we find ourselves reluctant to call that act "suicide," but if persons with a terminal illness take their life by active means we do refer to that act as one of suicide. Yet to only describe those acts that involved a direct action as suicide is misleading since we are not sure how we should describe cases where "a patient with a terminal condition might easily avoid dying for a long time but might choose to end his life immediately by not taking cheap and painless medication."[7]

Beauchamp and Childress suggest the reason we have difficulty deciding the meaning of suicide is that the term has an emotive meaning of disapproval that we prefer not to apply to certain kinds of ambiguous cases. The very logic of the term therefore tends to prejudice any pending moral analysis of the rightness or wrongness of suicide. As a means to try to deal with this problem they propose an "uncorrupted" definition of suicide as what occurs "if and only if one intentionally terminates one's own life—no matter what the conditions or precise nature of the intention or the causal route to death."[8]

As sympathetic as one must feel with their attempt to provide a clear and non-prejudicial account of suicide, however, the very idea of an "uncorrupted" definition of suicide distorts the very grammar of such notions. Beauchamp and Childress are quite right to point out that the notion itself cannot settle how and why suicide applies to certain kinds of behavior and not others. But what must be admitted, as Joseph Margolis has recently argued, is the culturally variable character of suicide. There are many competing views about the meaning and nature of suicide, "some religious, some not, some not even significantly so characterized. . . . There is no simple formula for designating, except trivially, an act of taking, or yielding, or making likely the end of, one's life that will count, universally as suicide. No, some selection of acts of this minimal sort will, in accord with an interpreting tradition, construe what was done as or as not suicide; and, so judging, the tradition will provide as well for the approval or condemnation of what was done. In short, suicide, like murder itself, is an act that can be specified only in a systematic way within a given tradition; and that specification itself depends on classifying the intention of the agent. We can say, therefore, that there is no minimal act of commission or omission that counts as suicide, except relative to some tradition; and, within particular traditions, the justifiability of particular suicides may yet be debatable."[9]

So the very way one understands "suicide" already involves moral judgments and requires argument. So I shall contend that if we rightly understand what life is about, suicide should be understood negatively and should not therefore be recommended as an alternative for anyone. This is not to deny that from certain perspectives suicide can be considered rational—as an institution, that is a way of characterizing a whole range of behavior, as well as an individual act. That it can be so understood, however, reveals how little the issue turns on the question of "rationality." We must rather ask whether the tradition through which we understand the meaning and nature of suicide is true.

3. Why Suicide is Prohibited

I have argued elsewhere that suicide as an institution must be considered morally doubtful. That conclusion is based on the religious understanding that we should learn to regard our lives as gifts bestowed on us by a gracious Creator.[10] That such an appeal is explicitly religious is undeniable, but I would resist any suggestion that the religious nature of this appeal disqualifies it from public argument. Rather it is a reminder of Margolis' contention that any account of suicide necessarily draws on some tradition. Therefore my appeal to this kind of religious presupposition is but an explicit avowal of what any account of suicide must involve—though I certainly would not contend that the only basis for disapproving suicide is religious.

It is important, however, that the significance of the shift to the language of gift be properly appreciated. For it is a challenge to our normal presumptions about the way the prohibition of suicide is grounded in our "natural desire to live." Indeed it is not even clear to me that we have a "natural desire to live," or even if we do what its moral significance entails. The very phrase "natural desire to live" is fraught with ambiguity, but even worse it seems to suggest that when a person finds they no longer have such a desire there is no longer any reason for living.

In contrast the language of gift does not presuppose we have a "natural desire to live," but rather that our living is an obligation. It is an obligation that we at once owe our Creator and one another. For our creaturely status is but a reminder that our existence is not secured by our own power, but rather requires the constant care and trust in others. Our willingness to live in the face of suffering, pain, and sheer boredom of life is morally a service to one another as it is a sign that life can be endured as well as a source for joy and exuberance. Our obligation to sustain our lives even when they are threatened with or require living with a horrible disease is our way of being faithful to the trust that has sustained us in health and now in illness.[11] We take on a responsibility as sick people. That responsibility is simply to keep on living as it is our way of gesturing to those who care for us that we can be trusted and trust them even in our illness.

There is nothing about this position which entails that we must do everything we can do to keep ourselves alive under all conditions. Christians certainly do not believe that life is inherently sacred and therefore it must be sustained until the bitter end. Indeed the existence of the martyrs is a clear sign that Christians think the value of life can be overriden.[12] Indeed I think there is much to be said for distinguishing between preserving life and only prolonging death, but such a distinction does not turn on technical judgments about when we have in fact started dying, though it may involve such a judgment.[13] Rather the distinction is dependent on the inherited wisdom of a community that has some idea of what a "good death" entails.[14]

Such a death is one that allows us to remember the dead in a morally healthy way—that is, the manner of death does not prevent the living from remembering the manner and good of their life. To be sure we can train ourselves to remember a suicide as if the suicide said nothing about their life, but I think we would be unwise to do so. For to face the reality of a death by suicide is a reminder how often our community fails to offer the trust necessary to sustain our lives in health and illness. Suicide is not first a judgment about the agent, but a reminder that we have failed to embody as a community the commitment not to abandon one another. We fear being a burden for others, but even more to ourselves. Yet it is only by recognizing that in fact we are inescapably a burden that we face the reality and opportunity of living truthfully.

It is just such a commitment that medicine involves and why the physician's commitment to caring for the sick seems so distorted by an ethics of autonomy. Medicine is but a gesture, but an extremely significant gesture of a society, that while we all suffer from a condition that cannot be cured, nonetheless neither will we be abandoned. The task of medicine is to care even when it cannot cure.[15] The refusal to let an attempted suicide die is only our feeble, but real, attempt to remain a community of trust and care through the agency of medicine. Our prohibition and subsequent care of a suicide draws on our profoundest assumptions that each individual's life has a purpose beyond simply being "autonomous."

4. Reasons for Living and "Rational Suicide": an Example

However, the kind of religious appeals I have made as well as this kind of talk about "purpose" can easily be misleading. For it sounds as though suicide is religiously prohibited because people who believe in God really know what life is about. But that is not the case—at least in the usual sense a phrase such as "what life is about" is understood. Indeed the very reason that living is an obligation is that we are to go on living even though we are far from figuring out what life is about. Our reason for living is not that we are sure about the ultimate meaning of life, but rather that our lives have been touched by another and through that touch we believe we encounter the very being that graciously sustains our existence.

Indeed one of the problems with discussions of "rational suicide" is they seem to be determined by the assumption that the decision to live or to die turns on whether life, and more importantly, one's particular life, has meaning or purpose. Thus, Margolis, for example, suggests that a relatively neutral understanding of the issue raised by suicide is whether the deliberate taking of one's life in order simply to end it, not instrumentally for any ulterior purpose, can ever be rational or rationally justified. He suggests a rational suicide is when a person "aims overridingly at ending his own life and who, in a relevant sense, performs the act. The manner in which he suicides may be said to be by commission or omission, actively or passively, directly or indirectly, consciously or unconsciously, justifiably or reprehensibly—in accord with the classificatory distinctions of particular traditions."[16] According to Margolis such suicide is more likely to be justified if the person "decided that life was utterly meaningless" or "sincerely believed life to have no point at all."[17]

My difficulty with such a suggestion is that I have no idea what it would mean to know that life, and in particular my life, was "utterly meaningless" or had "no point at all." In order to illustrate my difficulty about these matters let me call your attention to one of the better books about suicide—John Barth's *The Floating Opera.*[18] Barth's book consists of Todd Andrews' account of how one day in 1937 he decided to commit suicide. There was no particular reason that Andrews decided to commit suicide and that, we discover, is exactly the reason he decided to do so—namely there is no reason for living or dying.

The protagonist has written the book to explain why he changed his mind and in the process we discover quite a bit about him. Most people would describe him as a cynic, but there is more to him than that. Andrews makes his living by practicing law in a small backwater town in the Chesapeake tidewater country. He became a lawyer because that is what his father wanted, but he is later stunned by his father's suicide. What bothered him was not that his father killed himself, but that he did so because he could not pay his debts due to the Depression.

Andrews has chosen to live free from any long term commitments since the day in WW I when he killed a German sergeant with whom he had shared a foxhole through a terrible night of shelling. His lack of commitment extends even to his arrangement for living—he lives in a hotel room where he registers on a day to day basis. He has, however, been involved in a long term affair with Jane Mack, his best friend's wife. Harrison Mack not only approved but actually arranged this as a further extension of their friendship. However by mutual agreement they have recently decided to end this form of their relation.[19] This is partly the result of the recent birth of Jeannie, who, even though her paternity remains unclear, has given the Macks a new sense of themselves as a couple.

Andrews also suffers from two diseases—subacute bacteriological endocarditis and chronic infection of the prostate. He was told thirty-five years ago that the former could kill him any time. The latter disease only caused him to cease living a wastrel's existence he had assumed during law school and begin what he claims is almost a saintly life. And indeed his life is in many ways exemplary, for he is a man who lives his life in accordance with those convictions he thinks most nearly true.

Even though he is not a professional philosopher, Andrews is a person with a definite philosophical bent. For years he has been working on notes, suitably filed in three peach baskets, for the writing of a Humean type *Inquiry* on the nature of causation. For if Hume was right that causes can only be inferred, then his task is to shorten as much as possible the leap between what we see and what we cannot see. That is, to get at the true reasons for our actions.[20]

This becomes particularly relevant if we are to understand Andrews' decision to commit suicide. He fully admits that there are abundant psychological reasons, for those inclined for such explanations, to explain his suicide—a motherless boyhood, his murder of the German sergeant, his father's hanging himself, his isolated adulthood, his ailing heart, his growing sexual impotency, injured vanity, frustrated ambition, boredom—the kinds of things psychoanalysts identify as "real" causes.[21] But for him the only reasons that interest him in dying are philosophical.

These he states in five propositions which constitute his completed *Inquiry.* They simply are:

I. Nothing has intrinsic value. Things assume value only in terms of certain ends.
II. The reasons for which people attribute value to things are always ultimately arbitrary. That is, the ends in terms of which things assume value are themselves ultimately irrational.
III. There is, therefore, no ultimate 'reason' for valuing anything.
IV. Living is action in some form. There is no reason for action in any form.
V. There is, then, no 'reason' for living.[22]

And so Todd Andrews decided to kill himself one day in 1937.

However before doing so he decides to go see *The Original and Unparalleled Floating Opera,* a local minstrel show on a rundown showboat. The absurdity of the show matches perfectly Andrews' view of the absurdity of life. During the performance, Andrews goes to the ship's galley, turns on the gas only to be interrupted and saved by a workman who angrily calls him a damn fool—not because he tried to take his life, but because he could have blown up the ship.

More importantly, however, just as he is recovering, the Macks, who had also been attending the opera, rush into the galley with Jeannie who had suddenly taken sick and fainted. Though appealed to for help, Andrews suggests he is no good at such things and advises the Macks to rush to the hospital. However, the local doctor arrives and advises an alcohol rub reassuring everyone nothing is seriously wrong. In the emergency, however, and the concern Andrews felt about Jeannie, he discovers he no longer wants to commit suicide even though he could still easily jump into the Choptank river. For as he tells us, "something was different. Some qualitative change had occurred, instantly, down in the dining room. The fact is I had no reason to be concerned over little Jeannie, and yet my concern for that child was so intense, and had been so immediately forthcoming, that (I understood now) the first desperate sound of Jane's voice had snapped me out of a paralysis which there was no reason to terminate. No reason at all. Moreover, had I not, in abjuring my responsibility for Jeannie, for the first time in my life assumed it—for her, for her parents, and for myself? I was confused, and I refused to die that way. Things needed explaining; abstractions needed to be straightened out. To die now was simply out of the question, though I hated to spoil such a perfect day."[23]

Andrews suspects most philosophizing to be rationalization, but nonetheless his experience requires him to return to the propositions of his *Inquiry* to make a small revision of the fifth: V. There is, then, no 'reason' for living (or for suicide).[24] For now he tells us that he realized that even if values are only relative there are still relative values. "To realize that nothing has absolute value is surely overwhelming, but if one goes no further from that proposition than to become a saint, a cynic, or a suicide on principle, one hasn't gone far enough. If nothing makes any final difference, that fact makes no final difference either, and there is no more reason to commit suicide, say than not to, in the last analysis. Hamlet's question is, absolutely, meaningless. A narrow escape."[25]

The Christian prohibition of suicide is clearly based in our assumption that our lives are not ours to do with as we please. But that prohibition is but a reminder of the kind of commitments that make suicide which appears from certain perspectives and at particular times in our lives so rational, so wrong. It reminds us how important our commitment to be the kind of people who can care about a sick little girl and in the process learn to care for ourselves. That kind of lesson may not give life meaning, but it is certainly sufficient to help us muddle through with enough joy to sustain the important business of living.

Notes

1. For example T. Beauchamp and J. Childress (*Principles of Biomedical Ethics* [New York: Oxford University Press, 1979], 90) suggest, "If the principle of autonomy is strongly relied upon for the justification of suicide, then it would seem that there is a right to commit suicide, so long as a person acts autonomously and does not seriously affect the interests of others."

2. "British 'Right to Die' Group Plans to Publish Manual on Suicide," *New York Times.*

3. T. Beauchamp and J. Childress, *Principles of Biomedical Ethics,* 93.

4. See F. Bergman, *On Being Free* (Notre Dame: University of Notre Dame Press, 1977); and G. Dworkin, "Moral Autonomy," in *Morals, Science, and Sociality,* ed. H. Engelhardt and D. Callahan (Hastings-on-Hudson, New York: Hastings Center Publications, 1978).

5. Augustine, *The City of God,* trans. Henry Bettenson (Harmondsworth: Penguin, 1977), 856-57.

6. Ibid., 857. Earlier Augustine had argued, "There were famous heroes who, though by the laws of war they could do violence to a conquered enemy, refuse to do violence to themselves when conquered; though they had not the slightest fear of death, they choose to endure the enemy's domination rather than put themselves to death. They were fighting for their earthly country; but the Gods they worshipped were false; but their worship was genuine and they faithfully kept

their oaths. Christians worship the true God and they yearn for a heavenly country; will they not have more reason to refrain from the crime of suicide, if God's providence subjects them for a time to their enemies for their probation or reformation. Their God does not abandon them in that humiliation, for he came from on high so humbly for their sake," pp. 35-36.

7. Beauchamp and Childress, *Principles of Biomedical Ethics,* 86.

8. Ibid., 87. Elsewhere Beauchamp provides a fuller account arguing suicide occurs when "a person intentionally brings about his or her own death in circumstances where others do not coerce him or her to the action, except in those cases where death is caused by conditions not specifically arranged by the agent for the purpose of bringing about his or her own death," T. Beauchamp, "Suicide," in *Matters of Life and Death,* ed. T. Regan (New York: Random House, 1980), 77.

9. J. Margolis, *Negativities: The Limits of Life* (Columbus: Merriall, 1975), 25-26.

10. S. Hauerwas, *Truthfulness and Tragedy* (Notre Dame: University of Notre Dame Press, 1977), 101-15.

11. See S. Hauerwas, "Reflections on Suffering, Death, and Medicine," *Ethics in Science and Medicine* 6 (1979): 229-37.

12. See S. Hauerwas, *Community of Character* (Notre Dame: University of Notre Dame Press, 1980).

13. S. Hauerwas, *Vision and Virtue* (Notre Dame: Fides Claretian, 1974), 166-86.

14. S. Hauerwas, "Religious Conceptions of Brain Death," in *Brain Death: Interrelated Medical and Social Issues,* ed. J. Korein (New York: New York Academy of Sciences, 1978), 329-36.

15. S. Hauerwas, "Care," in *Encyclopedia of Bioethics,* ed. W. Reich (New York: Free Press, 1978), 1: 145-50.

16. Margolis, *Negativities,* 29.

17. Ibid., 24.

18. J. Barth, *The Floating Opera* (New York: Avon, 1956). For a similar approach from which I have learned much see H. Nielsen, "Margolis on Rational Suicide: An Argument for Case Studies in Ethics," *Ethics* 89, no. 4 (1979): 394-400. The fact that we must resort to example when considering such matters is an important indication how easily abstract discussions of the rightness or wrongness of suicide, for which there is no substitute and must certainly be done, can as easily mislead as they can help us clarify why the suicide is rightly understood in a negative manner. Seldom are any of us sure why it is we act and do not act as we do. We may say we would rather die than live with such and such disease, but how can we be so sure that is the reason. Beauchamp and Childress' suggestion that ideally a person contemplating suicide would consider all the variables is as much a formula for self-deception as one for self-knowledge. I suspect that is why Barth's book is so helpful—namely it is only by telling a story that we come to understand how the prohibition against suicide is meant to shape the self.

19. Andrews admits that this turn of affairs made him reconsider briefly his decision to commit suicide since the Macks might interpret his suicide as caused by their decision. But he says that this lasted only a moment since it occurred to him "What difference did it make to me how they interpreted my death? Nothing, absolutely, makes any difference. Nothing is ultimately important. And, that, at least partly by my own choosing, that last act would be robbed of its real significance, would be interpreted in every way but the way I intended. This fact once realized, it seemed likely to me that here was a new significance, if possible even more genuine," Barth, *The Floating Opera,* 224.

20. The full title is actually *An Inquiry into the Circumstances Surrounding the Self-Destruction of Thomas F. Andrews, of Cambridge, Maryland, on Ground-Hog Day, 1930 (More Especially into the Causes Therefor).* For Andrews tells us his aim is simply to learn why his father hanged himself. Andrews admits the real problem was one of "imperfect communication" between him and his father as he could find no adequate reason for his father's act. His *Inquiry,* however, became primarily a study of himself since he realized to understand imperfect communicatives requires perfect knowledge of each party. Andrews suggests at the end of the book if we have not understood his change of mind he is again cursed with imperfect communication—but the suggestion seems to be we have a better chance at communication than he had with his father as now at least we have Todd Andrews' story.

21. Barth, *The Floating Opera,* 224.

22. Ibid., 238-43.

23. Ibid., 266.

24. Ibid., 270.

25. Ibid.

74. Integrity, Humility, and Heroism: May Patients Refuse Medical Treatment?

ALLEN VERHEY

Despite a perhaps flippant-sounding title, the film *Whose Life Is It, Anyway?* (starring Richard Dreyfuss, John Cassavettes, and Ken McMillan; screenplay by Brian Clark and Reginald Rose) raises a serious moral issue and deserves a Christian response. What follows is not a cinematic assessment of *Whose Life Is It, Anyway?,* but an effort to look at the question of a patient's right to refuse medical treatment, using the story of this film to uncover the important ethical questions involved.

To videotape a symposium in which first-rate philosophers and theologians debated whether—and if so under what circumstances—patients have the right to refuse medical treatment would, I suppose, make for an extraordinarily dull film. *Whose Life Is It, Anyway?* gets at this same moral question by way of drama, by developing narrative and character, not by way of rational analysis and applying abstract principles. That may be due to the constraints of the art, but it is also morally illuminating, because ordinary people who confront such choices typically discern their way through them less on the basis of abstract principles than their own narratives and character. Their own history and the communities in which they now live are more decisive than are "rational" and "impartial" principles to be applied deductively.

Viewing a movie like *Whose Life Is It, Anyway?* of course becomes part of our personal "history." It shapes character as well as depicting it; and it can form a readiness to live and die in certain ways. That is why it is of some moral importance to think about whether it is morally appropriate to applaud the characters in this drama as well as the actors who play them.

To the movie's dramatic and moral credit there is more than one character vividly developed. The story centers on Ken Harrison (Dreyfuss), a young sculptor who is left a quadriplegic by an automobile accident. Harrison asserts his right to refuse the continuing dialysis treatments on which his life depends. Dr. Michael Emerson (Cassavettes) is the masterful physician who first saves Harrison's life and then fights to keep him living it. Judge Wyler (McMillan) is the conscientious jurist who has to decide whether or not Harrison's refusal of treatment must be honored.

To these three characters, the two protagonists and the one called in to adjudicate their conflict, to their stories and virtues, this review will mainly attend. But it is important also to acknowledge an assortment of other impressive characters: Harrison's lover Pat, cast off by Harrison, ostensibly for the good of them both; Dr. Claire Scott, a woman physician torn between that role and her respect and affection for Harrison; a couple of nurses, both of whom care *about* Harrison as well as *for* him (one of them wishes him "good luck" as he leaves to appear before the judge; the other refuses to); a carefree orderly who wheels Harrison around the hospital and, on one occasion, stealthily out of it for a clandestine audience of his musical group; a well-meaning but offensive social worker; a stuttering lawyer; a couple of psychiatrists; and a little girl whom Harrison meets on dialysis and helps and encourages.

This cast of characters is important for reasons besides the fact that there are a number of good performances. The story remains, of course, Harrison's story, Harrison's life and dying, but his acting it out (I do not mean Dreyfuss' performance), his authoring it (I do not mean Clark's and Rose's screenplay), is constrained by other actors (I do not mean the cast but the persons they play), other agents with narratives and identities of their own. Once again the dramatic approach is morally illuminating. Moral decisions are intelligible and meaningful, not simply as discrete decisions made by a solitary individual and governed by abstract rational principles, but also as part of a person's narrative, as expressive of a person's character, in a setting of other persons with their own stories and characters.

Moralists need to be reminded of that, for a good deal of moral analysis is done in abstraction from the historical and communal contexts of a decision and simply applies the principle of utility or the categorical imperative or Rawls' theory of justice. Just because a decision is intelligible, of course, it does not necessarily follow that it is justifiable: there can be morally better or worse stories and characters.

Indeed, that is the possibility I want to examine in this essay. Before we applaud Harrison's decision or the doctor's resistance to it or the judge's adjudication of their conflict, we must ask whether the characters and stories which make those actions intelligible are in fact morally praiseworthy. The virtue of *Whose Life Is It, Anyway?*—morally and cinematically—is

From *The Reformed Journal* 32 (March 1982): 18-21. Used by permission.

that it enables and indeed constrains the viewer to make that sort of examination.

Dr. Emerson's character has been shaped by the tradition and community to which he belongs. "Doctor" describes who he is as well as what he does; it is his identity as well as his title. He understands himself as enlisted on the side of life, fighting a messy and losing—but heroic—battle against death. Unable to accept defeat easily, he will not tolerate any indifference to death among his medical students. Nor can he understand or accept his patient's decision to refuse the therapy that would enable him to live. Emerson's passion and that to which he devotes himself are understandable in terms of his own narrative and character, and they are commendable. Life is a good; and if it is not the only good, it is the good which is prerequisite for valuing other goods. God intends life for people; his creative and redemptive will chooses life; the signs of it are a commandment and a rainbow and an empty tomb. A character formed to protect and sustain life is a commendable character.

But Dr. Emerson's character is also flawed. The military images in the previous paragraph describe his commendable commitment to human life but also hint at his flaw. He is a crusader; his passion for a righteous end blinds him to the injustice of certain means. He lacks the virtue of justice. Not that he is uncaring; he is prepared to care for Harrison even when he cannot (or may not) cure him. It is not that he is a liar; he tells Harrison the truth about his prospects. But he lacks justice; he is prepared to override Harrison's will, to dominate him when he will not cooperate, to take advantage of his powerlessness in order to achieve the good of life. A critical scene is played out early in the film when Harrison refuses a valium prescribed to calm him after he first begins to question the wisdom of continuing life. Dr. Emerson takes advantage of Harrison's quadriplegia to inject the valium against his will. This is a violent, unjust act, well-motivated, well-intentioned, and intelligible in terms of the doctor's narrative and character, but unjust all the same.

Ironically, this powerful act against the powerless quadriplegic seems to determine Harrison's course. The injection and his inability to resist it so repel him that he begins to investigate and then to assert his legal power to stop the doctor and to render him powerless to "save" him. The doctor's response, in turn, is to crusade to have his patient declared "incompetent," to render him finally powerless and without options, so that the doctor can achieve his good cause.

Dr. Emerson's narrative and character could have been better. If we may applaud his passion for preserving life and his commitment to sustaining it, we must also despise his lack of justice. And it is tragic that his relationship with Harrison is reduced to a confrontation of power, in which one has to end up powerless and the other powerful.

Into that confrontation Judge Wyler must step. The film provides little characterization of the judge as a person. He is conscientious, to be sure, and compassionate, but his person is overshadowed by his role. And the virtue of his role is justice—at least an impartial fairness which is disposed to protect the equal freedom of each one and ready to protect anyone against being unwillingly used in the pursuit of another's "good."

The judge sees and praises the moral good the doctor seeks, but he also sees the injustice of imposing it on Harrison against his will. It is Harrison's life—to answer the question posed by the title—and the decision to refuse treatment is his to make on the basis of his own values, even if they are wrong, even if the decision leads to his death. (The judge's ruling, incidentally, is faithful to recent court decisions—some of which are cited in the film—acknowledging the right of competent patients to refuse treatment and discrediting the Catch-22 which would treat as incompetent anyone who refused treatment.)

Whether the character of justice and of the judge's role could be better is, of course, an ancient and enduring question. "Justice" can be made to serve "the good" or "the cause"; or it can be made blind to any cause and passion except impartiality. The strength—the virtue, if you will—of "blind" justice, of justice as impartiality and fairness, is the protection it provides against arbitrary dominance, even well-intentioned arbitrary dominance. Its weakness is its minimalism. "Blind" justice tells us not so much what goods to seek as what restraints to exercise in seeking them. It tends to reduce covenantal relationships to contracts between independent individuals. Its minimalism can be seen in its emphasis on procedural questions, especially on the question of who decides, rather than on substantive questions, especially the question of what should be decided.

If the minimalism of "blind" justice is acknowledged, it sometimes makes it possible for people with different loyalties to cooperate, enabling adjudication of conflicting interests without arbitrary dominance. That is no small service. But if its minimalism is not recognized, it can distort the moral life, reducing it to a matter of what the law allows, so that legal permission is mistaken for moral license (witness the incidence of abortion).

Neither Judge Wyler nor the movie, however, makes too much of justice; neither reduces morality to legality.

Justice is not the whole of morality here. The judge reveals his personal conflict, for he is at least sympathetic with the doctor concerning what should be done. But in his character, in his role, the decision rests on the more restricted procedural question. On that question he decides that it is neither the doctor nor the judge but Harrison who should decide what should be done or left undone. The viewer, therefore, is confronted with the question of the proper character of justice and protected from mistaking legal permission for moral license. The viewer is not relieved from having to make a judgment on Harrison's decision by the fact that the judge has rendered his; and that is to the film's credit.

It is also to the film's credit, as we have said, that it sets Harrison's own judgment in the context of his narrative and character. He is a sculptor or, rather, he was, for the accident and his quadriplegia have made it impossible for him to be that any longer. There is the tragedy: "sculptor" is not simply what he *did* but what he *was,* and no longer that, he is alienated from himself. The story he was authoring has already, therefore, in some sense at least, come to an end. And *he* cannot begin again, for *he* is a sculptor. His imagination is bound to his hands. With his hands he imaged and shaped new form. With his hands he could begin again. But his hands no longer respond to either his brain or his world.

Harrison's refusal of treatment is not simply based on his "autonomy," on an arbitrary freedom to will what he will. Rather, it is based on his integrity, his faithfulness to his own identity, his consistent exercise of freedom to create one unified life within which his choices are quite predictable (but no less free). The arbitrary freedom of autonomy, I judge, provides an insufficient basis for demanding assent to a patient's refusal of treatment, if only because the very arbitrariness of autonomy makes it possible that the decision would be different tomorrow. But integrity, a person's faithfulness to his established self, does provide an adequate basis for demanding assent to refusals of treatment. And so, I judge, one must assent to Harrison's decision.

That is not to say that his decision or the story and character which make it intelligible are praiseworthy. We can understand Harrison's decision to refuse treatment in terms of his integrity with his own narrative and character, and we must acquiesce to it, but we need not applaud it.

Harrison's character is unveiled and his story takes a decisive turn in the moving scene in which he cuts off his relationship with his lover Pat. He wants, he says, not to burden her, not to bind her; he wants her to be free for a normal life and a normal love. There is no reason to doubt the sincerity of his concern about her future. Moreover, Harrison says, he himself wants to be free from the memory of their relationship, from the torment each time he looks at her of remembering what had been and knowing what could never be again. Again, we have no reason to doubt his anguish at his impotence. But he makes the decision for her; he writes her narrative. Her protestations fall on deaf ears. The fact that her narrative is bound inalienably to his and that her character involves faithfulness to him is no longer allowed to shape their story. His very powerlessness is used powerfully to dominate her. He casts her out; she has no recourse but to treat him as dead already, as a memory, and to begin again a separate narrative.

At the procedural level, this decision of Harrison's was not his alone to make—any more than the decision for him to continue therapy was the doctor's alone. As Dr. Emerson's concern for Harrison's good led Emerson to violate justice, so Harrison's concern for Pat's well-being led Harrison to violate justice. At the substantive level, Harrison's decision was, I judge, a tragic one, neither good nor evil. It was a situation in which goods conflict and to choose one good is to reject others, a decision in which virtues conflict and where to follow one is to disown others. Harrison's decision is a choice for charity, but it is also a decision which will not own humility or heroism as part of his own character and narrative. Refusing gratuitous support, nurturance, and affection, Harrison cuts off past relations which, although changed, might nevertheless provide some continuity, some integrity, for an heroic attempt to begin again, to continue his story.

Harrison's decision to refuse treatment can be understood in terms of the same tragic choice about who he would be, about his character and narrative. His decision to die is neither humble nor heroic. It is not that he is a braggart or a coward. But he is not disposed to rely on the care and gifts of another or to submit to their gratuitous kindness. He is not disposed—in the face of the fragility of life and the vulnerability of persons—to take the risk of living the kind of life that is given to one to live.

What may finally be necessary to nurture and sustain the virtues of humility and courage in situations like this is a religious sense of our dependence on God. Humility, after all, really submits to God and his gracious reign. It would answer the question of this film's title in the words of the Heidelberg Catechism: ". . . I am not my own, but belong—body and soul, in life and in death, to my faithful Savior. . . ." Humility, let it be noted, is not Stoic resignation. It is not fatalism. It does not deny the brokenness of our world or of Harrison's body. It does not glibly identify automobile accidents with God's intention. It does not call for an end to passion; it calls rather for us to share the passion of Christ. It disposes persons to bear the brokenness, sadness, and tragedy of our world in hope and faith and love.

When humility is joined with gratitude it leads to small acts of kindness which do not repay the generosity of those on whom we rely but embody it and extend it to still others. Such kindnesses were not beyond Harrison; and the episode in which he befriends the little girl on dialysis is demonstration enough that this way is open to him. But he lacks the humility (not the charity) to undertake the way which would provide opportunities also for his own charity.

Humility is also joined with heroism. The catechism describes its answer to the question "whose life is it, anyway?" as our only comfort, our *cum-fortis,* that which strengthens and enables us so that we are "wholeheartedly willing and ready . . . to live for him." Our comfort is our courage; our humility is our heroism. It disposes us not only to receive with gratitude the gracious gifts of others but to risk new beginnings, new stories, new lives, which are less ours than God's. It disposes us to bear and share the burden and sadness of our world and of our lives for the sake of God's cause and someone's good.

To the extent that Harrison's decision had integrity with his narrative and character, one must acquiesce in his refusal of treatment. But his decision lacked humility and heroism, and so I think one need not applaud it or hold it up as a model. It was a tragic choice, and so one may not blame it. But the story to tell if we want to think Christianly about such decisions is finally not Harrison's but Christ's, the story of one who endured tragedy for the sake of God's cause and turned the greatest evil to good by bearing it with humility and heroism in faith and hope and love.

I am not sure that I would have the resources of character to make any decision other than the one Harrison made. The film's dramatic approach suggests, moreover, that the fundamental question is not simply what sort of discrete decision one would make about treatment but what kind of story one writes for oneself, what kind of character one forms. For a Christian viewing the film, then, the question is not just whether one could make a decision about treatment with humility and heroism but whether one's whole narrative and character have integrity with one's confession.

75.

"Whose Life Is It, Anyway?" Ours, That's Whose!

GLORIA MAXSON

In this national year of the disabled, I take strong exception to the film *Whose Life Is It, Anyway?* for its underlying false premise: that the life of a disabled person could not be worth living, and should thus be "mercifully" terminated by suicide or euthanasia. As a chairbound victim of polio and arthritis, I strongly protest that the life I and my many disabled friends lead has genuine value in the sight of God—and humanity.

In the film, Richard Dreyfuss plays Ken, a young sculptor who has become a "quad" (quadriplegic—a person who is paralyzed in all four extremities) in a car accident, and decides in the initial period of trauma—never an auspicious time to make major decisions—that suicide is the only "rational" choice for a man severely disabled. In its one-sided argument in favor of Ken's death, the film denies the value of the lives we disabled persons live.

Whose Life Is It, Anyway? stacks the deck in favor of its position by failing to present the options available to a quadriplegic. It is shockingly untypical that Ken is kept for six months in intensive care before any rehabilitation is begun; actually, most quads have *completed* their rehabilitative training by that time. Glib doctors and social workers tell Ken he will "feel better" when his therapy starts—but it never does; nor is Ken ever taught to use such adaptive devices as reading machines and special typewriters. He is never introduced even to an electric wheelchair but is wheeled passively about, which deepens the sense of immobility and total dependency that makes him long for death.

What a difference an electric chair (covered by Medicare) has made in my own life! Gone is that awful sense of being preyed upon, the "sitting duck" syndrome that kept me weeping on the porch in driving rain, terrified to enter the house where I imagined that Something huge, mindless, nameless and malign awaited me. Now my husband says *I* am the Something mindless and malign as I careen at full tilt down our block, terrorizing the "fluffy old pussies"

(Agatha Christie's phrase for little old ladies). I could have told the Ken character that if we can't have wings-at-our-heels, we can at least have wheels-at-our-hips. But no one tells him that or anything else that could alter his death wish.

Another inadequately treated aspect of Ken's trauma is his bitter sense of lost virility and conviction that he is "not a man anymore." Again, those around him fail to give him the insights provided by any good SCI (spinal cord injury) specialist, namely, that 70 per cent of quads can have normal genital intercourse, and that there are many other satisfying ways of making love, as the disabled veteran in *Coming Home*—a much more honest film—showed. No one examines Ken's sexuality to determine what sensory avenues are still open to him. Through those parts that confirm the popular assumptions about quadriplegics' sexuality, the man I saw the film with—himself a quad—kept muttering such things as: "There's more sex between the ears than between the extremities! As much warmth *north* of the Masters-Johnson line [the waistline] as *south* of it!"

We were both unnerved by Ken's insistence that death is "the only way out" since he is "dead already." The poet Robert Frost, and any of us "black-eyed ones" (Thomas Mann's phrase; the healthy-and-wealthy are "the blue-eyed ones"), could have told Ken that "the only way out is through," and to "learn what to make of a diminished thing." In the real world, any good doctor would have introduced Ken to SCI patients whose successful coping would have helped him navigate his dark passage back to life. But in the film no one helps him through the initial stages of grief and despair to self-acceptance. It is never explained to Ken that even a quadriplegic on dialysis, like himself, need not be hospitalized for life; with modern techniques and attendants, a person can live at home with the family and friends who can help him or her learn a new way of life based on "viable alternatives." All these tragic omissions strengthen Ken's case for taking his life—a case carefully manipulated by the film.

Although sculpting was Ken's life, he is not shown the many other ways his thwarted creativity could be expressed; only teaching is suggested, and he angrily rejects it. I, too, felt the awful anguish of losing my artistry with piano and guitar when my hands became crippled with arthritis. I could not have foreseen then, in the midst of my moist jeremiads, that one day I'd have an electric keyboard on which I could play melody with the two remaining, dancing fingers on my right hand, and automatic chords and rhythms with a dancing thumb on the left. Now, as I dash off "Für Elise," "Minuet in G" and "Turkish March," Beethoven no longer turns over in his grave, but sits bolt upright and bellows, "Ach Du Lieber, Meine Gloria—das ist gut!" I could not see in that dark night of the soul, when all problems became "soul-sized," that I would be able to transfer my guitar skills to a large ukulele, and bawl out the same old ballads and naughty calypsos I did before. Furthermore, when I could no longer type at 90 wpm, or even handwrite, I didn't know I'd soon type with two fingers and find an orthopedic gripper that would enable me to write again, in so neat a hand my husband says it is "one of the graphic arts," and calls me "the Picasso of the ballpoint pen!"

As my friend and I viewed the film, we grew nervous on hearing the audience murmur assent to all the nihilisms about the disabled life, and remembered all the times people had said to us, "If I were you, I'd kill myself." It's just a small step from that to, "And why *don't* you?" In the audience, we sensed a latent antagonism to our vulgar tenacity in preserving our lives, our precious "space" on this crowded planet—a space which may be hotly contested in the future, with elderly and ill-derly classed as expendables. Many films and plays still perpetuate the false notion that a disabled life is not worth living—a misperception that is still killing people, through suicide and misguided "mercy killings."

The film *Whose Life?* traffics in the current political mood that is dangerously cutting back vital aid to the severely disabled. At one point in the film, a character grumbles that "we are spending thousands on people like Ken, with little return, when with a few cents we could save Third World children!" How dare people force us to choose between our lives and those of Third World children! True, much money *is* wasted keeping Ken alive and hospitalized; for much less he could have been cared for at home, safely and with better results.

This film reflects the negative views about disability that are gaining wide acceptance in the many "wrongful life" suits against doctors for allowing babies born with defects to live. More hospitals now routinely offer parents of disabled babies the option of "mercy killing," even if the baby's defect is only deafness. A TV film told the story of a man who shot his quadriplegic brother on request, again reinforcing the misconception that a disabled life is worthless. *Whose Life?* purports to be an honest drama about an important social and ethical dilemma of our time, but in its shrinking from the moral obligation of treating the issue factually, the film is irresponsible. It was puzzling to hear such film critics as Gene Shalit of the "Today" show praise it as "life-affirming"—an enigmatic phrase, indeed, to use about a film that advocates suicide. To us of the black-eyed community, Mr.

Shalit, "life-affirming" means body-retraining and body-retaining. Anything less is mere wordplay and sophistry.

As the film ended, my friend and I joined the crowd in the lobby to munch popcorn and chat, and received so many glances—some openly hostile—that we felt we might have to stand (sit) our ground or we'd be rushed and strung up between features! No matter what the public feels, *I* will never willingly relinquish a life that contains my husband, family, friends, a home, lobster thermidor, music and P. G. Wodehouse! Even in my handicapped childhood, I would have chosen to live. I read somewhere that all of nature's young things are valiant—they do not whine or bargain, but despite their wounds fight fiercely to live, and revel in being—and I know it is true. Perhaps I've "just compensated," as an atheistic college friend used to tell me. My reply is, "Yes, I have compensated—Christ is my compensation." For just as in my blinded early childhood I developed the "facial perception" that set every hair vibrating when someone was near, so now my nerve ends vibrate with the sense of that Presence who stands near but outside my harsh circumstances, and molds them into coherence and beauty.

Whose life is it, Ken? It's all of ours—and it should have been yours.

Chapter Fifteen
CARE OF NEONATES

Introduction

The Long Dying of Baby Andrew is an account by Robert and Peggy Stinson of the birth and dying of their infant son in 1977.[1] Baby Andrew was born at 24 weeks gestation, weighing 1 lb. 12 oz. He was taken to a neonatal intensive care unit, and all of the sophisticated resources of modern neonatal technology were used to keep him alive in spite of a multitude of medical problems, an uncertain prognosis for mental development, and the Stinsons' wishes that "heroic" measures not be taken.

The Stinsons recounted this response to the neonatal unit's power to intervene in their child's dying:

> What threatened to be a simple, private horror has changed unexpectedly into something so altogether different, so altogether complicated that thoughts and feelings tangle hopelessly and give no guidance.
>
> Andrew is not our baby anymore—he's been taken over by a medical bureaucracy. The bureaucracy controls Andrew—access to Andrew, information about Andrew, decisions about what will happen to Andrew. It rolls inexorably onward, oblivious to our attempts to communicate, participate. . . .

When Andrew finally died, Mrs. Stinson wrote in her journal, "Modern medicine makes possible a sad new epitaph: He died too late for grief."

The sophisticated medical technology of neonatal care sometimes enables a child not only to live but to flourish, but sometimes to live with no hope of human flourishing, sometimes to live with no hope of even human communication, sometimes only to suffer its way in a long dying toward death. The care of the newborn presents special medical and moral difficulties because diagnosis and prognosis are often obscure and uncertain and because neonates are mute about their preferences. Someone must make decisions about their care, but who and on what basis? These two questions—who should make decisions of this kind and what criteria should be used in making them—demand answers if we are to use our new powers in morally responsible ways. Theological reflection concerning them is also required if we are to use these powers with Christian integrity and speak of them with Christian conviction.

Theologians have long reflected on these issues, sometimes on the basis of an impartial perspective, sometimes on the basis of a candidly theological perspective. Once again, the question of the appropriate mode of moral reflection and the relation of Christian moral reflection to an impartial perspective are relevant. And again the application of even impartial principles will depend upon dispositions and biases shaped by one's fundamental convictions and loyalties.

It is recognized, for example, that an infant is not and has not ever been a rational autonomous individual, able to give free and informed consent. This is what necessitates a decision by someone else about care. But should the procedural decision about who should decide be based on "substituted judgment"—what the infant would be likely to decide if it were rational and autonomous—or the interdependency of members of communities, including and especially families? Again, one's disposition toward medical technology subtly effects discernment in such cases. Is medical technology simply a value-free assortment of tools accessible to consumers who can decide either to use them to get what they want or, failing that, not to use them at all? Or is medical technology to be considered a part of medical practice and profession with its own ethos and commitment to benefit the patient, even a tiny patient? Is technology, including medical technology, not just the power of people over natural processes but necessarily also the power of some people, the medical community, for example, over other people, say, an infant's parents? Our answer to this will influence how we answer the first overriding question given above: Who is to make the decisions about the care and treatment of neonates? If we see neonatal technology as tied to a concern to benefit the patient, we may work to nurture a role for the physician in the decision-making process; whereas if we see the technology as inevitably resulting in a power imbalance, we may work to restrain the role of the physician.

With respect to our second overarching question, what criteria are to be used in deciding on care and treatment of neonates, theological reflection may supply, support, qualify, or reject criteria advanced to guide the decision, whoever is to make it. The value of physical life, for example, can be given theological backing. But is life the only value—in the whole constellation of values involved in such decisions—which can be given theological backing? How, for example, should Christians think about suffering? May we *choose* suffering for another? How shall we weigh unavoidable suffering, if we do keep an infant alive, against unavoidable death, if we refrain from technological intervention? Can theological reflection help order the goods which cannot all be chosen? Can it help order the evils which cannot all be avoided? Can theological reflection help us to be truthful about the genuine conflict of genuine goods? Can it help us acknowledge tragic choices in the care of neonates?

Besides illuminating the questions of who should decide about the care of neonates and what criteria for deciding we ought to use in such cases, theological reflection may point us toward a third question, that of character: no matter who decides, what sort of person should they be? If parents make decisions about and for their infants, their decision will be made not only in terms of a rational application of a more or less abstract principle, but also in terms of their identity and integrity as parents. Then the question of a normative understanding of being a parent is reopened.

If physicians decide, they will rely not only on technical skill in making diagnoses and prognoses but also on their understanding of the moral significance of their role. They will decide in ways that cohere with their self-understanding, that have integrity with their professional identity, and that are faithful to their moral passions. So the question of a normative understanding of being a physician is reopened. What is the relation of character and conduct, of integrity and principles; and how should theological reflection or religious conviction qualify either?

Religious faith may at least remind us that we are talking not just about "defective neonates" but about our own children. It may remind us of ways other than technology to respond to their life and their death, to the threats to their flourishing, and to their sometimes long dying. A religious response to children and the loss of children may provide an important context in which to think about the appropriate technological, professional, parental, and social responses to the demands of neonatal care.

Notes

1. Peggy Stinson and Robert Stinson, *The Long Dying of Baby Andrew* (Boston: Little, Brown, 1983).

Suggestions for Further Reading

Hauerwas, Stanley. "The Demands and Limits of Care: On the Moral Dilemma of Neonatal Intensive Care." In *Truthfulness and Tragedy,* by Stanley Hauerwas and Richard Bondi. Notre Dame, Ind.: University of Notre Dame Press, 1977.

McCarthy, Donald B. "Care of Severely Defective Newborn Babies." In *Moral Responsibility in Prolonging Life Decisions,* edited by Donald G. McCarthy and Albert S. Moraszewski. St. Louis: Pope John Center, 1981.

McCormick, Richard A. "To Save or Let Die: The Dilemma of Modern Medicine." *Journal of the American Medical Association* 229 (1974): 172-76.

McCormick, Richard A. and John J. Paris. "Saving Defective Infants: Options for Life or Death." *America* 146 (1983): 313-17.

Meilaender, Gilbert. "If This Baby Could Choose. . . ." *Linacre Quarterly,* November 1982, 313-21.

Smith, David H. "On Letting Some Babies Die." *Hastings Center Studies* 2 (May, 1974): 37-46.

Veatch, Robert M. *Death, Dying and the Biological Revolution: Our Last Quest for Responsibility.* New Haven: Yale University Press, 1976.

Weber, Leonard J. *Who Shall Live?* New York: Paulist Press, 1976.

76. Mongolism, Parental Desires, and the Right to Life

JAMES M. GUSTAFSON

The Problem

The Family Setting

Mother, 34 years old, hospital nurse.
Father, 35 years old, lawyer.
Two normal children in the family.

In late fall of 1963, Mr. and Mrs. _____ gave birth to a premature baby boy. Soon after birth, the child was diagnosed as a "mongoloid" (Down's syndrome) with the added complication of an intestinal blockage (duodenal atresia). The latter could be corrected with an operation of quite nominal risk. Without the operation, the child could not be fed and would die.

At the time of birth Mrs. _____ overheard the doctor express his belief that the child was a mongol. She immediately indicated she did not want the child. The next day, in consultation with a physician, she maintained this position, refusing to give permission for the corrective operation on the intestinal block. Her husband supported her in this position, saying that his wife knew more about these things (i.e., mongoloid children) than he. The reason the mother gave for her position—"It would be unfair to the other children of the household to raise them with a mongoloid."

The physician explained to the parents that the degree of mental retardation cannot be predicted at birth—running from very low mentality to borderline subnormal. As he said: "Mongolism, it should be stressed, is one of the milder forms of mental retardation. That is, mongols' IQs are generally in the 50-80 range, and sometimes a little higher. That is, they're almost always trainable. They can hold simple jobs. And they're famous for being happy children. They're perennially happy and usually a great joy." Without other complications, they can anticipate a long life.

Given the parents' decision, the hospital staff did not seek a court order to override the decision (see "Legal Setting" below). The child was put in a side room and, over an 11-day period, allowed to starve to death.

From *Perspectives in Biology and Medicine* 16 (Summer 1973): 529-57.

Following this episode, the parents undertook genetic counseling (chromosome studies) with regard to future possible pregnancies.

The Legal Setting

Since the possibility of a court order reversing the parents' decision naturally arose, the physician's opinion in this matter—and his decision not to seek such an order—is central. As he said: "In the situation in which the child has a known, serious mental abnormality, and would be a burden both to the parents financially and emotionally and perhaps to society, I think it's unlikely that the court would sustain an order to operate on the child against the parents' wishes." He went on to say: "I think one of the great difficulties, and I hope [this] will be part of the discussion relative to this child, is what happens in a family where a court order is used as the means of correcting a congenital abnormality. Does that child ever really become an accepted member of the family? And what are all of the feelings, particularly guilt and coercion feelings that the parents must have following that type of extraordinary force that's brought to bear upon them for making them accept a child that they did not wish to have?"

Both doctors and nursing staff were firmly convinced that it was "clearly illegal" to hasten the child's death by the use of medication.

One of the doctors raised the further issue of consent, saying: "Who has the right to decide for a child anyway? . . . The whole way we handle life and death is the reflection of the long-standing belief in this country that children don't have any rights, that they're not citizens, that their parents can decide to kill them or to let them live, as they choose."

The Hospital Setting

When posed the question of whether the case would have been taken to court had the child had a normal IQ, with the parents refusing permission for the intestinal operation, the near unanimous opinion of the doctors: "Yes, we would have tried to override their decision." Asked why, the doctors replied: "When a retarded child presents us with the same problem, a different value system comes in; and not only does the staff acquiesce in the parents' decision to let the child die, but it's probable that the courts would also. That is, there is a different standard. . . . There is this tendency to value life on the basis of intelligence. . . . [It's] a part of the American ethic."

The treatment of the child during the period of its dying was also interesting. One doctor commented on "putting the child in a side room." When asked about medication to hasten the death, he replied: "No one would ever do that. No one would ever think about it, because they feel uncomfortable about it. . . . A lot of the way we handle these things has to do with our own anxieties about death and our own desires to be separated from the decisions that we're making."

The nursing staff who had to tend to the child showed some resentment at this. One nurse said she had great difficulty just in entering the room and watching the child degenerate—she could "hardly bear to touch him." Another nurse, however, said: "I didn't mind coming to work. Because like I would rock him. And I think that kind of helped me some—to be able to sit there and hold him. And he was just a tiny little thing. He was really a very small baby. And he was cute. He had a cute little face to him, and it was easy to love him, you know?" And when the baby died, how did she feel?—"I was glad that it was over. It was an end for him."

The Resolution

This complex of human experiences and decisions evokes profound human sensibilities and serious intellectual examination. One sees in and beyond it dimensions that could be explored by practitioners of various academic disciplines. Many of the standard questions about the ethics of medical care are pertinent, as are questions that have been long discussed by philosophers and theologians. One would have to write a full-length book to plow up, cultivate, and bring to fruition the implications of this experience.

I am convinced that, when we respond to a moral dilemma, the way in which we formulate the dilemma, the picture we draw of its salient features, is largely determinative of the choices we have. If the war in Vietnam is pictured as a struggle between the totalitarian forces of evil seeking to suppress all human values on the one side, and the forces of righteousness on the other, we have one sort of problem with limited choice. If, however, it is viewed as a struggle of oppressed people to throw off the shackles of colonialism and imperialism, we have another sort of problem. If it is pictured as more complex, the range of choices is wider, and the factors to be considered are more numerous. If the population problem is depicted as a race against imminent self-destruction of the human race, an ethics of survival seems to be legitimate and to deserve priority. If, however, the population problem is depicted more complexly, other values also determine policy, and our range of choices is broader.

One of the points under discussion in this medical case is how we should view it. What elements are in the accounts that the participants give to it? What elements were left out? What "values" did they seem to consider, and which did they seem to ignore? Perhaps if one made a different montage of the raw experience, one would have different choices and outcomes.

Whose picture is correct? It would not be difficult for one moral philosopher or theologian to present arguments that might undercut, if not demolish, the defenses made by the participants. Another moralist might make a strong defense of the decisions by assigning different degrees of importance to certain aspects of the case. The first might focus on the violation of individual rights, in this case the rights of the infant. The other might claim that the way of least possible suffering for the fewest persons over the longest range of time was the commendable outcome of the account as we have it. Both would be accounts drawn by external observers, not by active, participating agents. There is a tradition that says that ethical reflection by an ideal external observer can bring morally right answers. I have an observer's perspective, though not that of an "ideal observer." But I believe that it is both charitable and intellectually important to try to view the events as the major participants viewed them. The events remain closer to the confusions of the raw experience that way; the passions, feelings, and emotions have some echo of vitality remaining. The parents were not without feeling, the nurses not without anguish. The experiences could become a case in which x represents the rights of the infant to life, y represents the consequences of continued life as a mongoloid person, and z represents the consequences of his continued life for the family and the state. But such abstraction has a way of oversimplifying experience. One would "weigh" x against y and z. I cannot reproduce the drama even of the materials I have read, the interviews with doctors and nurses, and certainly even those are several long steps from the thoughts and feelings of the parents and the staff at that time. I shall, however, attempt to state the salient features of the dilemma for its participants; features that are each value laden and in part determinative of their decisions. In the process of doing that for the participants, I will indicate what reasons might justify their decisions. Following that I will draw a different picture of the experience, highlighting different values and principles, and show how this would lead to a different decision. Finally, I shall give the reasons why I, an observer, believe they, the participants, did the wrong thing. Their responsible and involved participation, one must remember, is very different from my detached reflection on documents and interviews almost a decade later.

The Mother's Decision

Our information about the mother's decision is secondhand. We cannot be certain that we have an accurate account of her reasons for not authorizing the surgery that could have saved the mongoloid infant's life. It is not my role to speculate whether her given reasons are her "real motives"; that would involve an assessment of her "unconscious." When she heard the child was probably a mongol, she "expressed some negative feeling" about it, and "did not want a retarded child." Because she was a nurse she understood what mongolism indicated. One reason beyond her feelings and wants is given: to raise a mongoloid child in the family would not be "fair" to the other children. That her decision was anguished we know from several sources.

For ethical reflection, three terms I have quoted are important: "negative feeling," "wants" or "desires," and "fair." We need to inquire about the status of each as a justification for her decision.

What moral weight can a negative feeling bear? On two quite different grounds, weight could be given to her feelings in an effort to sympathetically understand her decision. First, at the point of making a decision, there is always an element of the rightness or wrongness of the choice that defies full rational justification. When we see injustice being done, we have strong negative feelings; we do not need a sophisticated moral argument to tell us that the act is unjust. We "feel" that it is wrong. It might be said that the mother's "negative feeling" was evoked by an intuition that it would be wrong to save the infant's life, and that feeling is a reliable guide to conduct.

Second, her negative response to the diagnosis of mongolism suggests that she would not be capable of giving the child the affection and the care that it would require. The logic involved is an extrapolation from that moment to potential consequences for her continued relationship to the child in the future. The argument is familiar; it is common in the literature that supports abortion on request—"no unwanted child ought to be born." Why? Because unwanted children suffer from hostility and lack of affection from their mothers, and this is bad for them.

The second term is "wants" or "desires." The negative feelings are assumed to be an indication of her desires. We might infer that at some point she said, "I do not want a retarded child." The status of "wanting" is different, we might note, if it expresses a wish before the child is born, or if it expresses a desire that leads to the death of the infant after it is born. No normal pregnant woman would wish a retarded child. In this drama, however, it translates into: "I would rather not have the infant kept alive." Or, "I will not accept parental responsibilities for a retarded child." What is the status of a desire or a want as an ethical justification for an action? To discuss that fully would lead to an account of a vast literature. The crucial issue in this case is whether the existence of the infant lays a moral claim that supersedes the mother's desires.

If a solicitor of funds for the relief of refugees in Bengal requested a donation from her and she responded, "I do not want to give money for that cause," some persons would think her to be morally insensitive, but none could argue that the refugees in Bengal had a moral claim on her money which she was obligated to acknowledge. The existence of the infant lays a weightier claim on her than does a request for a donation. We would not say that the child's right to surgery, and thus to life, is wholly relative to, and therefore exclusively dependent upon, the mother's desires or wants.

Another illustration is closer to her situation than the request for a donation. A man asks a woman to marry him. Because she is asked, she is under no obligation to answer affirmatively. He might press claims upon her—they have expressed love for each other; or they have dated for a long time; he has developed his affection for her on the assumption that her responsiveness would lead to marriage. But none of these claims would be sufficient to overrule her desire not to marry him. Why? Two sorts of reasons might be given. One would refer to potential consequences: a marriage in which one partner does not desire the relationship leads to anxiety and suffering. To avoid needless suffering is obviously desirable. So in this case, it might be said that the mother's desire is to avoid needless suffering and anxiety: the undesirable consequences can be avoided by permitting the child to die.

The second sort of reason why a woman has no obligation to marry her suitor refers to her rights as an individual. A request for marriage does not constitute a moral obligation, since there is no prima facie claim by the suitor. The woman has a right to say no. Indeed, if the suitor sought to coerce her into marriage, everyone would assert that she has a right to refuse him. In our case, however, there are some differences. The infant is incapable of expressing a request or demand. Also, the relationship is different: the suitor is not dependent upon his girl friend in the same way that the infant is dependent upon his mother. Dependence functions in two different senses; the necessary conditions for the birth of the child were his conception and *in utero* nourishment—thus, in a sense the parents "caused" the child to come into being. And, apart from instituting adoption procedures, the parents are the only ones who can provide the necessary conditions for sustaining the child's life. The infant is dependent on them in the sense that he must rely upon their performance of certain acts in order to continue to exist. The ethical question to the mother is, Does the infant's physical life lay an unconditioned moral claim on the mother? She answered, implicitly, in the negative.

What backing might the negative answer be given? The most persuasive justification would come from an argument that there are no unconditioned moral claims upon one when those presumed claims go against one's desires and wants. The claims of another are relative to my desires, my wants. Neither the solicitor for Bengal relief nor the suitor has an unconditioned claim to make; in both cases a desire is sufficient grounds for denying such a claim. In our case, it would have to be argued that the two senses of dependence that the infant has on the mother are not sufficient conditions for a claim on her that would morally require the needed surgery. Since there are no unconditioned claims, and since the conditions in this drama are not sufficient to warrant a claim, the mother is justified in denying permission for the surgery.

We note here that in our culture there are two trends in the development of morality that run counter to each other: one is the trend that desires of the ego are the grounds for moral and legal claims. If a mother does not desire the fetus in her uterus, she has a right to an abortion. The other increasingly limits individual desires and wants. An employer might want to hire only white persons of German ancestry, but he has no right to do so.

The word "fair" appeals to quite different warrants. It would not be "fair" to the other children in the family to raise a mongoloid with them. In moral philosophy, fairness is either the same as justice or closely akin to it. Two traditional definitions of justice might show how fairness could be used in this case. One is "to each his due." The other children would not get what is due them because of the inordinate requirements of time, energy, and financial resources that would be required if the mongoloid child lived. Or, if they received what was due to them, there would not be sufficient time, energy, and other resources to attend to the particular needs of the mongoloid; his condition would require more than is due him. The other traditional definition is "equals shall be treated equally." In principle, all children in the family belong to a class of equals and should be treated equally. Whether the mongoloid belongs to that class of equals is in doubt. If he does, to treat him equally with the others would be unfair to him because of his particular needs. To treat him unequally would be unfair to the others.

Perhaps "fairness" did not imply "justice." Perhaps the mother was thinking about such consequences for the other children as the extra demands that would be made upon their patience, the time they would have to give the care of the child, the emotional problems they might have in coping with a retarded sibling, and the sense of shame they might have. These consequences also could be deemed to be unjust from her point of view. Since they had no accountability for the existence of the mongoloid, it was not fair to them that extra burdens be placed upon them.

To ask what was due the mongoloid infant raises harder issues. For the mother, he was not due surgical procedure that would sustain his life. He was "unequal" to her normal children, but the fact of his inequality does not necessarily imply that he has no right to live. This leads to a matter at the root of the mother's response which has to be dealt with separately.

She (and as we shall see, the doctors also) assumed that a factual distinction (between normal and mongoloid) makes the moral difference. Factual distinctions do make moral differences. A farmer who has no qualms about killing a runt pig would have moral scruples about killing a deformed infant. If the child had not been mongoloid and had an intestinal blockage, there would have been no question about permitting surgery to be done. The value of the infant is judged to be relative to a quality of its life that is predictable on the basis of the factual evidences of mongolism. Value is relative to quality: that is the justification. Given the absence of a certain quality, the value is not sufficient to maintain life; given absence of a quality, there is no right to physical life. (Questions about terminating life among very sick adults are parallel to this instance.)

What are the qualities, or what is *the* quality that is deficient in this infant? It is not the capacity for happiness, an end that Aristotle and others thought to be sufficient in itself. The mother and the doctors knew that mongoloids can be happy. It is not the capacity for pleasure, the end that the hedonistic utilitarians thought all men seek, for mongoloids can find pleasure in life. The clue is given when a physician says that the absence of the capacity for normal intelligence was crucial. He suggested that we live in a society in which intelligence is highly valued. Perhaps it is valued as a quality in itself, or as an end in itself by some, but probably there is a further point, namely that intelligence is necessary for productive contribution to one's own well-being and to the well-being of others. Not only will a mongoloid make a minimal contribution to his own well-being and to that of others, but also others must contribute excessively to his care. The right of an infant, the value of his life, is relative to his intelligence; that is the most crucial factor in enabling or limiting his contribution to his own welfare and that of others. One has to defend such a point in terms of the sorts of contributions that would be praiseworthy and the sorts of costs that would be detrimental. The contribution of a sense of satisfaction to those who might enjoy caring for the mongoloid would not be sufficient. Indeed, a full defense would require a quantification of qualities, all based on predictions at the point of birth, that would count both for and against the child's life in a cost-benefit analysis.

The judgment that value is relative to qualities is not implausible. In our society we have traditionally valued the achiever more than the nonachievers. Some hospitals have sought to judge the qualities of the contributions of patients to society in determining who has access to scarce medical resources. A mongoloid is not valued as highly as a fine musician, an effective politician, a successful businessman, a civil rights leader whose actions have brought greater justice to the society, or a physician. To be sure, in other societies and at other times other qualities have been valued, but we judge by the qualities valued in our society and our time. Persons are rewarded according to their contributions to society. A defense of the mother's decision would have to be made on these grounds, with one further crucial step. That is, when the one necessary condition for productivity is deficient (with a high degree of certitude) at birth, there is no moral obligation to maintain that life. That the same reasoning would have been sufficient to justify overtly taking the infant's life seems not to have been the case. But that point emerges later in our discussion.

The reliance upon feelings, desires, fairness, and judgments of qualities of life makes sense to American middle-class white families, and anguished decisions can very well be settled in these terms. The choice made by the mother was not that of an unfeeling problem-solving machine, nor that of a rationalistic philosopher operating from these assumptions. It was a painful, conscientious decision, made apparently on these bases. One can ask, of course, whether her physicians should not have suggested other ways of perceiving and drawing the contours of the circumstances, other values and ends that she might consider. But that points to a subsequent topic.

The Father's Decision

The decision of the father is only a footnote to that of the mother. He consented to the choice of not operating on the infant, though he did seek precise information about mongolism and its consequences for the child. He was "willing to go along with the mother's wishes," he "understood her feelings, agreed with them," and was not in a position to make "the same intelligent decision that his wife was making."

Again we see that scientific evidence based on professional knowledge is determinative of a moral decision. The physician was forthright in indicating what the consequences would be of the course of action they were taking. The consequences of raising a mongoloid child were presumably judged to be more problematic than the death of the child.

The Decision of the Physicians

A number of points of reference in the contributions of the physicians to the case study enable us to formulate a constellation of values that determined their actions. After I have depicted that constellation, I shall analyze some of the points of reference to see how they can be defended.

The constellation can be stated summarily. The physicians felt no moral or legal obligation to save the life of a mongoloid infant by an ordinary surgical procedure when the parents did not desire that it should live. Thus, the infant was left to die. What would have been a serious but routine procedure was omitted in this instance on two conditions, both of which were judged to be necessary, but neither of which was sufficient in itself: the mongolism and the parents' desires. If the parents had desired the mongoloid infant to be saved, the surgery would have been done. If the infant had not been mongoloid and the parents had refused permission for surgery to remove a bowel obstruction, the physicians would at least have argued against them and probably taken legal measures to override them. Thus, the value-laden points of reference appear to be the desires of the parents, the mongolism of the infant, the law, and choices about ordinary and extraordinary medical procedures.

One of the two most crucial points was the obligation the physicians felt to acquiesce to the desires of the parents. The choice of the parents not to operate was made on what the physicians judged to be adequate information: it was an act of informed consent on the part of the parents. There is no evidence that the physicians raised questions of a moral sort with the parents that they subsequently raised among themselves. For example, one physician later commented on the absence of rights for children in our society and in our legal system and on the role that the value of intelligence seems to have in judging worthiness of persons. These were matters, however, that the physicians did not feel obligated to raise with the distressed parents. The physicians acted on the principle that they are only to do procedures that the patient (or crucially in this case, the parents of the patient) wanted. There was no overriding right to life on the part of a mongoloid infant that led them to argue against the parents' desires or to seek a court order requiring the surgical procedure. They recognized the moral autonomy of the parents, and thus did not interfere; they accepted as a functioning principle that the parents have the right to decide whether an infant shall live.

Elaboration of the significance of parental autonomy is necessary in order to see the grounds on which it can be defended. First, the physicians apparently recognized that the conscientious parents were the moral supreme court. There are grounds for affirming the recognition of the moral autonomy of the principal persons in complex decisions. In this case, the principals were the parents: the infant did not have the capacities to express any desires or preferences he might have. The physicians said, implicitly, that the medical profession does not have a right to impose certain of its traditional values on persons if these are not conscientiously held by those persons.

There are similarities, but also differences, between this instance and that of a terminal patient. If the terminally ill patient expresses a desire not to have his life prolonged, physicians recognize his autonomy over his own body and thus feel under no obligation to sustain his life. Our case, however, would be more similar to one in which the terminally ill patient's family decided that no further procedures ought to be used to sustain life. No doubt there are many cases in which the patient is unable to express a preference due to his physical conditions, and in the light of persuasive medical and familial reasons the physician agrees not to sustain life. A difference between our case and that, however, has to be noted in order to isolate what seems to be the crucial point. In the case of the mongoloid infant, a decision is made at the beginning of his life and not at the end; the effect is to cut off a life which, given proper care, could be sustained for many years, rather than not sustaining a life which has no such prospects.

Several defenses might be made of their recognition of the parents' presumed rights in this case. The first is that parents have authority over their children until they reach an age of discretion, and in some respects until they reach legal maturity. Children do not have recognized rights over against parents in many respects. The crucial difference here, of course, is the claimed parental right in this case to determine that an infant shall not live. What grounds might there be for this? Those who claim the moral right to an abortion are claiming the right to determine whether a child shall live, and this claim is widely recognized both morally and legally. In this case we have an extension of that right to the point of birth. If there are sufficient grounds to indicate that the newborn child is significantly abnormal, the parents have the same right as they have when a severe genetic abnormality is detected prenatally on the basis of amniocentesis. Indeed, the physicians could argue that if a mother has a right to an abortion, she also has a right to determine whether a newborn infant shall continue to live. One is simply extending the time span and the circumstances under which this autonomy is recognized.

A second sort of defense might be made: that of the limits of professional competence and authority. The physicians could argue that in moral matters they have neither competence nor authority. Perhaps they would wish to distinguish between competence and authority. They have a competence to make a moral decision on the basis of their own moral and other values, but they have no authority to impose this upon their patients. Morals, they might argue, are subjective matters, and if anyone has competence in that area, it is philosophers, clergymen, and others who teach what is right and wrong. If the parents had no internalized values that militated against their decision, it is not in the province of the physicians to tell them what they ought to do. Indeed, in a morally pluralistic society, no one group or person has a right to impose his views on another. In this stronger argument for moral autonomy no physician would have any authority to impose his own moral values on any patient. A social role differentiation is noted: the medical profession has authority only in medical matters—not in moral matters. Indeed, they have an obligation to indicate what the medical alternatives are in order to have a decision made by informed consent, but insofar as moral values or principles are involved in decisions, these are not within their professional sphere.

An outsider might ask what is meant by authority.

He might suggest that surely it is not the responsibility (or at least not his primary responsibility) or the role of the physician to make moral decisions, and certainly not to enforce his decisions on others. Would he be violating his role if he did something less determinative than that, namely, in his counseling indicate to them what some of the moral considerations might be in choosing between medical alternatives? In our case the answer seems to be yes. If the principals desire moral counseling, they have the freedom to seek it from whomsoever they will. In his professional role he acknowledges that the recognition of the moral autonomy of the principals also assumes their moral self-sufficiency, that is, their capacities to make sound moral decisions without interference on his part, or the part of any other persons except insofar as the principals themselves seek such counsel. Indeed, in this case a good deal is made of the knowledgeability of the mother particularly, and this assumes that she is morally, as well as medically, knowledgeable. Or, if she is not, it is still not the physician's business to be her moral counselor.

The physicians also assumed in this case that the moral autonomy of the parents took precedence over the positive law. At least they felt no obligation to take recourse to the courts to save the life of this infant. On that issue we will reflect more when we discuss the legal point of reference.

Another sort of defense might be made. In the order of society, decisions should be left to the most intimate and smallest social unit involved. That is the right of such a unit, since the interposition of outside authority would be an infringement of its freedom. Also, since the family has to live with the consequences of the decision, it is the right of the parents to determine which potential consequences they find most desirable. The state, or the medical profession, has no right to interfere with the freedom of choice of the family. Again, in a formal way, the argument is familiar; the state has no right to interfere with the determination of what a woman wishes to do with her body, and thus antiabortion laws are infringements of her freedom. The determination of whether an infant shall be kept alive is simply an extension of the sphere of autonomy properly belonging to the smallest social unit involved.

In all the arguments for moral autonomy, the medical fact that the infant is alive and can be kept alive does not make a crucial difference. The defense of the decision would have to be made in this way: if one grants moral autonomy to mothers to determine whether they will bring a fetus to birth, it is logical to assume that one will grant the same autonomy after birth, at least in instances where the infant is abnormal.

We have noted in our constellation of factors that the desire of the parents was a necessary but not a sufficient condition for the decisions of the physicians. If the infant had not been mongoloid, the physicians would not have so readily acquiesced to the parents' desires. Thus, we need to turn to the second necessary condition.

The second crucial point is that the infant was a mongoloid. The physicians would not have acceded to the parents' request as readily if the child had been normal; the parents would have authorized the surgical procedure if the child had been normal. Not every sort of abnormality would have led to the same decision on the part of the physicians. Their appeal was to the consequences of the abnormality of mongolism: the child would be a burden financially and emotionally to the parents. Since every child, regardless of his capacities for intelligent action, is a financial burden, and at least at times an emotional burden, it is clear that the physicians believed that the quantity or degree of burden in this case would exceed any benefits that might be forthcoming if the child were permitted to live. One can infer that a principle was operative, namely, that mongoloid infants have no inherent right to life; their right to life is conditional upon the willingness of their parents to accept them and care for them.

Previously we developed some of the reasons why a mongoloid infant was judged undesirable. Some of the same appeals to consequences entered into the decisions of the physicians. If we are to seek to develop reasons why the decisions might be judged to be morally correct, we must examine another point, namely, the operating definition of "abnormal" or "defective." There was no dissent to the medical judgment that the infant was mongoloid, though precise judgments about the seriousness of the child's defect were not possible at birth.

Our intention is to find as precisely as possible what principles or values might be invoked to claim that the "defectiveness" was sufficient to warrant not sustaining the life of this infant. As a procedure, we will begin with the most general appeals that might have been made to defend the physician's decision in this case. The most general principle would be that any infant who has any empirically verifiable degree of defect at birth has no right to life. No one would apply such a principle. Less general would be that all infants who are carriers of a genetic defect that would have potentially bad consequences for future generations have no right to life. A hemophiliac carrier would be a case in point. This principle would not be applicable, even if it were invoked with approval, in this case.

Are the physicians prepared to claim that all genetically "abnormal" infants have no claim to life? I find no evidence that they would. Are they prepared to say that where the genetic abnormality affects the capacity for "happiness" the infant has no right to live? Such an appeal was not made in this case. It appears that "normal" in this case has reference to a capacity for a certain degree of intelligence.

A presumably detectable physical norm now functions as a norm in a moral sense, or as an ideal. The ideal cannot be specified in precise terms, but there is a vague judgment about the outer limits beyond which an infant is judged to be excessively far from the norm or ideal to deserve sustenance. Again, we come to the crucial role of an obvious sign of the lack of capacity for intelligence of a certain measurable sort in judging a defect to be intolerable. A further justification of this is made by an appeal to accepted social values, at least among middle- and upper-class persons in our society. Our society values intelligence; that value becomes the ideal norm from which abnormality or deficiencies are measured. Since the infant is judged not to be able to develop into an intelligent human being (and do all that "normal" intelligence enables a human being to do), his life is of insufficient value to override the desires of the parents not to have a retarded child.

Without specification of the limits to the sorts of cases to which it could be applied, the physicians would probably not wish to defend the notion that the values of a society determine the right to life. To do so would require that there be clear knowledge of who is valued in our society (we also value aggressive people, loving people, physically strong people, etc.), and in turn a procedure by which capacities for such qualities could be determined in infancy so that precise judgments could be made about what lives should be sustained. Some members of our society do not value black people; blackness would obviously be an insufficient basis for letting an infant die. Thus, in defense of their decision the physicians would have to appeal to "values generally held in our society." This creates a different problem of quantification: what percentage of dissent would count to deny a "general" holding of a value? They would also have to designate the limits to changes in socially held values beyond which they would not consent. If the parents belonged to a subculture that valued blue eyes more than it valued intelligence, and if they expressed a desire not to have a child because it had hazel eyes, the problem of the intestinal blockage would not have been a sufficient condition to refrain from the surgical procedure.

In sum, the ideal norm of the human that makes a difference in judging whether an infant has the right to life in this case is "the capacity for normal intelligence." For the good of the infant, for the sake of avoiding difficulties for the parents, and for the good of society, a significant deviation from normal intelligence, coupled with the appropriate parental desire, is sufficient to permit the infant to die.

A third point of reference was the law. The civil law and the courts figure in the decisions at two points. First, the physicians felt no obligation to seek a court order to save the life of the infant if the parents did not want it. Several possible inferences might be drawn from this. First, one can infer that the infant had no legal right to life; his legal right is conditional upon parental desires. Second, as indicated in the interviews, the physicians believed that the court would not insist upon the surgical procedure to save the infant since it was a mongoloid. Parental desires would override legal rights in such a case. And third (an explicit statement by the physician), if the infant's life had been saved as the result of a court order, there were doubts that it would have been "accepted" by the parents. Here is an implicit appeal to potential consequences: it is not beneficial for a child to be raised by parents who do not "accept" him. The assumption is that they could not change their attitudes.

If the infant had a legal right to life, this case presents an interesting instance of conscientious objection to law. The conscientious objector to military service claims that the power of the state to raise armies for the defense of what it judges to be the national interest is one that he conscientiously refrains from sharing. The common good, or the national interest, is not jeopardized by the granting of a special status to the objector because there are enough persons who do not object to man the military services. In this case, however, the function of the law is to protect the rights of individuals to life, and the physician-objector is claiming that he is under no obligation to seek the support of the legal system to sustain life even when he knows that it could be sustained. The evidence he has in hand (the parental desire and the diagnosis of mongolism) presumably provides sufficient moral grounds for his not complying with the law. From the standpoint of ethics, an appeal could be made to conscientious objection. If, however, the appropriate law does not qualify its claims in such a way as to (*a*) permit its nonapplicability in this case or (*b*) provide for exemption on grounds of conscientious objection, the objector is presumably willing to accept the consequences for his conscientious decision. This would be morally appropriate. The physician believed that the court would not insist on saving the infant's life, and thus he foresaw no great jeopardy to himself in following conscience rather than the law.

The second point at which the law figures is in the determination of how the infant should die. The decision not to induce death was made in part in the face of the illegality of overt euthanasia (in part, only, since also the hospital staff would "feel uncomfortable" about hastening the death). Once the end or purpose of action (or inaction) was judged to be morally justified, and judged likely to be free from legal censure, the physicians still felt obliged to achieve that purpose within means that would not be subject to legal sanctions. One can only speculate whether the physicians believed that a court that would not order an infant's life to be saved would in turn censure them for overtly taking the life, or whether the uncomfortable feelings of the hospital staff were more crucial in their decision. Their course of decisions could be interpreted as at one point not involving obligation to take recourse to the courts and at the other scrupulously obeying the law. It should be noted, however, that there is consistency of action on their part; in neither instance did they intervene in what was the "natural" course of developments. The moral justification to fail to intervene in the second moment had to be different from that in the first. In the first it provides the reasons for not saving a life; in the second, for not taking a life. This leads to the last aspect of the decisions of the physicians that I noted, namely, that choices were made between ordinary and extraordinary means of action.

There is no evidence in the interviews that the language of ordinary and extraordinary means of action was part of the vocabulary of the medical staff. It is, however, an honored and useful distinction in Catholic moral theology as it applies to medical care. The principle is that a physician is under no obligation to use extraordinary means to sustain life. The difficulty in the application of the principle is the choice of what falls under ordinary and what under extraordinary means. Under one set of circumstances a procedure may be judged ordinary, and under another extraordinary. The surgery required to remove the bowel obstruction in the infant was on the whole an ordinary procedure; there were no experimental aspects to it, and there were no unusual risks to the infant's life in having it done. If the infant had had no other genetic defects, there would have been no question about using it. The physicians could make a case that when the other defect was mongolism, the procedure would be an extraordinary one. The context of the judgment about ordinary and extraordinary was a wider one than the degree of risk to the life of the patient from surgery. It included his other defect, the desires of the family, the potential costs to family and society, etc. No moralists, to my knowledge, would hold them culpable if the infant were so deformed that he would be labeled (nontechnically) a monstrosity. To heroically maintain the life of a monstrosity as long as one could would be most extraordinary. Thus, we return to whether the fact of mongolism and its consequences is a sufficient justification to judge the lifesaving procedure to be extraordinary in this instance. The physicians would argue that it is.

The infant was left to die with a minimum of care. No extraordinary means were used to maintain its life once the decision not to operate had been made. Was it extraordinary not to use even ordinary procedures to maintain the life of the infant once the decision not to operate had been made? The judgment clearly was in the negative. To do so would be to prolong a life that would not be saved in any case. At that point the infant was in a class of terminal patients, and the same justifications used for not prolonging the life of a terminal patient would apply here. Patients have a right to die, and physicians are under no moral obligation to sustain their lives when it is clear that they will not live for long. The crucial difference between a terminal cancer patient and this infant is that in the situation of the former, all procedures which might prolong life for a goodly length of time are likely to have been exhausted. In the case of the infant, the logic of obligations to terminal patients takes its course as a result of a decision not to act at all.

To induce death by some overt action is an extraordinary procedure. To justify overt action would require a justification of euthanasia. This case would be a good one from which to explore euthanasia from a moral point of view. Once a decision is made not to engage in a life-sustaining and lifesaving procedure, has not the crucial corner been turned? If that is a reasonable and moral thing to do, on what grounds would one argue that it is wrong to hasten death? Most obviously it is still illegal to do it, and next most obviously people have sensitive feelings about taking life. Further, it goes against the grain of the fundamental vocation of the medical profession to maintain life. But, of course, the decision not to operate also goes against that grain. If the first decision was justifiable, why was it not justifiable to hasten the death of the infant? We can only assume at this point traditional arguments against euthanasia would have been made.

The Decisions of the Nurses

The nurses, as the interviews indicated, are most important for their expressions of feelings, moral sensibilities, and frustrations. They demonstrate the importance of deeply held moral convictions and of profound compassion in determining human responses to ambiguous circumstances. If they had not known that the infant could have survived, the depth of their frustrations and feelings would have not been so great. Feelings they would have had, but they would have been compassion for an infant bound to die. The actual range of decision for them was clearly circumscribed by the role definitions in the medical professions; it was their duty to carry out the orders of the physicians. Even if they conscientiously believed that the orders they were executing were immoral, they could not radically reverse the course of events; they could not perform the required surgery. It was their lot to be the immediate participants in a sad event but to be powerless to alter its course.

It would be instructive to explore the reasons why the nurses felt frustrated, were deeply affected by their duties in this case. Moral convictions have their impact upon the feelings of persons as well as upon their rational decisions. A profound sense of vocation to relieve suffering and to preserve life no doubt lies behind their responses, as does a conviction about the sanctity of human life. For our purposes, however, we shall leave them with the observation that they are the instruments of the orders of the physicians. They have no right of conscientious objection, at least not in this set of circumstances.

Before turning to another evaluative description of the case, it is important to reiterate what was said in the beginning. The decisions by the principals were conscientious ones. The parents anguished. The physicians were informed by a sense of compassion in their consent to the parents' wishes; they did not wish to be party to potential suffering that was avoidable. Indeed, in the way in which they formulated the dilemma, they did what was reasonable to do. They chose the way of least possible suffering to the fewest persons over a long range of time, with one exception, namely, not taking the infant's life. By describing the dilemma from a somewhat different set of values, or giving different weight to different factors, another course of action would have been reasonable and justified. The issue, it seems to me, is at the level of what is to be valued more highly, for one's very understanding of the problems he must solve are deeply affected by what one values most.

The Dilemma from a Different Moral Point of View

Wallace Stevens wrote in poetic form a subtle account of "Thirteen Ways of Looking at a Blackbird." Perhaps there are 13 ways of looking at this medical case. I shall attempt to look at it from only one more way. By describing the dilemma from a perspective that gives a different weight to some of the considerations that we have already exposed, one has a different picture, and different conclusions are called for. The moral integrity of any of the original participants is not challenged, not because of a radical relativism that says they have their points of view and I have mine, but out of respect for their conscientiousness. For several reasons, however, more consideration ought to have been given to two points. A difference in evaluative judgments would have made a difference of life or death for the infant, depending upon: (1) whether what one ought to do is determined by what one desires to do and (2) whether a mongoloid infant has a claim to life.

To restate the dilemma once again: If the parents had "desired" the mongoloid infant, the surgeons would have performed the operation that would have saved its life. If the infant had had a bowel obstruction that could be taken care of by an ordinary medical procedure, but had not been a mongoloid, the physicians would probably have insisted that the operation be performed.

Thus, one can recast the moral dilemma by giving a different weight to two things: the desires of the parents and the value or rights of a mongoloid infant. If the parents and the physicians believed strongly that there are things one ought to do even when one has no immediate positive feelings about doing them, no immediate strong desire to do them, the picture would have been different. If the parents and physicians believed that mongoloid children have intrinsic value, or have a right to life, or if they believed that mongolism is not sufficiently deviant from what is normatively human to merit death, the picture would have been different.

Thus, we can redraw the picture. To be sure, the parents are ambiguous about their feelings for a mongoloid infant, since it is normal to desire a normal infant rather than an abnormal infant. But (to avoid a discussion of abortion at this point) once an infant is born its independent existence provides independent value in itself, and those who brought it into being and those professionally responsible for its care have an obligation to sustain its life regardless of their negative or ambiguous feelings toward it. This probably would have been acknowledged by all concerned if the infant had not been mongoloid. For example, if the pregnancy had been accidental, and in this sense the child was not desired, and the infant had been normal, no one would have denied its right to exist once it was born, though some would while still *in utero,* and thus would have sought an abortion. If the mother refused to accept accountability for the infant, alternative means of caring for it would have been explored.

To be sure, a mongoloid infant is genetically defective, and raising and caring for it put burdens on the parents, the family, and the state beyond the burdens required to raise a normal infant. But a mongoloid infant is human, and thus has the intrinsic value of humanity and the rights of a human being. Further, given proper care, it can reach a point of significant fulfillment of its limited potentialities; it is capable of loving and responding to love; it is capable of realizing happiness; it can be trained to accept responsibility for itself within its capacities. Thus, the physicians and parents have an obligation to use all ordinary means to preserve its life. Indeed, the humanity of mentally defective children is recognized in our society by the fact that we do not permit their extermination and do have policies which provide, all too inadequately, for their care and nurture.

If our case had been interpreted in the light of moral beliefs that inform the previous two paragraphs, the only reasonable conclusion would be that the surgery ought to have been done.

The grounds for assigning the weights I have to these crucial points can be examined. First, with reference simply to common experience, we all have obligations to others that are not contingent upon our immediate desires. When the registrar of my university indicates that senior grades have to be in by May 21, I have an obligation to read the exams, term papers, and senior essays in time to report the grades, regardless of my negative feelings toward those tasks or my preference to be doing something else. I have an obligation to my students, and to the university through its registrar, which I accepted when I assumed the social role of an instructor. The students have a claim on me; they have a right to expect me to fulfill my obligations to them and to the university. I might be excused from the obligation if I suddenly become too ill to fulfill it; my incapacity to fulfill it would be a temporarily excusing condition. But negative feelings toward that job, or toward any students, or a preference for writing a paper of my own at that time, would not constitute excusing conditions. I must consider, in determining what I do, the relationships that I have with others and the claims they have on me by virtue of those relationships.

In contrast to this case, it might be said that I have a contractual obligation to the university into which I freely entered. The situation of the parents is not the same. They have no legal contractual relationship with the infant, and thus their desires are not bound by obligations. Closer to their circumstances, then, might be other family relationships. I would argue that the fact that we brought our children into being lays a moral obligation on my wife and me to sustain and care for them to the best of our ability. They did not choose to be; and their very being is dependent, both causally and in other ways, upon us. In the relationship of dependence, there is a claim of them over against us. To be sure, it is a claim that also has its rewards and that we desire to fulfill within a relationship of love. But until they have reached an age when they can accept full accountability (or fuller accountability) for themselves, they have claims upon us by virtue of our being their parents, even when meeting those claims is to us financially costly, emotionally distressing, and in other ways not immediately desirable. Their claims are independent of our desires to fulfill them. Particular claims they might make can justifiably be turned down, and others can be negotiated, but the claim against us for their physical sustenance constitutes a moral obligation that we have to meet. That obligation is not conditioned by their IQ scores, whether they have cleft palates or perfectly formed faces, whether they are obedient or irritatingly independent, whether they are irritatingly obedient and passive or laudably self-determining. It is not conditioned by any predictions that might be made about whether they will become the persons we might desire that they become. The infant in our case has the same sort of claim, and thus the parents have a moral obligation to use all ordinary means to save its life.

An objection might be made. Many of my fellow Christians would say that the obligation of the parents was to do that which is loving toward the infant. Not keeping the child alive was the loving thing to do with reference both to its interests and to the interests of the other members of the family. To respond to the objection, one needs first to establish the spongy character of the words "love" or "loving." They can absorb almost anything. Next one asks whether the loving character of an act is determined by feelings or by motives, or whether it is also judged by what is done. It is clear that I would argue for the latter. Indeed, the minimal conditions of a loving relationship include respect for the other, and certainly for the other's presumption of a right to live. I would, however, primarily make the case that the relationship of dependence grounds the claim, whether or not one feels loving toward the other.

The dependence relationship holds for the physicians as well as the parents in this case. The child's life depended utterly upon the capacity of the physicians to sustain it. The fact that an infant cannot articulate his claim is irrelevant. Physicians will struggle to save the life of a person who has attempted to commit suicide even when the patient might be in such a drugged condition that he cannot express his desire—a desire expressed already in his effort to take his life and overridden by the physician's action to save it. The claim of human life for preservation, even when such a person indicates a will not to live, presents a moral obligation to those who have the capacity to save it.

A different line of argument might be taken. If the decisions made were as reliant upon the desires of the parents as they appear to be, which is to say, if desire had a crucial role, what about the desire of the infant? The infant could not give informed consent to the nonintervention. One can hypothesize that every infant desires to live, and that even a defective child is likely to desire life rather than death when it reaches an age at which its desires can be articulated. Even if the right to live is contingent upon a desire, we can infer that the infant's desire would be for life. As a human being, he would have that desire, and thus it would constitute a claim on those on whom he is dependent to fulfill it.

I have tried to make a persuasive case to indicate why the claim of the infant constitutes a moral obligation on the parents and the physicians to keep the child alive. The intrinsic value or rights of a human being are not qualified by any given person's intelligence or capacities for productivity, potential consequences of the sort that burden others. Rather, they are constituted by the very existence of the human being as one who is related to others and dependent upon others for his existence. The presumption is always in favor of sustaining life through ordinary means; the desires of persons that run counter to that presumption are not sufficient conditions for abrogating that right.

The power to determine whether the infant shall live or die is in the hands of others. Does the existence of such power carry with it the moral right to such determination? Long history of moral experience indicates not only that arguments have consistently been made against the judgment that the capacity to do something constitutes a right to do it, or put in more familiar terms, that might makes right. It also indicates that in historical situations where persons have claimed the right to determine who shall live because they have the power to do so, the consequences have hardly been beneficial to mankind. This, one acknowledges, is a "wedge" argument or a "camel's nose under the tent" argument. As such, its limits are clear. Given a culture in which humane values are regnant, it is not likely that the establishment of a principle that some persons under some circumstances claim the right to determine whether others shall live will be transformed into the principle that the right of a person to live is dependent upon his having the qualities approved by those who have the capacity to sustain or take his life. Yet while recognizing the sociological and historical limitations that exist in a humane society, one still must recognize the significance of a precedent. To cite an absurd example, what would happen if we lived in a society in which the existence of hazel eyes was considered a genetic defect by parents and physicians? The absurdity lies in the fact that no intelligent person would consider hazel eyes a genetic defect; the boundaries around the word defect are drawn by evidences better than eye color. But the precedent in principle remains; when one has established that the capacity to determine who shall live carries with it the right to determine who shall live, the line of discussion has shifted from a sharp presumption (of the right of all humans to live) to the softer, spongier determination of the qualities whose value will be determinative.

Often we cannot avoid using qualities and potential consequences in the determination of what might be justifiable exceptions to the presumption of the right to life on the part of any infant—indeed, any person. No moralist would insist that the physicians have an obligation to sustain the life of matter born from human parents that is judged to be a "monstrosity." Such divergence from the "normal" qualities presents no problem, and potential consequences for its continued existence surely enter into the decision. The physicians in our case believed that in the absence of a desire for the child on the part of the parents, mongolism was sufficiently removed from an ideal norm of the human that the infant had no overriding claim on them. We are in a sponge. Why would I draw the line on a different side of mongolism than the physicians did? While reasons can be given, one must recognize that there are intuitive elements, grounded in beliefs and profound feelings, that enter into particular judgments of this sort. I am not prepared to say that my respect for human life is "deeper," "profounder," or "stronger" than theirs. I am prepared to say that the way in which, and the reasons why, I respect life orient my judgment toward the other side of mongolism than theirs did.

First, the value that intelligence was given in this

instance appears to me to be simplistic. Not all intelligent persons are socially commendable (choosing socially held values as the point of reference because one of the physicians did). Also, many persons of limited intelligence do things that are socially commendable, if only minimally providing the occasion for the expression of profound human affection and sympathy. There are many things we value about human life; that the assumption that one of them is the *sine qua non,* the necessary and sufficient condition for a life to be valued at all, oversimplifies human experience. If there is a *sine qua non,* it is physical life itself, for apart from it, all potentiality of providing benefits for oneself or for others is impossible. There are occasions on which other things are judged to be more valuable than physical life itself; we probably all would admire the person whose life is martyred for the sake of saving others. But the qualities or capacities we value exist in bundles, and not each as overriding in itself. The capacity for self-determination is valued, and on certain occasions we judge that it is worth dying, or taking life, for the sake of removing repressive limits imposed upon persons in that respect. But many free, self-determining persons are not very happy; indeed, often their anxiety increases with the enlargement of the range of things they must and can determine for themselves. Would we value a person exclusively because he is happy? Probably not, partly because his happiness has at least a mildly contagious effect on some other persons, and thus we value him because he makes others happy as well. To make one quality we value (short of physical life itself, and here there are exceptions) determinative over all other qualities is to impoverish the richness and variety of human life. When we must use the sponge of qualities to determine exceptions to the presumption of the right to physical life, we need to face their variety, their complexity, the abrasiveness of one against the other, in the determination of action. In this case the potentialities of a mongoloid for satisfaction in life, for fulfilling his limited capacities, for happiness, for providing the occasions of meaningful (sometimes distressing and sometimes joyful) experience for others are sufficient so that no exception to the right to life should be made. Put differently, the anguish, suffering, embarrassment, expenses of family and state (I support the need for revision of social policy and practice) are not sufficiently negative to warrant that a mongoloid's life not be sustained by ordinary procedures.

Second, and harder to make persuasive, is that my view of human existence leads to a different assessment of the significance of suffering than appears to be operative in this case. The best argument to be made in support of the course of decisions as they occurred is that in the judgment of the principals involved, they were able to avoid more suffering and other costs for more people over a longer range of time than could have been avoided if the infant's life had been saved. To suggest a different evaluation of suffering is not to suggest that suffering is an unmitigated good, or that the acceptance of suffering when it could be avoided is a strategy that ought to be adopted for the good life, individually and collectively. Surely it is prudent and morally justifiable to avoid suffering if possible under most normal circumstances of life. But two questions will help to designate where a difference of opinion between myself and the principals in our drama can be located. One is, At what cost to others is it justifiable to avoid suffering for ourselves? On the basis of my previous exposition, I would argue that in this instance the avoidance of potential suffering at the cost of that life was not warranted. The moral claims of others upon me often involve emotional and financial stress, but that stress is not sufficient to warrant my ignoring the claims. The moral and legal claim of the government to the right to raise armies in defense of the national interest involves inconvenience, suffering, and even death for many; yet the fact that meeting that claim will cause an individual suffering is not sufficient ground to give conscientious objection. Indeed, we normally honor those who assume suffering for the sake of benefits to others.

The second question is, Does the suffering in prospect appear to be bearable for those who have to suffer? We recognize that the term "bearable" is a slippery slope and that fixing an answer to this question involves judgments that are always hypothetical. If, however, each person has a moral right to avoid all bearable inconvenience or suffering that appears to run counter to his immediate or long-range self-interest, there are many things necessary for the good of other individuals and for the common good that would not get done. In our case, there appear to be no evidences that the parents with assistance from other institutions would necessarily find the raising of a mongoloid child to bring suffering that they could not tolerate. Perhaps there is justifying evidence to which I do not have access, such as the possibility that the mother would be subject to severe mental illness if she had to take care of the child. But from the information I received, no convincing case could be made that the demands of raising the child would present intolerable and unbearable suffering to the family. That it would create greater anguish, greater inconvenience, and greater demands than raising a normal child would is clear. But that meeting these demands would cause greater suffering to this family than it does to thousands of others who raise mongoloid children seems not to be the case.

Finally, my view, grounded ultimately in religious convictions as well as moral beliefs, is that to be human is to have a vocation, a calling, and the calling of each of us is "to be for others" at least as much as "to be for ourselves." The weight that one places on "being for others" makes a difference in one's fundamental orientation toward all of his relationships, particularly when they conflict with his immediate self-interest. In the Torah we have that great commandment, rendered in the New English Bible as "you shall love your neighbour as a man like yourself" (Lev. 19:18). It is reiterated in the records we have of the words of Jesus, "Love your neighbor as yourself" (Matt. 22:39, and several other places). Saint Paul makes the point even stronger at one point: "Each of you must regard, not his own interests, but the other man's" (1 Cor. 10:24, NEB). And finally, the minimalist saying accredited both to Rabbi Hillel and to Jesus in different forms, "Do unto others as you would have others do unto you."

The point of the biblical citations is not to take recourse to dogmatic religious authority, as if these sayings come unmediated from the ultimate power and orderer of life. The point is to indicate a central thrust in Judaism and Christianity which has nourished and sustained a fundamental moral outlook, namely, that we are "to be for others" at least as much as we are "to be for ourselves." The fact that this outlook has not been adhered to consistently by those who professed it does not count against it. It remains a vocation, a calling, a moral ideal, if not a moral obligation. The statement of such an outlook does not resolve all the particular problems of medical histories such as this one, but it shapes a bias, gives a weight, toward the well-being of the other against inconvenience or cost to oneself. In this case, I believe that all the rational inferences to be drawn from it, and all the emotive power that this calling evokes, lead to the conclusion that the ordinary surgical procedure should have been done, and the mongoloid infant's life saved.

77. The Death of Infant Doe: Jesus and the Neonates

ALLEN VERHEY

I imagine it was a hot and sunny day, the kind of day when kids seem to have such boundless energy and grownups seem to wilt. The disciples, I suppose, were quite glad for the rest; at least they were a little peevish when women and children threatened to interrupt it. They rebuked them, the story in Mark 10 says. "Can't you see Jesus is an important person. What business do you have bothering him? Get back to your ovens, women! Return to your toys, children! Stay out of our way."

The disciples' response was conventional enough; surely understandable. Women and children were just not that important. They were numbered among the heathen and illiterate, with sinners and those who do not know the law, with slaves and property. They were not numbered at all when the members of the synagogue were counted. You needed ten *adult males* for a synagogue. Nine plus all the women and children of Galilee would not make a synagogue. Women and children just did not count for much. The disciples knew that and told them to go away.

Jesus gets angry too, but not with the women, not with the children. He gets angry with the disciples. He turns the conventional rules of pomp and protocol upside down. Those who don't count do count with him; he makes the last first! When will his disciples ever learn that? He says to them, "Let the children come to me. Do not hinder them. To them belongs the kingdom of God." The disciples must have been more than a little dumbfounded. Other strange behavior of this Galilean teacher had hardly prepared them for this.

There must have been babies there, and more than one dirty diaper, and Jesus takes them in his arms. There must have been toddlers and youngsters, curious and energetic, crying occasionally and interrupting often. "Women are meant to deal with them," the disciples thought, but Jesus blesses them. There must have been boys and girls, taking a break from playing tag and catch, and some who stood on the sidelines because of a limp or a disease or something else that made them unwelcome in the game, and Jesus lays his hands on them.

From *The Reformed Journal* 32 (June 1982): 10-15. Used by permission. Revised by the author for this volume.

And as though all this is not enough, Jesus says, "If you want to enter the kingdom become like one of these children." People have speculated endlessly about how we are supposed to be like children. It is their *trust* some say; their *dependence* others say; their *joy* still others say; or their *simplicity.* There is perhaps some truth in each of those comparisons, but I really think they are beside the point. Jesus says in other places, "If any would be first of all, let him be last of all and the servant of all." And that's what he says here too. "Become like one of these children" means simply "become last—for such are first with me." That's the shocking thing. Jesus exalts the humble and humbles the exalted. He makes the last first. Those who don't count count with him. He blesses kids: dirty-diapered, sweaty, silly, obnoxious kids. He rebukes the disciples, impressed with their own importance and conventional prestige. And he makes it clear that to be his disciple, to welcome the kingdom, will mean to welcome, to serve and to help, these little children. Who is greatest in the kingdom? These little children and those who bless and serve them.

Soon after the death and resurrection of Jesus, that story was being told again and again in the young church. Pentecost had convinced the people of the church that Jesus continued to abide with them and that he continued to address them in their memory of what he had once said or done. Even as the church awaited the new creation, the redemption of their bodies and their adoption as sons, as Paul says, it was constantly informed and reformed by the stories about Jesus. Imagine, for example, Peter telling the story to settle the question of whether the children of believing parents should be baptized. Or Andrew telling the story in a slightly different way to exhort his hearers to a childlike faith. Or again, imagine some unknown preacher telling the story to protest the neglect and abandonment of children that was practiced in the Roman empire. The story found its way finally into Mark's gospel alongside sayings about marriage and riches to provide guidance for a Christian household.

The story continues to be told in the churches, of course. It is told in countless stained glass windows. We have all seen them. The only thing wrong with these windows is that the kids are too angelic. There are no runny noses or bruised knees or imperfections to be found in the stained glass representations of the story. The story has indeed become so familiar that we have to make an effort to stop and think about it, to contemplate what it would mean to make this story our story, to be informed and reformed by this story. I invite you to make that effort, specifically to think about what this story might mean for our care of neonates.

To do that there is another story that I want you to think about. It is a familiar story, too, the story of Infant Doe. It happened in Bloomington in 1982. Now Bloomington is a pleasant little city set in the lovely hills of southern Indiana. Bloomington Hospital is typical of hospitals in pleasant little cities; the daily human events of giving birth, suffering, and dying are attended to with the ordinary measure of professional competence and compassion. It seems unlikely that the story of birth, suffering, and death of a baby in Bloomington would capture national attention.

On April 9, 1982, a boy was born in Bloomington Hospital with Down's syndrome and esophageal atresia. Down's syndrome is a fairly common genetic defect which causes varying degrees of mental retardation and physical deformity. Esophageal atresia is a malformation of the esophagus, so that food taken orally cannot enter the stomach and instead causes choking.

The parents of this baby refused to consent to the surgical procedure necessary to correct the esophageal atresia. The obstetrician who had initially presented such "benign neglect" as one of the medical options supported the parents in that decision. A pediatrician who had been consulted to confirm the diagnosis dissented from such a course of "treatment." The Circuit Court in Bloomington and subsequently the Indiana Supreme Court in Indianapolis refused to override the parents' decision and to order the surgery to correct the esophagus of "Infant Doe." The baby lay in Bloomington Hospital for six days until his starving yielded to his death on April 15.

The obstetrician and the pediatrician disagreed not only about the recommended treatment but also about the chances for successful esophageal surgery, about the likelihood of other serious physical problems, and about the prognosis of retardation. The obstetrician, in presenting the options to the parents, said that the chances for successful surgery were about fifty-fifty, that other physical defects, including congenital heart disease, would subsequently have to be surgically corrected, and that the child would certainly be severely retarded. The pediatrician insisted that the likelihood of successful surgery was more like ninety percent, that there was no evidence of congenital heart disease, and that it was impossible to determine the severity of the retardation Infant Doe would have. The conflicting medical opinions and recommendations weighed heavily in the courts' decisions not to intervene, not to play either doctor or parent to the child.

The courts' hesitancy to pretend to either medical competence or parental compassion can be appreciated (especially by those schooled in something called "sphere sovereignty"). Moreover, the competence of the doctors and the compassion of the parents were widely attested. Still, the medical recommendation of the obstetrician and the decisions by the parents and by the justices were morally wrong—not just tragic, but wrong.

Decisions are tragic when goods come into conflict, when any decision brings in its train some wrong. This was not such a decision. The right decision would have been to do the surgery. I will undertake to defend that judgment in ways that are standard in medical ethics, in ways that rely on "impartial rationality" to formulate judgments and to solve dilemmas. One need not be a Christian to see that the decision not to treat Infant Doe was wrong. But I will also undertake to show that impartial rationality is inadequate, that it can provide only a minimal account of morality, and that when its minimalism is not acknowledged it can distort the moral life. Finally, because the conventional approach is inadequate, I will undertake another approach, a candidly Christian approach, an approach which owns the Christian story, including the story of Jesus and the children, as *our* story also in cases like Infant Doe's.

First, then, one need not be a Christian to see that the right decision would have been to perform the surgery to correct the esophagus so that Infant Doe could be fed. The impartial rational justification for saying this might be provided in a number of different ways. The most telling in my view is that if a "normal" child had been born with esophageal atresia, the surgery would have been performed—even if the obstetrician were right about the risks and the additional physical problems. The reason for "treating" Infant Doe differently was an irrelevant one, Infant Doe's Down's syndrome. (Furthermore, the obstetrician was simply wrong about the ability to predict so early the extent of retardation caused by Down's syndrome.)

Suppose that on April 9 two other babies were born in Bloomington. Suppose "Infant Smith" was born without Down's syndrome but with esophageal atresia. The consent to operate would surely have been given or ordered, and Infant Smith would probably be alive today. Suppose "Infant Jones" was born with Down's syndrome but without any life-threatening malformations of the esophagus. No consent to operate would have been necessary, and Infant Jones would probably be alive today. The difference between Infant Doe and Infant Smith, the difference between life and death, is that Infant Doe had Down's syndrome, nothing else. The difference between Infant Doe and Infant Jones, also the difference between life and death, is that Infant Doe had esophageal atresia in addition to Down's syndrome. If we ought to preserve and cherish the life of Infants Smith and Jones, then we ought also to have preserved and cherished the life of Infant Doe. The differences among these infants are irrelevant to the obligation to sustain their lives and to nurture their bodies and spirits.

This is not to deny that different conditions among infants may indicate different treatments or even in some cases the cessation of treatment. If a condition is terminal and if treatment would only prolong the child's dying and exacerbate his or her suffering, then treatment is not indicated. Anencephalic newborns are a clear case of legitimate neglect. There are tragic cases where a child's suffering from a disease and from the treatment of the disease is so profound as to put it outside the reach of human caring, let alone human curing. Such, however, was not the case with Infant Doe or other Down's syndrome youngsters. Down's syndrome is not a terminal condition; and if people who have it suffer more, it is not because surgery pains them more but because "normal" people can be cruel and spiteful. A Down's child can experience and delight in the reach and touch of human caring.

The neglect of Infant Doe was morally wrong. His death was caused by "natural causes," to be sure, but it was both possible and obligatory to interfere with those "natural causes." If a lifeguard neglected a drowning swimmer whom he recognized as his competition for his lover's affection, we would say he did wrong. That the drowned man died of "natural causes" would not prevent us from seeing the wrong done to him—or from invoking the category "murder." If the same lifeguard neglected a drowning wader whom he recognized as an infant with Down's syndrome, we should also say he did wrong. That the infant died of "natural causes" should not prevent us from seeing the wrong done to him—or from invoking the category "murder."

Someone may argue that "lifeguard" is a well-defined role with specific responsibilities and a tradition involving certain technical skills and moral virtues, and that the obligation to rescue the swimmer and the wader is really a role-obligation. Two replies might be made to this objection to our analogy. First, we might say that any person—lifeguard or not—who sees an infant stumble and fall face down in the water is obliged to attempt to rescue the child, Down's syndrome or not. The decision to neglect Infant Doe, by analogy, is simply morally wrong. The second reply is to acknowledge that "lifeguard" is a special role with special responsibilities and a tradition, and to insist that "physician" and "parent" are also such roles.

But here impartial rationality begins to fail us, for it tends to reduce role relations—for example, the relation of the doctors to Infant Doe or his parents or the relation of the parents to Infant Doe—to *contractual* arrangements between independent individuals. That is a minimal account of such roles at best, and when its minimalism is not acknowledged, it is an account which distorts the moral life and the covenants of which it is woven. The stance of impartial rationality cannot nurture any moral wisdom about these roles or sustain any moral traditions concerning them. And it is our confusion about these roles, our diminishing sense of a tradition concerning them, that accounts for the failure of a competent physician, compassionate parents, and duly humble justices to make the morally right decision with respect to the care of Infant Doe.

There are other inadequacies in the stance of impartial rationality which bore on the story of Infant Doe. The stance of impartial rationality tends to emphasize the procedural question, the question of who decides, rather than the substantive question of what should be decided. The first and final question in the care of Infant Doe was who should decide, and the answer was consistently that the parents should decide. I am not saying that that question or that answer is wrong, but I am saying that it provides only a minimal account of the moral issues, and that if its minimalism is forgotten or ignored, the moral life and particular moral issues can be distorted. I am saying that a fuller account of morality would focus as well on substantive questions—on the question of *what* should be decided—and on questions of character and virtue—on the question of *what* the person who decides should *be.*

Let me call attention to one other weakness (or inadequacy) of the approach of impartial rationality. This approach requires alienation from ourselves, from our own moral interests and loyalties, from our own histories and communities in order to adopt the impartial point of view. We are asked, nay, obliged, by this approach to view our own projects and passions as though we were objective outside observers. The stories which we own as our own, which provide our lives a narrative and which develop our own character, we are asked by this approach to disown—and for the sake of morality. Now, to be asked to pause occasionally and for the sake of analysis and judgment to view things as impartially as we can is in certain contexts not only legitimate but salutary, but neither physicians nor parents nor any Christian can finally live their moral lives like that with any integrity.

These remarks about the inadequacies of impartial rationality allow us to turn an important corner in this paper. My concern is not merely to make a moral judgment about the care of Infant Doe. The decision not to treat him was wrong, but the more interesting questions—and finally the more important questions, from my point of view—are, How could a competent physician, compassionate parents, and duly humble justices make such a decision? What stories and traditions make sense of such a decision? And how can the Christian story, explicitly the story of Jesus and the children, be brought to bear on such decisions? Can we begin to write a story of Jesus and the neonates? Let us examine briefly the stories and traditions of medicine, of parenting, and of society's attitude toward the handicapped.

The obstetrician, however competent and skillful he may have been, had apparently not been initiated into the tradition of medical care which insists that the practice of medicine involves more than techniques and skills, that it serves and embodies certain intrinsic goods. According to one witness to that tradition, the Hippocratic Oath, the end of medicine is "the benefit of the sick," not some extrinsic good like money or fame or the wishes of the medical "consumer."

The benefit of the sick does not stand as a motive for taking up certain ethically neutral skills. It does not identify an extrinsic good to be accomplished by means of ethically neutral technical means. Rather, the benefit of the sick is the *intrinsic* good of medicine. It governs the practice of medicine and entails certain standards which define medicine as a moral art. Medicine in this tradition intends to heal the sick, to protect and nurture health, to maintain and restore a measure of physical well-being. All the powers of medicine are guided and limited by those ends, and they may not be used to serve alien ends—and death is an alien end. In this sad world death will win its victories finally, but medicine which has identified with the tradition to which the Hippocratic Oath witnesses will not serve death or practice hospitality toward it. This tradition has its own stories, of course, stories about the great Hippocrates initiating his students into the art with an oath that they will indeed practice medicine for "the benefit of the sick," stories about dedicated physicians braving the elements or the opposition to help some sick scoundrel without worrying about the social utility of his patient or of his profession.

Medicine truly in the tradition formed and informed by such stories would and should have stood in the service of Infant Doe, the sick one, the patient, and braved the claims of any and all who wanted him dead. A physician initiated into such a tradition would not present the choice between possible life with Down's syndrome or certain death without esophageal surgery as an option to be contemplated, nor would he or she support the choice of death.

The obstetrician's failure to embody this tradition is symptomatic of our entire society's diminishing appreciation of this view of medicine and a growing confusion about the physician's role. These stories of medicine are today considered naive, sometimes foolish, both by physicians and by society. Properly impressed by modern medicine's technological accomplishments, we are tempted to view medicine as a collection of skills to get what we want, as a value-free enterprise which may be bought and sold to satisfy consumer desires, hired to do the autonomous bidding of the one who pays. Thus, a new model has taken over the understanding of medicine—that omnipresent model of the marketplace, where you get rich by supplying what the buyer wants.

The decision about Infant Doe is understandable, I think, within the marketplace model, but we are justifiably uncomfortable with this way of understanding medicine, for medical skills alone, removed from their original tradition, can make one either a good healer or a crafty murderer. The skills alone cannot provide the wisdom to make a morally right decision. Medicine formed by the model of the marketplace cannot and will not sustain the disposition of care and trust which have defined the characters of doctor and patient in the Hippocratic tradition. On the contrary, the marketplace model will end with medicine in the service of the rich and powerful, while the poor and weak watch and pray.

Infant Doe was too young to pray but not too young to groan with the rest of us "as we wait for . . . the redemption of our bodies" (Rom. 8:23). That eschatological vision of Christianity—and the entire Christian story, including the story of Jesus and the children—provides a resource to support the fragile Hippocratic tradition of medicine, for it enlists us on the side of life and health in a world where death and evil still apparently reign. It makes us suspicious of and repentant for human capacities for pride and sloth with respect to medical technology. And it calls us to identify with and to serve especially the sick and the poor, the powerless and the despised, and all those who do not measure up to conventional standards.

A note must be added with respect to another community that evidently has the resources to support the fragile tradition of medicine—nurses. The nurses at Bloomington Hospital who were first charged with the "care" of Infant Doe refused to participate in his non-treatment masquerading as care. It violated the ends of nursing as they understood them; it compromised their integrity as members of a nursing community and as heirs of a medical tradition. The immediate consequence of their protest was not great: Infant Doe was simply moved from the nursery to a private room on a surgical floor. But a worthy tradition of medicine was represented and protected by their action. These nurses and others like them are a precious resource if the medical professions and society are to remember and relearn the medical moral tradition.

Our society is also confused about the role of parent. The parents of Infant Doe, however compassionate they may have been, had apparently not been initiated into a tradition of parental care which insists that parents have a duty not only to care *about* their children but to care *for* them, to tend to their physical, emotional, moral, and spiritual needs, not because they "measure up," but because they are their children.

The parents' failure to represent this tradition is symptomatic of our society's growing confusion about parenting. The tradition has always been challenged by the contrary opinion (now usually unstated) that children are the property of parents to be disposed of as they wish, that children exist for the happiness of parents. Today, however, especially among the compassionate, the tradition is being challenged by a contrary opinion: the view that parents have the awesome responsibility to produce "perfect" children and to assure them a happy and successful life or at least the capacity to attain to and conform to the American ideal of "the good life."

All of us who are parents know we desire our children to be perfect. And all of us who are children know the pain that can be caused by that desire. The responsibility of making perfect children and making children perfect, which is now entering and forming a new model of medicine, will allow—or finally require—the abortion of the unborn who do not meet our standards and the neglect of newborns with diminished capacities to achieve *our* ideal of "the good life." Such a view of parenting will finally reduce our options to a perfect child or a dead child. The Infant Doe decision is understandable, I think, within a model of medicine that requires making perfect children and making children perfect, but that model will not and cannot coexist with the disposition of uncalculating nurturance and basic trust which have defined the relation of parent and child within the Christian story.

It is a commonplace to assert that the institution of the family is in crisis, but it can receive little support from conventional modern moral theory, whether utilitarian or formalist. Both have some power in dealing with our relation with strangers, but neither can deal adequately with the family or sustain it in a time of crisis. Family loyalties are an embarrassment to our calculations of "the greatest happiness for the greatest number" and to our assertions of autonomy. The tradition of the family—and experience in a family—reminds us both that "happiness" is not what it's all about and that we are not as independent, self-sufficient, and autonomous as we sometimes claim.

The fragile tradition of the family, too, may be and should be supported by the Christian story, for the Father's uncalculating nurturance is still the model from which to learn parenting. In the Christian vision the family is seen as a gift and a vocation, providing opportunities to learn to love the *im*perfect, the runny-nosed, and the just plain obnoxious. The story of a Lord who welcomed little children (along with the sick and women and sinners and all others who did not measure up) is a resource foı that sort of uncalculating nurturance that can love the child who is there, that would and should insist on the support of others to enable that child to live and—within the limits of his condition and the world's fallenness—to flourish. Infant Doe's groans awaited not only "the redemption of our bodies" but "our adoption as sons." Parental nurturance formed and informed by the story of Jesus and the children would think it curious—at best—to be told that it was *optional* to do the surgery necessary for the child's life and flourishing, as though one has a choice whether to attend to those things necessary for one's child's life and flourishing or to neglect and starve one's child.

The fundamental point is this: although the parents were, by all accounts, compassionate individuals, love is *not* all you need—no matter what popular songs and popular preaching may tell us. Compassion exercised outside the moral tradition of parenting is quite capable of pitying and killing ("mercy-killing," some would call it) those who do not measure up to the perfection we want for and from our children. Joseph Fletcher—whom no one may accuse of not emphasizing love enough—has (in spite of himself) at least one moral rule: "No unwanted child should ever be born." Compassion by itself may be quite capable of formulating another rule: "No unwanted child need be fed."

The Indiana judges were properly hesitant to intervene in the private arena of medical and parental decisions about the appropriate care of "defective neonates" (a neologism to help us forget that it is our children we are talking about). As we have observed, the decision not to treat is sometimes perfectly legitimate and sometimes legitimately controverted. In such cases that decision is best left to the parents and to the advice of physicians. The decision not to treat Infant Doe, however, was immoral; yet the court did not have the resources to call it illegal.

In part the court could not judge the decision illegal because of the simple lack of law governing such cases. But it is also true that the predominant legal theory today, quite self-consciously impartial and rational, emphasizes autonomy and privacy and contract in ways which make it difficult to give legal support to the interdependencies of a family or to the moral traditions of certain roles in which there is no formal contract. I do not deny the moral importance of this legal theory or the pluralism it sponsors and sustains, but I do claim that it can give only a minimal account of the moral life, and also that society and the courts dangerously distort the moral life and endanger our life together when they reduce morality to such legality.

The courts might still have intervened in the case of Infant Doe if not for our confusion about the rights of the retarded and the otherwise handicapped and the rights of others to be free from contact with them. On the one hand, there is physical evidence everywhere—ramps, special bathrooms, barrier-free doorways—of legislation to integrate the handicapped into our social life. On the other hand, many such people remain segregated in institutions acknowledged to be inhumane; and in fact a 1981 Supreme Court decision, *Pennhurst v. Haldemann,* overturned a state court's order to close one such institution and to establish smaller facilities integrated into the state's residential communities.

Integration versus segregation, the rights of a minority versus the rights of a majority not to be confronted with them—it all has a dismally familiar ring. In the case of Infant Doe and others like him, integration would entail welcoming their life without celebrating or romanticizing their condition. It would mean recognizing their right to equal treatment by the law and by medicine. It would mean acknowledging that even if we call them "defective neonates" they remain our children and that attempts to cut off emotional and role relations with them are self-deceptive. And it would mean a willingness to pay the additional taxes necessary to support the care and nurturance of such children. Segregation, on the other hand, would mean a refusal to practice hospitality toward them or toward their lives, seceding from the obligations of community with them, and asserting our independence from them. The duly humble decision of the justices not to rule in the case is understandable in terms of the segregationist position, and—however unwittingly—it strengthened that tradition for the future.

The Christian story—including the story of Jesus and the children—would support and sustain a tradition of including and welcoming society's outcasts, of serving and helping those who are last. If we keep telling the story of Jesus we may yet learn and live a life of joyful acceptance of people, including little people, who in other stories and other views don't count for much.

A competent physician, compassionate parents, and humble justices failed to make the right decision. The problem was not that the decision was extraordinarily difficult, a real moral dilemma. The problem was not that these people were mean-spirited or evil. The problem was rather that they had—however unwittingly or unconsciously—accepted the wrong models of medicine and parenting and relations with the handicapped. This is not altogether their fault: the traditions of caring and nurture and respect are fragile in contemporary culture. But those traditions have not completely broken down. Witness the statement of the pediatrician, "As a father and physician I can't make the decision to let the baby die." Witness the response of the nurses. Witness the offers to adopt Infant Doe.

Yet the traditions are weak. Babies are not even as fragile as the moral traditions that protect them. And the courts are apparently powerless to preserve these traditions. Infant Doe and all of us are dependent on moral traditions and communities, on covenants which can neither be reduced to contracts nor rendered legally enforceable means to legally enforceable ends.

Infant Doe now rests in peace. The sleep of many others is still disturbed by thoughts of his brief but real suffering and his calculated death. To judge these parents or these physicians will not ease our restlessness. But to resist the erosion of some ancient traditions about medicine and parenting and to establish a tradition of including the handicapped in our community is today part of our Christian vocation and our cultural mandate. Christians can, sometimes do, and should preserve and cherish a tradition about medicine that gives to doctors the worthy calling of healer, not the demeaning role of hired hand to do a consumer's bidding. Christians can, sometimes do, and should preserve and cherish a tradition about the family that gives parents the vocation of uncalculating nurturance and rescues them from the impossible obligation of making their children either perfect or "happy." Christians can, sometimes do, and should welcome and include those whom it is too much our impulse to shun and neglect.

Such medicine and such families and such a community may not always be "happy," but they will always be capable of being surprised by joy in caring for one they cannot cure. They will learn to tell and live a story of Jesus and the neonate. And when the groanings of all creation cease, they may hear, "As you did it to one of the least of these my brethren, you did it unto me."

78. Selective Nontreatment of Defective Newborns: An Ethical Analysis

PAUL R. JOHNSON

In the Oct. 25, 1973 issue of the *New England Journal of Medicine* Raymond Duff and A. G. M. Campbell reported on 299 deaths in the special-care nursery of the Yale-New Haven Hospital from January, 1970 through June, 1972. Of this number, 43, or 14%, were the result of withholding treatment.[1] The report brought public attention and analysis to procedures which previously had been practiced quietly, inconsistently, and not always with careful rationale. In the intervening years, the topic of selective nontreatment of defective newborns has been receiving increased popular and professional attention. The issues raised by this subject are manifold. Answers remain ambiguous, in part because the questions are so new and are not themselves yet clearly formulated. Nonetheless, three issues come forward for special consideration: basic assumptions concerning human life, ethical analysis and formulation, and methods of implementation of policy developed.

Assumptions

Confrontation with death forces concern with life and its meaning. Thus, in the matter of selective nontreatment of defective newborns, we are compelled to bring to conscious examination our basic assumptions about human life. The ethical analysis which follows is built on four premises.

First, defective newborns are human beings. Those who, like Joseph Fletcher in his statements on the topics,[2] formulate their discussion around the "humanhood" of the neonate, obscure matters and intensify visceral rather than rational response by abusing the normal sense of words. The neonate can be no other kind of being than human. The discussion is more properly set in terms of the "personhood" of this human life, the quality or potential quality of this

Reprinted with permission from *Linacre Quarterly,* vol. 47 (February 1980), pp. 39-53. 850 Elm Grove Road, Elm Grove, WI 53122. Subscription rate: $20 per year; $5 per single issue.

human life.[3] This distinction is no mere semantic quibble, for while the designation of defective newborns as human does not lead us directly to clear decisions on appropriate treatment, acknowledgement of the humanity of the neonate prevents us from dismissing the infant with little reflection. Human beings merit respect. The obligation to respect requires that careful moral deliberation takes place.

Secondly, human beings have value. Thus, the defective newborn is of value. In the discussion of the possibility of selective nontreatment, there is no necessary implication that such infants are of lesser or no value compared with other newborns. To recognize the value of the neonate is to assert its fundamental worth and indicate a preference for its protection. But once again, the recognition of value does not itself dictate which decisions are to be made with regard to the object of value. Values exist within a context of interrelated values, sometimes subordinate, sometimes superior, sometimes supplementary, sometimes competitive. Thus one is led to ask, valuable in relation to what? This points to my third premise.

Life is valued in relation to the attainment and exercise of other values. Richard McCormick quotes a 1957 statement of Pope Pius XII regarding the moral obligation to use ordinary means of life preservation: "A more strict obligation would be too burdensome for most men and would render the attainment of the higher, more important good too difficult. Life, death, all temporal activities are in fact subordinated to spiritual ends."[4] McCormick proceeds to argue—correctly, I think—that this means that life is valuable in its relation to higher values, in particular to the values of human relationships and relation to the transcendent, through relation to neighbor. On another occasion, McCormick carries his analysis further. We often confuse two meanings of the term "life," he points out. We may mean either "the existence of vital and metabolic processes" or a state of or potential human personhood. The former is not valued for its own sake, but as a foundation for the latter.[5] To argue to the contrary that the "basic" value of biological life must always take precedence over considerations of "higher values" of personal life is to risk collapsing the wholistic view of man in which both physicality and spirituality are integral to personhood. In analysis of decisions regarding the treatment or nontreatment of defective newborns, therefore, life must be viewed within a wider constellation of personal human values.

Fourth, just as reductionistic vitalism is questioned by an understanding of human being which places highest emphasis on a network of personal values, so death itself is relativized by the religious perspective. Death, as biological cessation, is not the Ultimate Enemy. Because death is not the final negation, it cannot be reified into a demonic god who is to be avoided at all costs. This has long been recognized in the honoring of sacrifices for higher principles and loyalties. In recent years we have seen increasing acceptance of death as a natural and, at times, suitable part of life. Despite some demur about "the indignity of death with dignity,"[6] most theologians and philosophers, as well as psychological therapists, have seen the contemporary openness to acceptance of death as a good and appropriate human attitude. Acceptance of one's own death as appropriate appears in the current literature of counseling the dying as a legitimate goal of personal adjustment for the terminally ill person. Acceptance of the appropriateness of the death of another is also proposed when, for such reasons as discussed below, prolongation of the life of the other is seen as meaningless. Thus, the death of defective newborns cannot, *a priori,* be rejected as an absolute evil.

Paul Ramsey has argued that, viewed religiously, life is a gift and a trust. Thus it is immoral, he claims, to choose death as an end. One may allow death and choose how to live while dying, but should not opt directly for death.[7] His point should be kept in mind. It reminds us, as will be developed below, that western religious ethics has a bias toward life. Though the conclusions of this essay differ from those of Ramsey, acceptance of death, as described here, is neither refusal of a gift nor violation of a trust. It is a recognition that gifts and trusts are to be acted on responsibly. In the ethical analysis which follows, the nature of this responsibility will be outlined.

Ethical Analysis

Basic to the humanistic ethical analysis which is rooted in the western religious heritage is a bias toward life. While death is not necessarily to be thought of fearfully, life is not to be considered lightly. Human life in all its personal qualities is a value to be maintained. It is to be given up only in carefully considered situations and for proportionate reasons. Like Ramsey, Leonard Weber proposes an ethical viewpoint from which life is viewed as a gift: "When life is viewed as a gift . . . there are limits to what one may do to it and with it. To see life as a gift . . . means to have an attitude of acceptance and protection rather than of control."[8] This gift analogy, provided it does not lead to a hesitance to question or make decisions regarding experiences which come to us,[9] provides a useful perspective. Appreciation and cultivation rather than rejection are responses appropriate to gifts. Thus, a bias toward life is a natural corollary of a world view which recognizes the world and human existence as, in a general sense, a gracious bestowal.

Two implications follow from this bias toward life. First, care should be taken that if we err in judgment with regard to selective nontreatment, we err on the side of life. We cannot avoid decisions; and error is an unavoidable part of human decision-making. But we can develop guidelines to fault, when necessary, in conservation of life. A second implication, one to which we shall return later, is that commitment to life logically should entail commitment to provision of means to support and enhance life. As a society we are committing ourselves to the preservation of lives of neonates who, under past circumstances, would have died. We are doing so by furnishing increasingly sophisticated neonatal intensive care and other advanced forms of lifegiving therapy. It is reasonable to assert, however, that to give only existence to defective newborns, without provision for necessary life-long maintenance and life enhancement, is only a partial commitment to life.

Because the choice between maintaining or letting go the lives of defective newborns is of relatively recent origin, moralists have found it difficult to establish specific ethical criteria by which to guide decisions. Assistance has been found, however, in a tradition which has been developed to deal with a closely related issue. This is the traditional distinction between ordinary and extraordinary or heroic means of life preservation. Widely accepted by physicians and philosopher-theologians alike, this distinction provides guidance as to which actions are morally mandatory (ordinary means) and which are elective (heroic means). Although the content of these two designations is not without some ambiguity,[10] most would use a person-centered rather than procedure-centered definition. According to the person-centered approach, two characteristics are central to declaring a proposed means heroic and therefore elective: 1) lack of benefit, and 2) excessive personal or social burden accompanying the attainment or use of these means.[11]

In his *Ethics at the Edges of Life,* Ramsey argues that, at least in relation to the dying, the ordinary-extraordinary analysis can and in most cases should be reduced to a "medical indications" policy.[12] He concludes that the first characteristic just cited, lack of benefit, is sufficient as a criterion of judgment. When treatment is no longer medically indicated, i.e., beneficial, it may be ceased. One may choose to live until death without this superfluous treatment. Even where death is not imminent and some might talk about a patient's right to refuse treatment, Ramsey prefers to avoid the ordinary-heroic terminology in favor of a medical indications approach. He sees referring the decision-maker to objective elements in the context of the decision to be made as the prime value in not entirely jettisoning the terminology.

Though medical indications, as Ramsey defines them, are integral to the analysis which follows, especially at the first level of applying the ordinary-extraordinary distinction, it is too narrow a base for the topic as described here. This is seen even in Ramsey's presentation. He recognizes some right to refuse treatment by conscious persons not imminently dying. He acknowledges in this regard that the traditional ordinary-heroic distinction has been applied to those persons "whose lives could not be *meaningfully* prolonged. . . . "[13] Further, to speak as Ramsey does of the possibility of refusing "life-prolonging" as contrasted with "life-saving" treatment when no more "curative" treatment is indicated does not avoid the quality of life considerations he obviously wishes to turn aside. Life quality factors are surely a part of life-prolongation decisions, and unless "cure" means only thorough or substantial recovery, such considerations may be part of the definition here as well. Finally, it is not entirely accurate to call a medical indications policy solely a *medical* indications policy. Strictly speaking, there is medical benefit to treatment which, though it cannot cure, can extend life even briefly. To choose, in one's way of dying, to refuse such treatment is to do so not because it lacks benefit, but because it lacks *sufficient* benefit. This matter of *sufficient* benefit opens the door once again to indications which are not strictly medical. Ramsey's argument cautions us to define terms carefully. But the traditional ordinary-extraordinary categories are still useful in consideration of the topic at hand and can be followed as proposed below.

Ordinary-Heroic Distinction

The traditional context for the application of the ordinary-heroic distinction differs in some ways from the problem faced by those considering treatment of newborns. The guidelines have been developed to assist judgment regarding persons both seriously and terminally ill. They have come to be applied to those imminently approaching death. Though this may be true of some defective newborns, it is not always so. Procedures, sometimes sophisticated, sometimes rather common, which reverse or significantly postpone drawing near to death, can often be carried out. But the question may be raised as to whether the procedures *should* be employed. Thus, the question with defective neonates is not *can* death be postponed without significant burden, but *should* it be? Can the ordinary-extraordinary distinction be useful as a moral guide in that question? The answer appears to be yes, with varying degrees of precision and certitude, at three levels.

At one level the analysis can be applied directly in a more traditional form. Some infants may be born with such extreme physical defectiveness that death is imminent. Any procedures of life preservation followed would simply be a matter of prolongation of dying, rather than restoration to living. In such situations, treatment would clearly fall under the category of heroic, and therefore elective, means. Ramsey's identification of extraordinary with "not medically indicated" would be most applicable here. The "benefit" of such treatment is negligible. Selective nontreatment of newborns in that context would generally be morally acceptable.[14]

The ordinary-extraordinary reasoning can be extended to a second level, suggested by Leonard Weber. He raises the questions: when does the *treatment* of an infant impose an excessive burden on the child? on the family? on society? When possible benefit to the infant can be obtained only by means in which the burden imposed by the treatment becomes excessive, he argues, such means may morally be omitted.[15] Applied to the child, this would appear to mean that when the treatment itself brings extended subjection to pain beyond that of the underlying condition, or so concentrates all energies on the sheer struggle to survive that personal qualities are minimized, or would result in severe treatment-induced disability or disease,[16] such treatment may not necessarily be mandated.

This application is more difficult to use in the case of a possible burden imposed by the treatment on family or society. Weber himself recognizes this and is certain that in many instances the family could be, at least in part, relieved of the burden by external assistance and support. He also sees little likelihood of society being totally bereft of resources. Such considerations have led David Smith to come to an almost total prohibition of selective nontreatment when family or social burden is the prime factor of deliberation.[17] Nonetheless, given the lack of accessibility to sufficient assistance to all families and given the competition for scarce monetary and manpower resources in society, the application of the principle under consideration cannot be absolutely set aside. Severe strain and dislocation can be brought on families. And minimal provision of resources may not be sufficient to assure extensive and adequate care. This concern with the burden on family and society is important not so much with a view to its effect on them, but insofar as it reflexively creates a burden on the infant as well. Thus, concern with the effect of treatment can properly be considered in the case of the neonate, the family, and society. The further one proceeds from the immediate burden placed on the infant, however, the more caution is called for.

The third level of application of the ordinary-extraordinary moral reasoning is the most problematic in current discussion. It is at this level that the most obvious questions of "quality of life" arise. Unlike the second level, at which the *procedures* of life preservation are questioned, it is the *quality of life* itself which is at issue here. Weber, who avoids committing himself to the quality of life ethic, notes the difficulty of dismissing the issue. His answer, as we have seen, is to focus on the treatment rather than the underlying condition. Yet clearly it is the negative quality of life to which the treatment leads that causes him to admit such procedures as non-obligatory.

Ramsey's preference for a medical indications policy for treatment of the dying is in part based on his suspicion of quality of life judgments. This is amplified when he distinguishes between the dying and those who are perhaps incurable but not yet terminal. "Sometimes . . . infants are not born dying. They are only born defective and in need of help."[18] As pointed out above, one of the implications of a life-biased ethic is the obligation to provide such help. But one needs to consider the possibility that not all help will be helpful. Ramsey acknowledges this in the case of "non-curative" treatment of the dying. He also considers the possibility of the "exception" of those who are inaccessible to care, in states in which "care cannot be conveyed."[19] Perhaps to such possibilities there needs to be added another—the infant who, through treatment, could be kept from imminent death but whose life quality is so minimal that it renders "help" not helpful and therefore extraordinary.

The argument of Richard McCormick is helpful.[20] He proposes a line of thought which sees quality of life judgments as an appropriate implication of traditional ordinary-heroic moral analysis. Examining past applications of this tradition, he finds that the *type* of life a person would have to live was often determinative of whether certain actions were morally obligatory or not. He argues further that the moral tradition within which the ordinary-extraordinary analysis is set assumes that biological life "is a value to be preserved precisely as a condition for other values, and therefore insofar as these other values remain attainable."[21] It is the quality of life which finally renders means ordinary or heroic. Discussion of selective nontreatment must therefore take this issue under serious review.

Quality of Life Considerations

Recognizing the need for quality of life considerations is far easier, however, than actually providing specific content to that formal criterion. Attempts at definition have varied. Joseph Fletcher's 15 positive human criteria build out from neo-cortical functioning to include such variables as minimal intelligence, a sense of time, concern for others, curiosity, and idiosyncrasy.[22] James Nelson points to socialness, capacity to experience limitation and freedom, and religiosity or intentionality.[23] Michael Tooley focuses on self-consciousness.[24] The debate among these moralists and others indicates the need to proceed with caution in this matter.

The line of reasoning proposed by McCormick provides such a cautious but useful starting point. As seen earlier, McCormick places special emphasis on relational potential. Life is a good insofar as it affords access to higher goods, in particular to the goods of social relatedness and relationship to the transcendent through relationship to neighbor. Thus, this relational potential would be the touchstone of quality of life judgments. McCormick argues, "It is neither inhuman nor unchristian to say that there comes a point where an individual's condition itself represents the negation of any truly human—i.e., relational—potential. When that point is reached, is not the best treatment no treatment?" He answers his own question: "When in human judgment this potential is totally absent or would be, because of the condition of the individual, totally subordinated to the mere effort for survival, that life can be said to have achieved its potential."[25]

Absence of minimal relational potential could probably be ascribed to the anencephalic neonate. Such infants currently cannot ultimately be kept from dying. Should technical means beyond those now available be developed which would sustain their lives, indefinitely or for an extended period of time, these newborns would be rather clear cases of appropriate candidates for nontreatment. On the other hand, as Gustafson argues,[26] it is the capacity for relationship that is one of the strong reasons for the life preservation of Down's Syndrome infants. The judgment for other infants is not so clear. Early diagnosis and, even more so, prognosis[27] are difficult. Moralists can point to the criteria. Medical and psychological science will have to help fill out these criteria with specificity. Individual decisions will be made with risk, but cannot be avoided. Caution and courage are called for.

It may be more difficult yet to determine when the condition of the individual subordinates all else to "the mere effort for survival" and thereby minimizes the capacity for relationship. Constant severe pain, incapacitating response to treatment, or enduring nonconsciousness may be elements of such a condition. Some moralists have drawn upon the established maxim of medical ethics *primum non nocere* (first do no harm) in this context. H. Tristram Engelhardt, Jr., for example, proposes the concept of "the injury of continued existence" to apply where conditions of continuing life would not be tolerable.[28] In the same fashion, participants in a conference sponsored by the University of California, San Francisco, included as one ethical proposition of their moral policy, "Life-preserving intervention should be understood as doing harm to an infant who cannot survive infancy, or will live in intractable pain, or cannot participate even minimally in human experience."[29]

The interaction of human potential and the level of care and support provided are demonstrated in prognosis of the infant's future relational ability within the context of subordinating all else to the effort for survival. Relational potential may be kept at a low level if initial and life-long support is not adequate. This fact in turn directs us toward a closer look at the inference drawn earlier from the ideal of "bias toward life." Commitment to life logically entails commitment to provision of means to support and enhance life. Our assessment of quality of life potential is based in part on our expectation of benefits from treatment we are willing or able to provide. John A. Robertson points out that the low quality of life expectation of some defective newborns is due to the absence of provision made by society to bring these children to their fullest capability. This lack of provision, which is "the fault of social attitudes and the failings of healthy persons," rather than congenital defectiveness in the infants alone, is often a subtle factor in the judgment that the neonate has little potential.[30]

Two implications can be drawn from these observations. First, in following out the bias toward life, we must be assured that those whom we keep alive are given full opportunity to maximize their potential. Continuing research and development in neonatal, pediatric, and adult medical care of persons with defects should be supplemented with provision of extensive social support services. If children are now kept alive who would previously have died, we are obliged to help them achieve their highest quality of life. Families who care for these children need the assistance of such services as special education, physical therapies, and family counseling. Financial relief and respite care may be necessary. Institutions for raising such children need to be fully funded and staffed so as to be compassionate rather than custodial care. It is not fair to the newborn to choose a life he would not otherwise have to suffer and not choose to allocate the resources to make that life livable.[31]

Thus, a second implication which could be suggested is that some possible criticism of selective nontreatment is unjustified unless we provide the personal life enhancement to follow the biological life preservation. The more we provide for life support and enhancement, the less appropriate will selective nontreatment be. The converse may also be true. The less often means of increasing life quality are made available, the more choices not to maintain life may be justified. While ethical and/or medical decisions ought not simply reflect current structures of social justice, neither ought they be made without any reference to them. Recognizing that financial and personnel resources are not inexhaustible, allocation decisions will have to be made and consequences faced honestly.

We have seen, then, that life-biased ethics will incline us toward caution in judgment about selective nontreatment and that it urges us to expand life-enhancing services, thus increasing the number of neonates for whom a life preservation decision is appropriate. Recognizing that avoidance of death is not always the most suitable stance, we have found help in decision-making in the tradition of the ordinary-extraordinary means analysis. This has led us to see that selective nontreatment may be a moral decision when dying is irreversibly proximate, when the means of life maintenance themselves create excessive burden, and when relational potential is negligible or unable to be exercised.

Implementation

Although a complete analysis is beyond the scope of this essay, directions of thought regarding implementation of the foregoing moral analysis are offered. Issues are complex here, especially in light of excesses which are to be avoided. Two major concerns come to mind: Who is to make the decision? What legal status should such decisions have?

There is little moral or legal question over the necessity or propriety of proxy consent in the treatment of defective newborns. Paul Ramsey has recently focused attention, however, on the parameters of the acceptable range of decisions to be made as he questions the criteria used in the deliberation process. He states that both covenant loyalty to others and familial, medical, and legal obligations "require that a medical indications policy alone be applied where another, voiceless, human life is at stake."[32] To do otherwise, he argues, is to open the door to quality of life judgments, to risk circularity of reasoning in the "reasonable man" approach to proxy consent, and to chance ascribing rather than discovering the best interest of the patient. Although the caution which prompts Ramsey's concern must not be set aside, we have already seen that criteria other than medical indications might morally be applied. Thus, we must cautiously enter the domain of substituted judgment.

There are at least four possible loci of decision-making: the parents, the physician, a review committee, and the courts. Each has its benefits and drawbacks. Each does, in fact, have a role to play, but the preponderance of opinion among moralists has given priority to parents. Parents, of course, do not *own* their children. They are not free morally or legally to do whatever they wish with their children. Weber correctly observes that "it is better to speak of the obligations rather than the rights of parents." Where obligation lies, there lies also a degree of priority in decision-making. "They have the obligation to care for their children and the obligation to make decisions that seriously affect the future of their children."[33] The relationship of decision and nurturing can also be noted here. Engelhardt points out that "the decisions in these matters correctly lie in the hands of the parents, because it is primarily in terms of family that children exist and develop. . . . "[34] Both the general obligation of parents to children and their specific role in nurturing direct us to the parents as having primary claim on the role of decision-maker.

Although at an earlier point in the development of neonatal medicine, the press of very limited time often forced physicians into the decision-making role, modern procedures make this decreasingly true. This being so, Daniel Maguire argues that the doctor may be an inappropriate person to be given a primary role in decisions due to such factors as traditional professional roles, the trend toward mixing experimentation and care, lack of specific ethical training, and fear of legal complications.[35] The physician does, however, have medical information necessary to make an informed decision. Facts about the infant's current status and probabilities regarding future developments must be shared with the parents. Thus, the first role of the doctor in this process is as a source of information.[36]

A hospital review committee, made up of institutional personnel, possibly including community representatives, has the disadvantages of emotional abstraction and the compromise nature of decision-by-committee. Such a committee, nevertheless, might play a useful role in establishing general hospital guidelines within which parents and physicians could work. Similarly, the courts represent the wider interests of society. Not always equipped to be the first voice of decision, the courts play a role in appeal of decisions at a lower level. However, if other courts follow the recent decision of the Massachusetts Supreme Judicial Court in the case of Joseph Saikewicz,[37] they will play a more central role than proposed here. Some ambiguity remains about the exact implications of the Saikewicz decision, but it did intend to claim to the court's jurisdiction primary decision-making prerogative in at least certain nontreatment contexts. Although it now appears to include fewer cases than first feared by many physicians and ethicists,[38] this ruling will result in more decisions in the courts. The more this is restricted to conflict of judgment situations mentioned below, the less will the court involve itself in actions outside its special competence.

Thus we return to the parents as primary locus of decision. Some argue that the emotional involvement of parents makes them unfit for decision. Deliberation would be swayed by rejection of the infant, growing out of shock or disappointment,[39] or by need to compensate due to feelings of guilt. Studies are mixed on this matter. While some show the danger does exist, others have shown it can be less of a problem than anticipated. Raymond Duff has observed that "if families regardless of background are heard sympathetically and at length and are given information and answers to their questions in words they understand, the problems of their children as well as the expected benefits and limits of any proposed care can be understood clearly in practically all instances."[40] Duff found the parental decisions to have been thoughtful and reasonable. Rosalyn Darling also found data suggesting that parents can be responsible in their judgments. Her study showed that though many parents admitted disappointment, the typical attitude came to be "realistic acceptance." In fact, she found physicians to define the situation as a tragedy more often than parents.[41] Considering this possibility for careful and thoughtful decision-making by parents and noting that parental reaction may be correlated with the nature of the defect and options of community support perceived to be available,[42] we recall the point made earlier. If we as a society wish to establish a bias toward life, we must also make commitments to provision of support and enrichment resources.

Priority in the decision-making process and the generally responsible action of parents would not, of course, guarantee that choices will always be correct. Here is the second point at which physicians and society, through review committees or the courts, may play an important role. We have seen their role in provision of information and guidelines. Here the issue is intervention. When the parents' decision can reasonably be construed as acceptable, no steps should be taken to counter that choice. Three points of intervention may be appropriate, however: one opposing nontreatment, two pursuing it. Engelhardt argues that "society has a right to intervene and protect children for whom parents refuse care . . . when such care does not constitute a severe burden and when it is likely that the child can be brought to good quality of life."[43] Engelhardt views such intervention as necessary both for the sake of the specific child and with the social impact in mind that selective nontreatment in such cases could have in undermining respect and care for children in a more general sense. The link between intervention and responsibility for nurturing should be called to mind. To overrule the parents' decision may require us to provide them with counseling and community support to help them fulfill the role we are asking of them. Or we must make available adequate institutional care for children whose parents cannot or will not raise them. To intervene without such provision is unfair both to parents and children.

To intervene in favor of nontreatment may be more difficult to justify, given the recognition of parental obligation to protect and care for their children and covenantal moral and legal obligations to continue care once it is begun. Two possibilities for such intervention have been suggested and should at least be mentioned. Engelhardt proposes that a challenge to the decision to continue treatment might be appropriate where extended life for the infant would lead to enduring pain, etc., which has been lightly considered by the parents.[44] This circumstance would seem rare. Also possible is the situation brought about by the problem of allocation of scarce resources. One of the propositions put forward by the Sonoma Conference states: "In cases of limited availability of neonatal intensive care, it is ethical to terminate therapy for an infant with poor prognosis in order to provide care for an infant with a much better prognosis."[45] Such a stance is not above moral challenge.[46] We have noted above the general acceptance of the principles of parental obligation to care and the covenantal obligation of care which has begun. Applied to the situation under consideration, this would seem to mean that intervention in favor of nontreatment in such cases will probably also be infrequent. While intervention in favor of nontreatment cannot be excluded out of hand, challenge against nontreatment is more easily justified and would no doubt be the more common.

A thorough and clear legal review of selective

nontreatment of defective newborns has been provided by John Robertson[47] and will not be treated extensively here. A few remarks will suffice. Direct, active taking of the life of the newborn (*not* under consideration in this essay) is clearly defined legally as murder. But participants in selective nontreatment, family or medical personnel, could also be held criminally liable, for charges ranging from homicide to neglect to violation of child abuse laws. Although prosecution has been rare and conviction even more so, there is no assurance that it will always be so. The spotlight thrown by more public discussion of this issue may encourage legal action. With increased legal action or without it, the threat of prosecution may inhibit parents and medical personnel in their decision-making. These deliberations are difficult to carry out apart from legal considerations which affect them. If we accept as moral the decision for selective nontreatment, we must allow those who make the decisions to do so without excessive fear of the law.

Carte blanche in decision-making is neither legally nor morally acceptable. Drafting of clear and useful legislation has not moved far with regard to other contexts of decisions to allow death. There is no reason to believe it will prove easier with regard to newborns. Some argue that any legislation would prove restrictive to decisions currently made quietly in the absence of specific law. This overlooks the possible prosecution under existing law and the effect on decision-making of fear of this possible legal action, but it does caution us to proceed carefully in this matter. Two suggestions are in order. First, laws which *permit* rather than *mandate* decisions are preferable. This would maintain respect for a bias toward life, avoid the spectre of assigning certain infants to death, and still allow for decisions that should be made. Second, legislation and the courts can look after the processes by which decisions are made to assure that full deliberation has taken place.[48] To involve the courts in all initial deliberations would be cumbersome, time-consuming, and counterproductive to the process being pursued. Development of fair yet cautious laws will not be necessary. But as Duff and Campbell urged in their 1973 article, "If working out these dilemmas . . . is a violation of the law, we believe the law should be changed."[49]

Conclusion

Each year parents, physicians, and courts are facing questions of treatment or nontreatment of defective newborns. Developing ethical reflection, changing medical possibilities, and increasing court rulings render the decision-making process, already painful and difficult for those involved, even more complicated. Against the background of personal anguish and perplexing deliberation for those who must come to the point of decision, continued effort must go into ethical analysis and policy formulation.

Notes

1. Duff, Raymond S. and Campbell, A. G. M., "Moral and Ethical Dilemmas in the Special-Care Nursery," *New England Journal of Medicine,* 289 (Oct., 1973), pp. 890-894.

2. Fletcher, Joseph, "Indicators of Humanhood: A Tentative Profile of Man," *Hastings Center Report,* II (Nov., 1972), pp. 1-4. See also his "Four Indicators of Humanhood—The Enquiry Matures," *ibid.,* IV (Dec., 1974), pp. 4-7.

3. Cahill, Lisa S., "Correspondence," *ibid.,* V (April, 1975), p. 4; James Nelson, *Human Medicine* (Minneapolis: Augsburg, 1973), pp. 17-27.

4. McCormick, Richard, "To Save or Let Die: The Dilemma of Modern Medicine," *Journal of the American Medical Association,* 229 (July 8, 1974), p. 174.

5. McCormick, Richard, "The Quality of Life, The Sanctity of Life," *Hastings Center Report,* VIII (Feb., 1978), pp. 34-35.

6. Ramsey, Paul, "The Indignity of Death with Dignity," *Hastings Center Studies,* II (May, 1974), pp. 47-62.

7. Ramsey, Paul, *Ethics at the Edges of Life: Medical and Legal Intersections* (New Haven: Yale University Press, 1978), pp. 146-148. As will be evident, Ramsey's line of thought is different than that taken in this essay. His position, argued in this volume, is an important counter statement to the one proposed here. Though I shall refer to a couple of his central ideas, his whole analysis merits the attention of the interested reader. See especially chapters 4-6 of *Ethics at the Edges of Life.*

8. Weber, Leonard, *Who Shall Live? The Dilemma of Severely Handicapped Children and Its Meaning for Other Moral Questions* (New York: Paulist Press, 1976), p. 40.

9. See, for example, Stanley Hauerwas's overextension of this analogy in his chapter "Having and Learning to Care for Retarded Children" in his *Truthfulness and Tragedy* (Notre Dame: University of Notre Dame Press, 1977), pp. 147-156. Hauerwas moderates his position somewhat in later chapters.

10. Ramsey, Paul, *The Patient as Person* (New Haven: Yale University Press, 1970), pp. 118-124; Daniel Maguire, *Death by Choice* (New York: Schocken, 1970), pp. 122-125.

11. Examples of the breadth of application of such criteria by traditional moralists are found in Charles J. McFadden, *Medical Ethics,* 6th ed. (Philadelphia: F. A. Davis Co., 1967), pp. 239-261.

12. Ramsey, *Edges,* pp. 153-160.

13. *Ibid.,* p. 155; emphasis mine. Application to nonconscious persons will be discussed below.

14. Hauerwas, *Truthfulness and Tragedy,* p. 178; Weber, *Who Shall Live?* pp. 90-91.

15. *Ibid.,* pp. 90-98.

16. Jonsen, Albert R. and Lester, George, "Newborn Intensive Care: The Ethical Problems," *Hastings Center Report,* VIII (Feb., 1978), p. 16.

17. Smith, David H., "On Letting Some Babies Die," *Hastings Center Studies,* II (May, 1974), pp. 37-46.

18. Ramsey, *Edges,* p. 194.

19. *Ibid.,* pp. 214-217; Ramsey, *Patient as Person,* pp. 161-162.

20. McCormick, "To Save or Let Die," pp. 172-176.

21. *Ibid.,* p. 175. McCormick's interpretation and application of Pope Pius XII's teaching in this regard (see above under "Assumptions") has not gone unchallenged. See, for example, Ramsey, *Edges,* pp. 172-173, footnote 33.

22. Fletcher, "Indicators of Humanhood"; "Four Indicators."

23. Nelson, *Human Medicine,* pp. 19-24.

24. Tooley, Michael, "Abortion and Infanticide," *Moral Problems in Medicine,* ed. by Samuel Gorovitz *et al.* (Englewood Cliffs: Prentice-Hall, 1976), pp. 297-317.

25. McCormick, "To Save or Let Die," p. 175.

26. Gustafson, James, "Mongolism, Parental Desires, and the Right to Life," *Perspectives in Biology and Medicine,* XVI (Summer, 1973), p. 550.

27. Jonsen and Lester, "Newborn Intensive Care," p. 17; Jane V. Hunt, "Mental Development and the Survivors of Neonatal Intensive Care," *Ethics of Newborn Intensive Care,* ed. by Albert R. Jonsen and Michael J. Garland (Berkeley: Institute of Government Studies, 1976), pp. 47-52; Robert Veatch, "The Technical Criteria Fallacy," *Hastings Center Report,* VII (Aug., 1977), pp. 15-16.

28. Engelhardt, H. Tristram, Jr., "Ethical Issues in Aiding the Death of Young Children," *Beneficent Euthanasia,* Marvin Kohl, ed. (Buffalo: Prometheus Books, 1975), pp. 180-192.

29. Jonsen, A. R., *et al.,* "Critical Issues in Newborn Intensive Care: A Conference Report and Policy Proposal," *Pediatrics,* LV (June, 1975), p. 760. See also Albert R. Jonsen and Michael J. Garland, "A Moral Policy for Life/Death Decisions in the Intensive Care Nursery," *Ethics of Newborn Intensive Care, op. cit.,* pp. 147-149. This application of the "do no harm" principle is recent and has not met universal acceptance. See Ramsey, *Edges,* pp. 239-241.

30. Robertson, John A., "Involuntary Euthanasia of Defective Newborns: A Legal Analysis," *Stanford Law Review,* XXVII (Jan., 1975), pp. 252-255.

31. This implication is not to be interpreted as the general demand for social justice, the case for which can be made on other grounds. It is not being argued that every child has as its birthright a fulfilled life in a just society. It is, rather, a call to provide access to a decent minimal level of personal human life for those who without aid would have little opportunity to achieve even that.

32. Ramsey, *Edges,* p. 161; see his full discussion, pp. 160-171. See also his "The Saikewicz Precedent: What's Good for an Incompetent Patient?" *Hastings Center Report,* VIII (Dec., 1978), pp. 36-42.

33. For example, Weber, *Who Shall Live?,* pp. 115-116. See also F. Raymond Marks, "The Defective Newborn: An Analytic Framework for a Policy Dialog," *Ethics of Newborn Intensive Care, op. cit.,* pp. 122-123.

34. Engelhardt, "Ethical Issues," p. 184.

35. Maguire, *Death by Choice,* pp. 177-184.

36. Weber, *Who Shall Live?,* pp. 106-110.

37. Annas, George J., "The Incompetent's Right to Die: The Case of Joseph Saikewicz," *Hastings Center Report,* VIII (Feb., 1978), pp. 21-23.

38. Annas, George J., "After Saikewicz: No-Fault Death," *ibid.,* June, 1978, pp. 16-18; Ramsey, "The Saikewicz Precedent."

39. Fletcher, John, "Attitudes Toward Defective Newborns," *Hastings Center Studies,* II (Jan., 1974), pp. 24-28; Marrianna A. Cohen, "Ethical Issues in Neonatal Care: Familial Concerns," *Ethics of Newborn Intensive Care, op. cit.,* pp. 55-62.

40. Duff and Campbell, "Moral and Ethical Dilemmas," p. 893. See also Beverly Kelsey, "Which Infants Shall Live? Who Should Decide? An Interview with Dr. Raymond S. Duff," *Hastings Center Report,* V (April, 1975), pp. 5-8.

41. Darling, Rosalyn Benjamin, "Parents, Physicians and Spina Bifida," *ibid.,* VII (Aug., 1977), pp. 10-14.

42. Cohen, "Ethical Issues in Neonatal Care," pp. 57-63.

43. Engelhardt, "Ethical Issues," p. 185.

44. *Ibid.*

45. Jonsen, *et al.,* "Critical Issues," p. 761.

46. Childress, James, "Who Shall Live When Not All Can Live?" *Soundings,* LIII (Winter, 1970), pp. 347-354; Ramsey, *Edges,* pp. 232-234.

47. Robertson, "Involuntary Euthanasia," pp. 213-269. A summary can be found in John A. Robertson and Norman Fost, "Passive Euthanasia of Defective Newborn Infants: Legal Considerations," *Journal of Pediatrics,* LXXXVIII (May, 1976), pp. 883-889.

48. *Ibid.,* pp. 888-889.

49. Duff and Campbell, "Moral and Ethical Dilemmas," p. 894.

79.
How Much Should a Child Cost? A Response to Paul Johnson

JAMES BURTCHAELL

Paul Johnson begins his inquiry into the ethics of letting defective infants die by rejecting the position of Joseph Fletcher that they may not, in some instances, be humans at all. In his well-known pieces on "indicators of humanhood" Fletcher has offered a checklist of qualities one might require of a being for him/her/it to qualify (and be protected) as a human: e.g., neocortical function, curiosity, a sense of time, self-awareness. Minimal intelligence, for instance, would be demanded: "Any individual of the species *homo sapiens* who falls below the I.Q. 40-mark in a standard Stanford-Binet test, amplified if you like by other tests, is questionably a person; below the 20-mark, not a person. *Homo* is indeed *sapiens,* in order to be *homo.*"[1] Johnson disagrees. The question, he says, is not whether defective newborns are human children; all live progeny of women and men must be human. The question is, rather, what their relative value as humans might be.

I shall be arguing that the position Johnson takes is considerably more savage even than the barbarities Fletcher espouses.

To reckon the value of a given infant's life, Johnson explains, we must estimate the quality, realized or potential, that this life possesses. A child's value is related to the degree to which he or she can be expected to attain those higher functions which are most characteristic of human personhood and which distinguish humans from lower species of animal life. Since the purpose of human life is not merely biological existence, not simply to metabolize, we must calculate it as valuable to the extent that it attains higher goods, by being actively and fruitfully inter-personal. Relying on Richard McCormick, the distinguished Jesuit moralist, Johnson argues that it is an ability to relate to other humans which is the essential and validating activity for human persons. "McCormick places special emphasis on relational potential. Life is a good insofar as it affords access to higher goods, in particular to the goods of social relatedness and relationship to the transcendent through relationship to neighbor. Thus, this relational potential would be the touchstone of quality of life judgments. McCormick argues, 'It is neither inhuman nor unchristian to say that there comes a point where an individual's condition itself represents the negation of any truly human—i.e., relational—potential. . . . When in human judgment this potential is totally absent or would be, because of the condition of the individual, totally subordinated to the mere effort for survival, that life can be said to have achieved its potential.' "

The problem faced by parents, physicians, public servants and the ethicists who advise them is that the resources and attention needed for the survival of infants can vary greatly. Some seriously defective or damaged or diseased children need therapeutic care well beyond the means of most families, thus bringing a private need into the jurisdiction of public policy. Are we ethically obliged to nurture every infant, whatever the cost, whatever the benefit? Fletcher would relieve us of some burden by declaring some of the most crippled infants to be non-humans. Johnson is anxious to find some way, while insisting that all newborn children are humans, to assess their claims on our care according to some reasonable scale.

He begins by stipulating that all humans have value, and follows this with assurances that we should treat an infant with a "preference for its protection," and that this "bias toward life" should give a newborn the benefit of the doubt when we are deliberating whether he or she should live or be let die. What this seems to mean is that the burden of proof lies, not with the child struggling to live, but with anyone disposed to decide it should die. While this "bias toward life" is perhaps not so ardent that any of us would confidently entrust our own life or health to a medical staff so mildly motivated, it is difficult to quarrel with those who assert at the outset that all human life has value. Yet that is exactly where one needs to take issue, for there is a lethal error at the very threshold of this argument.

So many things can be valuable to us: a week's holiday from work, a loving parent, a collection of books, a garden with lawn and flowers, strong athletic dexterity, a fine education, a full head of hair, a true friend, shoes that do not leak, a symphony concert, an air conditioner. Even social institutions like the state deal in many varied valuables: a park system, peace between nations, secure retirement benefits, prenatal care, stable banking, clean waterways, reliable pharmaceuticals. The thing about valuable things is that they have such different values. Not only are they unequal; they are sometimes incommensurable. How compare the value of a faithful, loving husband to that of a

Reprinted with permission from *Linacre Quarterly,* vol. 47 (February 1980), pp. 54-63. 850 Elm Grove Road, Elm Grove, WI 53122. Subscription rate: $20 per year; $5 per single issue.

legal career . . . or of a second car in the garage? How assess the relative values of full employment and of better railway roadbeds? Or the relative disvalues of juvenile, drug-related crime and a soybean crop failure? How compare the incomparable? Yet we do this all the time, as anyone knows who has deliberated whether to move the family in order to secure a professional promotion, or has sat long on a budget committee.

Dealing with Values

When we deal in values we are treating of "lesser" and "greater" and "different." And yet we can choose among them. It is said that every thing has its price, and that every person can be bought. But the fundamental measure of value is neither money, nor the work that money represents, nor the portion of our life and time and energy given to the work. The basic measure of our value is our own self: how much do I value this thing, this opportunity, this person? What other valued things am I willing to give for it, for her, for him? The medium of barter among valuable things may not always be money, but they all can be and are traded off against one another.

What I mean when I accord you value is that you have a worth for me. Other humans are valued insofar as they serve needs or wants. We possess a calculus whereby to reckon who is worth what. To the scale of other persons' needs I can apply the scale of my own resources, and also the scale of how generously I would yield the resources to meet others' needs, according to how valuable those persons are to me.

The Johnson-McCormick argument on selective withholding of treatment from defective newborn children appears to pivot around what value such treatment might have for the infants themselves. But a close examination of this value-theory discloses that the pivotal value is not internal to the lives and interests of the infants, but what value those children have to others.

Let me try to illustrate this first by comparisons. A short while ago a young orderly in a Swedish home for the elderly was accused of killing a dozen or more of the residents by offering them carbonated drinks laced with corrosive acid. These old people, he later explained, were leading meaningless lives. What did this "meaningless" mean? Was the young man stating that, in his judgment, the relational potential of these old people was now totally used up, or that it had become totally subordinated to the mere effort for survival? Or was he saying simply that they were now more trouble than they were worth? Whatever his drift, he was making a life-and-death judgment that appears to involve three variables: how much care the old people required; how much relational or spiritual activity so much care would make possible, and how dear these persons were to him. For himself as a staffer, or for the Swedish public whose interests he decided to assert, there seemed to be no adequately "meaningful" outcome from institutional care. The old folks' lives may have had some fundamental value, but now no longer enough value to justify continued care. Now, although his statement may appear to have considered the matter from the standpoint and interests of the old men and women, the decisive variable was related, not to them (how much meaningful outcome), but to himself and the public he claimed to represent (how meaningful it was having them around to care for). The measure of meaning was not the victims, but the one who sent them to their deaths.

One remembers similar applications of this value-theory. The orderly's judgment about "meaningful life" put me in mind of the Nazi formula, *lebensunwertes Leben* (life not worth living), which was frequently used when the Third Reich had recourse to judgments of relative value on human lives. The Slavs, they decided, were *Untermenschen,* sub-humans fit only for slave labor. Well below them on the value scale were Gypsies and, lower still, Jews, the bacilli of society. Values at this lowest level were finely calculated. There were Jews, and *Mischlinge* (cross-breeds) first-class, and *Mischlinge* second-class. These categories could be subdivided into "productive" and "nonproductive." Bolshevik commissars in the Soviet army were also quite unvaluable, as were other "useless eaters" and "anti-socials": mental patients, the enfeebled elderly, unrecoverably wounded soldiers, "racially valueless children" and, to come full circle to what we are presently considering, defective newborn children (the very first of all these categories for whom Hitler approved an extermination order). It cannot be said that the Nazis assigned no value to human life. Their programs were grounded precisely on an elaborate scale of values. At its base the value system was quite simple. As Hitler once explained to a gathering of general officers, he decided upon the "removal of the Jews from our nation, not because we would begrudge them their existence—we congratulate the rest of the world on their company—but because the existence of our own nation is a thousand times more important to us than that of an alien race."[2]

A few decades earlier, liberal reformers in England had been proposing and legislating social policies that, in their way, were also value-responsive. "It was, to illustrate, the law of the land that upon certification of any two doctors, any person might be incarcerated indefinitely for feeblemindedness. Charles Wicksteed

Armstrong was saying: 'the nation which first begins to *breed for efficiency*—denying the right of the scum to beget millions of their kind . . . is the nation destined to rule the earth. . . . To diminish the dangerous fertility of the unfit there are three methods: the lethal chamber, segregation and sterilization.' The professor of eugenics at London University was proposing that paupers, tramps, and the insane be left to starve; otherwise the fertile but unfit would continue to reproduce and prevent England from continuing as a world power. A physician with governmental authority who was concerned with mental deficiency tested his theory that it was due to small skulls by operating on children's heads; a fourth of them died. When the National Insurance Act required compulsory contributions from all workers, it provided that workmen could be denied unemployment compensation if they had been discharged for misconduct—insolence, for example. Pensions were withheld from those who had been in prison or had 'persistently failed to work.' "[3]

Assigning a Variable Value

When one is prepared to assign a variable value to other human beings according as they are expected to rise to a high level of social performance, and then to allot to them a corresponding measure of life's sustenance, this is no ethical refinement. It is the same old business of the runt of the litter getting pushed away from the teat. All too often when we apologize that it would be too unkind to make some creature face so unsatisfying an existence, what we really mean is that we don't want to pay his or her bills.

By evaluating human beings insofar as they are "relational," or by "what they can come to be," or by their "personal or social consciousness," their "quality of life," their "access to higher goods," their potential for attaining a "truly human life," we assign to our fellows a value measured by their active participation in our society. The ideally valuable, "truly human life" at its best appears to belong to a taxpaying adult who earns a living. To the extent that one falls short of this ideal, by infancy or senility or criminality or retardation or infirmity, one slips down the value scale. Behind all this calculation lurks a readiness to appraise others according as they are pleasant or congenial or contributory towards ourselves, and then to act on this appraisal.

I discern two ethical impediments here. First, in this business of applied values, one appears to be considering three distinct factors: how much this other person needs (burden on the benefactor), how much good it would do this person if helped (benefit to the beneficiary), and how dear this other person is to me (relationship of beneficiary to benefactor). The interplay of all these factors would seem to promise a fair judgment. I must consider how much claim on my own life and resources is being made, how much proportionate gain this will bring my neighbor, and how dear to me my neighbor is or how beholden or bound to him or her I am. But when one calculates the anticipated benefits to the other person by that person's anticipated social response, then the factor supposedly respecting my neighbor's welfare is turned around and becomes, in effect, an indicator of how pleasant it is to have that person around. The benefits anticipated are measured, not intrinsically with respect to him or her, but extrinsically with respect to myself and others who stand to gain from a grudging judgment. The calculation is no longer an interplay of interests; it is put entirely at the pleasure of the one in power. The neighbor and the neighbor's future are cast into dependence on how useful I reckon him to be to the rest of us. So when H. Tristram Engelhardt, Jr. wants to relieve some infant of the "injury of continued existence" or SS Gruppenführer Prof. Karl Brandt describes the elimination of "useless eaters" and "undesirable individuals" as an "act of grace," I suspect that this is an injury I should pray for and a grace I should shun. This concern for "quality of life" is a self-concern bearing the likeness of other-concern.

The second ethical impediment is raised by the readiness to treat persons according as it would be valuable for them. I do not wish to question the way in which persons are evaluated. Quite clearly others are more or less valuable according as they become socially valuable, or as they realize their "relational potential." What I would dispute is that we have any ethical warrant to make this value the first basis for our treatment of others.

Let me suggest another way of approach. Rather than designating all human life as valuable, I would propose that all human beings are not valuable. They are invaluable. Our fellow humans are not merely the most valuable things around; they are off the scale, truly incommensurable, not even to be introduced into the rate of exchange whereby we convert the relative values of other things. A human being can be valued, as has been described. But a human being ought also, and more importantly and fundamentally, be reverenced. Possibly this would support the way some folks have of calling life sacred: not because of any necessary relationship to God, but because it seems an appropriate category in which to shelter those very precious beings of transcendent goodness. As Simon Peter explained to Simon Magus, there are some things too valuable to have a price. The governing insight in this assertion that human persons are beyond value—legitimate without recourse to religious premises—is that mankind is obliged, if they are to live and grow in spirit, to deal with others not simply according to what good it may produce, what use it serves, what response it subsidizes.

Corrupted Morally, Destroyed Spiritually

We are corrupted morally and destroyed spiritually if we treat others only as they are valuable. We have of course only limited goods and service to dispose of, and fellow humans whose needs and claims far exceed our wherewithal. In matching our resources to their needs we are presented with a most rudimentary moral option: whether to exert ourselves to meet those endless neighbor-needs, or whether to adjudicate those needs and claims to serve our pleasure by calculating their social benefit potential. There is obviously no congruence or conformity between the invaluable persons we confront and the value-benefits we might afford them. But there is a telltale and deep-cleft difference whether they are the measure of our lives or we the measure of theirs.

This is not, as I say, a religious position, though it might be. The injunction that mankind is to be provided for, from each according to means and to each according to need (an injunction more gracious than all this calculation of values), may be ascribed either to first century Jerusalem Christians or 19th century Russian-German atheists. Both were of the mind that it is not enough to run a cost-benefit analysis on one's neighbor (though that is exactly what most Communist powers and some Christian institutions are now doing). In any case, what I know of Christian faith reinforces the conviction that no follower of Jesus, holding in his or her hand the powers of life and death over those less advantaged, should begin to wield such powers by asking how much social yield there will be from any given material investment. We owe things of value to persons beyond value. Indeed, we live by a belief that it is the least able, the least forthcoming who have strongest claim on our lives and substance.

One is often reminded that, whatever our disposition to treat our fellows as invaluable, there are still certain situations in which it is both allowable and dutiful to appraise others in a strictly utilitarian way. Triage is the typical situation put forward. At a field hospital in a combat zone, battle will produce casualties that swamp the capacity of the hospital. It becomes an inexorable fact that some must be saved and some left to die. A triage officer stands at the entry, sorting casualties so that the medical facility can accomplish the most practical good. One soldier disastrously wounded has to be set aside in favor of five others who, in the same amount of time, can have their lives saved. The battalion commander is sent in and the assistant cook held back. Officers have priority over enlisted men. Enemy wounded are given last place after one's own comrades whose survival will help the war effort. Faced with life-and-death needs and inadequate resources, the triage officer does his duty precisely by being ruthlessly utilitarian. The wounded are evacuated; they are treated in accordance with their value to the group and to the struggle. People are sent for saving treatment or are left to die on grounds of the payoff a given amount of care will produce.

About triage as a paradigm of ethical choice I would make several observations. First, even when it seems quite justified, it has a way of consuming a person. For a doctor, the fibers of whose self are braided into lifelines of generous concern, it snarls the soul, not simply to lose a patient to death, but to mark him or her for death. It may require uncommonly high and durable virtue to perform this task without making a vice out of necessity. To illustrate: during the Holocaust, certain Jewish community leaders, after agonizing at the Nazi order, consented to select numbers of their own communities to be sent to their destruction, in the hope that some others—the right others—might be spared. One such *Alteste,* leader of the ghetto in Lodz, Poland, explained: "Now, when we are deporting 10,000 people from the ghetto, I cannot pass over this tragic subject in silence. Unfortunately, in this respect, I received a ruthless order, an order which I had to carry out in order to prevent its being carried out by others. Within the framework of my possibilities . . . I have tried to mitigate the severity of the decree. I have settled the matter so that I assigned for deportation that portion which was for the ghetto a suppurating abscess. So the list included the ousted operators of the underground, scum, and all sorts of persons harmful to the ghetto."[4] Another in Upper Silesia argued that the Jews should accept from the Gestapo the onus of selecting the contingents for extermination, so as to preserve for the community its most helpful elements. First to go, on his lists, were informers, thieves, and "undesirables"; next went the insane, the sick, and the defective children.[5] The victims had, by acquiescing in the work, somehow been contaminated by the minds of the oppressors. Even when necessity seems to call for it, can a person long deal with his or her neighbors in this way, calculating their "worth to society," their relational potential, without soon acquiring the perverse habit of mind which one wants to resist but perhaps cannot?

Triage Easily Invoked

Another thing about triage: it is so easily invoked. A few years back one had to decide which patients could have use of the few kidney dialysis machines and which could not. There was much evaluating then. And there could be little argument, and little misgiving, for there simply were no more machines to be had. But in a world where medical resources are never likely to satisfy medical needs, is not every day one of triage? Are not all medical practitioners who administer life and death likely to calculate the relative value of their patients? And will this reckoning not be heavily influenced by what this treatment, what this survival would mean to them, the medics? It goes far beyond medicine. Johnson reminds us of "the competition for scarce monetary and manpower resources in society," and Garret Hardin is arguing from that that the United States had better leave the poorer nations to starve if it wants to preserve the good life.

A recent newspaper canvass of citizen comment on the "boat people" from Southeast Asia who were frantically seeking asylum elicited a wave of hostile statements from Americans who insisted that our country could not harbor endless waves of feckless refugees. Knowing the devastation the United States has visited upon the homelands of these people, and that their predecessors have been some of America's most industrious and self-reliant immigrants, and that our country enjoys such relative abundance among the nations of the earth, what is one to think of these claims that a welcome for these refugees would be wasted? Why is it that the powerful and affluent and engorged of this world are always the most aware that there is not enough to go around and that there are so many people who will make poor use of what is given them?

And as for the necessity that imposes triage on us: granted the battle, it may be justified to pick some wounded to die because they are less worthwhile. But why grant the battle in the first place? Granted the inadequacy of medical care in poor communities, some people must be left to ail and to die who might otherwise be saved. But why grant the inadequacy? So often we consent to participate in what we lament as "tragic" decisions that cost other people their lives or well-being without challenging the social injustice that has imposed the tragedy. One is reminded of a proposal submitted to Adolf Eichmann: "There is an imminent danger that not all the Jews can be supplied with food in the coming winter. We must seriously consider if it would not be more humane to finish off the Jews, insofar as they are not fit for labor mobilization, with some quick-acting means. In any case this would be more agreeable than to let them die of hunger."[6] There is no triage when the same people who offer humane death are the ones who cause the imminent danger. And so it often is.

There is, behind this application of value-theory, the possibility of great mischief (though I see Johnson and McCormick as willing parties to none of it). This can be seen perhaps by considering the canon drawn up at the conference at the University of California, San Francisco: "Life-preserving intervention should be understood as doing harm to an infant who cannot survive infancy. . . . " Compare this to the medical experience in Holland during the Second World War. "When Seiss-Inquart, Reich Commissar for the Occupied Netherlands Territories, wanted to draw the Dutch physicians into the orbit of the activities of the German medical profession, he did not tell them 'You must send your chronic patients to the death factories' or 'You must give lethal injections at Government request in your offices,' but he couched his order in most careful and superficially acceptable terms. One of the paragraphs in the order of the Reich Commissar of the Netherlands Territories concerning the Netherlands doctors of 19 December 1941 reads as follows: 'It is the duty of the doctor, through advice and effort, conscientiously and to his best ability, to assist as helper the person entrusted to his care in the maintenance, improvement and re-establishment of his vitality, physical efficiency and health. The accomplishment of this duty is a public task.' The physicians of Holland rejected this order unanimously because they saw what it actually meant—namely, the concentration of their efforts on mere rehabilitation of the sick for useful labor, and abolition of medical secrecy. Although on the surface the new order appeared not too grossly unacceptable, the Dutch physicians decided that it is the first, although slight, step away from principle that is the most important one. The Dutch physicians declared that they would not obey this order. When Seiss-Inquart threatened them with revocation of their licenses, they returned their licenses, removed their shingles and, while seeing their own patients secretly, no longer wrote death or birth certificates. Seiss-Inquart retraced his steps and tried to cajole them—still to no effect. Then he arrested 100 Dutch physicians and sent them to concentration camps. The medical profession remained adamant and quietly took care of their widows and orphans, but would not give in. Thus it came about that not a single euthanasia or non-therapeutic sterilization was recommended or participated in by any Dutch physician."[7]

Truly human, relational potential was the guiding star over San Francisco. In Holland they seem to have held—with costly stubbornness—that as doctors they would often have to tend patients who could never be cured. They knew their job was not to produce a healthy, working population, nor to eliminate the stunted; it was their profession to heal whom they could, alleviate the affliction of those they could not, and stand by all whom they served. They would have agreed with Johnson that death is not the ultimate enemy (though perhaps abandonment is). Their dedication, though, would be not to human life, as Johnson would say, but to human beings whose lives we heal if we can, but still serve if we cannot.

Does it follow that all defective infants must, because reverenced as our invaluable human comrades, be given every available medical treatment, no matter what the cost? I am not arguing that this must necessarily follow. What I am asking is that the issue be remanded for further and different consideration. One would require that when parents, physicians and statesmen look into a crib to ask themselves whether it be right to let death claim a blighted child, they not consider what measure of potential the infant has to become truly human. For their purposes, that stunted, afflicted fellow human of theirs is already as invaluably valuable as he or she ever will or would be, and is far more dependent on them than are most children for the protection of its person and its life.

Notes

1. Fletcher, Joseph, "Indicators of Humanhood: A Tentative Profile of Man," 2 *The Hastings Center Report,* 5 (Nov., 1972), p. 1.

2. Dawidowicz, Lucy S., *The War Against the Jews 1933-1945* (New York: Holt, Rinehart & Winston, 1975), p. 163.

3. Burtchaell, James, "Reheating the Mutton Chop of Chesterton," *The Review of Politics* XL, 4 (Oct., 1978), p. 550, reviewing Margaret Canovan, *G. K. Chesterton: Radical Populist.*

4. Dawidowicz, *op. cit.,* pp. 291-292.

5. *Ibid.,* p. 299.

6. *Ibid.,* p. 162.

7. Alexander, Leo, M.D., "Medical Science Under Dictatorship," 241 *New England Journal of Medicine* 2 (July 14, 1949), pp. 44-45.

80. Justice and Equal Treatment

PAUL RAMSEY

Let us consider one moral aspect of the practice of neglect: the question of justice. Some physicians who have reported that they let some babies die (perhaps hasten their dying) also report that they make such life or death decisions not only on the basis of the newborn's medical condition and prognosis, but on the basis of familial, social, and economic factors as well. If the marriage seems to be a strong one, an infant impaired to x degree may be treated, while an infant with the same impairment may not be treated if the marriage seems about to fall apart. Treatment may be given if the parents are wealthy; not, if they are poor.[1] Now, life may be unfair, as John Kennedy said; but to deliberately make medical care a function of inequities that exist at birth is evidently to add injustice to injury and fate.

Wiser and more righteous is the practice of Dr. Chester A. Swinyard of the New York University medical school's rehabilitation center. Upon the presentation to him of a defective newborn, he immediately tries to make clear to the mother the distinction between the question of ultimate custody of the child and questions concerning the care it needs. The mother must consent to operations, of course. But she is asked only to make judgments about the baby's care, while she is working through the problem of whether to accept the defective child as a substitute for her "lost child," i.e., the perfect baby she wanted. In the prism of the case, when the question is, Shall this open spine be closed? Shall a shunt be used to prevent further mental impairment? the mothers can usually answer correctly. In the case of spina bifida babies, Dr. Swinyard also reports very infrequent need of institutionalization or foster parents. That results from concentrating the mother's attention on what medical care requires, and not on lifelong burdens of custody.[2] One must entirely reject the contention of Duff and Campbell that parents, facing the prospect of oppressive burdens of care, are capable of making the most morally sensible decisions about the needs and rights of defective newborns. There is a Jewish teaching to the effect that only disinterested parties

From Paul Ramsey, *Ethics at the Edges of Life* (New Haven: Yale University Press, 1978), pp. 201-6.

may, by even so innocuous a method as prayer, take any action which may lead to premature termination of life. Husband, children, family and those charged with the care of the patient may not pray for death.[3]

One can understand—even appreciate—the motives of a physician who considers an unhappy marriage or family poverty when weighing the tragedy facing one child against that facing another; and rations his help accordingly. Nevertheless, that surely is a species of injustice. Physicians are not appointed to remove all life's tragedy, least of all by lessening medical care now and letting infants die who for social reasons seem fated to have less care in the future than others. That's one way to remove every evening the human debris that has accumulated since morning.

There is a story that is going around—in fact I'm going around telling it—about how the pope, the chief rabbi of Jerusalem, and the general secretary of the World Council of Churches arrived in heaven the same day. Since they had been spiritual leaders here below and ecclesiastical figures to take notice of, they had some difficulty adjusting. Such was the equality there that everyone had to take his place and turn in the cafeteria line. After some muttering protest they fell into the customs of the place, until one day a little man dressed in a white coat came in and rushed to the head of the line. "Who's that?" asked the pope resentfully. "Oh, that's God," came the reply. "He thinks he's a doctor!"

If physicians are going to play God under the pretense of providing relief for the human condition, let us hope they play God as God plays God. Our God is no respecter of persons of good quality. Nor does he curtail his care for us because our parents are poor or have unhappy marriages, or because we are most in need of help. Again, a true humanism also leads to an "equality of life" standard.

A policy of selectively not treating severely defective infants appeals ultimately, it is true, to whatever constitutes the greatness and glory of humankind to give us a standard by which to determine the bottom line of life to be deemed worth living. Thus Joseph Fletcher proposed fifteen "positive human criteria" and five "negative human criteria" as an ensemble quality-of-life index.[4] Then he reduced the number in an article entitled "Four Indicators of Humanhood—the Enquiry Matures."[5] There is no need for us to examine Fletcher's criteria—three of which seem to declare anyone who does not have a Western sense of time to be a non-person. Fletcher is simply a sign of our times. Many, more serious ethicists have joined in the search for "indicators of personhood." The fundamental question to be faced is whether the practice of medicine should be based on any such set of criteria (presuming they can be discovered and agreed upon).

To that question I want first to say that that's no way to play God as God plays God. That was not the bottom line of his providential care. When the prophet Jeremiah tells us, "Before I formed thee in the belly I knew thee; and before thou camest forth out of the womb I sanctified thee; and I ordained thee" (1:5), he does not mean to start us on a search for the "indicators of personhood" God was using or should have used before calling us by name. Neither did the psalmist when he cried, "Behold . . . the darkness and the light are both alike to thee. For thou hast possessed my reins: thou hast covered me in my mother's womb. I will praise thee; for I am fearfully and wonderfully made: marvelous are thy works; and that my soul knoweth right well" (139:12b, 13, 14). No more did God, at the outset of his Egyptian rescue operation, look around for "indicators of peoplehood," choosing only those best qualified for national existence. "The Lord did not set his love upon you, nor choose you, because you were more in number than any people; for you were the fewest of all people. But because the Lord loved you, and because he would keep the oath he had sworn unto your fathers, hath the Lord brought you out with a mighty hand" (Deuteronomy 7:7, 8a).

Many of God's life and death decisions are inscrutable to us. People are born and die. Nations rise and fall. Doubtless God in his official governance does—or at least permits—lots of things (as the Irishman said) which he would never think of doing in a private capacity. Nor should we, who are not given dominion or co-regency over humankind. But there is no indication at all that God is a rationalist whose care is a function of indicators of our personhood, or of our achievement within those capacities. He makes his rain to fall upon the just and the unjust alike, and his sun to rise on the abnormal as well as the normal. Indeed, he has special care for the weak and the vulnerable among us earth people. He cares according to need, not capacity or merit.

These images and shadows of divine things are the foundation of Western medical care, together with that "Pythagorean manifesto,"[6] the Hippocratic oath. As *John* Fletcher has written:

> If we choose to be shaped by Judeo-Christian visions of the "createdness" of life within which every creature bears the image of God, we ought to care for the defective newborn as if our relation with the creator depended on the outcome. If we choose to be shaped by visions of the inherent dignity of each member of the human family, no matter what his or her predicament,

> we ought to care for this defenseless person as if the basis of our own dignity depended on the outcome.[7]

Care cannot fall short of universal equality.

Indicators of personhood may be of use in psychology, in educational theory, and in moral nurture, but to use such indices in the practice of medicine is a grave mistake. Even the search for such guidelines on which to base the care of defective newborn infants would launch neonatal medicine upon a trackless ocean of uncertainty, directly into arbitrary winds. Thus, one of the physicians at Yale-New Haven Hospital, explaining on television the newly announced policy of benign neglect of defective infants in that medical center, said that to have a life worth living a baby must be "lovable."[8] Millard S. Everett in his book *Ideals of Life* writes that "no child should be admitted into the society of the living" who suffers "any physical or mental defect that would prevent marriage or would make others tolerate his company only from a sense of mercy. . . . "[9] Mercy me, to that we must say no. Medical criteria for care should remain physiological, as should also the signs by which physicians declare that a patient has died. Decisions to treat or not to treat should be the same for the normal and the abnormal alike. Searching for an index of personhood to use (comparing patient-persons, not treatments or treatment with no treatment) is rather like founding medical care on theological judgments about when God infuses the soul into the human organism.

Notes

1. In a published interview, Dr. Raymond S. Duff seems to me to be ambiguous on these points, even contradictory. On the one hand he says, "My guess is that neither social nor economic considerations influence the decisions we are talking about to any significant degree. I never felt that a troubled marriage or the economics of the family has really had a major influence. Parents may fight with one another but they still adhere to what they both consider is fair to the child." Yet two or three paragraphs later he reported the case of a couple who had to decide "how many lives would be wrecked: one of dubious value plus four others, *or* the one of dubious value. There was no real choice the family felt" primarily because of space, money, time, and personal resources. That couple of modest means noted that the wealthy can "buy out" of the choice. Yet, again, a few paragraphs later, when asked whether there would be "a substantive difference in the number of infants allowed to die" if society was equipped with uniformly excellent, well-staffed custodial institutions, Dr. Duff replied, "I doubt it," citing "several parents who felt it is not right for their child to exist primarily to provide employment for others." He also distinguished the decision to "let die" in Yale-New Haven Hospital from the treatment accorded defective children in Nazi Germany by saying that in the current cases "family and physicians took into account not only the child's right (to live or to die) but the needs of the family and society, and, to some extent, future generations," protesting that "if we cannot trust these persons to do justice here, can anyone be trusted?" (Beverly Kelsey, "Shall These Children Live?"; reprinted in the *Hastings Center Report* 5, no. 2).

The more technical and presumably well-considered article by Duff and Campbell is quite clear on these points ("Moral and Ethical Dilemmas in the Special-Care Nursery," *New England Journal of Medicine* 289, no. 17). There, the references to "the family economy," "siblings' rights to relief from the seemingly pointless, crushing burden," "the strains of the illness . . . believed to be threatening the marriage bonds and to be causing sibling behavioral disturbances," "fear that they and their other children would become socially enslaved, economically deprived, and permanently stigmatized, . . . [in] a state of 'chronic sorrow,' " stand without modulation, or without the claim that the family-physician decision was made simply for the sake of the defective child.

2. Swinyard's practice, as I understand it, is quite different from withholding prognosis of the child's condition. The parents of a child with meningomyelocele are not "simply told that the child needed an operation on the back as the first step in correcting several defects . . . while the activities of care proceeded at a brisk pace" (Duff and Campbell, "Moral and Ethical Dilemmas").

3. R. Chaim Palaggi, Chikekei Lev., I, Yoreh De'ah, no. 50.

4. "Medicine and the Nature of Man," in *The Teaching of Medical Ethics,* ed. Robert M. Veatch, Willard Gaylin, and Councilman Morgan; *Hastings Center Report* 2, no. 5 (November 1972): 1-4. See also the correspondence in vol. 3, no. 1 (February 1973), p. 13.

5. *Hastings Center Report* 4, no. 6 (December 1974): 4-7. These accordion concepts of "meaningful/meaningless," "humanhood," "relationships that can be considered human," and "man's ability to relate" (called, incorrectly, "minimal" criteria) are used throughout *Dying: Considerations Concerning the Passage from Life to Death,* an Interim Report by the Task Force on Human Life of the Anglican Church of Canada (Office of the General Secretary, 600 Jarvis Street, Toronto, Canada, June 1977; presented to the 1977 session of the Synod on August 11-18, 1977). Representing no official or authoritative views of the Anglican church of Canada, the report proceeds to address our duties toward defective newborns as if they are "human-looking shapes" or at most "sentient" creatures: " . . . the only way to treat such defective infants humanly is not to treat them as human" (p. 14). A widening controversy over the report was reported in *The New York Times,* July 28, 1977. The Synod sent the report back to committee.

6. *Roe v. Wade,* 410, U.S. 113.

7. John Fletcher, "Abortion, Euthanasia, and Care of Defective Newborns," *New England Journal of Medicine* 292 (January 9, 1975): 75-78.

8. CBS News, January 2, 1973. In their landmark article ("Moral and Ethical Dilemmas") Drs. Raymond S. Duff and A. G. M. Campbell used the expression "meaningful humanhood." Dr. Duff in a subsequently published interview explained that criterion to mean "the capacity to love and be loved, to be independent, and to understand and plan for the future" (Beverly Kelsey, "Shall These Children Live?"). Asked whether a mongoloid child may have "meaningful humanhood," Dr. Duff seemed to hedge, leaving the decision to parents who "pay the fiddler to call the tune," while the physician and hospital policy need only sometimes decide "whether the family's God is fair to the child."

9. Cited by Daniel C. Maguire, *Death by Choice,* p. 7. Here Maguire indicates no disagreement with such criteria.

81. Our Religious Traditions and the Treatment of Infants

DAVID H. SMITH

I

The babies I want to discuss in this paper are not those that we call "normal" babies; rather, they are those that have problems and cause problems. They can only make the heart ache, and commentary written by outsiders can easily chafe the wounds. This may be especially true when the commentary is said to reflect the religious sensibilities or traditions of our people, for religion means to be about life and death and truth. We are sometimes outraged by religious claims and arguments, but usually that is because our expectations for religious insight and principle are so high. We chastise the goddess who has failed us. I understand my role to be to offer one ordering of religious perspectives on the care of impaired infants. Because the issues are so powerful and so complex, I shall strike at them in several different ways. I hope the result has a kind of unity or continuity, but I think it is more likely to be the coherence of a symphony rather than the logical tightness of a Euclidean proof. Indeed, I shall play several of the same notes that Professor Arras has struck in his discussion of this topic, but they are important notes, and my chord structure is rather different.

My general plan in the remarks that follow goes something like this. I shall begin by discussing some of the images or portraits of children and parents that rest in the consciousness of Western religious people. These portraits, I think, have informed our thinking about human relationships in profound ways. They provide some of the data from which theological moralists should begin their reflection. Of course, like all portraiture, they reflect the perspective of the painter; these are not value-neutral descriptions. Moreover, the "morals" of the incidents I am about to mention are not always clear and unambiguous. This ambiguity may well be part of their greatness, but it is also a limitation for purposes of moral analysis. The portraits are not a sufficient moral framework, nor even a

---

This article appears in Thomas H. Murray and Arthur L. Caplan, eds., *Which Babies Shall Live?* (Clifton, N.J.: Humana Press, 1985). Used by permission of the Hastings Center and the author.

sufficient basis for such thinking. Still, they are illuminating and constitutive of the life of our central traditions.

With these data spread out before us, I shall presume to extract some general principles from them. And I will apply these principles to some of the moral issues that may well have challenged many of us already.

II

At age 40 Isaac married Rebekah; their sons Esau and Jacob were born soon thereafter. "When the boys grew up, Esau was a skilful hunter, a man of the field, while Jacob was a quiet man, dwelling in tents. Isaac loved Esau, because he ate of his game; but Rebekah loved Jacob" (Genesis 25:27-28). Children here, and elsewhere in the Bible, have a kind of particularity, and parents respond to them with partiality. They like and dislike; they pick favorites. This human tendency, the stuff of great literature and soap-opera, is treated as an inevitable fact in the scriptural narratives.

In fact throughout our history the individuality of a child is related to the child's lineage. This is not always fortunate, however. In the book of Judges, Jephthah swears to kill the first person he sees on returning home if only the Lord will help him to triumph over the Ammonites. When he does come home victorious, "behold his daughter came out to meet him with timbrels and with dances; she was his only child; beside her he had neither son nor daughter." With her agreement he sacrifices her, "for I have opened my mouth to the Lord and I cannot take back my vow" (Judges 11:29f). We shall return to the question of parental vows shortly; for the moment I note that the fate of Jepthah's daughter is appropriately—if unhappily—determined by the behavior of her parent. Children are often victims in the biblical narratives and images (cf. Psalm 137:9—"Happy shall be he who takes your [i.e., Babylonian] little ones and dashes them against the rock"). They are victims of a particularity, or peculiarity, over which they have no control. This is a not altogether happy or benevolent aspect of reality, in the biblical portraits.

This stress on particularity has not always been reflected in Western consciousness about children. In his rich study, *Centuries of Childhood,* Philippe Aries notes that hundreds of years passed before Western Europeans really discovered the special characteristics of childhood. Before the 17th century, he writes,

> No one thought of keeping a picture of a child if that child had either lived to grow to adulthood or had died in infancy. In the first case, childhood was simply an unimportant phase of which there was no need to keep any record; in the second case, that of the dead child, it was thought that the little thing which had disappeared so soon in life was not worthy of remembrance: there were far too many children whose survival was problematical. . . . One had several children in order to keep just a few. . . . People could not allow themselves to become too attached to something that was regarded as a probable loss.[1]

Increasingly, Aries observes, people began to realize that childhood was a special stage of life, valuable in its own right. This led to treating children as pets, to coddling, but increasingly to a notion that children had to be educated or disciplined so as to grow up into happy adults. Ultimately, however, only increased medical success as well as contraception has been able in the past 200 years to bring about a time in our society in which children are valued in and for themselves. Really taking particularity seriously was a long time coming.

This mention of education gets at another religious image of the child—the child as one whose future must be prepared for and whose character and education therefore matter. Beginning with the embryonic passover traditions in Exodus 12 and continuing right through the passover haggadah of the present time, Jewish life has always wanted to help the child situate himself as part of a people with a destiny, to have a sense of himself as part of a community with a past, present, and future. The great 20th century Protestant theologian Karl Barth expresses this idea very well. Children, he says, "are not by nature their [parents'] property, subjects, servants or even pupils, but their apprentices, who are entrusted and subordinated to them in order that they might lead them into the way of life."[2] Jewish or Christian parenthood inevitably looks to the child's future with a vision of the good life.

Thirdly, and most centrally for our purposes, the religious images of childhood and parenting that we know are—as the quotation I just cited from Barth suggests—images of *limited* parental authority and dominion. When the baby Moses was three months old his mother put him in a basket and let him be taken over by others for his well-being (Exodus 2). At age twelve Jesus in the temple is not a very good boy, straying from his parents and telling them that he really has more important things to do than go home with the family. Mary and Joseph's authority over him is distinctly limited—indeed, if he is *the* paradigmatic child he vividly illustrates the ambivalence of parent/child relations, for he both is, and is not, *their* child.

This limitation of parental authority is nowhere more vivid than in the story of the binding (*akedah*) of Isaac by Abraham in Genesis 22. We are used to thinking of this story in terms of Isaac's loss of life, but of course it would have been Abraham's sacrifice in more ways than one. He is being asked to give up that which means the very most to him; it is a story of letting go. Abraham looks up and sees the ram and God explains "now I know that you fear God, seeing you have not withheld your son, your only son, from me" (Genesis 22). Isaac's life is not, ultimately, Abraham's to dispose of as he may see fit, for Abraham would never have chosen this sacrifice. As a planning parent Abraham serves a master, and his parental power is limited.

This brings us to a fourth image of childhood that we find in our heritages. Elijah the Tishbite stays with a widow whose son dies. Elijah "stretched himself upon the child three times" and the child revived (1 Kings 17). The earliest history of Christianity tells the story of a boy named Eutychus (Lucky) who fell asleep in a third story window while listening to a long sermon. He falls out of the window and dies, but Paul (the preacher) revives him with an embrace (Acts 20:8-12). Children are presented as having access to Jesus, and his contact with them in at least one version of the story is wonderfully physical and bodily: he takes them in his arms and blesses them (Mark 10:16 and parallels). It is not the child's personality alone, nor his future, but his body that is the focus of concern in these images. And for Christians this image is intensified even more in the extraordinary claim for an identification of God with the body of a crying, soiled, human baby. The *baby* Jesus is one of the two or three dominant Christian portraits.

Children in these images—and I have not pretended to give an encyclopedic account—are embodied human beings with a particular past and future. They create responsibilities for their parents. These parents, however, are not given complete dominion over their children, only a "slight seniority."[3]

III

These images do not of themselves lead us to moral conclusions. They only inform us; they require an ordering. I propose to use the notion of fidelity as an ordering principle. I shall assume that the great theme of Western religion is God's loyalty to us—a loyalty responded to with betrayal and disobedience, occasionally with trust and love. A life of passionate devotion to God should involve compassionate loyalty to other persons: this is the central theme of Western religious morality. What does a faithful working out of the images I have sketched entail?

When we try to figure out how to be faithful to people, one thing these images push us to think about is the things that they live for, what—as we say—makes them tick. Thus when it comes time to shop for presents for a birthday or Christmas or Chanukah we look for presents that relate to the interests of a person. A set of records of Beethoven symphonies is marvelous for one person, a waste for someone else. Someone likes jewelry, someone else a set of golf clubs. People's interests or, as I would prefer to say, their loyalties vary. Loyalty to someone means respecting this kind of particularity. And the respect may go quite far; my love for my friend may well bring me to love what he loves, to care for those things that matter to him.

Usually we know something of a person's specificity from his or her explicitly stated preferences. We know that Dad likes to play golf because he says he does, and he says he doesn't care for classical music. In fact, however, this correlation between what people really are and who or what they say they are is not one to one. Many people *say* they like to do things which in fact it is clear that they do not much enjoy; anyone who has ever lived in a family can write a book about the various kinds of self-deception that human beings indulge in. Still, throughout most of our lives, we are willing to acknowledge that a person's decisions about his or her own life ought, at least, to have a preferred place. Medical decisions are no exception. Thus we support a right to refuse treatment and stress the importance of a requirement of informed consent.

The striking thing about babies, however, is that part of this stress on moral particularity cannot exist for them. They have never had a chance to care about or live for anything. They have not established a style of life or character. And some infants will never be able to do these things. It's not just that because of great defects some babies will never have the kind of personality that a normal person would have. It's rather that they have never got off the launching pad. The effect on our moral reasoning about them is that an important variable simply drops out of the picture. We see them as children whose individuality has not yet emerged.

They also begin with a minimal medical history. Their prognosis is at best uncertain. We don't know what degree of retardation a child with Down's syndrome will have, or how serious the deformity and hydrocephalus associated with myelomeningocele will turn out to be. Some premature babies have terrible and short lives; others do not. It is never possible to be absolutely sure of the outcome.

I draw from these facts the conclusion that for the most part we owe it to these babies to get them started. They are cursed by powers in their lineage over which no one has control. But the arguments of personal style and preference that might justify a decision for the death of an adult can never be applied directly to newborns, and it takes time to establish a kind of pattern of biological functioning such that we can extrapolate to future events and responses with some fairly good degree of plausibility.

A second thing that loyalty to another person means is interest in or concern for what he or she may become. Hence the power of the image of parent as educator. The idea perhaps is difficult. We think of people as set in their ways: "Oh, he could do it if he wanted to, but he will never skip Monday night football." And we tend to form and hold set pictures of people: he is punctual, she is stubborn, they are argumentative. It is true that the characters people have have a kind of constancy, but it is also true that people change and grow. Saints fall away, sinners convert, Prince Hal becomes Henry IV.

When we look into the future for our friends we find that we want many things for them. One of these is *happiness.* This is a notoriously hard term to define, and I am not capable of producing a statement that will instantly persuade everyone. But I think it obvious that happiness is something that we want for those that we care about. We would describe as sick someone who wanted his child or spouse or parents to be *un*happy. Naturally I don't mean that we want happiness of any kind for them—we may well feel that some kinds of happiness are better than others. Certainly our religious traditions suggest the importance of piety before God as an ingredient in true happiness.

A second thing that we want for our friends is *excellence.* We hope that they will do something well. This something may be athletic, intellectual, or social. Some are good runners, others good thinkers, others are, as we say, good people. Yet however we define it, excellence is something that we want for our friends, and for religious persons it is associated with some kind of relation to God.

Given these goals the question becomes whether they are attainable. Seldom do we know the answer to this. This is particularly true with handicapped babies. We may be certain that they will *not* have the kinds of happiness or excellence that are open to normal children, *but this is scarcely the issue.* We are not trying to compare them with others, for not all children of God play the same role in the kingdom. Who of us would survive some great assize trying to decide if his own life, with all its defects, was worth living? The issue is, is some kind of happiness or excellence open to this child? As the custodians of their future we may act with hope. Our role is to help them know themselves and God, whatever their future may hold.

Related to this, I should mention that this stress on hope and the future is especially important when families are stretched and torn as they are in the cases we have been discussing. On the one hand, the parents need to stick with the child; on the other hand, the medical staff needs to stick with the family. Care is not an episodic or momentary thing. To be genuine it must involve a commitment to what is to come. Follow-up is very important. The uncertain character of the future is frightening, especially to parents whose dreams and expectations have been smashed. Loyal medical care for families in this situation involves living through this uncertainty with them and, through one's presence, giving them hope.

Third, loyal care for persons involves care for their *bodies.* Children in the religious images are not just personalities, nor bundles of potentiality; they are living, struggling bodies. There are two aspects of this obvious point to which I wish to call attention. One of them is that the body has a kind of life of its own. It is not altogether malleable to human desire, whether we speak of the desire of its "owner" or of someone else. And health is comparably objective.

Let me put the issue a little differently. Bodies are not just things we have, they are things we *are.* The requirements of a healthy body can be generalized—they are not completely relative to cultural prejudices or values. And medical care involves care for bodies in a special way—not to the exclusion of everything else, not in some scientific way that excludes the caress and the cuddle—but oriented to the body all the same. My lawyer is a consultant on my rights, my tax man on my money, and my doctor on my body and its health. Medical care for a baby means making him comfortable.

A second important feature of bodies is that they change. Bodies pass through stages, regardless of the desires of anyone. These include infancy, adolescence, middle age, aging, and dying. Proper forms of care should be adjusted to these various stages or moments in a life span. Pediatrics is not just medicine on small adults; we rightly use different terms to describe a highway accident to children, other adults, and the aged. Fidelity to a patient will always require optimal care, but as we change, so do the requirements of care. Throughout most of our lives medical loyalty to us means keeping us alive, but this ceases to be true at some point in our lives. Then we may actually speak of a need to die. Dr. Anna Fletcher has referred to a baby who was "trying to die."

Paul Ramsey has made this point with characteristic force. He says that the determination of when a person enters dying is a "medical" decision.[4] This means that there are changes in the ill person himself that determine what the right forms of treatment are. When a person starts to die our responsibilities shift. Ramsey's idea, which is rooted in religious images, is that a person's life trajectory at some point enters a dying phase. When that happens moral responsibility changes. Then the issue is, "Is he dying?" or, more generally, "What forms of treatment are optimal care for her in whatever time she has left?"

If the discernment of when someone begins to die—a determination that is relevant to the choice of appropriate forms of care—is a matter of what Eric Cassell has called the "healer's art," the substance of the point is best captured not in argument but in metaphor. A couple invite friends to dinner. Food and drink are pleasant; the conversation bubbles. The good host is hospitable and courteous to his guest, no matter what his shifts in mood. But there comes a time when the party "winds down"—a time to acknowledge that the evening is over. At that point, not easily determined by clock, conversation or basal metabolism, the good host does not press his guest to stay, but lets him go. Indeed he may have to *signal* that it is acceptable to leave. A good host will never be sure of his timing and will never kick out his guest. His jurisdiction over the guest is limited to taking care and permitting departure.

Analogously, loyalty to other persons involves care for them of the best possible sort, and changing the forms of care as needs change. It means recognizing that a time comes when we can care for them no longer, only bid them Godspeed. We may, as it were, show them the door. But we should not kill a patient because that would be to betray him, to assume the kind of jurisdiction over his fate that is incompatible with being a good host. And we can never be sure of our timing.

Loyalty to the dying, in other words, is compatible with a choice of palliative clinical care and personal human support over life-extending technologies. It is of the greatest possible importance that this shift be seen as a shift to an alternative *medical* form of care and it is the great strength of the hospice movement to have refined and institutionalized these alternative forms of medical care. Loyalty to the dying not only tolerates but positively mandates this shift; making a guest stay longer than is good for him is very bad manners.

Many people will recognize the possibility that some children are born dying. This may be simply in virtue of prematurity. Thus I think we should simply comfort some newborns as they die. On the other hand, I have meant to suggest that any predictable defect, in particular retardation, is not a sufficient reason for saying a child is dying. It is especially important not to yield to pressure to come to a quick and efficient decision in order to spare people's feelings. It takes time to discern what is going on with a young and small patient's body.

This brings us to the last point I wish to make. *Loyalty to a defective baby requires involvement in a decision-making procedure of integrity and credibility.*

Some writers on medical ethics see this as the only issue. In the case of adults they stress the patient's right to die; for children they assert an absolute right of parents to make the decision. However, it is clear that in the biblical images the gift of a child does not entitle parents to unlimited sovereignty over it. Abraham has to let go, despite his plans and hopes. Even if parents are the child's best proxy in virtue of their identification with it, their power should not be unchecked. There are other reasons for this. Parental judgment is finite and it is possible that the parent's identification and stake in the issue will produce excessive bias. Further, the communal nature of human existence implies that we do not live by ourselves; the family is not an island. Desertion of the family—and simply leaving the decision in their hands may amount to desertion—is a form of betrayal.

In effect I am saying that loyalty in these situations requires patience. There is no rushing the decision-making procedure, and no substitute for involvement of the physician throughout it. What is needed is a lot of talking among parents, physicians, nurses, and appropriately concerned others.

This is no panacea. Even a good process can go wrong or be misused. I can well understand—indeed I largely share—the impulse to establish minimal standards in the law. For in this area discretion abused is not just indiscreet; it is immoral. I do not think babies should be let go simply in virtue of Down's syndrome—as I hope I have suggested. But at the moment I cannot imagine a regulatory net or law that would ensure a discriminate result or that could be fine tuned to the whole variety of cases we want to acknowledge. Thus I fall back on moral education and a process of listening, learning, and support.

In sum, loyalty is what the people of God owe defective babies. We owe them respect and hope, care and comfort for their body, fair play and due process. Sometimes this will mean we have to kiss them goodbye—but never without having made them welcome, never without a hug, and never without regret.

Notes

1. Philippe Aries, *Centuries of Childhood: A Social History of Family Life* (New York: Random House, 1965), p. 38.
2. Karl Barth, *Church Dogmatics,* III/4 (Edinburgh: T. & T. Clark, 1960), p. 243.
3. Ibid., p. 246.
4. Sometimes Ramsey suggests that it is a strictly objective and factual matter. This is mistaken. While there are clinical signs that one is dying (as there are of the onset of puberty), the actual discernment of the beginning of the process is largely a matter of art. Experience and skill are relevant to the determination, of course. Many of us (including some physicians) are tone deaf to what is happening in the body of another. But there is no escaping the factor of judgment, of discerning perception. People's judgments will differ, to be sure, but this fact in no way proves the nonexistence of dying as a last stage of life.

82. Biblical Faith and the Loss of Children

BRUCE C. BIRCH

Death always comes as an offense. Death is the end of life. For most of us life is good; death is the ultimate end of the touching, the sharing and the struggling together that make for wholeness. There has been much recent effort in the church to understand and deal with death, and we have been blessed by a great deal of helpful literature and attention in the communities of faith to the issues of death and dying.

There is something about the death of a child, however, which heightens the offense; we have not often faced that matter very directly in our churches. The death of a child is felt to be unacceptable. It seems unnatural. We can't use some of those bromides that we sometimes use to reassure ourselves: for example, "She lived a full life." Often a child's death becomes the occasion for a crisis of faith. Not only a matter of the psychology of grief, a child's death is a challenge to our own deepest faith understandings. What kind of God would allow this to happen? What could faith possibly have to say to this experience?

These questions have been my own. In the fall of 1970 we were told that our daughter Christine had acute lymphocytic leukemia. This diagnosis came at the end of a difficult year for us. I had been fired from my first college teaching job because of antiwar activities. We had been unable to find a job and were forced to move out of our house. There was no place to go. We stored our furniture in a friend's basement and headed for parts unknown. I finally found a teaching job in August, one month before the beginning of school, and moved from Iowa, out on the plains where we had family close by, to South Carolina, a region of the country where we knew no one.

Six weeks after we arrived in South Carolina, we learned that our daughter had a potentially fatal illness. The nearest treatment center was in Atlanta, the Henrietta Eggleston Children's Hospital at Emory University. We traveled there to begin the arduous course of treatments which we hoped would put our daughter's disease into remission. A remission might have allowed her to receive the benefits of advancing medical knowledge in dealing with leukemia. But before Christine could be put into remission, she broke out in chicken pox, to which she had been exposed in the church nursery before we knew she had leukemia. Her diseased blood cells could not fight the infection and she went into shock. One month after the diagnosis, she died, on her third birthday. The precipitating cause of her death and its timing seemed cruel ironies.

We were filled with anger and grief. Where was God? Where was justice? Where was meaning? I can only share with you out of my own knowledge of the power of those questions—and my conviction that in the biblical tradition of the Christian faith, we do have some resources which help us, even in times of such loss.

We can begin by talking about the problem of God. God is the easiest hook on which to hang blame. Many instinctively feel that God must somehow be punishing them. "Why did God do this to me? I must have done something to deserve this." Unfortunately, that notion is reinforced by a good deal of popular religion; but the punisher God is not a helpful concept. It either produces guilt that is undeserved and unrelated to the situation, or it leads to angry rejection of God altogether.

This concept of a punisher God does sometimes appear in the Bible, however, In the Old Testament, particularly in Deuteronomy and in the Wisdom literature, we find a God who dispenses rewards and punishments for every human action, as if life could be reduced to such mechanical blessings and curses. But a corrective to this view also appears in the Bible; the entire Book of Job is a protest against it, sweeping away its irrelevant and monstrous blasphemy. Job is a righteous man who has suffered great and grievous loss. In the traditional story (chapters 1-2; 42:7 ff.) he is patient and long-suffering, and God finally restores everything to him. This traditional tale of the patient sufferer was surely known widely in the ancient world of Israel. That is not the total picture in the Book of Job, however. The author has split the old story in half, inserting into the middle of it, alongside the traditional picture of the patient Job, the hurt, angry and rebellious Job. This Job argues with the friends and challenges God. The friends say all the pious things: "God's purposes are too great for us. You must have deserved this, so accept it." But Job argues that all people, whether righteous or not, are vulnerable to suffering, and that a hidden, uncaring God is no help at all.

The Book of Job helps us to reject the notion of the punisher God as inadequate. It calls us to look further for a God who does care and who identifies with our pain. Perhaps the God who finally appears to Job in a whirlwind at the end of the book is a pointer toward a deity who at least engages and is present with those who suffer—but the Book of Job is not intended to give us easy answers to that struggle. By sweeping away glib responses to the problem of God in times of deep pain and suffering, the book points to our own struggles and our own engagement with an even wider biblical tradition in which there does appear a caring God who is central to our faith tradition. I want to describe three aspects of this divine image over against that of the punisher God.

The first is *God as hearer.* Over and over again in Scripture, we find lines like these: "I have heard their cries. Their cries have come to me. Their cries have fallen on my ears." Dorothee Sölle, in her important book *Suffering* (Fortress, 1975), suggests that the outcry is the beginning of healing. Israel knew the importance of expressing pain and despair to God, and in the midst of the community. Nowhere is this seen more eloquently than in the laments of the Psalter. We think of the Psalter as a book of praises, but the largest number of Psalms are songs of lamentation. One cannot read those laments without being impressed that Israel had a rather different concept of worship than we commonly do. The Psalms are gutsy and honest; they don't pull any punches. They express despair: "Out of the depths have I cried to thee, O Lord" (Ps. 130). They express doubts: "My God, my God, why hast thou forsaken me?" (Ps. 22). They express anger and bitterness. The 137th Psalm, which begins, "By the waters of Babylon we sat down and wept," ends with lines so terrible in their expression of anger and bitterness that we almost never read them in public worship: "O daughter of Babylon, you devastator! . . . Happy shall he be who takes your little ones and dashes them against the rock!" Anger, bitterness, despair, doubt—it is all there, not because the tradition desires to affirm those expressions as ends in themselves but because if the pain is not exposed the healing cannot begin. These Psalms are often shocking to us because so much of our own worship tries to conceal our deepest wounds. Our own worship so often takes place at the level of the lowest common denominator of our corporate experience.

The role of the pastor as counselor can also serve to hide our deepest wounds from the wider community. I once was in a church in which someone expressed very deep hurt and anger during the time set aside for the sharing of concerns in the worship service—only to have the pastor remark at the end of the service, "Well, Fred, if you had brought that to me we could have talked about it without imposing on everyone else's worship experience." If the hurt is not exposed, the healing word cannot be spoken.

My wife and I found many in the church especially reluctant to deal with the death of a child. One can speak of one's recently deceased parent for years; it is not unusual and is widely acknowledged as healthy. But to speak of one's lost child is often to evoke responses like "Hasn't he gotten over that yet?" One of the most frequent pieces of advice given to people who lose small children is to have another child as soon as possible—as though that could mask the hurt or take away the loss. Out of our own experience we came to understand that the death of a child is threatening to all in a way that our own death as adults is not. Thus many prefer to hide their pain.

The Hebrews understood instinctively that such pain had to be shared. They believed God heard; if our cries were not expressed, then they could not come to God. Their response to pain and loss was dialogic. It was offered up to God in the belief that God cared and would respond. The interesting thing about the laments of the Psalter is that with one exception (Ps. 88), all the laments move toward praise. They begin with lines of despair and anguish such as "My God, my God, why hast thou forsaken me?" and move to expressions of confidence and trust. This was not because Israel thought God heard simply in order to grant our wishes. Israel knew that what we sometimes wish for in painful situations does not always take place—but it believed that God *would* respond. The Israelites ended their laments in praise, anticipating that out of God's response, new life could come from any crisis as God's gift, sometimes in unexpected ways.

This brings us to a second image of God which can aid us in times of loss: *God as life-giver.* Both the Hebrew Scripture and the New Testament know that God is the one who makes new life possible where only death seems to reign. It is important not to misunderstand this assertion. It does not remove the reality and the pain of death. That pain remains an offense. There are two great biblical symbols of God as life-giver out of the experience of death, which are also the great central symbols of salvation: the Exodus event in the Old Testament and the resurrection of Christ in the New Testament. Each of these central events witnesses to the faith conviction that life wins out over death, not because death is unreal or to be ignored or submerged but because God acts as the life-giver beyond death.

The deliverance from bondage in Egypt was a moment of birth for Israel as a people. They had come into being not out of their own efforts but as a result of God's gracious activity of deliverance. In bondage in Egypt and in the dramatic moment at the sea, death seemed to be the only possibility. Life came unexpectedly as God's gift, enabling a new future where none had seemed possible. To Israel this moment became a symbol of possibilities for new life beyond any experience of death. To be an Exodus people was not to live in a world without death; only God was without death. Exodus was a sign of God's gift of life despite death, beyond death, in the midst of death. One can give praise for life as God's gift even when the life of a child is ended prematurely, as was our daughter's. The three years of her life were a gift which her death cannot erase.

The resurrection symbol which is central to the Christian faith in the New Testament witness points to a message similar to that of Exodus. For the church, the resurrection has often lost its power because it is used to obscure the reality of death shown forth in the crucifixion. Our daughter's death came to us as a terrible offense and brought to us an immense sense of aloneness. No meaningful word could ever obscure that reality. It is present within me at this very moment. The disciples also knew the experience of pain and loss in Christ's crucifixion. The power of the resurrection is not in removing the offense of death but in saying, "This is not the final word." This is the good news which the community of faith is charged to carry to each new age.

The community of faith we knew in a house church in Iowa gathered around us again in Wichita, Kansas, to support us at the time of our daughter's death. Its members shared and received our sense of loss. With their support we chose to write a service of thanksgiving for Christine's life because we believed that her death could not be the final word, obscuring all that she had been in life. Her death could not be the final word for our lives either, and in the days after her death, church people helped us see the life that God makes possible beyond such painful moments.

Finally, I want to speak about *God as sufferer.* The biblical picture of God is of a God who suffers with us. This God not only hears and offers us the possibility of life-giving ways into the future; this God has shared our sufferings.

In the account of Moses' encounter with God in the burning bush, God says to Moses, "I have seen the affliction of my people, I have heard their cries. I know their sufferings" (Ex. 3:7). The Hebrew verb we translate as "know" is much broader than can be captured by any English word. It does not indicate "cognitive knowledge, knowledge in the head." Its meaning is closer to our verb "experience." It indicates interaction with and participation in the reality of that which is known. God's statement to Moses is one of the earliest points at which we can see the beginning of the tradition of a God who not only sees and hears from on high but who also chooses to enter into and experience our suffering with us.

The concept of the suffering God reaches a culmination in the crucifixion. There the divine Self shares our ultimate aloneness in pain and death in the form of the cross. Then God can say in the resurrection that death is not the final word, and say that not as a word from on high but as a word from our very midst. And we can better hear that word as meaningful.

We have been speaking of the problem of God. The Scriptures also address us at the point of affirming the life of a child. Our response to the death of a child often suggests that his or her death was more important than his or her life, however short. But Scripture is absolutely clear that all life is of God; all life should be valued as fully participating in God's creation.

One way the faith community can assist grieving parents is by honoring children in the first place. We need to examine our communities of faith in this regard. If we are attentive to the full personhood of our children, then when death tragically takes a child from our midst, we can celebrate the gift which has been among us and not just the life that might have been.

Finally, we must say a word about the role of the covenant community. It seems to me that the Scriptures uniformly witness to the importance of the corporate body of faith as the context of support in times of crisis. This was certainly our experience. In South Carolina, where we knew not a soul, people rose up to claim the privilege of ministering to our hurt. Even though we had no history with that community, we were part of the wider community of faith, and we received unqualified support. People also gathered to be with us in Kansas, where we went for our daughter's burial. If we had been alone, we might not have seen how important it was to affirm our daughter's life and not simply her death.

There seem to be three roles that the community of faith plays in such crises. First, the community helps to relieve the isolation suffered along with the anger and pain. A terrible sense of aloneness comes in the midst of such hardships; the community should surround us in those moments with a presence that is a witness to the presence of God.

Second, the church should pass on and hold up symbols of our faith so that they are available to us in time of trauma as ways of seeing God's gift of life even beyond the offense of the moment. This function cannot be left until a crisis occurs. We have to labor constantly at the task of preparing people with the great symbol resources of our faith, in anticipation of the crises that come to us all.

We must know of Exodus and resurrection. We must learn of the God who hears, gives life to and suffers with us. In stories, hymns, liturgies and studies we equip ourselves with the resources of our faith. These resources will also help us bring the grief and pain out of the counselor's study and into the wider community, so that we all begin to draw on the faith symbols and words that speak to these experiences. We can then have recourse to those traditions when pain descends on us.

Finally, the community of faith mediates the healing word. The community helps to show us pathways into the future when we do not see them ourselves. It does this by receiving our pain and our loss, but also by refusing to believe that such pain and loss constitute the final word.

Out of these perspectives from Scripture and experience, has my daughter's death been made more acceptable? No! But is there a further word of meaning about her life and the life which goes forward for us? Through the grace of God and the support of the people of God, Yes!

Chapter Sixteen

THE PHYSICIAN–PATIENT RELATIONSHIP: ADVISE AND CONSENT

Introduction

There is much talk in our society about how destructive relationships of dependency can be. Many people are concerned about the relationship between the patient and the physician because they see it as one of dependency. At the same time, others in our society are concerned because they see medicine becoming more and more impersonal and see the physician-patient relationship of the "good old days" becoming less and less possible.

What is at stake in these discussions? Those who take part in them often raise two points that appear to center upon the effect of technology on the physician-patient relationship. First, they claim that technology can lead to a depersonalization in that relationship: the patient becomes a "case" instead of a person. Second, they state that the new technology that gives physicians power to cure disease also gives them a capacity to control patients. They argue that we must be protected from this new power, or else physicians will use it to in fact encourage patient dependency.

As a response to the power imbalance between patients and physicians, some have suggested that physicians and patients should understand themselves as independent actors, each free to enter into or to leave the relationship. Recognition of the patient's freedom would act as a constraint upon the physician's power and would consequently boost the patient's own power. As the two actors approach each other with a greater degree of equality, many of the problems stemming from the original imbalance would be ameliorated. Critics of this approach charge that it is false to the reality of illness. Ill people *are* unfree; in fact, illness is experienced as a lack of freedom, at least initially. Thus the patient is, initially and almost by definition, dependent. What the physician is trying to do is to restore that patient to the freedom and independence that is the absence of illness.

It is clear that one of the contested issues here is the authority of the physician. All agree that the physician has an authority of a certain kind, but there is disagreement about the basis of that authority, what kind of authority it is, and the limits upon its legitimate exercise.

We are familiar with a number of different models of authority in our culture. In one model, people have authority by virtue of some skill they possess. Thus automobile mechanics have the skill that gives them the authority to make recommendations about what should be done to a car, but they may not impose their will. In another model, people have authority because they have been elected to public office or are responsible to elected officials. Within the limits of law, these people not only recommend, they also decide and can impose their will. We are all familiar with a third model, too: the authority of the parent, who is assumed to have the child's best interest at heart and who can, again within limits, direct the child in certain ways. Corporate authority, based on the assumption that those who invest and risk their money may decide how it is spent, provides yet another model. Consumers are the authority in the marketplace, deciding what will be produced by their choices. Finally, teachers are authorities in the transmission of knowledge. Our problem is not that we do not have enough different models of authority; we may have too many. What can we learn from the models we have about the authority of the physician and his or her relationship to the patient?

Most of us would want the physician to have our best interest in mind, to be especially interested in our welfare—the kind of concern demanded of the parent in the parent-child model. Yet adult patients are not children; they ought to have more say in their treatment than do children in their upbringing, something that must be expressed by any model which emphasizes the independence of the patient. But we can learn from other models as well. Physicians have been given certain responsibilities and authority by public officials, and they, and they alone, can perform certain actions for the public good. Rightfully, we expect them to live up to this public trust. Further, they have learned certain skills so that they may proceed on the basis of facts. Thus they have part of their authority because of their skill. Finally, physicians not only make recommendations to patients about what should be done, but they are expected to make decisions themselves and to teach the patient. This teaching takes place on two levels: first, there are basic facts about health and disease; and second the physician teaches what patients may expect, both of others and of themselves. In short, physicians appear to have unique roles with respect to the truth of our *lives,* not just the truths about our disease.

It is this fact among others which makes truth telling in medicine so complicated. In the first place, truths about disease are often avoided, so say some physicians, in order to make it easier for the patient. But that very justification opens up a new area of inquiry. Do we avoid telling any truth that will be difficult for the patient, or are there truths that all ought to hear, including the truth that they will die? The question becomes even more troublesome when we recognize that Christians believe that suffering and death are not the last word about human life; consequently the prevention of suffering and the amelioration of the fear of death cannot stand by themselves as good reasons for evading the truth.

There is one further point to be made. Christians are called upon not simply to tell the truth but to build communities which will sustain truthfulness. What does this mean in the context of medicine? Does it change the question about telling the truth into something more complicated? Is it possible that some of the discussion about telling the truth stems from a fear about our inability to sustain truthfulness with the patient?

Thus far, the discussion of the relationship has focused upon the responsibilities of the physician. Are there obligations that are owed by the patient to the physician? For example, what about the patient's obligation to be truthful to the physician? Do they have an obligation to follow the doctor's orders or at least to inform the doctor if they are not going to do so? Physicians "practice" upon patients. Do we have an obligation to make ourselves available to novice medical practitioners so that the art of medicine may continue? Some suggest that patients teach their physicians. Is this part of what it means to be a patient? Further, is this something that the physician must remember in order to keep from becoming arrogant about the source of his or her knowledge?

Note that the more we discuss the mutual responsibilities of patients and physicians, the more we make it possible for both parties to acknowledge that each is indebted to the other for something that only the other can give. If that is the case, then both patients and physicians are dependent upon each other. And if that is the case, then the assumption of many that dependency is always to be avoided is called into question. Christians have a stake in this discussion. Is the very image of the independent actor who can make decisions apart from—indeed, even in opposition to—others a seductive image to all of us in our culture, seductive in that it does not say enough about the relationship of the patient and the physician while pretending to say all?

Decisions in medicine are often struggles—not only between those involved in the process of deciding but also within us—to discover what ought to be done. The process may depend as much upon imagination as upon the available medical and other resources, as much upon who we think we are and what we wish to be as upon rational principles of right and wrong or the objective values of the goods to be accomplished or the evils to be avoided. Medical decisions are such that we are at stake, and this is why we have to think carefully about the context in which they take place, the relationship between the physician and the patient.

Suggestions for Further Reading

Augustine, "Against Lying." In *Treatise on Various Subjects,* edited by R. J. Deferrari. Fathers of the Church, vol. 16. New York: Catholic University of America Press, 1952.

Bok, Sissela. *Lying: Moral Choice in Public and Private Life.* New York: Random House, 1979.

———. *Secrets.* New York: Pantheon, 1982.

Burt, Robert A. *Taking Care of Strangers: The Rule of Law in Doctor-Patient Relations.* New York: Free Press, 1979.

Childress, James F. *Who Should Decide? Paternalism in Health Care.* New York: Oxford University Press, 1982.

May, William F. *The Physician's Covenant: Images of the Healer in Medical Ethics.* Philadelphia: Westminster, 1983.

Pellegrino, Edmund D., and David C. Thomasma, *A Philosophical Basis of Medical Practice: Toward a Philosophy and Ethic of the Healing Professions.* New York: Oxford University Press, 1981.

Thomas Aquinas, *Summa Theologica* 2.2 q. 110.

Walters, LeRoy. "Ethical Aspects of Medical Confidentiality." In *Contemporary Issues in Bioethics,* edited by Tom L. Beauchamp and LeRoy Walters, 2d ed. Belmont, Cal.: Wadsworth Publishing Co., 1982.

83. Authority and the Profession of Medicine

STANLEY HAUERWAS

To develop the argument about the nature of authority in medicine necessitates nothing less than a philosophy of medicine that makes credible certain claims about the nature of medical practice. Edmund Pellegrino and David Thomasma have provided some insight as to what an adequate philosophy of medicine entails. They reiterate that medicine is a complex activity and as such is difficult to characterize philosophically. For example, they argue that medicine is neither art nor science, but a *tertium quid* involving both but distinct from each. Medicine is the "cognitive art of applying science and persuasion through a complex human interaction in which a mutually satisfactory state of well-being is sought, and in which the uniqueness of values and disease, and the kind of institution in which care is delivered, determine the nature of the judgments made." Or medicine is "a relation of mutual consent to effect individualized well-being by working in, with, and through the body."[1]

One aspect of Pellegrino and Thomasma's account which is crucial to any understanding of the kind of authority medicine does or at least should have is the insistence that whatever else medicine may involve, the overriding commitment of physicians is to care for individuals who come to them with complaints of illness. They conclude that "medicine *as* medicine is a process aimed at an action taken in the interest of a specific patient. Its chief aim is not discovery of laws of nature. The end of medicine, its justifying principle, is, in the final analysis a moral one: the good of a person seeking help."[2]

Pellegrino and Thomasma thus make the interesting suggestion that medicine is not only science and art, but also a virtue. They argue that what constitutes medicine is the accumulated wisdom of well-reasoned and concrete judgments about the "capacity to act with regard to the things that are good or bad for man." The practice of medicine is thus "a habit of the mind" that embodies the good inherent in the process of healing. Since health is a good, it follows that medicine must be a virtue, because a virtue "must make right choices about the ends and purposes for which the decisions and actions are produced. Medicine must not only perform well but also act well. It must choose what should be done to heal a particular whose good is the true end of the whole activity."[3]

Surely the claim that medicine is a virtue is an odd one, because a virtue is a disposition of a particular agent. Pellegrino and Thomasma, on the other hand, interpret medicine to be a relation. Of course, it is true that Aristotle called justice and friendship virtues, though each is clearly a quality of a relation rather than a good inherent to the self. Tha a relation may be subject to virtuous formation is but a reminder that all virtues require formation through the practical judgments shaped by the wisdom of a community's translations. Medicine, therefore, is a virtue insofar as it is the name for a tradition of wisdom concerning good care of the body. As such it is not a "means" to health, but rather is part of the activity of health—an activity that involves as much the participation of the patient as the physician.

Pellegrino and Thomasma's case for medicine as a moral profession goes well beyond the notion that health is a normative category.[4] The issue is not simply that medicine involves values in decisions concerning the care of particular patients, but that medicine is an activity which requires as well as enhances a virtuous life.[5] In this context, the physician is not the sole participant in the activity; rather, medicine becomes a relation that inextricably involves patient and physician. This does not mean that patients need to possess the skills of their physicians; it is sufficient that patients have moral reasons to trust physicians to support their patients' life projects insofar as those projects involve a well-functioning body.

The very willingness of patients to permit physicians to be present as well as to lay hands on them in times of crisis is a telling indication of physician dependence on patients. In this respect, perhaps the best way of thinking about the medical relation is to see it as fundamentally an educational process both for doctor and patient, in which each is both teacher and learner.[6] It is from patients that physicians learn the wisdom of the body. Both physicians and patients must learn that each of them is subject to a prior authority—the authority of the body. The form and practice of medicine may change throughout history and differ from one cultural setting to another, but these differences in the end are merely reflections of different attitudes toward the body and are regulated finally by the body. Medicine thus represents a transcultural practice of learning to live with finitude.[7]

From *Responsibility in Health Care,* ed. George J. Agich (Dordrecht: D. Reidel, 1982), pp. 90-97.

Pellegrino and Thomasma, however, properly insist that "the body" is by no means a straightforward category.[8] Each person is not simply a physical body, but a "lived body" which organizes a whole field of perceptions in addition to being the subject of a history of experiences. The body sets the norm for medicine because it is the "artist of its own healing."[9] The task of medicine is to aid that process so that individuals may better learn to live in and through their bodies, since they cannot successfully live beyond or without their bodies. Medicine is therefore a tradition of inherited wisdom and practices through which physicians acquire the responsibility to remember, learn, and pass on the skills of learning to live with a body.

As mentioned before, there is little evidence to support the claim that the health of a population is a result of the practice of medicine. Except for the contentions of those persons who try to justify the special privileges of medicine in this light, the claim should not be viewed as a judgment against medicine. Those who justify privileges are responsible in part for the eventual perversion of medicine, since medical authority cannot long be sustained by promising more and more cures through technological advances.[10]

Wise physicians, on the other hand, have learned their craft better. As Eric Cassell notes, the primary task of physicians is to remove the world of illness from the unknown to the known world where it can become subject to human care.[11] Their task, however, is not limited to those who become ill. By steadfastly identifying with the ill, physicians become teachers also for the healthy. Part of the physician's vocation, therefore, is to serve as a bridge between the world of the sick and the world of the healthy.

The sick constitute a threat to us by making us aware of the frailty of our own connectedness, the thinness of our shield of reason and the limit of our control over the world. By segregating the sick in hospitals having special rules of behavior, the threat for us and the sick is somewhat mitigated, if not entirely eliminated. It is not surprising that we do not often discuss or even secretly recognize the essential characteristics of sickness, because it would be too frightening to do so. This carries over into medicine itself. Cassell points out: "Ostensibly, the physician deals only with disease elements of the illness. His manifest function is the cure of disease, but his latent function, healing, which involves restoring the sick to the world of the healthy, is a secret even to himself."[12] Because physicians have this task, they stand as a constant reminder that the worlds of the sick and the healthy are actually one world joined by common destiny.

In his book *The Healer's Art,* Cassell provides impetus for the contention that medicine is primarily an educational process by showing how physicians act as arbitrators between patients and their bodies.[13] Yet as important as Cassell's explicit thesis is the way in which he uses examples to make his case. These examples nicely reveal how he was in fact educated by his patients to understand what medicine is about.[14] The wisdom manifest in Cassell's book is therefore a witness to the wisdom of the body that teaches "what life is really about underneath the social conventions."[15]

This point is exemplified in Cassell's observation that it is possible, and even a duty, for a physician to teach patients how to die—"to give his patients in this final stage of life the same kind of control that can be taught in earlier stages of living."[16] This is not to say that teaching patients how to die is the first priority. Cassell admits that the primary duty of a physician is to aid in patients' recovery. He is not suggesting that the physician can give the patient control for which the patient does not already have the resources. Patients cannot and should not be made to die better than they have lived. Likewise, medicine should refrain from substituting technology for a patient's lack of moral resources. Physicians, however, can help their dying patients to acquire the "innate ability to command the body, and then enlist the aid of those who surround him—family, friends, and physician. It is dependent on what humans have within themselves; to that extent it is a lonely thing, as is death itself. But the dying are also dependent on others and relationship is based on trust. Both inner resources and trust in others are required because the enemy of control is fear."[17]

It is ironic, though, that what people fear is loss of control. That fear is so all-consuming an indication of the common misunderstanding of what control of the body entails. To control the body does not mean to "manage" or even, as Cassell suggests, to "soar" over the body,[18] but rather to appreciate how the body's limitations are also the source of the most creative and interesting possibilities available to us.[19] Cassell concludes:

> I think that those who die well and in control have something to teach the living about the body and about living. They show us that it is possible to come to peace with the body, both to be controlled by its limitations and to control it to a far greater extent than unlearned existence would suggest. They teach us that control is not denial or repression. That which we deny or repress about ourselves or within ourselves controls us by the very fact of our constant need to deny rather than to come to terms. Control implies

> acceptance of limitations plus an awareness that the limitations provide room for the continued exercise of self, even into death. The beauty and potential of growth lie not only in intellectual transcendence and the formation of transcendent emotional bonds, but also in the possibility of dynamic unity with the body. In that state the fear of death, an essentially backward look, becomes unimportant.[20]

Medicine is therefore a learned profession because it literally learns from patients the skills necessary for acceptance of the possibilities and limits of the body. It is a tradition comprised of the skills of caring for, and sometimes even curing, those who are ill. Medicine is a profession because it has learned how to teach and initiate new agents into that tradition and how to govern the practice of their skills. That even neophyte physicians have authority indicates that medicine as a practice does not begin *ex nihilo* with each new generation. On the other hand, young physicians acquire their skills in a manner that makes them their own. Learning is thus fundamentally a moral training because the skills are of the sort that can be mastered only by watching a master perform them. Such learning is necessary not only in order to pass on tradition, but also because it is the source of critique and innovation of tradition.

In summary, medicine constitutes a community formed by an authority. People are participants in a community based on common bodily existence that has the potential to sustain the authority of medicine as an educational practice. Specialization, or, preferably, the calling of some members of the community to become physicians, is justified by the community's need to have some of its members committed to practicing the wisdom of the body. That such a calling is required and justified indicates the kind of knowledge which can be gained through learning from the body, as well as the kind of skills necessary to care for individuals who are ill. This knowledge and these skills are not universal truths that can be known by just anyone. Rather, they are matters of learned judgments and wisdom which can only be sustained by those willing to place themselves under the guidance of an acknowledged master.

Even if this account of medicine is persuasive (and there obviously are powerful challenges to the arguments raised here), one might argue that what is lacking is a wider community and/or morality sufficient to sustain and support such a medicine. This response probably would be apropos, but it is important to understand why.

As suggested earlier, physicians like Cassell insist that one of medicine's tasks is to teach us how to die. This task is drawn from the authority of the body. But in the absence of any consensus of what an appropriate death morally involves, how can any profession be entrusted with such an important task? It is no wonder that in the absence of such consensus or community the medical profession is tempted to become a self-protective interest group which tries to secure unwarranted power over our lives by claiming to be in possession of a knowledge peculiar to itself. It tries to justify its power by being what it cannot—a science that frees us from, rather than teaching us, the limits of our bodies. This is not really the result of increasing technological power. Instead, increasing technological power is an attempt to maintain the moral coherence of medicine in a morally incoherent society—that is, medicine gains its moral coherence by drawing on the fear of death, the one thing people still seem to have in common. As a result, rather than a profession which provides assistance in living with the body, medicine becomes the modern analogue to the gnostic heresy.[21]

Put differently, a medicine which assumes that its first task is educative in the sense I suggested here cannot help but appear as a sectarian community and challenge to a pluralistic society. This point can be illustrated by calling attention to the difficulty as well as necessity of physicians avowing their fallibility. That such an avowal is necessary is implied in the commitment to care for individual patients. This commitment involves contingent judgments which in principle exclude certainty.[22] Of course, some judgments can be more assured than others, but in principle physicians know they are making judgments for which they cannot claim infallibility.[23] Therefore, the physician's pledge to the patient (or perhaps more appropriately, the *covenant* that the physician and patient enter) does not include a guarantee of errorless judgment, but rather a pledge of steadfast presence and care.

The avowal of fallibility required of physicians is also necessitated through their commitment to learning how better to care for their patients, which is not the same thing as the growth of medical knowledge. Good patient care, as well as good science, depends on the willingness to expose what does not work as readily as that which works. Failure is actually more important than success. Consequently, what is good for medicine as a profession may be disquieting to the patient who sees the physician as savior. Patients have to learn that they cannot put themselves under the care of physicians and in doing so assume that such care can be without error.[24] Indeed, patients must face the possibility that the best possible medicine of the day may be the wrong thing for them.[25] This is no reason to reject the care the physician can offer, but it does change decisively the attitude with what care should be approved.

Yet as this essay suggests, the practice of fallible medicine cannot help but appear as a sectarian alternative in our society. Medicine as a profession only exists because it is also supported by an equally sectarian community formed by essential convictions. Such a community must not presuppose that the task of medicine is to keep illness and death at bay as if such a task were an end in itself. Rather, the community should recognize that medicine involves those skills which allows its members to continue pursuing the goods of that community. These benefits naturally will be offset by some members suffering from illness and finally dying. Thus, a fallible medicine is sustained not only because this medicine serves the common good, but also because participation is a form of service for the whole community.

The absence of such a community in actuality, however, has meant that medicine increasingly has been forced to take the form of a contract between patient and physician. Contracts are the moral substitutes for modern society's lack of shared moral tradition. Of necessity medicine continues to insist that it is a self-sufficient institution, at least in part as an attempt to preserve its past commitment to the service of individual patients. As a result:

> . . . it develops and maintains in the profession a self-deceiving view of the objectivity and reliability of its knowledge and the virtues of its members. Furthermore, it encourages the profession to see itself as the sole possessor of knowledge and virtue, to be somewhat suspicious of the technical and moral capacity of other occupations, and to be at best patronizing and at worst contemptuous of its clientele. Protecting the profession from the demands of interaction on a free and equal basis with those in the world outside, its autonomy leads the profession to so distinguish its own virtue from those outside as to be unable to even perceive the need for, let alone undertake, the self-regulation it promises.[26]

Until now the only solution to this dilemma has been to demand more patient "autonomy", that is, to use the disease to try to cure the disease. This strategy is doomed to fail since the contract between physician and patient can never be "voluntary" in that the very condition which encourages patients to seek their physicians' help is coercive. Physicians are also bound to this contract by the fact that in their state of submission, patients expect the impossible. Once physicians fail, as they inevitably will, patients will blame them.

There seems to be little possibility of breaking this vicious cycle of false expectations and correlatively distorted forms of authority and power. At least for awhile the practice of medicine probably will remain better than critics of medicine allege. A. MacIntyre suggests that one possible strategy would be to work with "those with whom one does share sufficient beliefs to rescue and to recreate authority within communities that will break with the pluralist ethos. In medicine it means working for a variety of new forms of medical community, each with its own shared moral allegiance. With these the notion of authority could again begin to find context and content."[27]

This strategy might also have the unexpected effect of aiding in understanding the relationship between religious and medical communities. The ability of a community to sustain a fallible medicine, a medicine that understands its first task to be mediating between us and our bodies, is ultimately dependent on convictions about goods that set the task of medicine within a larger framework. When these goods are not seen to exist, or at least can be safely ignored, medicine is tempted to become an end in itself. It thus becomes a pseudo-salvific institution.

In other words, medicine requires the existence of another institution to be able to keep its extremely significant, but limited, task *limited.* This does not mean that religious convictions should be supported in order to sustain medicine. Indeed, such functional justifications of religious beliefs are ill-advised. (If religious beliefs are false, then they should not be entertained no matter what good results they might engender.) Yet the fact that medicine as a practice requires convictions and institutions beyond itself to sustain its activity at least helps us understand why we are constantly tempted to ask too much of medicine in our secular times.

Notes

1. Edmund D. Pellegrino and David C. Thomasma, *A Philosophical Basis of Medical Practice* (New York: Oxford University Press, 1981), pp. 69, 80.
2. Ibid., p. 147.
3. Ibid., p. 148.
4. See, for example, Eric Cassell's claims in this respect (*The Healer's Art: A New Approach to the Doctor-Patient Relationship* [Philadelphia: Lippincott, 1976], pp. 87, 113). Of course, I am not denying that various illnesses involve normative judgment, but I am suggesting the idea of "health" as a clear and distinct idea is a chimera. Health is an activity with a shifting meaning. The current attempt to limit the

province of medicine by developing a firm definition of health is thus doomed to failure.

5. From this perspective one of the most overlooked aspects of our current situation is how medical schools continue to function as schools of virtue. They are among the few institutions in our society that have coherent enough purpose that enables them to form character. I only wish we could exhibit the same kind of self-confidence in our seminaries.

6. See William F. May, "Code and Covenant or Philanthropy and Contract," in Chapter 3 of this book.

7. This fact may be one of the reasons that medicine and religion are always interrelated. Each deals with the same subject, but in different ways. Both are tempted to deny the special task of the other in hopes of being the sole authority. In truth, neither can be helpful without the other.

8. Pellegrino and Thomasma, *A Philosophical Basis of Medical Practice,* pp. 73–74.

9. Ibid., p. 79.

10. Again the church provides a useful illustration in this respect. The more specialized the function of the priest became from that of the layman, the more the potential for the delegitimation of the priesthood itself. The more laymen viewed their priests' roles as foreign to their own lives, the more likely it became that the roles of the priests would be associated with magic and/or arbitrary power. This would result finally in either rejection or legitimacy, the latter by making Christianity a mystery cult. With rejection laymen are no better off because too often priestly authority is rejected in the name of an equally destructive authority which offers a bogus salvation. The technological form of contemporary medicine involves many of the same dangers. The more laymen are prevented from understanding what is being done to them in the name of science, the more likely they are to turn to alternative forms of care. Quackery and purely technological medicine are but two sides of the same coin. From the laymen's perspective they are judged by the same criterion—results.

11. Cassell, *The Healer's Art,* p. 131.

12. Ibid., p. 46.

13. Ibid., p. 47.

14. Cassell's examples are not just illustrations—they are the argument, and rightly so. Contrary to the most contemporary accounts of argument, I assume that good arguments cannot be separated from the context that makes them intelligible in the first place. It would take me too far afield to develop this point, but stated briefly it involves the contention that there exists no foundational point on which arguments as such rest. Rather, all arguments begin in the midst of things and are proved true or false exactly by how plausibly they display the narratives on which they depend.

15. No doubt Cassell means that when people are faced with illness or death they exhibit what they want and what they are. But I think it wrong to suggest this is a challenge to social convention, since what we really want and are is itself a convention. Conventions are sometimes lies but they are also just as likely to be the way to truth.

16. Cassell, *The Healer's Art,* p. 203.

17. Ibid., p. 204.

18. Ibid., p. 146.

19. Cassell's way of putting this is an interesting case of someone's insight fighting against its own expression. Although Cassell uses the word "soar", the very examples he uses (polio victims' struggles to retain some control over their bodies) suggest that "soaring" is really more a matter of learning to live at peace with the body. The same kind of problem occurs in Cassell's defense of the importance of the "omnipotence" of physicians for helping patients recover their own omnipotence. Yet Cassell's own critique of the dangers of such omnipotence for physician and patient alike suggests that the control patients seek is not so much omnipotence as simply the power to make their lives their own. See *The Healer's Art,* pp. 142–45.

20. Ibid., p. 228.

21. Gnosticism was not only a Christian heresy, but a widespread and extremely complex phenomenon in the ancient world. No simple generalization can be sufficient to characterize gnostic beliefs or practices. By suggesting that some aspects of modern medicine bear close analogy to gnosticism I mean no more than: (1) medicine, like gnosticism, is often seen, at least implicitly, as offering a form of salvation; (2) that such salvation is obtained through esoteric knowledge possessed by those who have a special training; and (3) that the salvation offered is basically an attempt to free us from the limits of our bodies.

22. See Pellegrino and Thomasma, *A Philosophical Basis of Medical Practice,* p. 124. Actually, Charles L. Bosk (*Forgive and Remember* [Chicago: University of Chicago Press, 1979]) presents the most complete analysis of error in medicine. He distinguishes between *technical errors,* which are expected to happen to everyone and which must thus be quickly reported, *judgmental errors,* which involve clinical judgments, and *normative* and *quasi-normative errors,* which involve a failure to fulfill the moral expectations of the physician's role. In medicine the former must be exposed and forgiven, since only in that way can the failure be prevented from happening again (p. 128). Thus Bosk notes that Grand Rounds and Mortality and Morbidity Conferences are actually elaborate rituals "the entire congregation of surgeons have evolved for witnessing them [errors], resolving the confusion they create, and incorporating them into the group's history and the individual's biography" (p. 121).

23. Pellegrino and Thomasma's account of clinical judgments is particularly worth reading, as is their argument for the necessity of discretionary space in professional judgments (see *A Philosophical Basis of Medical Practice,* pp. 155–69). For a particularly biting critique of the model of the clinician as requiring personal judgment to justify the "autonomy" of the physician, see Eliot Freidson, *The Profession of Medicine: A Study of the Sociology of Applied Knowledge* (New York: Harper and Row, 1970), pp. 346–49. However, Bosk's study of how medical students are trained to assume the moral role of "professional self-control" at least qualifies Freidson's critique. Bosk points out, "The problem is not, as some have claimed, an absence of any socialization, controls, or ethical sense in the profession; the problem is rather a system which celebrates individual conscience as a control while ignoring corporate responsibility.

The profession of medicine needs to develop structural remedies—or structure socialization—in a way that brings into balance both the corporate and the individual dimensions of control" (p. 188).

24. I have not discussed the implication of my analysis of the authority of medicine for the specification of and/or relation between the various roles in medicine—i.e. physician, nurse, counselor. I think no *a priori* formula exists by which this can be done. Different roles develop historically as part of medicine's conversation with itself or are governed by changing needs of patients. However, the current dominance of the physician, in part justified by their technical expertise, or the attempt of the physician to usurp all other roles, is dangerous for the physician as well as the patient. If the physician is "first among equals," he is so because of the need to have someone morally responsible, not simply because of his expertise.

25. It is interesting that Bosk only treats the necessity of surgeons to expose errors among themselves—he does not ask if error should also be exposed to the patient and, if so, what would be the implication of such exposure.

26. Freidson, *Profession of Medicine,* p. 370.

27. A. MacIntyre, "Patients as Agents," in *Philosophical and Medical Ethics: Its Nature and Significance,* ed. H. T. Engelhardt, Jr., and S. F. Spicker (Dordrecht, Holland: D. Reidel, 1977), p. 212.

84. Principles of Professional Communication

BENEDICT M. ASHLEY
AND KEVIN D. O'ROURKE

Listening and Truth Telling

In health care, as in all professional relations, adequate communication between professional and client is a fundamental ethical requirement. In the medical model, opportunities for such communication may be rather sharply restricted, but they are still crucial. Within these limits, what are the duties of physicians and nurses?

The first obligation is to listen to the patient. Yet often in the medical model while professionals concentrate on filtering out medically significant information, patients are attempting to express their malaise in a rhapsody of symptoms, fears, fantasies, evasions, cries for attention, and so forth. The work-pressured professional cannot afford to sit and hear a long and rambling discourse from a self-pitying patient. Even the psychotherapist, who has a special interest in all sorts of behavioral clues, must insist that patients "get to work" without evading the therapeutic process. Somehow professionals must cut through the noise and get at the real message; but they need to remember that "the medium *is* the message," that is, the way patients are (or are not) communicating may be the most significant symptom.

Therefore, no matter how busy they may be, health care professionals may not ethically rush through interviews or simply rely on laboratory tests. They have the responsibility to acquire the art of medical dialogue by which they can help patients say what needs to be said. The first rule of this art is for the professional to repeat back to the patient what the professional has heard that seems significant and to ask whether it is what the patient meant. This feedback not only reassures the patient, but can also gradually train the patient in giving relevant information. A second rule is to obtain the patient's cooperation by explaining the purpose of questions, since unexpected and cryptic questions are threatening and confusing to many patients. If physicians are unable

Reprinted from *Health Care Ethics,* second edition, by Benedict M. Ashley and Kevin D. O'Rourke, The Catholic Health Association of the United States, 1982, pp. 103–8.

or unwilling to learn this art of dialogue, then they must learn to work in a team which includes other professionals with such communication skills.

A professional must not only hear but also *believe* patients who have the basic right to be believed until they lose that right by clearly proved deception. Hence the temptation of some busy physicians and exasperated nurses to jump to the conclusion that a patient is malingering has to be resisted. While what a patient reports may not be objectively true, it is subjectively so because it expresses what the patient really *feels* and is therefore medically significant and important.

Of course, professionals also have the right to require honesty and frankness from clients. When they suspect deliberate deceit, they should deal with the situation explicitly and directly as a breach of the patient's contract with the professional. In most illnesses, however, psychological factors may cause communication to be distorted by unconscious elements of self-deceit, denial, confusion, or panic. Psychotherapists in particular have to deal with this perplexing inability of some patients to communicate openly, but therapists also experience in themselves something of the same ambiguity. William Appleton is of this opinion.

> Psychiatrists advocate honest and open communication by physicians with patients but too often do not practice what they preach. Their reasons for silence include uncertainty about the cause, treatment, and prognosis of psychiatric illnesses and unwillingness to depress, demoralize, anger, or alienate their patients.[1]

This observation applies to all health care professionals, who cannot expect truth from their patients unless they are equally truthful with them. Lack of frankness by professionals is usually excused as concern to spare the patient, but is just as often the result of unconscious fear on the part of the professional. Chapter 13 of our book *Health Care Ethics* discusses the problem of telling the truth to the incurable or dying patient.[2] Here it suffices to say that the fundamental principle in all such situations is that the patient has the right to the truth, however difficult it may be for the professional to communicate it.

Confidentiality

Patients have the right to the truth about their health because they have the primary responsibility for their health. They also have the right to privacy about those aspects of life which do not directly affect others. Human community is based on free communication which is impossible if confidences cannot be shared. Hence health care professionals have a serious obligation to maintain such confidences that protect the patient's right of privacy.

How is a professional to act when questioned by others about a patient's condition? Can confidentiality be protected by lying? All Catholic moralists agree that it is always wrong to "lie," even to protect confidentiality, but not all agree on how to define *lying.* Some[3] distinguish between a *falsehood,* that is, a false statement, and a *lie,* which is not only a false statement but also one made to someone who has the right to a true answer. Consequently, they hold that someone who has a duty to keep a secret can answer falsely to inquirers. It seems better to say with Peter Knauer[4] that the meaning of any human statement must always be determined from the context in which communication occurs. Consequently, when persons ask questions which they have no right to ask, the context renders any answer given essentially *meaningless,* so that it is ethically inconsequential whether that answer in a normal context would be true or false. Thus health care professionals who are questioned about confidential matters may without lying or even falsehood reply in any way that protects confidentiality. This fact, however, cannot excuse a physician from frankly answering questions put by a patient or the patient's guardians, because these persons have the right to know. Whether one has the obligation to reply to a question with unambiguous and accurate information then depends upon the questioner's right to such information.

It is not easy to draw the line between what individuals have the right to keep private and what they may have the duty to make public. Hence, the contract between professional and patient should determine this as exactly as possible. If professionals are convinced that in order to do the best for a patient they need to discuss the case with consultants or before other members of a team or of the professional staff, the professionals must obtain the informed consent of the patient. Generally, this consent is implicitly contained in the contract. Thus in most mental hospitals it is assumed that voluntary (or even involuntary) commitment implies the right to discuss the patient's condition and progress with other members of the therapeutic staff.

Such assumptions, however, are easily open to abuse. Books have been published by physicians and psychiatrists about their famous or notorious patients, living or dead. In our opinion much greater care must be taken to obtain explicit consent from patients with regard to matters that may be embarrassing to them, especially in the present age of medical teamwork and computerized records. Most patients (when they are incompetent, their guardians) readily permit the therapeutic use of information, but they should have the opportunity to restrict the use of this information when entering into contractual relations with the professional. It should not be too difficult for a physician or for a health care institution to work out a regular procedure by which patients are informed of their rights to privacy and asked for explicit consent for any necessary use of confidential information. One of the most difficult problems, however, is the need of researchers to have access to records, especially when doing epidemological studies; yet even here it should be possible to guard the privacy of individuals from public knowledge.

Nevertheless, the right of privacy, sacred as it is, is limited by the rights of other persons and by the individual's own limited rights of self-disposal. Patients may behave in ways which directly injure themselves and indirectly or directly injure others. For example, patients may commit suicide, seek ways to continue their chemical dependency, spread contagious diseases, or commit acts of theft or aggression against other patients or the staff. Some may become so seriously incompetent as to become a public danger on release from an institution, for example, the epileptic bus driver who refuses to change his job. In the case of *Tarasoff v. Regents of University of California* the court held a therapist responsible for not warning third parties that his client might be dangerous.

In all these cases, the family or society has an obligation to prevent harm both to the patient and to the public because all are members of a community which exists for the good of each of its members in relation to all others. Hence, generally speaking, professionals have not only the right but also the duty to communicate information necessary to prevent serious harm to the patient or to others, even when it is given to them in confidence, to those who may be able to prevent this injury.

Thus, professional secrecy is not as absolute as the secrecy demanded of a Catholic priest who may not reveal what he has learned in confession regarding the sins or defects of a penitent even to prevent harm to a third party. Nor is it even as absolute as that given by law to the confidences between accused criminals and their lawyers. In the first case the penitent is revealing personal moral responsibility before God which is beyond human judgment. In the second case the accused is protected in his or her rights by the adversary process. In medical matters, however, patients seldom need to reveal to the professional anything which is essentially incriminating but usually only what at worst might be a matter of embarrassment. Moral fault, however, may incidentally be revealed: for example, when the patient voluntarily admits an intention to commit a crime and when the medical condition has moral implications (addiction, venereal disease, illegitimate pregnancy).

When what is revealed is an intention to commit a crime (including suicide), the professional has the obligation to reveal to appropriate persons whatever information is necessary to prevent such a crime. When no crime is contemplated, but there is probable danger of harm which can be prevented, the professional should discreetly do what is likely to be helpful in preventing such harm. Ordinarily this should not be done without first warning the patient of exposure if the patient refuses to desist. For example, the professional should keep the fact of addiction confidential if the patient is willing to cooperate with treatment, but may be forced to make it known to the family if cooperation is refused. A professional should protect the confidence of someone illegitimately pregnant unless the intention to secure an abortion is evident, in which case, in spite of recent deplorable court decisions declaring the "right" of minors to free choice of abortion, professionals may be forced to inform the parents of a minor or the father of the child. This will at least permit parents to discuss the decision with their child and attempt to protect the rights of their grandchild. In the case of venereal disease of a minor, confidentiality should be maintained unless the minor refuses treatment. In other situations professionals should first seek to obtain the cooperation of the patient, and only proceed to inform the third party when this cooperation is refused and the damage feared is both serious and probable, since the benefit of the doubt is in favor of confidentiality, which influences the dependence of the patient or the professional.

Certain very serious problems about confidentiality have been raised recently by the computerization of health records and also by the requirement of private and government health insurance plans that physicians report the nature of a patient's illness as a condition of receiving payment. It is clear enough that a physician does not have the right to give information of this sort without the patient's permission. This, however, leaves the larger question of how patients are to obtain the benefits to which they are entitled without giving such permission. The insurance or public agency has the right to ask proof from patients that they have used funds for a legitimate medical purpose, but the agency also has the duty to design adequate controls which do not require detailed information which might be embarrassing or injurious to the patient. Computerization of health records should always require the patient's permission, and even when permission is given, care must be taken to limit the availability of these records to a few definitely authorized persons.

Some professionals[5] argue for an extreme individualistic and libertarian position. For example, they contend that addicts should be permitted free access to alcohol and drugs, and some even believe that suicidal persons should be permitted to take their own lives if they wish. This opinion is based on such notions as: "Freedom is doing what you want with your own life," and "Immorality is only doing harm to another, nonconsenting adult." However, the very nature of personhood implies involvement in a community. Self-destructive behavior is not merely of concern to the person in question, but to all with whom his or her life is intertwined. In fact, psychology seems to show that such behavior is an often unconscious cry for help.[6] To let such persons destroy themselves because they claim that is what they want is actually to ignore this cry that comes from the true self. The real answer must be a social concern for persons in their real liberty, which consists in becoming more open to others, not more closed. To achieve openness, the trust of the alienated must be gained.

In view of this discussion, the *Principle of Professional Communication* can be formulated as follows:

In order to fulfill their obligations to serve the patient's health, health care professionals have the responsibility:

1. To strive to establish and preserve trust at both the emotional and rational levels;
2. To share the information they possess with those who legitimately need it in order to have an informed conscience;
3. To refrain from lying or giving misinformation;
4. To keep secret information which is not legitimately needed by others, but which if revealed might either harm the patient or others or destroy trust.

Notes

1. William S. Appleton, "The Importance of Psychiatrists' Telling Patients the Truth," *American Journal of Psychiatry* 129 (1972): 743.
2. Ashley and O'Rourke, *Health Care Ethics: A Theological Analysis* (St. Louis: The Catholic Health Association of the United States, 1982).
3. E.g., J. A. Dorszynski, *Catholic Teaching About the Morality of Falsehood* (Washington, D.C.: Catholic University of America Press, 1949).
4. "The Hermeneutic Function of the Principle of Double Effect," *Natural Law Forum* 12 (1967): 132–62.
5. E.g., Thomas Szasz, *Ceremonial Chemistry: The Ritual Persecution of Drugs, Addicts, and Pushers* (New York: Doubleday, 1974).
6. Edwin S. Schneidman and Robert E. Litman, *The Psychology of Suicide* (New York: Science House, 1970).

85. Thorn-in-the-Flesh Decision Making: A Christian Overview of the Ethics of Treatment

RICHARD J. MOUW

The ethical perspectives which get employed in medical ethical discussions often seem rather narrow in scope. Sometimes the methodology seems closely linked to a "values clarification" approach, in which the people involved are encouraged to get clearer about the value commitments with which they operate. Or, ethical issues are introduced within a framework of a kind of "systems analysis," and the questions are put in this way: How can we plug our values into the procedures of medical care? How can we best fit the ethical component into the system of medical decision making?

From a Christian point of view there is something deeply unsatisfactory about these ways of dealing with the issues. This sense of dissatisfaction was expressed to me recently by a medical professional who had been involved in a discussion of ethical issues at a seminar in the hospital where she works. At this seminar she experienced a profound frustration: "I just didn't know where to *begin* in bringing my own beliefs to bear on that discussion. I felt like those questions were very important to me, but I also felt that I had to come at those questions in a very different way!"

This experience of frustration is based—or so I judge—on a proper assessment of typical discussions of medical ethics. Very often those discussions move on to casuistry before getting clear about the principles which must inform casuistical deliberation. Nor can the moral principles proper to medical decision making be arrived at merely by explicating our intuitions or by systematizing our hunches. Medical ethical discussion must be rooted in a broad-ranging, self-conscious awareness of the larger moral and more-than-moral contexts in which medical questions arise.

Take, for example, the systems-analysis approach to which I have already alluded. This approach seems to work on the following model. There is a system of medical decision making that encompasses various diagnostic, prognostic, and therapeutic options. This system is taken as a given. The question then is asked whether this system or set of procedures and options is fully adequate without some ethical components being added to it. The view that the system by itself is inadequate seems to be what Ivan Illich has in mind when he complains that in a highly "medicalized" culture "medical ethics have been secreted into a specialized department that brings theory into line with actual practice" (*Medical Nemesis: The Expropriation of Health* [New York: Bantam, 1977], p. 40). Illich's own view calls for an evaluative critique of that system of medical care itself; he is convinced that the basic assumptions of our medicalized society must be called into question. Whatever our own assessment may be of the details of Illich's critique, he does seem to be correct in insisting that we must be sensitive to the basic presuppositions which shape the discussion of medical ethics.

We must recognize the limitations of the medical perspective by looking at the ways in which formulations of that perspective relate to other kinds of concerns, including ethical concerns. But lest that sound like a self-serving statement coming from an ethicist, let me go one step further. We must also recognize the limitations of the ethical perspective by looking at the ways in which formulations of *that* perspective relate to other kinds of concerns, concerns which range more broadly than the issues of ethical rightness and wrongness.

Medical ethics as an area of scholarly and professional inquiry must be tamed—put into its proper place—by the recognition that neither medical nor ethical nor medical ethical discussion is adequate for dealing with the issues which arise in the context of medical decision making. My basic contention here will not be shocking to Calvinists. Medical ethics must itself function within the context of a larger world-and-life view. As Christians we cannot discuss a perplexing medical dilemma for very long without sensing the need to discuss our views of human nature, our perspectives on the society in which we live, and our concepts of health and healing and human well-being and eternal destiny.

For as long as any of us can remember there have been groups around that have reminded us of the role of basic presuppositions in dealing with medical issues. Jehovah's Witnesses have refused blood transfusions; Christian Scientists have rejected conventional definitions of "disease" and "cure"; Seventh Day Adventists have questioned accepted traditions regarding nutrition; the Old Reformed have eschewed preventative medicine. Few of us are convinced by the exegetical and theological cases which these groups offer in defense of their departures from conventional medical wisdom. But, like Ivan Illich's more recent heterodoxies, they do

---

Used by permission of the author.

remind us of a *level* of critical concern which we must attempt to maintain—a reminder that has also been reinforced by recent interest in Chinese acupuncture, "indigenous" medicine, the hospice movement, and other phenomena.

Some rather harsh recent criticisms of medical orthodoxy have alleged that there are perverse psychological, social, political and economic forces which have shaped the attitudes and patterns at work in medical decision making. These criticisms have a direct bearing on a consideration of the processes of medical treatment. Elisabeth Kübler-Ross and others have argued that the alleged "objectivity" of medical practitioners is often a coverup for the insecurity and fear in the presence of suffering and death on the part of those professionals. Others have argued that the medical care professions are tainted by sexism, racism, classism, ageism, and elitism.

As I have said, these latter considerations—which we might think of as having to do with, roughly speaking, the sociology of medicine—bear very directly on the ethics of treatment. It is not necessary here to decide the degree to which these sociological criticisms of medical orthodoxy are correct. But we can allow the sensitivities from which they stem to inform our own discussion. At the very least this means that we ought not construe the treatment process in too narrow a fashion. There is, for example, a distressing tendency in much of the literature dealing with the ethics of treatment to focus almost exclusively on the physician-patient relationship, as if these were the only two roles which have an important place in medical treatment. The fact is that the treatment process encompasses many relationships involving a number of different roles: for example, the relationship between physician and nurse, nurse and patient, physician and family, clergy and patient.

How should we as Christians view these relationships in the context of the treatment process? In a 1956 article published in the *A.M.A. Archives of Internal Medicine,* Thomas Szasz and Marc Hollender distinguished among three basic models of the physician-patient relationship in the hope of showing "that certain philosophical preconceptions associated with the notions of 'disease,' 'treatment,' and 'cure' have a profound bearing on both the theory and practice of medicine." Their first model is that of "Activity-Passivity," which they judge to be the oldest model operating in medical care. Here the physician is viewed as active, the patient as acted upon. " 'Treatment' takes place irrespective of the patient's contribution and regardless of the outcome. There is a similarity here between the patient and a helpless infant, on the one hand, and between physician and parent, on the other."

The second model is that of "Guidance-Cooperation." Here the patient takes on a more active role than in the previous model. But the decision-making power resides with the physician. The physician "guides"; the patient "cooperates." If the earlier model can be likened to the relationship between parent and helpless infant, this one more closely parallels that between parent and adolescent child.

The third model is given the label of "Mutual Participation," and it is based on "the postulate that equality among human beings is desirable." Patient and physician have roughly equal power, they are mutually interdependent, and they search for decisions which will be satisfactory to both parties.

Several observations are necessary concerning the intentions of Szasz and Hollender in presenting these models. First, they make it clear that no one single model is adequate to all situations involving medical decisions. For example, the Activity-Passivity model may be quite appropriate to a situation where a physician must treat a comatose patient. Second, Szasz and Hollender obviously do think that the third model, Mutual Participation, is the ideal to be strived for. They tell us that "in an evolutionary sense, the pattern of mutual participation is more highly developed than the other two models of doctor-patient relationship." And third, we must highlight the fact that Szasz and Hollender are presenting these models as ways of sorting out different patterns or distributions of power and authority in medical decision making. In the first model, all power resides with the physician; in the second, the patient at least has the right or power to consent to the physician's decision; in the third, power is distributed along egalitarian lines.

I want to comment further on some of these matters. But before doing so, I must briefly observe that Szasz and Hollender themselves manifest the syndrome, which I mentioned earlier, of discussing the treatment process as if it were exclusively an affair between *physician* and patient. I will attempt to remedy that pattern by referring more generally to the relationship between medical professional and patient.

I daresay that many of us in the Christian community would never think of attempting to understand the relationship between medical professional and patient along the lines suggested by the third model proposed by Szasz and Hollender. Nor would we find the first model, that of Activity-Passivity, to be appropriate, except in unusual circumstances. Most of us would take the second model, in which the patient cooperates with the expert guidance of the professional, as quite proper—even the ideal way of viewing medical situations. But of course it is precisely the notion of the "expertise" of the professional which is under attack from the perspective of the egalitarian.

The denial of the expertise of the medical professional comes in two forms today. First, there are those who hold to a pluralistic or relativistic view of medical theory. They reject the notion of a "neutral" or "objective" medical science. Medical theories and technologies are shaped by cultural perspectives, and their formation and formulation are guided by culturally embedded understandings of such things as "health," "disease," and "cure." The Navajo medicine man, the faith healer, the Eastern guru, the shaman, the surgeon from Cincinnati, the practitioner of acupuncture—each is rooted in a different form of social organization embodying a different normative understanding of human nature. To evaluate these perspectives in terms of "primitive" or "modern" or "advanced" is already to be adopting a given cultural archimedian point. There can be no question of whether one system is better than another; each is simply different from the rest. Or, if comparative evaluations *can* be made, they cannot be made superficially: they must be based on an assessment of the larger cultural context from which given perspectives and technologies derive their meaning and effectiveness.

There are important and fascinating issues here—issues which bear directly on questions in the philosophy of science and epistemology. But the second form of the challenge to medical expertise has closer links to medical ethics and the sociology of medicine, so we will look at that version more closely.

The second way in which people challenge the expertise of the medical professional focuses on the role of what are considered to be significant nonmedical factors in medical decision making. Those who issue this kind of challenge may or may not have sympathies with the first form of challenge. Nonetheless they are inclined to view situations of medical decision making in such a way that careful attention is given to various nonmedical features of those situations. The medical professional may be viewed as having some degree of expertise with regard to medical science and technology; but it is argued that the benefits of medical expertise are outweighed by the professional's lack of expertise regarding other, more important, factors at work in situations of medical decision making. Sometimes it is even suggested that medical professionals manifest a systematic bias regarding these nonmedical factors, a bias which distorts and perverts their appeals to medical expertise. For example, a feminist writing under a pseudonym and describing herself as a "fat Radical Therapist" (Aldebaran, "Fat Liberation," in *Love, Therapy and Politics,* ed. Hogie Wyckoff [New York: Grove Press, 1976], pp. 197-212) has argued that the medical establishment and the insurance companies have conspired to suppress and distort accurate information regarding fatness and health. In the course of making her case she refers to "the mystification of medical knowledge which has oppressed fat people for so long," and she alleges that "the hostility of doctors toward fat people is well-documented." This oppression, she suggests, is especially directed toward women: the medical and mental-health professions are committed to the ideals of "beauty, poise and health." In foisting these ideals on women in the name of medical "objectivity" they force many people into lives of "anxiety, self-hatred, and, ultimately, more failure."

This line of argument is an extreme case in point for a pattern of thinking which others are inclined to pursue in more modest tones: the medical professions are organized along lines which promote insensitivity to what it means to be a woman, a black, a homosexual, a ghetto-dweller. Yet characteristics of this sort are crucial elements in medical situations. A patient possessing such characteristics is in fact the "expert" regarding the medical situation in which he or she is involved. Prescriptions concerning what is "best" for a person in that situation must be made from the point of view of the patient.

It should be obvious from the little that I have said about this line of criticism of medical professionals that this is an area of discussion where a number of different dynamics are at work. Some critics attribute to medical professionals a systematic bias against certain groups of people; others view medical orthodoxy as a manifestation of a perverse ideology; still others limit themselves to pointing out certain widespread social and psychological insensitivities associated with medical practice.

But underlying some of the criticisms in this area are assumptions which are closely related to the third model described by Szasz and Hollender, the egalitarian model. This does seem to me to be what is going on in Ivan Illich's critique of what he considers our "medicalized society." I offer as evidence the concluding paragraph of his book, *Medical Nemesis:*

> Man's consciously lived fragility, individuality, and relatedness make the experience of pain, of sickness, and of death an integral part of his life. The ability to cope with this trio autonomously is fundamental to his health. As he becomes dependent on the management of his intimacy, he renounces his autonomy and his health *must* decline. The true miracle of modern medicine is diabolical. It consists in making not only individuals but whole populations survive on inhumanly

> low levels of personal health. Medical nemesis is the negative feedback of a social organization that set out to improve and equalize the opportunity for each man to cope in autonomy and ended by destroying it.

Here we have a clear example of someone who pits human "autonomy" against the "dependency" fostered by medical orthodoxy. According to Illich, the most significant factors at work in a situation of medical decision making are these: as a fragile individual, the questions of how I am going to cope with *my* pain, *my* sickness, *my* death, are an integral part of my life. The autonomous exercise of my ability to cope with these matters is central to my own health. "Health" is not something which can be defined in purely physiological terms, such that a professional intervention on my behalf, an intervention over which I have no control and which brings about a certain state of physiological equilibrium, can make me "healthy." Health *includes* my autonomous coping with my own pain and sickness. Any medical care system which attempts to bypass my active involvement in the decisions which affect these most intimate matters in my life is, as Illich puts it, diabolical: it inevitably reduces my personal health; it makes me dependent on its own alleged expertise. The fact is that the professional is attempting to manage a situation in which I alone am the true expert; for I alone am qualified to decide how my pain, my sickness, and my death will function in my life plan.

I must confess that my own response to this line of argument is an ambivalent one. Let me first explain the negative side of my reaction. As an orthodox Calvinist I bristle when I hear the word "autonomy." I cut my own theological and philosophical teeth on the writings of Carl Henry, Cornelius Van Til and Herman Dooyeweerd, and I learned my lessons well. "Autonomy" means "self-legislating"; an autonomous agent makes his or her own laws. And from a biblical perspective this simply will not do. People are not their own lawmakers; they cannot produce their own norms for living. The plea for autonomy is a vain boast, a boast which echoes the arrogance of the serpent in Genesis 3: "when you eat of [the fruit of the tree] your eyes will be opened, and you will be like God."

This is not to say that the word "autonomy," whenever it is used, always means something devilish. Even some orthodox Calvinists have been known to speak of the need for an "autonomous Christian school system"—by which they mean a school system whose direction is not decided by a government or a church but which sets its own course. I do not know whether Illich himself means to use the term in a way that I would consider to be completely perverse. But I do know that sinful autonomy—the prideful desire to set one's own course, thereby refusing to recognize God's sovereign rule—is a very real tendency in the human heart. And it is a tendency which manifests itself in all areas of living and decision making, including those areas having to do with medicine and health. So it is never silly for us to raise the question whether we are hearing echoes from the Garden in contemporary pleas on behalf of autonomous decision making.

But even when we are sure that a given plea for autonomy is diabolical in nature, that does not decide the matter. Even the serpent of Genesis 3 must be given his due. We know that the serpent always lies, that he is always wrong; but we must take pains to discern the nature of his error in a given context. The Bible makes it clear that while the serpent was thoroughly evil, he was not thoroughly stupid. Genesis 3 begins, after all, with the observation that "the serpent was more subtle than any other wild creature that the Lord God had made." The serpent's lie was in fact a perversion of the truth. He was trading on a subtlety. In tempting Eve, the serpent told her that she could become "like God." Now that is not just a simple falsehood—it is a perversion of the truth. In Genesis 1 we learn that Adam and Eve were in fact created in the image and likeness of God. There is a perfectly proper sense in which human beings are "like God." We are God-imagers. The serpent in Genesis 3 was twisting that truth into a falsehood. He was telling a God-imager that she should become a God-pretender; he was encouraging someone who was already made in the image of God to try to *be* a god. In doing so the serpent was trading on a subtlety: he was, as I have already said, twisting the truth.

Now, what does all of this have to do with Ivan Illich's plea for autonomy? I want to suggest that even if we were convinced that Illich was encouraging persons to be autonomous in the straightforwardly sinful sense of Genesis 3, he still might not be *all* wrong. He might be twisting the truth. And then it would be our job to see the truth that might reside in his perversion of the truth.

Let me try to illustrate my contention here by going through a few lines of Illich's paragraph again, but this time substituting references to the image of God for his uses of the concept of autonomy.

> Man's consciously lived fragility, individuality, and relatedness make the experience of pain, of sickness, and death an integral part of his life. The ability to cope with this trio in a God-imaging manner is fundamental to his health.

> As he becomes dependent on the management of his intimacy, he renounces the divine image and his health *must* decline. . . .

I am of the opinion that this formulation does not sound so off-base to Christian ears. To be healthy in a Christian sense is to be capable of exercising God-given capacities; it is to be able to fulfill one's calling. If conventional medical practice creates the kind of dependency that reduces this capacity in a patient then it would seem that we must say Christian things about that medical practice which are as harsh as the things being said by Illich and others.

But there is an important "if" in what I just said: "*if* conventional medical practice" reduces God-imaging activity. . . . The important question here is, *Does* it?

A fully adequate answer to this question would, of course, require the sifting of much empirical data. But we can get at the question in a slightly different way by expanding it in this manner: Does it *necessarily?* That is, given the fact that conventional medical practice creates certain kinds of dependencies in patients, are these dependencies necessarily detrimental to God-imaging?

Dependency as such is not a bad thing, viewed from a Christian perspective. Indeed, in a rather basic and crucial way, human beings are radically dependent upon God. Nor is dependency upon the *expertise* of others a bad thing, since the God on whom we are dependent is overwhelmingly expert about everything. Is it, then, that dependency upon the expertise of other *human beings* is something to be avoided? I think not. The notions of individual callings and mutual service suggest that different human beings will develop different kinds of expertise, and that we each must respect the gifts of others and rely on others for guidance in different areas of life. We might put the point this way with reference to medical expertise: dependence on the expert guidance of medical professionals is good and proper if that dependence is an image-promoting dependence. Similarly, expert medical guidance is a good thing for a professional to provide, if that guidance is image promoting.

This way of putting the case is neither trivial nor misleading. The apostle Peter instructs believers to "be subject for the Lord's sake to every human institution" (1 Peter 2:13); and although the immediate context of his remarks seems to be political in nature, I do not think that we violate the spirit of this instruction when we apply it to patterns of authority in other spheres of life. But if this legitimately applies to subjection to medical authority, we must also draw parallels between what the Bible says about the proper exercise of political authority and the proper exercise of authority in the medical sphere. Romans 13 makes it clear that God calls rulers to serve as his ministers, rewarding those who perform good works and punishing evildoers. Similarly, if we extend this pattern of biblical teaching to medical practice, those who would exercise medical authority must minister to those under their care.

If the desire to exercise sinful autonomy is to be condemned in the patient, it must also be condemned in the medical professional. In neither case may a person act like a "self-legislator," pretending that he or she is the sole source or reference point for decision-making norms. Patient and professional alike stand *coram deo,* before the face of God.

But of course the situation is complicated by the fact that not all human beings agree about matters pertaining to the relationship of people to God. Some people, both professionals and patients, do not believe in God. And even among Christians there is much diversity in beliefs concerning what it means to live before the face of God. Even under the best conditions possible in a sinful society, some degree of conflict is to be expected.

The professional-patient relationship can be characterized by four possible distributions of belief and unbelief: Christian professional and Christian patient; Christian professional and non-Christian patient; non-Christian professional and Christian patient; non-Christian professional and non-Christian patient. For our purposes here, let us concentrate on the roles of Christian professional and Christian patient under some of these distributions.

Consider first the role of the Christian patient. I am convinced that the Christian patient ought to have a strong interest in being knowledgeably involved in basic decisions regarding his or her medical treatment. This flies in the face of the attitudes of many professionals, especially in the pre-Kübler-Ross era. For example, in a 1961 study of physicians' attitudes toward "truth telling" in cancer cases (reprinted in *Moral Problems in Medicine,* pp. 109-16), Donald Oken reported that many physicians favored a policy of telling "as little as possible in the most general terms consistent with maintaining cooperation in treatment. . . . Questioning by the patient almost invariably is disregarded and considered a plea for reassurance unless persistent, and intuitively perceived as 'a real wish to know.' Even then it may be ignored. The vast majority of these doctors . . . approach the issue with the view that disclosure should be avoided unless there are positive indications, rather than the reverse."

The language used here is clearly that of power and control. The professional controls information about the patient's condition, dispensing it only when it is judged to be in the "real" interests of the patient to do so. From a biblical point of view, this attitude seems to be clearly unsatisfactory. In almost every case there are prima facie reasonable grounds for thinking that it *is* in the best interests of the Christian patient to struggle knowledgeably with the issues of pain, suffering, and death. In 2 Corinthians 12, the apostle Paul describes his own struggles before the Lord regarding his "thorn in the flesh"; three times he bargained with God in the hope of having the affliction removed. Whether his bargaining process was characterized by emotional maturity and stability is not revealed. But it is obvious that his struggle had an important spiritual outcome, namely, the recognition that God's power could be made perfect in his own weakness. This episode, along with the account of King Hezekiah's negotiations with the Lord regarding the time of his own death, reveals, I think, a biblical pattern for viewing the role of suffering in the life of the believer: we must allow pain, suffering, and the expectation of death—even though these are usually very agonizing factors to confront—to visit us as sanctifying forces in our lives. No medical professional has the unqualified right to deny us these struggles by withholding information from us. Perhaps there are extenuating circumstances in which information may be withheld from a Christian patient, but the bias must clearly be in favor of truth telling, even if such disclosures require educating the patient regarding complex medical analyses. There is, I suggest, a Christian "right to know" about the facts concerning one's physical condition.

But what of the role of the Christian professional in situations in which there is real or potential conflict between professional judgment and the wishes and beliefs of the patient? There is an increasing body of medical and legal literature which argues strongly for the rights of patients to refuse life-saving treatment or even to commit what we might think of as "active suicide." For example, Norman Cantor comes to this conclusion in a 1973 *Rutgers Law Review* article after reviewing a wide variety of medical and legal considerations. He suggests that professional deference to the desires of the patient in refusing treatment must be based on a "sensitivity toward personal interests in bodily integrity and self-determination."

I'm not sure exactly what Cantor means by "bodily integrity," but his appeal to the importance of "self-determination" is clearly related to the "autonomy" theme which we have already discussed. My own hunch is that we as Christians can arrive at a similar conclusion to Cantor's by traveling quite a different route.

It is unfortunate that the phrase "playing God" is often used to describe a pattern whereby professionals override the wishes and desires of a patient in prescribing certain kinds of treatment. This is unfortunate because the biblical God in important respects does not himself "play God" in this manner. The God of the Scriptures is patient with unbelief and sin. He does not override the human will in some tyrannical fashion in order to bring people into conformity with his plans. Even the Canons of the Synod of Dort—which many consider to be the harshest of Calvinist documents—insist that God "does not treat men as senseless stocks and blocks, nor take away their will and its properties, or do violence thereto." The Canons then go on to use the language of "wooing" or courtship to describe God's electing procedures, and they regularly treat the unsaved as being *allowed* by God to remain in the condition of unbelief which they *themselves* have chosen. The biblical God does not "play God" by manipulating people with a disregard to their own choices and convictions.

The Christian professional must imitate God's patience with sinners, refusing to coerce, but choosing instead to invite, to persuade, to educate, and to reason—all of which presupposes a respect for the sincerely held convictions and desires of others. The patient's right to know must be supplemented by the professional's right to attempt to persuade.

In a profoundly Christian sense, medical decision making is a "thorny" business; our decisions must be wrestled with in a world that is presently full of thorns. And our struggles are complicated by the fact that these thorns come in several varieties, from the point of view of theological taxonomy. There are, first of all, the thorns of the curse: "Cursed is the ground because of you; in toil you shall eat of it all the days of your life; thorns and thistles it shall bring forth to you" (Genesis 3:17-18). Surrounded by these thorns, human beings issue forth the groans of their physical suffering, they chafe under the yoke of a host of oppressors, and they are drenched with the sweat of their own labors—sensing in all of this that they are made of dust, and to dust they shall return.

But if we survey the thorn-infested landscape of the fallen world with the eyes of faith, we can also discern the thorns of our redemption. Those thorns, which drew blood when pressed into the Savior's brow, were worn as a crown of victory over the cursedness of the creation: for "he was wounded for our transgressions, he was bruised for our iniquities; upon him was the chastisement that made us whole, and with his stripes we are healed" (Isaiah 53:5). And because of the thorns which were worn on Calvary, we can carry the thorns which become embedded in our own flesh as thorns of sanctification, knowing that in our own weakness, we are made strong in the power of God (2 Corinthians 12:10).

A thorny business indeed. And it is made no easier by the difficulties at times of sorting out the thorns of our cursedness from the thorns of our sanctification. When do I resign myself to suffering and disease and when do I pray confidently for the removal of a thorn lodged in my flesh? In a given encounter with pain, into which garden is the Savior leading me: the Garden of Gethsemane or the garden which surrounds the empty tomb?

The Christian, whether as patient or professional, must face these questions in their complexity and troublesomeness: not in the loneliness of a pretended human autonomy, but with the responsibility of a God-imager, called to share in the exercise of dominion over all that the Lord has placed in the world. In the present age, this necessitates thorn-in-the-flesh decision making. But it is decision making that must take place in the context of the kind of community described so well by Father Henri Nouwen in his excellent little book, *The Wounded Healer* (New York: Doubleday, 1972, p. 96):

> A Christian community is . . . a healing community not because wounds are cured and pains are alleviated, but because wounds and pains become openings or occasions for a new vision. Mutual confession then becomes a mutual deepening of hope, and sharing weakness becomes a reminder to one and all of the coming strength.

86.
The Truthfulness of a Physician

HELMUT THIELICKE

It is impossible to make lying even a subject of ethical discussion, if the person who tells the lie is acting on the maxim that the purpose of his speaking alone determines the truth or falsity of what he says. Voltaire has something to this effect in his letter of October 21, 1736, to Thiriot: "Lying is a vice only when it effects evil; it is a great virtue when it accomplishes good. So be more virtuous than ever! One must lie like the devil, not timorously or only occasionally, but confidently and constantly. Lie, my friend, lie!"[1] Lying can be the subject of ethical discussion only when we are clear on two points.

In the first place, we must acknowledge that there is genuine conflict between truth and love, between truth and practical necessity. A well-known example used by such diverse writers as F. H. R. Frank,[2] Fichte,[3] and N. H. Søe,[4] involves the question of what one should do when a critically ill woman asks about her dying child, and there is a strong possibility that a full disclosure of the truth will kill the mother. For our present purposes the important thing is not to resolve the conflict but simply to point out that a real conflict exists.

As a matter of fact, the three authors cited give very different answers, in accordance with radically different criteria. Søe thinks that the duty of love takes priority; as a test he commends the consideration that if I withhold the truth from someone, he will come to know this later on when the situation changes, and will then lose all confidence in me. Frank says that the truth should not be withheld because the death of the child is from God, and God can spare the mother any harmful consequences of the disclosure. Fichte says abruptly: "If the woman die of the truth, then let her die!" Though the solutions differ so widely, they are all at one in seeing that what is required here is decision rather than casuistic calculation.

A real conflict always raises the question of compromise, namely, which of the two colliding postulates should be given priority over the other. In

---

From Helmut Thielicke, *Theological Ethics,* vol. 1, ed. William H. Lazareth (Philadelphia: Fortress, 1966), pp. 520-21, 551-66.

certain circumstances, therefore, there is in fact a relation between the truth and a specific situation, a relation which I cannot overlook.

The second point on which we must be clear is that there is a relation between "truth and the person" as well as between "truth and the situation." A statement may be objectively correct and still not be "true," if the one who utters it is not qualified to do so. When a schoolboy writes in his essay that Goethe is the greatest of all poets, this may be correct, but as stated by these lips or by this pen it is not "true." That is doubtless what Nietzsche meant when he said that "a toothless mouth no longer has the right to the truth."

In this connection we may also remember Kierkegaard's comparison. When, at the end of a life devoted to the pursuit of knowledge, Faust asserts, "I now see that we can know nothing," this conclusion, formulated at the end of his development, is qualitatively very different from the same statement taken over by a student in his first semester to justify his indolence. What is "correct" about the utterance in both cases is too trivial to deserve being called "truth." Correctness becomes truth only when it is so related to existence as to become the confessional expression of existence, its self-declaration. This is why proverbial truths, when uttered by school children or indolent freshmen, do not stand under the sign of truth. They are characterized either by "precocity" or by trickery, and in either case by an element of mendacity which is the very opposite of truth. . . .

We shall proceed by analyzing closely a typical situation which can reliably serve to illustrate a larger complex of questions. To illustrate the conflict between the duty of sparing others and the duty of telling the truth, we shall examine here the problem of the physician at the bed of his patient. We shall begin with certain basic insights which either were expressed in our earlier deliberations or may be deduced from them.

We have stated that truth is not adequately defined simply in terms of the agreement between a statement and objective reality. On the contrary, it became clear to us that, if we are to define a statement as true, account must also be taken of the sphere within which that statement is made. In fulfilling my duty to tell the truth I cannot abstract myself from the situation in which I speak.

It is also clear, however, that truth depends on the person who does the speaking. Naturally this is not true of the statements of exact science.[5] But it does apply to truths which belong to the human and personal sphere. I can communicate only that which I have and am. I can state a truth only in the act of confessing, i.e., only as I am myself related to the truth in question.

He who himself lives in untruth covertly changes even the objective truths which he happens to speak into untruths. What is formally true, true in form, can be falsified by what it is that actually dwells in this form. Pornographic literature, for example, may contain objectively correct statements concerning erotic and sexual processes.[6] Yet in pornography the parcels of truth are integrated into a perverse system of values and thus become unequivocal lies. Pornography falsifies the place of sex in humanity. It depersonalizes, biologizes, and psychologizes it. Out of the "true" stones of individual processes it makes a perverted mosaic. It uses "truths" but tells lies. It does so because the pornographer, although he uses correct and in some sense "true" details, is not personally related to the truth of the whole. In his own person he has missed its real meaning and purpose. So it is that the untruth of the person makes the statement to be untrue.

An analogous process may be seen in the temptation of Jesus in the wilderness. The tempter appeals to the words of Holy Scripture. He thus appeals to "truths," to things which are correct in detail. But on the lips of the satanic liar these become lies because they are spoken in the context of a false relationship. To use an arithmetical figure, these individual truths are set within a bracket before which there stands a minus sign. The negative thus robs them of their positive value as truths. The devil who so uses them is falsehood in person. Hence that which is originally correct becomes false; the truth becomes a lie.

The general statement of Luther that it is "the person who makes the works"[7] may here be reformulated to the effect that it is the person who makes the statement true or false. Only he who is subject to truth tells the truth. The liar always lies, even when he uses truth. Either way, man is always making confession of the ultimate relationship in which he stands. Confession is the only way in which "human" truth can be stated.

These preliminary but very basic observations, which in part take up and develop points already made, will serve then to introduce us to the specific problem of this section: What should the physician do when his patient is incurably ill or at the point of death? Does he owe his patient the truth or should he practice deception?[8]

It is obvious that this situation creates a genuine conflict. In the weakened condition of those who are seriously ill, information concerning the gravity of the sickness may come as a shock and really prove fatal. If we assume that there is still a slight hope of improvement, this prospect may be shattered by the imparting of such information, whereas the encouragement afforded the patient by a positive, though untrue, diagnosis of his condition may in fact spark his will to recover, and thus snatch him back from the critical point.

To recognize this possibility is to come directly up against a fundamental fact in the whole problem of truth. In certain circumstances truth is not just the sum and substance of a correct determination and delineation of the facts. On the contrary, the statement of a very questionable truth can itself conceivably bring into being facts which were not really present at the moment they were proclaimed in the name of truth, facts which could not at that time have comprised the content of a "true" statement. This is what happens, for example, in "fortune-telling." Here the significance of the pronouncement is not objectively to state something, but magically to bring it to pass. In other words, the prognosis in fortune-telling, while it does not state an existing truth concerning the future (since to do so would be to presuppose the existence of the future itself), it often does make the stated facts true. It causes them, as it were, to become true. This may happen, for example, when the one who is under the influence of such a prognosis actually reckons with the facts contained in it, whether by looking forward hopefully to something which is welcome, or by allowing some fearful prospect to gain magical power over him, like a tree which has such power over someone learning to ride a bicycle that he is magnetically attracted by it.

Only when we grasp this point do we appreciate the full severity of the problem by which we are confronted. If there is some chance that the optimistic, though dubious, prognosis of the doctor may become true, ought he not to risk it? Ought he not to tread the narrow and slippery ridge which separates truth from falsehood?

How then is the doctor to decide between the constructive lie and the destructive truth? The deception of patients has, in fact, made its way into the stronghold of medical practice to some extent under the rubric of "suggestion therapy." We need only think of the saline injections given in lieu of a drug which has to be withheld, like morphine. Psychosomatic interaction may make it imperative that certain psychical preconditions be created in order to make somatic effects possible. These preconditions are impossible unless wool is pulled, as it were, over the eyes of the psyche, i.e., unless it is deceived. This is undoubtedly a working rule of the doctor's art which the patient, without any loss of confidence, will regard as justified once he is in condition again to make appropriate judgments. Indeed the deception is practiced precisely in order to bring the patient to this condition. In the situation of the patient it certainly does not amount to a lie, because it does not affect the person in the central core of his being, as it would if he were misled about his proximity to death, or if during a long siege of cancer he were deceived into neglecting important internal or external matters which he would have wanted to care for had he been given a more realistic appraisal of his situation.[9]

Then too in the latter case concealment of the true situation is inevitably followed by a chain reaction of further deceptions, so that finally we have, not a single structure of lies, but a whole colony of such structures. A pact of secrecy and deception must be sworn by a whole group of nurses, attendants, relatives, and friends. To avoid the terrible collapse of these finely spun illusions, and the attendant shock and radical collapse of confidence which must go with it, the deception is sometimes sustained even in the very last stages of the illness by means of narcotics, a chemically induced kind of personal irresponsibility.

These examples show that the concept of "a working rule of the doctor's art" cannot be a blanket authorization for all the various deceptions which, rightly or wrongly, are advanced as being necessary for medical reasons. The line between what is permissible and what is impermissible is very difficult to determine. Indeed this cannot be done a priori. There are, however, certain indications that this line does not lie merely at the point where the deception relates to the issue of life and death. This is shown, for example, by the therapeutically as well as morally dubious mock operations which are sometimes performed on neurotics under the category of "suggestion therapy."[10]

In our further discussion of this medical conflict between telling the truth and sparing the patient we shall now apply to the situation of the physician what we have laid down concerning the dependence of the truth that we speak on the truth that we are as persons. We may begin with the negative proposition that the untruth in which a person, in this case the doctor, may find himself can show itself at the sickbed of one who is on the point of death, or very likely to die, in the following forms.

The physician may be motivated by fear in respect of the dying person or his relatives. The anguish, the psychologically understandable reluctance, which keeps him from "shattering" the other person with a grave pronouncement, leads to out and out lying if in fact it triumphs over the truth. For in this case the motive is not to spare the other; it is to spare oneself. Hence the doctor does not merely speak untruth; he speaks out of untruth, i.e., out of a situation which is itself untrue. In appearance he seems to be impelled by the motive of a love which desires to spare; in fact, however, he is impelled by the very opposite.

It is again the untruth of the person which is involved when the doctor fears that he may have to share these last moments with a patient who is incurably ill and knows it. In other words, the doctor is afraid that he will have to disclose the secret of his own failure. This particular fear is twofold.

In the first place, there is the natural and understandable defensive reaction against the fact that in every visit and consultation and treatment he must publicly demonstrate the limits of his ability, and perhaps even his human failure. Any concession to this defensive reaction is obviously a concession to untruth. What is involved here is not only an untruth of speech but also an untruth of being. The reaction is not merely psychological but also philosophical. It is based on the fact that the doctor does not clearly understand the fundamental relation between medical treatment and the nature which is treated, between medical ability and its limits, between the courage to act and the humility to surrender. It is based too on ignorance of the fact that sickness and death are not just a fate which befalls a man but a task to be taken up—by doctor and patient together. When the doctor is not clear about these basic questions he stands in a false and illusory relationship to the fundamental realities of existence. It is no wonder, then, that what he says on the basis of this untruth should also be untrue.

In the second place, and closely related to what has just been said, there is the fear that in face of death, and of the mystery of life therein declared, he can only betray his complete "inner" helplessness, and so be forced to give a false hope instead of saying something which conveys real help, enlightenment, and "knowledge." Not to know the truth about death always means lying in face of death. If the physician has not himself faced the mystery of death, he must evade the dying. None of us can give more than he himself has.

Having stated the matter negatively, we may now put it in positive terms and say that the doctor is in the truth, first, if he himself has a relation to death, or, more accurately, if he has the true relation to death, i.e., if he knows the Lord of life and death. The man who is clear about the basic realities of life and death, who has faced up to these realities, will also be able to find the word of truth. There are no routine statements which can fill the gap when this existential condition is not met. Truth is constitutively linked with the confession of that which we have come to know in our own existence.

Second, the doctor is in the truth if he sees the "true man" in the other person. This "true man" is characterized by the fact that he is not merely the activating center of certain vital functions, a physiological "it," a bundle of woes which must be spared as many pains and disturbances as possible. On the contrary, his life between birth and death is one of decision and responsibility; in face of the borderline situation of death he is thus summoned to win his life, or to lose it, to hold on or to fail, in short, to face the basic realities of his existence. Only when the physician respects this situation does he stand in a relation of truth to the other person. If he does not, the relation is one of falsehood, whether he actually tells lies or merely follows the evasive tactic of silence.

Third, the doctor is in the truth if he respects the truth of illness and of the fact that man must die, i.e., if he does not regard sickness merely as a physiological and somatic event but realizes that man, the whole man, is sick. He must note well the terminology of the sufferer, which more often than not says quite specifically "I am sick," rather than just that "something is wrong with" this or that particular part of the anatomy; and he must know the reason for such phraseology. The patient's use of the first person means that man is the subject of his illness. Sickness is not a calamity which befalls him, reducing him to the level of an object. We need not call upon psychosomatic medicine—which is of course very emphatic, determined, and perhaps even extreme on this score—to find medical men who appreciate this point and who interpret the phenomenon of illness along these lines even from the medical standpoint.

This understanding means that being sick is a matter of the whole person. Consequently the truth of sickness can be grasped only when it is regarded not as a hostile force from without, but as a component part of man himself with which man must grapple and come to terms as he does with himself.

For the doctor this means that he must be ready to help the patient to accept illness, and in certain instances its incurability, and also death, and to understand these things as a task to be tackled. The truth of sickness and death is not perceived if we simply allow the instinct of self-preservation to dominate the field, and hence take a purely negative attitude toward illness. There is of course an unnatural element in it which must be combatted. Yet illness also has about it a providential aspect which is to be accepted and brought into harmony with the person.

The struggle which is demanded of the patient in face of sickness and death can never be an externally oriented insistence that this cannot and must not happen to me. It must be rather an inwardly oriented struggle with oneself, a struggle for an answer to the question who and what this person is who is thus stricken, how to deal with the new demands that such a blow brings, how through endurance and acceptance it can be made meaningful and hence differentiated from an accidental calamity. The question is not merely why did this have to happen to me, but for what purpose.

Fourth, the doctor is thus in the truth to the degree that he knows the truth, i.e., to the degree that he knows the meaning and purpose of the blow and lives it out in his own life. Only according to the measure of his relation to this truth can he give true information on the actual situation of the patient in respect of the blow that has befallen him. Where the doctor is not related to this truth, or where the relationship is a negative one, he will be forced to lie, and at the same time to resort to the false excuse that he does so out of a desire to spare the patient, that he is acting out of a love which is here in conflict with the duty of truth. In face of death there can be no openness and honesty unless at least one of the two parties, doctor or patient, knows the meaning of that which is about to happen. In such a case, however, experience repeatedly confirms the fact that the truth makes free (John 8:32), and that fear of the unknown gives way to peace. Truth and peace indeed belong together. . . .

Now that we have stated the basic points—but not before!—we can turn to the pedagogical question of how in the borderline situation of incurable illness or death those who know the "truth" can impart it to the patient. If we tackle this question too soon, we fail to see the existential problem of the physician, which is the main point at issue, and treat the matter instead as one simply of tactics or technique. Something which touches the very roots of our understanding of man is thus reduced to a matter of simple working rules.

Even here, however, we again do only partial justice to the situation if the final result of our wisdom is only the recommendation of a certain method or technique, or if we speak merely of the required tact and necessary sympathy. For here too the problems are not just psychological but existential.

We come up against this problem when we ask why a certain method is needed at all. There are obviously some truths which can be communicated by means of a method which is wholly factual and not at all psychological. The question as to the truth of the Pythagorean theorem requires proof, and hence also a method of "proving" it, whereas the truth about death clearly demands a method of "communication" which embraces the human element.

Obviously this must mean that this particular truth is not one I can just blurt out at any time. The physician may come right out with it, of course, when he is dealing with a colleague who is called in as consultant; to him he can discreetly communicate the realization that there is nothing more to be done. In relation to the patient, however, such directness of communication is not possible. Whereas the colleague who takes part in a medical consultation can receive such news with factual objectivity, or with emotion but of a very different kind, for the patient himself it could entail a fatal shock.

The fact that the same truth can have such very different effects on different individuals is clear indication of the fact that in respect of this kind of truth—as distinct from that of the Pythagorean theorem!—men can have very different relationships to it. We may formulate the distinction as follows. Relationship to the Pythagorean theorem is timeless and hence unhistorical; that which relates to this truth is the abstract understanding which is independent of situations and of a particular existence. Relationship to the truth of death and of whatever else befalls me, however, is historical. This truth becomes free only in concrete encounters with the blows that strike, in the conflict and experienced problems of life. It is a truth which in the course of things either comes to light or is increasingly obscured. Its corollary, then, is either a developing knowledge or a hardening ignorance.

The development of this knowledge is expressed in the concept of "enlightenment" or "wisdom," that which lies at the end of the process. Wisdom is not something that can be imparted at any moment, like the Pythagorean theorem. It has its own time, its own hour and moment. To the degree that it is the object of wisdom, therefore, the truth cannot be taken over from others, like the truths of mathematics, or even like certain communicated facts, e.g., of history. Truth can only be appropriated. It can be attained to only in the process of growth. It becomes free only as I am confronted with it, only as these confrontations actually take place in my life. A child can, of course, repeat the sayings of Plato or of Paul concerning death. He can even bring to them a measure of intellectual apprehension. But he cannot "appropriate" them because he has not yet been confronted by death or by our "being unto death." He must simply wait upon this knowledge until it is released within him.

But this means that we have departed from the purely psychological level of how to tell the patient and have pressed on to the heart of the matter itself, namely, the truth which is to be communicated. The truth at issue here is the truth of death, not the fact that a certain concrete event is about to take place, but the truth about death itself: the truth that we must die, we must depart this life, and that our life has a goal (Ps. 39:4–6).

This is a truth which I cannot communicate to the one concerned in a direct way, or at any time whatever, as I might communicate truth to a colleague who is not personally involved. The inability to do so obviously means that in practice I must to some extent withhold and conceal the truth, giving it only slowly and in small doses. Am I lying, then, when I do this?

We can make headway with this question only if we distinguish sharply between the psychological and the existential standpoints involved in the situation. The psychological answer to the question why a direct and unmitigated communication is impossible is that the suddenness of the communication (since it could presumably take place "at any time") does not befit the psychical state of the patient and could produce quite a shock. The existential answer is that such a communication would not be in keeping with the nature of this truth. By its very nature, the truth about life and death is a developing and ripening truth; it is not timeless and hence accessible at any time. The communication of this truth must consequently include that process in the course of which the truth can become free and the physician can contribute to its becoming free. Our concern here is with a truth to which we must be led, a truth which is not a presupposition but a goal.

For this reason it is not a lie, nor is it sabotage of the truth, if the doctor is at first very slow and hesitant about communicating, if he steers clear of the subject of death in order to approach the patient from a wholly different angle and prepare him for the real theme of his situation. Whether the physician lies or not does not depend on whether he momentarily avoids the situation or directly acknowledges it. It depends rather on whether he regards his first momentary denial as the initial or preliminary stage of that process which ultimately leads to the truth, a process into and through which he is determined to lead his patient *or* whether the denial is final, made with the intention of "sparing" the patient to the very end any certainty as to his condition, so that he can finally be conjured over the last threshold in a state of unconsciousness, with the help of narcotics as a chemical means of concealment.

In the latter case the method can only be the expression of a particular matter, the actual relationship to death. In terms of the specific relationship in question, it is held that beyond death there is nothing but unconscious nothingness. Hence it is deemed appropriate on this side of the threshold too to induce unconsciousness. A man's life has no specific significance since it bears no relation to anything beyond itself which could force him to make certain basic decisions. As a result, the last phase of a man's life is filled up entirely with the wounded and hence anguished impulse of self-preservation. Since man is helpless in face of death to forestall that lethal attack upon his instinct to survive, the only remaining possibility is to put an end to those final torments which it causes. Logically, then, the acute problem is one not of existence but of chemistry. The question of death has been reduced to zero.

If, on the other hand, the doctor is resolved to lead the patient into that process of disclosure, into that borderline theme of existence, then his action is not out of keeping with the truth even if in the first instance he conceals rather than reveals. The doctor does honor to the truth by making himself a companion of the patient in this entire process, and by therewith deciding to communicate with him in face of the ultimate reality. . . .

We are thus confronted by an important and basic fact of human existence which we have now observed in many different connections. Man's special prerogative of being endowed with personal freedom is wholly ambivalent. It is oriented toward genuine responsibility before the divine Thou, toward man's relationship with God; but on the dark side it also possesses the other possibility of using a gift of grace to evade the claim of that which is sent and ordained by God.

We have said that the truth of death really becomes free only when I can speak in the first person: "I die." And we have tried to explain this statement in terms of its negative counterpart. Only when the death at issue is my death does it cease to be a general and hence only half-true phenomenon and become a personal event in which I experience the mystery of my existence. Thus death is something that must grow upon me. In the words of Rainer Maria Rilke, it must grow "in me."

It was in this sense that Karl Holl, when he lay on his death bed and the doctor wanted to help him over the last hour with narcotics, stated in reply, "I will not be robbed of *my death!*" It goes without saying that what moved him in this desire to remain conscious was not the curiosity of a scientist wanting to observe the extinction of life "from within," but the mystery of existence, to which one's own death belongs and which is experienced in this personal and intimate way. Because love, the meaning of life, and human extremity all reach their end and climax in death, it is here that the real substance of life first becomes fully apparent. A person really comes to know himself at death. This is why death is not merely physical or natural but quite "personal." Its truth is revealed fully only when "*I* die."

It is important to bear in mind this fact that the

truth about death is something which "grows" in life. It is not something that we always have at our disposal and can communicate at any time. It is also important to realize that in this process of growth there is always a gap between knowledge of "death in general" and knowledge of "my own death" in particular.

Now the relation to death—or lack of relation—in which the patient stands is something which cannot be known in advance. Consequently the character of the disclosures which the doctor must make is linked with the situation, with the person addressed, with the doctor's own knowledge of death, and in all of these with that particular form of truth which is involved in man's "being unto death." Certainly the fact that this truth is one which grows and develops must be expressed also in the character of the communication made to the person who is incurably ill or on the point of death. This communication must itself be a gradual disclosure, a preparatory leading of the patient into a discovery of his own.

On these grounds compromise—the merely temporary compromise!—between the postulate of "sparing" the patient, i.e., the postulate of a gradual process, on the one side, and factual diagnostic truth, on the other, is perfectly legitimate. This must be said even though the suspension of factual truth remains a genuine burden for the conscience which is constantly at war with itself and always tempted to yield to illusion. Even in this case the rift in the structure of the world is too obvious to miss, namely, the divergence and conflict between the different forms of truth. If the peace with God which prevailed at the beginning were still extant, there would be no conflict as there is now between the privilege of going home and the necessity of departing. There would be no painful severing of ties, because there would really be only one tie. And we would not be wandering between two worlds, existing in a state of cleavage. But then no "preparatory leading" would be needed, and consequently no compromise such as that involved in the suspension of factual truth. Thus in the depths of every human situation we discover evidence of the fact that our world is a fallen world still awaiting its redemption.

In conclusion, we may repeat the decisive point of all we have been saying. No man can bring another to what he himself does not have. No man can liberate in another a truth which he himself does not share. The final issue is not the psychological technique used in such disclosures nor the problem of formal factual truth, i.e., the agreement between what the doctor says and the actual state of things at a given moment. What is ultimately at stake is the appeal to the fact that the physician is himself a human being who must come to truth and to maturity. This is his task.

There is much talk about the patient being a person, a whole man who is to be treated therapeutically in his personal being, in his humanity, and whose illness is not to be regarded as a somatic or biological accident, something which has merely come upon him. All this is true. But it is equally true—and unfortunately this has not been seen with the same clarity—that the physician too is a person, a whole man, and that his skillful deeds of diagnosis and therapy are not merely a matter of technique, but are expressive of his humanity, which is herewith challenged to its very foundations.

Notes

1. The quotation from Voltaire's *Oeuvres complètes* (Paris, 1818), XXXI, 446, is cited in Victor von Cathrein, *Moralphilosophie* (Leipzig, 1924), II, 90, n. 8.

2. See F. H. R. Frank, *System der christlichen Sittlichkeit* (Erlangen: Deichert, 1884), I, 421.

3. This question was put to Fichte by H. Steffens, according to H. Martensen, *Christian Ethics* (Special Part, First Division: Individual Ethics), trans. William Affleck (4th ed.; Edinburgh: T. & T. Clark, n.d.), p. 217.

4. See N. H. Søe, *Christliche Ethik* (Munich: Kaiser, 1949), pp. 277-278.

5. See Kierkegaard's "Reflections on Christianity and Natural Science," in his *Eine Literarische Anzeige,* trans. Emanuel Hirsch (Düsseldorf: Diederichs, 1959), pp. 125-129.

6. This is true even of the various Kinsey reports, which stand on the three-corner frontier of zoology, pornography, and anthropology.

7. *WA* 39^{I}, 283.

8. The same question could of course be put to the pastor, but for reasons of method which will emerge later the example of the physician is more suited to our present purposes, since it forces us to consider how the situation of illness works out in terms of a variety of philosophical positions.

9. This example is suggested by Richard Siebeck, *Medizin in Bewegung* (Stuttgart, 1949).

10. The case reported by Jores, for all the humor of its outcome, nonetheless illustrates the point. A very wealthy and pampered woman, severly neurotic, constantly complained about headaches caused by the sofa in her head. Various remedies were tried but without success. Finally a mock operation was performed. When the patient awakened from the anesthetic, back in her room with her head generously wrapped in bandages, she noticed on her night stand a tiny doll-house size sofa. Looking at it but a moment she said merely, "My sofa was green." Arthur Jores, "Arzt und Lüge," *Universitas,* X (1949), 1198 f.

87. The Physician-Patient Relationship

BERNARD HÄRING

The doctor-patient tie is a covenant of persons. In times of serious illness and in the total ordering of the medical profession, the contribution of the doctor can never be severed from personal concern. The privacy and intimate reactions of the ailing person transcend by far the impersonal basis of many other relationships. While the seller-buyer contract is founded on commutative justice, the relationship between doctor and patient is distinguished and characterized by such personal attitudes as fidelity, reverence, respect, truthfulness and mutual trust. If the doctor wants to do justice to the patient by caring for his total health and helping him to accept his illness and discover its personal meaning, he must regard the sick human being in his uniqueness, with inviolable personal rights and expectations. He must also take into account the patient's relationship to God, his fellowmen and society, particularly his family.

A physician's fidelity and responsibility towards his patient entail a correlative responsibility towards his fellowmen and society, although it is not always simple to reconcile the interests of the patient with those of society. At times the dilemma of medical ethics seems insoluble because of the need to consider the patient on the one hand, as a distinct individual, and on the other, as a constituent member of a society which sets claims upon him. The physician's resolution not to depart from the concept of the patient as a person is decisive ethically; such a stance necessarily includes his essential relationships and responsibilities to his fellowmen. In this frame of reference, the doctor does not violate the fidelity of his covenant if he fails to accede to a patient's selfish and irresponsible wishes but acts according to the best interests and personal calling of the patient. In grave cases, after having exhausted all means of persuading a patient to responsible action, the physician may be compelled to protect the just expectations and rights of his fellow-citizens and of society even against the patient's will.

I have already mentioned the importance of an atmosphere of truthfulness and trust in the crucial matter of the doctor's deportment when faced by the prospect of a patient's death. Only if we understand fully the import of these qualities in the covenant between physician and patient can we realize the attitude proper to a doctor as death approaches. On the other hand, we have also seen how a guarded truthfulness in this extreme situation influences the patient-physician relationship in the matter of therapy. Truthfulness and trust from both patient and doctor are needed, but it is chiefly the veracity and trustworthiness of the physician that condition responsiveness and confidence in the patient.

The significance of the covenant of trust linking doctor and patient becomes most critical in the matter of confidentiality. Professional secrecy is an essential component of the medical ethos. The oath of Hippocrates says: 'If it be what should not be noised abroad I will keep silence thereon.' The American Medical Association code declares: 'Confidence . . . should never be revealed unless the law requires it or it is necessary to protect the welfare of individuals or communities.'

In almost all countries, the law requires that contagious diseases be reported. Such a request is absolutely justified by the common good in spite of the fact that it may be most unpleasant for the diseased person. Beyond the legal obligation and on the grounds of his medical ethos, the doctor will evince concern that other persons be not unnecessarily exposed to the danger of contagion. Even in highly developed countries, the general population is not yet sufficiently protected against contamination by communicable diseases, open tuberculosis for instance. The immediate family should be informed of proper methods of protecting itself and friends. Care should be taken that contagious persons do not use any public facilities as long as they constitute a considerable threat as 'carriers'.[1]

It is first of all the patient's obligation to show responsibility towards the people with whom he lives. The doctor or, where available, the social worker or member of the community medical team, ought to explain to him the situation and the consequences of irresponsible behaviour. The adult patient should then be expected to act responsibly, but if he cannot, or if he proves unwilling to do so, the physician must assume his part of the responsibility in keeping with the principle of subsidiarity, so as to protect the patient and society.[2]

In cases where the physician cannot motivate or convince the patient of his duty to communicate what he should, the doctor himself becomes accountable. But before informing others because of special responsibilities, the doctor has to ponder well all the values at stake. There are situations, for example, in cases of

From Bernard Haring, *Medical Ethics* (South Bend: Fides, 1973), pp. 199–205. Used by permission.

venereal disease, when even though others may be exposed to some danger or damage, it may be better to keep silent than to make use of information which has been obtained professionally, with the inevitable risk of diminishing the patient's trust. It is not just the relationship of this one patient to this one doctor that is in jeopardy. One doctor's imprudent use of confidence, should it come to the knowledge of others, can impair the relationship of many doctors with their patients. Only when there is serious danger for others is the doctor allowed or obliged to speak when a patient refuses to fulfil an obvious obligation to make known his infectious disease.

Every patient should be aware that when he reveals his condition to a physician, the doctor can never be a willing accomplice to crime by an unjustified silence. Secrecy can never become a taboo. Observance or non-observance must always be judged with respect to the welfare of the patient and of all other persons involved. The saying, 'The sabbath was made for man and not man for the sabbath' applies also to secrecy. . . .

A trust-inspiring relationship between physician and patient demands, according to the situation, reliable information relative to the extent of risk attendant on certain treatments to be taken by the patient. It is understood that the doctor will first decide which treatment is most suitable so that he will not propose indifferently a number of possibilities which the patient himself would have to examine in order to find out which would best serve him. In most cases, it is incumbent on the physician to decide on the desirability of a treatment, but whenever a certain procedure or operation entails considerable risk, he will inform the patient adequately in view of the total situation of his health. Were the disclosure of such information to constitute a risk of grave harm to the patient, the doctor will renounce doing so directly. Instead he may choose to inform members of the family and await the final decision from them.

The physician will refrain from using new and yet unproven medication or therapeutic means when a better or equally good prospect with lesser risk is available. Similarly, the doctor will not prefer a very expensive treatment to a relatively less expensive one if both serve the same purpose unless the patient or his family, after accurate information, explicitly indicate preference for the more costly method. Whenever there is question of using very expensive treatments with no real prospect of success, the physician should not burden the patient or his family with a decision since they would not enjoy the full freedom of spirit to say 'no' although they might be resentful of the idea. He should unilaterally decide to renounce such a course of action; it would be against the physician-patient covenant to impose on the patient's family extremely high expenses for a treatment which holds no promise of substantial help.

The physician's responsibility is particularly great when he resorts to medication or treatment which can cause moral danger to the patient. The concept of full human health serving as a basis for ethical considerations obliges him to include in his diagnostic efforts all the elements of his patient's particular endowment and character, such as for instance, *abulia* or weakness of the will. He may have to renounce hormonal treatments which can stimulate sexual desire beyond the patient's capacity for self-control.

Should a therapist consider hypnosis as a part of treatment, he has then to inform the patient honestly and seek his permission. No one ever entrusts himself so totally to possible manipulation by a therapist without making an explicit judgment that the therapist is worthy of this great moral trust. The therapist must also ask himself whether such a procedure will truly serve his patient in terms of promoting his moral freedom.

Particular caution is to be exercised in the use of sedatives and other drugs likely to constitute for certain individual patients a danger of addiction. Especially serious in consequence would be to risk such treatment when a patient has previously manifested a propensity towards drug addiction.

The hormonal control of pregnancy in the case of unmarried women, especially of young girls, poses serious moral problems for the doctor. He can often foresee that his prescription will be a further step towards moral laxity. On the other hand, his refusal to prescribe may well result in an abortion in the case of an undesired pregnancy. His decision needs serious reflection. If by medical arguments he cannot change the patient's attitude, then a realistic approach may avoid the greater danger. Where law makes the permission of the parents mandatory, the doctor will not resort to any subterfuge. Even where there is no legal interdiction to the treatment of a minor without parental permission, the doctor will not forget his responsibility towards the family. He will consult the parents to the extent he can without abdicating his own responsibility.

Notes

1. R. Arnoldt, 'Seuchenhygienisch bedenkliche Verschwiegenheit bei ansteckungsfähiger Lungentuberkulose,' *Praxis der Pneumologie,* 22 (1968), 176–182.

2. Cf.: Henry A. Davidson, 'Professional Secrecy,' in *Ethical Issues in Medicine,* ed. E. F. Torrey (Boston: Little, Brown and Co., 1968), p. 193.

88. Teacher

WILLIAM F. MAY

Among several images one could use to describe the healer, the covenantal image alone demands that healers teach their patients. Other images—those of parent, technician, fighter, and contractor—may do so incidentally, but at best they usually generate ambivalence toward the teaching function.

The parental image tends to reduce patients to dependent children, stricken sheep. Compassionate care and vicarious decision-making rather than candid instruction characterize the professional's task. Only too often, parentalist healers, like Dostoevsky's Grand Inquisitor, have a low estimate of their charges and want to protect them from that turmoil which knowledge and freedom entail.

The location of many teaching hospitals and residency training programs in the inner city tends further to convince young professionals that preventive medicine and the teaching it requires are activities of low yield. Residents complain that patients often come in only when their diseases flare. Preventive medicine seems beside the point. Destructive habits so grip the patient as to make rehabilitation or stable chronic care difficult to sustain. After treatment, patients go back into the streets and fall into the same injurious habits again. They forget appointments; they don't comply with a regimen. Patients will say: "I don't know what medicines I take. It's in the chart. Read the chart." But the resident knows that the chart records what the physician prescribed, not what the patient is taking, if anything. Further, patients fear the truth or fail to assimilate it, or accept it but selectively. Some pounce on the bad news and panic; others dissolve the bad news in a blurry confusion and ignore the importance of compliance. In response, physicians retreat into a limited parentalist mode, making decisions on behalf of the patient in the sanctuary of the hospital, knowing that the world beyond the hospital walls will shortly defeat their childlike charges. Thus, early in their education physicians come to expect very little from patients. Cynicism, despair, and sometimes resentment infect the exhausted resident.

From *The Physician's Covenant: Images of the Healer in Medical Ethics,* by William F. May. Copyright © 1983 by William F. May. Used by permission of The Westminster Press, Philadelphia, PA.

And yet—even parentalism offers some moral warrant for teaching one's patients. The parent, after all, is committed to the being and well-being of the child, and the good parent recognizes education as an important ingredient in the child's flourishing. The main thrust of the image, however, condescends too much to encourage persistent teaching. Give what care you can to hurting charges and let it go at that.

To the degree that practitioners think of themselves only as contractors dispensing technical services they will also tend to depreciate the place of teaching in therapy. Contracted for and paid on a piecework basis, whether by the consumer personally or by a third-party payment system, the therapist offers discrete, itemizable services rather than taking continuous responsibility for the patient's improvement in self-care and health maintenance. Teaching takes time; it reduces the number of patients the physician can see; it complicates the question of patient management and exposes the physician to the possibility of making personal as well as technical errors. Both the specialist and the generalist can draw back from teaching the patient—the specialist offering encoded information to the attending physician, and the attending physician sometimes reneging on the task by defining himself or herself chiefly as the orchestrator of technical services. And yet the contractualist model retains a fragment of the teaching responsibility, to the degree that the seller of services accepts responsibility to inform the buyer about the services and the product offered for sale. Further, Health Maintenance Organizations (HMOs) draw up contracts with their patients that give professionals financial incentives to teach better.

The military model hardly emphasizes the physician as teacher. It conjoins the technical and contractual models with an adversarial setting to produce the mercenary who fights against disease and death. The patient has fallen victim to invasive powers. Amateurs mucking about with weapons that they hardly understand will only blow themselves up. A little knowledge is a dangerous thing. The expert in biological warfare should decide which drugs best counter the intricacies of the enemy's attack, its time, its place, and its force. Besides, under the conditions of battle, with the physician fighting on behalf of a thousand little principalities, explaining wastes time.

Both the economics of medicine and the structure of medical education reinforce the tendency of physicians, who live by the technical-contractualist-military models, to neglect teaching. The third-party payment system rewards physicians for discrete, piecework services to the sick. It does not reward them for teaching patients how to maintain their health or even for securing high levels of compliance with the doctor's regimen. Not surprisingly, a President's Committee on Health Care Education reported for 1973 that only one half of one percent of annual health care expenditures went for health education.[1] While HMOs make a good-faith effort to redirect the economic incentives toward preventive medicine, the high turnover rates of patient subscribers in HMOs (30 percent per year) do not suggest that those organizations have succeeded in giving the professional much financial incentive to practice pedagogically persuasive preventive medicine.[2]

Neither medical school education nor residency training programs prepare physicians adequately for teaching. Professional education prepares them as depositories of information, not sharers of what they know. "Medicine is the only graduate school to rely on multiple choice examinations," complains one academic physician.[3] Sadly enough, this subarticulate standard of testing fails to challenge the student to organize and teach effectively, or even to retain what he or she knows. According to a study of a second-year class at a distinguished medical school, the half-life of a retained factual item is about three weeks; 90 percent of factual items retained for true-false examinations have taken flight by graduation.[4]

Cumulatively, a professional education that centers in the mere acquisition of factual information converts education itself from a public trust to privately held property. The student soon assumes that he or she has acquired knowledge as a private stockpile of goods to be sold wholly as the certified possessor sees fit. The information that lab tests, X-rays, and biopsies yield belongs to the professional rather than to the patient whose destiny they foretell. And patients often submit to this view. They would feel as shy about reading the physician's workup of their case—while he or she is out of the office—as about reading any other papers or letters on the desk. Such information seems like private property, for the physician alone to divulge. Thus the very terms of professional education and clinical training and practice combine to obscure the communal origins of professional education and the duty to share generously what one knows.

The quarrel in medicine over whether physicians should teach their patients is not new; it dates back to the classical world. The "rough empirics" in ancient Greece (who, familiar with treatments but not with the scientific reasons for their success, practiced largely on slaves) used to ridicule the more scientifically oriented physicians (who, practicing largely on free men and their families, sought to teach their patients). The scientific physicians complained that the empirics offered little more than what Lain Entralgo has called a veterinary practice on men. But the empirics argued that patients don't want to become doctors, they want to be cured.

Modern technicians have argued *a fortiori* that the knowledge base of medicine has grown so complicated as to make the effort to teach patients today even more futile than in ancient Greece. Physicians do not share a common scientific understanding with even their most educated patients. The knowledge explosion has produced in our time a fallout of ignorance. And since knowledge confers power, the ignorant, to the extent of their ignorance, become powerless. For better or for worse, patients can only submit themselves to the superior knowledge, authority, good intentions, and technical ingenuity of the doctor.

And yet, modern technology itself has allowed us in many respects to break with the understanding of disease that heretofore has minimized the teaching role of the healer. Traditionally interpreted, disease seemed to erupt episodically, breaking health and suspending the normal discretion that the patient exercises over his or her life. Upon falling ill, one surrenders one's natural authority until, through the mysterious interventions of the physician, a return to the normal world becomes possible. As the analogy would have it, disease disrupts health the way war interrupts peace. This irruptive and episodic account of disease, however, overlooks what Horacio Fabrega of Michigan State University has called the processive character of both disease and health.[5] Long before symptoms appear, the cardiovascular system may be preparing for catastrophe. A processive understanding of disease (which sophisticated monitoring devices make accessible to the modern practitioner) argues for a more collaborative interpretation of the physician-patient relationship. The physician must function as teacher, sharing information with the patient and engaging the layperson more actively to maintain good health. The professional charged with care needs to serve as more than a technician; for technology itself provides the physician with early warning of diseases that may respond to professionally assisted self-care.

The covenantal image for the health care practitioner pushes the profession unequivocally in the direction of teaching. To the degree that physicians and institutions accept a covenantal responsibility for the being and well-being of their patients—above and beyond the delivery of technical services—they must engage in the delicate business of transforming their patients' habits. The prevention of disease, the recovery from a siege of illness, and the successful coping with chronic conditions require, in one form or another, the reconstruction of life-styles. Whenever healers engage in these activities, they transform rather than merely transact. They do not simply offer services to satisfy the wants and wishes of people as they are; they engage in transforming commitments, priorities, and life rhythms.

But any professional effort to transform patients flirts with danger. It can quickly deteriorate into a puritanical officiousness—a runaway parentalism—unless teaching becomes its chief instrument. Teaching offers one of the few ways in which one can engage in transformation while respecting the patient's intelligence and power of self-determination. Good teaching depends not only upon a direct grasp of one's subject, a desire to share it, and some verbal facility, it also requires a kind of moral imagination that permits one to enter into the life circumstances of the learner: to reckon with the difficulties the learner faces in acquiring, assimilating, and acting on what he or she needs to know. Good teachers do not attempt to transform their students by bending them against their will, or by charming them out of their faculties, or by managing them behind their backs. Rather, they help them see their lives and their habits in a new light and thereby aid them in unlocking a freedom to perform in new ways.

Teaching has a place in medical practice across a broad spectrum of activities. Obviously, preventive, rehabilitative, chronic, and terminal care include a teaching component. Since the educational task of the physician shows least obviously in those activities in which physicians intervene most, this brief tour of the horizon ought to begin with the physician's efforts to cure.

Acute Care Medicine

Except for the most aggressive of interventions, therapy requires some measure of cooperation from the patient. But noncompliance rates range from 30 to 60 percent of patients, and even higher in those cases in which patients suffer no painful symptoms.[6] Those percentages are extraordinarily high. A clinical drug test would probably disappoint if it failed to help 30 to 60 percent of patients treated. No obstacle looms quite so large as noncompliance in impeding effective intervention.

Strategies for enhancing compliance depend upon improving the physician's prowess as a teacher. One study shows that rates of compliance doubled from 29 to 54 percent depending upon whether instructors provided low or high levels of instruction.[7] "Words are to a prescription what a preamble is to a constitution," as Laín Entralgo, the Spanish historian of medicine, once argued. The Preamble to the Constitution of the United States ("We the people of the United States in order to form a more perfect union . . . ") provides a clarifying context that makes sense and provides purpose for the laws that follow. Without that preamble, the fundamental law of the land just sits there, opaque, arbitrary, and perhaps relatively unintelligible to subsequent generations. Even God provided a context for his commands. Before issuing the Ten Commandments, Scripture reports, God announced and explained to the Israelites the grounds for their obedience: "I am the LORD your God, who brought you out of the land of Egypt, out of the house of bondage" (Ex. 20:2). The reminder about these deeds explains the commandments that follow: "You shall have no other gods before me. You shall not . . . " When physicians issue prescriptions wordlessly, opaquely, without an earnest effort to clarify and persuade, they do not play God; they usurp another kind of privilege, high-handed, arrogant, and ultimately obtuse. One thinks of Kierkegaard's characterization of the demonic state in *The Concept of Dread.*[8] He describes it as "shut-upness," a dreadful taciturnity, unrevealing, unhelpful, withdrawn, and cruelly destructive to those who need a healing word.

Every profession depends upon an esoteric body of knowledge, encoded by specialists and relatively inaccessible to the layperson. What has been carefully encoded needs decoding; and that process requires adept teaching. Not surprisingly, then, the literature on compliance emphasizes those strategies prized by the good teacher. Physicians must teach early in the game (one of the most stubborn obstacles to compliance springs from the patient's conviction that the original diagnosis itself is wrong);[9] they must teach clearly in nontechnical language (decoding); they produce better results when they offer the explanation in both oral and written form; and whatever they say, they must organize well. They have to allow for a period of time in the course of which the patient internalizes the news. Doctors partly condemn the learning capacity of their patients because they fail to appreciate the patient's need for repetition and for time to assimilate the diagnostic and prognostic news, which is sometimes difficult to bear. Information simply unloaded on the patient sits like a parallel deposit in the mind; unassimilated and inert.

Compliance rates also improve when the physician teaches not only the patient but the patient's family. Efforts at weight loss or control of hypertension and arthritis, and recovery programs after heart attacks, show better results when the family actively supports the program.[10] Problems of compliance in these areas raise questions about the place of teaching in preventive and rehabilitative medicine.

Preventive Medicine

Physicians and the public at large, until recently, have held preventive medicine in low esteem. Hygeia, the goddess of health, has never been a match for the god of healing. Asclepius always appears in full feather, the quintessentially male, TV-spectacular agent of interventionist medicine. Since the discovery of penicillin and the antibiotics, money for research and health delivery has gone largely to acute care. Expenditures in the name of Asclepius rose 800 percent in the two decades following World War II.[11] The third-party payment system, under public and private insurance programs, has tilted in almost every detail toward curative medicine. The fraction of funds going into health education has remained constant and minuscule (about one half of one percent) while the portion of the GNP devoted to health care has risen astronomically during the period 1940–1,981.[12] Yet, during this same period—except for the success of antibiotics, mind-control drugs, and some surgical procedures—the actual advances in acute care have not been all that striking. The life expectancy of fifty-year-old white males during two decades rose only 8 months despite the most generous expenditure of funds and talent on acute care in world history.[13]

The goddess Hygeia symbolizes the condition of health rather than the activity of healing: the steadfast rule of reason in body care rather than the rule of ingenuity in body repair; the balanced classical concern for dietetics and gymnastics rather than the more occult appeals to special nostrums, insights, and powers. But, alas, Hygeia has always been, and ever will be, a dull gray goddess, without box-office draw or fund-raising appeal. W. Hutchinson saw the structural problem with a steady eye when he wrote:

> The system of remuneration makes the physician's income dependent upon the amount of sickness. Our system's philosophy might be condensed in the motto "millions for the care and not one cent for prevention." It seems to me that the weakness of our system lies in this one fact, that it gives [physicians] such exceedingly little opportunity for what has been called the practice of preventive medicine.[14]

Hutchinson wrote these lines in 1886.

The obstacles to the development of preventive medicine do not come entirely from physicians—either from their economic self-interest or from a special perception of role that discourages good teaching. Four types of patients, even under the best of circumstances, make the task of preventive medicine a slow boring through hard wood (Max Weber's phrase about another difficult vocation—politics). Patients of the first type assume their own de facto immortality. Someday they will die, but not yet. Disease and death for the moment remain abstract, deferrable, and remote. They feel the medicine of immortality already within them. They do not need preventive medicine. Patients of the second type seem less given to denial. They go to the doctor and listen to all the explanations. But the doctor discovers on the next visit that none of it sinks in. A kind of selective interferon seems at work, blocking out what the doctor has to say. The patient has internalized nothing.

At the opposite extreme are those patients given to what Robert Jay Lifton, in another connection, called nuclearism. Such persons solve the problem of threat by cozying up to the source of danger. Contact with the forbidden, the destructive, magnifies their life. The actor Slim Pickens, in the film *Dr. Strangelove,* portrays a country colonel who straddles a nuclear bomb and rides it ecstatically to his own destruction. Nuclearists feel drawn to the pull of the cigarette, the regular swell of liquor in the head, the helmetless ride on a motorcycle at high speed, the pressure cooker of a job, the brinkmanship with the psyche that goes with drugs and sleep deprivation. Recklessness in all its forms acquires a kind of demonic force that makes all the cautionary advice and counsel of preventive medicine seem beside the point and demeaning.

Finally, there are the hypochondriacs. Like the nuclearists, they preoccupy themselves with danger, but in this case they let danger provide them with an excuse for diminishing their life. Hypochondriacs see trouble on every side, risk at every corner, poison in the very food they eat, the blast of cancer in the sun, a dangerous depletion in every psychic exertion, and the potential for terminal disease in the most transient colony of germs to which they play host. Such persons frustrate preventive medicine. Health alone unhealthily obsesses them, miniaturizes their life, makes them too fearful to exude that health which a life well expended on matters of greater moment sometimes fosters. Encountering patients such as these in their daily experience must dampen physicians' hopes for preventive medicine. So much advice falls on stony ground.

Still, the rate of deaths due to heart attack and stroke has declined rapidly in recent years, and the evidence does not suggest that open-heart surgery, resuscitation techniques, and other improved interventions have made the difference in the huge decline. Rather, changes in diet (especially reduced salt intake), regular exercise, reductions in weight, drug compliance for control of hypertension, and other essentially preventive measures seem to account for the improvements in health. This progress hardly results from the teaching efforts of physicians alone. Deeper cultural changes are at work. The magisterial authority of the media and the networking of patient groups play their part in improving self-care. But it would be passing strange for physicians to withdraw from preventive work simply because others as well help to provide it.

The skepticism doctors often betray toward preventive work may result partly from their failure to be imaginative about the social setting in which it should take place. They too readily generalize from their own one-on-one curative work and take for granted the individual tutorial (a little too private to be fully effective) as the only appropriate setting for their teaching. As alternatives to the tutorial in the physician's office, society offers the even more private and isolating spot commercials on television, the bus advertisements, the newspaper columns, or the individual pamphlets distributed by the American Heart Association and American Cancer Society. Physicians largely ignore the fact that most teaching takes place in public classrooms—from the three R's to AA. Other, more communal, strategies for educating patients deserve attention.

The chief of clinical services in student health at a large Midwestern university saw just such an opportunity for communal preventive medicine at his campus. Ordinarily, jobs in student health are dull. (Either students seem radiantly healthy and need nothing medical that is more technically complicated than antibiotics and a good night's respite from the dormitory, or they are too sick to remain in school—in which case also the physician does not get to handle an interesting case. Psychiatrists, of course, are an exception in that they get to take care of young students just separated from home whose emotional problems respond best to treatment *in situ.*) But this young physician—not a psychiatrist—chose a career in student health because he was interested in preventive medicine and, given that interest, he explained, a university campus offered a splendid opportunity. In its preventive program, his clinic did a health profile of each student on arrival, including a projection of life expectancy on the basis of current habits and a second projection on the basis of an alternative set of habits. Then the clinic, taking advantage of a computer analysis and classification of problems, pulled the potentially hypertensive, the obese, et al., into a classroom where the health care practitioners taught and worked at their problems collectively.

The program had four advantages over conventional preventive efforts: it picked up patients at a relatively early age; it pulled them into a setting that kept them feeling normal and let them respond normally to their obligations; it provided them with a support group of fellows with a similar problem, thus overcoming the discouraging isolation that young people with special problems feel; and finally, the classroom provided for economies of scale as compared with conventional, expensive tutorial contact with a professional. When a visitor to the campus asked why a similarly motivated health care team could not work with other institutions—such as corporations, unions, service organizations, and churches—the young physician reported that his own group in student health was on the verge of signing a contract with the local Presbyterian church.

A few health care groups have similarly allied themselves with religious communities, but on the whole, the helping professions have not thought through the ways in which they might link with so-called intermediate institutions to offer services directed to prevention and rehabilitation. The dominant model of health care defined by the delivery of services in a freestanding hospital or in a private office has—in addition to its other disadvantages—emphasized the individual at the expense of the communal, and the manipulative at the expense of the cognitive in the task of healing.

Rehabilitative and Chronic Care

In preventive medicine, the physician faces the difficult task of persuading patients that they face real threats to their health. In rehabilitative medicine, few patients can doubt for long the reality of the assault. The patient has just suffered a massive blow to body confidence. An accident maims or disfigures and imposes a catastrophic change on the patient's very self-perception—his or her movement and looks. A coronary suddenly throws the mainspring of life itself into terrible disarray. A stroke slurs speech, renders useless one side of the body, confuses memory and vision, and depresses the spirit. A burn scorches the skin and tightens movement, leaving the victim like a countryside charred and crippled by the firestorm of war; and kidney failure poisons every river in the system, subjecting the victim to impotence and depression.

Patients pass through three stages: (1) their life brutally changes and they plunge into shock, numbness, and grief; (2) they suffer a period of perilous transition; until at length (3) they make their way into a new life under the terms and conditions of their disability. The entire process compares structurally with the great rites of passage in traditional societies.

Similarly, the ritual "turning points" in traditional

societies—the events associated with puberty, marriage, birth, death, seedtime, sickness, and war—included three moments, all of them important to a successful passage. The first moment imposed a radical separation of the participant from his or her past life. Young people undergoing a puberty rite suffered, at the outset, perhaps segregation, a whipping, a tattooing, or the pulling of a tooth. The mutilation visibly signified a death to one's former life. Second, the novitiate underwent a period of transition, with its appropriate regimen and ordeal under the tutelage of specialists. Third, the candidate eventually entered into a new estate. One could not view this new identity as something added on to one's previous life by way of peaceful annexation. A radical alteration had occurred, affecting habits, demands, regimen, and core identity. The relation between old and new resembled a kind of death and resurrection. Calendars reflect this sacral dimension as they order and measure time before and after the event.

Similarly, in the case of personal catastrophe, we measure time before and after—the accident, the heart attack, the stroke, the operation, or the birth of the retarded child.

The role of the modern healer both resembles and differs from that of the religious specialist who presides over traditional rites of passage. First, the healer does not, like the traditional priest, make the first "moment" occur. But he or she has special knowledge of what has taken place and of its convulsive impact on the patient. If the healer served as the attending physician in the case, he or she helped set a limit to its destructive consequences. That special knowledge and service provides a basis for the second role as tutor and guide during the transition period. Or, by referral, the healer helps legitimate those who will take over rehabilitative therapy. Depending on the severity of the accident or the disease, the patient will need to engage in a drastic reconstruction of habits. One must perhaps learn all over again how to walk, exercise, eat, rest, and pace oneself in daily work.

In addition to helping in the reconstruction of skills, the healer has to reckon with the psychological perils of the transitional period. The sufferer, to be sure, cannot doubt the reality of the problem; the heart attack overwhelms, palpably, beyond compare, but all outsize events, whether good or bad, have their own kind of unreality. "Has this really happened to me? It hardly seems possible. It won't be there when I wake up in the morning." Alternatively, the patient descends into despair—another kind of unreality that obscures the resources of both therapy and the gathering inner resources that the passage of time places at the patient's own disposal. Or again, the patient passes beyond the confusion and disorientation of the original assault into the ordered procedures of the institution that has provided treatment, but this alien order still seems unreal because so patently not his or her own.

When the patient begins tentatively, almost experimentally, to take hold of the rehabilitating regimen, then that person may move suddenly out of numbness, despair, and confusion and be inclined to overestimate touchingly and pathetically the speed of recovery—expecting rapid strides back into the old familiar world—only to experience a setback, physical and psychological, that signals a far more protracted period of recovery. And then, still later, there is the discovery that one recovers not only slowly but incompletely. The patient will never become again the person he or she once was, "as good as new," but a different human being, permanently limited in one way or another, and inwardly altered by this ordeal.

And yet a third stage eventually comes when the patient reenters the world, a world itself not quite the same, shadowed in some ways, poignantly heightened in others, as skills once taken for granted now seem almost miraculous, and as sounds and smells hitherto unnoticed seem a grace note in life. Friendships and family bonds stretch and rearrange—in some cases deepen, in others tragically weaken—until at length one's powerful link with the attending physician, physical therapist, or occupational therapist, one's mentor and guide, as it were, ends.

The company of those who serve as tutors to patients may include not only the attending physician and nurse but also physical therapists, occupational therapists, workers on various outpatient services, and, last but hardly least, other patients who have themselves survived a similar ordeal.

Most healers other than the physician, both by training and conviction, acknowledge the importance of teaching. In fact, the best teaching I witnessed across a year as an observer at a hospital came from a family health care practitioner who worked under the auspices of an inner-city clinic with links to the teaching hospital. This paraprofessional grew up in the ghetto himself and worked under the direction of sophisticated nurses (who warned me before I set out on home visitations with the practitioner that the chief medical problem in the neighborhood was no particular disease but inadequate housing). The family practitioner took me on his rounds to overcrowded, sometimes windowless, vermin-infested apartments, largely occupied by old couples or young mothers and children who either seemed temporarily quelled by visitors or squirmed in the dark. He painstakingly taught his patients and worked just as conscientiously with their family caretakers. The head physician administering the program recognized the social value of this service to the hospital, above and beyond its value to the individual patient. She observed with pride that the hospital-clinic was one of the few buildings in the area spared in the last spate of neighborhood riots. Apparently the institution had kept covenant with the neighborhood. And ghetto residents, even teenagers, respected this fact.

The physician's general neglect of teaching increases the burden on other health care professionals. This substitution sometimes seems an improvement. Training programs in other fields usually emphasize the professional's responsibility to teach not only in rehabilitation but in preventive, curative, and chronic care. But when the physician defaults from teaching and hands on the patient to persons with less clout, the legitimation of authority sometimes suffers. The physician needs to lay the groundwork for what follows even if he or she does not execute in every detail the therapeutic regimen.

Nurses particularly find themselves in a delicate position, in dealing with acute care cases, if they must teach the patient—yet the physician retains full authority over disclosure and neglects the responsibilities that go with that authority. Since the nurse sees the patient constantly while the physician ducks in and out, the emotional strain of failing to level with the patient and the patient's family falls on the nurse's shoulders. Other professionals need the legitimation of authority and direction and technical guidance that the physician can provide, and the physician needs the kind of information that only those who have day-to-day contact with the patient can furnish.

Selected former patients, organized and unorganized, also serve a teaching function. Admittedly, the company of other patients in a similar plight has its risks. They sometimes exhibit a tedious missionary zeal, a paternal officiousness that seeks to dominate through greater experience, a half-baked professionalism or a strained cheerfulness. Leaders of support groups usually try to weed out those former patients who have failed to effect successful passage through the illness (sometimes for reasons not at all related to their ordeal). But even those who have reconstructed their life despite catastrophe can depress the newly arrived patient, as they soberly remind that person of the severe handicaps he or she must eventually accept. The pitfalls await, yet the active mentoring performed by former alcoholics, burn victims, heart attack and cancer patients remind us, in an age that tends to reduce healing to the limited alternatives of professional care or self-care, that instruction often goes on among a company of peers.

Terminal Care and the Question of Style

The forms of medical care covered so far—curative, preventive, and rehabilitative—demand that the physician teach; terminal care, less obviously so. Teaching seems irrelevant to the ultimate crisis. Indeed, the truth itself appears, at best, out of place; at worst, crushing. In the last chapter, I argued for the truth, but the truth in the context of fidelity. In this context, the truth expands beyond true assertions to the professional's more extended vocation as a teacher. The issue of terminal care now returns us again to the further question of the teacher's style. Clearly, teaching in medical crisis differs from ordinary academic instruction. The teacher deals with a profoundly troubled listener. The news the teacher brings can devastate. One must be wise and tactful in how one tells the truth.

The delicacy of crisis and terminal care forces a further look at the language used in communicating with patients. Our resources in language fall into several categories: (1) direct, immediate, blunt talk; (2) circumlocution or double-talk; (3) silence; and (4) discourse that proceeds—partly, at least—by way of indirection.

Silence, of course, can lead to sharing, but also to evasion. The technical nature of the medical vocabulary provides plenty of opportunities for a second form of evasion—elusive double-talk. Evasion is more difficult to achieve than it appears. Body language and countenance blurt out more than words reveal. Even though physicians manage information, family members cannot do so deftly. The face betrays what the tongue cannot say. So the patient lives with the knowledge, without benefit of whatever additional help the physician might offer. We may deny death but cannot avoid it.

The last decade has seen a huge reaction against the response of silence. Death courses have out-enrolled their competitors in elective offerings at American colleges. Dr. Kübler-Ross achieved celebrity with her book *On Death and Dying.* Broadway has brought forth several plays on the subject. Direct talk on the subject abounds. Too often, however, we assume (especially as Americans) that we can only tell the truth directly, immediately, bluntly. Such talk seems the only alternative to evasive silence or circumlocution. On the subject of sex, for example, we assume that as the only alternative to the repressions of the Victorian Age is the tiresome, gabby, explicit discussion of sex imposed upon our adolescents from junior high forward.

However, we can also talk *indirectly* on the weighty subjects of death, religion, and love. Obviously, gabby bluntness in the presence of one dying is wholly inappropriate. It reckons in no way with the solemnity of the event. The physician owes the truth, but not all patients want the truth in exhaustive clinical detail. In such cases, we can surely find some alternatives to blunt talk other than double-talk, a condescending cheerfulness, or a frightening silence.

Perhaps examples of what I mean by indirection will suffice. One doctor reports[15] that many patients brought up the question of their own death in an indirect form: some asked him, for example, whether he thought they should buy a house, marry, or undergo plastic surgery. The doctor realized that the answer "Yes—surely, go ahead" in a big cheerful voice evaded. On the other hand, the answer "No" stopped discussion. He found it important to tell them that he recognized the importance of the question. From that point on, he could discuss with them their uncertainties, anxieties, and fears. The doctor and the patient could share. The doctor need not dwell on the subject for long; after its acknowledgment, he could proceed to the details of daily life without the change of subject becoming an evasion.

We can achieve indirection in another way. Although it sometimes imposes too much to approach the subject frontally under the immediate pressure of its presence, we can achieve indirection if we discuss death in advance of a crisis. Rabbis, priests, or ministers who suddenly feel tongue-tied and irrelevant in the sickroom get what they deserve if they have not worked through the problem with their people in a series of sermons or in work sessions with lay groups. Words too blunt and inappropriate in the crisis itself may, if spoken earlier, provide an indirect basis for sharing burdens. Physicians may similarly discover that the truth shared earlier provides a basis for weathering subsequent events without having to impose it suddenly in a later crisis.

Professionals should not use the option of indirect language as an excuse for delivering signals so remote as to evade or mislead. At its best, indirect discourse verbally respects rather than avoids reality. A kind of double respect comes into play: a respect both for the solemnity of the event and for the distance that the patient chooses to maintain in his or her relationship to the event. A man who knew that he had cancer once said to his middle-aged son, a writer on the subject of death and dying, "Go easy, Don." The man knew he had cancer. But at the same time, he wanted to establish the distance he wished to maintain between himself, his son, and the imminent event of his death. He did not want his son to favor him with seminar-length discussions on the subject. Only a fool would not have respected this request. Some distancing and indirection occurs in our relationship to death.

The language of indirection treats death decorously as a sacred event. Indirection often best suits our approach to the sacred. The Jews did not attempt to look directly on Yahweh's face. They dared not approach God casually and directly. But they also could not avoid God's presence. Jews could hold their ground before their Lord in a relation that was genuine but indirect. So also, we need not dwell directly on the subject of death interminably or avoid it by a condescending cheerfulness wholly inappropriate to the event. Still, two human beings can acknowledge death, if ever so indirectly, and hold their ground before it until parted.

Medical Education

If physicians must teach their patients well, then it may be necessary to recast premedical and medical education and clinical training. Tucking away the subject of teaching strategies in the Department of Public Health and Community Medicine hardly atones for an education that generally aspires to bestow on its graduates no more articulateness than the hieroglyphs on a prescription bottle.

Until the twentieth century, almost all medical education took place in an apprenticeship system. At the turn of the century, only 10 to 12 percent of physicians had a liberal arts education before entering medical schools. The Flexner report of 1910, however, eventually sited medical education in the university and therefore exposed young premedical students to the liberal arts.[16] Theoretically, at least, this new institutional location, which required that every candidate for medical school acquire some background in the humanities, should have helped produce professionals more pedagogically skilled than the "rough empirics" of whom Plato complained. But in fact, an undergraduate liberal arts education today hardly prepares students to write or teach well. The liberal arts faculty at large—not just science teachers—bear responsibility for this failure. Unfortunately, academicians have assumed that only some of their graduates become teachers; the rest do not. Therefore, they have treated teaching as a segregated profession. Nonacademic professionals will merely dispense technical services. Teaching is, of course, a special profession, but at the same time a liberal arts education ought to turn out good teachers whether students go into teaching or not. Nonacademic professionals must teach, even as they dispense esoteric services. The lawyer, the statesman, and the business leader, as well as the physician, must teach. Accordingly, the teacher in the humanities and the social sciences should learn how to set requirements for reports, papers, and examinations so as to produce people who know how to share what they know (a discipline which at its best also increases the sharer's own grasp of the subject matter).

Similarly, residency training programs need to encourage good teaching. In a "teaching hospital" today, doctors use patients as teaching material; patients are not themselves taught. The very structure of morning rounds discourages the teaching of patients. The attending physician on the floor is accompanied by a small platoon of young clerks and residents, all of them bristling with good health. They stop by a bed under a very considerable time pressure. Twenty patients must be seen in an hour and fifteen minutes, a ration of but three or four minutes to a bed. The patient, meanwhile, has just awakened. He has spent the night mulling over the five or six things that he wanted to discuss, when suddenly he finds himself confronted by these inspectors, jacked like a deer in the glare of headlights. He has remembered and voiced but one or two things on his list when they move the procession on into the hallway. There the serious teaching takes place as the attending physician and retinue rapidly discuss the case, *sotto voce,* before traveling on to the next room. Young physicians-to-be, of course, surely need the hallway instruction. Patients do serve as teaching material in a teaching hospital. But if residents are to practice competently in their own right, and if teaching is an important part of medical practice, then the teaching hospital should structure education so as to produce professionals who, rather than mutely performing procedures, genuinely profess what they know.

Teaching Among Professional Colleagues

Throughout this chapter the emphasis has fallen on teaching the patient. Only a fraction of physicians, however, deal with patients. Others function as specialists who abet the work of their colleagues with patients. Such specialists must teach their attending colleagues—discreetly. In the course of delivering technical information, specialists engage in a kind of continuing education. This delicate relationship to colleagues generates opposing moral dangers. Specialists can display, on the one hand, a too-officious, judgmental, and pompous style that condescends toward the generalist and, on the other hand, an obsequiousness that fails in candor, often for the sake of referrals. Particularly specialists at university tertiary care centers face important moral and political issues of style as they relate to outlying practitioners. A kind of town-gown tension can grow up between the two sets of professionals. The staff at a teaching hospital must teach in such a way as to empower rather than humiliate their colleagues who have responsibility for primary care. Otherwise, the mediocre and defensive practitioner may fail to refer for fear of exposing his or her own inadequacies. This outcome produces not only inconvenient business consequences for the specialist but also more than inconvenient results for future patients who fall into the hands of inadequate caretakers.

Some of the dangers that go with the pomp of hierarchy would abate if the specialist remembered his or her professional debt to the generalist. To be sure, the specialist normally instructs and advises the general practitioner, but often the teaching role is reversed. The specialist needs to learn from, and sometimes to be corrected by, the generalist. The specialist requires, in the first place, the proper flow of information. Further, in case of ambiguous symptoms the specialist sometimes needs to be protected from the tendency to pull a diagnosis in the direction of his or her own particular field of expertise. The generalist alone may possess both the information and the broader perspective crucial to developing the correct differential diagnosis.

Notes

1. Carter L. Marshall, "Prevention and Health Education," in *Maxcy-Rosenau Public Health and Preventive Medicine,* 11th ed., ed. by John M. Last et al. (Appleton-Century-Crofts, 1980), pp. 1114-1115.
2. Duncan Neuhauser, "Don't Teach Preventive Medicine: A Contrary View," *Public Health Reports* 97 (May–June 1982): 222.
3. Ibid., p. 221.
4. Ibid.
5. Horacio Fabrega, "Concepts of Disease: Logical Features and Social Implications," *Perspectives in Biology and Medicine* 15 (Summer 1972): 605-615.
6. Marshall Becker and Lois Maiman, "Strategies for Enhancing Patient Compliance," *Journal for Community Health* 6 (Winter 1980): 113.
7. Ibid., p. 114.
8. Søren Kierkegaard, *The Concept of Dread,* tr. by Walter Lowrie (Princeton University Press, 1944), pp. 110-115.
9. Becker and Maiman, "Strategies for Enhancing Patient Compliance," p. 119.
10. Ibid., pp. 127-129.
11. Marshall, "Prevention and Health Education," p. 1114.
12. Daniel R. Waldo (ed.), *Health Care Financing Trends* 3, No. 1 (June 1982): 2.
13. Marshall, "Prevention and Health Education," p. 1114.

14. W. Hutchinson, "Health Insurance, On Our Financial Relation to the Public," *Journal of the American Medical Association* 7 (Oct. 30, 1886): 477–481. Quoted by Duncan Neuhauser, "Don't Teach Preventive Medicine," p. 222.

15. Samuel L. Feder, "Attitudes of Patients with Advanced Malignancy," in *Death and Dying: Attitudes of Patient and Doctor,* Symposium No. 11, Group for the Advancement of Psychiatry (New York: Mental Health Materials Center, 1965), p. 619.

16. Abraham Flexner, *Medical Education in the United States and Canada* (1910; repr. Arno Press, 1972).

Chapter Seventeen
PSYCHIATRIC CARE: PROFESSIONAL COMMITMENTS AND SOCIETAL RESPONSIBILITIES

Introduction

Psychiatry is formed from two Greek words, *psyche* (soul) and *iatreia* (healing). The derivation itself raises the question of the relation of religion to the new knowledge and skills of scientific psychology because the cure of souls has long been considered a part of the task of the people of God,[1] even though today a "psychiatrist," a "soul healer," is a specially trained physician, not a specially trained cleric.

There are still many practitioners of the "cure of souls" besides psychiatrists, of course. A psychologist is not a medical doctor but one who holds a Ph.D. in psychology and has put in at least a year of supervised practice. The psychiatric social worker, the professional counselor, the family therapist, the pastoral counselor, and still others all practice the "cure of souls." Some of these are not professionally trained; some of them are not professionally committed to the benefit of the client; some of them nevertheless have—or claim to have—the "gift" of healing. The presence (and competition) of so many different practitioners raises the issue of regulation. This is an important issue because many of those who need counseling may be especially vulnerable to exploitation; yet it is also a complicated issue because there are so many different assumptions, therapies, and loyalties among the different practitioners. The psychologist working on the biochemical bases of schizophrenia may have very little in common with a colleague studying small-group behavior. The therapist utilizing behavior modification techniques may have little interest in logotherapy or gestalt therapy or hypnotherapy or psychodrama or transactional analysis or EST or the primal scream. The disciples of Freud may have a polemical relation with the disciples of Jung or Rogers or Skinner or Frankel.

But what about Christian practitioners; what about the relationship of Christianity to contemporary psychiatric care? On the one hand, there are those who would wholly reject secular psychiatric knowledge and skills in favor of the religious practices of prayer, confession, absolution, and even exorcism. On the other hand there are those who would test and exercise religious practices in terms of their therapeutic benefits alongside other psychiatric methods. Religion may be advocated as instrumental to human happiness and peace of mind, but it may also be disregarded as secondary or irrelevant. If such consolations as religion does provide come only from a profound consent to the will of God, then a utilitarian account of religion (hardly a "profound consent") may well fail to even recognize those consolations—and it will surely fail to honor the struggles of Job and Jeremiah, the passion of Christ, and the laments of the psalmists and of some honest, pious believers today. One may examine Seward Hiltner's piece, for example, with these questions in mind.

From Job's "miserable comforters" to this day, people have sought to provide not only help to those sick of soul but also advice to the helpers, challenging their assumptions, their therapies, and their loyalties. The assumption of Job's comforters that was challenged was that there was a neat fit between piety and well-being. That challenge remains relevant to any utilitarian account of religion, but it may also provide a model for theological reflection about the cure of souls today. Perhaps we need neither wholly reject psychological knowledge and skills nor reduce religion to merely another therapeutic tool; perhaps we can and must rather challenge and qualify certain assumptions, reflect about the goals and means of particular therapies, and both nurture and order certain loyalties on the basis of theological reflection.

One controversial assumption is whether there is any such thing as mental illness. Thomas Szasz, for example, has challenged this assumption, acknowledging certain diseases of the brain but rejecting "mental illness" as an explanation of behavior which deviates from social and ethical norms. This challenge sustains Szasz's critique of certain goals and means in psychiatry, notably his criticism of the involuntary hospitalization of the "mentally ill" as a form of imprisonment without due process. The challenge also forces a reevaluation of the self-understanding and loyalty of the psychiatrists, for one must ask whose agent they understand themselves to be—the patient's, the relatives', the community's, the institution's?[2] Morris Kaplan's review of the play *Equus* raises similar questions. Is the young man Alan who blinded the horses "mentally ill"? Is the medical model appropriate to care for his soul, or would the criminal model recommended by the owner of the stables be better? What about the religious model utilized by Alan's mother; is it an alternative or a correlative explanation? Can a religious explanation be given which honors the compassion and skills of the doctor as well as the patient's need for transcendence? To whom is the psychiatrist loyal—to Alan, to the profession, to the community, to God? How should these loyalties be ranked and ordered? Are a patient's suffering and a doctor's compassion sufficient legitimation for the exercise of psychological powers?

Behaviorists sometimes make the assumption that freedom is illusion and dignity is "reinforced behavior."[3] One need not make such an assumption, of course, to find the experimental work in behavioral psychology useful to therapy; but if one does make it, does it render questionable any moral reflection about the goals and means of therapy? (For example, is Skinner's utopian vision in *Walden Two* then simply conditioned nostalgia for small-town America at the turn of the century?)

One need not accept a rugged individualism in order to challenge the behaviorist assumption, but once challenged, questions may and will be raised about goals and means and professional identity and loyalty whenever we attempt to influence ideas and behavior, and especially when we use the expanding human powers to control and manipulate patients and their behavior. It has, of course, always been the intention of parents, teachers, pastors, and all those charged with the "cure of souls" to influence human behavior, but the means of influence have typically utilized speech and gesture and so acknowledged and honored as distinctively human beings even those they wanted to change. New powers, including behavior modification techniques, mood-altering drugs, electrical stimulation of the brain, and brain surgery, by contrast, make it possible to bypass the distinctively human capacities not only of speech and gesture but also of understanding and willing.

The fundamental issue here may be control. Indeed, Perry London describes behavior modification technologies as a form of social power, as the ability of X to get Y to do Z.[4] Then, as he says, "the moral problem of behavior control is how to use power justly."[5] Within that general concern, however, more particular questions may be focused upon: by whom, on whom, by what means, and for what ends.

The concern about "by whom" may be extended to the question, Who controls the controllers? Whose agent is the therapist? Who decides what behavior is to be modified—the patient, the parent, the state, the military, the warden, the teacher, the institution? The therapist often finds himself with conflicting responsibilities, as a double agent with conflicting interests at heart.

The concern about "on whom" is raised especially with respect to involuntary participants in therapy and with respect to those whose consent is given in deeply ambiguous contexts.[6]

Concerns about means are raised when people question whether the use of contingency contracting as a means fosters a manipulative exchange orientation to social interaction—for example, whether the use of such a means in marriage counseling reduces the meaning of marriage to contract, or whether the use of token economies in schools and institutions fosters a materialistic and reductionistic evaluation of human acts. Again, some have been concerned that the use of drugs like Anectine, which produces a sensation of drowning, or aversive treatment in general can tempt controllers in prisons or other settings to misuse it as retribution for real or imagined lack of cooperation, as a way to keep recalcitrant people in line.

The concern about ends is raised when people warn about the imposition of "orthodox" behavior in a community or about the possibility of using manipulative powers to silence dissent or to eliminate "social deviancy" or simply to preserve control in a prison, a classroom, an institution, or a society. Perhaps here we come back to the question about loyalties of psychiatrists—to the question of whose agents they really are and to the meaning of professional integrity when both patients and society make demands on their skills to serve their private or their social goods.

The articles by Wayne Oates and James Gustafson in this section raise some of these questions and more besides with respect to behavior control and brain research respectively, and they should invite and enable theological reflection and response. The articles by Robert Burt and Stanley Hauerwas focus on those we cannot cure but for whom we are still obliged to care, the retarded. The piece by Burt is interesting for its use of the Christian tradition not only to call Christians to care about and for the retarded but also to advise judges in the secular realm of possibilities and opportunities in their role. The readiness of Burt to use the Christian tradition to address a wider public stands in some contrast to Hauerwas's self-consciously restricted address to the Christian community and his insistence on Christian integrity within that community. It nicely serves to raise again the issue of the relation of a Christian perspective to an impartial moral perspective and to social policy.[7]

Notes

1. John T. McNeill, *A History of the Cure of Souls* (New York: Harper & Brothers, 1951).

2. Thomas Szasz, *Ideology and Insanity: Essays on the Psychiatric Dehumanization of Man* (Garden City, N.Y.: Doubleday, 1970).

3. B. F. Skinner, *Beyond Freedom and Dignity* (New York: Knopf, 1971).

4. Perry London, "Behavior Control, Values and the Future," in *Modifying Man: Implications and Ethics,* ed. Craig Ellison (Washington, D.C.: University Press of America, 1977).

5. Perry London, *Behavior Control* (New York: Harper & Row, 1969), p. 199.

6. See, for example, Robert A. Burt, "Why We Should Keep Prisoners from the Doctors: Reflections on the Detroit Psychosurgery Case," *Hasting Center Report,* Feb. 1975, 25-34.

7. We have not paid any special attention in this section to the responsibilities of confidentiality or truth telling, although psychiatric care confronts these issues in case after case. (In addition to the selections from the previous section, interested readers may consult the famous case *Tarasoff v. Regents of the University of California* and commentary on it.)

Suggestions for Further Reading

Burt, Robert. "Why We Should Keep Prisoners from the Doctors." *Hastings Center Report* 5 (1975).

———. *Taking Care of Strangers: The Rule of Law in Doctor-Patient Relations.* New York: Free Press, 1979.

Kanoti, G. A. "Ethical Implications of Psychotherapy." *Journal of Religion and Health* 10 (1971): 180-91.

Shore, Milton E., and Stuart E. Golann, eds. *Current Ethical Issues in Mental Health.* Rockville, Md.: National Institute of Health, 1973.

Szasz, T. S. *Law, Liberty, and Psychiatry: An Inquiry into the Social Uses of Mental Health Practice.* New York: Macmillan, 1963.

89. Some Contributions of Religion to Mental Health

SEWARD HILTNER

Mental hygiene teaches something to religion and the church. But religion and the church make contributions to mental health whose full significance is not always realized. "There is no integration which compares with that which comes from religious faith or a religious goal," says Dr. Earl D. Bond.[1] "I am convinced that the Christian religion is one of the most valuable and potent influences that we possess for producing that harmony and peace of mind . . . needed to bring health and power to a large proportion of nervous patients," reports Dr. J. A. Hadfield.[2]

Fortunately we are not wholly dependent upon the personal testimony of scientists for our conviction that religion does have a constructive influence for health in the widest and deepest sense. Such quotations as these, which could be multiplied, perform the service, however, of indicating how we may look for the kind of contribution which religion in practice makes to health. . . .

In approaching the contributions which religion makes to mental health in a practical sense, we must accept two points as preliminaries. The first is that religion is not interested merely in health. Theologians would say that health, even considered in the modern sense as relating to body, mind and spirit, is not the same as salvation because health is "temporal" or in time, and salvation is "eternal" or beyond time. As George A. Buttrick puts it in reference to prayer, for example, "The integration wrought by prayer goes far beyond health of body and 'mind'—as it must to be convincing, for all men must die."[3] Assertions of this kind are true in the basic sense in which they are intended. It is also true that Kagawa in the slums of Tokyo spent his physical health, perhaps to the advancement of his spiritual health—yet that which he enhanced can hardly be completely circumscribed under the idea of health. Christianity says there are other things than health which man should seek. But it does not say that one should seek ill-health. . . .

The second introductory point we must make is that not all interpretations (and living out) of religion,

---

From Seward Hiltner, *Religion and Health* (New York: Macmillan, 1943), pp. 22-35, 41. Used by permission of the Hiltner family.

or of Christianity, are healthy, in the sense of health of the whole personality. We have not spoken of "healthful" or "unhealthful" religion. This is because use of the latter words would imply a discussion of the relative soundness of something before the individual got hold of it (or before it got hold of him). It is certainly true that healthful and unhealthful religions exist. We believe that a religion glorifying the state as a substitute for the Christian God is possessed of, to say the least, unhealthful tendencies. We believe that a group which, wittingly or not, emphasizes but one aspect of the nature of God to the exclusion of all others is unhealthful, as for instance sentimental groups which say that because God forgives, he never judges. Yet our concern will not basically be with the healthfulness or unhealthfulness of religions; that has been well written about in other places.[4]

What we must also recognize is that a Christianity sound in ideas can be so interpreted by an individual that its total influence upon his personality may be progressive or regressive, healthy or unhealthy.[5] This fact has always been recognized by the church in some measure. As early as Cyprian's time, and probably earlier, we find church leaders counseling against those who went out to seek martyrdom. Heinrich Suso, the great mystic of the Middle Ages, was refused canonization because he had "punished" himself too much and too severely. Thus the basic impulse to sacrifice for the sake of the Christian cause was recognized as sound, but the church had to be sure it was "for the Christian cause" and not for something else of which even the individual might be unaware. Catholic theology in particular has paid a good deal of attention to such matters.

But in recent years we have been aided to more basic standards for judging whether or not an individual is interpreting his religion soundly. A few suggestions about the criteria for distinguishing healthy from unhealthy religion are in order at this point. We suggest six criteria.

A healthy interpretation of religion must be related to the whole personality. To put it one way, it cannot profess to deal only with the soul or spirit and neglect the mind and body. There are still people who believe that because Christianity deals with the eternal and the hereafter it has no relevance to the state of things today. There are literalists who are concerned with salvation of the "soul" to the neglect of the individual's total welfare, which includes neglect of what is, from our point of view, his spiritual welfare. Much moralistic interpretation of religion belongs in this class. One might of course point out kinds of religion which emphasize the body out of proportion to the mind and spirit, and even some which emphasize the mind out of proportion to the body and spirit. But the danger of confusing the soul with the personality is more common in Christianity. That indicates both its high state and its great danger. The thing that we are forced to call the total personality is that to which our interpretation of religion must be related.

Religion must grow up intellectually and emotionally along with other aspects of the personality. This is not done by interpreting religion after the Alice in Wonderland fashion, believing seven impossible things before breakfast. If religion sometimes means dealing with the impossible, it is never *because* it is impossible. The great lawyer, Clarence Darrow, used to make annual trips to the Chicago Theological Seminary to discuss religion with the students. With his keen mind, he would nevertheless spend these sessions explaining why he did not believe in a religion that none of his hearers had believed in since their earliest childhood. An interpretation of religion which insists on remaining at a childhood level can only be rejected. There is no more point in "disbelieving" in a childish conception of God than there would be in disbelieving in what such concepts as "earth" or "art" meant to one as a child. There is no point in disbelieving in the existence of one's father merely because the early belief in the father's omnipotence has changed with the growth of the personality. Religious ideas and feelings must grow up.

Emotional interpretations of religion must be non-substantive. Religion, for example, which replaces the need for earthly friends by supplying heavenly friends may be more healthy than no religion at all, but it is still rather far down the scale. Religion brings something which nothing else can bring; it is not a substitute for something else. It is not even a substitute for relaxation, for work, for clear thinking, for making autonomous decisions, or for suffering. It is not an automatic solver of problems. In the basic sense it does aid in the solution of problems, but not as a substitute for hard work, clear thought or courageous decision. It strengthens the resources with which problems may be solved, though it may at times heighten the urgency of the problems.

Religion must be interpreted in a non-compulsive manner. There are some types of individual attitudes which are often incorrectly praised as fine religious outlooks. One of these is submissiveness, which is essentially a strategy of trying to get what we want by making the other fellow sorry for us. Mental hygiene has told us enough about the dangers of the model child to indicate where the danger lies. Power-getting through the institutions of religion is also sometimes, though not so frequently, mistaken for a sound religious outlook. There is the church worker who expresses his craving to lead or to boss only in church activities because there he does not expect to meet with the open rejection of his ambition which he would find elsewhere unless it were curbed by social interests.

More subtle than either of these compulsive ways in which religion may be used is trying to coerce others into loving us. Love and security are fundamental needs. The only proper way in which to get them is first to give them, as they are first given us in childhood. If the child is not given them, he will—indeed he must—try somehow to get them. Parents who have themselves been frustrated in receiving affection and basic psychological and spiritual security may not be able to receive spontaneous affection from their children because they cannot give it; and they may use coercive methods without any awareness of what they are doing. They may bribe, threaten, appeal to pity or to duty—and all of these techniques may be bound up with religion. Where religion is interpreted in this way, the soundest of Christian ideas will be badly warped. The compulsive element lies in the fact that, although the strategy is self-defeating, under the circumstances it seems impossible to do anything else. This is the spiritual vicious circle at work, and it scarcely makes for a healthy interpretation of religion.

Religion must be interpreted in an outgoing manner. It must have a social as well as a divine object. "Emotional atheists" are usually people who feel so defensive about themselves, who have so little real regard or affection for what they feel themselves to be, that they cannot possibly have regard or reverence for anything outside themselves. Love and regard (which are akin to reverence in the high Christian sense) are not quantities; and in their deepest respects are not to be compared with energy concepts. For one cannot love others (or God) more as he loves (or has regard for) himself less. Without some self-affirmation there can be little affirmation of others or of God which is not spurious.[6] Religion is sometimes interpreted in such highly individualistic terms that it has no real social reference. To call religion "what man does with his solitariness," as A. N. Whitehead does, is one thing which in a deep sense is true.[7] To say that religion has no social reference is quite another, as is the common attempt to separate a mythical "individual" from a "social" gospel. Religion will furnish no technical answers to questions of social organization, politics, and the like; but it will have reference to change in social organization as much as it will to the basic concerns for the status of others represented in all welfare movements. Religion must be interpreted in an outgoing manner.

There are other ways of approaching the standards by which healthy and unhealthy interpretations of religion may be judged. Those which are exploitative are unhealthy. Those which condemn the sinner as well as the sin are unhealthy; those which insist that the sinner is always more and greater than the sin are healthy. Those which are sentimental are unhealthy; as are those which are purely rationalistic or voluntaristic. Religion is not all idea, not all will. Those religions which make the personality equivalent to consciousness are unhealthy; those which see the whole personality as something both greater and deeper are not. Those which refuse to face the potentialities for evil in men as well as in man are unhealthy; but so are those which refuse to recognize the potentialities for creation and for good.

These criteria are not purely those of mental hygiene, nor yet of religion. They represent the infusion of mental hygiene discoveries into the pattern of critical Christian thinking. Without first accepting some basic Christian notions, it would be difficult to accept them all. It is beyond our scope to go much into their background; yet their character is sufficiently self-authenticating for us to recognize the validity of most of them even as they are stated. The fact that mental hygiene reinforces most of them indicates only the increased necessity for religion and mental hygiene to work co-operatively together.

It is useless, however, to consider the contributions which religion makes to health without this prior attention to the relative healthiness or unhealthiness of the interpretations of religion. Religious ideas themselves are important; and various criteria, including those of healthfulness or unhealthfulness, may be used to evaluate them. One idea is not as good as another. But there has rarely been any danger of forgetting that fact, while there is a constant danger of forgetting the importance of the emotional interpretation. Hence this introduction.

If we suppose that a person has a healthy emotional interpretation of religion, in what ways specifically does his religious life support and enhance the health of his whole personality? Though it is valuable to put our question in this way, we should not forget that none of us have "perfect" interpretations of religion. What we do is to share certain insights into the nature of reality and our relationship to it. We are speaking, then, as much of religious outlooks and practices that may be used for improving health as of simple examination of the influence of fine religious insights that are already present.

Religion can help us to integrate our lives around the reality in the universe which is both rational and meaningful—the only worshipful reality. We have already hinted that a lack of reverence or regard for what we mean when we say "God" is a kind of blocking of natural trends toward socialization, and that it is caused by a feeling of lack of psychological safety and security within ourselves, however unconscious this feeling may be. If a person is tied up in knots inside himself, will power will not get him out. But if religion can give him a vision of something in the universe that he can actually trust, whose counterpart is within him, he is on the road to finding himself. In such a person's background we usually find that he has not been able to trust—that his mother, for example, sometimes slapped him and sometimes gave him a stick of candy when he disobeyed instead of being consistent about his emotional education. How can such a person be other than tied up in knots? Of course he may take religion and tie it up inside himself along with everything else. But if he gets any vision of that meaningful reality which does protect and bring safety and security, it may help him so that he will look for the evidences of security and affection that exist all about him and even in himself.

In the second place, religion may help to get a person away from egocentricity, infantilism, and the avoidance of responsibility. We know today that most stages in the development of the emotional life are accompanied by more pain than we later remember. Once the transition is made—for example, from the gang period to adolescence—the rewards of growth and new responsibility normally outweigh the pains. But in some persons the pains are so great as to retard the progress, and in none of us is the process entirely smooth or complete. And it is so easy to relapse into infantilism or avoidance of responsibility about some things that are especially important. Here religion may enter. Suppose that one's particular infantilism is to ridicule the prevalence of great social needs, to feel at least that paying attention to them is none of one's own business. And suppose that such a person somehow gets a vision that the brotherhood of man is the other side of the coin of the fatherhood of God? His social conscience can no longer be so dull or so dulled.

If we had a text, it would be this story from Luke:[8] "When a foul spirit goes out of a man, it roams through deserts in search of rest, and when it finds none, it says, 'I will go back to my house that I left.' And it goes and finds it unoccupied, cleaned and in order. Then it goes and gets seven other spirits more wicked than itself, and they go in and live there, and in the end the man is worse off than he was before." The search for health cannot be merely negative. Mental hygiene cannot be merely a process of chasing out evil spirits. For if the devils are chased out and nothing constructive takes their place, the person may indeed be worse off than before. Never take away a man's crutch unless you can say, "Take up thy bed and walk." And religion can say this, metaphorically speaking. Healthy religion ought to furnish the constructive occupant of the house. The evil spirits must be driven out, to use the ancient language, but that is only half the story. Health in our usage is not merely negative—it is also positive; but it cannot be truly positive unless the perspective and the insights of religion are a part of it.

There are two ways to reach a goal. The first is by keeping one's eyes fixed on the goal and ignoring the obstacles. This should be known as the cracked-shin method. The other is by keeping one's eyes on the obstacles and failing to look at the goal. We may call this the wander-in-circles method. Neither is adequate in itself. The great contribution of mental hygiene to religion is the pointing out of the real nature of the obstacles; the great contribution of religion to mental hygiene is the vision of the goal.

Healthy religion makes a person less dependent upon mere cultural standards, upon keeping up unconsciously with the Joneses. We live in a culture in which a man's worth is too often judged by his skill in competition, and especially in economic competition. The spiritual danger arises at the point where a man has no other standard of judgment of his own worth than that which this cultural pattern, as one example, can give him. We know of the suicides that followed the beginnings of the depression in 1929. Though there were individual factors involved, we could see in the lives of such persons the confusion of their success in competition with their very selves. They had no concept of themselves except that which they accepted from their culture; hence they had no resources when the crisis came. We are not implying that personal worth should be independent of what one does, but that one should have standards in reaching an estimate of one's personal worth which go deeper than that of keeping up with the Joneses. If religion gives anything at all, it is this. What but this can give the magnificent courage to our brother religionists and others who are being persecuted in many lands? This is what we mean by the religious statement that every man is a child of God. There is something in the nature of the universe that in itself gives life meaning and value. We call recognition of this freedom, but it is not merely freedom of the will. We would do better to call it freedom of the whole personality.

We thought once that "human nature" was what we saw in people around us and in ourselves, that is, that our culture was the only possible expression of inherent "human nature." Those sciences which have contributed to mental hygiene, and in this case anthropology in particular, have shown us how false this is. Through the comparative study of different cultures, we have seen that inherent human nature is a great deal more flexible than anyone fully realized even a half-century ago.[9] Such conclusions suggest an additional reason why religion is not simply something to reinforce the prohibitions or commands laid upon the individual by the prevailing environment. Underlying assumptions become more necessary than ever. Science can make clear to us what the prevailing assumptions are, and that these are not the only possible ones; but only religion can furnish the kind of assumptions needed to transform the unsatisfactory elements in our own culture. Religion can speak of what life ought to be as well as pass judgment on what it is.

We know, too, that religion may actually have a marked influence upon the processes of healing. With mental and spiritual symptoms this scarcely needs proof. But there is also some evidence that religion has an influence upon bodily symptoms and processes.

Worship is a religious method that helps to develop healthy persons, though this is of course not the only aim of worship. Worship ought to and does mean many things; but prominent among them is the sense that an individual thereby becomes one of a community on the level of aspiration. He bows before that which he reverences, not so much to honor it as because it is natural to do so, and he thereby gets a sense of "communion" with all mankind. All high religions believe that this community is not artificial or merely sociological, but that it goes deep into the nature of reality. Worship is, then, a discovery in some measure of the reality of that community. It makes a great difference what one worships. We know now why the early Christians could not worship the symbols of the Roman Empire. For only in religions of the quality of Christianity and Judaism do we find a God who is truly worshipful. Worship itself is a natural activity of man, one of the motivating forces toward which is the desire for fellowship and communion; but it makes a great difference what one worships. For religion cannot be satisfied with reverence of that which is not worshipful, and cannot be interested merely in an integration of personality around ideals that are temporarily successful or efficient but that in the long run are destructive. The integration that brings real health must in the long run be one that corresponds with the nature of the highest reality of which we are aware.

Still another contribution that religion can make to health is in developing what has been called "tension capacity." Children want what they want when they want it. As adults we have to learn that the fulfilment of some needs or wishes must be postponed or even renounced. Thus we must learn to live in situations that would ordinarily produce tension without being tense. This is an inner achievement. No one else can do it for us. This emphasis on self-discipline (which does not mean bowing the head in defeat) rather than discipline from outside is an essential part of all healthy religion. Such religion can help us attain it.

Finally, religion appreciates and helps us to face what may be called the irreducible mystery of life. Fortunately life is not all a mystery; and religion performs a poor service to health if it tries, as has often been done, to create a mystery where none exists, or to seek allegiance by claiming a special hold on mystery. But when all that is said, much of life and experience is still a mystery. One may ignore or deny the mystery, which is blind. Or one may think only of the day when it may be past, which is romantic. Or one may work as the scientist does to make the mystery intelligible at specific points, which is praiseworthy, of course, so far as it goes. But some mystery still remains. Religion first of all faces this mystery as such. At its best, the mystery is never reverenced. We do not worship God because we have no idea of what He is. But the mystery is there.

In the ordinary experiences of life we know that problems must be faced as problems, not evaded or ignored. If one is to have health of spirit as well as of body and mind, one must apply the same principle in this cosmic realm. Emerson said of the great historian, Gibbon, "That man Gibbon had no shrine." A man with no consciousness of the mystery within his existence is ignoring or evading a problem. The proper attitude is, of course, not to magnify the mystery nor to worship it, but to face it as such. . . .

We have been able only to suggest some of the contributions which religion can and does make to health. We believe that these contributions are among the most significant, though not the only, functions of religion. In so far as religion helps persons to face realities, and especially realities which are actually or potentially evil, and provides strength or wisdom or courage to deal with them—it leads toward health as well as toward Christian character. Not all religion, not all Christianity, and not all interpretations of sound Christian ideas accomplish this; and one of our first steps in attempting to make the Christian contribution to mental health larger is to recognize this fact. Armed with some comprehension of what kinds of religious interpretations and practices tend to make for health and which do not, we are in a position to consider both the general and the specific contributions of religion to health.

Notes

1. Earl D. Bond, M.D., Quoted in "Aims," Commission on Religion and Health, Federal Council of Churches.
2. J. A. Hadfield, M.D., "The Psychology of Power" in *The Spirit,* ed. by B. H. Streeter, The Macmillan Co., 1919, p. 110. Quoted by George A. Buttrick in *Prayer,* Abingdon-Cokesbury, 1942, p. 50.
3. *Ibid.,* p. 51.
4. See for instance Charles T. Holman, *The Religion of a Healthy Mind,* N.Y., Round Table Press, 1940.
5. See Carroll A. Wise, *Religion in Illness and Health,* N.Y., Harper and Bros., 1942.
6. See Erich Fromm, "Selfishness and Self-Love," *Psychiatry,* November, 1939.
7. A. N. Whitehead, *Religion in the Making,* N.Y., The Macmillan Co., 1926.
8. Luke 11:24-26.
9. See for example Ruth Benedict, *Patterns of Culture,* Boston, Houghton Mifflin Co., 1934.

90.
Equus—A Psychiatrist Questions His Priestly Powers

MORRIS BERNARD KAPLAN

One of the current Broadway phenomena is the startling success of a play concerned with issues more commonly debated at conferences on the ethical and social implications of psychiatry. The play in this instance is *Equus,* by British playwright Peter Shaffer. The issues about which it provokes reflection include the adequacy of the medical model, the values implicit in concepts of normality and mental health, the use of therapy to deal with socially deviant behavior, and the possibility of a human need to transcend the limits of secular rationality.

Equus is a powerful theatrical presentation of the personal and professional crisis of Martin Dysart, a psychiatrist in a provincial British hospital: accomplished in his profession, unhappy in his marriage, fascinated by the passions that animated ancient Greece. Alan Strang is a seventeen-year-old printer's son. Estranged from family and society, unskilled and without much prospect of any accomplishment in the world, he has deliberately blinded six horses in the stables where he works weekends. Brought to Dysart for treatment in place of a long prison sentence, Strang becomes the focus for the psychiatrist's searching of himself which moves from an acknowledgment of "professional menopause" to a fundamental questioning of the doctor's role in his encounter with the patient.

The major conflict of the play is not that between doctor and boy, but within the consciousness of the doctor. Dysart's articulate and literate monologues alternate with dramatic re-enactments of the therapeutic sessions and the boy's own history. The setting is a spare square space encircled by the audience. It is at once an operating theater and a boxing ring, doctor's office and the arena of his struggle with himself.

Alan Strang is a boy possessed. The frenzied outburst in which he blinded the horses is a departure from years of quiet desolation and secret nursing of a private passion, an obsession with horses that rises to a quasi-religious service of the indwelling equine god-slave "Equus." It is a self-abasing devotion, forged from a deep confusion of thwarted psychosexual energy

From *The Hastings Center Report* 5 (February 1975): 9-10. Used by permission of the publisher and the author.

and images of Christian suffering. Working in a stable, riding out secretly one night every three weeks for orgiastic communion with his private god, Alan appears to Martin Dysart the embodiment of his own intellectual preoccupation with pagan worship:

> "Oh the primitive world," I say. "What instinctual truths were lost with it." And while I sit there, baiting a poor unimaginative woman [Dysart's wife] with the word, that freaky boy tries to conjure the reality. I sit looking at pages of centaurs trampling the soil of Argos—and outside my window he is trying to *become one* in a Hampshire field!

Dysart feels himself lost—he admires a world animated by the worship of dark, departed gods, and he finds meager the secular norms which have taken their place. In his own dreams the doctor sees himself as a priest: not the benevolent listener of the Christian confessional, but the pagan practitioner of human sacrifice.

The Limits of Psychiatry

Yet the criminal act that brought the boy to the law and to Dysart, the blinding of the horses, Alan had done in furious revolt against his god's hold on him. He is in pain. Adjustment to the workaday world promises the boy escape from his pain; yet such adjustment, Dysart suspects, brings with it a shrinking of human possibilities, a loss of worship and mystery:

> The normal is the good smile in a child's eyes—all right. It is also the dead stare in a million adults. It both sustains and kills—like a God. It is the Ordinary made beautiful; it is also the average made lethal. The Normal is the indispensable, murderous God of Health, and I am his Priest. My tools are very delicate. My compassion is honest. I have honestly assisted children in this room. I have talked away terrors and relieved many agonies. But also—beyond question—I have cut from them parts of individuality repugnant to the God in both his aspects. Parts sacred to rarer and more wonderful gods.

The spirit of Equus addresses Dysart: "Why me? Account for me!" and the psychiatrist cannot answer. He senses that his science may trace the source of the boy's disturbance; it may be able to undo his deviant attachment; but it can neither explain nor replace the power and passion which Equus calls forth. For Dysart, the boy's obsession, painful and disturbing as it is, becomes a challenge to his own belief in the power of his science and the social norms which it serves. What then is Dysart's responsibility—"not socially, not clinically, but fundamentally?"

Three other characters offer competing interpretations of the boy's predicament and the treatment he is owed. Alan's devout mother sees in her son's act the hand of the Devil, a view which converges with the doctor's belief that psychiatric explanations cannot finally account for the boy, but which also bespeaks a Christian theology which Dysart rejects. The owner of the stables sticks with the criminal model, unvarnished, unqualified: "In my opinion the boy should be in prison, not in a hospital at the taxpayer's expense." The compassionate woman magistrate who has in fact kept Alan out of prison and brought him to Dysart insists on the hard reality of the boy's suffering, "He's been in pain for most of his life. . . . And you can take it away. . . . That simply has to be enough for you, surely?"

Neither Dysart nor the play follows the leads offered by the mother or the stable owner, but Dysart does accept the magistrate's reminder that there are priorities—"Children before grown-ups, things like that." Finally, uncertainly, Dysart submerges his own doubts and yearnings and undertakes to relieve the boy of his pain. And yet the doctor's own questions are not resolved but intensified by the play's end. He denies the adequacy of his science to explain life, and of society's norms to guide it:

> Essentially I cannot know what I do—yet I do essential things. Irreversible, terminal things. I stand in the dark with a pick in my hand, striking at heads. . . . I need—more desperately than my children need me—a way of seeing in the dark. What way is this? . . . *What dark is this?* . . . I cannot call it ordained of God. I can't get that far.

The Need for Transcendence

Some critics have seen in *Equus* the romanticizing of madness identified with the work of R. D. Laing and other "anti-psychiatrists." Martin Dysart is certainly tempted by such a view. ("At least he has galloped. I have not.") But his friend the magistrate condemns this as self-indulgence, insisting on the superior importance of "your thoughts, your ways of connecting with people." Dysart's action in following through with his cure of the boy repudiates the theory that sees psychosis as access to a higher Truth. Nevertheless, the play does invite reexamination of our ordinary notions of normality and mental illness. In the play's opening speech, Dysart comments, "In a way, it has nothing to do with this boy. The doubts have been there for years, piling up steadily in this dreary place. It is only the extremity of this case that's made them active." Dysart's dissatisfaction with the normal and routine and his fascination with Alan Strang's bizarre worship reflect a deeper malaise which may be shared by the audiences which have so enthusiastically received the play.

The comforts which modern technology and social organization make possible have been perceived by many modern thinkers as exacting a considerable cost. Both secular instrumental rationality and conventional modes of social behavior have been seen as diminishing the range of human possibility, as denying a deep need for transcendence. Blake sought liberation from the "mind-forged manacles" of the spirit; Nietzsche denounced the triumph of "the last men, who make everything small." In our own day, this concern has found expression both in widespread experimentation with physical, psychological, and spiritual techniques of altering ordinary experience and in a revival of religious movements including traditional Eastern faiths, primitive forms of Christianity, diverse messianisms, even astrology, witchcraft, and satanism.

There are plausible social and psychological explanations of this apparent spiritual hunger. Surely the failure of community and the breakdown of traditional institutions of authority are important factors. But an interpretation based on the appearances themselves may be the most adequate. Martin Heidegger has called ours a time of need: the old gods have died, and the new have not yet appeared. The need to orient one's self in relation to a transcendent source of meaning and value may be an irreducible aspect of the human condition.

Legitimation Despite Ambiguity

The absence of such orientation and the very denial of the need may be definitive of the culture of modernity. In relation to civilization and its discontents, psychiatry plays an ambiguous role. On the one hand, it recognizes the importance of nonrational factors like feelings, fantasies, and dreams in shaping human life, and has explored the implications of ancient myth and ritual for understanding the human psyche. On the other, it aspires to the status of science, has allied itself with medicine, and can function as an instrument of adjustment to conventional norms. These tensions provide the central problematic of Shaffer's *Equus*.

Psychiatrists have already gone on record criticizing the play's lack of realism in portraying their art and have even analyzed the fantasies about therapy and therapists they see the play as promoting. No doubt the public portrayal of a very private and complex relationship raises many conflicting responses among patients and professionals alike. The verisimilitude of Dysart's techniques is less important than the fact that they are presented as working only because the boy trusts him and wants to be helped. Alan resists Dysart's stratagems, yet his desire to escape his entrapment is a premise of the play.

But to focus on realism and technique only is to overlook the play's embodiment in symbolic form of more general conflicts and ideas. Perhaps the play's most moving moment occurs after the boy has reenacted the violent scene in the stable, when the doctor gathers up in his arms the terrified, exhausted child, and carries him to rest. Psychiatry may be caught in the conflicting currents of our time of need, but finally its practice requires no legitimation beyond the suffering of the patient and the capacity of the doctor to help.

91. Bioethical Issues in Behavior Control

WAYNE E. OATES

Immanuel Kant said that "the universal law of right may be expressed thus: 'Act externally in such a manner that the free exercise of your will may be able to coexist with the freedom of all others, according to a universal law.' Ethics imposes upon me the obligation to make the fulfillment of right a *maxim* of my conduct."[1] The application of "the universal law of right" to the differential diagnoses of biomedical decision making involves a molecular, interacting field of persons. Their freedom has to coexist with each other in order that right may be exercised. The purposes of this article are as follows: (1) To identify the specific tools of behavior control now in use in the fields of psychology and psychiatry, (2) to clarify and state some major ethical issues involved in the use of these tools insofar as the inherent ambiguity of human life will permit, (3) to relate these tools and issues to our knowledge of God as we have been enabled to know God in Jesus Christ.

What Is Behavior Control?

Behavior control refers to the personal or technological power to intervene in the functions of another person. The emotional functions of the other person, the behavioral patterns of another person, and even the belief patterns of another person are interfered with in such ways as to cause that person to conform to the prechosen emotions, behaviors, and beliefs of the person or persons doing the intervening. In short, behavior control refers to the use of psychological and/or psychiatric technology to alter the thought and behavior of individuals.[2] Earlier the issues concerning behavior control, concerned with the involuntary and indeterminate commitment of mentally ill patients, were the focus of the issues of human rights. This concern still exists. More recently, a new climate of concern has arisen over the powers of psychologists and psychiatrists (to say nothing of the media and advertisement industries) to shape behavior. However, we grope with the fear that technologists of behavior control will exercise their will freely without regard to the freedom of persons whom they treat. Thus patients will be subtly or forthrightly deprived of their human freedom.

Wayne E. Oates, "Bioethical Issues in Behavior Control," pp. 32-49 from *A Matter of Life and Death: Christian Perspectives,* edited by Harry Hollis (Nashville: Broadman Press, 1977).

The Technologies of Behavior Control

The specific technologies of behavior control can be identified and described as follows:

Milieu Therapy

Milieu therapy is the scientific programming of the environment of the hospital situation. The objective is to change the personality of the patient. Schedules of activities such as picnics, buffet suppers, dances, and card games, et cetera, are arrayed around other treatment modalities such as drug therapy, shock therapy, and individual psychotherapy. Critical issues arise in this kind of therapy. It can become an unreal environment so different from the demands of the patient's workaday world that the patient is prone to stay in treatment indefinitely. The contemporary support of patients with insurance aids and abets this by taking the edge off the financial motive for getting back into the nonhospital world. The ethical issue of the weight of the cost of this kind of treatment on the rest of the family is a second issue. Milieu treatment can be a means for doctors paying less personal attention to the patient. Staff indecision about the treatment plans while physicians spend considerable amounts of time in private psychotherapy with nonhospitalized patients is probably the most critical issue. As one patient put it, "I spend all of my week with people who are least responsible for and equipped to treat me. I rarely get to see the person who makes the decision as to whether I am to be kept in the hospital or discharged."

Individual Psychotherapy

The individual psychotherapist depends upon the conversational relationship between the patient and himself. He employs devices and strategies which meet the person at his own level "for the explicit intent of reaching mutual understanding through the process of insightful learning. The therapist may, at times, focus on removing symptoms, but not as an end in itself. He may employ ventilation, reeducation, clarification, interpretation, modeling, and many other modalities for the purpose of alleviating an undue degree of suffering, such as, feelings of alienation, rejection, sadness, guilt, aggression and sexual unrest."[3]

The critical issues involved in individual psychotherapy are the length of the treatment process, the emotional exploitation of the client for sexual or power purposes, the expense for the treatment in terms of the actual removal of the symptoms which bring the patient into treatment, and the way in which the more or less rational approaches to the problems may substitute talk for action. The heavy criticisms of these issues have been most responsibly stated by William Glasser in his book, *Reality Therapy.*[4]

Group Psychotherapy

The central hypothesis of group psychotherapy is that the isolation, brokenness, and behavioral deviance of a given individual have sprung from his/her relationship to significant groups. Therefore, if the person's behavior and values are to be changed, the group itself is the medium of control. Leadership style has much to do with the ethical quality of the group life. A leader may range all the way from a dictatorial personality upon whom the group members depend and by whom they are subjected to forced indoctrination to a completely laissez-faire leader who insists that all issues be dealt with and resolved by the group. Critical issues arise (1) as to the relationship of the group to other groups and to the larger milieu, (2) as to the right of a member of the group to discuss matters with persons whose lives are affected who are not members of the group, such as a spouse or a parent, (3) as to the degree to which the use of groups becomes an easy answer to the shortage of personnel in the institution where group therapy is the method of choice. Probably, however, the most critical issue is whether the leader is a competent and experienced person, which is the criterion of selecting group leaders.

Drug Therapy

Probably the most widely used technology for behavior control today is psychotropic drugs. The galaxy of different drugs is overwhelming to the lay person. A classification of drugs and their uses in behavior control can be briefly presented here.

Maintenance control drugs are used in rather commonly known instances. For example, in epilepsy dilantin and phenobarbital are used on a regular, maintenance basis. In diabetes, insulin is a maintenance medication of choice. In withdrawn, senile persons, as well as hyperkinetic children, Ritalin (Methylphenidate hydrochloride) is used. Minor tranquilizers such as Librium (Chlordiazepoxide) or Valium (Diazepam) are used in controlling muscle spasms, controlling hysteria in acute grief reactions, and in enabling highly compulsive people to work more effectively.

Antidepressants are also commonly used. Mood changing drugs are administered on several hypotheses, one of which is that catecholamines (epinephrine, noreprenephrine, and dopamine) are deficient in supply and therefore disrelate the neurotransmitters to each other causing depression. The introduction of such drugs as Tofranil (imipramine), Elavil (amitriptyline), and other closely related compounds, allowed physicians to estimate that 32 to 80 percent improvement occurs depending upon the criterion for diagnosis and improvement.

A longer term, more nearly maintenance kind of medication for persons suffering from bipolar or manic-depressive illness is lithium carbonate. I have seen at least two patients hitherto nonfunctional able to work and be remarkably creative as long as they "stayed on" lithium. The chemical formula and hypotheses of this medication are different from the MAO inhibitors.

Phenothiazine derivatives, over two dozen in number, are used to treat schizophrenic disorders, reducing thought disorders, loss of self-care motivation, and paranoid symptoms. The "workhorse" medication is chlorpromazine (Thorazine). As in the case of lithium as a long-term maintenance drug, prolixim has similar effects for schizophrenics. The present issue of treatment seems to revolve around the low-dosage-high-dosage concepts. Some of those who have the facilities to keep a patient in longer term psychotherapy and to maintain extensive milieu therapy tend to rely upon low-dosage approaches. Some of those who have limited facilities and less affluent patients tend to move toward high dosage treatment. In fact some studies indicate that as one moves higher up the social ladder, the treatment of choice tends to rely less and less upon medication therapy and more upon milieu therapy and psychotherapy.[5] One critical ethical issue rests at the point of the ways in which more rapid and intensive forms of therapy are provided for the poor against the more leisure expensive forms of treatment for the affluent. To what extent do private hospitals *need* the affluent patient more than the patient needs them?

Aversion Therapy

Aversion therapy is the attempt to change and/or control undesirable behavior by presenting an exceptionally unpleasant stimulation in conjunction with or as a result of the behavior. For example antabuse is an aversive treatment for alcoholism. If the person is on antabuse, and if that person ingests alcohol, then the person becomes nauseated, vomits, has throbbing headaches, has a fall in blood pressure, and develops labored breathing and blurred vision. Sexual deviants may be treated in another aversive form of therapy. Pornographic pictures may be presented and an electric impulse presented at the same time as a shock device. The temporary results of such treatment are the most outstanding characteristic, in my opinion.

Electroconvulsive Therapy

Electroconvulsive therapy, commonly known as "shock therapy," has been in use since the early 1940s. Originally thought to be a counteragent for schizophrenic behavior, it is now largely focused on the treatment of depressive patients. Hamilton and others place ECT above drug therapy for depression, but considerable numbers of clinicians feel that drug therapy is the treatment of choice. I work in two psychiatric facilities. In Louisville General Hospital, shock therapy is not used at all. In the Norton Psychiatric Clinic, a private hospital, it is used only occasionally. In the early years of the use of ECT, it was almost a panacea, because little else was available at the somatic level of treatment except custodial care and such things as hydrotherapy. Rather than being a panacea, it was probably a form of desperation.

Psychosurgery

With the advent of the psychotropic drugs, psychosurgery went into a decline. We are experiencing a resurgence of the art now because of the refining of the procedures, the claimed successes with the drug addicts, homosexuals, patients with intolerable pain, severe obsessional neurotic behavior, and other conditions. The common feature of all psychosurgical inventions is reduction of response to unpleasant stimuli. It does not remove the symptoms but reduces the responses to the symptoms. A patient hearing voices may continue to do so, but pays less attention to them.[6] Psychosurgery is done, not by psychiatrists, but by neurosurgeons. The psychiatrists select the patients, however. It is a *last* treatment, after all other methods have been used. Therefore, it is impossible to compare and contrast it effectively with other forms of treatment.

Electronic Stimulation of the Brain

A technique of behavior control has been developed in which tiny electric drills are used to bore holes in the skull. Then electrical conductors are placed at strategic locations in the brain with the objective of inducing the thought, feeling, or behavior associated with that section of the brain. A clinic has been established in Boston to treat patients who have uncontrollable rage periods. The important issue to consider here ethically is that the rage may be evoked or terminated, as determined by the physician.

Stereotaxic psychosurgery is a form of treatment used at the fringes of psychiatric and psychological practice to control behavior. It consists of placing the patient's head in a firm and stable position, drilling a hole in the skull from a specific angle indicated by the knowledge of the neurosurgeon about the function and location of specific areas of the brain. A knife or an electrode may be used to accomplish the results intended. The most used and reliable results of this surgery have been with parkinsonism in operations on the thalamus of the patient. Dramatic relief of symptoms has been achieved. However, more recent uses of this kind of surgery have been aimed at the alteration of certain parts of the brain to control violent, aggressive behavior. Also, homosexuals have allegedly been turned straight by surgical changes in what is known as Cajal's nucleus in the brain, the section supposedly governing the sexual behavior of persons.

Two Japanese neurosurgeons initiated stereotaxic surgery in 1951. Their initial efforts were to devise surgical procedures to correct temporal lobe epilepsy. Then it was extended to include patients with combined electroencephalogram abnormalities and marked behavior disturbances. These doctors were Hirataro Narabayashi and Y. Uchimura. The cases cited by them were all accompanied by neurological pathology such as mental retardation, extreme lack of control of aggressive behavior, and post-encephalitic behavior. None of these cases were used to demonstrate that criminal or deviant behavior without concomitant neurological abnormalities were the targets of such surgery.[7] Valenstein in commenting upon such operations as a deterrent to aggressive behavior and/or undesirable sexual behavior says: "The changes that can follow . . . can be very unpredictable and far reaching. Characterizing the total effects of these operations by such phrases as 'taming' and 'hypersexuality' can be very misleading . . . different and opposite behavior changes can be expressed under other circumstances."[8]

Anectine Therapy

Anectine (Succynlcholine Chloride) is a powerful muscle relaxant used in anesthesia and as an adjunct to administering electroconvulsive therapy. Apparently a patient remains conscious throughout the time of the drug's effects, but the main effect is immobilized skeletal musculature. During the entire time the patient receives supplemental oxygen, he is conscious and can comprehend what is going on around him. The patient is "counseled while he is under the drug." This drug has been used in one experiment at least at the Vacaville, California facility for treating sociopathic offenders against the law as well as at a state hospital and a prison for women in California. They are persons who had attacked others, been extremely self-destructive, and were generally extremely angry persons. Under the influence of the drug they were counseled to realize how dangerous their behavior was to themselves and others and to learn to be as free of the impulse to violence as they were while under the influence of anectine. The anectine treatment is a combination of hypnosis, operant conditioning, classical conditioning, and even punitive treatment. It has been discontinued in California treatment facilities because it does not accomplish anything that forms of behavioral modification can accomplish without chemical intervention.

Behavior Modification

Most of the previously mentioned forms of behavior control have been the province of psychiatrists. The contribution of psychologists to behavior control has been through various forms of behavior modification and/or behavioral therapy. Such treatment modalities may be either of a classical conditioning variety or of an operant conditioning variety. Classical conditioning is "respondent" or Type S conditioning. In it a person responds positively or negatively to a given stimulus. When that stimulus is repeated, then the person responds similarly. "Extinguishing" an undesirable trait may consist of "flooding" the patient with stimuli such as a thing he may fear until the fear is extinguished; or, it may consist of intermittently presenting the patient with the stimulus.

The other kind of behavioral therapy is operant conditioning, which works on behavior that is strengthened or weakened by its consequences rather than its antecedents. B. F. Skinner refers to the Christian teachings concerning heaven and hell as subsequent consequences to behavior. "The power achieved by the religious agency depends upon how effectively certain verbal reinforcements are conditioned—in particular the promise of heaven and the threat of hell."[9]

In hospitals a "token economy" is developed in which persons are rewarded or deprived of things they want in proportion to the way they accomplish the simpler tasks of socialization, such as arising at a certain time, bathing themselves, attending and participating in certain activities, et cetera. Tokens or script can be used to buy things for themselves, to admit them to movies, et cetera.

Several therapeutic and ethical concerns have been raised by the American Psychiatric Association concerning behavioral therapy. (1) The inadequate and partial training of many persons doing the therapy is likely to reduce the therapy to techniques without broader understanding. (2) The lack of supervisors with clinical experience may cause the therapist to overlook or ignore personal relationships to the patient and fail to provide the patient with support, guidance, advice, encouragement, reassurance, and clarification. (3) The possibility that sociopolitical and ethnic behaviors will become the target of treatment as a latent form of social control or forced indoctrination. (4) The ethical problem of coercive manipulation is another form of the third threat. (5) The possibility that the programs will become nontherapeutic ways of punishing behavior and rationalizing sadistic behavior. These are legitimate ethical concerns. Any one of them could be true of psychiatric methods of therapy such as shock therapy, drug therapy or lobotomies. Any one of them can be applied to pastoral counseling, use of the Bible, prayer, and church participation. The hand and motive of the user shape the efficacy of any form of treatment.[10]

Critical Issues of Human Rights

After such a labyrinthine survey of technologies of behavior control, we need to face the critical issues in human freedom and dignity involved in the use of these methods in controlling human behavior.

1. The Issue of Survival. Psychiatrists and psychologists and other specialists working in the treatment settings are concerned with minimal function for effective survival. B. F. Skinner defines values this way: "Things are good (positively reinforcing) or bad (negatively reinforcing) presumably because of the contingencies of survival under which the species evolved."[11] Survival is a powerful motive for behavior. A young person working in a Louisville Boatworks finds after two years that there must be some better way to make a living and decides to go to college. This is an everyday, normal example of what Skinner means. However, the clinician psychiatrist, psychologist, and clinically expert minister are concerned with such elemental survival as a person being willing to eat, as in the case of the mental patient who is starving himself to death (anorexia nervosa). We are interested in patients being able to tell what time of day it is, where they are, and what their names are. We are interested in their being clothed and in their right minds. We are interested in their being able to feed themselves, shelter themselves, and to pay for these things through having been gainfully employed.

The measures of behavior control that I have previously described here have these minimal goals in mind. The issues of values at this point of survival are minimal. However, when these technologies are applied to more complex values, such as the appropriate response to injustice, the nature of one's political behavior and one's religious beliefs, the peril increases.

When a staff is concerned with whether the patient is going to kill himself or someone else if discharged, then the goals of behavior control are much more concrete, circumscribed, and desperate. Persons who have never struggled with these issues of survival with patients can afford the luxury of being abstract and debonair about the rights of persons. But the clinician needs to lift his head up from such problems long enough to ask some more philosophical and ethical questions.

A case in point: an upper middle-class woman comes to the emergency psychiatric center of a hospital. She is saturated internally with alcohol and permeates the air with the smell of it. She is medically on the verge of delirium tremens. She has no adult relatives in the city; only a daughter who is a minor. She has had an automobile accident in the last twelve hours with only property damage. She will not voluntarily be admitted to the hospital. The staff uses its legal authority to hold her for forty-eight hours against her will. She is placed in the acute room and given Valium intramuscularly to offset delirium tremens. She is prevented from killing herself or someone else or both in an auto accident until her adult relatives can come and take responsibility for her. We require her to act externally in such a manner that her exercise of her will will coexist with the freedom of others to live and do well, too.

However, if we were to use the power to control her life in such a way as to determine her political, religious, and economic beliefs, her capacity to use what autonomy of judgment she does have, then, as Philip Roos says, "the ethical question can be raised as to what degree and under what conditions is the shaping of social behavior to be sanctioned?"[12] Similarly, the use of religious sanctions outside a hospital setting to overcontrol the behavior of persons was questioned early by Freud. He accused families of having conditioned children to fit into the parents' programs when they were too young to defend themselves. Such could be exemplified in the provision of hamburgers and money given to children who are bused by churches who aspire to be the world's largest church. The same ethical conditions prevail.

Where we as Christians would challenge the behavior modification theorists is exactly at the point that they become theorists. The issue is *the selection of goals* for the conditioning. What are the goals and what was the due process in the selection of the goals? It is one thing to prevent a person from driving a car when on the verge of delirium tremens. It is another to administer Valium if she has objections on the grounds that she is a Christian Scientist. This is seen by Bruce J. Ennis, a lawyer, as an unnecessary concomitant of hospitalization.[13] Furthermore, we had to have data beyond a reasonable doubt that she was indeed dangerous to the lives of the children on her street. We had the eyewitness account of three neighbors as well as the account of her minor daughter.

What, therefore, are the goals of behavior control and who selects them? What are the values of those doing the selecting? In the name of scientific objectivity, some behavioral therapists will plead that they are neutral and have no values. One feels they protest too much. Charlotte Buhler, a therapist herself, says that "knowingly or unknowingly the therapist conveys something to the patient about values." Carrera and Adams say that "operant conditioning with children lends itself to the endorsement of what the parents want, without formal or ritualized appeal to any canons regarding the child's best interests."[14]

2. The Issue of the Patient's Best Interest. In the article by Carrera and Adams just quoted, a basic ethical issue is made of "the patient's best interests" in any kind of behavior control measure. In the Helsinki Declaration of the World Health Organization, special stress is laid upon the precariousness of the use of any means that weakens the physical or mental resistance of a person. They expect the physician to use only those means that are in "the best interest of the patient himself/herself."[15] In explaining this further, Seymour Halleck, M.D., insists that the patient's best interest consists in (1) *never* deceiving the patient, (2) taking care that overdiagnosis of dangerousness of the patient to himself and others is not done, (3) and of asking for a board of consultants in such cases as the prolonged use of tranquilizers, the use of irreversible procedures such as lobotomies, and the decision for long-term psychiatric hospitalization.

I personally would add that cases in which patients have been under treatment for more than six months be reviewed by a group of outside peers to see what the diagnosis is, what the treatment has been, and what the treatment plan is. Champus Insurance Company gives a foretaste of governmental monitoring of pastoral counseling and psychiatric treatment. The first eight interviews, a written diagnosis, plan of treatment, and prognosis are required. Beyond twenty interviews, a peer review organization report is required.

The iatronic disasters that occur in long-term psychiatric treatment become knowledge too often by accident and not plan. I myself have seen patients who have been in treatment for as many as twelve years, in one instance, and twenty-two in another. I am confident that the psychiatrist today has often become a sort of lifelong private chaplain of a secular nature to wealthy families. Much good has been done by these persons; however, descriptions of this treatment rarely appear in the literature. Nor is it held up to the light by day in answerability of one physician to his or her peers. The question one raises here ethically and practically is: "To what extent do such families need such care and to what extent does the psychiatrist need such patients?" Also, the same question could be raised about the pastoral care of such families.[16]

3. The Patient's Threat of Legal Action. The patients treated by psychologists and psychiatrists would not be candidates for such treatment if they were thoroughly rational persons. The dilemma arises when we insist that the ethical responsibility of the physician is to help the patient make a rational choice as to the desirability of the treatment. A reverse backlash has occurred at the clinical level of decision making about treatment as a result of the cancellation of malpractice insurance policies, the elevation of costs of such insurance, and so on.

Exceptional amounts of publicity have been given to professions who have a tradition of privacy—no advertisement for patients, and no public utterances that can be avoided. For example, a family member of a patient called me recently and asked that I see her daughter, a twenty-four-year-old woman. She said that she had seen five psychiatrists, and they all refused to treat her daughter. I asked her to tell me something of what she, the mother, felt was wrong with her daughter. She said that her daughter kept threatening suicide. I asked her if she felt her daughter needed around-the-clock attention to prevent this from happening. She said that she did and that she was worn out from doing so. I told her that I work as a professor in a department of psychiatry and that I would be legally culpable if I took her daughter as a counselee unless she was willing to go into a hospital.

The mother then said: "I don't think she ought to be in a hospital, and I refuse to see that happen." I then gently referred her to another pastoral counselor who is *not* a member of a department of psychiatry. The critical issue here is that of *defensive medicine.* Physicians and those associated with them are refusing to take the risks involved in many treatment situations because *they* do not have the right to use their own judgment in treatment situations.

There is another side to this, however, in that culture has become psychiatrized to such an extent that conditions that were previously assimilated in communities are now diagnosed as psychotic conditions. In reverse, too, behaviors that were previously considered abnormal, such as deviant sexual practices, are now considered alternative life-styles. For example, a patient in one hospital discovered for himself that the thing that kept him in the hospital was his insistence that he regularly experienced mystical visions of the "light of God" guiding his actions. No adverse social effects were associated with these visions hindering the freedom of others. Yet, when asked, he obediently told his physician that he had these visions, until one day he discovered that this was his own private business. Then he ceased to tell the doctor. Much to his surprise he was dismissed within five days after he ceased to tell his physician about his visions of God. The problem of informing the physician is the obverse side of the physician informing the patient!

4. The Patient's Right to Privacy. The reference to the patient's discovery that his eccentric patterns of thinking were his own private business raises a basic ethical issue being debated among psychotherapists of the existential tradition as over against the behavioral therapists of the Skinnerian tradition: Does a human being have a private self, or is a human being the sum total of his "external" behaviors, to paraphrase Kant. Kant spoke often of the "privatus intellectus" which characterizes the human person. Skinner rejects this idea as he says: "It is tempting to attribute the visible behavior to another organism inside—to a little man or homunculus. The wishes of the little man become the acts of the man observed by his fellows. The inner idea is put into words." Concepts such as the "soul" and "the self" are ways of describing the "little man" or the "homunculus."[17]

When we view this debate between Skinner and Carl Rogers, we are likely to be drawn into the great battle as to whether man is a living soul. I believe that man is, not has, a soul. In the Hebrew tradition I believe that this involves mankind's total, unified being with integrity. That is not the issue, here, however. The issue in terms of a person's freedom is: Does a person have a right to his or her own private thoughts? The patient described above discovered that his own private relationship to God was his own private business! We cannot effectively discuss the ethics of the invasion of a person's privacy through behavioral control methods described in this paper until we come to the conclusion that the patient *has* privacy by the nature of his or her own thought process. I have not seen this issue discussed in the literature on the ethics of behavior control.

5. Minimal versus Maximum Goals for Human Behavior. Another critical issue in the ethics of behavior control concerns the quality or extent of goals for the human person. In treatment situations, the goals are minimal and have been stated as the survival of the person as one who is able to behave in such a way that he or she is able to survive at a minimum in terms of eating, sleeping, housing, clothing for himself, and working to such an extent that these needs are

met without undue dependency on others. However, these are least-common-denominator goals for human existence, albeit they are prerequisite to any others. The Christian faith subordinates these minimal needs to a supreme, maximal goal. That goal is placing the survival of our neighbor above that of ourselves, that is loving one's neighbor as oneself (a Jewish ideal) and even more, loving one another as Christ loved us and gave himself for us.

The maximum goal of psychotherapy at its best is, as Harry Stack Sullivan put it, to enable a person to the kind of maturity in which he or she can love another person as much as, or almost as much as, oneself. When we read this, we think that this person is not far from the kingdom of God. As I have experienced psychiatrists, psychotherapists, and behavioral therapists in the setting in which I work, I find a quiet, nondenominational commitment to this higher goal for therapy. As a Christian, I would explicitly say that an even higher expectation of self-sacrificing love over and above simply providing freedom in coexistence, according to Kant, is the summum bonum of goal selection for behavior modification, even for churches themselves.

6. The Restoration of Creation. Some of the somatic therapies which have been described in this paper can specifically be seen as restoring the organism of a person to the original purpose of its creation. For example, the diabetic, with insulin supplementation wisely administered and conscientiously taken, can live a normal life. The question is being raised as to whether some of the symptoms of chronic depression and mania may not be in this same way treated. If a given psychotropic drug is a specific and demonstrable supplement to the body chemistry, then is this a restoration of the creation as it was originally intended to work?

When we ask such questions, the answer is yet a mystery. We have been formed in the secret wisdom of God whose eyes beheld our unformed substance when as yet there was none of them. Such knowledge is too wonderful for us. Yet, we have been given the technology to search after the knowledge of the true state of our own being.

As we see the mysteries of the human organism being revealed to us, we can say: "O God, these are your thoughts we are thinking after you!" Or, we have other more self-centered options. God grant that we will know that knowledge is surpassed by self-sacrificing therapeutic wisdom and our best humanity lies beyond our own survival.

Notes

1. Immanuel Kant, *The Science of Right.* Great Books Series, vol. 49, p. 398.

2. "Conditioning and Other Technologies Used to 'Treat?' 'Rehabilitate?' 'Demolish?' Prisoners and Mental Patients," *Southern California Law Review* (1972) 45:616–684.

3. Frank Carrera, III, M.D., and Paul L. Adams, M.D., "An Ethical Perspective on Operant Conditioning," *Journal of American Academy of Child Psychiatry,* vol. 9 (October, 1970), no. 4, p. 609.

4. William Glasser, *Reality Therapy* (New York: Harper & Row, 1965).

5. Jerome K. Myers and Lee L. Bean, *A Decade Later: A Follow-Up of Social Class and Mental Illness* (New York: John Wiley, 1968), pp. 97–98.

6. Freedman, Kaplan, and Sadock, *Comprehensive Psychiatry II.* Second Edition (Baltimore: William Wilkins), vol. 2, p. 1982.

7. Eliot S. Valenstein, *Brain Control: A Critical Examination of Brain Stimulation and Psychosurgery* (New York: John Wiley, 1973), pp. 210 ff..

8. Ibid., p. 142.

9. B. F. Skinner, *Science and Human Behavior* (New York: Free Press, 1953), p. 353.

10. The American Psychiatric Association, *Task Force Report on Behavior Therapy in Psychiatry* (New York: Jason Aaronson, 1974), pp. 97–105.

11. B. F. Skinner, *Beyond Freedom and Dignity* (New York: A. A. Knopf, 1971), p. 104.

12. Philip Roos, "Human Rights and Behavior Modification," *Mental Retardation,* vol. 12, no. 3 (June 1974), pp. 3–6.

13. Bruce J. Ennis, "Civil Liberties and Mental Illness," *Criminal Law Bulletin,* vol. 7, no. 2 (1971), pp. 101–127.

14. Frank Carrera and Paul Adams, "An Ethical Perspective on Operant Conditioning," *Journal of the American Academy of Child Psychiatry,* vol. 9, no. 4 (October 1970), pp. 607–623. Buhler quoted here also.

15. World Medical Association, 1964, *Declaration of Helsinki: Human Experimentation.*

16. Seymour L. Halleck, "Legal and Ethical Aspects of Behavior Control," *The American Journal of Psychiatry,* 131:4 (April 1974), pp. 381–385.

17. T. W. Wann, ed., *Behaviorism and Phenomenology* (Chicago: University of Chicago Press, 1964), pp. 79–80.

92. Christian Humanism and the Human Mind

JAMES M. GUSTAFSON

'We are evolution.' So wrote the French Jesuit, Pierre Teilhard de Chardin.[1] Making the point more poignantly, he said, 'We have become aware that, in the great game that is being played, we are the players as well as being the cards and the stakes.'[2] Christopher Mooney, SJ, in a faithful exposition of Teilhard's passage says, 'For it is not only *in* man that the movement of evolution is now carried on, but *by* man. . . . Through man evolution has not only become conscious of itself but free to dispose of itself,—it can give itself or refuse itself. Upon man therefore falls the awful responsibility for his future on earth.'[3] Evolution can now be carried on *in* man *by* man. The topic of this Nobel Conference, like those of the previous two, faces this awesome point. What was formerly shrouded in mystery, interpreted by myths, assumed to be under the determinative powers of Providence or Fate, or the effects of random chance, is becoming known and manageable through the research of molecular biologists. With the more accurate and intricate explanations of the electrochemical system of the brain comes a heightened sense of man's freedom and power to control the minds of men. This new knowledge does not in itself determine the use that will be made of it, any more than the knowledge of nuclear physics in itself determines the uses made of it. But the growing recognition of its potential uses intensifies our sense of responsibility and obligation. The *sense* of responsibility and obligation, however, is not in itself determinative of the answers to the questions: 'Responsible to whom? Obligated to whom? Responsible for what? Obligated for what?' This new knowledge intensifies our awareness of human freedom in the sense that we are not as enslaved to ignorance as we have been, and in the sense that we realize that men can now direct the course of human development rather than be the more passive reactors to processes over which they have little control. Men need not be the accidental effects of generations of genetic development; their knowledge of genetics moves them toward liberation from determination by random development to the liberty and power to direct future development. Men need no longer simply adapt to their natural environments, but can culturally and technically achieve the liberty to control their environments, indeed to create environments adapted to man. Men need no longer assume that their brains are stable 'givens' upon which register the impressions to which they happen to become subject; they are beginning to perceive that the brain itself is subject to development, as a result of the neuro-biological experiments and potential uses of them. Thus, while men have for ages assumed that they could develop their 'minds' by training and study, they now see that they can control and develop their 'brains' in such a way that their 'minds' are capable of new responses and new achievements.

It is this kind of knowledge, with its accompanying senses of both liberation and responsibility, both power and obligation, that Teilhard de Chardin had in mind when he made that statement, so clear that any card player can understand it: 'We have become aware that, in the great game that is being played, we are the players as well as being the cards and the stakes'. The cards are more complicated: molecular biology gives us an increasingly complex deck that requires elite capacities and training to understand fully. The stakes are higher: the future of man itself. But the players in many respects are the same: morally there has been no progress to compare with scientific and technical progress among the players, whether they be theologians or scientists, humanists or technologists, politicians or investors, business managers or philosophers.

Some Basic Observations

I would like to make some simple observations about this situation and about some responses that have been made to it, before proceeding to suggest some concerns and some lines of activity I believe we ought to consider. First, the *values* of human life have not appeared more clearly because we have a more accurate account of the *facts* of life. Neuro-biologists move toward giving us more and more accurate accounts of memory, but these accounts themselves do not tell us what is *worth* remembering and what is *worth* forgetting. It is worth remembering the things I have learned in reading about the research of the molecular biologists, and it is worth remembering what I learn in this conference, but it is not worth remembering what I had for breakfast this morning, or what the name of the stewardess was on the flight that carried me to Minnesota. To introduce the word 'worth' is to introduce a realm of discourse that has a considerable autonomy from the realm of scientific

From *The Human Mind,* ed. J. Roslansky (Amsterdam: North-Holland, 1967), pp. 85–109. Used by permission.

discourse. How would I decide what is worth remembering? This could be answered by referring to many values, not all of which are necessarily in harmony with each other, and not all of which I might consider to be praiseworthy. Let me suggest a couple of them in a random way. I might say it is worth remembering what I read about molecular biology so that I can make a favorable impression on people I talk to at parties and over lunch tables; I could impress them as being a person who seems to have some knowledge outside of his own field of specialization, and thus if they value 'learned men' my memory of these things would redound to my glory. Appealing to the most commonly accepted standards of moral values, however, that would not be a very *good* reason. I might say that it is worth remembering because it will be *useful* to me in my future teaching and research in ethics. Then the next question is, 'what constitutes utility?' I could answer in various ways: My students and I would be forced to deal more concretely with specific issues that are very complex, and thus we would not be able to get away with platitudes and high level abstractions in a way that we have. This is an appeal to the value of 'realism', of facing honestly and directly the hard questions. Or I might say that material that suggests the potentially most important consequences for man is more useful to remember than such trivial but useful information as where in the library stacks I will find Aristotle's works and the secondary materials on them. This latter reason would appeal to the values we would affirm about the continuation and development of life itself; it is more useful to retain information about materials that will have potential effects on the life of the universal human community. This, most men would agree, would be a *better* reason for remembering than would the desire to impress people with one's erudition. Why? Because life is valued, and its continuity and development is thus worthy of more attention than any one man's vanity. But in each instance I appeal to a *value* that does not immediately emerge from biological facts themselves.

My second observation is that this gap between facts about life and the values of life moves toward some closure if certain assumptions are made. These assumptions might be stated as follows. First, to know is itself of value. Why would this be? Because man has developed into the kind of being who has insatiable curiosity about himself and the world around him, and thus in the fulfillment of this drive for knowledge there is a fulfillment, development, and extension of man's existence itself. This assumption presupposes that it is good simply to be, and that to be human is in part to be curious about life, and this curiosity is good. But it does not yet face the question of the uses of knowledge.

Second, in penetrating the molecular biology of the brain, we discern (with reference to other animals, and with reference to man's own past) a direction of development, and *that this direction is on the whole worthy of sustaining and promoting.* The latter phrase jars us a little, it seems to me, because there is a kind of leap of faith involved in it. Teilhard de Chardin makes the leap in a double move: he extrapolates from where he ascertains the evolutionary process has come to where he thinks on the basis of speculative reason it is going, with its 'hominization', 'personalization', etc., moving toward an Omega point. At the same time that this extrapolation is made he is impregnating it with ideas derived from Christian faith about a 'Christification' of the process, its 'amorization' because God entered history and nature in the person of Jesus Christ. But Teilhard's double move is questionable, and he himself was not a blind optimist about life, as our introductory quotations suggest. We can ask on factual grounds: How much extrapolation is warranted on the basis of evidence from the past? With man's new liberty and power to give direction to evolution, can we assume continuities based on projections from the most primitive forms of life? Or do we have to be prepared for radical discontinuities as a result of the new power to interpose in the developments, and thus be more modest in our projections. We could ask, on theological grounds, whether affirmations about the redemption of life by a gracious deed of God properly pertain to an impregnation of the natural evolutionary process. Molecular biologists I have read are not theologians, but they are moral men; the second move of Teilhard's would not be persuasive, but the first could at least be discussed. Is there a discernible direction in the development of the brain? That is a factual matter, and subject to verification. Is that direction *good?* The answer to that suggests that the convergence of fact and value diverges again. How it would be answered would involve at crucial points 'leaps of faith' on the part of the biologists; it would involve at some point a move beyond empirical and rational support to an affirmation that: (a) the continuation of life is of value; and (b) that the development of life in the direction it is moving and could move is of value. It is the latter that is jarring, and uncertainties about it locate the moral questions we all now face together.

My third observation is of a different order. It pertains to religious and theological responses that have been made, not to any things as particular as the work of neuro-biologists, but to the awareness of man's new freedom and power to give direction to human development. This awareness has to a considerable extent been embraced as a cultural fact of great theological significance, or at least one that has implications for theology and for religious life. Among the notions overworked and imprecisely developed in recent Christian thinking are those of 'maturity' and 'a world come of age'. If 'maturity' is used analogously to its use as a chronological and biological term with reference to the growth processes from infancy to childhood, to adolescence to adulthood, it will be as misleading as other biological analogies have been for the interpretation of historical developments. Do we move into old age and death? No one knows. If maturity is used analogously to a psychological process, suggesting that in infancy there is almost absolute dependence on support from others, and that one gradually grows to greater autonomy, there might be some warrant for its use. Man has some greater autonomy with reference to nature through his knowledge and his power, though he is still dependent on many things. If maturity suggests a growth in moral wisdom, a fulfillment of potential qualities for excellence, so that religious men now heartily and indiscriminately embrace scientific and technological developments in the culture as worthy of joyful celebration, its use is dubious indeed. I believe that popular, avant-garde, religious discourse has made some mistakes in its broadside and indiscriminate celebration of the 'new age' in which we are supposed to be living, mistakes that morally conscientious scientists themselves are not making. These mistakes are several. If what is celebrated is liberation from determination by nature and ideas about nature that have in some sense crippled men spiritually and intellectually, there is some propriety to the mood. If, however, in the celebration it is assumed that this new liberty and power are somehow going to be directed by moral wisdom to the well-being of man, the joy and praise are premature. If the celebration assumes that now religious men can see that the world is good and it is for man in some simple way, whereas formerly they felt it had to be denied, they have grounds for celebrating a recovered theological belief (that God the creator of the world is graciously good and is together with his creation good *for* men). But there are no grounds for confusing this theological affirmation with the facts of historical and scientific development. What religious men believe about God (his goodness, the goodness of creation, the Omega toward which it is moving) can rightfully tell them something about what they *intend* that scientific developments be used for. It may tell them that their attitude toward scientific developments ought to be open rather than closed. But there is no warrant for assuming that the new power, and new freedom are being or will be used unambiguously for human good, or for the good even of biological development. The possibilities of new freedom and new power do not either by natural endowment or by some grace of God bring with them a quality of *moral* maturity. The hard issues are not even addressed by the celebration of science and technology; celebration is an expression of an attitude, in this case an affirmative one. It does not help either the molecular biologist, or the technician, solve the problems of the ends to which knowledge and power ought to be put, the values to be served, the means of both control and development to be instituted in the use of knowledge. If the celebrative theme is to say something to the biologists, I cannot imagine what it is. I doubt if they care one whit whether Christians have now decided to embrace what some of them formerly feared. I suspect they might appreciate more understanding and hard work on the part of people primarily concerned with the ends of human existence as these ends pertain to the wider range of choice that their research now presents to men.

My fourth observation pertains to the impact on theological thinking and religious life of our awareness that we are the players, as well as the cards and the stakes. Both man's thinking about the nature of ultimate being, and his disposition in life are being altered by the awareness that we are *participants in creativity,* rather than the tenders and caretakers of something that has been created. We are shapers rather than conformers to static established shapes. The move from thinking about things as static to thinking about them as dynamic has been in the making for many decades. Philosophers like Bergson, Whitehead, and Hartshorne, and such a religious thinker as Henry Nelson Wieman, have been pointing the way in their different patterns of thought and expression. Recently in Catholic thought as well, this notion has taken hold; not only in Teilhard de Chardin, but among others. The American Jesuit Robert Johann in his Aquinas Lecture, *The Pragmatic Meaning of God,* makes the point in this way: 'Instead of separating man from his environment, personal transcendence, as presently conceived [by which Johann means something of the new freedom and power I have been indicating], means a new intimacy and a more significant involvement with it. It marks the release of limitless possibilities and opens the door to a more truly human and genuinely *creative* participation of man in the world.'[4] God, for Johann, is the 'essential condition' for this creative participation and interaction, he is the one who enables all things to come into coherence and community as they interact in experience, if I understand him correctly. This is neither the time nor the place to examine critically various doctrines of God as they correlate with our new awareness of creativity. It is proper, however, to underline a trend in theological and religious reflection; namely, that man is an actor and innovator, responding and interacting with the actions of other beings, including the activity of God himself. I would be remiss if I did not recall that biblically oriented theology has found grounds in the Scriptures for more dynamic interpretations of the nature of God and his relations to men and the world. Joseph Sittler, a master of theological aphorisms, put it this way, 'God simply *is* what God manifestly does.'[5] Gustaf Wingren, in expounding the meaning of God's law, says that 'God's demand that men should continue to 'have dominion' over Creation is part of *His continuing Creation of the world.*'[6] This suggests that the meaning of God the Creator is to be developed in terms of a continuous creative activity of God, and that man's scientific and technological pursuits are part of the dominion over the world that man is to have and are part of God's own creative activity in the world. H. Richard Niebuhr moves from the indicative language of God's action in the world to its consequent imperative for man in his famous sentences, 'God is acting in all actions upon you. So respond to all actions upon you as to respond to his action.'[7]

From all this, it can at a minimum be observed that theological thought, and religious interpretation of life are affirming not static models of being (although the dynamic ones do have order and structure as part of them), but models that conceive of both God and man in active terms. They do not make man *the* Creator, however, any more than the molecular biologist claims that he or any other man has created the neurons he examines. Rather man is seen as the creative responder and innovator in interaction with development and activity that is already there, that is going on. But creative interaction is not an end in itself; what the religious man has the audacity to suggest is that he has some insight into what the outcome of that creative interaction ought to be, the direction in which it ought to go in the course of development. He has a source to which he turns for insight into the *values* that are worthy of acceptance, sustenance, and development. I have no interest here in claiming that this source is a 'revelation' of God, or how it might be considered to be a 'revelation' of God. We can find in the Western cultural tradition some of these values; many of them have apparently been confirmed both by reason and by experience as worthy of appropriation, or at least consideration, in thinking about what uses the freedom and power of man ought to be put to, what ends they ought to serve. We can find in them some clues about the value and meaning of existence, man together with other men.

These observations and the commentary on them are not random in choice, but are the bases from which I shall now move to more particular considerations of the human and moral potentialities and threats that the research of molecular biologists on the brain seem to portend.

A Christian Humanistic Response

What I have said before can be restated as a way of proceeding. The question that the molecular biologists are proceeding to answer is this one: 'How does the brain function?' But this is not the same question as: 'What does it mean to be a person?' But the two questions are related. They are related existentially for all of us, biologists, theologians, humanists alike, because we are persons who have been exposed to the knowledge that scientists have given us. Biologists are persons, living in community with others; we non-biologists, like them, are persons, whose understanding of life is altered by the knowledge that they give us. The relation between the questions, however, is not just an existential one. Whatever qualities or dimensions we might wish to include in our understanding of what it means to be a person are biologically dependent upon our having the intricate brains that human beings have in contrast to other animals. We could not even wonder about what it means to be a person, what the ends and values of man's life are, if we did not have the memory, the ability to reflect, the cells and fluids that biologists are now describing for us. We could not ask the question of values if we did not have the brains that have developed over the long course of evolution from other forms of life, if there were not similarities between us and the rats on which so much research is done, and about which many humanists make snide comments.

Given the brain that we are now coming to know and understand in biological terms, the Christian humanist can raise three general areas for reflection. First, how are we to be *disposed* toward this knowledge and its potential use? Second, what are the 'functional requisites' for maintaining *human* (personal) life? Third, are there any principles that can be formulated that will give direction to ends and means in the use of this research for the well-being of life?

Disposition toward Research

How are we to be disposed toward the research of the molecular biologists who explore the brain, and to the potential uses of this research? I wish to stress the notion of 'disposition' here, for it has proper references and limits. It refers to our fundamental *attitudes* toward, in this case, the research and its use. In themselves, as we have noted, attitudes do not tell us what to do; something more is needed; namely, intellectual reflection and the will to act in accord with the ends that are formed by both attitude and intellect. But attitudes are important, and we sense their significance especially in the situation to which this conference is addressed.

It would not be difficult to stack the cards of knowledge, and of man's potential use of this knowledge so that a disposition of fear could be evoked. Indeed, the evocation of fear has often been the response of both scientists and humanists to new developments in scientific research. We need recall only the response of many humanists and scientists to the unleashing of nuclear energy to see how fear is not only a rather 'natural' moral disposition, but also a very proper one. I recall, for example, not only the early numbers of the *Bulletin of the Atomic Scientists,* but addresses given by Professor Harold Urey at the University of Chicago after World War II, as efforts to awaken the moral sensitivities of other intellectuals to the potential dangers of atomic warfare. There was no ringing apocalypticism in these presentations by responsible scientists; there was, however, an appeal to dread: the dread of possible unintended alteration of human life, and indeed of its destruction. Such dread is fitting, now as it was then. It is not dread of biological information but dread of man's inability to organize and use it in such a way that certain fundamental values on which almost all men agree, namely, the values of life as we now know it and its continuation, would be sustained. The appeal to dread—an attitude or disposition—was not the end in itself, fortunately. In cooperation with many others, efforts were made to protect life, and to channel the uses of nuclear research so that a measure of order has persisted, though in the eyes of many of us that order remains fragile enough to warrant continued vigilance.

With reference to brain research, there has also been some publicity that evokes dread and fear in men. Essays through the years on the work of Dr. José Delgado and others have persistently raised the question of who controls the electronic devices that in turn control the electrodes that can be placed in certain areas of the brain so that behavior itself is in turn controlled. The dread is not so much of potential destruction as in the case of nuclear war, as it is in the possibilities of the accumulation of power that could be used to determine and control the behaviour of men in ways that are not possible at the present time. The latter phrase is important. There are and always have been ways in which the minds of men have been directed—by teaching, by indoctrination, by propaganda, by control of the kinds of information and ideas that men can have. Every such effort has been to train minds to respond in particular ways (and the ways themselves have varied greatly, particularly in terms of certain moral values). Perhaps the new element of dread comes in with the possibilities of determination through drugs and electrical stimulations; these possibilities portend the diminution of the liberty of individuals without power to reject or accept the stimulations of those who have power. What is dreaded is that new knowledge, which gives potential capacities to control the brain, will fall into the power of those whose values we might not approve of.

With most knowledge that evokes new dread, there is also new hope. Whether dread or hope is evoked depends upon many things, including the sophistication of knowledge about potential uses, the availability of resources to protect against misuses and to foster 'good' uses. We have already seen how some drugs can be used to still the potential violence of psychotics, how many persons whose humanity and productivity in the human community have been crippled by mental illness have been able to resume fruitful and quite normal human activities. I have not found, however, any evangelistic utopians among neurobiologists who are sounding the coming of a new age as the result of their research—a new age in which men will find some absolute good, and persistent euphoria. Even where one might find hints of a new sense of peace and harmony emerging, this is seen to raise other questions about the meaningfulness and productivity of life under such potential conditions.

What kinds of dispositions seem proper in the light of neuro-biological research? On what grounds might they be deemed to be proper? The morally ambiguous possibilities of the use of knowledge are clear; one does not need a theologian to remind men of them. Though it sounds terribly like a 'middle way', a case can be made for realism without despair, for hope without illusions, for avoiding the attitudes of apocalypticism on the one hand and utopianism on the other. Some bases for this can be briefly adumbrated.

First, the moral conscientiousness of the researchers themselves gives some ground for confidence. While their scientific work proceeds without immediate justification by the social and humane values that are the more professional concerns of some of the rest of us, they are men who themselves love life, defend the conditions in life which enable them to exercise their intelligence and freedom, and envision the potential possibilities for and threats to human order and life that might be forthcoming from their work. They existentially unite the humane and the scientific, and often are more aware of the relations of one to the other than some are who embody only the humane.

Second, in free societies there is a social pluralism that gives grounds for confidence, that enables men to be realistic and hopeful at once. Social pluralism in free societies, while it creates tensions and abrasiveness that make human relations complex, keeps alive a diversity of values since various communities in the society attend to the cultivation of different values. It also keeps alive a diversity of institutionalized centers of power that prohibit any one center from absolutely dominating. The normative moral concerns of religious communities, for example, are never simply embodied by universities or business establishments or the state. There is always abrasion between the interests and values of these and other groups. But, there are also centers of loyalty and commitment that they share in common which enable them to live together not only in peace, but in some creative interaction with each other. In this interaction with each other, it is possible for each to learn from the other, each to restrain and limit the other, each to make its contribution to the general direction that the society itself takes. Very often the fear that one interest or value community in the society creates in the minds of members of another is the result of absence of interaction and communication between them. It is my judgment that we can be realistic and hopeful about the uses of the knowledge that we now are getting about the ways that the brain works as long as we have a plurality of value communities and social institutions in significant interaction with each other in free societies. If an imperative is to be drawn from this, it is twofold: to keep alive various humanistic centers for interpretation of the values of life together with the scientific centers that explore its facts, and to maintain the avenues of interaction between them and other centers, such as business and the state so that policy and the exercise of power are affected by the interaction. (More on this later.)

Third, the nature of man as a moral being is such that while he is able to be 'nasty, mean, brutish and small', to quote from Hobbes, he also inclines away from the evil and toward the good, to follow St. Thomas. The 'evil' and the 'good' are terribly vague terms in such a statement, but can minimally be given content sufficient for our purposes here. At least inclination away from evil can be transposed into 'abhorrence at the destruction of what seems to make human life worth living'. Historically, for example, we have seen the persistence of men's chafing under conditions that drastically limit their freedom—to choose, to act, to believe. We have seen resuscitation again and again of human longing for a better life—free from needless suffering, searching for order and peace, enlarging of the ranges of human choice. To be sure, the contrary tendencies have emerged persistently enough to prohibit a bland optimism or a blind utopianism, but countervailing tendencies to these seem also to persist, and to become correctives to what many men would consider to be aberrations from what it means to be human. Perhaps, under possible totalitarian conditions research on the brain could be used to implement the domination of man's destructive tendencies; but on the basis of man's deep longing for life, for peace, for the good, we can have some confidence that such a possibility will be limited.

Fourth, Christians and Jews particularly have certain convictions about God, the source and power of life itself, that ought to bring confidence tempered by a realistic assessment of potential human misuses of knowledge and power. There is, to quote again from Father Robert Johann, a 'bearing or import of belief in God on the qualities of our lives.'[8] That import or bearing is dependent upon the nature and content of those beliefs, as well as our appropriation of their significance for dispositions and attitudes toward human development. Christian doctrine, and its significance for our bearing toward life cannot be more than pointed to here. But it is at least this: that God is worthy of our confidence, and the God who is worthy of our confidence is the one who has given and continues to give life, its development and its order, the one who makes possible the restoration of brokenness in the human community, who makes possible the restraints of man's moral evil as well as the newness of life and knowledge that he enjoys, indeed the God who is himself love and power, goodness and power. The significance for our lives of such beliefs of trusting in God whom confessionally we know in Jesus of Nazareth, ought to be, can be, and often is one of confidence without either despair or illusion, as we face the human uses of human knowledge.

Men are prone to extremes in dispositions all too often. They flutter like birds between despair and illusion. They fear a world that will destroy all that they value, or they dream of a world that will realize all that they cherish. They forget that they participate in creativity, and that this makes possible both new good and new evil. Despair results from the absence of confidence and hope; it is a resignation to fatedness (as if things will be inexorably what they will be without human initiative and activity). Confidence and hope come from 'a sense of *the possible*',[9] from those certainties of experience and belief that enable men to be participative and creative interactors with the processes of life itself, knowing that mistakes will be made, but also that many of them can be corrected.

Requisites for Personal (Human) Life

What seem to be the 'functional requisites' for human life, in the sense not only of biological preservation and development, but in the sense of personal meaningfulness? We can begin this exploration by looking at the lists of such requirements that have been made by others. Bronislaw Malinowski[10] was one creative analyst of human culture who stipulated several adumbrations of such requisites. On one occasion he listed seven basic needs of man, each of which is the basis for a 'cultural response', an institutionalization. Metabolism requires a 'commissariat', reproduction requires a kinship system, bodily comforts require shelter, safety requires protective institutions, movement requires the organization of activities, growth requires 'training', and health requires 'hygiene'. The Princeton sociologist, Marion J. Levy, Jr.,[11] raised the question with reference to the needs for a human society to exist, and listed ten 'requisites': adequate physiological relationships for biological survival, differentiation and assignment of social roles, communication, a shared 'cognitive orientation', or way of knowing, a shared articulated set of goals, some regulation of the choice of means, a regulation of emotional expression, adequate procedures for education or socialization, effective control of disruptive behavior, and adequate institutionalization. Such lists are subject to refinement, elaboration, and revision, but for our purposes can be accepted as pointing to minimal conditions necessary for minimal continuation of human life. They do not, without extension and revision, account for many of the things that we, as human persons, find to be most valuable and rewarding in life. Just as the question 'What makes the brain function?' is not the same as the question, 'What does it mean to be a person?' so the question, 'What conditions are necessary for basic survival of man?' is not the same question as 'What makes life *worth* living?' If some of the things that make life *worth* living can be indicated, we are on the way to understanding what values ought to be preserved, sustained, and developed in the uses of neuro-biological research.

I shall not attempt a full delineation of all the things that men strive for and live for. Rather, I shall isolate only a few that seem to be crucial to the enhancement of the human 'spirit', to use a term that has no precise neuro-biological references. The first is freedom, which has been alluded to as an aspiration that is persistent enough in men to give us some confidence that men will resist uses of knowledge that destroy it, and promote uses that enhance it. The preservation and development of human liberty, within the bounds necessary for order which itself sustains liberty, comes to the fore again and again in moral responses to political developments. We see it in anticolonialism, we see it in the reform of the Catholic church, and we see it in the concerns men have about the uses of human beings for scientific experimentation. Edward Shils, in a passionate critique of some of the research of his fellow social scientists, for example, raises three ethical issues that arise from experimentation itself, not to mention the uses of knowledge derived from it. Each of the three, but primarily the first, has reference to freedom. They are 'the propriety of the manipulation of adult, normal human beings, even for their own good, by other human beings; the propriety of possible injury to a human being on behalf of scientific progress and the progress of human well-being; and the depth and permanence of the effects of the experiment on the individual subject.'[12] Absolutized in the abstract such concerns would seem to falsify many other concerns that we have for the worthiness of life. Human beings are influenced, if not manipulated, by other human beings all their lives; indeed, culture would not persist if this were not so. The liberty and rights of some men are limited, if not injured, for the sake of progress that has moral value over and over again (for example the limitation of the liberty of a landlord to designate to whom he will rent an apartment that is involved in the progress in civil rights). But Shils is pointing to some almost primitive moral sensitivities that crop up whenever personal liberty is threatened. Men resent being 'manipulated', there seems to be a betrayal of trust and confidence in it, a diminution of one's control over his own responses. Human life seems to be worth living only if the value of personal freedom is attended to, though obviously other values of equal or almost equal importance are not always in perfect harmony with it.

Another requisite that needs to be met to keep life worth living is 'trust'. As such perceptive thinkers as Marcel and Royce have shown, men live to a great extent by reliance upon the trustworthiness of others, and must themselves be trustworthy in order to live in community with others. Trust becomes important only when we have the development of the human brain that enables personal liberty to be meaningful, and personal relations to be determined not simply by biological interactions and necessities, but by responses and commitments consciously made. To be sure, some analogies might be drawn between the reliance of chemical agents upon the functioning of each other in the workings of the brain on the one hand, and the reliance of persons upon each other for the sustenance and meaningfulness of life on the other. But 'trust' as something valued in personal interrelations or in the relations between groups and even nation states, can be withdrawn, betrayed, broken, by willful acts of men. Trust, like the assurance of a significant domain of personal freedom, is a moral requisite for human life. It involves honesty, compliance with promises and commitments, conformity to rules and procedures of life that set the boundaries and directions within which human interactions occur, as well as personal confidence that others will sustain rather than betray the self. Uses of knowledge that make life and other persons untrustworthy will denigrate personal existence; uses which enhance the phenomenon and value of trust will sustain and develop it.

Personal existence in the human community depends upon relationships of love. Love is one of the looser terms in common human discourse; it refers to sexual relations in which there is an affection of the persons for each other; it refers to utter self-sacrifice as symbolized by the cross in the Christian community; it refers to the relationship of friendship; and it refers to a profound longing for various objects as potential sources of self-fulfillment. As a moral requisite for personal life, however, we might use more restricted references. It involves joyous and thankful response for the existence of other, and for the relationship between us. It directs a relation of respect for the autonomy of others, so that in love there is neither a swallowing up of others for the sake of self-aggrandizement, nor a blind submissiveness to others for the sake of the loss of identity. There is loyalty to others, not for the sake of their utility to the self, but for their very existence as others. There is trustworthiness in love; fidelity to each other is part of the order of love.[13] The possibility for the fulfillment of relations of love is a requisite for human personal existence. Research that is now being done on the human brain might very well lead to developments which make such relationships more possible rather than less possible; at least insofar as such relationships are dependent upon neuro-biological functions, men may be able to check some of the basically physical conditions that cripple some persons, that do not enable them to respond freely in loving relationships. Certainly, the use of new knowledge for the sake of human and personal life will have to consider the importance of maintaining and enhancing the possibilities of love as one of its touchstones. Uses that deter such possibilities will have to be guarded against.

Many other requisites, in part related to freedom, trust, and love, could be developed, such as hope, justice, order, joy, opportunity for achievement, and others. I shall limit consideration to these three, for they illustrate the kinds of 'moral requisites' that are dependent upon biological survival and upon the intricacies of the human brain, but take some flight from this dependence as values or concerns to be attended to in themselves. I would not claim that these values are any more dependent upon religious beliefs about God, or upon the cultivation of the religious life than they are upon the neurological structure and function of man. I would, however, indicate that freedom, trust, love, justice, joy, and hope have been nourished by humanistic Christianity and Judaism, and that in the pluralism of the society that is to come, it will be the function of religious communities, or their secular alternatives, to nourish these needs of man, and to keep their importance alive in an increasingly technically-oriented culture. If fewer and fewer men will appropriate traditional religious beliefs out of doubts about their credibility, they will nonetheless have to recognize the importance of religious faith and life in providing and cultivating the sense of the numinous, and the qualities of life that make scientific and technical life worth pursuing. While I, no more than any other theologian, would wish to justify religious belief exclusively on the basis of its bearing and import on the 'quality of life' that it can bring into being, I am prepared to assert that renewed religious life, dependent upon certain beliefs, does make a contribution to humanization by sustaining, and fostering the moral requisites for personal human life. Like the uses of scientific knowledge, the uses of religion are morally ambiguous: there is no absolute certainty that traditional religion will function for humanization just as there is no certainty that new knowledge of the brain will. But the pangs of criticism and renewal through which religious communities are now going give some expectation that the recognition that God is for man and his well-being will strengthen man's own ability to be for man and his well-being.

Principles for Direction

Finally, some attention needs to be given to a risky effort, namely the development in more concise form of some directives, moral and social, that can be considered with reference to the uses of our new knowledge about the brain.

(1) The scientific community has responsibility to

man, to life (and in theological terms) to God the giver of life, to be vigilant in its own reflection about the potential uses and misuses of knowledge. This vigilance can be exercised in interaction with humanists.

(2) Religious and other communities concerned with human values have a responsibility to scientists and to all men, and to God, to participate in the interactive processes out of which institutionally and culturally the uses of new knowledge will be determined. This means clearly that humanists need at least a layman's knowledge of the crucial research and its potentialities.

(3) All of us have an obligation to keep active a concern for human values in the culture as a whole, through churches, educational institutions, mass media of communications, and other agencies. If such work is not done, some of the values themselves might atrophy in the consciences of men. This requires public moral discourse, not for the sake of evoking fear, but for the sake of developing the awareness of man's own worthwhileness in the light of which knowledge can be put to the service of man. I wish to underscore this third point, for all too often our immediate response to new developments that pose threats as well as possibilities for good is to think in terms of legal restraints and direction, with sanctions of political power. To such we will turn, but even legal directives will depend for their efficacy on that nebulous 'moral ethos' that will or will not exist.

(4) All of us have an obligation to maintain pluralism in and through free societies, pluralism of activities (sciences, religion, arts, etc.), pluralism in institutionalization of moral concerns, and pluralism in concentrations of power. No one group is sufficient in itself to provide 'answers' to existing and potential questions. There is need of others for information, insight, restraint, support, and development.

(5) New institutionalizations are necessary to make possible the significant interaction between groups with particularized interests and knowledge that can give direction to the development of man. Some such seminars and centers are coming into being, but all too often the interaction is on a random basis. There are centers for the study of population problems and for international policy that bring together the knowledge, ideas and insights of various disciplines that bear upon such problems. Further developments of this sort are in order, whether under the auspices of states, universities, churches, business, or various combinations of them.

(6) Some boards or agencies with technical competence and power are needed to set limits through law and other means to potentially destructive uses of knowledge. We face this on an issue that may be in the long run of limited significance in comparison with potential uses of knowledge developed from molecular biology; namely, in the whole business of electronics and 'bugging'. Ways of protecting human rights to privacy, and of enforcing such protection are much the order of the day. Something comparable may be necessary with reference to other areas.

(7) The freedom to do research needs to be distinguished sufficiently from the use of research so that man's right to knowledge is preserved. This involves its own risks; new knowledge may enable a development of man into something quite different from what we know in our thin slice of history. Man is no more a static part of the process of creativity and development than are some other organisms. The right to know what is involved in human development needs to be protected.

(8) Much more detailed and clearer formulation of those values to be preserved and developed in human existence needs to be made so that these might function both to indicate the direction that uses of research ought to take, and the limitations of those uses that ought to be firmly formed. Biological survival is only the beginning of such a formulation, and its form is itself subject to change. To confine myself to previous remarks made in this paper, I would say that uses which preserve and foster freedom, trust, love, justice, joy and hope are to be supported; those that deprive men of these are to be prohibited. Intensive and continuous dialogue need to be sustained to solve the harder questions as to what new use would have what effect on what values. Amendment of possible legal restrictions will have to be possible so that prohibitions can be revised in the light of worthy new possibilities. But law and morality have a necessary conservative function in the preservation of life and what makes it worthwhile.

'In the great game that is being played, we are the players as well as being the cards and the stakes'.

Notes

1. Teilhard de Chardin, *The Phenomenon of Man* (New York: Harper Torchbook, 1961), 231.
2. Ibid., 229.
3. Christopher Mooney, *Teilhard de Chardin and the Mystery of Christ* (New York: Harper and Row, 1966), 50.
4. Robert Johann, *The Pragmatic Meaning of God* (Milwaukee: Marquette University Press, 1966), 6.
5. Joseph Sittler, *The Structure of Christian Ethics* (Baton Rouge: Louisiana State University Press, 1958), 4.
6. Gustaf Wingren, *Creation and Law* (Philadelphia: Muhlenberg Press, 1961), 150; italics mine.

7. H. Richard Niebuhr, *The Responsible Self* (New York: Harper and Row, 1963), 126.

8. Johann, *The Pragmatic Meaning of God,* 1.

9. William Lynch, *Images of Hope* (Baltimore: Helicon, 1965), 32.

10. Bronislaw Malinowski, *A Scientific Theory of Culture and Other Essays* (Chapel Hill: University of North Carolina Press, 1944), 91ff.

11. Marion J. Levy, Jr., *The Structure of Society* (Princeton: Princeton University Press, 1952), 141ff.

12. Edward Shils, "Social Inquiry and the Autonomy of the Individual," in *The Human Meaning of the Social Sciences,* ed. Daniel Lerner (New York: Meridian Books, 1959), 141.

13. This follows loosely the more beautiful passage of H. Richard Niebuhr in *The Purpose of the Church and Its Ministry* (New York: Harper and Row, 1956), 34-36.

93.

Constitutional Rights of Handicapped People and the Teaching of the Parables

ROBERT A. BURT

During the past fifteen years or so, considerable public attention has been focussed on the needs and the rights of handicapped people. This attention is a dramatic reversal of the public attitudes that had dominated social policy during the preceding fifty years or more—the policy of assuring the effective invisibility of handicapped people. This change in public attitude is apparent regarding all kinds of handicaps, physical and mental. Consider, for example, the extensive reconstruction of public facilities mandated by congressional action in 1968 to assure access for people in wheelchairs and for blind people.

In this essay I intend to pay particular attention to the situation of retarded people; but the trends that I will discuss and the conclusions that I will offer are not restricted to retardation. The question whether handicapped people should be excluded from or included in communal relations with others has particularly vivid application regarding retarded people, but the basic issues underlying this question are the same for all manner of handicaps.

The most striking expression of the social policy of excluding retarded people from any communal relation was in the creation, in the late nineteenth and early twentieth centuries, of isolated rural residential institutions for the lifetime confinement of retarded people and the subsequent expansion of the resident population in these institutions during this century until by 1966 they held almost 200,000 people across the country. The conditions in these institutions were, to put it mildly, less than benign; to put it less mildly and more accurately, they were horrifying, nightmarish places. As one prominent retardation professional put it, on entering one of these institutions you walked into "purgatory, the land of the living dead." But these institutions and their horrifying conditions remained virtually unknown, invisible to the general public—and even invisible to most of the families who put their retarded relatives into these institutions and effectively severed all relations with them. Many of these families were, of course, forced to institutional

---

Used by permission of the author.

placements because there were no alternative facilities to assist them in the burdens of caring for these relatives at home or in some community setting. Public policy at that time—even just a decade ago—offered nothing for retarded people but exclusion from public schools and from community residence: nothing but exclusion and invisibility.

Since that time there has been an extraordinary shift in public policy. Litigation in federal courts played a critical instrumental role in fostering this change; beginning in 1970, public interest attorneys brought suit in various states challenging conditions in retardation institutions. Federal judges, beginning with Judge Frank Johnson in Alabama, were stunned at the evidence of inhumane treatment set out before them and ruled in various ways that the states were violating the constitutional rights of retarded people. These lawsuits were followed by two significant acts of Congress, both passed in 1975. The most obviously far-reaching was the Education for All Handicapped Children Act which required all states, as a condition for receiving any federal education assistance, to provide a "free, appropriate public education" for all children no matter how severely disabled, whether physically or mentally. The second act was less obviously sweeping in its implications but nonetheless had considerable potential impact on state retardation institutions; this was the Developmental Disabilities Assistance and Bill of Rights Act which, among other things, proclaimed that retarded people had a right to state-supported residence in home-like community facilities rather than in isolated, large-scale institutions.

Each of these acts had high price tags attached to it; in the last fiscal year alone, for example, the Education for All Handicapped Children Act cost the federal government some $3.5 billion and required at least an equal matching expenditure of state education funds for handicapped children. The costs involved were, moreover, more than simply financial. Many communities were fiercely resistant to sharing their neighborhoods and their schools with apparently strange and even seemingly frightening retarded people; and many parents of institutionalized retarded people were deeply troubled at the fearful prospects (as they saw them) of removing their children from institutions into newly created community facilities, particularly in communities that did not seem hospitable to their children.

Thus, as with many social change movements, resistance appears after the first flush of reform activity. The costs of change suddenly seem too high; the forces that supported the old ways reassert themselves with renewed vigor. This understandable reaction has not yet led to a full-scale reversal of the new social policies, but new questions, new doubts, have been raised. In part, these doubts have focussed on whether the new emphasis on community-based services and residential facilities in fact serves the best interests of retarded people; the basic concern on this score comes from suspicions that retarded people will not be truly welcomed in these settings so that adequate efforts will not be made to respond to their special needs. These doubts gather force from a more fundamental source of misgivings—a growing belief that the overall social costs are simply too great, that even if retarded people will benefit from inclusion in ordinary community life, nonetheless the provision of these benefits is too costly for everyone else—too costly just simply in financial terms (though perhaps in psychological terms as well).

These doubts are visibly at work in the most recent court cases, and particularly in recent Supreme Court decisions. In 1980 the Supreme Court took its first case challenging conditions in state retardation institutions. In this case, which involved a Pennsylvania residential institution known as Pennhurst, the federal District Judge had found that conditions were so outrageous, so abusive, that there was no way that the institution could be reformed or improved. He found that the constitutional rights of these retarded people could only be adequately protected if Pennhurst were completely closed and the state provided home-like, therapeutic community residences for all the retarded people living in Pennhurst. The Court of Appeals essentially affirmed this District Court order, though it found the right to community placement in the 1975 congressional Bill of Rights Act and thus didn't have to reach the more basic constitutional question. The Supreme Court, however, reversed this reading of the congressional act; and though it didn't reach the underlying constitutional issue, the Court (in an opinion by Justice Rehnquist) conveyed considerable skepticism and spoke fervently on behalf of a countervailing principle of state autonomy—the right of states to decide what public funds, if any, should be made available to retarded people and, by implication, the right of individual citizens in each state to decide whether they wanted to share their tax resources or their neighborhoods with retarded people.

I want to explore two related questions that are posed by this Supreme Court ruling. The first is the question of how the competing social costs and social benefits should be calculated when anyone—whether judge, legislator, or any of us as citizens—deliberates whether it is worthwhile to expend the considerable resources that are required to adequately welcome and support retarded people in community settings and to end the previous social policy of their exclusion and isolation. In exploring this question, I want to assume that this new inclusive policy would benefit retarded people; my central inquiry is whether this new policy would benefit the rest of us sufficiently to justify whatever burdens might fall on us from implementing that policy. The second question that I want to explore is whether courts in our constitutional scheme are obliged to favor one side or the other in the communal deliberations about the costs versus the benefits of special social efforts to include rather than to exclude retarded people.

The first question, then, first. How do we go about the cost-benefit calculation? Many of the costs of the communal-inclusive policy are obvious; $3.5 billion each year of federal funds for educating handicapped children is one obvious cost. What are the countervailing benefits? I want to dwell today on one benefit in particular, as I see it. This is not a dollars-and-cents financial benefit; it is, in the jargon of economists, a "soft" benefit—a social-psychological benefit. If we give adequate weight to this "soft" benefit, as I will describe it, then I think we will be led to see how our most fundamental interests—the interests of non-retarded people, of so-called "normal" people—are served by making special efforts to include retarded or other handicapped ("not normal") people in our community. Indeed, if I am correct in my perception of this basic interest, then we will change the very way that we frame the question at issue. The question will no longer be, "Should we permit retarded people to share our community—our resources and our residential neighborhoods?" We will instead see the question in a different light. If I am correct, the true questions will be, "Should we admit the fact that we are all members of the same community, whether we are retarded or not, 'normal' or not? Should we abandon the false belief that we can choose to exclude retarded people from our community because in fact we have no choice, because we and they have an inescapable communal relationship whether we like this fact or not?" If these are the real questions, then Justice Rehnquist was wrong in fact—and not simply wrong as a matter of moral or constitutional principle—when he suggested in the *Pennhurst* case that a state or its citizens might exercise supposedly autonomous choice to break off all social relations with retarded people.

My assertion may seem implausible to you, or at most metaphorical. What kind of true social relationship is really possible with retarded people—or, to put the issue most starkly, with a profoundly retarded person who has a measured I.Q. less than thirty-five and lacks capacity to speak or even to think in any way that resembles ordinary human social intercourse? What can I mean in referring to a communal relationship with such a person?

Let me set out a hypothesis. I cannot conclusively prove the truth of this hypothesis here, but I hope to persuade you that it is a plausible hypothesis, for which empirical verification could emerge if we look in the correct places and with the correct investigational methodology. Let me suggest at least two ways that a social relationship, a genuinely communal relationship, can exist with even the most profoundly retarded person.

Both ways paradoxically take root in the mind of only one participant in the relationship. The first and perhaps the most easily understood way depends on hope—the optimistically imagined prospect that some future relation on some terms is possible, even with the most profoundly retarded person. In some circumstances, of course, this hope may seem wholly improbable to most observers. But this improbability does not diminish and may even intensify the hope of some people.

This is a common attitude of many parents of retarded children and is reflected in their intense, prolonged efforts to elicit even the most minimal social responses from them. This attitude most likely reflects an intensely felt identification of parent with child based on the fact of biological linkage, a tie that the parent does not view as severable by any unilateral act of choice. When these parents demand that others view their children as they do—as disabled but potentially less so and in any event as fundamentally equal participants in the human community—others can refuse this demand only by disparaging the deepest-held convictions of these parents and thereby denying the essential terms of a communal relationship with these parents as well as with their children. This is one way, then, that those who are not themselves parents of retarded children nonetheless are drawn to enter into a communal relation with those children—because we do acknowledge a clear social relation with the parents and these parents in turn lead us to see our relationship with them as necessarily including their children.

This formulation of a communal relationship depends on empathy—on parents' feeling for their children and others' regard for those parents. There is, however, another way to consider relations with a profoundly retarded person that does not so ostentatiously depend on this benign, altruistic view. Hope is not the only wellspring from which mentally normal people draw a conception of social relations with profoundly retarded people. Fear is another. This fear can grip parents and others as deeply as hope, and it can also distort rational capacities by creating a fantastic image of retarded people, even the most remote and helplessly retarded person. This fear and the imagery it spawns may be irrational, but they are nonetheless passionately real for those gripped by them. Let me cite one example of this phenomenon—an observation written in a Supreme Court opinion in 1927 by one of the most revered Justices ever to sit on the Court. Note these words written by Justice Oliver Wendell Holmes, speaking for a unanimous Supreme Court to uphold compulsory sterilization of mentally retarded people:

> We have seen more than once that the public welfare may call upon the best citizens for their lives. It would be strange if it could not call upon those who already sap the strength of the State for these lesser sacrifices ... in order to prevent our being swamped with incompetence. It is better for all the world, if instead of waiting to execute degenerate offspring for crime, or to let them starve for their imbecility, society can prevent those who are manifestly unfit from continuing their kind.... Three generations of imbeciles are enough.

It is clear today that these fears were wildly exaggerated, as were the then-dominant beliefs in the biological heritability of retardation and its amenability to reproductive control. But the sense of vast threat from retarded people and the consequent embattled stance of Holmes and his contemporaries were real enough for them. If the threat of "degenerate ... crime," of "being swamped with incompetence," did not come from retarded people, it must have come from the imagination of those who viewed them. Perhaps Holmes and his contemporaries painted their darkest fears about themselves and their vulnerability in the world as they saw it onto the temptingly empty faces (as they saw them) of retarded people. From this perspective, it was not retarded people who were feared; they were not seen except for what they were fearfully imagined to represent.

This same projective process may be at work today, even in the more benign attitude currently apparent toward retarded people. I mentioned the *Pennhurst* case earlier; you will recall that the District Judge in that case had ordered this residential retardation institution wholly closed because its very existence necessarily violated the constitutional rights of any resident. Note this indictment of all such institutions by the District Judge, Raymond Broderick, in his opinion in that case:

> At its best, Pennhurst is typical of large residential state institutions for the retarded. These institutions are the most isolated and restrictive settings in which to treat the retarded. Pennhurst is almost totally impersonal. Its residents have no privacy—they sleep in large overcrowded wards, spend their waking hours together in large day rooms and eat in a large group setting. They must conform to the schedule of the institution which allows for no individual flexibility.... The environment at Pennhurst is not conducive to normalization. It does not reflect society. It is separate and isolated from society and represents group rather than family living.

Judge Broderick is undoubtedly correct in his portrayal of the harm this institution works on its residents. But I hear an added force behind his words, an attitude toward and fear of institutions that is not restricted to their impact on retarded people. I hear this force in one aspect of the judge's indictment that is surely wrong: his conclusion that Pennhurst "does not reflect society." It *does* reflect society—frightening aspects, that is, of contemporary American society in its impersonality, its threats to individual privacy, its demands for conformity "which allow for no individual flexibility." Retarded residents of Pennhurst are more patently afflicted by these institutional characteristics, more obviously disabled from developing their capacities for self-sufficiency than ordinary people. But Pennhurst is nonetheless a nightmare reflection of the powerful social institutional constraints on anyone's capacity to achieve self-sufficient autonomy.

To see fears that afflict most people, "mentally normal" people, in the injuries inflicted on retarded people does not disprove the reality of those injuries. To see a pervasive fear of institutional depersonalization in contemporary American society as adding intensity to Judge Broderick's wish to close down Pennhurst does not show the error of this course. I draw these linkages for a more limited purpose, to suggest that this kind of projective identification itself significantly shapes the conception of a social relationship. The claims of retarded people may owe their recent public visibility and salience to widespread (and newly intense) fears among mentally normal people about personal independence and vulnerability. From these fears alone, a conception of a relationship can occur in the minds of mentally normal people regarding even the most profoundly, the most remotely uncommunicative retarded person. Indeed, the very remoteness of this person can feed the image of a relationship that arises from a belief and fear that interpersonal isolation is a characteristic affliction of our time.

This troubling image of retarded people can have a

paradoxical impact. The fear that lies behind this image can lead those gripped by it to deny its force in their own minds, to wish that they could conquer the fear by banishing the imagined embodiment of that fear. This impulse to isolate and even to abuse the embodied expression of one's own fears can take many forms. The history I sketched earlier regarding the origins and expansive use of isolated residential institutions for retarded people is one such form. But whatever social form this impulse takes, its underlying implication is the same. In one sense this effort to banish retarded people is a kind of warfare with them—often waged with extraordinary brutality, as the history of residential institutions testifies. But in a related sense, those who wage this brutal warfare are also at war with themselves. They are not only battling retarded people; they are fighting against, running away from, that part of their own minds that suggests a common identity with retarded people. This effort to banish retarded people—to sever all imaginable relationship with them—is thus an exhausting pursuit because it has no end; it cannot be achieved but only endlessly pursued. This pursuit harms its retarded victims of course. But it is also paradoxically experienced by the non-retarded perpetrators as a self-inflicted wound—an injury that only adds to their fury and frustration. This endless effort to banish retarded people, to deny any common bond with them, thus in itself feeds a viciously escalating circle of fear, hatred and brutalization.

If all of this is true, then the question of how to interrupt this escalating cycle is of considerable social importance. The question is important, moreover, not simply to save its retarded victims from the brutal consequences of this cycle. The question is equally important in order to save the non-retarded perpetrators from their own self-inflicted injuries, from the warfare they are waging against themselves. If this warfare could be ended, retarded people would benefit of course. But everyone would benefit because each could be led to accept his own vulnerabilities, his own fears, his own sense of common identifications with retarded people, rather than endlessly and exhaustingly running from them. All of this social benefit, this new-found social peace and inner psychological harmony, could follow—*if* this hypothesis is correct.

I stated earlier that I cannot prove the truth of this hypothesis. But it seems plausible to me. And it seems potentially worthwhile and important for us, as a society, to explore in some systematic fashion whether this hypothesis is true, whether the benefits that I see are truly available to us if we admit that retarded people and mentally normal people are inescapably members of the same human community and if we act accordingly to acknowledge that communal relationship.

Here, in this testing process, is the special role and special obligation that I see for judges in our society. I do not have in mind here the conventional conception of judges as impartial fact-finders. I do not envision a fact-finding trial at which experts will testify to the truth or falsehood of the social psychological forces I have sketched, and a judge will then make a definitive decision. The basic question is not whether some federal judge, or even whether all federal judges including the Justices of the Supreme Court, believe the truth of these propositions. The basic question is whether all of us—judges and citizens alike—can test for ourselves whether these forces are at work in our own minds, whether we have the psychological (and I would say the moral) strength to acknowledge these forces and act accordingly. No judge—no one at all—can authoritatively decide the truth of this proposition for another person. A judge can, however, preside over a social process which will lead all of us to explore its possible truth, to consider it as a serious possibility, and to deny its truth, to find it false, only after prolonged and intensive deliberation.

This is a somewhat unconventional view about the role of judges in our society—or at least a view that is not yet clearly understood or widely accepted. The more conventional view is that on questions of individual rights, such as the constitutional rights of retarded people, judges announce the truth—the true meaning of the Constitution, that is—and the rest of us are obliged to obey. But this view seems simplistic and ultimately wrong to me. I have a different view. In order to set out a cogent argument for my view, I want to turn for the remainder of this essay to an example—a precedent, if you will—that in itself is not usually invoked in discussions about judicial conduct in our society. The example is in the New Testament and specifically in the parables taught by Jesus.

It is of course possible and plausible to invoke the parables, and the New Testament generally, as authoritative support for the hypothesis I set out in the first part of this lecture—the hypothesis that all people, retarded and mentally normal alike, are members of the same community and that, no matter how fervently some people want to deny this universal brotherhood, it is a deep and inescapable truth. But it is not my purpose to invoke the parables for this substantive evidentiary purpose. I mean instead to examine the methodology of the parables—to explore the way that Jesus undertook to teach this lesson of universal community rather than to consider the truth or falsehood of the lesson. I want to focus on the methodology of the parables because once we have identified the distinctive characteristics of that methodology we will then see how this same methodology is available to judges in the secular realm, and we should also see reasons that oblige judges to use this pedagogic methodology regarding the question whether an inescapable communal relation exists between retarded and mentally normal people.

To pursue this purpose, I will consider just one parable at some length: the parable of the prodigal son from Luke 15. This parable has special relevance to the issues posed in the lawsuits regarding institutional placement of retarded people and, in particular, the question whether family members or community residents generally are obliged to accept (what appear to them as) extraordinary financial and emotional burdens as a result of the integration of retarded people into ordinary schools and residential neighborhoods.

We all know the familiar outlines of the parable: the father divides his inheritance between his two sons; the younger son takes his share away from the family home and squanders it, then returns in abject poverty and disgrace; but the father welcomes him joyously, kills the fatted calf for a feast of homecoming and proclaims to everyone, "Let us eat and make merry; for this my son was dead, and is alive again; he was lost, and is found."

But what of the elder son and his attitude? What kind of burden did the return of this younger prodigal put on him? Why should he welcome the prodigal's return? The parable continues:

> Now [the] elder son was in the field; and as he came and drew near to the house, he heard music and dancing. And he called one of the servants and asked what this meant. And [the servant] said to him, "Your brother has come, and your father has killed the fatted calf, because he has received him safe and sound." But [the elder son] was angry and refused to go in. His father came out and entreated him, but he answered his father, "Lo, these many years I have served you, and I never disobeyed your command; yet you never gave me a kid, that I might make merry with my friends. But when this son of yours came, who has devoured your living with harlots, you killed for him the fatted calf!" And [his father] said to him, "Son, you are always with me, and all that is mine is yours. It was fitting to make merry and be glad, for this your brother was dead, and is alive; he was lost, and is found." (Luke 15:25-32)

The parable ends here; we are not told whether the elder brother was persuaded by his father's injunction to join in the rejoicing. But this, it seems to me, is the crucial aspect of the story. Should the elder brother rejoice? And why? Is it because the father has *ordered* him to rejoice, has invoked his superior authority? And is the further implicit message that Jesus in telling the parable has invoked his extraordinary authority, his divine authority, to establish the correctness of the father's command that we all should rejoice?

But how does anyone *order* rejoicing; grudging acquiescence, perhaps, can be ordered, but not joy. Yet it is joyfulness, merrymaking, that the father enjoins. He cannot expect the elder son to comply—to feel joy, to "make merry and be glad"—unless his words have struck a resonant chord, unless they touched a deeper feeling already in the elder brother's heart, a feeling that this younger son, this unworthy prodigal, was in fact his brother—his brother whom, in spite of everything, he did love; who was "dead, and is alive; [who] was lost, and is found"; so that the elder brother also finds joy in his heart that, initially and from a distance, when he was "in the field," he had not recognized in himself.

Perhaps the elder brother did not feel this; perhaps he never would join in the general rejoicing. The parable tells us nothing of this; it leaves the question open (quite pointedly so, I believe). What we do know from the parable is that the father's authority is insufficient to obtain the result he wants. All that the father's authority can command—but this it clearly can command—is a hearing for this point of view. The father can command that the elder son *listen* to the lesson but not that he obey it. And this is the heart of the methodology of the parable.

Jesus said this explicitly to his disciples. Matthew recounts that Jesus explained, "This is why I speak to them [the crowds of people who flocked to him] in parables, because seeing they do not see, and hearing they do not hear, nor do they understand." Jesus then invoked Isaiah's prophecy in the Old Testament—which, he said, had now been fulfilled—that "this people's heart has grown dull, and their ears are heavy of hearing, and their eyes they have closed, lest they should perceive with their eyes, and hear with their ears, and understand with their heart, and turn for me to heal them." (13:13, 15). Thus Jesus meant by the parables to open people's hearts so that they could understand what is already there but had become inaccessible, "closed," "dull" to their senses. His authority did not compel obedience; it commanded a hearing.

This is also the implicit underlying message of Christ's weakness. He had no force, he had no troops to command obedience. He has only the Word—his words—and his capacity to command a hearing for those words.

In all of this I find a parallel with judges today in our society. Their authority is not divine, of course. But it is, I think, appropriate—it is far from sacrilege—to suggest that the source of judges' authority in our society is a secular equivalent of a divine force—the Constitution as the founding document (in our beginning as a national community, this was our Word) and the remote, black-robed and sanctified role of judges in safekeeping this special document. And, as specially sanctified as this role is in our society, judges are also extraordinarily weak in their direct power to command secular force. The armed forces are under the command of others in our society—the President as Commander-in-Chief and the Congress as the controller of the purse. Judges only speak to these powerful authorities to tell them their duties under the Constitution. Judges cannot directly command obedience; they can only command attention—so that their words will be heard but not necessarily followed.

This is the same power that Jesus invoked in his parables—the only power he truly invoked, as I read the gospel. Jesus used this power in the parable of the prodigal son and in others (the Good Samaritan, the lost sheep and shepherd, for example) to teach the lesson of the universal brotherhood of man, the indissolubility of communal relations in the kingdom of God. Secular judges may have a similar power to command attention; but here we must face a further question. Why should judges use this attention-commanding power to teach the same lesson of universal brotherhood that the biblical parables taught? Or, to put the question in a more complicated but I think analytically correct way, why is it not a proper lesson to teach that each person must be free to refuse to engage in relations with others who are regarded as making excessive, unfair, unworthy demands? Why is it not a proper application of the lesson of universal community, at least in a secular society, to say that everyone must respect the autonomous rights of others to withdraw from relations?

Can the answer to this question, for our national community, be found in the Civil War? I think not—at least not directly. The war was fought to preserve the Union and to deny the right of some members of the community to withdraw at will—that is true. But the lesson we can draw from this war is uncertain, ambiguous. The cost imposed by the war in lost lives, in persistent bitterness afterward, and in other ways seemed so excessive at the time that the abolitionist cause was directly abandoned and the principle against the right of secession was undercut by the widespread acceptance and Supreme Court ratification of racial segregation—of an implicit secession from relations between blacks and whites.

Brown v. Board of Education reversed both of these results. But we cannot confidently say that *Brown* has conclusively resolved the question, even regarding race relations, whether blacks and whites are free to refuse any relationship with one another, whether they are free to deny the existence of common community between them. *Brown* appeared to stand against this proposition, but we may be in the process today of abandoning it just as we abandoned it in the generation that followed the Civil War. And for the same reason: because the costs of communal relations appear excessive, at least to one party—recessive and fearful, filled with apparently unresolvable conflict and violent potential. We may in race relations today be drawing distinctions between some blacks and whites who share common ground, on the one hand, and others who are divided by residence, income, family structure, and prospects for employment and who, by this viewpoint, have so little in common that they are not members of the same community. This same kind of line drawing is currently offered by some as a way for thinking about relations between mentally retarded and normal people—the idea that at least some retarded people lack sufficient indicia of human status to be included within a universal conception of human community.

I do not think we can conclusively resolve the question whether this kind of line drawing between retarded and normal people, or between blacks and whites, is permissible in our society under our Constitution and our national experience. The Civil War and the Civil War amendments to the Constitution have relevance—but inconclusive relevance. And there is another tradition that seems to favor the secessionist principle—a tradition that the white Southerners invoked in 1860 when they claimed the right to withdraw from the Union. That tradition can be drawn from the events that led to the founding of the country as an act of secession from Great Britain, in our Declaration of Independence. The very language of our hallowed Declaration has an ironic relationship to the principle of secession as it came to be expressed in black-white relations. The opening words of the Declaration have become so familiar that we have almost stopped hearing them; but listen to them again: "When in the course of human events it becomes necessary for one people to dissolve the political bands which have connected them with another, and to assume among the powers of the earth, the separate and equal station to which the Laws of Nature and of Nature's God entitle them . . . " Here was the introduction into our political vocabulary of the formula which came ironically to justify the division of blacks and whites in the South into supposedly "separate but equal" stations.

This is not the whole message of the Declaration, however, nor in my view its most important message. This is only the introductory phrase of the famous first sentence. The full sentence continues, however, to state that when the dissolution of the political bands becomes necessary, "a decent respect to the opinions of mankind requires that they [this seceding people] should declare the causes which impel them to the separation." Here is the methodological heart of the parables: the obligation to explain one's reasons, to acknowledge this much of a continuing communal relationship even though the explanation itself is offered to justify refusing any closer or more enduring ties. And with an obligation to explain comes a reciprocal obligation to *listen*—and also the possibility that persuasion will come on one side or the other, and that thereby at least a common language will emerge from this discord, a shared set of meanings. And thus there is a possibility, in this very basic way, that these discordant parties will discover or uncover or rediscover their common humanity, the ties that truly bind them together notwithstanding their many divisive conflicts.

This is the heart of the judicial role in our society as I would see it: to insist that if conflict arises, neither party quickly or automatically assume that all relations must be severed. And even if one party reaches this conclusion—that the cost of a continuing relationship is so burdensome that all ties must be broken—nonetheless that party must explain this reasoning, and be prepared at least to listen to the other party's perspective that the costs of secession are so great and that this party's need and desire for a continuing relationship are so powerful that the seceder should reconsider and affirm their enduring brotherhood. This process of explanation and justification is not simply process for its own sake. It is process with a substantive implication—that no one can or should or truly wants to dissociate himself from others without having a good reason that this other must acknowledge and respect. If carried out in this spirit, the act of secession itself can become transformed, by this very process of explanation and justification, into a celebration of common understandings, of communal obligations acknowledged and respected on both sides.

Thus the principle of individual autonomy, of the right to refuse to enter relations, need not be a repudiation of an underlying sense of community—so long as this act of refusal is seen as carrying an obligation to explain, to justify, to debate for as long as the other party insists on the injustice and wrongfulness of this act of secession. This is the one basic underlying communal bond that I believe judges in our society should command. Without this bond between us, we have no common language, no community of discourse—and no way to talk meaningfully about rights or mutual obligations, even the obligation peacefully to respect one another's wishes to be left alone. Without this basic bond of persistent obligatory dialogue, each of us is truly alone and defenseless, destitute in our isolation.

This is not, however, the vision which the current majority of the Supreme Court holds out; this is not the way in which Justice Rehnquist and his colleagues interpret the principle of autonomy in social relations. The current Court majority appears to read the autonomy principle as self-justifying, as a conclusive trump card and conversation-stopper. Thus, for example, when a state claims autonomy in the operations of its retardation institutions, the current Court majority appears ready to accept this claim as an absolute barrier to any further challenge or inquiry—whether in a judicial forum, or in Congress. This is the essential attitude that the Court majority, in an opinion by Justice Rehnquist, adopted in the *Pennhurst* case. This vision of states' rights and of the underlying claim for individual autonomy from relations with others, treats the simple assertion of freedom to avoid association as intrinsically justified without any need to account for, or to listen to, competing claims. And this vision of autonomy thus does not give a fair opportunity for those who might be able to persuade, to touch the hearts of those who would otherwise abandon future relations with them. Conflict between these two parties may in fact be so deep that this broader sense of community might never emerge: and so separation would come. But the current Court majority assumes this result too quickly.

Of course social resources are scarce; of course the claims of retarded and other handicapped people conflict with the claims of others to keep their scarce resources for themselves; of course there is considerable prospect that these conflicting claims will end in irreconcilable and open hostility. Courts should nonetheless hold out the possibility for sustained serious deliberation that these claims are not truly in conflict, that as the father in the parable suggested to his elder son, the return of these lost brothers will be an occasion for rejoicing because everyone will have regained a lost part of himself.

Courts in our constitutional scheme can play a significant role in giving life to this aspiration, in repeatedly resurrecting it from apparent defeats inflicted in majoritarian political institutions. Ultimately this is the great gift that the institution of judicial review offers our society—the opportunity for a majority to undo an action whose consequences appear on "sober second thought" (as Chief Justice Harlan Fiske Stone put it) to harm the majority and the minority, the perpetrator and the victim. The majority will make good use of this gift only if, when forced to this "sober second thought," it finds more in common with the previously defeated and excluded minority than it earlier had been prepared to acknowledge. If the majority finds this, it will then seek to affirm this common ground, this communal fellow-feeling, with the previously subordinated minority. Judges cannot force this result. But by identifying the values impeached by the majority's prior action and by forcing the majority to reconsider its action in the light of those values, judges can lead the majority toward embracing this result.

This is what Judge Broderick did in ordering that the Pennhurst institution be closed and that ordinary communities must make room for—that they must welcome—retarded people in their residential neighborhoods, in their schools, in their community service facilities. And this is why the Supreme Court was wrong, why it should have affirmed Judge Broderick's order in the *Pennhurst* case. The communities may of course reject Judge Broderick's order, and he has no effective power to enforce it on them. But he was forcing them to consider—to explore seriously and intensively—whether they *truly* wanted to reject retarded people. And he was thus forcing them to consider the possibility that if they do reject these people they are rejecting part of themselves.

Let me illustrate this same pedagogic process by returning to biblical exegesis. What I have ascribed to Judge Broderick was the ultimate pedagogic goal of the father toward his elder son in the prodigal son parable. The father invoked his authority only to demand that this son consider the possibility that he had more reason to welcome than to regret his brother's return. He left it for the elder son to discover the truth of this conclusion for himself. But though the father did not spell out the reasons, the elder son could find them if he accepted the premise that he and his brother shared common interests—that both were equally vulnerable and that neither could find a safe haven unless each was willing to embrace the other. But once he had seen this identity of interest with his brother, the elder son might also see his own true identity.

The father did not openly assert the true identity of his elder son nor does the parable explicitly reveal this for us as listeners or readers. But there are many hints that the true identity of the elder son was Cain, who had once murdered his younger brother Abel. In the Old Testament, Cain was impelled to murder after God had favored Abel's offerings of the "fat portions" of slaughtered lambs and had rejected Cain's offerings of produce. Then, Genesis recounts, "Cain was very angry, and . . . said to Abel his brother, 'Let us go out to the field.' And when they were in the field, Cain rose up against his brother Abel, and killed him." Genesis continues that God then cursed Cain to "be a fugitive and a wanderer on the earth." In the New Testament parable, the elder son was "in the field" when he first appears in the narrative and when he later complains of his father's favoritism in killing the "fatted calf" to welcome his brother. The parable thus suggests that the younger son Abel has been brought back to life—he "was dead and is alive; he was lost, and is found"—so that the elder son Cain is given the chance to end his own fugitive status and return home. But he can grasp this opportunity to repent, this chance for a "sober second thought," only if he understands and acknowledges both his true identity and the wrongfulness of his past inflictions on his brother.

The father did not force this lesson on the elder son in the New Testament parable. The lesson is hidden, embedded in the narrative of the parable. The elder son could find this lesson only if he exerted effort to search for it. But if he discovered this lesson, and saw how directly it applied to him, then he would have clear reason to rejoice at his younger brother's return, for this would now mark the end of his own wandering and permit his own safe return home.

The parable thus gives the same opportunity for repentance, for "sober second thought" regarding the fraternal infliction of harm, to which Chief Justice Stone referred in 1936 in his characterization of the function of judicial review. Like the father in the parable, judges cannot force anyone to take advantage of these opportunities. But, also like the father, judges can and must show how these opportunities for communal reconciliation might be grasped. When judges understand this lesson, they can force others to attend to its truth in the same way that Jesus commanded attention when he told his first parable, saying "Listen! . . . If you have ears to hear, then hear."

94. The Christian, Society, and the Weak: A Meditation on the Care of the Retarded

STANLEY HAUERWAS

As a meditation, this short essay neither provides comprehensive analysis nor suggests all the ethical issues raised by the care of the retarded. The arguments presented here are not designed to satisfy those skilled in ethical and theological matters. This is a personal attempt by one weak Christian—who incidentally happens to be a theologian and ethicist—to understand what it means to live in a world peopled by those born retarded.

Therefore this is not written for everyone; it is written for men and women who find themselves both Christian and confronted by the retarded. Those who do not share the Christian conviction may find what I say here at best incredible and at worst morally irresponsible. For some, including many Christians, the fact that unbelievers will stumble over the Christian perspective is a decisive argument against any attempt to understand the obligation to care for the retarded from a "narrowly" Christian viewpoint. There seem to be at least two reasons for this reluctance: (1) Christians are increasingly aware of their obligation to avoid the scandal of the inhumanity and self-righteousness often associated with those who claim special "religious" obligation; and (2) Christians feel a duty to serve the needy; in a pluralist society, this seems to entail downplaying our differences in order to join in a common effort for human betterment. Thus, in the interest of a good society, Christians impressed by the bad faith of our own society have tended to write their ethics from a broadly humanistic perspective; thereby, they hope to be able to formulate for institutional structures clear policy entailments that all men of good will can jointly pursue.

Even though I am not unsympathetic to every aspect of this style of ethical reflection, I do not think it adequately permits the Christian to articulate his obligation to care for the retarded. For the humanism which the Christian accepts in the name of the good society all too quickly seduces him into accepting the good which is humanly possible rather than the good we must do as Christians. Thus, in the name of humanity we begin to entertain the sacrifice of the few for the many, the weak for the strong. We try to calculate the "rights" of the "retarded" against the "rights" of the "normal," or to determine who shall live and who shall die in terms of the "quality" of their lives. Moreover, by accepting the humanism of the day, Christians betray their unique contribution to the good society; this leaves unchallenged the humanist assumption that there is no good beyond what can be accomplished in this existence. The question of the care of the retarded is the most compelling example illustrating this general contention. (However, the care of the retarded in many ways is but an aspect of our care for all children. Any full attempt to treat the ethics of the care of the retarded should be a subdivision of the more general ethics of responsible parenthood. Our inability to face the retarded is but a specific and intense form of our society's distaste for children and its failure to properly respect and care for them.)

For the presence and necessary care of the retarded raise harder and deeper problems than the optimism necessary to sustain any humanism can entertain. These harder questions were best articulated for me by a young man through a song he sang during the reception of the Eucharist at the University of Notre Dame. He had written the song after a friend had shared his agony about learning to live with a retarded brother. It goes like this:

(For Rick)

I. I have a brother, forgotten child
I ask myself why? I get no answers.
Does anyone know, in God's name, why
Some are retarded?

Refrain
Give me strength to face the madness.
To be able to say there was some purpose.
Give me strength to face the madness.
Why? No it's happened.
Why? No it's happened.

II. He's older than I, I've always thought
We should have grown up together
Playing baseball, going swimming
Enjoying summer, like other brothers.

III. He does not know me, He can say nothing.
I have no reasons, but I love him.
We could have been friends, learned together
I only ask, *where is he?*

(Steve Campbell)

Reprinted, with permission, from Stanley Hauerwas, *Vision and Virtue* (Notre Dame: University of Notre Dame Press, 1981), pp. 187-94.

We are seldom able to ask the questions raised by this song; they remind us too much of the fragility and ambiguity of our existence. Therefore, it is not accidental that such a song was sung in the presence of the sacrifice of the Mass. For only if such a sacrifice is good, only if such a sacrifice sustains and constitutes our own existence and the existence of the world, can we be free from our fear of meaninglessness to look honestly at our retarded brothers. The sacrifice of the Son of God affirms that our existence is bounded by a goodness we can trust; Calvary reveals that we, even the weakest among us, are valued in ways not dependent on our human purposes and strengths.

The God we Christians worship is the God of the sacrifice, the God of weakness and suffering, who draws us to his table not by coercive power but by sacrificial love. Such love is formed by a weakness that is not of this world. God's weakness is strong enough to resist the temptation to be just another (more subtle) method of controlling others. For we know from our experience that as men we cannot even will to be weak without using that weakness to gain power over another person; this power is even more destructive than force since it has the form of a renunciation of power that controls completely since it does not appear to control at all. But the weakness of God is no sham; this is fully manifest in the absolute commitment which leads him to become a man and to suffer even to dying on a cross. Such weakness lures us from our pretentious attempt to make our lives meaningful through power and violence; it draws us to trust in him who has suffered much in order to make peace possible for us.

In his weakness, God comes to us not to dominate in the name of the good, but to serve in the reality of goodness, to reveal the nature of the good. Jesus did not come with new political alternatives in the sense that Caesar or those that opposed Caesar would understand; he came proclaiming a new Kingdom where men would share in the very life of God. He came not to the rich and the powerful, but to the poor, the weak, the dying, and the sinner. Through such as these the nature of his kingdom is revealed as the freedom to feed the poor and forgive the sinner. God, therefore, refused to establish himself through the violent power of this world with its many deceptions; his rule can be established only through the gentleness that comes from genuinely being weak and not just from taking the form of the weak. Only such a God could be the God of the Mass; through his Church, he continues to give himself in weakness so that his people will have the strength to renounce the power of this world.

When we have been joined to this God through this meal of weakness, we cannot get up as the same people. This meal fills us with the power to trust God and to serve the weak of the world who are his special concern. In each other, in the weak, we find Christ; like him, they love us even though they do not have the power to preserve themselves. We become transformed exactly to the extent we learn to accept this love without letting it turn to self-hate because of what it reveals of our wretchedness.

The Christian's task to care for the weak is but an aspect of his call to love God. Serving the weak in the name of man is not enough; God calls us to love and care for the weak just as He has loved and cared for us. Surely this is the force of Jesus' admonition to be perfect as his Father is perfect.

The Christian songwriter who asks "Where is he?" knows his retarded brother is in Christ, but this "answer" does not provide an easy explanation that can relieve the anxiety of the question. Rather, this answer provides the pattern of obedient love and care in conformity to the one on whom any genuine purpose in this life must be dependent. The retarded are the sign that all men have significance beyond what they can be for us—our friend, our playmate, our brother; each of us is previous and significant because his being is grounded in God's care. The retarded, the poor, the sick, are but particularly intense forms of God's call to every man through the other. Thus, God calls us to regard each other as significant as we each exist in Him, as we are each God's gift to the other.

Thus to see the retarded honestly is to remind ourselves that we cannot earn significance for our lives; it is a gift of God. In this context it makes sense to say that I must live in such a way that only one thing matters: that my life manifest God's glory. I do not gain significance by trying to relieve all suffering; that would be another form of trying to establish my power. Rather, my hard task is to learn to love this one retarded brother who can never understand the very opportunity of love he offers. From his presence I learn the radicalism of refusing to deny love and care for him; I cannot deny this care for my retarded brother even in the name of creating a better world for all "humanity" or for "my already existing family." A world so created or a family so sustained cannot be "better"; it deafens me to the call to humanity this one retarded child offers me.

Christ makes it possible for me to love my retarded brother in a way radically different from the possessive love that thrives on the need to be needed. Christ's love creates the conditions for respect of the retarded. A respect that frees us to care without stifling sentimentality. For it is sentimental love which builds the uncaring institutions where we enclose the retarded in invisibility in the name of their own good. To love the weak in Christ is to dare to free the weak from our dependency on their need. This love respects the being of the retarded so much that it is willing to allow them to experience the pain and frustration of using their capabilities to come to terms with the world. I do not need to protect my retarded brother with the smothering care that only reinforces his retardation; I can love him with the love that sustains his efforts. He knows this love will not abandon him when he has gone through the struggle to fashion a will independent of mine.

Moreover, such love reveals the perversity of those theodicies which try to save God's honor by attributing the existence of the retarded to his will. It is certainly true that the existence of such children may provide the occasion for producing much good; they call us to a fuller humanity by challenging our notions of what makes life meaningful. But these possible good fruits do not warrant the implication that God wills these children for such purposes; this would make the Lord of this world into a weak and petty monarch who would stop at nothing to get his way. Such children are not directly willed by God; rather he is the kind of God who makes it possible for them to be present among us in a nondestructive way. In their presence we learn how difficult, how terrible, and how wonderful it is to say that God is love and that his love is most perfectly revealed on a cross.

Please note that I have not attempted to base the Christian obligation to the retarded on such principles as the "right to life" or "respect for life." Such principles embody moral wisdom that the Christian has an interest in preserving, but these very principles are sometimes used to justify forms of life foreign to the gospel. But the Christian is not obligated to protect human life as if life were an end in itself. To do so would belie the affirmation that because God gives life, the existence of ourselves and others is but a relative good within his providential care for us. Divorced from this proper theological context, principles such as "right to life" tend to become ideologies supporting some men's feverish attempts to sustain their existence at all cost in preference to others. It is, therefore, the Christian's task to care for the retarded in ways that make clear that there are much worse things in this life than death.

I am aware that some will interpret my insistence on the care of the weak as a religious justification for societal irresponsibility. It seems unjust to argue such care of the retarded in a society with so many needs. For example, in an article discussing the genetic aspects of therapeutic abortion, Dr. James Neel describes the tremendous and exorbitant cost to society that the care of the retarded and other genetically deficient children entails. Moreover, despite this expenditure, these children can have only a "very marginal performance in our complex society. While I do not for one moment wish to place a price tag on a human life, I cannot help wondering how that same sum spent on normal children might advance the interests of society." ("Some Genetic Aspects of Therapeutic Abortion," *Perspectives in Biology and Medicine,* Autumn, 1967, pp. 133-134.)

Dr. Neel's question is not unfair. It is not inhuman; the question embodies much humanness and charity. But it is a charity run wild and gone crazy because it is unable to totally relieve the world of its suffering. This charity tries to join hands with the powers created by men; thus it is willing to destroy some in the name of the "quality" of life. This charity no longer has the patience to attempt to act justly in a world racked with suffering. This charity blinds itself to the existence of the one retarded child in the name of a better way of life for the many; but this way of life can only be empty if it fails to meet the needs of such a child. Neel's question assumes that there is nothing to live for apart from relieving the suffering we experience in this life. For all of its great humanity, it is therefore a godless question.

It is not a question we can contemplate as Christians. For the Lord who spreads his table before us requires more than this question even envisions. The Christian's duty is to care for the weak, and no limits can be placed on that demand. The Christian can hold nothing back in his care for the weak; he may even have to sacrifice his dream of "advancing the interests of society." If the Christian must sacrifice even his own life so that the weak may be cared for, he will do so; for he does not live as if he were placed on earth to exist forever. The Christian cares little for existing; his aim is to learn to live. Nor must he care for others as if their care were but a means to the existence of an even-higher quality of the human species. The Christian's care for the weak embodies no grand humanistic vision, but only the idea that regardless of its accomplishments, no society that fails to care for retarded will be worthy or humane. It is just this kind of vision that exposes the sinful and power-hungry pretensions we hide behind our claims to serve others in the name of humanity. No such humanity exists except as it is found in a child who must struggle to speak his name.

We Christians must admit that we have hesitated to recognize this demand plainly, because we know how unfaithful we have been to it. We have tried to help the poor and the weak through the philanthropy of thanksgiving baskets or government programs, programs which do not require us to give of ourselves. We have deluded ourselves that opposing the repeal of abortion laws was sufficient even though we were unwilling to sacrifice to meet the needs of the child born in poverty. We have so trapped ourselves through our bad faith that we eagerly grasp the latest technique that does some good as if it expressed the full demand of Christ. By so doing we buy cheaply into the reigning humanism; we turn the uncompromising Christian demand to love all men into the possibility of being kind and helpful to some men. And Christians wonder why men no longer think belief in God relevant to learning to live in this life! Only as Christians refuse to avoid the existence and care of the retarded will men realize faith makes a difference. For we have failed to realize how radical our position is for even though we help the retarded we do not embody the implications of that kind of help for our total existence. To genuinely support the care of the retarded as Christians is bound to put us in much greater tension with our society than we now envisage.

It is therefore the Christian's task and the Church's responsibility to provide care for the retarded beyond what is considered to be "socially responsible" at the time. For in its faithful worship the Church provides the vision of existence within which we can articulate our obligation to care for others; this clarity of vision is radically different from the blindness produced by our attempts to avoid self-hate. Only thus will we be able to admit that it is our own uncare and self-assertion which often produce the retarded (environmental retardation is more prevalent than genetic), yet such knowledge need not force us deeper into the defenses of our self-interest. For the demand of Christian love can be radical exactly because it frees the self from defensiveness; we are freed from the necessity of creating and sustaining the significance of our own lives.

What I have said does not mean the Christian must refuse to support what can be done through the wider society; it does mean he must recognize that the demands laid on a member of the human species or a citizen of a nation are not the same as the demands laid on him as a member of the church. It seems a trivial observation that the church and Christians feel deeply at home in the civilization created by them. But I suspect that the more Christians consider the fundamental issues raised by the care of the retarded, the stranger they will feel as they go about amid the glories and the ruins of their own building. As we live with such strangeness, perhaps we will be better able to comprehend and love those who exist as strangers among us; they cannot understand as we understand, but these retarded brothers are no less members of God's kingdom.

Chapter Eighteen
RESEARCH AND EXPERIMENTATION

Introduction

After the Second World War the world was horrified to learn that Nazi physicians had conducted experiments upon human beings against their will. Jews, gypsies, and others were subjected to painful and often lethal experiments, ostensibly for the sake of information useful to the war effort. Many were outraged and disappointed that physicians had taken part in these experiments. Physicians are supposed to have the special interest of patients in mind, but these doctors used the patients for their own or other's purposes. In reaction to this Nazi activity, the Nuremberg Code was published in 1946, a declaration in which some minimal protections were proposed for human beings who were experimental subjects.

The real-life horror stories about the Nazi research took their place in our cultural tradition alongside the fictional horror stories of the "mad scientist" who creates a human being and tries to keep his creation under his will. Knowledge can be power, and power can be used unjustly. Knowledge can also be costly, and the costs can be distributed unfairly.

Experimentation upon human beings has always raised many troublesome questions. One question, surely not the least important, is the identity of the physician. In the past, physicians were expected to put the patient's interests before their own acquisition of knowledge. Experimentation seemed a violation of the physician's commitment to the patient. Things are not nearly so simple today, though. The modern scientific physician demands not only that experimentation may be done but that it must be done. Only through experimentation can we evaluate new therapies and insure that only truly effective therapies make their way into the marketplace and into the hands of physicians. Too often in the past, unproven therapies have been brought forward with great fanfare, only later to be found of little or no therapeutic value. The rigorous demands of experimentation would limit all of this potential harm to patients. Even assuming that the experimentation is done for a beneficial purpose, a conflict is always possible between the need to advance knowledge so that many patients may benefit and the need to help *this* patient at the lowest possible risk.

To what is a physician loyal? Experimentation only exacerbates a problem already present in patient care today. Numerous commentators have noted how fragmented modern medical care has become. Specialist upon specialist sees the patient and often it is unclear who is in charge of the case. Experimentation simply increases the possibility of that fragmentation of care, not only in terms of the potentially divided identity and loyalty of the physician-researcher but also in terms of the extra personnel who will be involved with the patient.

If the responsibility to benefit the patient above all else is no longer professed by all physicians or is too diffuse among caretakers, how can the patient/subject be protected? Modern technology has given physicians enormous power over patients; that power can only increase when physicians seek to use those patients for their own purposes.

This is potentially very serious because patients are so dependent upon physicians; often they acquiesce to a physician's requests out of fear of losing care or because they trust in the physician's commitment to their well-being. Now patients may wonder to whom and to what the physician is truly committed. It has been suggested by some that the only way in which patients may be protected is to insist upon free and informed consent for all experimentation. In that fashion, all patients will know what is being proposed and will have the opportunity to accept or refuse participation in the experiment.

Thus two moral imperatives confront one another. The first might be framed, "Give no untested therapy" while the second might read, "No testing without consent." It would appear that these two demands are in fact the starting point of the discussion. They state what *must* be done but they do not point up what *may* be done. The impartial perspective may be of little help at this juncture. One might urge some complex cost-benefit analysis to determine the potential good from experimentation, or one might urge that a consideration of the rights of patients would lead to a situation in which no experimentation would be done without a careful consent procedure.

If experimentation is to go forward, there are a number of important questions to be asked. The first concerns the meaning of "free and informed" consent. There have been occasions when captive populations—prisoners, children in institutions, and the mentally retarded—have been experimental subjects. There is some question about their ability to give the kind of consent necessary for participation in experimentation.

The second and related question is, "Who will have the benefits and who will bear the burdens of experimentation?" If we are not candid about this question, poor people in the wards of teaching hospitals will be the ones who will be experimented upon while the middle and upper class will benefit from the research. Hans Jonas, in his essay in this chapter, suggests an alternative approach to risk and benefit which would demand that those who have the knowledge and whose loyalty is to the experimental process be the ones who volunteer as experimental subjects. Whatever one thinks of Jonas's proposal, the discussion of the benefits and burdens of experimentation makes one point clear: it is not enough to talk about the informed consent of the experimental subject. Indeed, in some areas of human experimentation, it may not be relevant at all.

There are at least two areas in which the ethics of experimentation and other issues overlap—in behavioral research and genetic research. Here we encounter questions not only about how the research should proceed but about whether certain kinds of research should be done at all. The second of these issues revolves around the potential power over other human beings that is being developed by research in genetics and behavior control. We are not speaking of power being developed for evil purposes, such as that of the Nazis. Most troubling here is research in genetics which opens up the possibility of manipulating entire groups of people before they are in a situation where they might be able to make choices themselves. There is the possibility that one generation may attempt to determine what is "good" for future generations and so become the controller for the future.

The important point about the development of this power is that it proceeds under the umbrella of science, which is supposed to be concerned with the search for truth—"pure" research detached from pragmatic drives. It turns out that the truth sought in genetic research is often the truth that has immediate application, either in the prevention of disease or in some eugenics proposal—a different kind of truth that may be turned to self-seeking ends. The scientific inquiry might not always be as disinterested as it first appears. The knowledge that we gain today becomes the power that we can exercise over others in the future. Yet the *use* of the power might be only a consequence of the inquiry, not inherent in it; then the knowledge is both promise and threat to human flourishing. We have yet to decide whether this kind of truth is a legitimate subject of societal control in a way that the pursuit of other kinds of truth is not.

Suggestions for Further Reading

Bondeson, William B., et al., eds. *New Knowledge in the Biomedical Sciences.* Boston: D. Reidel, 1982.

Childress, James F. *Priorities in Biomedical Ethics.* Philadelphia: Fortress, 1981. See pp. 51-73.

———. "Love and Justice in Christian Biomedical Ethics." In *Theology and Bioethics,* edited by Earl E. Shelp. Dordrecht: D. Reidel, 1985.

Fried, Charles. *Medical Experimentation: Personal Integrity and Social Policy.* Amsterdam: North-Holland Publishing, 1974.

Freund, Paul A., ed. *Experimentation with Human Subjects.* New York: George Braziller, 1970.

Lebacqz, Karen. "Controlled Clinical Trials: Some Ethical Issues," *Controlled Clinical Trials,* May 1980, 29-36.

Levine, Robert J. *Ethics and the Regulation of Clinical Research.* Baltimore: Urban and Schwarzenberg, 1981.

McCormick, Richard A. "Experimental Subjects: Who Shall They Be?" *Journal of the American Medical Association,* May 17, 1976, 2197.

Ramsey, Paul. *The Ethics of Fetal Research.* New Haven: Yale University Press, 1975.

Walters, LeRoy. "Some Ethical Issues in Research Involving Human Subjects." *Perspectives in Biology and Medicine,* Winter 1977, 193-211.

95. Vivisection

C. S. LEWIS

It is the rarest thing in the world to hear a rational discussion of vivisection. Those who disapprove of it are commonly accused of 'sentimentality', and very often their arguments justify the accusation. They paint pictures of pretty little dogs on dissecting tables. But the other side lie open to exactly the same charge. They also often defend the practice by drawing pictures of suffering women and children whose pain can be relieved (we are assured) only by the fruits of vivisection. The one appeal, quite as clearly as the other, is addressed to emotion, to the particular emotion we call pity. And neither appeal proves anything. If the thing is right—and if right at all, it is a duty—then pity for the animal is one of the temptations we must resist in order to perform that duty. If the thing is wrong, then pity for human suffering is precisely the temptation which will most probably lure us into doing that wrong thing. But the real question—whether it is right or wrong—remains meanwhile just where it was.

A rational discussion of this subject begins by inquiring whether pain is, or is not, an evil. If it is not, then the case against vivisection falls. But then so does the case for vivisection. If it is not defended on the ground that it reduces human suffering, on what ground can it be defended? And if pain is not an evil, why should human suffering be reduced? We must therefore assume as a basis for the whole discussion that pain is an evil, otherwise there is nothing to be discussed.

Now if pain is an evil then the infliction of pain, considered in itself, must clearly be an evil act. But there are such things as necessary evils. Some acts which would be bad, simply in themselves, may be excusable and even laudable when they are necessary means to a greater good. In saying that the infliction of pain, simply in itself, is bad, we are not saying that pain ought never to be inflicted. Most of us think that it can rightly be inflicted for a good purpose—as in dentistry or just and reformatory punishment. The point is that it always requires justification. On the man whom we find inflicting pain rests the burden of showing why an act which in itself would be simply bad is, in those particular circumstances, good. If we find a man giving pleasure it is for us to prove (if we criticise him) that his action is wrong. But if we find a man inflicting pain it is for him to prove that his action is right. If he cannot, he is a wicked man.

Now vivisection can only be defended by showing it to be right that one species should suffer in order that another species should be happier. And here we come to the parting of the ways. The Christian defender and the ordinary 'scientific' (i.e. naturalistic) defender of vivisection, have to take quite different lines.

The Christian defender, especially in the Latin countries, is very apt to say that we are entitled to do anything we please to animals because they 'have no souls'. But what does this mean? If it means that animals have no consciousness, then how is this known? They certainly behave as if they had, or at least the higher animals do. I myself am inclined to think that far fewer animals than is supposed have what we should recognise as consciousness. But that is only an opinion. Unless we know on other grounds that vivisection is right we must not take the moral risk of tormenting them on a mere opinion. On the other hand, the statement that they 'have no souls' may mean that they have no moral responsibilities and are not immortal. But the absence of 'soul' in that sense makes the infliction of pain upon them not easier but harder to justify. For it means that animals cannot deserve pain, nor profit morally by the discipline of pain, nor be recompensed by happiness in another life for suffering in this. Thus all the factors which render pain more tolerable or make it less totally evil in the case of human beings will be lacking in the beasts. 'Soullessness', in so far as it is relevant to the question at all, is an argument against vivisection.

The only rational line for the Christian vivisectionist to take is to say that the superiority of man over beast is a real objective fact, guaranteed by Revelation, and that the propriety of sacrificing beast to man is a logical consequence. We are 'worth more than many sparrows',[1] and in saying this we are not merely expressing a natural preference for our own species simply because it is our own but conforming to a hierarchical order created by God and really present in the universe whether any one acknowledges it or not. The position may not be satisfactory. We may fail to see how a benevolent Deity could wish us to draw such conclusions from the hierarchical order He has created. We may find it difficult to formulate a human right of tormenting beasts in terms which would not equally imply an angelic right of tormenting men. And we may feel that though objective superiority is rightly claimed for man, yet that very superiority ought partly to *consist in* not behaving like a vivisector: that we ought to prove ourselves better than the beasts precisely by the fact of acknowledging duties to them which they do not acknowledge to us. But on all these questions different opinions can be honestly held. If on grounds of our real, divinely ordained, superiority a Christian pathologist thinks it right to vivisect, and does so with scrupulous care to avoid the least dram or scruple of unnecessary pain, in a trembling awe at the responsibility which he assumes, and with a vivid sense of the high mode in which human life must be lived if it is to justify the sacrifices made for it, then (whether we agree with him or not) we can respect his point of view.

But of course the vast majority of vivisectors have no such theological background. They are most of them naturalistic and Darwinian. Now here, surely, we come up against a very alarming fact. The very same people who will most contemptuously brush aside any consideration of animal suffering if it stands in the way of 'research' will also, on another context, most vehemently deny that there is any radical difference between man and the other animals. On the naturalistic view the beasts are at bottom just the same *sort* of thing as ourselves. Man is simply the cleverest of the anthropoids. All the grounds on which a Christian might defend vivisection are thus cut from under our feet. We sacrifice other species to our own not because our own has any objective metaphysical privilege over others, but simply because it is ours. It may be very natural to have this loyalty to our own species, but let us hear no more from the naturalists about the 'sentimentality' of anti-vivisectionists. If loyalty to our own species, preference for man simply because we are men, is not a sentiment, then what is? It may be a good sentiment or a bad one. But a sentiment it certainly is. Try to base it on logic and see what happens!

But the most sinister thing about modern vivisection is this. If a mere sentiment justifies cruelty, why stop at a sentiment for the whole human race? There is also a sentiment for the white man against the black, for a *Herrenvolk* against the non-Aryans, for 'civilized' or 'progressive' peoples against 'savage' or 'backward' peoples. Finally, for our own country, party, or class against others. Once the old Christian idea of a total difference in kind between man and beast has been abandoned, then no argument for experiments on animals can be found which is not also an argument for experiments on inferior men. If we cut up beasts simply because they cannot prevent us and because we are backing our own side in the struggle for existence, it is only logical to cut up imbeciles, criminals, enemies, or capitalists for the same reasons. Indeed, experiments on men have already begun. We all hear that Nazi scientists have done them. We all suspect that our own scientists may begin to do so, in secret, at any moment.

The alarming thing is that the vivisectors have won the first round. In the nineteenth and eighteenth century a man was not stamped as a 'crank' for protesting against vivisection. Lewis Carroll protested, if I remember his famous letter correctly, on the very same ground which I have just used.[2] Dr Johnson—a man whose mind had as much *iron* in it as any man's—protested in a note on *Cymbeline* which is worth quoting in full. In Act I, scene v, the Queen explains to the Doctor that she wants poisons to experiment on 'such creatures as We count not worth the hanging,—but none human.'[3] The Doctor replies: 'Your Highness / Shall from this practice but make hard your heart.'[4] Johnson comments: 'The thought would probably have been more amplified, had our author lived to be shocked with such experiments as have been published in later times, by a race of men that have practised tortures without pity, and related them without shame, and are yet suffered to erect their heads among human beings.'[5]

The words are his, not mine, and in truth we hardly dare in these days to use such calmly stern language. The reason why we do not dare is that the other side has in fact won. And though cruelty even to beasts is an important matter, their victory is symptomatic of matters more important still. The victory of vivisection marks a great advance in the triumph of ruthless, non-moral utilitarianism over the old world of ethical law; a triumph in which we, as well as animals, are already the victims, and of which Dachau and Hiroshima mark the more recent achievements. In justifying cruelty to animals we put ourselves also on the animal level. We choose the jungle and must abide by our choice.

You will notice I have spent no time in discussing what actually goes on in the laboratories. We shall be told, of course, that there is surprisingly little cruelty. That is a question with which, at present, I have nothing to do. We must first decide what should be allowed: after that it is for the police to discover what is already being done.

Notes

1. Matthew x. 31.
2. 'Vivisection as a Sign of the Times', *The Works of Lewis Carroll,* ed. Roger Lancelyn Green (London, 1965), pp. 1089-92. See also 'Some Popular Fallacies about Vivisection', *ibid.,* pp. 1092-1100.

3. Shakespeare, *Cymbeline,* I, v, 19–20.
4. *Ibid.,* 23.
5. *Johnson on Shakespeare: Essays and Notes Selected and Set Forth with an Introduction by Sir Walter Raleigh* (London, 1908), p. 181.

96. The Necessity, Promise and Dangers of Human Experimentation

EDMUND D. PELLEGRINO

"In every field of twentieth century development there comes a point of technical perfection beyond which man finds himself in the shadow of his own creations."[1]

New technologies by their very nature must challenge existing social values and institutions. The opening up of new options for human action must call the old ones into question. As man gains control of the process of change, he is forced to decision on the ends to which he will direct his own future.[2]

Characteristically, the enthusiasm for innovation far outstrips the conscious decision-making essential to the humanization of technologic advances. Society is inevitably forced to a more conscious choice between what *can be* done and what *should be* done. It is also required to reexamine the dominant assumption that human happiness will be had if only we can apply more technical knowledge to human problems.

These tensions are exquisitely epitomized in modern medicine which owes its prodigious advances to the avid absorption of technology. For here, in the most human of sciences, technology has forced two profound transformations, the consequences of which are still to be understood. First, the physician is called upon increasingly to be a scientist as well as a helper of the patient, and second, medicine itself promises to become increasingly an instrument of applied biology and sociology.

These two trends are altering the traditional character of the relationship of the physician to the person and to society. They impart the features of a technological transaction to what must remain an intensely human relationship and they intrude the features of a public and social transaction into what must also be a personal and individual confrontation. These transformations challenge the ethical codes and values as well as the decision-making mechanisms which have served medicine for so long.

From *Experiments with Man: Report of an Ecumenical Consultation,* World Council of Churches Studies no. 6, ed. Hans-Ruedi Weber (New York: Friendship Press, 1969), pp. 31–56. Published by the World Council of Churches and used by permission.

Human experimentation is a special case of this conflict of technological possibility and human values. Indeed, it is the paradigm of the larger question of how man deals with the value decisions induced by technologic progress and the powers it confers. Examination of the questions raised by the use of human beings to advance the technology of medicine and biology can illumine the larger question of how best to institutionalize and socialize the decisions which will determine if new technologies are truly to serve human ends. It is within this larger frame that we must examine the necessity, promise and problems of human experimentation.

Emergence of the Physician as Scientist

Medicine has advanced through most of its history by careful observation of largely uncontrolled and fortuitous clinical events. Through rigorous reasoning and careful attention to the rules of evidence, the natural history of diseases was formulated from these observations. Our vast storehouse of clinical wisdom was collected in this way by consummate clinicians from Hippocrates to Sydenham and Osler to the present day. Such experiments as occurred were the "experiments" of nature, perceptible as such to only the most astute clinicians. Deliberate and controlled modification of the clinical situation as part of an orderly advance of knowledge was virtually unknown.

As long as the acquisition of knowledge remained thus essentially observational, the physician did not face a conflict in values or functions. But, as soon as the spirit of experimental science becomes a part of medicine, the doctor is faced with serious conflicts in his role as helper of other humans in distress. Experimental science means the collection of verifiable, quantifiable data in a controlled way and usually to test an hypothesis derived from prior observations and reasoning. In clinical medicine, this requires that the patient become a subject as well as a patient and the doctor must simultaneously be a scientist as well as a helper. In addition to being an ailing person, the patient becomes a complex experimental system in which multiple variables must be controlled and manipulated if valid information is to be derived.

The patient-subject and physician-helper dichotomies are an irremediable complexity of human experimentation and the distinctions between them must not be blurred out. They imply an essential tension in values and a paradox of function and roles for both doctor and patient. Individual good is necessarily counterpoised against the common good; scientific values are placed against personal and human values; and, even the rights of future generations are potentially compromised by the rights of those living today. The expectations of society can only be fulfilled by a critical ordering of these conflicting values in such a way that experimentation on humans can be used to advance the good of man without violating his humanity in the process.

Levels of Human Experimentation

There is a continuum of ways in which humans may participate in the acquisition of useful medical knowledge, each associated with ethical questions of differing complexity. Recognizing the arbitrary nature of such divisions, it is nonetheless essential to break the continuum into a few categories.

First, is the level of unconscious and unintentional experiment which is part of everyday medical practice. Each patient possesses a personal and physiological uniqueness which is the admiration and the frustration of every clinician. Even routine treatment can become an experimental venture, since the variables are never the same and the outcome always in doubt.

A major function of scientific medicine is to reduce this form of experimentation to an absolute minimum and to make ordinary clinical decisions as rational as possible. Much of what we accept as standard practice has not been subjected to the same scrutiny accorded a new procedure. The ethically sensitive physician will keep this fact always before him and remember that the rights of his patients can be as much compromised by propagation of an accepted but untested procedure as by a new one. A clinician contributes much to medical progress if he demonstrates the dangers or inadequacies of an accepted procedure.

A second level of medical research, not necessarily experimental, is the observational alluded to above as the major source of medical advances in the past. The collation of clinical observations from charts, examination of patients, autopsy material, epidemiologic studies, tests on blood and body fluids obtained in the normal course of clinical management are examples of this type of research.

The ethical problems here are relatively simple. They involve such matters as how much additional discomfort one can ask a patient to undergo to obtain extra samples of blood, whether it is proper to impose extra days of hospitalization and expense necessary for a clinical study, whether data obtained in one situation can be used for another purpose, etc. These are important ethical questions which are not given the consideration they deserve. The dangers to the patient, however, are usually minor and the invasion of personal rights is minimal. Hence, the ethical issues are generally resolvable by a weighing of benefits and risks.

The third level of research is human experimentation properly speaking. It involves the conscious manipulation of the patient's clinical situation, altering some aspect of his management to gather information, answer some specific question or devise a new treatment. Here, the rules of scientific procedure and evidence can come squarely into conflict with the rights of the patient. Such experimentation is usually of three types:

(a) therapeutic research aimed at some benefit to the patient himself, trial of a new drug or operative procedure.

(b) experimentation designed to answer physiological or clinical questions about a disease process with results only remotely of benefit to the patient.

(c) physiological observations, assessment of drug effects on normal volunteer subjects with no personal benefit accruing to the subject, but of potential value in the general advance of medicine.

In type (a) the patient is a patient primarily and a subject secondarily. In type (b) he is a subject primarily and in type (c) the subject is not a patient at all unless something goes awry with the experiment.

There is a fourth level of experimentation which derives from the possibilities inherent in genetic engineering and it will be discussed later.

It might be well to illustrate more specifically some of the distinctions between these different levels of medical research by alluding to hypertension. In this disorder, we are interested in the nature of elevation of the blood pressure beyond certain norms set for a given population of a specific age and sex.

At the observational level of research we can study hypertension by a variety of simple non-injurious manoeuvres—measurement of the blood pressure, study of family history, life span, autopsy finds and cause of death, blood chemical findings, etc. Except for the potential invasions of privacy inherent in the use of certain details of the patient's life, there is little threat to personal rights. Much useful information has been gathered in this way on the natural history of high blood pressure.

Another level of investigation would involve attempts by drugs or operative procedures to treat the elevated blood pressure in the hope of preventing damage to heart, brain and kidney. Here, all the ethical problems of drug trials would be faced. There is potentiality of benefit to the patient, but also possibility of harm in the use of an untried drug whose toxic effects are as yet unknown.

A more complex problem is the study of the disorders of function of heart, brain or kidney in patients with hypertension. To do this, the patient is subjected to manipulations and studies which have no promise of immediate benefit to him, but would add to our knowledge of the disease. They might be helpful to others at a future date. These manipulations, like cardiac catheterization, kidney function studies or cerebral blood flow measurement carry certain risks and discomforts and, hence, pose certain threats to the rights of the patient. Even more difficult ethically is the situation in which these same studies are performed on normal volunteers with the hope of providing information of ultimate benefit to those with hypertension.

The most difficult level of research involving manipulation of genetic chemistry is still only a very remote possibility in hypertension. Yet, we do know that there is a high incidence of hypertension in certain families and, hence, some genetic defect as yet undescribed probably exists. If the biochemical genetic defect were to be described, we would wish to eradicate this defect in the fetus during pregnancy by appropriate chemical alteration of the genetic material. Even more appropriate would be prevention of the defect by altering the genetic constitution of the germ cells of mother or father, or both. The dangers of such experimentation are not at all clear. The total effects of manipulation of so delicate and so vital a mechanism as the gene and its subunits are so complex that they cannot be accurately assessed in advance.

To these legitimate forms of experimentation we can add examples of two spurious varieties—pseudo-research and unrecognized experimentation. A physician would be engaged in the former if he "tried out" a new drug on twenty-five patients in his practice, without controls of any kind and then drew conclusions on its effectiveness. The latter kind is more common. It involves, for example, accepting a new preparation or procedure for routine use in one's practice before it had received adequate evaluation for effectiveness and danger.

The Necessity of Human Experimentation

Human experimentation in practice usually poses a mixture of these several levels of ethical complexity. Each raises special questions which in the actual situation are closely intermingled and difficult to dissect free of each other. The complexities of the ethical problems and their analysis cannot vitiate the importance of continuing to develop the scientific and experimental basis of medical practice. For, lacking this, we would be compelled to indulge in unrecognized experimentation or what is worse, a variety of pseudo-research, which gives the benediction of validity to unsubstantiated conclusions.

There can be no substitute for observations in humans to obtain reliable information ultimately to be used in treating human disease. Animal experiments, comparative physiology, artificial organ systems and computer models are all useful preliminary adjuncts to prevent the premature initiation of human experimentation or the pursuit of a trivial problem. The human response to a drug or an operation must finally be assessed and in this assessment scientific and moral probity must both be preserved.

This being the case, the focal issue is a more precise definition of the conditions under which human experimentation is legitimate and the extent to which the individual can be permitted to yield up some of his rights as a person for potential benefits to himself and his fellows. This is the ground upon which physicians, moralists, lawyers, theologians and others can meet to resolve the conflicts inherent in the use of humans for individual and social good.

There are certain values essential to the moral health of the individual and of society which cannot be sacrificed without peril—the right of privacy and dignity, of informed consent, of freedom to participate in any experiment, of veracity on the part of the investigator and of justice which guarantees redress and compensation to the subject of an ill-advised or immoral experiment. The Nazi example of unprincipled experimentation on humans in the name of science or the state is still fresh in our minds and stands for ever as the extreme denial of those personal rights we must guard at all cost. A more absolute repudiation of the physician's role as helper cannot be imagined.

Yet, even the rights we regard as absolutes must be placed within a social context. Here, we have the classical ethical problem of a potential conflict of two values, both classified as good and impinging upon each other. Resolution cannot be achieved by exalting one or by complete abnegation of the other. Instead, we are compelled to a critical ordering of individual and social good to each other. This is the central ethical requirement in making human experimentation serve truly human ends. In a highly organized and complex society all rights are interdependent and few are absolute. Each right must be operationally and situationally conditioned by the social matrix within which it occurs.

We can now examine some of the dangers to personal rights which are inherent in human experimentation. Which of these can be yielded up, for what reasons, to what extent and under what scientific, social and ethical controls? Some rights endangered in all types of human experimentation are: the rights of privacy, of consent and disclosure, of life and of redress for wrong.

Dangers to the Rights of Privacy

Every person has the right to choose what parts of his interior life and personality he will expose to others and under what conditions. This right is fundamental to his dignity and integrity as a person; his social effectiveness and emotional health depend upon it. Protection of this right is a mandate in medical and other professional ethical codes. Without it the person cannot confidently enter transactions with lawyer, physician or psychologist.

The right to privacy is so intrinsic to human dignity and freedom that we can violate it only for the highest social and public purposes. In the interests of public health and safety we already permit some invasions of the right to privacy as in census-taking, registering for a passport and professional licensure. As the dependence of society upon an individual increases, even more infringement on privacy is tolerated as in security clearances, for national defense, and in law enforcement and the certification of pilots and operators of public vehicles.

In human experimentation, too, there are gradations of permissible forfeiture of the right to privacy. Clinical records, laboratory tests, x-rays, interviews, results and details of operations and sundry other data collected in the ordinary care of patients are universally used to advance medical knowledge and teaching. As long as anonymity is preserved, there is only a small danger to privacy in such activities. The use of such data is implicit and is sanctioned by society in every teaching hospital.

The problem is more complex where more specific identifying data are essential to the research such as photographs, family background and other intimate personal data. Certain examinations may be undertaken for research purposes unrelated to the needs of the patient and thus expose him to revelations he would not sanction. Specimens of blood or body secretions, biopsies or x-rays examined for research purposes unrelated to treatment constitute potential violations of privacy. The danger to privacy is still quite indirect in these situations.

The really serious threat to privacy, however, lies in behavioural research in which the patient's own beliefs and emotional responses are the subject of study.[3] The social utility of such research is hardly contestable in a world beset by individual and national social maladjustments. While the social benefits are great, the threats to privacy are equally great and sometimes very subtle. The gadgetry of an electronic age—microphones, tapes, concealed cameras, one-way mirrors, computer storage and retrieval of data, as well as behaviour modifying drugs and hypnosis—all provide serious temptations even to the scrupulous investigator. Irresponsibly used, these devices can frustrate the subject's freedom to decide what he shall reveal, to whom and for what purpose.

Even the more traditional research tools, like the interview, the psychological test, the observation and interpretation of behaviour by others often leads to unwitting revelations by the patient. In many studies deception is an essential part of the protocol and is deliberately used to unmask the subject's deeper attitudes, beliefs and fears. Unconscious or subtle deception, coercion and exploitation of the subject are constant threats and these are accentuated when the data are stored and recalled later for uses different than those originally intended. Moreover, long term storage of data makes them available to investigators who did not make the original agreement with the subject and can unwittingly violate privacy.

The ethical accommodation between the social benefits of behavioural research and the threats it poses to privacy centre on the issues of consent and confidentiality. Under conditions which guarantee understanding and free assent by the patient, the right to privacy can be forfeited for social benefit. We shall speak of the intricacies of consent more specifically later.

The assurance of confidentiality is a minimum requirement if the right to privacy is to be licitly invaded. Confidentiality must be protected as fully as the aims of the research will permit. Whenever possible the research design must incorporate anonymity. Even more important is the assumption by the responsible investigator of the personal duty to safeguard the information he collects from present and future usages which might violate privacy. Highly personal data must not be made available to other investigators without prior consent of the subject. Personal identifications with research data should be destroyed as soon as the purposes of the research have been attained.

There may well be situations in which the public interest in certain data transcends the individual right to privacy. Such situations should be unusual and the decision to violate confidentiality in such instances must be made only after the most careful deliberation and only with some definite expression of social sanction.

There is promise that part of the ethical problem of confidentiality created by electronics can be ameliorated by this same means. Newer methods of data retrieval built on special codes or even the specific voice pattern of the investigator might well be used to protect privileged data against improper use.

Public anxiety about the misuse of privileged information of all kinds is mounting. If the merits of behavioural research are to be preserved, the investigator must provide a very clear statement of his ethical code underscoring the importance of personal privacy and the conditions for its preservation. The alternative is a restrictive public response inimical to research as well as the public good.

The Right of Consent and the Responsibility of Disclosure

In a democratic society, the right to integrity of the psychological sphere contained in the notion of privacy is paralleled by the right to bodily integrity. The right to determine what shall be done with one's own body is a fundamental posit of human personality. Every medical intervention, experimental or therapeutic, carries some risk of bodily injury or discomfort and, hence, every medical intervention potentially threatens this human right no matter how promising it might be for the individual or society.

The ethical safeguards against loss of the right of privacy as well as bodily integrity reside in the investigator's obligation to obtain the consent of the subject and to disclose the information requisite to that consent. This is a complicated and vexatious subject which will engage most people who think about human experimentation. I will emphasize only a few points which, as a physician, I consider fundamental.

Consent has a variety of definitions. The most useful operational condition for consent in my opinion is the agreement on the part of the subject, the investigator and subsequent reviewers that the subject has been afforded maximum opportunity to determine what shall be done to him in every kind of medical transaction, experimental or therapeutic. In short, the subject must be a partner in the decision and the final determinant of whether he participates and under what conditions. For consent to be valid it must be free of coercion and comprehending of the dangers and alternatives as well as the benefits of the proposed intervention. Absolutely stated then, no procedure can be justified which does not achieve agreement by a subject who is free and informed.

An overly rigid and literal interpretation of this principle would impede experimentation to the detriment of both the individual and society. We face again the intersection of a fundamental human right with the need to "invade" that right in a controlled way in order to advance knowledge for the benefit of all. The right must be protected maximally while impediments to legitimate research are minimized.

An extensive array of dangers to freedom of consent is subtly intermingled in any clinical investigation. These centre usually on hidden duress or the difficulty of communicating the investigator's knowledge to a layman so that the latter can make a truly informed decision.

Obviously, in certain situations free and knowledgeable consent is impossible in infants, young children, the aged, the feeble, the unconscious or the mentally retarded. Here, consent must be delegated to some other person or agency who can act as advocate on behalf of the subject. The greatest care must be exerted in experimentation with these groups. Social utility can too easily be adduced as a reason for performing an experiment. Prior social sanction by some of the mechanisms to be described later is an absolute necessity.

Concealed coercion, often unrecognized by the physician or his subject, is a more subtle but more frequent danger to be guarded against assiduously. We have but to consider the effects on consent of such factors as the excessive awe of the unsophisticated for science, the overwhelming zeal of the investigator and his need to advance himself academically, the disproportion in technical information between investigator and subject, the peculiar susceptibility of students, prisoners, the underprivileged or the fear of loss of regard among one's peers by not "volunteering". Misplaced efforts to protect the patient from "anxiety" or to "spare" him complicated explanations can become unrecognized justifications for feeble and superficial attempts at "consent". Then, too, there are the legalistic few who use a signed permission as a substitute for full and adequate explanation.

Free consent is impossible without the chance to weigh the risks involved, the alternatives to a given intervention, the benefits to be derived and discomforts to be borne. The responsibility for disclosure of all significant information affecting the subject's well-being rests firmly on the physician investigator. Zeal for the experiment can too easily obfuscate this duty and the temptation to easy consent is an ever present threat. Even where deception is part of the experimental design as in drug trials, responsibility for disclosure still remains. The subject must be told that certain information is being withheld and its general nature identified, e.g. that some patients will get a placebo and others a drug and that he may be in either group.

I wish to express a strong personal bias in favor of total or near-total disclosure. In my own experiences, I have found few patients who did not prefer candour if delicately handled, to deception, however slight or well-meaning. Without adequate disclosure consent becomes a meaningless justification for medical interventions and an insult to the dignity of a free person.

Even prior to valid consent is the question of whether it is morally proper to ask the patient to run the risk at all. If the subject is a grievously ill patient and the new procedure or observations are designed to help him even remotely, a crude cost-benefit analysis is usually possible. Weighing knowledge of the disease, its prognosis, the utility of standard methods of treatment, patient and doctor can jointly arrive at a valid decision to run the risks. Most medical advances, including the much discussed organ replacement procedures, involve such decisions. If all the dimensions of consent are scrupulously attended to, such research need not violate the rights of the person though it may raise other social questions.

But, the really delicate situation is the one in which the experiment is designed to gain knowledge of potential benefit to others, but not to the subject as in non-therapeutic research on volunteers. Here, the issues of morality are most complex. When a normal volunteer allows himself to be infected with hepatitis virus or the malarial parasite, takes a new drug or undergoes cardiac catheterization, he exposes himself to considerable risk and discomfort with no benefit to himself.

While such experiments are necessary for the good of all, they do most sharply juxtapose the individual and social good. In such circumstances, the investigator must rigidly respect the right of the subject to full disclosure, including the fact that the information obtained may be of dubious or even trivial significance. The advance of science is too freely used as a justification for such experiments especially when uninformed subjects are used. Man can legitimately be a means to helping other men, but not a means to the mere advancement of science.

The voluntary exposure of the subject to some hazards under such circumstances appears to be justifiable. Subject and investigator are on the frontiers of exploration just as much as if they were embarking on a voyage into space. Our current system of morality permits the voluntary risking of life in battle, or in emergencies to save another's life. Is not a similar principle involved in human experimentation for the potential benefit of mankind? Provided the volunteer is not foolhardy or psychotic or under duress and the investigator has devised a significant experiment with appropriate safeguards, experiments on normal volunteers for the general good are consistent with the values we hold as individuals and as a society.

In any kind of human experimentation, with patients or well volunteers, attempts to weigh risks against benefits in arriving at consent become meaningless if the research question is trivial, the control inadequate or the investigator incompetent. The investigator cannot ask himself too often whether the experiment is worth doing, whether it has already been done adequately or whether his methods will answer the question at issue. As one reviews experimental protocols involving human subjects, it becomes only too apparent that this is an oft-neglected dimension of morality. More surveillance over experimental design is necessary if we wish to reduce our vulnerability to informed public criticism. It is certainly immoral to ask a subject to run even the slightest risk to obtain information that is redundant or trivial.

It is appropriate at this juncture as we consider the matter of consent to note some of the very powerful, but often sublimated pressures which modulate the investigator's behaviour as he seeks to obtain the consent of his subject. The clinical investigator is an academic physician whose advancement is contingent upon the quality of research he produces. His drives to make significant discoveries, to design and effect "elegant" experiments and to mimic the rigor of the physical scientist can obfuscate the small light of conscience under a cloud of justifications. The scientist, after all, shares with other humans the drives for power, glory and preferments.

Indeed, there is some basis for the fear of some humanists that scientific investigations in humans may constitute the most acute form of human "Hubris". Current widespread discussion of the necessity for ethical criteria and social sanctions for human investigations should result in reasonable constraints on these subtle temptations peculiar to the physician-scientist.

The Right of Life—A Specific Challenge

The most fundamental of human rights, the right to life, may be endangered in human experiments although this danger is usually remote. The ethical questions in these instances focus on the right of disposition of one's own body and life. The traditional limitations of this right imposed on the investigator and the subject have long been the subject of much consideration and will not be reviewed here.

There is, however, a new and specific challenge to this right which is inherent in the current experiments and therapeutic procedures involving organ replacement. A diseased vital organ in one person is replaced by one removed from another person supposedly dead. By this act, in the case of heart transplantation, for example, one person gains the privilege of life and the donor loses it. The matter is complicated by the fact that technical success is enhanced by maintaining organ viability which may mean sustaining "life" in the donor by artificial means.

The crucial danger lies in the temptation to "update" the moment of death to ensure better results for the recipient with the resultant danger of removing a vital organ from a donor still "alive". Thus, some surgeons have even suggested that in cardiac transplantation the heart of the donor should be "beating" for best results.[4] The ethical issues are clearly dependent upon a more generally accepted definition of death than is now available.

On this point some physicians are willing to define death in terms of a configuration of objective observations.[5] They base the diagnosis on such things as: total unawareness of external stimuli, absence of spontaneous muscular movements or breathing for one hour, absence of eye movements, swallowing, yawning or vocalization and loss of all tendon reflexes. When these observations are repeated in 24 hours death is diagnosed and all measures are discontinued. Other physicians, as in the "Sydney Declaration", prefer to leave the diagnosis to the "clinical judgment" of the physician and are disinclined to a more specific definition.[6]

All authorities are, however, increasingly in agreement that death is a gradual process in which there are successive steps of increasing reversibility or stripping away of boundary conditions.[7] The ethician here must depend upon the physician's expert testimony and the physician must combine ethical and scientific judgements in providing his answer. The matter is of more than academic interest since cardiac transplantation is becoming more widespread and, in one hospital at least, approaches the cost of an ordinary surgical procedure.[8]

I am of the opinion that a more specific and objectively stated definition of death is necessary for moral and legal purposes. A definition is needed which can receive social sanction and which can be used to define the boundaries of invasion of the right to life which society will permit. More importantly, it is an absolute requisite if certain types of experimentation and new forms of therapy are to be made morally tolerable. Any such definition will still need applicability in an individual case and here the physician's clinical judgement is brought into play. His burden is still a fearful one, but he can make the decision within a specific and objective framework, continually redefined and clarified by new knowledge.

The Right of Redress for Patient and Investigator

A society which expects to reap the benefits of new technologies should sanction experimentation explicitly enough to protect the subject and the investigator against the liabilities they may incur even in morally acceptable and carefully planned experimentation. The subject is in justice entitled to compensation for injury or disability he may suffer in experiments designed to benefit others. The investigator has the right to be protected against legal actions or damage to his reputation from alleged or actual injury to the subject in valid experimental situations.

Legitimate investigators are becoming increasingly sensitive to mounting public sensitivity and may be dissuaded from morally proper and important studies by fear of legal action. The investigator must not be allowed to bear the responsibility for advancing the general good alone. Hospitals, research institutions, universities must provide legal and insurance protection to the participants in legitimate research. Many technical, legal and economic issues are raised but the moral requisite for compensation seems indisputable.

Stresses on the Physician-Patient Relationship

The absorption of effective technologies into medicine and the emergence of the physician as scientist have induced stresses in the most important features of the medical transaction—its intensely personal nature. Until the emergence of scientific medicine, the physician's behaviour was dictated solely by the good of his individual patient and this was above all other considerations. The whole thrust of traditional codes of medical ethics has been to protect this right.

Clinical investigation dilutes the physician's responsibilities. His duties to science and society become admixed with his mandate to be the helper, advocate and protector of the patient. Some hold that it is unreasonable to expect the same physician to be both scientist and helper.[8] One physician, it is asserted, should be assigned the care of the patient and another the care of the experiment.

This suggestion would introduce another danger to the physician-patient relationship—that of divided responsibility. The physician in charge of the care of the patient needs the fullest understanding of the experimental protocol. Without it, he cannot act in the patient's best interest which sometimes is better served by continuing the experiment and sometimes by discontinuance. The patient will be better protected when responsibility for his care and for the experimental protocol are in the same hands. Our efforts must be directed more strenuously to preparing clinical investigators for double responsibilities as helpers and scientists. By institutionalizing the policies governing research on humans and by providing surveillance by professionals and laymen, the subtle dangers of a double responsibility can be minimized but not entirely eliminated.

The team nature of most clinical investigations is an additional factor tending to dilute responsibility. Many persons—physicians, nurses, technicians, basic scientists and non-professionals—may be involved in carrying out some part of the experimental procedure. How do we allocate responsibility equitably when something goes awry with the experiment? There must be a leader of the experimental team who can assume responsibility for its actions. It is difficult to conceive how this peculiar combination of responsibilities can be optimally fulfilled by other than a single physician—one capable of clinical judgement, scientific expertise and ethical consciousness.

There are two additional violations of the trust implicit in the physician-patient transaction which may occur. One of these is pseudo-research, in which a physician attempts to evaluate some new drug or procedure in his own practice without controls, experimental design or means for objective evaluation. The other is to be found in the unrecognized research which accompanies the use of long accepted procedures or new diagnostic methods which have never been properly evaluated. In both instances the patient is unwittingly the participant in an experiment which can serve no useful purpose and which may be useless, costly or even risky. These two spheres of "research" can hardly be dignified as scientific but they do represent a neglected realm of medical morality upon which each practitioner should periodically examine himself.

Medicine as Social and Applied Biology

We have dealt up to now with the dangers to certain individual human rights which grow out of our efforts to make medicine a more rational discipline through experimentation. More complex threats are faced when we begin to apply the potentialities of modern biology on a large scale for social purposes which may transcend individual rights. The range of possibilities grows each day as discoveries succeed each other in genetics, the behavioural sciences, immunology and sex and population biology. We can consider here only a few illustrative situations to epitomize the varieties of ethical questions we must confront even now.

Among the possibilities opened up by modern biology, manipulation of the genetic material by chemical or mechanical means is the most spectacular. It offers man the possibility of predetermining the number, kind, quality, and behaviour of present and future generations. The species for the first time could determine its own evolution. We must deal then, with compromise of the rights of the unborn or of future generations whom we shall never meet. Consent in the usual sense is meaningless.

Genetic engineering, that is, manipulation of the genetic material by chemical or physical means may be "primary" or "secondary", each type with different ethical dimensions. In the "secondary" variety some genetically induced metabolic or structural abnormality in an unborn fetus could be modified or corrected during intrauterine life for example. The experimental subject—the fetus—cannot consent but the parents can at least act as its advocates and can enjoy the privilege of free and informed consent on its behalf. Such genetic manipulation, if it can be made to yield predictable results, might be a very useful tool. It would pose the same problems as other types of experimentation in which a valid therapeutic goal is sought. A cost-benefit analysis would at least be possible since the results would be immediate enough to be studied in one generation.

A more exquisite threat to human rights is posed in "primary" genetic engineering. Here, the genetic material of individuals or groups might be manipulated in order to produce some ideal or more desirable human being in future generations. New and unparalleled freedom is thus open to the race, but new constraints would be imposed on future individuals who would have no opportunity to participate in the decision. The temptations in such human engineering are enormous for utopians all of whom have a favourite plan for the improvement of the species. We can hardly deny that the recorded behaviour of the human race is susceptible to improvement. But unfortunately, the scientific and moral deterrents to the use of genetic engineering as a solution to man's problems are formidable.

First, genetic engineering, while much talked of, is still barely a promise. Then, the predictability of a given genetic manipulation has yet to be appraised. Thirdly, we have no way of guaranteeing the wisdom of our genetic engineers.

More disturbing are the moral questions involved in usurping the rights of the unborn and imposing upon them our own version of the good life—a version our young people everywhere are already rejecting. Man's wisdom to determine the ends to which his new powers will be directed is highly questionable.

Granting the limitations of our scientific knowledge of genetic engineering, we already have potent methods of altering the number and distribution of humans. The principles of human eugenics have been known for some time. Long-term contraception is a reality. Sperm banks and thus controlled fertilization are already a possibility. The reproductive process is being brought under explicit control so that the right to procreate might be limited to those with the most favorable confluence of genes. To ensure the emergence of this "genetic aristocracy", the reproductive function might even be separated from marriage and the family. The more effective these methods become the more urgent will be the pressures to apply them.

The control of human behaviour by psychologic, pharmacologic and electronic means constitutes the penultimate threat to human freedom. It is possible experimentally to modify behaviour, change anger to pacificity, aggression to submission and increase intellectual productivity. Such potent instruments for good and evil are perhaps more dangerous than an atomic bomb. Annihilation might be preferable to certain kinds of manipulation which could divest man of the things which make him human, and uniquely a person.

The ethical questions in behavioural manipulation are of the most fundamental sort. How much diversity in personality and behaviour will society tolerate? Are the social virtues of the termitary or the ant hill sufficient to outweigh the less directed, but hazardous play of personal choices? What indeed is mind, personality and spirit? Are these realms as inviolate as we thought? Or, are they too as manipulable as the body, for what appear to be socially desirable goals?

There is little doubt that man will explore these and other potentialities inherent in the new biology. When he does so man will undoubtedly turn to the physician as the agent through whom to apply his new technology. As the physician of the future increasingly delegates his technical functions to nonphysicians, he will be drawn into a new role as a practitioner of social biology. The public will expect him to assume this role, since he has traditionally dealt with man in the totality of his existential experiences.

This role as an applied biologist will immerse the physician more deeply in ethical problems than ever before. He will be required to answer for himself as a person, and for his patients such frustrating questions as: Who shall be permitted to procreate to ensure a "better" species? Who shall determine the desirable characteristics of future humans? What physical and behavioural characteristics should be bred in and which ones bred out? How many males do we need and how many females? Who will make the policy decisions?

These are not fanciful questions given the present directions of biological investigations. A collision course seems inevitable between the physician's responsibility to protect individual and personal rights and the possible goals society may select from the expanding armamentarium of the new biology. As a practitioner of social biology the doctor will be compelled to re-examine all the assumptions which underlie his traditional relationship with the patient. If relevant guidelines are to be developed a deeper discourse than has hitherto been the case will be demanded in medical ethics. Presumptuous indeed would be the physician or the profession which attempted to solve these dilemmas alone. Medicine must enter into continuing and respectful conversations with the social and humane disciplines—law, theology, philosophy, political science. The doctor will remain the expert witness in matters medical, but his policy decisions must be modulated within a broader social frame than he has ever experienced before.

Some Implications in Philosophy and Theology

It would be inappropriate before an audience of theologians to dilate at length on some of the deeper but more important implications in human experimentation and the new biology. Yet, it may be useful as a clinician to make two points which I feel are particularly relevant.

First, it is clear that answers to the new questions posed in medical ethics must be based in a renewed inquiry into the metaphysics and ontology of man. This is the central problem of modern philosophy. We cannot hope for a final "definition" of man, but we can expect a continuing refurbishment of what we think he is and what his destiny should be. Medical thinking has been too exclusively normative and not enough ontological in its perspectives.[9]

Secondly, a few words on charity are essential. We have throughout this essay emphasized the rights of the person as they have emerged in the philosophy of the western world. The language of rights necessarily imposes certain limitations on our actions. These limitations can be ameliorated in theological discourse which deals with the possibilities of surrender of these rights voluntarily and out of love for one's fellows. Indeed, there are imaginable instances in which participation as a subject in human experiments can be regarded as a duty as well as a charitable act. It is for the physician to define the promise and dangers of experimentation in man; it is for the ethician to dissect the intersecting rights of person and society; it is for the theologian to temper their findings with the theology of charity and of duty.

Some Educational Implications

To function within the matrix I have described and to deal effectively with the newer dimensions of medical ethics the education of physicians will require considerable modification. With such powerful tools at his disposal, the doctor's ethical sensibilities and perceptions really become critical determinants of whether man will indeed fall under "the shadow of his own creations".

The physician's acts grow finally out of his personal conception of what he thinks man is and society should be. Medical education, at least in the United States, is largely technical, pragmatic and geared to the development of competence—all essential and ethically defensible goals. But, they are not sufficient to meet the ethical questions physicians face even today, to say nothing of tomorrow's problems. Too many clinical faculty members eschew discussion of critical, ethical and philosophical issues or feel that they can be pragmatically resolved. The antispeculative bias of medical education has served it well, but not sufficiently.

Fortunately, students themselves are generating pressures for freer discussion of these matters and I am certain that their interest will make medical education more responsive to social and ethical issues. Educators are examining a variety of ways to introduce ethical and social perspectives into medical education. I should like to enumerate a few of my personal preferences in this regard.

(a) "Courses" in medical ethics have been notoriously nonproductive for today's students, who are disinclined to abstract discussions. Such courses might have validity as electives in depth after a student has seen the problems in a concrete situation.

(b) The most effective means of eliciting student interest in ethical issues is to discuss them in the clinical situation, at the "bedside" and as part of his daily clinical experience. Interdisciplinary conferences, built around a specific patient with whom the student has worked, have proven in my personal experiences to be well received. This requires that theologians, philosophers and lawyers be willing to enter the clinical situation, participate in a concrete dialogue and make their points in a "give and take" atmosphere. It also requires too that clinical teachers be themselves better prepared for ethical discourse.

(c) A more formal education in ethics and philosophy should be afforded for small numbers of students who may wish to specialize in the newer questions posed by medical advances. We need a core of individuals educated in medicine and philosophy or the relevant disciplines to do scholarly work in this field, be teachers for the rest of us and provide a more effective liaison with the other university disciplines.

(d) Admission committees must seek out more applicants with a sincere interest in the social responsibilities of medicine. Premedical scientific preparation will continue to be important. But, an orientation to the social sciences and the humanities is as significant for most of tomorrow's doctors.

(e) Obviously we cannot wait solely for a new generation to improve the perceptions of physicians to these questions. Efforts along the lines I have outlined above, are urgently needed to bring the practising physician into closer contact with the social and ethic effects of his daily medical acts.

Social and Institutional Control of Experimentation

My major purpose has been to fulfil my assignment to outline the necessity and dangers of human experimentation. *Clearly,* human experimentation is a necessity; *clearly,* it threatens certain individual rights; *clearly,* in permitting it, society sanctions certain graded limitations on the absolute rights of individuals for the good of all. What mechanisms can we elaborate to assure that the partial invasion of human rights is carried out in conformity with our system of moral values and in a rational and balanced way?

I do not believe, as some of my colleagues have argued, that the stewardship can be assigned solely to the physician investigator. To do so would encourage an increasingly restrictive public policy which would restrain the responsible investigator and impede the development of judicious social sanctions for therapeutics as well as experimental medical acts.

Instead, I see the physician acting as an indispensable part of a socialized and institutionalized system, the totality of which is directed to reasonable control of the delicate ethical algebra involved in human experimentation. Let us examine briefly, the several levels of responsibility and control in this system.

1. The physician is the final instrument for attaining health aspirations of society. In human experimentation he must combine ethical science and ethical behaviour. The first safeguard, then, is his adherence to the ethics of good science which in itself can reinforce other social and institutional means for protecting the rights of patients. I refer to the mandates of good science—personal competence, careful formulation of the questions, careful design of the experiment, reliable observation, honesty in reporting results, willingness to expose one's work to peer criticism and surveillance, and willingness to explain it to the public.

Good scientific ethics will prevent the initiation of frivolous or faulty protocol. It must be combined with the strictest attention to ethical behaviour in the traditional professional sense. Medical ethical codes have recently been expanded and refined to deal more explicitly with the questions of human experimentation. They are not immutable guides but statements of ideals to be preserved. To be living documents they need constantly to be refurbished in the light of new technologies and the evolution of ethical and legal thought.

To this groundwork of unassailable scientific and professional ethics, the physician must add humanity and compassion in dealing with his subject as both work their way through the intricacies of consent, disclosure and the conduct of the experiment.

2. The next level of control is the assumption by each institution of its corporate ethical responsibility for the conduct of all research within its walls. Ethical review committees, as now required by the United States Public Health Service, must be the instruments of institutional guarantee for the rights of patients studied in universities and hospitals.

These committees have two clear functions—Firstly, the values of the community in which they reside. Thus, they define operationally the degree to which certain rights can be invaded for the common good and under what conditions. Secondly, they provide a first point of appeal for the patient who is wronged. Such committees must separate out morally trivial experiments from those which significantly threaten personal rights. In the review of protocols such committees could make on-the-spot decisions in cases of doubt within a certain measure of freedom from strict adherence to any particular code.

The membership of such committees should be widely representative, consisting of physicians and other health professionals, lawyers, theologians, and members of the educated public. They should be chosen for their sensitivity and empathy for both the patient and investigator. They must utilize relevant scientific information and enjoy some sophistication in the psychology and sociology of decision making.

Such committees must appreciate their own moral responsibilities. The members necessarily share some of the investigator's responsibilities. Careless review of a proposal is morally indefensible. The committee members thereby become abettors of an injustice and are morally and legally culpable if they do not carry out their work conscientiously.

3. The highest level of control should reside in a national or governmental body which sets the policies and the moral climate within which local committees and individuals work. This body should set long range policies, anticipate dangers and maintain proper balance between the concern for human rights and for legitimate scientific investigation. This group could act as the advocate of cultural values at the national level. It should provide social sanctions for experimentation and the legal machinery for protecting the subject and the investigator from the risks they incur. It could serve as an appeal mechanism for unusual cases or when a new technology introduces new ethical dimensions.

Lastly, a potent means of control for the whole process lies in the non-regulatory but highly essential dialogue between ethicians, physicians, sociologists, theologians on the ontological bases for the rights of man. After all, the entire process of decision making rests on a proper metaphysic of man. This, too, must undergo continuing development and refinement as biology and medicine reveal new insights into body, mind and spirit.

Responsibility exerted at each of these levels would provide a matrix for reasonable and just decision making which could simultaneously advance the social good and protect the precious rights and dignity of the individual human person.

Society, the Individual and Medicine

Our age is characterized by the most strenuous effort thus far to expand man's experiences as a free individual and a social being. A crisis between these values is inevitable, but it must not be resolved as an antinomy of individual *versus* society. Indeed, as Teilhard de Chardin has so admirably suggested, the interdependence and convergence of human life which he envisioned can presage an even more precious kind of individual life: "The socialization whose hour seems to have sounded for mankind does not by any means signify the ending of the era of the individual on Earth, but far more its beginning."[10]

Medicine, posited between the sciences and the humanities, is one of man's most potent instruments for enlarging both his individual and his social being. To serve this purpose, medicine must respond to the current challenges by creating a new unity of its scientific, ethical and social perspectives. If it does, it might become the genius of that new humanism the world so desperately needs to make technology ever the servant of human purpose.

Notes

1. P. Gascar, "Putting Technology in its Place," *World Health,* March 1968, 50.

2. E. G. Mesthene, "How Technology Will Shape the Future," *Science,* 161 (12 July 1968): 135-143.

3. O. M. Ruebhausen and O. G. Brim, "Privacy and Behavioral Research," *Columbia Law Review,* 65 (November 1965): 1184 ff.

4. Harold M. Schmeck, Jr., "Symposium Hears Transplant Plea," *New York Times,* 9 September 1968, 23.

5. Robert Reinhold, "Harvard Panel Asks Definition of Death Based on Brain," *New York Times,* 5 August 1968, 1, 35.

6. The Declaration of Sydney, *Medical Journal of Australia,* 24 August 1968, 364.

7. M. Polanyi, "Life's Irreducible Structure," *Science,* 160 (21 June 1968): 1308-1312.

8. O. Guttentag, "The Physician's Point of View," *Science,* 117 (1953): 207-210.

9. E. D. Pellegrino, "Medicine, Philosophy and Man's Infirmity." *Conditio Humana, Festschrift for Professor Erwin Straus,* Springer Verlag, October 1966, 272-284.

10. P. Teilhard de Chardin, *The Future of Man* (New York: Harper and Row, 1964), p. 47.

97.
A Jewish Approach to the Issue of "Experiments with Man"

ROLAND GRADWOHL

Any Jewish approach must take its bearings from the Tenach (the Old Testament) and its later interpretation, the extensive Talmudic writings. This source material is very meagre for our problem—as might be expected—because it does not give any concrete indications concerning experiments on human beings. Nevertheless the situation is not a hopeless one. Aided by the old maxim "*hafoch ba vahafoch ba dechola va*" ("turn it [the doctrine] round and turn it over, for everything is contained in it", *Sayings of the Fathers* V, 25) one can recognize in the biblical-talmudic view of the world and of man certain guidelines which can make a contribution to this modern problem in all its complexity. Therefore it seems advisable to begin with an outline of the basic ideas about Creation and the nature of Man and his rôle within Creation, and then to try to deduce some criteria for man's experimentation on his fellow human beings.

I. Creation

The first verses of the book of Genesis contain the decisive statements:

1. The world has been created by God, not out of a kind of original matter but—according to the Talmud—out of nothingness, *ex nihilo,* in Hebrew: *yesh me-ayin.* (It is interesting to note that the biblical account of the Creation does not begin with the creation of the primeval ocean. This is presupposed to exist already—by which presupposition one must not, however, be misled into assuming that water was the primeval matter out of which the world developed.)

2. The process of creation advanced from chaos to cosmos, from disorder to order. Order with its regularity and its pattern is the striking sign of the divine action.

3. As the account of the flood shows, this order is jeopardized. Chaos—today conjured up by atomic war—can break through again and destroy the existing order.

II. Man

1. Man, created in God's last act of creation, is the "crown of Creation", for the biblical account of Creation exhibits a certain evolutionist tendency: from the simple to the complex (plants, fishes, birds, mammals, man). "The different works of creation are related to man. Nature is not observed 'per se', but in relation to man" (Werner H. Schmidt, *Die Schöpfungsgeschichte der Priesterschaft* [The Creation Account According to the Priestly Document], Neukirchen, 1967, p. 193).

2. Man has been created in the image of God (*imago Dei,* Hebrew: *zelem elohim,* Genesis 1:27). How this expression is to be understood, has been explained for example by Friedrich Horst ("Der Mensch als Ebenbild Gottes" [Man as the Image of God], in *Gottes Recht,* Theologische Bücherei, No. 12, Munich 1961, p. 227 f.): "The notion that man is created in the image of God is not intended to say something about God—His shape, His appearance, His nature or His being; on the contrary, it is meant to express the uniqueness of man, his special human quality, as a mystery coming from God."

3. Man stands in a perennial struggle between good and evil, which results in his approaching, or falling away from, God. His most decisive task is to overcome evil. This task cannot be realized by eliminating evil but rather through a self-education of each individual man, mastering his inclination to do evil. The interpretation given by the wise men of Israel to the verse in Deuteronomy 6:5, "Love the Lord your God with *all* your heart . . . " is "Love God with *both* your desires, the good *and* the evil one" (*Midrash Sifre*).

III. Man's Role in Creation

This is characterized by the following:

1. Man, endowed with reason, can and must explore the world, for such an exploration of the created world brings him closer to the Creator and to worship Him (Psalm 19).

2. Man possesses supremacy over the earth (Genesis 1:28), but is not its owner. This is the reason for the prohibition to eat or drink blood: "Only be sure that you do not eat the blood; for the blood is the life, and you shall not eat the life with the flesh" (Deuteronomy 12:23). Man has no right to dispose of the "soul of the animal", i.e. of life in general.

3. Man's supremacy is only legitimate if it serves

From *Experiments with Man: Report of an Ecumenical Consultation,* World Council of Churches Studies no. 6, ed. Hans-Ruedi Weber (New York: Friendship Press, 1969), pp. 57-60. Published by the World Council of Churches and used by permission.

the *well-being* of the whole of creation. Based on the prohibition to cut down fruit trees, i.e. organisms which maintain life, when besieging a city (Deuteronomy 20:19, 20), talmudic law formulates the prohibition "*bal tashchit*", "do not destroy!" According to this prohibition no *experiments on animals* should be conducted which are not absolutely necessary for the progress of science.

4. The biblical prohibition to cross or mix different species of plants or animals (Leviticus 19:19) seems to be based on some notion of "nature protection": the existing species are to be preserved. Any arbitrary intervention into the natural order would be a sign of the arrogant pride of man.

IV. Experiments on Human Beings

A. Therapeutic Aspects

1. Judaism has always stressed the *responsibility of the physician* towards the patient and his duty to be conscientious. As, however, not every therapeutic attempt succeeds, the saying: "The best among the physicians is condemned to hell" was in circulation already some 2000 years ago (*Mishna Kiddushin* IV, 14). However, we must stress that ever since talmudic times the medical sciences were highly esteemed by the Jews (in the talmudic academies of Babylon, in the 3rd to the 5th centuries, medical sciences were taught—cf. I. Jakobovits, *Jewish Medical Ethics,* 3rd edn New York, 1967, p. 343). Outstanding Jewish scholars, as e.g. Maimonides (1135-1204), were at the same time acknowledged physicians.

2. The *most important principle* of therapeutic measures is the duty to preserve and protect life. Any therapeutic intervention is not only permitted but even required if it is a case of preserving life or health. If life is at stake, even for the most orthodox Jew religious prohibitions are null and void, e.g. the prohibition to work on the Sabbath, if an urgent operation is needed.

3. We know from the Talmud that *autopsies* occasionally occurred (*Babli Bechorot* 45a). We do not know, however, whether they served medical purposes. The question of autopsies is at present one of the most debated issues in Judaism, especially in Israel. The following guide-lines are advocated by orthodox Jews: autopsies are permissible for determining the cause of death, for saving a severely sick person who suffers from the same disease as the one who died, and for diagnosing cases of hereditary disease which may prove fatal, because such autopsies may make it possible to save other persons whose lives are directly threatened. (This problem is treated in detail in a symposium written in Hebrew, *Tora shebeal pe,* ed. Izchak Raphael, Jerusalem 1964 [= 5724]).

4. The question of organ transplantation has so far been disapproved by orthodox circles—contrary to liberal Judaism—in so far as they are of the opinion that a dead person (i.e. in this case the donor of an organ) must be buried intact. The final word, however, has not yet been spoken (cf. again *Tora shebeal pe*).

5. Following the principle that any person threatened by another person must be saved under all circumstances, even if this can only be done by killing the persecutor, the Talmud permits saving the life of a pregnant woman, at the expense of the foetus, even if this involves an abortion. (For more details see I. Jakobovits, *op. cit.,* p. 179 ff.) In certain cases the Talmud also allows for contraceptive measures (*Babli Jebamot* 12b). Today birth control is accepted by liberal Judaism without restriction. Orthodox and conservative circles have not yet taken a final stand.

B. Clinical Research

Whoever ventures to set up binding theses in this field is on dangerous ground. I personally think that, based on the considerations stated under III, 1-4, clinical research must be welcomed if it increases our knowledge of nature and serves mankind. All experiments, however, which by means of genetic manipulation would result in a mutation of the species "man", must be rejected from the ethical point of view as unjustifiable.

98. Basic Reflections on the Right Criteria for Experiments on Human Beings

PAUL LABOURDETTE

Any moral reflection of a Catholic theologian naturally wants to remain faithful to a certain number of principles and data which, to my mind, however, do not prevent him from being open and responsive towards all experimental findings.

This reflection is placed, right from the beginning, in the perspective of the *creation of man in the image of God.* In this perspective the Church Fathers and the Christian tradition found much depth; in my treatise, however, I shall only take up that dimension which enables man to dominate the world and to possess it, because he is first of all capable of a dialogue with God: man acts according to his own discretion, he is free. He came into this world as a land-lord, a lieutenant of God; he is like a channel of Providence.

This first biblical presupposition is taken up and reinforced, by our faith in the divinity of Jesus Christ, the son of God, made man in order to save man and to grant him to regain even more fully the image of God, disfigured by sin. For, ever since the first fall, all men, both Jews and Gentiles, are under sin from which they can only break away by their faith in Jesus Christ. Thus saved, our mortal bodies become "a temple of the Holy Spirit" (I Cor. 6:19).

As human life has been given by God, it can only be accomplished in Him: it is aimed at nothing less than eternal life, a life which implies, after the second coming of the Lord, the resurrection of the body.

Whatever were the vacillations of theological or spiritual formulations between a platonian dualism on the one side and the aristotelian affirmation of the unity of the human make-up on the other, this first set of principles fosters a great respect of man, of the whole of man, and of his life in which, at least in this world, body and spirit are indissociable.

In the light of this faith in God the Creator, a notion is set in the right perspective; a notion in which the obscure and primitive perceptions and pre-Christian attitudes can be revived, i.e. that of the sacred: Everything is sacred as a creation, for nothing stands outside this fundamental relationship to God; everything comes from Him and bears witness to Him; but at the same time nothing is more sacred than anything else.

Then, there is another understanding of the "sacred", which belongs to the realm of religion proper, and which is opposed to the profane, for here, by its symbolism, "sacred" serves to point out the sovereign lordship of God. In a religion inspired by faith, this second meaning of the "sacred" must always be kept clear and pure from any superstition, magic or taboos which a natural religiosity only too often attributes to this notion. Therefore, it is necessary to keep this distinction in mind (when one says that man, his life, his blood, his functions are "sacred") in order to preserve them from the "profanations" of human investigation.

Although the idea of creation underlines the relationship with God, it nevertheless emphasizes the *selfhood of the created being.* There is no room for either pantheism, cosmic illusion, emanatism or occasionalism. The created being exists, it acts, it causes. God does not take the place of any agents in this world. His all-comprising action is of entirely another category and cannot be discerned by any method of scientific observation. The created nature has its own laws; this has made scientific research possible.

These assertions account for the importance attributed to the notion of *nature,* understood as meaning this created being with its own resources and capacities of self-realization and enrichment. The will of God, therefore, must not be conceived as primarily a more or less arbitrary commandment, inflicted upon man from the outside, but as something which is inherent to the structure and the process of self-tulfilment. Therefore, when we speak of the *human nature,* a notion maintained by natural law, we must underline the following points:

1. It is "natural" that man has to fulfil himself. He realizes himself only by developing his own being and his God-given capacities. This is done on two different levels: (a) on that of art and technology: man is the architect of his induction and life in this world; and (b) on that of the development of his inner self: as man is free to decide in his actions he is an ethical being; his culture is necessarily an ethical one. There is an ethics of his development, his research work and his technical activity, at the basis of which there is an ethics of thought.

From *Experiments with Man: Report of an Ecumenical Consultation,* World Council of Churches Studies no. 6, ed. Hans-Ruedi Weber (New York: Friendship Press, 1969), pp. 61-64. Published by the World Council of Churches and used by permission.

2. Man neither is nor develops alone; he lives in a group, he belongs to communities. Personalization and socialization do not oppose but attract each other. Just as personalization does not mean individualism, so socialization does not mean the levelling down of the masses, but it attributes to everybody his appropriate value. "Union differentiates" (Teilhard de Chardin). Research, work, and technology concern indissociably both the individual person and the community.

3. Man develops in time. His life is *history.* This holds even more true for a group, concrete human groups and, finally, through their encounter, for the whole of mankind.

Research and Experiments

Generally speaking, scientific research, the development of technology and, consequently, experiments, represent for man, for the whole of mankind, a fundamental duty, namely the duty to become what they are, amongst other things, the architects of their induction into the world which thus itself becomes hominified.

Now, can these experiments be carried out on man himself? There is no reason why not. This has happened ever since man existed. The choice and the dressing of his food, the search for shelter and clothing, the search for remedies: all this is made possible by his skill. Every case of administering a medicament is an embryo of an experiment on man.

This, however, must obviously be kept *within certain limitations:*

1. There were limitations drawn which we would consider today as irrelevant, e.g. those connected with a primitive notion of the "sacred" or with a false "providentialism", etc. (prohibition to dissect a dead body).

2. I would call permanent limits—and these are not so much limits, but must be considered as an intrinsic dimension of all research on man: never to treat the human person as a simple object, a thing; never to make man a simple means. Man's life (and with it his corporal and psychical integrity) belongs to himself alone. He cannot directly renounce it by committing suicide, for his life has been given to him by God in order to fulfil it in Him. Man possesses his life by right (human rights before civic rights). Man can *accept* even the serious danger of death or mutilation provided he does so for an end which is worthy of himself. If this is allowed in the case of trying out a new type of aeroplane or of conquering space, why should it be forbidden when the question is, for example, to try and find a remedy for cancer?

3. Finally, we must emphasize that the fixing of limitations for experiments must be conceived in such a way that they allow for progress in research: an operation which before Pasteur might have been quite risky can be a minor one today. Therefore, the limitation must not be fixed on individual cases.

Conclusion

I wish to conclude by pointing out that for any new case ethics cannot provide us with a preconceived solution. New information must continuously be fed into our ethics. And I add that theology alone will never be able to provide the complete answer: all questions are so complex that they can never be solved by theology alone.

99. Ten Theses Concerning Human Beings

J. ROBERT NELSON

I. *The primary datum for understanding man's nature is the awareness of each person that he is an individual self, a psycho-somatic being.*

This comes first for psychological and epistemological reasons, although it is not first in theological statement. Ego-consciousness, self-love and self-hatred are mental and emotional evidences of each person's perception of his identity, but they can be isolated neither from the recognition of his physical body's make-up nor from the often unrecognized genetic and chemical influences. Yet, the mystery of human personhood cannot be fully known. Introspection and scientific knowledge tell only part of the whole truth.

II. *Intrinsic to human selfhood is the necessity for some degree of freedom over against external conditions and restraints.*

To think and act according to the self-determination of his own will may never be unconditionally possible. A perfectly free and unconditioned person would be an isolated monster. Physical and social environment impose restraints in numerous ways. In experimentation, therefore, the completely free "informed consent" of the subject may never be possible. Freedom is indispensable to humanness, even though it is always measured in degrees.

III. *In recognizing both the limits of his freedom and the results of the misuse of freedom, man perceives the evil of the world and state of his own inner contradiction.*

Every man's daily confrontation with the external forces of confusion, frustration and destruction is matched by his introspective awareness of the inner distortions of his own best inclinations. The fact that no person is exempt from involvement with evil and with the contradiction of selfhood (called "sin") has utmost meaning for morality and law. Thus with respect to experimentation there are evidences of evil: (a) The very existence of disease, deformity and death; (b) man's abuse of his knowledge and skill with harmful consequences; (c) avaricious motivations of some persons who experiment; and (d) the moral dilemmas wherein a relative good is purchased at the cost of a relative evil.

IV. *The firmest ground for holding human life in awe and reverence is known theologically as belief in the image of God in man.*

Man alone can violate the nature of his species. Thus his self-awareness requires the vocabulary of "inhumanity" and "subhumanity". He can measure behaviour by the standard of "humanity" because it is the distinct gift granted to the species *homo sapiens* by the Creator, making man both free and responsible. This distinguishes our concern for human experimentation from that done on animals; but any needless pain inflicted upon the animal debases the humanity of the experimenter. The image of God is seen in every person, and yet in a damaged and imperfect form, needing repair and healing.

V. *While all persons participate in the common unity of humanity, each one who ever lives is an individual self.*

There can be no exact duplication of any person, whether physically (biologically), psychologically or spiritually. No person is replaceable.

VI. *Equal in importance to man's individuality is his inescapable existence in community.*

The male-female relation is not merely the condition for reproducing the species, but is the necessary basis for authentic humanity. Likewise, man's existence in family and society is not only desirable but indispensable. The wholeness of a person, toward which scientific inquiry is directed, consists not only in individuality. It is experienced in his social relations and corporate life. Both the doctrine of creation (for the "covenant community") and of redemption (in the "Body of Christ") point beyond the individual's identity to his social character.

VII. *Equality in worth and rights of all persons, as distinct from unequal abilities and values for society, is acknowledged as an inevitable corollary of the image of God in man.*

All persons stand before God—and should be regarded by men—as being of intrinsically equal worth.

VIII. *Existing in relation to the rest of creation, both animate and inanimate, man is given by the Creator a relative dominion over it.*

From *Experiments with Man: Report of an Ecumenical Consultation,* World Council of Churches Studies no. 6, ed. Hans-Ruedi Weber (New York: Friendship Press, 1969), pp. 61-64. Published by the World Council of Churches and used by permission.

Man is a creature and thus bound to live in the creation of which he is part; but his given nature is such that the increasing mastery of his environment is bound up with his destiny. This rapidly developing mastery is also subject to abuse, causing destructiveness to nature and to himself. However, it still provides some empirical evidence that man plays a significant role in his own evolution.

IX. *Man's true identity, his humanum, can be known only proximately by reference to descriptions of his physical, psychological, social and spiritual properties. Beyond these his humanity is measured in terms of conformity to the person of Jesus Christ, who is the full image of God.*

Christians especially need to reconceive their idea of salvation in the light of contemporary scientific knowledge of man and the world. But faith in Jesus Christ as the complete image of God, and thus of the full and proper manhood toward which the whole race is drawn, is not vitiated or cancelled by this scientific knowledge.

X. *Knowing that all men must die, human beings cannot be satisfied to regard death as the cessation and annihilation of personal life; therefore they hope for immortality.*

The hopes shared by most persons are set either upon infinite survival of the personal identity, or soul, or else upon God's creative act of resurrecting the whole person in a transfigured state. Awareness of this ultimate mystery of man's life opposes all concepts of man as a finite mechanism. Even the body of a subject of experimentation, then, is related to man's participation in an infinite realm of being which is of God.

100. Philosophical Reflections on Experimenting with Human Subjects

HANS JONAS

Experimenting with human subjects is going on in many fields of scientific and technological progress. It is designed to replace the over-all instruction by natural, occasional experience with the selective information from artificial, systematic experiment which physical science has found so effective in dealing with inanimate nature. Of the new experimentation with man, medical is surely the most legitimate; psychological, the most dubious; biological (still to come), the most dangerous. I have chosen here to deal with the first only, where the case *for* it is strongest and the task of adjudicating conflicting claims hardest. . . .

I. The Peculiarity of Human Experimentation

Experimentation was originally sanctioned by natural science. There it is performed on inanimate objects, and this raises no moral problems. But as soon as animate, feeling beings become the subjects of experiment, as they do in the life sciences and especially in medical research, this innocence of the search for knowledge is lost and questions of conscience arise. The depth to which moral and religious sensibilities can become aroused over these questions is shown by the vivisection issue. Human experimentation must sharpen the issue as it involves ultimate questions of personal dignity and sacrosanctity. One profound difference between the human experiment and the physical (beside that between animate and inanimate, feeling and unfeeling nature) is this: The physical experiment employs small-scale, artificially devised substitutes for that about which knowledge is to be obtained, and the experimenter extrapolates from these models and simulated conditions to nature at large. Something deputizes for the "real thing"—balls rolling down an inclined plane for sun and planets, electric discharges from a condenser for real lightning, and so

From *Experimentation with Human Subjects,* ed. Paul A. Freund (New York: George Braziller, 1970), pp. 1-30. Used by permission.

on. For the most part, no such substitution is possible in the biological sphere. We must operate on the original itself, the real thing in the fullest sense, and perhaps affect it irreversibly. No simulacrum can take its place. Especially in the human sphere, experimentation loses entirely the advantage of the clear division between vicarious model and true object. Up to a point, animals may fulfill the proxy role of the classical physical experiment. But in the end man himself must furnish knowledge about himself, and the comfortable separation of noncommittal experiment and definitive action vanishes. An experiment in education affects the lives of its subjects, perhaps a whole generation of schoolchildren. Human experimentation for whatever purpose is always *also* a responsible, nonexperimental, definitive dealing with the subject himself. And not even the noblest purpose abrogates the obligations this involves.

This is the root of the problem with which we are faced: Can both that purpose and this obligation be satisfied? If not, what would be a just compromise? Which side should give way to the other? The question is inherently philosophical as it concerns not merely pragmatic difficulties and their arbitration, but a genuine conflict of values involving principles of a high order. May I put the conflict in these terms. On principle, it is felt, human beings *ought not* to be dealt with in that way (the "guinea pig" protest); on the other hand, such dealings are increasingly urged on us by considerations, in turn appealing to principle, that claim to override those objections. Such a claim must be carefully assessed, especially when it is swept along by a mighty tide. Putting the matter thus, we have already made one important assumption rooted in our "Western" cultural tradition: The prohibitive rule is, to that way of thinking, the primary and axiomatic one; the permissive counter-rule, as qualifying the first, is secondary and stands in need of justification. We must justify the infringement of a primary inviolability, which needs no justification itself; and the justification of its infringement must be by values and needs of a dignity commensurate with those to be sacrificed. . . .

II. "Individual Versus Society" as the Conceptual Framework

The setting for the conflict most consistently invoked in the literature is the polarity of individual versus society—the possible tension between the individual good and the common good, between private and public welfare. . . . I have grave doubts about the adequacy of this frame of reference, but I will go along with it part of the way. It does apply to some extent, and it has the advantage of being familiar. We concede, as a matter of course, to the common good some pragmatically determined measure of precedence over the individual good. In terms of rights, we let some of the basic rights of the individual be overruled by the acknowledged rights of society—as a matter of right and moral justness and not of mere force or dire necessity (much as such necessity may be adduced in defense of that right). But in making that concession, we require a careful clarification of what the needs, interests, and rights of society are, for society—as distinct from any plurality of individuals—is an abstract and, as such, is subject to our definition, while the individual is the primary concrete, prior to all definition, and his basic good is more or less known. Thus the unknown in our problem is the so-called common or public good and its potentially superior claims, to which the individual good must or might sometimes be sacrificed, in circumstances that in turn must also be counted among the unknowns of our question. Note that in putting the matter in this way—that is, in asking about the right of society to individual sacrifice—the consent of the sacrificial subject is no necessary part of the *basic* question.

"Consent," however, is the other most consistently emphasized and examined concept in discussions of this issue. This attention betrays a feeling that the "social" angle is not fully satisfactory. If society has a right, its exercise is not contingent on volunteering. On the other hand, if volunteering is fully genuine, no public right to the volunteered act need be construed. There is a difference between the moral or emotional appeal of a cause that elicits volunteering and a right that demands compliance—for example, with particular reference to the social sphere, between the *moral claim* of a common good and society's *right* to that good and to the means of its realization. A moral claim cannot be met without consent; a right can do without it. Where consent is present anyway, the distinction may become immaterial. But the awareness of the many ambiguities besetting the "consent" actually available and used in medical research[1] prompts recourse to the idea of a public right conceived independently of (and valid prior to) consent; and, vice versa, the awareness of the problematic nature of such a right makes even its advocates still insist on the idea of consent with all its ambiguities: an uneasy situation either way.

Nor does it help much to replace the language of "rights" by that of "interests" and then argue the sheer cumulative weight of the interest of the many over against those of the few or the single individual. "Interests" range all the way from the most marginal and optional to the most vital and imperative, and only those sanctioned by particular importance and merit will be admitted to count in such a calculus—which simply brings us back to the question of right or moral claim. Moreover, the appeal to numbers is dangerous. Is the number of those afflicted with a particular disease great enough to warrant violating the interests of the non-afflicted? Since the number of the latter is usually so much greater, the argument can actually turn around to the contention that the cumulative weight of interest is on *their* side. Finally, it may well be the case that the individual's interest in his own inviolability is itself a public interest, such that its publicly condoned violation, irrespective of numbers, violates the interest of all. In that case, its protection in *each* instance would be a paramount interest, and the comparison of numbers will not avail.

These are some of the difficulties hidden in the conceptual framework indicated by the terms "society-individual," "interest," and "rights." But we also spoke of a moral call, and this points to another dimension—not indeed divorced from the social sphere, but transcending it. And there is something even beyond that: true sacrifice from highest devotion, for which there are no laws or rules except that it must be absolutely free. "No one has the right to choose martyrs for science" was a statement repeatedly quoted in the November, 1967, *Daedalus* conference. But no scientist can be prevented from making himself a martyr for his science. At all times, dedicated explorers, thinkers, and artists have immolated themselves on the altar of their vocation, and creative genius most often pays the price of happiness, health, and life for its own consummation. But no one, not even society, has the shred of a right to expect and ask these things in the normal course of events. They come to the rest of us as a *gratia gratis data.*

III. The Sacrificial Theme

Yet we must face the somber truth that the *ultima ratio* of communal life is and has always been the compulsory, vicarious sacrifice of individual lives. The primordial sacrificial situation is that of outright human sacrifices in early communities. These were not acts of blood-lust or gleeful savagery; they were the solemn execution of a supreme, sacral necessity. One of the fellowship of men had to die so that all could live, the earth be fertile, the cycle of nature renewed. The victim often was not a captured enemy, but a select member of the group: "The king must die." If there was cruelty here, it was not that of men, but that of the gods, or rather of the stern order of things, which was believed to exact that price for the bounty of life. To assure it for the community, and to assure it ever again, the awesome *quid pro quo* had to be paid over again.

Far should it be from us to belittle, from the height of our enlightened knowledge, the majesty of the underlying conception. The particular *causal* views that prompted our ancestors have long since been relegated to the realm of superstition. But in moments of national danger we still send the flower of our young manhood to offer their lives for the continued life of the community, and if it is a just war, we see them go forth as consecrated and strangely ennobled by a sacrificial role. Nor do we make their going forth depend on their own will and consent, much as we may desire and foster these. We conscript them according to law. We conscript the best and feel morally disturbed if the draft, either by design or in effect, works so that mainly the disadvantaged, socially less useful, more expendable, make up those whose lives are to buy ours. No rational persuasion of the pragmatic necessity here at work can do away with the feeling, a mixture of gratitude and guilt, that the sphere of the sacred is touched with the vicarious offering of life for life. Quite apart from these dramatic occasions, there is, it appears, a persistent and constitutive aspect of human immolation to the very being and prospering of human society—an immolation in terms of life and happiness, imposed or voluntary, of few for many. What Goethe has said of the rise of Christianity may well apply to the nature of civilization in general: *"Opfer fallen hier, / Weder Lamm noch Stier, / Aber Menschenopfer unerhoert."*[2] We can never rest comfortably in the belief that the soil from which our satisfactions sprout is not watered with the blood of martyrs. But a troubled conscience compels us, the undeserving beneficiaries, to ask: Who is to be martyred? in the service of what cause and by whose choice?

Not for a moment do I wish to suggest that medical experimentation on human subjects, sick or healthy, is to be likened to primeval human sacrifices. Yet something sacrificial is involved in the selective abrogation of personal inviolability and the ritualized exposure to gratuitous risk of health and life, justified by a presumed greater, social good. My examples from the sphere of stark sacrifice were intended to sharpen the issues implied in that context and to set them off clearly from the kinds of obligations and constraints imposed on the citizen in the normal course of things or generally demanded of the individual in exchange for the advantages of civil society.

IV. The "Social Contract" Theme

The first thing to say in such a setting-off is that the sacrificial area is not covered by what is called the "social contract." This fiction of political theory, premised on the primacy of the individual, was designed to supply a rationale for the *limitation* of individual freedom and power required for the existence of the body politic, whose existence in turn is for the benefit of the individuals. The principle of these limitations is that their *general* observance profits all, and that therefore the individual observer, assuring this general observance for his part, profits by it himself. I observe property rights because their general observance assures my own; I observe traffic rules because their general observance assures my own safety; and so on. The obligations here are mutual and general; no one is singled out for special sacrifice. Moreover, for the most part, *qua* limitations of my liberty, the laws thus deducible from the hypothetical "social contract" enjoin me from certain actions rather than obligate me to positive actions (as did the laws of feudal society). Even where the latter is the case, as in the duty to pay taxes, the rationale is that I am myself a beneficiary of the services financed through these payments. Even the contributions levied by the welfare state, though not originally contemplated in the liberal version of the social contract theory, can be interpreted as a personal insurance policy of one sort or another—be it against the contingency of my own indigence, be it against the dangers of disaffection from the laws in consequence of widespread unrelieved destitution, be it even against the disadvantages of a diminished consumer market. Thus, by some stretch, such contributions can still be subsumed under the principle of enlightened self-interest. But no complete abrogation of self-interest at any time is in the terms of the social contract, and so pure sacrifice falls outside it. Under the putative terms of the contract alone, I cannot be required to die for the public good. . . .

But in time of war our society itself supersedes the nice balance of the social contract with an almost absolute precedence of public necessities over individual rights. In this and similar emergencies, the sacrosanctity of the individual is abrogated, and what for all practical purposes amounts to a near-totalitarian, quasi-communist state of affairs is *temporarily* permitted to prevail. In such situations, the community is conceded the right to make calls on its members, or certain of its members, entirely different in magnitude and kind from the calls normally allowed. It is deemed right that a part of the population bears a disproportionate burden of risk of a disproportionate gravity; and it is deemed right that the rest of the community accepts this sacrifice, whether voluntary or enforced, and reaps its benefits—difficult as we find it to justify this acceptance and this benefit by any normal ethical categories. We justify it trans-ethically, as it were, by the supreme collective emergency, formalized, for example, by the declaration of a state of war.

Medical experimentation on human subjects falls somewhere between this overpowering case and the normal transactions of the social contract. On the one hand, no comparable extreme issue of social survival is (by and large) at stake. And no comparable extreme sacrifice or foreseeable risk is (by and large) asked. On the other hand, what is asked goes decidedly beyond, even runs counter to, what it is otherwise deemed fair to let the individual sign over of his person to the benefit of the "common good." Indeed, our sensitivity to the kind of intrusion and use involved is such that only an end of transcendent value or overriding urgency can make it arguable and possibly acceptable in our eyes.

V. Health as a Public Good

The cause invoked is health and, in its more critical aspect, life itself—clearly superlative goods that the physician serves directly by curing and the researcher indirectly by the knowledge gained through his experiments. There is no question about the good served nor about the evil fought—disease and premature death. But a good to whom and an evil to whom? Here the issue tends to become somewhat clouded. In the attempt to give experimentation the proper dignity (on the problematic view that a value becomes greater by being "social" instead of merely individual), the health in question or the disease in question is somehow predicated on the social whole, as if it were society that, in the persons of its members, enjoyed the one and suffered the other. For the purposes of our problem, public interest can then be pitted against private interest, the common good against the individual good. Indeed, I have found health called a national resource, which of course it is, but surely not in the first place.

In trying to resolve some of the complexities and ambiguities lurking in these conceptualizations, I have pondered a particular statement, made in the form of a question, which I found in the *Proceedings* of the earlier *Daedalus* conference: "Can society afford to discard the tissues and organs of the hopelessly unconscious patient when they could be used to restore the otherwise hopelessly ill, but still salvageable individual?" And somewhat later: "A strong case can be made that society can ill afford to discard the tissues and organs of the hopelessly unconscious patient; they are greatly needed for study and experimental trial to help those who can be salvaged."[3] I hasten to add that any suspicion of callousness that the "commodity" language of these statements may suggest is immediately dispelled by the name of the speaker, Dr. Henry K. Beecher, for whose humanity and moral sensibility there can be nothing but admiration. But the use, in all innocence, of this language gives food for thought. Let me, for a moment, take the question literally. "Discarding" implies proprietary rights—nobody can discard what does not belong to him in the first place. Does society then own my body? "Salvaging" implies the same and, moreover, a use-value to the owner. Is the life-extension of certain individuals then a public interest? "Affording" implies a critically vital level of such an interest—that is, of the loss or gain involved. And "society" itself—what is it? When does a need, an aim, an obligation become social? Let us reflect on some of these terms.

VI. What Society Can Afford

"Can Society afford . . . ?" Afford what? To let people die intact, thereby withholding something from other people who desperately need it, who in consequence will have to die too? These other, unfortunate people indeed cannot afford not to have a kidney, heart, or other organ of the dying patient, on which they depend for an extension of their lease on life; but does that give them a right to it? And does it oblige society to procure it for them? What is it that *society* can or cannot afford—leaving aside for the moment the question of what it has a *right* to? It surely can afford to lose members through death; more than that, it is built on the balance of death and birth decreed by the order of life. This is too general, of course, for our question, but perhaps it is well to remember. The specific question seems to be whether society can afford to let some people die whose death might be deferred by particular means if these were authorized by society. Again, if it is merely a question of what society can or cannot afford, rather than of what it ought or ought not to do, the answer must be: Of course, it can. If cancer, heart disease, and other organic, noncontagious ills, especially those tending to strike the old more than the young, continue to exact their toll at the normal rate of incidence (including the toll of private anguish and misery), society can go on flourishing in every way.

Here, by contrast, are some examples of what, in sober truth, society cannot afford. It cannot afford to let an epidemic rage unchecked; a persistent excess of deaths over births, but neither—we must add—too great an excess of births over deaths; too low an average life expectancy even if demographically balanced by fertility, but neither too great a longevity with the necessitated correlative dearth of youth in the social body; a debilitating state of general health; and things of this kind. These are plain cases where the whole condition of society is critically affected, and the public interest can make its imperative claims. The Black Death of the Middle Ages was a *public* calamity of the acute kind; the life-sapping ravages of endemic malaria or sleeping sickness in certain areas are a public calamity of the chronic kind. Such situations a society as a whole can truly not "afford," and they may call for extraordinary remedies, including, perhaps, the invasion of private sacrosanctities.

This is not entirely a matter of numbers and numerical ratios. Society, in a subtler sense, cannot "afford" a single miscarriage of justice, a single inequity in the dispensation of its laws, the violation of the rights of even the tiniest minority, because these undermine the moral basis on which society's existence rests. Nor can it, for a similar reason, afford the absence or atrophy in its midst of compassion and of the effort to alleviate suffering—be it widespread or rare—one form of which is the effort to conquer disease of any kind, whether "socially" significant (by reason of number) or not. And in short, society cannot afford the absence among its members of *virtue* with its readiness for sacrifice beyond defined duty. Since its presence—that is to say, that of personal idealism—is a matter of grace and not of decree, we have the paradox that society depends for its existence on intangibles of nothing less than a religious order, for which it can hope, but which it cannot enforce. All the more must it protect this most precious capital from abuse.

For what objectives connected with the medico-biological sphere should this reserve be drawn upon—for example, in the form of accepting, soliciting, perhaps even imposing the submission of human subjects to experimentation? We postulate that this must be not just a worthy cause, as any promotion of the health of anybody doubtlessly is, but a cause qualifying for transcendent social sanction. Here one thinks first of those cases critically affecting the whole condition, present and future, of the community we have illustrated. Something equivalent to what in the political sphere is called "clear and present danger" may be invoked and a state of emergency proclaimed, thereby suspending certain otherwise inviolable prohibitions and taboos. We may observe that averting a disaster always carries greater weight than promoting a good. Extraordinary danger excuses extraordinary means. This covers human experimentation, which we would like to count, as far as possible, among the extraordinary rather than the ordinary means of serving the common good under public auspices. Naturally, since foresight and responsibility for the future are of the essence of institutional society, averting disaster extends into long-term prevention, although the lesser urgency will warrant less sweeping licenses.

VII. Society and the Cause of Progress

Much weaker is the case where it is a matter not of saving but of improving society. Much of medical research falls into this category. As stated before, a permanent death rate from heart failure or cancer does not threaten society. So long as certain statistical ratios are maintained, the incidence of disease and of disease-induced mortality is not (in the strict sense) a "social" misfortune. I hasten to add that it is not therefore less of a human misfortune, and the call for relief issuing with silent eloquence from each victim and all potential victims is of no lesser dignity. But it is misleading to equate the fundamentally human response to it with what is owed to society: it is owed by man to man—and it is thereby owed by society to the individuals as soon as the adequate ministering to these concerns outgrows (as it progressively does) the scope of private spontaneity and is made a public mandate. It is thus that society assumes responsibility for medical care, research, old age, and innumerable other things not originally of the public realm (in the original "social contract"), and they become duties toward "society" (rather than directly toward one's fellow man) by the fact that they are socially operated.

Indeed, we expect from organized society no longer mere protection against harm and the securing of the conditions of our preservation, but active and constant improvement in all the domains of life: the waging of the battle against nature, the enhancement of the human estate—in short, the promotion of progress. This is an expansive goal, one far surpassing the disaster norm of our previous reflections. It lacks the urgency of the latter, but has the nobility of the free, forward thrust. It surely is worth sacrifices. It is not at all a question of what society can afford, but of what it is committed to, beyond all necessity, by our mandate. Its trusteeship has become an established, ongoing, institutionalized business of the body politic. As eager beneficiaries of its gains, we now owe to "society," as its chief agent, our individual contributions toward its *continued pursuit.* I emphasize "continued pursuit." Maintaining the existing level requires no more than the orthodox means of taxation and enforcement of professional standards that raise no problems. The more optional goal of pushing forward is also more exacting. We have this syndrome: Progress is by our choosing an acknowledged interest of society, in which we have a stake in various degrees; science is a necessary instrument of progress; research is a necessary instrument of science; and in medical science experimentation on human subjects is a necessary instrument of research. Therefore, human experimentation has come to be a societal interest.

The destination of research is essentially melioristic. It does not serve the preservation of the existing good from which I profit myself and to which I am obligated. Unless the present state is intolerable, the melioristic goal is in a sense gratuitous, and this not only from the vantage point of the present. Our descendants have a right to be left an unplundered planet; they do not have a right to new miracle cures. We have sinned against them, if by our doing we have destroyed their inheritance—which we are doing at full blast; we have not sinned against them, if by the time they come around arthritis has not yet been conquered (unless by sheer neglect). And generally, in the matter of progress, as humanity had no claim on a Newton, a Michelangelo, or a St. Francis to appear, and no right to the blessings of their unscheduled deeds, so progress, with all our methodical labor for it, cannot be budgeted in advance and its fruits received as a due. Its coming-about at all and its turning out for good (of which we can never be sure) must rather be regarded as something akin to grace.

VIII. The Melioristic Goal, Medical Research, and Individual Duty

Nowhere is the melioristic goal more inherent than in medicine. To the physician, it is not gratuitous. He is committed to curing and thus to improving the power to cure. Gratuitous we called it (outside disaster conditions) as a *social* goal, but noble at the same time. Both the nobility and the gratuitousness must influence the manner in which self-sacrifice for it is elicited, and even its free offer accepted. Freedom is certainly the first condition to be observed here. The surrender of one's body to medical experimentation is entirely outside the enforceable "social contract."

Or can it be construed to fall within its terms—namely, as repayment for benefits from past experimentation that I have enjoyed myself? But I am indebted for these benefits not to society, but to the past "martyrs," to whom society is indebted itself, and society has no right to call in my personal debt by way of adding new to its own. Moreover, gratitude is not an enforceable social obligation; it anyway does not mean that I must emulate the deed. Most of all, if it was wrong to exact such sacrifice in the first place, it does not become right to exact it again with the plea of the profit it has brought me. If, however, it was not exacted, but entirely free, as it ought to have been, then it should remain so, and its precedence must not be used as a social pressure on others for doing the same under the sign of duty.

Indeed, we must look outside the sphere of the social contract, outside the whole realm of public rights and duties, for the motivations and norms by which we can expect ever again the upwelling of a will to give what nobody—neither society, nor fellow man, nor posterity—is entitled to. There are such dimensions in man with trans-social wellsprings of conduct, and I have already pointed to the paradox, or mystery, that society cannot prosper without them, that it must draw on them, but cannot command them.

What about the moral law as such a transcendent motivation of conduct? It goes considerably beyond the public law of the social contract. The latter, we saw, is founded on the rule of enlightened self-interest: *Do ut des*—I give so that I be given to. The law of individual conscience asks more. Under the Golden Rule, for example, I am required to give as I wish to be given to under like circumstances, but not in order that I be given to and not in expectation of return. Reciprocity, essential to the social law, is not a condition of the moral law. One subtle "expectation" and "self-interest," but of the moral order itself, may even then be in my mind: I prefer the environment of a moral society and can expect to contribute to the general morality by my own example. But even if I should always be the dupe, the Golden Rule holds. (If the social law breaks faith with me, I am released from its claim.)

IX. Moral Law and Transmoral Dedication

Can I, then, be called upon to offer myself for medical experimentation in the name of the moral law? *Prima facie,* the Golden Rule seems to apply. I should wish, were I dying of a disease, that enough volunteers in the past had provided enough knowledge through the gift of their bodies that I could now be saved. I should wish, were I desperately in need of a transplant, that the dying patient next door had agreed to a definition of death by which his organs would become available to me in the freshest possible condition. I surely should also wish, were I drowning, that somebody would risk his life, even sacrifice his life, for mine.

But the last example reminds us that only the negative form of the Golden Rule ("Do not do unto others what you do not want done unto yourself") is fully prescriptive. The positive form ("Do unto others as you would wish them to do unto you"), in whose compass our issue falls, points into an infinite, open horizon where prescriptive force soon ceases. We may well say of somebody that he ought to have come to the succor of B, to have shared with him in his need, and the like. But we may not say that he ought to have given his life for him. To have done so would be praiseworthy; not to have done so is not blameworthy. It cannot be asked of him; if he fails to do so, he reneges on no duty. But *he* may say of himself, and only he, that he ought to have given his life. *This* "ought" is strictly between him and himself, or between him and God; no outside party—fellow man or society—can appropriate its voice. It can humbly receive the supererogatory gifts from the free enactment of it.

We must, in other words, distinguish between moral obligation and the much larger sphere of moral value. (This, incidentally, shows up the error in the widely held view of value theory that the higher a value, the stronger its claim and the greater the duty to realize it. The highest are in a region beyond duty and claim.) The ethical dimension far exceeds that of the moral law and reaches into the sublime solitude of dedication and ultimate commitment, away from all reckoning and rule—in short, into the sphere of the *holy.* From there alone can the offer of self-sacrifice genuinely spring, and this—its source—must be honored religiously. How? The first duty here falling on the research community, when it enlists and uses this source, is the safeguarding of true authenticity and spontaneity.

X. The "Conscription" of Consent

But here we must realize that the mere issuing of the appeal, the calling for volunteers, with the moral and social pressures it inevitably generates, amounts even under the most meticulous rules of consent to a sort of *conscripting.* And some soliciting is necessarily involved. This was in part meant by the earlier remark that in this area sin and guilt can perhaps not be wholly avoided. And this is why "consent," surely a non-negotiable minimum requirement, is not the full answer to the problem. Granting then that soliciting and therefore some degree of conscripting are part of the situation, who may conscript and who may be conscripted? Or less harshly expressed: Who should issue appeals and to whom?

The naturally qualified issuer of the appeal is the research scientist himself, collectively the main carrier of the impulse and the only one with the technical competence to judge. But his being very much an interested party (with vested interests, indeed, not purely in the public good, but in the scientific enterprise as such, in "his" project, and even in his career) makes him also suspect. The ineradicable dialectic of this situation—a delicate incompatibility problem—calls for particular controls by the research community and by public authority that we need not discuss. They can mitigate, but not eliminate the problem. We have to live with the ambiguity, the treacherous impurity of everything human.

XI. Self-Recruitment of the Community

To whom should the appeal be addressed? The natural issuer of the call is also the first natural addressee: the physician-researcher himself and the scientific confraternity at large. With such a coincidence—indeed, the noble tradition with which the whole business of human experimentation started—almost all of the associated legal, ethical, and metaphysical problems vanish. If it is full, autonomous identification of the subject with the purpose that is required for the dignifying of his serving as a subject—here it is; if strongest motivation—here it is; if fullest understanding—here it is; if freest decision—here it is; if greatest integration with the person's total, chosen pursuit—here it is. With the fact of self-solicitation the issue of consent in all its insoluble equivocality is bypassed *per se.* Not even the condition that the particular purpose be truly important and the project reasonably promising, which must hold in any solicitation of others, need be satisfied here. By himself, the scientist is free to obey his obsession, to play his hunch, to wager on chance, to follow the lure of ambition. It is all part of the "divine madness" that somehow animates the ceaseless pressing against frontiers. For the rest of society, which has a deep-seated disposition to look with reverence and awe upon the guardians of the mysteries of life, the profession assumes with this proof of its devotion the role of a self-chosen, consecrated fraternity, not unlike the monastic orders of the past, and this would come nearest to the actual, religious origins of the art of healing. . . .

XII. "Identification" as the Principle of Recruitment in General

If the properties we adduced as the particular qualifications of the members of the scientific fraternity itself are taken as general criteria of selection, then one should look for additional subjects where a maximum of identification, understanding, and spontaneity can be expected—that is, among the most highly motivated, the most highly educated, and the least "captive" members of the community. From this naturally scarce resource, a descending order of permissibility leads to greater abundance and ease of supply, whose use should become proportionately more hesitant as the exculpating criteria are relaxed. An inversion of normal "market" behavior is demanded here—namely, to accept the lowest quotation last (and excused only by the greatest pressure of need); to pay the highest price first.

The ruling principle in our considerations is that the "wrong" of reification can only be made "right" by such authentic identification with the cause that it is the subject's as well as the researcher's cause—whereby his role in its service is not just permitted by him, but *willed.* That sovereign will of his which embraces the end as his own restores his personhood to the otherwise depersonalizing context. To be valid it must be autonomous and informed. The latter condition can, outside the research community, only be fulfilled by degrees; but the higher the degree of the understanding regarding the purpose and the technique, the more valid becomes the endorsement of the will. A margin of mere trust inevitably remains. Ultimately, the appeal for volunteers should seek this free and generous endorsement, the appropriation of the research purpose into the person's own scheme of ends. Thus, the appeal is in truth addressed to the one, mysterious, and sacred source of any such generosity of the will—"devotion," whose forms and objects of commitment are various and may invest different motivations in different individuals. The following, for instance, may be responsive to the "call" we are discussing: compassion with human suffering, zeal for humanity, reverence for the Golden Rule, enthusiasm for progress, homage to the cause of knowledge, even longing for sacrificial justification (do not call that "masochism," please). On all these, I say, it is defensible and right to draw when the research objective is worthy enough; and it is a prime duty of the research community (especially in view of what we called the "margin of trust") to see that this sacred source is never abused for frivolous ends. For a less than adequate cause, not even the freest, unsolicited offer should be accepted.

XIII. The Rule of the "Descending Order" and Its Counter-Utility Sense

We have laid down what must seem to be a forbidding rule to the number-hungry research industry. Having faith in the transcendent potential of man, I do not fear that the "source" will ever fail a society that does not destroy it—and only such a one is worthy of the blessings of progress. But "elitistic" the rule is (as is the enterprise of progress itself), and elites are by nature small. The combined attribute of motivation and information, plus the absence of external pressures, tends to be socially so circumscribed that strict adherence to the rule might numerically starve the research process. This is why I spoke of a descending order of permissibility, which is itself permissive, but where the realization that it is a *descending* order is not without pragmatic import. Departing from the august norm, the appeal must needs shift from idealism to docility, from high-mindedness to compliance, from judgment to trust. Consent spreads over the whole spectrum. I will not go into the casuistics of this penumbral area. I merely indicate the principle of the order of preference: The poorer in knowledge, motivation, and freedom of decision (and that, alas, means the more readily available in terms of numbers and possible manipulation), the more sparingly and indeed reluctantly should the reservoir be used, and the more compelling must therefore become the countervailing justification.

Let us note that this is the opposite of a social utility standard, the reverse of the order by "availability and expendability": The most valuable and scarcest, the least expendable elements of the social organism, are to be the first candidates for risk and sacrifice. It is the standard of *noblesse oblige;* and with all its counter-utility and seeming "wastefulness," we feel a rightness about it and perhaps even a higher "utility," for the soul of the community lives by this spirit.[4] It is also the opposite of what the day-to-day interests of research clamor for, and for the scientific community to honor it will mean that it will have to fight a strong temptation to go by routine to the readiest sources of supply—the suggestible, the ignorant, the dependent, the "captive" in various senses.[5] I do not believe that heightened resistance here must cripple research, which cannot be permitted; but it may indeed slow it down by the smaller numbers fed into experimentation in consequence. This price—a possibly slower rate of progress—may have to be paid for the preservation of the most precious capital of higher communal life.

XIV. Experimentation on Patients

So far we have been speaking on the tacit assumption that the subjects of experimentation are recruited from among the healthy. To the question "Who is conscriptable?" the spontaneous answer is: Least and last of all the sick—the most available of all as they are under treatment and observation anyway. That the afflicted should not be called upon to bear additional burden and risk, that they are society's special trust and the physician's trust in particular—these are elementary responses of our moral sense. Yet the very destination of medical research, the conquest of disease, requires at the crucial stage trial and verification on precisely the sufferers from the disease, and their total exemption would defeat the purpose itself. In acknowledging this inescapable necessity, we enter the most sensitive area of the whole complex, the one most keenly felt and most searchingly discussed by the practitioners themselves. No wonder, it touches the heart of the doctor-patient relation, putting its most solemn obligations to the test. There is nothing new in what I have to say about the ethics of the doctor-patient relation, but for the purpose of confronting it with the issue of experimentation some of the oldest verities must be recalled.

A. The Fundamental Privilege of the Sick

In the course of treatment, the physician is obligated to the patient and to no one else. He is not the agent of society, nor of the interests of medical science, nor of the patient's family, nor of his co-sufferers, or future sufferers from the same disease. The patient alone counts when he is under the physician's care. By the simple law of bilateral contract (analogous, for example, to the relation of lawyer to client and its "conflict of interest" rule), the physician is bound not to let any other interest interfere with that of the patient in being cured. But manifestly more sublime norms than contractual ones are involved. We may speak of a sacred trust; strictly by its terms, the doctor is, as it were, alone with his patient and God.

There is one normal exception to this—that is, to the doctor's not being the agent of society vis-à-vis the patient, but the trustee of his interests alone: the quarantining of the contagious sick. This is plainly not for the patient's interest, but for that of others threatened by him. (In vaccination, we have a combination of both: protection of the individual and others.) But preventing the patient from causing harm to others is not the same as exploiting him for the advantage of others. And there is, of course, the abnormal exception of collective catastrophe, the analogue to a state of war. The physician who desperately battles a raging epidemic is under a unique dispensation that suspends in a nonspecifiable way some of the strictures of normal practice, including possibly those against experimental liberties with his patients. No rules can be devised for the waiving of rules in extremities. And as with the famous shipwreck examples of ethical theory, the less said about it the better. But what is allowable there and may later be passed over in forgiving silence cannot serve as a precedent. We are concerned with non-extreme, non-emergency conditions where the voice of principle can be heard and claims can be adjudicated free from duress. We have conceded that there are such claims, and that if there is to be medical advance at all, not even the superlative privilege of the suffering and the sick can be kept wholly intact from the intrusion of its needs. About this least palatable, most disquieting part of our subject, I have to offer only groping, inconclusive remarks.

B. The Principle of "Identification" Applied to Patients

On the whole, the same principles would seem to hold here as are found to hold with "normal subjects": motivation, identification, understanding on the part of the subject. But it is clear that these conditions are peculiarly difficult to satisfy with regard to a patient. His physical state, psychic preoccupation, dependent relation to the doctor, the submissive attitude induced by treatment—everything connected with his condition and situation makes the sick person inherently less of a sovereign person than the healthy one. Spontaneity of self-offering has almost to be ruled out; consent is marred by lower resistance or captive circumstance, and so on. In fact, all the factors that make the patient, as a category, particularly accessible and welcome for experimentation at the same time compromise the quality of the responding affirmation that must morally redeem the making use of them. This, in addition to the primacy of the physician's duty, puts a heightened onus on the physician-researcher to limit his undue power to the most important and defensible research objectives and, of course, to keep persuasion at a minimum.

Still, with all the disabilities noted, there is scope among patients for observing the rule of the "descending order of permissibility" that we have laid down for normal subjects, in vexing inversion of the utility order of quantitative abundance and qualitative "expendability." By the principle of this order, those patients who most identify with and are cognizant of the cause of research—members of the medical profession (who after all are sometimes patients themselves)—come first; the highly motivated and educated, also least dependent, among the lay patients come next; and so on down the line. An added consideration here is seriousness of condition, which again operates in inverse proportion. Here the profession must fight the tempting sophistry that the hopeless case is expendable (because in prospect already expended) and therefore especially usable; and generally the attitude that the poorer the chances of the patient the more justifiable his recruitment for experimentation (other than for his own benefit). The opposite is true.

C. Nondisclosure as a Borderline Case

Then there is the case where ignorance of the subject, sometimes even of the experimenter, is of the essence of the experiment (the "double blind"-control group-placebo syndrome). It is said to be a necessary element of the scientific process. Whatever may be said about its ethics in regard to normal subjects, especially volunteers, it is an outright betrayal of trust in regard to the patient who believes that he is receiving treatment. Only supreme importance of the objective can exonerate it, without making it less of a transgression. The patient is definitely wronged even when not harmed. And ethics apart, the practice of such deception holds the danger of undermining the faith in the *bona fides* of treatment, the beneficial intent of the physician—the very basis of the doctor-patient relationship. In every respect, it follows that concealed experiment on patients—that is, experiment under the guise of treatment—should be the rarest exception, at best, if it cannot be wholly avoided.

This has still the merit of a borderline problem. The same is not true of the other case of necessary ignorance of the subject—that of the unconscious patient. Drafting him for nontherapeutic experiments is simply and unqualifiedly impermissible; progress or not, he must never be used, on the inflexible principle that utter helplessness demands utter protection.

When preparing this paper, I filled pages with a casuistics of this harrowing field, but then scrapped most of it, realizing my dilettante status. The shadings are endless, and only the physician-researcher can discern them properly as the cases arise. Into his lap the decision is thrown. The philosophical rule, once it has admitted into itself the idea of a sliding scale, cannot really specify its own application. It can only impress on the practitioner a general maxim or attitude for the exercise of his judgment and conscience in the concrete occasions of his work. In our case, I am afraid, it means making life more difficult for him.

It will also be noted that, somewhat at variance with the emphasis in the literature, I have not dwelt on the element of "risk" and very little on that of "consent." Discussion of the first is beyond the layman's competence; the emphasis on the second has been lessened because of its equivocal character. It is a truism to say that one should strive to minimize the risk and to maximize the consent. The more demanding concept of "identification," which I have used, includes "consent" in its maximal or authentic form, and the assumption of risk is its privilege.

XV. No Experiments on Patients Unrelated to Their Own Disease

Although my ponderings have, on the whole, yielded points of view rather than definite prescriptions, premises rather than conclusions, they have led me to a few unequivocal yeses and noes. The first is the emphatic rule that patients should be experimented upon, if at all, *only* with reference to *their disease.* Never should there be added to the gratuitousness of the experiment as such the gratuitousness of service to an unrelated cause. This follows simply from what we have found to be the *only* excuse for infracting the special exemption of the sick at all—namely, that the scientific war on disease cannot accomplish its goal without drawing the sufferers from disease into the investigative process. If under this excuse they become subjects of experiment, they do so *because,* and only because, of *their* disease.

This is the fundamental and self-sufficient consideration. That the patient cannot possibly benefit from the unrelated experiment therapeutically, while he might from experiment related to his condition, is also true, but lies beyond the problem area of pure experiment. I am in any case discussing nontherapeutic experimentation only, where *ex hypothesi* the patient does not benefit. Experiment as part of therapy—that is, directed toward helping the subject himself—is a different matter altogether and raises its own problems, but hardly philosophical ones. As long as a doctor can say, even if only in his own thought: "There is no known cure for your condition (or: You have responded to none); but there is promise in a new treatment still under investigation, not quite tested yet as to effectiveness and safety; you will be taking a chance, but all things considered, I judge it in your best interest to let me try it on you"—as long as he can speak thus, he speaks as the patient's physician and may err, but does not transform the patient into a subject of experimentation. Introduction of an untried therapy into the treatment where the tried ones have failed is not "experimentation on the patient."

Generally, and almost needless to say, with all the rules of the book, there is something "experimental" (because tentative) about every individual treatment, beginning with the diagnosis itself; and he would be a poor doctor who would not learn from every case for the benefit of future cases, and a poor member of the profession who would not make any new insights gained from his treatments available to the profession at large. Thus, knowledge may be advanced in the treatment of any patient, and the interest of the medical art and all sufferers from the same affliction as well as the patient himself may be served if something happens to be learned from his case. But this gain to knowledge and future therapy is incidental to the *bona fide* service to the present patient. He has the right to expect that the doctor does nothing to him just in order to learn.

In that case, the doctor's imaginary speech would run, for instance, like this: "There is nothing more I can do for you. But you can do something for me. Speaking no longer as your physician but on behalf of medical science, we could learn a great deal about future cases of this kind if you would permit me to perform certain experiments on you. It is understood that you yourself would not benefit from any knowledge we might gain; but future patients would." This statement would express the purely experimental situation, assumedly here with the subject's concurrence and with all cards on the table. In Alexander Bickel's words: "It is a different situation when the doctor is no longer trying to make [the patient] well, but is trying to find out how to make others well in the future."[6]

But even in the second case, that of the nontherapeutic experiment where the patient does not benefit, at least the patient's own disease is enlisted in the cause of fighting that disease, even if only in others. It is yet another thing to say or think: "Since you are here—in the hospital with its facilities—anyway, under our care and observation anyway, away from your job (or, perhaps, doomed) anyway, we wish to profit from your being available for some other research of great interest we are presently engaged in." From the standpoint of merely medical ethics, which has only to consider risk, consent, and the worth of the objective, there may be no cardinal difference between this case and the last one. I hope that the medical reader will not think I am making too fine a point when I say that from the standpoint of the subject and his dignity there is a cardinal difference that crosses the line between the permissible and the impermissible, and this by the same principle of "identification" I have been invoking all along. Whatever the rights and wrongs of any experimentation on any patient—in the one case, at least that residue of identification is left him that it is his own affliction by which he can contribute to the conquest of that affliction, his own kind of suffering which he helps to alleviate in others; and so in a sense it is his own cause. It is totally indefensible to rob the unfortunate of this intimacy with the purpose and make his misfortune a convenience for the furtherance of alien concerns. The observance of this rule is essential, I think, to at least attenuate the wrong that nontherapeutic experimenting on patients commits in any case.

XVI. Conclusion

There would now have to be said something about nonmedical experiments on human subjects, notably psychological and genetic, of which I have not lost sight. But I must leave this for another occasion. I wish only to say in conclusion that if some of the practical implications of my reasonings are felt to work out toward a slower rate of progress, this should not cause too great dismay. Let us not forget that progress is an optional goal, not an unconditional commitment, and that its tempo in particular, compulsive as it may become, has nothing sacred about it. Let us also remember that a slower progress in the conquest of disease would not threaten society, grievous as it is to those who have to deplore that their particular disease be not yet conquered, but that society would indeed be threatened by the erosion of those moral values whose loss, possibly caused by too ruthless a pursuit of scientific progress, would make its most dazzling triumphs not worth having. Let us finally remember that it cannot be the aim of progress to abolish the lot of mortality. Of some ill or other, each of us will die. Our mortal condition is upon us with its harshness but also its wisdom—because without it there would not be the eternally renewed promise of the freshness, immediacy, and eagerness of youth; nor would there be for any of us the incentive to number our days and make them count. With all our striving to wrest from our mortality what we can, we should bear its burden with patience and dignity.

Notes

1. Cf. M. H. Pappworth, "Ethical Issues in Experimental Medicine" in D. R. Cutler (editor), *Updating Life and Death* (Boston, 1969), pp. 64-69.

2. *Die Braut von Korinth:* "Victims do fall here, / Neither lamb nor steer, / Nay, but human offerings untold."

3. *Proceedings of the Conference on the Ethical Aspects of Experimentation on Human Subjects,* November 3-4, 1967 (Boston, Mass.), pp. 50-51.

4. Socially, everyone is expendable relatively—that is, in different degrees; religiously, no one is expendable absolutely: The "image of God" is in all. If it can be enhanced, then not by anyone being expended, but by someone expending himself.

5. This refers to captives of circumstance, not of justice. Prison inmates are, with respect to our problem, in a special class. If we hold to some idea of guilt, and to the supposition that our judicial system is not entirely at fault, they may be held to stand in a special debt to society, and their offer to serve—from whatever motive—may be accepted with a minimum of qualms as a means of reparation.

6. *Proceedings,* p. 33. To spell out the difference between the two cases: In the first case, the patient himself is meant to be the beneficiary of the experiment, and directly so; the "subject" of the experiment is at the same time its object, its end. It is performed not for gaining knowledge, but for helping him—and helping him in the *act* of performing it, even if by its results it also contributes to a broader testing process currently under way. It is in fact part of the treatment itself and an "experiment" only in the loose sense of being untried and highly tentative. But whatever the degree of uncertainty, the motivating anticipation (the wager, if you like) is for success, and success here means the subject's own good. To a pure experiment, by contrast, undertaken to gain knowledge, the difference of success and failure is not germane, only that of conclusiveness and inconclusiveness. The "negative" result has as much to teach as the "positive." Also, the true experiment is an act distinct from the uses later made of the findings. And, most important, the subject experimented on is distinct from the eventual beneficiaries of those findings: He lets himself be used as a means toward an end external to himself (even if he should at some later time happen to be among the beneficiaries himself). With respect to his own present needs and his own good, the act is gratuitous.

101.
Ethical Considerations in Human Experimentation: Experimentation Involving Children

CHARLES E. CURRAN

It will be helpful to discuss in particular a significant and prismatic case of human experimentation—the use of children in nontherapeutic experimentation. The discussion will not descend to the level of proposing guidelines—for example, it will not even discuss the exact age of what is meant by children who are unable to give consent.

There has been a great divergence in the literature and proposed guidelines about the ethics of using children in medical experimentation understood in the strict sense. Many researchers have proposed the need to use children but have also recognized the role of proper safeguards. Louis Lasagna, a professor of medicine and experimental therapeutics, accepts the use of children and even justifies the famous experiment of the Willowbrook School in New York.[1] Franz J. Ingelfinger, an editor of the *New England Journal of Medicine,* argues against the absolute position of the World Medical Association statement that does not allow experimentation on children under any circumstances.[2] Charles Lowe, M.D., and associates point out all the advantages that have accrued through experimentation on children and accept its necessity but also recognize the need for some ethical restrictions which might very well prevent our obtaining some of the knowledge and technological progress which we could have obtained under the looser restrictions of the past.[3] The proposed Health, Education, and Welfare Department (HEW) guidelines also begin with the assumption that experimentation on children is necessary for medical advances for the good of other children. These guidelines conclude that substantial risk with children is never acceptable but that some risk is justified with the ultimate determination to be made by review committees.[4]

Some researchers have proposed that not even the parents should be allowed to consent to possibly risky research on their children. Henry K. Beecher and William J. Curran conclude that children under 14 may be involved in medical experimentation only when there is no discernible risk.[5] As might be expected, some philosophical and religious ethicists tend to be more reluctant or even opposed to the use of children in medical experimentation, but again this does not hold true of all ethicists. Paul Ramsey, basing his argument on the canon of loyalty by which the parent is related to the child, opposes any medical experimentation with children because the primary ethical consideration is not the risk or degree of risk but the offense of touching, which would be involved in any experimentation.[6] William F. May supports the same conclusion, since proxy consent by the parents in such cases involves a contradiction—it necessarily requires one to treat a child or other incompetent individual as a moral agent, something that a child or other incompetent actually is not.[7]

Richard A. McCormick disagrees with Ramsey and comes to a conclusion similar to Beecher's in allowing experimentation where there is no discernible risk (although he at times speaks of no notable disadvantages and accepts the concept of low risk if it means no realistic risk), undue discomfort, or inconvenience.[8] McCormick bases his conclusion on the fact that such an act is something that one ought to do for other members of the human community and is not merely a work of supererogation which would never be justified by proxy consent. Elsewhere McCormick rightly points out that his conclusion is quite similar to the one I have proposed on this question.[9]

In the light of further considerations, I have changed my earlier position, which, in reaction to Paul Ramsey's approach, proposed that experimentation on children is acceptable when there is no discernible risk.[10] Now I am willing to accept some risk, discomfort, or inconvenience. Theology and ethics have always had difficulty in dealing with children, primarily because of their inability to consent freely—the hallmark of the adult human. For example, Catholic theology at one time excluded children who died without baptism from the fullness of eternal life because they were unable to have baptism of desire. Recall, however, that in the ethical considerations I insisted that consent was not the only consideration, for consent itself must always be properly ordered.

McCormick and others claim that the HEW guidelines are utilitarian, but I do not think that conclusion is necessarily accurate. Unlike McCormick, I would see the individual human being in more relational terms rather than as an individual with certain basic human tendencies or human goods which are equally basic and self-evidently attractive and against which one must never directly choose.[11] A more relational understanding would not see all these goods as equally

From the *Duquesne Law Review* 13 (Summer 1975): 837-40. Used by permission.

basic and of equal value. Likewise, without unduly subordinating the individual or others, this view recognizes that in our relational existence with others we are often exposed to some risk which is not for our benefit—and this is so for children too. In a less complex and relational world, a child would be better off growing up in an environment where there is no air pollution, but other values are decisive in the choice of where the family lives, even though this redounds only secondarily to the good of the child and definitely causes some harm to the child. One might argue that even here the decision is made for the good of the child, but consider another example. I believe that individual children in some circumstances should undergo the inconvenience of busing in order to achieve the racial integration of schools—which is proximately and primarily for the good of others and only very indirectly redounds to the good of the individual child.

A more relational understanding recognizes that children are often exposed by parents and others to some risk or inconvenience which is not primarily and directly for their own benefit. I agree with McCormick and Lowe and associates that it is necessary here to distinguish two kinds of obligations.[12] A person may freely expose oneself to a greater risk than the parent can take with the child. The parent can, however, expose the child to some risk, low risk or slight risk for the good of others. My primary difficulty with the HEW guidelines is the failure to spell out what is meant by the some risk which is permitted as opposed to the substantial risk which is forbidden. As practical guidelines these would be much more helpful and less open to abuse if they would offer a more explicit understanding of what is meant by some risk and thereby give more detailed guidelines for the final decision to be made by review committees.

Although I would accept the ethical validity of parents giving proxy consent for experimentation which exposes their child to low risk, some risk, or slight risk (or discomfort or inconvenience), I still recognize the absolute need for practical vigilance in all areas of such experimentation. Above all, children should never be used in experimentation unless there is no other way to achieve the purpose of the experiment.

Notes

1. Lasagna, "Special Subjects in Human Experimentation," in *Reflections on Medical Experimentation in Humans,* ed. P. Freund (New York: George Braziller, 1970), p. 271.
2. Ingelfinger, "Ethics of Experiments on Children," *New England Journal of Medicine* 288 (1973): 791.
3. Lowe, Alexander, and Mishkin, "Nontherapeutic Research on Children: An Ethical Dilemma," *Journal of Pediatrics* 84 (1974): 468.
4. 38 Fed. Reg. 31, 740-42 (1973).
5. Curran & Beecher, "Experimentation in Children: A Reexamination of Legal Ethical Principles," *Journal of the American Medical Association* 210 (1969): 77, 82.
6. See P. Ramsey, *The Patient as Person* (New Haven: Yale University Press, 1970), pp. 1-58.
7. May, "Experimenting on Human Subjects," *Linacre Quarterly* 41 (1974): 238, 250.
8. McCormick, "Proxy Consent in the Experimentation Situation," in *Love and Society,* ed. J. Johnson & D. Smith (n.p., 1974), pp. 221-24 (hereinafter cited as McCormick).
9. McCormick, "Notes on Moral Theology," *Theological Studies* 36 (1975): 77, 117-28.
10. C. Curran, *Politics, Medicine and Christian Ethics* (Philadelphia: Fortress, 1973), pp. 132-35.
11. McCormick, "Proxy Consent," p. 218.
12. McCormick's thesis is that one may give proxy consent where it is a case of what the person ought to do but not if it is a work of charity that one could freely do for others. His explanation of this in terms of the parents deciding to allow the child to die (by withholding extraordinary means) seems weak, for ethicists do not usually claim that the child or person ought to die but that one *can* decide not to use extraordinary means.

Chapter Nineteen
ALLOCATION AND DISTRIBUTION

Introduction

The doctor in George Bernard Shaw's "The Doctor's Dilemma" had enough elixir to help only one patient. Who was it to be? The good man Blenkinsop or the rotten artist Dubedat? The doctor finds it a hard choice: "Blenkinsop's an honest decent man; but is he any use? Dubedat's a rotten blackguard; but he's a genuine source of pretty and pleasant and good things." Catching the drift of these remarks, the doctor's companion attempts to form from them a universal principle: "Suppose you had this choice put before you: either to go through life and find all the pictures bad but all the men and women good, or to go through life and find all the pictures good and all the men and women rotten. Which would you choose?"

The doctor's dilemma has been repeated many different times since then and with many different medical resources. When penicillin was first discovered and proven effective, hard choices had to be made about who would receive it. When hemodialysis was first clinically used, hard choices had to be made about who would receive the treatment. Organs for transplant do not match the demand or need for them, and hard choices are necessary concerning who will receive the available organs. The beds in intensive care units are sometimes in short supply, and hard decisions are required about who will get intensive care. Time and energy are also held in finite supply, and the limits on these resources, too, create dilemmas for doctors.

One suggestion in response to such hard choices is merely to increase the supply: Produce more elixir. Manufacture more penicillin. Make enough kidney dialysis units to treat everyone in need. Secure more organs for transplant. Build more intensive care units. Train more doctors.

Such a response, however, does not eliminate "the doctor's dilemma" with respect to developing technologies—for example, a totally implantable artificial heart—and increasing the supply of existing services requires a resource which is itself in short supply, money. Medical care is already costly, and becoming costlier still. There are a number of reasons for increasing medical costs, not the least significant of which is the increasingly sophisticated technology of medical care. The bill for the care of baby Andrew Stinson (the premature infant mentioned in the introduction to Chapter 15) was $104,403.20, for example. It is little wonder that the percentage of our gross national product that we spend on health care has climbed above ten per cent. The point is that even if we did secure more organs for transplant, perhaps by moving from a policy of organ donation to a policy of routine organ harvesting, it would not eliminate all limiting factors of scarcity; we would still have to find the money to pay the medical expenses for each transplant. If the transplants were unsupported by public monies, then only the rich would have access to such medical care, and the policy of organ acquisition, which in theory would allow more organ transplants, would end up serving only the rich. Is that fair allocation? If transplant surgery were paid for with public funds, the public would quickly encounter the problem of scarcity of funds and the resulting hard choices concerning allocation.

The decision to provide resources to meet the problems of scarcity in medical care thus creates hard choices for a society, for to allocate funds to organ procurement and transplant means to have less for the critical care of the hemophiliac, the diabetic, and the neonate. Suppose we increased funding for all critical care; then we would have less for the care of retarded and handicapped people, less for medical research, less for preventive medicine, less for providing access to a primary care physician for the indigent. Or suppose we increased funding for health-related needs, suppose we let the percentage of our gross national product spent on these needs move up to thirteen, fifteen, even twenty percent; then we would have less to spend on education, on security, on providing access to music and art and the humanities. Suppose you had this choice put before you: to go through life either to find all the men and women and children with the best health care available but ignorant of Shakespeare and Picasso and Mozart, or to find all the men and women and children knowledgeable and appreciative of the great artistic traditions but at risk of death should disease strike. Which would you choose?

How can or should public policy choices be made? Is the principle of justice enough? If so, what is justice and what does it require? If not, what vision of the sort of society we should be and become must supplement it, and how can it be justified? Again, what bearing does cost-effectiveness have? Preventive medicine is more cost-effective than crisis intervention. Should we, therefore, take resources from crisis intervention and put them into preventive medicine? But what if the sort of society we want to effect is not just a relatively healthy society but also a society in which the cries of the sick and helpless are heard and answered? Diagnostic Related Groups (DRGs) are an attempt to contain costs, but what if such a health care policy means patients go home sicker than they might otherwise? What if it prevents a hospital from shifting costs to cover the care of the indigent? What if it means that hospitals refuse to care for the poor or those so sick their care is likely to cost more than the DRG payment? What if they force the hospitals into business competition with each other in order to survive? Cost containment is a worthy goal, but must it not be joined to the pursuit of equitable access to health care or some form of guaranteed ordinary care if it is to be worthy social policy?

The doctor's dilemmas and the social policy questions usually take up most of our time and energy in discussions of allocation. But the churches are involved in this matter, too. Many hospitals were founded by churches as a signal of their loyalty to Christ the healer and a gesture of their care for the sick and helpless. Now the churches may have cause to reassert their interest in medicine, to assure the care of the poor and to give witness to society of their Lord and of their responsibilities. But churches and church members have limited resources, too. How can we rank health care and hunger relief and evangelism and securing justice and other needs all as part of the one mission of the one God? These are hard and costly choices for churches, too.

The essays below get to these issues—and more besides. Gene Outka's piece is justly considered a classic—not only because it is so often cited in the literature but also because it utilizes classic Protestant patterns of moral reflection, presupposing individualism, reflecting on the relation of love as the fundamental Christian principle and justice as the fundamental social principle, formulating standards for social policy makers, here the goal of equal access to health care for all. Joseph Boyle's piece is also concerned with social policy and with defending the claim to "a fair share" of health care. His argument is a classic Catholic one, not only because he appeals to papal pronouncements but more because he presupposes a more communal understanding of society and utilizes natural law arguments to identify certain basic goods not only as goods chosen by individuals but as communal goods. It is interesting to compare these two articles, to consider, for example, the differences between a right to equal access and a right to *ordinary* health care, or the differences in their treatment of individual responsibility for health, and to trace those differences, if possible, to the different perspectives of the authors.

The other two articles focus less on social policy issues and more on Christian and professional integrity. Edmund Pellegrino reflects about the church's role and the professional's role in an era when public policy focuses on cost containment and nurtures competition. Allen Verhey suggests that while considerations of justice and cost-effectiveness are necessary, they do not eliminate tragedy from hard allocation choices. To endure the tragedy without moral harm and, indeed, to sustain a morally acceptable public policy the profession must nurture certain virtues, and for that piety may be more important to the profession than technology.

Suggestions for Further Reading

Calabresi, Guido, and Philip Bobbitt. *Tragic Choices.* New York: Norton, 1978.

Childress, James F. "Who Shall Live When Not All Can Live?" *Soundings* 53 (Winter 1970): 339-55.

———. "Love and Justice in Christian Biomedical Ethics." In *Theology and Bioethics: Exploring the Foundations and Frontiers,* edited by Earl E. Shelp. Dordrecht: D. Reidel, 1981.

Gustafson, James M. *Ethics From a Theocentric Perspective.* Vol. 2, *Ethics and Theology.* Chicago: University of Chicago Press, 1984. See pp. 252-77.

Kilner, John F. "A Moral Allocation of Scarce Lifesaving Medical Resources." *The Journal of Religious Ethics* 9 (Fall 1981).

Ogelsby, William B., Jr. "Life or Death—Whose Decision? Theological Aspects," *Virginia Medical Monthly* 109 (Sept. 1975): 710-13.

Potter, Ralph B. "Labeling the Mentally Retarded: The Just Allocation of Therapy." In *Ethics in Medicine,* edited by Stanley Reiser, et al., 626-31. Cambridge: MIT Press, 1977.

Ramsey, Paul. *The Patient as Person.* New Haven: Yale University Press, 1970. See pp. 239-75.

Thielicke, Helmut. "The Doctor As Judge of Who Shall Live and Who Shall Die." In *Who Shall Live?* edited by Kenneth Vaux. Philadelphia: Fortress, 1970.

102.
Social Justice and Equal Access to Health Care

GENE OUTKA

I want to consider the following question. Is it possible to understand and to justify morally a societal goal which increasing numbers of people, including Americans, accept as normative? The goal is: the assurance of comprehensive health services for every person irrespective of income or geographic location. Indeed, the goal now has almost the status of a platitude. Currently in the United States politicians in various camps give it at least verbal endorsement.[1] I do not propose to examine the possible sociological determinants in this emergent consensus. I hope to show that whatever these determinants are, one may offer a plausible case in defense of the goal on reasonable grounds. To demonstrate why appeals to the goal get so successfully under our skins, I shall have recourse to a set of conceptions of social justice. Some of the standard conceptions, found in a number of writings on justice, will do.[2] By reflecting on them it seems to me a prima facie case can be established, namely, that every person in the entire resident population should have equal access to health care delivery.

The case is prima facie only. I wish to set aside as far as possible a related question which comes readily enough to mind. In the world of "suboptimal alternatives," with the constraints for example which impinge on the government as it makes decisions about resource allocation, what is one to say? What criteria should be employed? Paul Ramsey, in *The Patient as Person* thinks that the large question of how to choose between medical and other societal priorities is "almost, if not altogether, incorrigible to moral reasoning."[3] Whether it is or not is a matter which must be ignored for the present. One may simply observe in passing that choices are unavoidable nonetheless, as Ramsey acknowledges, even where the government allows them to be made by default, so that in some instances they are determined largely by which private pressure groups prove to be dominant. In any event, there is virtue in taking up one complicated question at a time and we need to get the thrust of the case for equal access before us. It is enough to observe now that Americans attach an obviously high priority to organized health care. National health expenditures for the fiscal year 1972 were $83.4 billion.[4] Even if such an enormous sum is not entirely adequate, we may still ask: how are we to justify spending whatever we do in accordance as far as possible with the goal of equal access? The answer I propose involves distinguishing various conceptions of social justice and trying to show which of these apply or fail to apply to health care considerations. Only toward the end of the paper will some institutional implications be given more than passing attention, and then in a strictly programmatic way.

Another sort of query should be noted as we begin. What stake does someone in religious ethics have in this discussion? For the reasonable case envisaged is offered after all in the public forum. If the issue is how to justify morally the societal goal which seems so obvious to so many, whether or not they are religious believers, does the religious ethicist then simply participate qua citizen? Here I think we should be wary of simplifying formulae. Why for example should a Jew or a Christian not welcome wide support for a societal goal which he or she can affirm and reaffirm, or reflect only on instances where such support is not forthcoming? If a number of ethical schemes, both religious and humanist, converge in their acceptance of the goal of equal access to health care, so be it. Secularists can join forces with believers, at least at some levels or points, without implying there must be unanimity on every moral issue. Yet it also seems too simple if one claims to wear only the citizen's hat when making the case in question. At least I should admit that a commitment to the basic normative principle which in Christian writings is often called *agape* may influence the account to follow in ways large and small.[5] For example, someone with such a commitment will quite naturally take a special interest in appeals to the generic characteristics all persons share rather than the idiosyncratic attainments which distinguish persons from one another, and in the playing down of desert considerations. As I shall try to show, such appeals are centrally relevant to the case for equal access. And they are nicely in line with the normative pressures agapeic considerations typically exert.

One issue of theoretical importance in religious ethics also emerges in connection with this last point. The approach in this paper may throw a little indirect light on the traditional question, especially prominent in Christian ethics, of how love and justice are related. To distinguish different conceptions of social justice will put us in a better position, I think, to recognize that often it is ambiguous to ask about "*the* relation." There may be different relations to different conceptions. For the conceptions themselves may some-

From *The Journal of Religious Ethics* 2 (Spring 1974): 11-32. Used by permission.

times produce discordant indications, or turn out to be incommensurable, or reflect, when different ones are seized upon, rival moral points of view. I shall note several of these relations as we proceed.

Which then among the standard conceptions of social justice appear to be particularly relevant or irrelevant? Let us consider the following five:

I. To each according to his merit or desert.
II. To each according to his societal contribution.
III. To each according to his contribution in satisfying whatever is freely desired by others in the open marketplace of supply and demand.
IV. To each according to his needs.
V. Similar treatment for similar cases.

In general I shall argue that the first three of these are less relevant because of certain distinctive features which health crises possess. I shall focus on crises here not because I think preventive care is unimportant (the opposite is true), but because the crisis situation shows most clearly the special significance we attach to medical treatment as an institutionalized activity or social practice, and the basic purpose we suppose it to have.

I

To each according to his merit or desert. Meritarian conceptions, above all perhaps, are grading ones: advantages are allocated in accordance with amounts of energy expended or kinds of results achieved. What is judged is particular conduct which distinguishes persons from one another and not only the fact that all the parties are human beings. Sometimes a competitive aspect looms large.

In certain contexts it is illuminating to distinguish between efforts and achievements. In the case of efforts one characteristically focuses on the individual: rewards are based on the pains one takes. Some have supposed, for example, that entry into the kingdom of heaven is linked more directly to energy displayed and fidelity shown than to successful results attained.

To assess achievements is to weigh actual performance and productive contributions. The academic prize is awarded to the student with the highest grade-point average, regardless of the amount of midnight oil he or she burned in preparing for the examinations. Sometimes we may exclaim, "it's just not fair," when person X writes a brilliant paper with little effort while we are forced to devote more time with less impressive results. But then our complaint may be directed against differences in innate ability and talent which no expenditure of effort altogether removes.

After the difference between effort and achievement, and related distinctions, have been acknowledged, what should be stressed I think is the general importance of meritarian or desert criteria in the thinking of most people about justice. These criteria may serve to illuminate a number of disputes about the justice of various practices and institutional arrangements in our society. It may help to explain, for instance, the resentment among the working class against the welfare system. However wrongheaded or self-deceptive the resentment often is, particularly when directed toward those who want to work but for various reasons beyond their control cannot, at its better moments it involves in effect an appeal to desert considerations. "Something for nothing" is repudiated as unjust; benefits should be proportional (or at least related) to costs; those who can make an effort should do so, whatever the degree of their training or significance of their contribution to society; and so on. So, too, persons deserve to have what they have labored for; unless they infringe on the works of others their efforts and achievements are justly theirs.

Occasionally the appeal to desert extends to a wholesale rejection of other considerations as grounds for just claims. The most conspicuous target is need. Consider this statement by Ayn Rand.

> A morality that holds *need* as a claim, holds emptiness—nonexistence—as its standard of value; it rewards an absence, a defect: weakness, inability, incompetence, suffering, disease, disaster, the lack, the fault, the flaw—the *zero.*
>
> Who provides the account to pay these claims? Those who are cursed for being non-zeros, each to the extent of his distance from that ideal. Since all values are the product of virtues, the degree of your virtue is used as the measure of your penalty; the degree of your faults is used as the measure of your gain. Your code declares that the rational man must sacrifice himself to the irrational, the independent man to parasites, the honest man to the dishonest, the man of justice to the unjust, the productive man to thieving loafers, the man of integrity to compromising knaves, the man of self-esteem to sniveling neurotics. Do you wonder at the meanness of soul in those you see around you? The man who achieves these virtues will not accept your moral code; the man who accepts your moral code will not achieve these virtues.[6]

I have noted elsewhere[7] that *agape,* while it characteristically plays down, need not formally disallow attention to considerations falling under merit or desert; for in the case of merit as well as need it may be possible, the quotation above notwithstanding, to reason solely from egalitarian premises. A major reason such attention is warranted concerns what was called there the differential exercise of an equal liberty. That is, one may fittingly revere another's moral capacities and thus the efforts he makes as well as the ends he seeks. Such reverence may lead one to weigh expenditure of energy and specific achievements. I would simply hold now (1) that the idea of justice is not exhaustively characterized by the notion of desert, even if one agrees that the latter plays an important role; and (2) that the notion of desert is especially ill-suited to play an important role in the determination of policies which should govern a system of health care.

Why is it so ill-suited? Here we encounter some of the distinctive features which it seems to me health crises possess. Let me put it in this way. Health crises seem non-meritarian because they occur so often for reasons beyond our control or power to predict. They frequently fall without discrimination on the (according-to-merit) just and unjust, i.e., the virtuous and the wicked, the industrious and the slothful alike.

While we may believe that virtues and vices cannot depend upon natural contingencies, we are bound to admit, it seems, that many health crises do. It makes sense therefore to say that we are equal in being randomly susceptible to these crises. Even those who ascribe a prominent role to desert acknowledge that justice has also properly to do with pleas of "But I could not help it."[8] One seeks to distinguish such cases from those acknowledged to be praiseworthy or blameworthy. Then it seems unfair as well as unkind to discriminate among those who suffer health crises on the basis of their personal deserts. For it would be odd to maintain that a newborn child deserves his hemophilia or the tumor afflicting her spine.

These considerations help to explain why the following rough distinction is often made. Bernard Williams, for example, in his discussion of "equality in unequal circumstances," identifies two different sorts of inequality, inequality of merit and inequality of need, and two corresponding goods, those earned by effort and those demanded by need.[9] Medical treatment in the event of illness is located under the umbrella of need. He concludes: "Leaving aside preventive medicine, the proper ground of distribution of medical care is ill health: this is a necessary truth."[10] An irrational state of affairs is held to obtain if those whose needs are the same are treated unequally, when needs are the ground of the treatment. One might put the point this way. When people are equal in the relevant respects—in this case when their needs are the same and occur in a context of random, undeserved susceptibility—that by itself is a good reason for treating them equally.[11]

In many societies, however, a second necessary condition for the receipt of medical treatment exists de facto: the possession of money. This is not the place to consider the general question of when inequalities in wealth may be regarded as just. It is enough to note that one can plausibly appeal to all of the conceptions of justice we are embarked in sorting out. A person may be thought to be entitled to a higher income when he works more, contributes more, risks more, and not simply when he needs more. We may think it fair that the industrious should have more money than the slothful and the surgeon more than the tobacconist. The difficulty comes in the misfit between the reasons for differential incomes and the reasons for receiving medical treatment. The former may include a pluralistic set of claims in which different notions of justice must be meshed. The latter are more monistically focused on needs, and the other notions not accorded a similar relevance. Yet money may nonetheless remain as a causally necessary condition for receiving medical treatment. It may be the power to secure what one needs. The senses in which health crises are distinctive may then be insufficiently determinative for the policies which govern the actual availability of treatment. The nearly automatic links between income, prestige, and the receipt of comparatively higher quality medical treatment should then be subjected to critical scrutiny. For unequal treatment of the rich ill and the poor ill is unjust if, again, needs rather than differential income constitute the ground of such treatment.

Suppose one agrees that it is important to recognize the misfit between the reasons for differential incomes and the reasons for receiving medical treatment, and that therefore income as such should not govern the actual availability of treatment. One may still ask whether the case so far relies excessively on "pure" instances where desert considerations are admittedly out of place. That there are such pure instances, tumors afflicting the spine, hemophilia, and so on, is not denied. Yet it is an exaggeration if we go on and regard all health crises as utterly unconnected with desert. Note for example that Williams leaves aside preventive medicine. And if in a cool hour we examine the statistics, we find that a vast number of deaths occur each year due to causes not always beyond our control, e.g., automobile accidents, drugs, alcohol, tobacco, obesity, and so on. In some final reckoning it seems that many persons (though crucially, not all) have an effect on, and arguably a responsibility for, their own medical needs. Consider the following bidders for emergency care: (1) a person with a heart attack who is seriously overweight; (2) a football hero who has suffered a concussion; (3) a man with lung cancer who has smoked cigarettes for forty years; (4) a 60 year old man who has always taken excellent care of himself and is suddenly stricken with leukemia; (5) a three year old girl who has swallowed poison left out carelessly by her parents; (6) a 14 year old boy who has been beaten without provocation by a gang and suffers brain damage and recurrent attacks of uncontrollable terror; (7) a college student who has slashed his wrists (and not for the first time) from a psychological need for attention; (8) a woman raised in the ghetto who is found unconscious due to an overdose of heroin.

These cases help to show why the whole subject of medical treatment is so crucial and so perplexing. They attest to some melancholy elements in human experience. People suffer in varying ratios the effects of their natural and undeserved vulnerabilities, the irresponsibility and brutality of others, and their own desires and weaknesses. In some final reckoning then desert considerations seem not irrelevant to many health crises. The practical applicability of this admission, however, in the instance of health care delivery, appears limited. We may agree that it underscores the importance of preventive health care by stressing the influence we sometimes have over our medical needs. But if we try to foster such care by increasing the penalties for neglect, we normally confine ourselves to calculations about incentives. At the risk of being denounced in some quarters as censorious and puritanical, perhaps we should for example levy far higher taxes on alcohol and tobacco and pump the dollars directly into health care programs rather than (say) into highway building. Yet these steps would by no means lead necessarily to a demand that we correlate in some strict way a demonstrated effort to be temperate with the receipt of privileged medical treatment as a reward. Would it be feasible to allocate the additional tax monies to the man with leukemia before the overweight man suffering a heart attack on the ground of a difference in desert? At the point of emergency care at least, it seems impracticable for the doctor to discriminate between these cases, to make meritarian judgments at the point of catastrophe. And the number of persons who are in need of medical treatment for reasons utterly beyond their control remains a datum with tenacious relevance. There are those who suffer the ravages of a tornado, are handicapped by a genetic defect, beaten without provocation, etc. A commitment to the basic purpose of medical care and to the institutions for achieving it involves the recognition of this persistent state of affairs.

II

To each according to his societal contribution. This conception gives moral primacy to notions such as the public interest, the common good, the welfare of the community, or the greatest good of the greatest number. Here one judges the social consequences of particular conduct. The formula can be construed in at least two ways.[12] It may refer to the interest of the social group considered collectively, where the group has some independent life all its own. The group's welfare is the decisive criterion for determining what constitutes any member's proper share. Or the common good may refer only to an aggregation of distinct individuals and considered distributively.

Either version accords such a primacy to what is socially advantageous as to be unacceptable not only to defenders of need, but also, it would seem, of desert. For the criteria of effort and achievement are often conceived along rather individualistic lines. The pains an agent takes or the results he brings about deserve recompense, whether or not the public interest is directly served. No automatic harmony then is necessarily assumed between his just share as individually earned and his proper share from the vantage point of the common good. Moreover, the test of social advantage *simpliciter* obviously threatens the agapeic concern with some minimal consideration due each person which is never to be disregarded for the sake of long-range social benefits. No one should be considered as *merely* a means or instrument.

The relevance of the canon of social productiveness to health crises may accordingly also be challenged. Indeed, such crises may cut against it in that they occur more frequently to those whose comparative contribution to the general welfare is less, e.g., the aged, the disabled, children.

Consider for example Paul Ramsey's persuasive critique of social and economic criteria for the allocation of a single scarce medical resource. He begins by recounting the imponderables which faced the widely-discussed "public committee" at the Swedish Hospital in Seattle when it deliberated in the early 1960's. The sparse resource in this case was the kidney machine. The committee was charged with the responsibility of selecting among patients suffering chronic renal failure those who were to receive dialysis. Its criteria were broadly social and economic. Considerations weighed included age, sex, marital status, number of dependents, income, net worth, educational background, occupation, past performance and future potential. The application of such criteria proved to be exceedingly problematic. Should someone with six children always have priority over an artist or composer?

Were those who arranged matters so that their families would not burden society to be penalized in effect for being provident? And so on. Two critics of the committee found "a disturbing picture of the bourgeoisie sparing the bourgeoisie" and observed that "the Pacific Northwest is no place for a Henry David Thoreau with bad kidneys."[13]

The mistake, Ramsey believes, is to introduce criteria of social worthiness in the first place. In those situations of choice where not all can be saved and yet all need not die, "the equal right of every human being to live, and not relative personal or social worth, should be the ruling principle."[14] The principle leads to a criterion of "random choice among equals" expressed by a lottery scheme or a practice of "first-come, first-served." Several reasons stand behind Ramsey's defense of the criterion of random choice. First, a religious belief in the equality of persons before God leads intelligibly to a refusal to choose between those who are dying in any way other than random patient selection. Otherwise their equal value as human beings is threatened. Second, a moral primacy is ascribed to survival over other (perhaps superior) interests persons may have, in that it is the condition of everything else. ". . . Life is a value incommensurate with all others, and so not negotiable by bartering one man's worth against another's."[15] Third, the entire enterprise of estimating a person's social worth is viewed with final skepticism. ". . . We have no way of knowing how really and truly to estimate a man's societal worth or his worth to others or to himself in unfocused social situations in the ordinary lives of men in their communities."[16] This statement, incidentally, appears to allow something other than randomness in *focused* social situations; when, say, a President or Prime Minister and the owner of the local bar rush for the last place in the bomb shelter, and the knowledge of the former can save many lives. In any event, I have been concerned with a restricted point to which Ramsey's discussion brings illustrative support. The canon of social productiveness is notoriously difficult to apply as a workable criterion for distributing medical services to those who need them.

One may go further. A system of health care delivery which treats people on the basis of the medical care required may often go against (at least narrowly conceived) calculations of societal advantage. For example, the health care needs of people tend to rise during that period of their lives, signaled by retirement, when their incomes and social productivity are declining. More generally:

> Some 40 to 50 per cent of the American people—the aged, children, the dependent poor, and those with some significant chronic disability are in categories requiring relatively large amounts of medical care but with inadequate resources to purchase such care.[17]

If one agrees, for whatever reasons, with the agapeic judgment that each person should be regarded as irreducibly valuable, then one cannot succumb to a social productiveness criterion of human worth. Interests are to be equally considered even when people have ceased to be, or are not yet, or perhaps never will be, public assets.

III

To each according to his contribution in satisfying whatever is freely desired by others in the open marketplace of supply and demand. Here we have a test which, though similar to the preceding one, concentrates on what is desired de facto by certain segments of the community rather than the community as a whole, and on the relative scarcity of the service rendered. It is tantamount to the canon of supply and demand as espoused by various laissez-faire theoreticians.[18] Rewards should be given to those who by virtue of special skill, prescience, risk-taking, and the like discern what is desired and are able to take the requisite steps to bring satisfaction. A surgeon, it may be argued, contributes more than a nurse because of the greater training and skill required, burdens borne, and effective care provided, and should be compensated accordingly. So too perhaps, a star quarterback on a pro-football team should be remunerated even more highly because of the rare athletic prowess needed, hazards involved, and widespread demand to watch him play.

This formula does not then call for the weighing of the value of various contributions, and tends to conflate needs and wants under a notion of desires. It also assumes that a prominent part is assigned to consumer free-choice. The consumer should be at liberty to express his preferences, and to select from a variety of competing goods and services. Those who resist many changes currently proposed in the organization and financing of health care delivery in the U.S.A. —such as national health insurance—often do so by appealing to some variant of this formula.

Yet it seems health crises are often of overriding importance when they occur. They appear therefore not satisfactorily accommodated to the context of a free marketplace where consumers may freely choose among alternative goods and services.

To clarify what is at stake in the above contention,

let us examine an opposing case. Robert M. Sade, M.D., published an article in *The New England Journal of Medicine* entitled "Medical Care as a Right: A Refutation" (1971). He attacks programs of national health insurance in the name of a person's right to select one's own values, determine how they may be realized, and dispose of them if one chooses without coercion from other men. The values in question are construed as economic ones in the context of supply and demand. So we read:

> In a free society, man exercises his right to sustain his own life by producing economic values in the form of goods and services that he is, or should be, free to exchange with other men who are similarly free to trade with him or not. The economic values produced, however, are not given as gifts by nature, but exist only by virtue of the thought and effort of individual men. Goods and services are thus owned as a consequence of the right to sustain life by one's own physical and mental effort.[19]

Sade compares the situation of the physician to that of the baker. The one who produces a loaf of bread should as owner have the power to dispose of his own product. It is immoral simply to expropriate the bread without the baker's permission. Similarly, "medical care is neither a right nor a privilege: it is a service that is provided by doctors and others to people who wish to purchase it."[20] Any coercive regulation of professional practices by the society at large is held to be analogous to taking the bread from the baker without his consent. Such regulation violates the freedom of the physician over his own services and will lead inevitably to provider-apathy.

The analogy surely misleads. To assume that doctors autonomously produce goods and services in a fashion closely akin to a baker is grossly oversimplified. The baker may himself rely on the agricultural produce of others, yet there is a crucial difference in the degree of dependence. Modern physicians depend on the achievements of medical technology and the entire scientific base underlying it, all of which is made possible by a host of persons whose salaries are often notably less. Moreover, the amount of taxpayer support for medical research and education is too enormous to make any such unqualified case for provider-autonomy plausible.

However conceptually clouded Sade's article may be, its stress on a free exchange of goods and services reflects one historically influential rationale for much American medical practice. And he applies it not only to physicians but also to patients or "consumers."

> The question is whether the decision of how to allocate the consumer's dollar should belong to the consumer or to the state. It has already been shown that the choice of how a doctor's services should be rendered belongs only to the doctor: in the same way the choice of whether to buy a doctor's service rather than some other commodity or service belongs to the consumer as a logical consequence of the right to his own life.[21]

This account is misguided, I think, because it ignores the overriding importance which is so often attached to health crises. When lumps appear on someone's neck, it usually makes little sense to talk of choosing whether to buy a doctor's service rather than a color television set. References to just trade-offs suddenly seem out of place. No compensation suffices, since the penalties may differ so much.

There is even a further restriction on consumer choice. One's knowledge in these circumstances is comparatively so limited. The physician makes most of the decisions: about diagnosis, treatment, hospitalization, number of return visits, and so on. In brief:

> The consumer knows very little about the medical services he is buying—probably less than about any other service he purchases. . . . While [he] can still play a role in policing the market, that role is much more limited in the field of health care than in almost any other area of private economic activity.[22]

For much of the way, then, an appeal to supply and demand and consumer choice is not quite fitting. It neglects the issue of the value of various contributions. And it fails to allow for the recognition that medical treatments may be overridingly desired. In contexts of catastrophe at any rate, when life itself is threatened, most persons (other than those who are apathetic or seek to escape from the terrifying prospects) cannot take medical care to be merely one option among others.

IV

To each according to his needs. The concept of needs is sometimes taken to apply to an entire range of interests which concern a person's "psycho-physical existence."[23] On this wide usage, to attribute a need to someone is to say that the person lacks what is thought to conduce to his or her "welfare"—understood in both a physiological sense (e.g., for food, drink, shelter, and health) and a psychological one (e.g., for continuous human affection and support).

Yet even in the case of such a wide usage, what the person lacks is typically assumed to be basic. Attention is restricted to recurrent considerations rather than to every possible individual whim or frivolous pursuit. So one is not surprised to meet with the contention that a preferable rendering of this formula would be: "to each according to his essential needs."[24] This contention seems to me well taken. It implies, for one thing, that basic needs are distinguishable from felt needs or wants. For the latter may encompass expressions of personal preference unrelated to considerations of survival or subsistence, and sometimes artificially generated by circumstances of rising affluence in the society at large.

Essential needs are also typically assumed to be given rather than acquired. They are not constituted by any action for which the person is responsible by virtue of his or her distinctively greater effort. It is almost as if the designation "innocent" may be linked illuminatingly to need, as retribution, punishment, and so on, are to desert, and in complex ways, to freedom. Thus essential needs are likewise distinguishable from deserts. Where needs are unequal, one thinks of them as fortuitously distributed; as part, perhaps, of a kind of "natural lottery."[25] So very often the advantages of health and the burdens of illness, for example, strike one as arbitrary effects of the lottery. It seems wrong to say that a newborn child deserves as a reward all of his faculties when he has done nothing in particular which distinguishes him from another newborn who comes into the world deprived of one or more of them. Similarly, though crudely, many religious believers do not look on natural events as personal deserts. They are not inclined to pronounce sentences such as, "That evil person with incurable cancer got what he deserved." They are disposed instead to search for some distinction between what they may call the conditions of finitude on the one hand and sin and moral evil on the other. If the distinction is "ultimately" invalid, in this life it seems inscrutably so. Here and now it may be usefully drawn. Inequalities in the need for medical treatment are taken, it appears, to reflect the conditions of finitude more than anything else.

One can even go on to argue that among our basic or essential needs, the case of medical treatment is conspicuous in the following sense. While food and shelter are not matters about which we are at liberty to please ourselves, they are at least predictable. We can plan, for instance, to store up food and fuel for the winter. It may be held that responsibility increases along with the power to predict. If so, then many health crises seem peculiarly random and uncontrollable. Cancer, given the present state of knowledge at any rate, is a contingent disaster, whereas hunger is a steady threat. Who will need serious medical care, and when, is then perhaps a classic example of uncertainty.

Finally, and more theoretically, it is often observed that a need-conception of justice comes closest to charity or *agape.*[26] I think there are indeed crucial overlaps.[27] To cite several of them: the equal consideration *agape* enjoins has to do in the first instance with those generic endowments which people share, the characteristics of a person qua human existent. Needs, as we have seen, likewise concern those things essential to the life and welfare of men considered simply as men.[28] They are not based on particular conduct alone, on those idiosyncratic attainments which contribute to someone's being such-and-such a kind of person. Yet a certain sort of inequality is recognized, for needs differ in divergent circumstances and so treatments must if benefits are to be equalized. *Agape* too allows for a distinction between equal consideration and identical treatment. The aim of equalizing benefits is implied by the injunction to consider the interests of each party equally. This may require differential treatments of differing interests.

Overlaps such as these will doubtless strike some as so extensive that it may be asked whether *agape* and a need-conception of justice are virtually equivalent. I think not. One contrast was pointed out before. The differential treatment enjoined by *agape* is more complex and goes deeper. In the case of *agape,* attention may be appropriately given to varying *efforts* as well as to unequal *needs.* More generally one may say that agapeic considerations extend to all of the psychological nuances and contextual details of individual persons and their circumstances. Imaginative concern is enjoined for concrete human beings: for what someone is uniquely, for what he or she—as a matter of personal history and distinctive identity—wants, feels, thinks, celebrates, and endures. The attempt to establish and enhance mutual affection between individual persons is taken likewise to be fitting. Conceptions of social justice, including "to each according to his essential needs," tend to be more restrictive; they call attention to considerations which obtain for a number of persons, to impersonally specified criteria for assessing collective policies and practices. *Agape* involves more, even if one supposes never less.

Other differences could be noted. What is important now however is the recognition that, in matters of health care in particular, *agape* and a need-conception of justice are conjoined in a number of relevant respects. At least this is so for those who think that, again, justice has properly to do with pleas of "But I could not help it." It seeks to distinguish such cases from those acknowledged to be praiseworthy or blameworthy. The formula "to each according to his needs" is one cogent way of identifying the moral relevance of these pleas. To ignore them may be thought to be unfair as well as unkind when they arise from the deprivation of some essential need. The move to confine the notion of justice wholly to desert considerations is thereby resisted as well. Hence we may say that sometimes "questions of social justice arise just because people are unequal in ways they can do very little to change and . . . only by attending to these inequalities can one be said to be giving their interests equal consideration."[29]

V

Similar treatment for similar cases. This conception is perhaps the most familiar of all. Certainly it is the most formal and inclusive one. It is frequently taken as an elementary appeal to consistency and linked to the universalizability test. One should not make an arbitrary exception on one's own behalf, but rather should apply impartially whatever standards one accepts. The conception can be fruitfully applied to health care questions and I shall assume its relevance. Yet as literally interpreted, it is necessary but not sufficient. For rightly or not, it is often held to be as compatible with no positive treatment whatever as with active promotion of other people's interests, as long as all are equally and impartially included. Its exponents sometimes assume such active promotion without demonstrating clearly how this is built into the conception itself. Moreover, it may obscure a distinction which we have seen agapists and others make: between equal consideration and identical treatment. Needs may differ and so treatments must, if benefits are to be equalized.

I have placed this conception at the end of the list partly because it moves us, despite its formality, toward practice. Let me suggest briefly how it does so. Suppose first of all one agrees with the case so far offered. Suppose, that is, it has been shown convincingly that a need-conception of justice applies with greater relevance than the earlier three when one reflects about the basic purpose of medical care. To treat one class of people differently from another because of income or geographic location should therefore be ruled out, because such reasons are irrelevant. (The irrelevance is conceptual, rather than always, unfortunately, causal.) In short, all persons should have equal access, "as needed, without financial, geographic, or other barriers, to the whole spectrum of health services."[30]

Suppose however, secondly, that the goal of equal access collides on some occasions with the realities of finite medical resources and needs which prove to be insatiable. That such collisions occur in fact it would be idle to deny. And it is here that the practical bearing of the formula of similar treatment for similar cases should be noticed. Let us recall Williams' conclusion: "the proper ground of distribution of medical care is ill health: this is a necessary truth." While I agree with the essentials of his argument—for all the reasons above—I would prefer, for practical purposes, a slightly more modest formulation. Illness is the proper ground for the *receipt* of medical care. However, the *distribution* of medical care in less-than-optimal circumstances requires us to face the collisions. I would argue that in such circumstances the formula of similar treatment for similar cases may be construed so as to guide actual choices in the way most compatible with the goal of equal access. The formula's allowance of no positive treatment whatever may justify exclusion of entire classes of cases from a priority list. Yet it forbids doing so for irrelevant or arbitrary reasons. So (1) if we accept the case for equal access, but (2) if we simply cannot, physically cannot, treat all who are in need, it seems more just to discriminate by virtue of categories of illness, for example, rather than between the rich ill and poor ill. All persons with a certain rare, non-communicable disease would not receive priority, let us say, where the costs were inordinate, the prospects for rehabilitation remote, and for the sake of equalized benefits to many more. Or with Ramsey we may urge a policy of random patient selection when one must decide between claimants for a medical treatment unavailable to all. Or we may acknowledge that any notion of "comprehensive benefits" to which persons should have equal access is subject to practical restrictions which will vary from society to society depending on resources at a given time. Even in a country as affluent as the United States there will surely always be items excluded, e.g., perhaps over-the-counter drugs, some teenage orthodontia, cosmetic surgery, and the like.[31] Here too the formula of similar treatment for similar cases may serve to modify the application of a need-conception of justice in order to address the insatiability-problem and limit frivolous use. In all of the foregoing instances of restriction, however, the relevant feature remains the illness, discomfort, etc. itself. The goal of equal access then retains its prima facie authoritativeness. It is imperfectly realized rather than disregarded.

VI

These latter comments lead on to the question of institutional implications. I cannot aim here of course for the specificity rightly sought by policy-makers. My endeavor has been conceptual elucidation. While the ethicist needs to be apprised about the facts, he or she does not, qua ethicist, don the mantle of the policy-expert. In any case, only rarely does anyone do both things equally well. Yet cross-fertilization is extremely desirable. For experts should not be isolated from the wider assumptions their recommendations may reflect. I shall merely list some of the topics which would have to be discussed at length if we were to get clear about the implications. Examples will be limited to the current situation in the United States.

Anyone who accepts the case for equal access will naturally be concerned about de facto disparities in the availability of medical treatment. Let us consider two relevant indictments of current American practice. They appear in the writings not only of those who attack indiscriminately a system seen to be governed only by the appetite for profit and power, but also of those who denounce in less sweeping terms and espouse more cautiously reformist positions. The first shortcoming has to do with the maldistribution of supply. Per capita ratios of physicians to populations served vary, sometimes notoriously, between affluent suburbs and rural and inner city areas. This problem is exacerbated by the distressing data concerning the greater health needs of the poor. Chronic disease, frequency and duration of hospitalization, psychiatric disorders, infant death rates, etc.—these occur in significantly larger proportions to lower income members of American society.[32] A further complication is that "the distribution of health insurance coverage is badly skewed. Practically all the rich have insurance. But among the poor, about two-thirds have none. As a result, among people aged 25 to 64 who die, some 45 to 50 per cent have neither hospital nor surgical coverage."[33] This last point connects with a second shortcoming frequently cited. Even those who are otherwise economically independent may be shattered by the high cost of a "catastrophic illness."[34]

Proposals for institutional reforms designed to overcome such disparities are bound to be taken seriously by any defender of equal access. What he or she will be disposed to press for, of course, is the removal of any double standard or "two class" system of care. The viable procedures for bringing this about are not obvious, and comparisons with certain other societies (for relevant alternative models) are drawn now with perhaps less confidence.[35] One set of commonly discussed proposals includes (1) incentive subsidies to physicians, hospitals, and medical centers to provide services in regions of poverty (to overcome in part the unwillingness—to which no unique culpability need be ascribed—of many providers and their spouses to work and live in grim surroundings); (2) licensure controls to avoid comparatively excessive concentrations of physicians in regions of affluence; (3) a period of time (say, two years) in an underserved area as a requirement for licensing; (4) redistribution facilities which allow for population shifts.

A second set of proposals is linked with health insurance itself. While I cannot venture into the intricacies of medical economics or comment on the various bills for national health insurance presently inundating Congress, it may be instructive to take brief note of one proposal in which, once more, the defender of equal access is bound to take an interest (even if he or she finally rejects it on certain practical grounds). The precise details of the proposal are unimportant for our purposes.[36] Consider this crude sketch. Each citizen is (in effect) issued a card by the government. Whenever "legitimate" medical expenses (however determined for a given society) exceed, say, 10 per cent of his or her annual taxable income, the card may be presented so that additional costs incurred will be paid for out of general tax revenues. The reasons urged on behalf of this sort of arrangement include the following. In the case of medical care there is warrant for proportionately equalizing what is spent from anyone's total taxable income. This warrant reflects the conditions, discussed earlier, of the natural lottery. Insofar as the advantages of health and the burdens of illness are random and undeserved, we may find it in our common interest to share risks. A fixed percentage of income attests to the misfit, also mentioned previously, between the reasons for differential total income and the reasons for receiving medical treatment. If money remains a causally necessary condition for receiving medical treatment, then a way must be found to place it in the hands of those who need it. The card is one such means. It is designed effectively to equalize purchasing power. In this way it seems to accord nicely with the goal of equal access. On the other side, the requirement of initial out-of-pocket expenses—sufficiently large in comparison to average family expenditures on health care—is designed to discourage frivolous use and foster awareness that medical care is a benefit not to be simply taken as a matter of course. It also safeguards against an excessively large tax burden while providing universal protection against the often disastrous costs of serious illnesses. Whether 10 per cent is too great a chunk for the very poor to pay, and whether by itself the proposal will feed price inflation and neglect of preventive medicine are questions which would have to be answered.

Another kind of possible institutional reform will also greatly interest the defender of equal access. This has to do with the "design of health care systems" or "care settings." The prevalent setting in American society has always been "fee-for-service." It is left up to each person to obtain the requisite care and to pay for it as he or she goes along. Because costs for medical treatment have accelerated at such an alarming rate, and because the sheer diffusion of energy and effort so characteristic of American medical practice leaves more and more people dissatisfied, alternatives to fee-for-service have been considered of late with unprecedented seriousness. The alternative care setting most widely discussed is prepaid practice, and specifically the "health maintenance organization" (HMO). Here one finds "an organized system of care which accepts the responsibility to provide or otherwise assure comprehensive care to a defined population for a fixed periodic payment per person or per family. . . ."[37] The best-known HMO is the Kaiser-Permanente Medical Care Program.[38] Does the HMO serve to realize the goal of equal access more fully? One line of argument in its favor is this. It is plausible to think that equal access will be fostered by the more economical care setting. HMO's are held to be less costly per capita in at least two respects: hospitalization rates are much below the national average; and less often noted, physician manpower is as well. To be sure, one should be sensitive to the corruptions in each type of setting. While fee-for-service has resulted in a suspiciously high number of surgeries (twice as many per capita in the United States as in Great Britain), the HMO physician may more frequently permit the patient's needs to be overridden by the organization's pressure to economize. It may also be more difficult in an HMO setting to provide for close personal relations between a particular physician and a particular patient (something commended, of course, on all sides). After such corruptions are allowed for, the data seem encouraging to such an extent that a defender of equal access will certainly support the repeal of any law which limits the development of prepaid practice, to approve of "front-aid" subsidies for HMO's to increase their number overall and achieve a more equitable distribution throughout the country, and so on. At a minimum, each care setting should be available in every region. If we assume a common freedom to choose between them, each may help to guard against the peculiar temptations to which the other is exposed.

To assess in any serious way proposals for institutional reform such as the above is beyond the scope of this paper. We would eventually be led, for example, into the question of whether it is consistent for the rich to pay more than the poor for the same treatment when, again, needs rather than income constitute the ground of the treatment,[39] and from there into the tangled subject of the "ethics of redistribution" in general.[40] Other complex issues deserve to be considered as well, e.g., the criteria for allocation of limited resources,[41] and how conceptions of justice apply to the providers of health care.[42]

Those committed to self-conscious moral and religious reflection about subjects in medicine have concentrated, perhaps unduly, on issues about care of individual patients (as death approaches, for instance). These issues plainly warrant the most careful consideration. One would like to see in addition, however, more attention paid to social questions in medical ethics. To attend to them is not necessarily to leave behind all of the matters which reach deeply into the human condition. Any detailed case for institutional reforms, for example, will be enriched if the proponent asks soberly whether certain conflicts and certain perplexities allow for more than partial improvements and provisional resolutions. Can public and private interests ever be made fully to coincide by legislative and administrative means? Will the commitment of a physician to an individual patient and the commitment of the legislator to the "common good" ever be harmonized in every case? Our anxiety may be too intractable. Our fear of illness and of dying may be so pronounced and immediate that we will seize the nearly automatic connections between privilege, wealth, and power if we can. We will do everything possible to have our kidney machines even if the charts make it clear that many more would benefit from mandatory immunization at a fraction of the cost. And our capacity for taking in rival points of view may be too limited. Once we have witnessed tangible suffering, we cannot just return with ease to public policies aimed at statistical patients. Those who believe that justice is the pre-eminent virtue of institutions and that a case can be convincingly made on behalf of justice for equal access to health care would do well to ponder such conflicts and perplexities. Our reforms might then seem, to ourselves and to others, less abstract and jargon-filled in formulation and less sanguine and piecemeal in substance. They would reflect a greater awareness of what we have to confront.

Notes

1. See, e.g., Richard M. Nixon, "President's Message on Health Care System," Document no. 92-261 (March 2, 1972), House of Representatives, Washington, D.C.; and Edward M. Kennedy, *In Critical Condition: The Crisis in America's Health Care* (New York: Simon and Schuster, 1972).

2. These writings include Hugo A. Bedau, "Radical Egalitarianism," in *Justice and Equality,* ed. Hugo A. Bedau (Englewood Cliffs, N.J.: Prentice-Hall, 1971); John Hospers, *Human Conduct* (New York: Harcourt, Brace and World, 1961); J. R. Lucas, "Justice," *Philosophy* 47 (July 1972): 229-48; C. Perelman, *The Idea of Justice and the Problem of Argument,* trans. J. Petrie (London: Routledge and Kegan Paul, 1963); Nicholas Rescher, *Distributive Justice* (Indianapolis: Bobbs-Merrill, 1966); John A. Ryan, *Distributive Justice* (New York: Macmillan, 1916); and Gregory Vlastos, "Justice and Equality," in *Social Justice,* ed. Richard B. Brandt (Englewood Cliffs, N.J.: Prentice Hall, 1962).

3. Paul Ramsey, *The Patient as Person* (New Haven: Yale University Press, 1970), 240.

4. Nancy Hicks, "Nation's Doctors Move to Police Medical Care," *New York Times,* 28 October 1973, 52.

5. See Gene Outka, *Agape: An Ethical Analysis* (New Haven: Yale University Press, 1972).

6. Ayn Rand, *Atlas Shrugged* (New York: Signet, 1957), 958.

7. Outka, *Agape,* 89-90, 165-67.

8. Lucas, "Justice," 321.

9. Bernard A. O. Williams, "The Idea of Equality," in *Justice and Equality,* ed. Bedau, 126-37.

10. Williams, "The Idea of Equality," 127.

11. See also Thomas Nagel, "Equal Treatment and Compensatory Discrimination," *Philosophy and Public Affairs* 2 (Summer 1973): 354.

12. Rescher, *Distributive Justice,* 79-80.

13. Quoted in Ramsey, *Patient as Person,* 248.

14. Ibid., 256.

15. Ibid.

16. Ibid.

17. Anne R. Somers, *Health Care in Transition: Directions for the Future* (Chicago: Hospital Research and Educational Trust, 1971), 20.

18. See Rescher, *Distributive Justice,* 80-81.

19. Robert M. Sade, "Medical Care as a Right: A Refutation," *New England Journal of Medicine* 285 (December 1971): 1289.

20. Ibid.

21. Ibid., 1291.

22. Charles L. Schultze et al., *Setting National Priorities: The 1973 Budget* (Washington, D.C.: The Brookings Institution, 1972), 214-15.

23. Outka, *Agape,* 264-65.

24. Perelman, *The Idea of Justice,* 22.

25. See John Rawls, *A Theory of Justice* (Cambridge: Harvard University Press, 1971), 104.

26. See, e.g., Perelman, *The Idea of Justice,* 23.

27. See Outka, *Agape,* 91-92, 309-12.

28. See also A. M. Honoré, "Social Justice," in *Essays in Legal Philosophy,* ed. Robert S. Summers (Oxford: Basil Blackwell, 1968).

29. Stanley I. Benn, "Egalitarianism and the Equal Consideration of Interests," in *Justice and Equality,* ed. Bedau, 164.

30. Anne R. Somers and Herman M. Somers, "The Organization and Financing of Health Care: Issues and Directions for the Future," *American Journal of Orthopsychiatry* 42 (January 1972): 122.

31. Anne R. Somers and Herman M. Somers, "Major Issues in National Health Insurance," *Milbank Memorial Fund Quarterly* 50 (April 1972): 182.

32. James Z. Appel, "Health Care Delivery," in *The Health of Americans,* ed. Boisfeuillet Jones (Englewood Cliffs, N.J.: Prentice Hall, 1970); and William N. Hubbard, "Health Knowledge," in *The Health of Americans,* ed. Jones.

33. Somers, *Health Care in Transition,* 46.

34. See some eloquent examples in Kennedy, *In Critical Condition.*

35. See Odin Anderson, *Health Care: Can There Be Equity? The United States, Sweden and England* (New York: Wiley, 1973).

36. For one much-discussed version, see Martin S. Feldstein, "A New Approach to National Health Insurance," *The Public Interest* 23 (Spring 1971).

37. Anne R. Somers, ed., *The Kaiser-Permanente Medical Care Program* (New York: The Commonwealth Fund, 1971), V.

38. See also Sidney R. Garfield, "Prevention of Dissipation of Health Services Resources," *American Journal of Public Health* 61 (1971).

39. Andrew Ward, "The Idea of Equality Reconsidered," *Philosophy* 48 (January 1973).

40. See, e.g., Stanley I. Benn and Richard S. Peters, *The Principles of Political Thought* (New York: The Free Press, 1965), 155-78; and Bertrand de Jouvenel, *The Ethics of Redistribution* (Cambridge: Cambridge University Press, 1952).

41. The issue of priorities is at least threefold: (1) between improved medical care and other social needs, e.g., to restrain auto accidents and pollution; (2) between different sorts of medical treatments for different illnesses, e.g., prevention vs. crisis intervention and exotic treatments; (3) between persons all of whom need a single scarce resource and not all can have it, e.g., Ramsey's discussion of how to decide among those who are to receive dialysis. Moreover, (1) can be subdivided between (a) improved medical care and other social needs which affect health directly, e.g., drug addiction, auto accidents, and pollution; (b) improved medical care and other social needs which serve the overall aim of community-survival, e.g., a common defense. In the case of (2), one would like to see far more careful discussion of some general criteria which might be employed, e.g., numbers affected, degree of contagion, prospects for rehabilitation, and so on.

42. What sorts of appeals to justice might be cogently made to warrant, for instance, the differentially high income

physicians receive? Here are three possibilities: (1) the greater skill and responsibility involved should be rewarded proportionately, i.e., one should attend to considerations of *desert;* (2) there should be *compensation* for the money invested for education and facilities in order to restore circumstances of approximate equality (this argument, while a common one in medical circles, would need to consider that medical education is received in part at public expense and that the modern physician is the highest paid professional in the country); (3) the difference should benefit the least advantaged more than an alternative arrangement where disparities are less. We prefer a society where the medical profession flourishes and everyone has a longer life expectancy to one where everyone is poverty-stricken with a shorter life expectancy ("splendidly equalized destitution"). Yet how are we to ascertain the minimum degree of differential income required for the least advantaged members of the society to be better off?

Discussions of "justice and the interests of providers" are, I think, badly needed. Physicians in the United States have suffered a decline in prestige for various reasons, e.g., the way many used Medicare to support and increase their own incomes. Yet one should endeavor to assess their interests fairly. A concern for professional autonomy is clearly important, though one may ask whether adequate attention has been paid to the distinction between the imposition of cost-controls from outside and interference with professional medical judgments. One may affirm the former, it seems, and still reject—energetically—the latter.

103. The Concept of Health and the Right to Health Care

JOSEPH M. BOYLE, JR.

The preamble of the Constitution of the World Health Organization states: "The enjoyment of the highest attainable standard of health is one of the fundamental rights of every human being. . . ."[1] Since 1946 when these words were written, the idea that health—or at least health care—is a matter of *right* has become so widely accepted as to be a commonplace.

Not the least of those who have joined in the affirmation of the right to health care is the Catholic Church. Pope John XXIII said "that every man has the right to life, to bodily integrity, and to the means which are necessary and suitable for the proper development of life; these are primarily food, clothing, shelter, rest, medical care, and finally the necessary social services."[2] Pope John's teaching has been reaffirmed by Pope Paul VI[3] and is present, at least implicitly, in the papal social teachings back to Pope Leo XIII.[4] More recently, the United States Catholic Conference, the National Conference of Catholic Charities, and the Catholic Hospital Association have invoked this right.[5]

However, within the last few years, thoughtful observers of American medical practice have raised important questions and serious objections to the claim that there is a right to health. The issues raised by these objections and questions also have application to the less extravagant and more easily justified claim that there is a right to health *care.*

The most common of these objections is based on the fact that being healthy is primarily a matter of individual responsibility. How can one claim as a right that which only his own efforts can achieve? As Leon Kass says:

> Health is a state of being, not something that can be given, and only in indirect ways something that can be taken away or undermined by other human beings. It no more makes sense to claim a right to health than a right to wisdom or courage. These excellences of soul and of body require natural gift, attention, effort, and disci-

From *Social Thought* 3 (Summer 1977): 5-17.

> pline on the part of each person who desires them. To make my health someone else's duty is not only unfair; it is to impose a duty impossible to fulfill.[6]

The line of inquiry suggested here deserves to be taken seriously. It is not based on a "rugged individualist" view of man and society which denies all societal concern for people's welfare. On the contrary, it is based on a serious effort to balance the moral demand that individuals take responsibility for their own lives—and particularly for those aspects of their lives which *only* their own effort can determine—with the equally serious demand that the community be concerned with the welfare of all its members. Victor Fuchs has pointed out that we have seen the dangers of the "jungle" of excessive individualism but must avoid the "zoo" of a security which is purchased at the expense of individual freedom and responsibility:

> From the idealization of individual responsibility and the neglect of social responsibility we have gone, in some quarters, to the denial of individual responsibility and the idealization of social responsibility. The rejection of any sense of responsibility for one's fellow men is inhuman, but the denial of any individual responsibility is also dehumanizing.[7]

Moreover, this concern is one that Catholics especially cannot disregard; the same Popes who affirmed the right to health care also affirmed—in the very same encyclicals—the importance of individual responsibility and initiative. This concern is embodied in the famous "principle of subsidiarity." According to this principle, "one should not withdraw from individuals and commit to the community what they can accomplish by their own enterprise and industry."[8]

In *Mater et Magistra,* Pope John XXIII points out the trend towards greater complexity and interdependence in modern society.[9] This trend has both good and bad features, he says,[10] and he gives as one of his examples the care of health.[11] The dangers he sees are those features of modern social life which diminish the "opportunity for free action by individuals" and thus violate the principle of subsidiarity.[12]

The challenge, then, is to understand the right to health care in such a way that it is not inconsistent with a recognition of the individual responsibility required for healthy living. Such an understanding will guarantee that the claim to the right to health care will not be a claim to what it is impossible for society to provide. As a consequence, the invocation of the right to health care in discussions of public policy for health care matters will be seen as more than an appeal to a persuasive slogan; it will be seen to provide an illuminating prescription which can settle some—but not all—of these issues and throw light on others.

The Concept of Health

To begin to respond to the challenge I have formulated, it is necessary to consider the object of the right in question. What is it to which we can be said to be entitled by this right? Do we have a right to health—that is, to whatever is necessary *and sufficient* to make us healthy? Or do we have a right to health care—to certain care which may be necessary but is not, by itself, sufficient to guarantee health?

The right to health can be understood negatively as the immunity from having one's health attacked or undermined. This right—like the right to life—needs little justification. A person's human dignity places an obligation on himself and others—taken both individually and corporately—to refrain from those acts which either directly or by neglect undermine his health. This right is absolute and negative—it requires of all people that they not do certain things.

However, if the right to health is understood as a positive right—that is, as a right to be provided with all that is necessary to guarantee health, then the right to health is very problematic as the quotes from Fuchs and Kass suggested. Even if unlimited medical care were available it could not guarantee health. Whatever else health may be, it is a feature of a living organism. Therefore, certain conditions on the part of the organism must obtain if what is provided is to contribute to health; the possibility of accidents cannot be removed, nor can a person's genetic make-up be substantially changed, nor can the deterioration that accompanies aging be stopped.

I will proceed, therefore, on the assumption that the only right to health which people have is the negative right that our health not be destroyed. The positive right in question is the right to health care—the right to be provided with certain necessities for healthy living without the guarantee that providing them will be sufficient to make one healthy.

Starting with this assumption, however, does not eliminate all the difficulties. We need to know how much care we are entitled to and what sort of care it is. To answer these questions we need to know the object of the care in question. We must define "health," and this is a matter of some difficulty and considerable controversy.[13]

The World Health Organization defines health as "a state of complete physical, mental and social well-being and not merely the absence of disease or infirmity."[14]

This very inclusive definition of health is open to many criticisms.[15] The identification of health with complete well-being implies that one will be healthy if and only if one is happy. And it is obvious that, however one conceives of happiness, one can be healthy and unhappy.[16] Furthermore, if one considers happiness or well-being to include the fulfillment of all one's wants and desires, then one will be entitled as part of the right to health care to whatever care he wants. On this conception, abortions, cosmetic surgery, and other medical and quasi-medical treatments will be a matter of right, as will be such things as exercise programs, psychological counseling of various sorts, and so on. Some such activities are thought by many people to be essential to their overall well-being.

Moreover, even if well-being is defined more narrowly than as the fulfillment of desires and wants, the WHO definition has the effect of making all problems health problems. Problems of war and peace, hunger and social justice, clearly affect the overall well-being of people. But although these problems may cause health problems or follow from them, they are not themselves health problems, and their remedies are not, on the face of it, similar to the remedies for health problems. Regarding these problems as health problems, besides stretching the concept of health beyond all recognition, has important social consequences. It is one of the factors leading to the over-medicalization of society about which there has been much concern in recent years.[17] If all problems are regarded as health problems, then we are likely to look for medical solutions in areas where perhaps they are inapplicable or even oppressive.[18]

It seems reasonable, then, to look for a narrower definition of health. In 1970 the House of Delegates of the American Medical Association proposed the following definition: "Health is a state of physical and mental well-being."[19]

This is narrower than the WHO definition in two respects: it omits reference to complete well-being and drops altogether the category of *social* well-being. These restrictions seem to be appropriate but they are not, I believe, sufficient. The main difficulty is with the meaning of "mental well-being." Does one have mental well-being just in case he is happy? An affirmative answer to this question returns us to the difficulties of the WHO definition. A negative response forces two further questions. How are we to define "mental well-being?" And is mental well-being sufficiently like physical well-being that the two can be the components of the same thing? In other words, does the word "health" differ in meaning when used in the phrase "mental health" from when it is used in the phrase "physical health?"

It appears that these questions have not as yet been answered in a definitive way.[20] For this reason, I propose to set aside the question of mental health and deal only with physical health. In doing this, I do not mean to imply that there is no right to mental health which is coordinate with physical health, or even that it cannot be shown that mental health is a part of physical health. I regard these as open questions. It goes without saying, however, that justifying a right to mental health care will be more difficult than justifying a right to physical health care. Questions concerning the responsibility of the mentally ill person are very complex. They arise in understanding of the genesis of the illness and in the treatment of it.

Having set aside the controversial question of the nature of mental health, we might try to understand bodily health along the lines suggested by the AMA—that is, as "physical well-being." This appears promising because health seems to be a bodily state—a qualitative feature of some organisms. But "well-being" is troublesome: it could mean the satisfaction of all bodily wants and desires. Thus to be healthy is to have all one's bodily wants satisfied. But this is at odds with common sense: the hungry person who is not starving is not thereby unhealthy and his having a good meal does not make him healthier. One who is exhausted by a hard day's work needs sleep but is not thereby unhealthy, nor does his night's sleep restore his health.

These difficulties suggest that we should understand physical well-being as the proper functioning of the body—that is, as a state of an organism whereby the organism is disposed to function well.[21] This understanding of health presupposes that it makes sense to think not only of the proper functioning of organs and organ systems but also of the proper functioning of the whole organism. This presupposition is reasonable: an organism's functions are those actions or behaviors which it performs to fulfill its biological potentialities or to achieve its biological goals, for example, individual and species survival.[22] A healthy plant, then, is a plant which can grow, photosynthesize, and reproduce without internal difficulty or hindrance. A healthy animal is one which can get food, ingest it, avoid predators, etc. without being constrained in these activities by the state of its own body. Human health is one kind of animal health. Thus, a human is unhealthy when he cannot perform—or can perform only with difficulty—his bodily functions. Human bodily functions, of course, are not ordered only to survival but also to the performance of those acts whereby man pursues those properly human goals which are often referred to as the object of human rationality: truth, beauty, religion, friendship, peace, and so on. But not every inability to pursue these goals is due to a lack of health; such inabilities constitute a lack of health only if they are rooted in biological malfunction. These "higher" activities, although based on a biological matrix, are not completely explained by it. If someone cannot carry out a research project or say his prayers because of distractions or grief, this person is not unhealthy as he would be if he could not do these things because his brain was not functioning properly, or because he was starving.

This understanding of health has several implications which accord well with common sense. First, health is something which an organism can have in some degree—one can have more or less of it. Second, health as thus understood is not identical with what medical care can produce—a point often made by critics of the health care system. Not every medical procedure contributes to the proper functioning of the organism. For example, most abortions do not contribute to health; likewise, much cosmetic surgery does not contribute to the proper functioning of the organism. Moreover, medical care is only one of the things which lead to health and there is no supposition that by itself medical care should be expected to guarantee health. Medical care can prevent and cure some of the effects of disease and trauma.[23] But there is no presumption that this type of care can substitute for the individual's efforts to make his body function well and to avoid what impairs this functioning. Consequently, some degree of this type of medical care—i.e., that medical care whose goal is the proper functioning of the body—is something which could be claimed as a right without denying the individual's responsibility for his own health.

However, in spite of the attractions of this narrow definition of health, there are objections to it. Bernard Haring, the prominent Catholic moralist, expresses some of these:

> Health cannot be defined from a mere study of the body; we must consider the whole person in his human vocation and final destiny . . . True health is revealed in the self-actualization of the person who has attained that freedom which marshals all available energies for the fulfilment of his total human vocation.
>
> Purely physiological health, viewed as exuberant vitality and freedom from pain, is too narrow and even too dangerous a concept; it would suitably describe the health of animals. This limited definition of health may actually stunt human well-being in its full sense since it reveals and promotes a lamentable imbalance and underdevelopment of man as an embodied spirit.[24]

Haring's argument contains a number of intuitions that are true. There is much more to human life than health. Like any other value, health can be absolutized in a way that demeans other values and prevents the carrying out of other obligations. But Haring's considerations do not require that one give up a narrow, bodily definition of health.

As Haring points out, the definition proposed refers to the health of animals. But what is supposed to follow from this? That this type of health is not valuable? Hardly. When used to refer to *human* health, it refers to what is a component of the basic good of human life. Unless we were *rational* animals we would not perceive the goodness of health, nor would we pursue health by deliberations, choice, and human actions. But we are *rational animals* and thus we recognize bodily health as part of what we are to be. If we are to flourish as human beings we must be healthy in the sense defined, for we are, on the face of it, animals, and not, as Haring thinks, spirits that happen to have bodies. Perhaps Haring supposes that health is merely a means to the more properly human flourishing of men—a flourishing that is spiritual, not physical. But this view is implicitly dualistic—it denies that man is a physical reality. The theoretical difficulties of this position are well known. Moreover, even if bodily health had only a limited instrumental value, it does not follow that one cannot define what it is that has this value.

Haring's remarks suggest another line of argument: the physician does not treat the disease or even the body; rather, he treats the whole person. These statements, however, can be understood in a way consistent with the narrow definition proposed. The physician's interest in disease is a function of his interest in bodily health—a genuine good for man. Since this good is not the only good for man, the physician must respect these other goods. He must respect the aspects of his patient's personality which are not of immediate biological concern. Moreover, since the physician's efforts by themselves are not sufficient to achieve the goal of bodily health, he must engage the patient as a responsible agent in a kind of partnership for promoting this goal—a partnership which must recognize that there is more to human life than health. Locating the goal of health care in proper bodily functioning does not, therefore, devalue health care; it focuses health care and presents a definite goal for the common responsible activity of patient and doctor.

In short, if health care is to be something to which

we can claim the entitlement of a right, it must be narrowly defined. It cannot be whatever we want it to be; it cannot be every procedure which could be called medical. But the health care to which we have a right can be some degree of that medical care which is directed towards proper bodily functioning. Such care is directed towards a basic human value and provides an essential part of what even the most responsible individual needs to maintain his health and cannot provide for himself. To answer the question of how much medical care one has a right to we must consider further the nature and justification of the right in question.

The Right to Health Care

The understanding that someone has a certain right plays an important role in ethics. The claim that someone has a right also plays an important role in political discourse. If one has an unqualified right, that right must be honored; other moral and social considerations are cut short. Deliberation must stop. The right must be honored.[25] However, claims to rights are often in conflict and in recent years the claims to rights have become extravagant.[26] These facts suggest that claims to rights need justification. Such claims are not self-evident[27] nor is the application of these claims in particular situations.

There are a number of ways to justify rights. I will briefly sketch only one of these—a kind of natural law justification.[28]

Human beings recognize that certain basic goods or values are worthy of their allegiance and that the pursuit of these goods constitutes human flourishing. Life and health, friendship and peace, truth and beauty are some of these. We also recognize that these goods are the object not only of individual pursuit but are the goals of our common activity. The obligation placed on us by these goods is not only individual but also common. The community of men—like individuals—ought to pursue and respect these values. The community *respects* these values in much the same way as individuals do. A community should not act against these values as they are realized in the lives of its members and other people and communities, nor should it allow individuals within the community to do so. Thus, we have the foundation of such negative rights as the right to life, the right to religious expression, and so on.

When it comes to the *pursuing* of these values by the community, however, things become more complex. Not all communities need pursue all that is good, and the pursuit of different values in a complex community is undertaken by dividing labor, separating tasks, and thus creating roles. Thus, not everyone in a community pursues the values of the community in the same way. Moreover, this pursuit of values which are common to the entire community by diversification of roles generates positive duties on the part of those who fulfill the various roles and entitlements on the part of others in the community. These roles are founded upon the common commitment of the community to the values which define the roles. This fact implies that the person who carries out a role does so on behalf of the community and for the good of its members insofar as they share in the commitment to the good in question. Thus, the person fulfilling a role has certain duties and members of the community have certain claims upon the benefits achieved through his specialized activities.

This brief and abstract sketch is sufficient to show why there is a right to a degree of health care. The aim of health care is health, which is a perfection of bodily life. As such, it is a component of human life—a basic good for man. Moreover, we live in a complex community which is committed to this value. The medical professions carry out this commitment in a specialized way and should do so for the common good. Thus, there is an obligation that the medical professions provide the results of their specialized activities to the members of the community. Similarly, the members of the community are entitled to a fair measure of these results: they have a right to health care, and especially to that care which—because they do not as individuals have the expertise of the medical professions—they cannot provide for themselves.

On this account, the right to health care is not a tendentious slogan or a mysterious ethical absolute; rather, it arises from the same source as individual obligations—the human good. Our entitlement to health care arises from the common commitment we have to the good of health. It follows that if a responsible moral agent's personal commitment to this good is lacking, his participation in the community of health seekers is, as it were, accordingly diminished, and his claim on the community's resources is to that extent weakened.[29] The need for health care is thus not sufficient by itself to generate the right to health care.[30] For those who are moral agents, a personal commitment to the good of health is also required.

Therefore, a practical policy for implementing the right to health care—National Health Insurance, for example—could justly include penalties or exclusions for those individuals whose illnesses arise primarily because of their own neglect of their health.[31]

These considerations do not immediately indicate how much health care one is entitled to by right.

They do, however, provide a basis for answering this question. One might suppose that the right to health care requires that the best care which is technologically feasible should be provided for all. This supposition is unreasonable. Societies such as our own pursue—and morally should pursue—many goals other than health. Defense, education, cultural enrichment, and aid to poorer societies are only some of these. The right to health care requires that the community's pursuit of health through the specialization of the medical professions be of benefit to each of the members of the community on a fair basis. It does not imply that health is the only important goal for the community or even that it is the most important goal. The ordering of a society's priorities is a matter of social choice which cannot be settled only by an appeal to rights. The community must consider the whole set of obligations by which it is directed and the whole set of values which it can pursue. Like a person it must constitute itself by choice; a people must decide what kind of people it will be.[32] Thus, even if health care should have a higher priority than it now has, this issue cannot be settled by the right to health care. Obviously, it would require such a reordering of priorities if the delivery of the maximal level of health care were considered a right.

It is perhaps more reasonable, therefore, to suppose that a minimally decent level of health care is what the right to health care guarantees.[33] Such a level of health care is certainly required by the right to health care in a society such as ours. But perhaps something more is required as well. If the resources committed to health care allow for more than a minimally decent level for all, then this too should be available to all as a matter of right. In other words, members of a community have a right to *ordinary* health care—that is, to a fair share of what is available to the community at a given time.

With one exception,[34] the basis for a fair distribution of health care resources is medical need—or, more precisely, that level of need compatible with the fulfillment of the similar needs of other persons in the community. There are other possible bases for a fair distribution, but in the case of health care, need is the most reasonable.[35] Other bases—such as merit or wealth—are only accidentally related to the community's goal of helping its members to promote their health. Merit, for example, can be a fair basis for distributing opportunities for higher education. Sophisticated training, however, is not based on an elemental need of the persons who may be given the opportunity. Deprivation of the benefits of such opportunities does not involve the pain, debility, and even the loss of life which may follow from the deprivation of health care.[36]

To sum up: there is a right to health care. This right does not by itself require that the community commit more of its resources to the health sector. Moreover, it does not demand that everything that some people regard as medical care be provided. Only that care which is directed to health is a matter of entitlement. To demand more is to demand what might not be part of the common good of the community and what might even be opposed to this good, or what might render impossible a common agreement about what constitutes this good. Nor does this right absolve individuals from responsibility for their own health; on the contrary, it presupposes this responsibility. What the right to health care *does* require is that the members of a community committed to health be provided on an equal basis with the medical care they need. This conclusion, although limited, has important practical implications, since what the right to health care demands clearly does not obtain in the United States today.[37] Justice thus requires that some community response—possibly but not necessarily National Health Insurance—be made.[38]

Notes

1. Quoted from William J. Curran, "The Right to Health in National and International Law," *The New England Journal of Medicine,* 284 (1971), p. 1258.
2. *Pacem in Terris,* paragraph 11; quoted from the Paulist Press edition, William J. Gibbons, S.J., editor (Glen Rock, N.J.: 1963), p. 8.
3. See *Progressio Populorum,* paragraphs 6, 18, 22-23, 33.
4. See Louis P. Buckley, "Catholic Social Thought Concerning the Right to Health and to Health Care," *Linacre Quarterly,* 37 (1970), pp. 72-83 for a survey of this literature.
5. Sister Virginia Schwager, Sister Mary Maurita Sengelaub, and Msgr. Laurence Corcoran, "Statement on National Health Insurance Before the Committee on Ways and Means" (Washington, D.C.: 1974), pp. 1-2.
6. Leon Kass, "Regarding the End of Medicine and the Pursuit of Health," *The Public Interest,* 40 (1975), p. 39; see also John H. Knowles, "The Responsibility of the Individual," *Daedalus,* 106 (1977), p. 59.
7. Victor R. Fuchs, *Who Shall Live? Health Economics and Social Choice* (New York: 1974), pp. 26-27.
8. *Mater et Magistra,* paragraph 53; here Pope John quotes *Quadragesimo Anno.* My quote is from the NCWC edition (Washington, D.C.: 1961), pp. 17-18.
9. *Ibid.,* paragraphs 59-60.
10. *Ibid.,* paragraphs 61-62.
11. *Ibid.,* paragraphs 60-61.
12. *Ibid.,* paragraph 62.

13. See Daniel Callahan, "Health and Society: Some Ethical Imperatives," *Daedalus,* 106 (1977), pp. 25-26.

14. Cited from Fraser Brockington, *World Health* (Harmondsworth, Baltimore: 1958), p. 19.

15. See Daniel Callahan, "The WHO Definition of Health," *The Hastings Center Studies,* 1 (1973), pp. 77-87 for an extended critique and discussion.

16. See Kass, *op. cit.,* p. 14: "That happiness, even in its full sense is different from *health* can be seen in considering whether it would ever make sense to say, 'Call no man healthy until he is dead'."

17. See Renee C. Fox, "The Medicalization and Demedicalization of American Society," *Daedalus,* 106 (1977), pp. 9-12.

18. The oppressive consequences of treating mental disorders as a kind of illness have been forcefully drawn out by Thomas Szasz; see his *Law, Liberty and Psychiatry* (New York: 1963). Relevant aspects of Szasz's work as well as that of other critics of mental health are surveyed by Peter Sedgwick, "Illness, Mental and Otherwise," *The Hastings Center Studies,* 1 (1973), pp. 19-29.

19. Cited from Paul Ramsey, "The Ethics of a Cottage Industry in an Age of Community and Research Medicine," *The New England Journal of Medicine,* 284 (1971), p. 701.

20. See the works by Szasz and Sedgwick cited above in footnote 18.

21. See Kass, *op. cit.,* pp. 19-29. Kass is indebted to Aristotle. See *Categories* 9a 21-24: "Men are called healthy in virtue of the inborn capacity of easy resistance to those unhealthy influences that may ordinarily arise unhealthy in virtue of a lack of this capacity."

22. Christopher Boorse, "On the Distinction Between Disease and Illness," *Philosophy and Public Affairs,* 5 (1975), pp. 49-62 defends a view like the one expressed here; he calls it "functionalism."

23. In putting the matter this way I hope to avoid a dispute between those who define health as an absence of disease and those who define it as the proper functioning of the organism. Medicine deals directly with cure and prevention of disease insofar as this effort leads to proper bodily functioning. Michael Gelfand, *Philosophy and Ethics of Medicine* (Edinburgh and London: 1968), p. 28, holds that the aim of medicine is "to help to restore the health of a person and to maintain it by preventing it from deteriorating or being attacked by disease." This understanding of the role of medicine is consistent with the definition of health proposed here.

24. Bernard Haring, ed. Gabrielle L. Jean, *Medical Ethics* (Notre Dame: 1973), p. 154.

25. See Charles Fried, "Equality and Rights in Medical Care," *The Hastings Center Report,* 6 (1976), p. 30: "A claim of right invokes entitlements, and when we speak of entitlements, we mean not those things which would be nice for people to have or which they would prefer to have, but which they must have, and which if they do not have, they demand whether we like it or not."

26. Some of the more extravagant of these claims are listed by the editors of *The Hastings Center Report,* 6 (1976), p. 33: the right to a tobacco-free environment, the right to sunshine, and the right to a sex break.

27. See Ruth Macklin, "Moral Concerns and Appeals to Rights and Duties," *The Hastings Center Report,* 5 (1975), pp. 31-38.

28. The approach taken here is based on the development of St. Thomas Aquinas's ethics worked out by Germain Grisez. Grisez's views are readily available in G. Grisez and R. Shaw, *Beyond the New Morality* (Notre Dame: 1974), especially chapters 11, 12, 13; for a contemporary Catholic understanding of rights which comports well with what I say here see Ronald Lawler, O.F.M. Cap. *et al.,* editors, *The Teaching of Christ: A Catholic Catechism for Adults* (Huntington, Indiana: 1976), Chapter 21, "Building a Just and Good Society," pp. 336-354.

29. This sentiment is analogous to that expressed by St. Paul in *2 Thessalonians* 3:10: "We gave a rule when we were with you: not to let anyone have any food if he refused to do any work."

30. But cf. Bernard Williams, "The Idea of Equality," in J. Feinberg, ed., *Moral Concepts* (London, New York: 1969), p. 163.

31. This is not to say that one can easily determine when such accountable neglect obtains: see Robert M. Veatch and Peter Steinfels, "Who Should Pay for Smokers' Medical Care?" *The Hastings Center Report,* 4 (1974), pp. 8-10.

32. There is an analogy here to one of the key theses of Victor Fuchs' important *Who Shall Live? Health Economics and Social Choice;* Fuchs contends that economics alone cannot settle the choices which must be made concerning health care. Neither can appeal to the right to health care.

33. This is proposed by Charles Fried, *op. cit.,* pp. 31-32.

34. It is in the common interest that some persons, for example, the President, be afforded the best possible health care.

35. See Gene Outka, "Social Justice and Equal Access to Health Care," *The Journal of Religious Ethics,* 2 (1974), pp. 11-32.

36. See Williams, *loc. cit.*

37. See Paul Starr, "The Politics of Therapeutic Nihilism," *The Hastings Center Report,* 6 (1976), pp. 27-29.

38. I wish to thank Richard Berquist, Germain Grisez, and James Reid for help in preparing this paper.

104.
Competition: New Moral Dilemmas for Physicians, Hospitals

AN INTERVIEW WITH
EDMUND D. PELLEGRINO

What changes do you foresee in acute and long term care delivery in the United States? How would you describe the American acute care facility of the year 2000?

By 2000 I think that the acute care facility will have become, for all intents and purposes, one large intensive care unit. Almost every patient will have needs comparable to those of patients who are presently in intensive or coronary care units. Persons with severe trauma, complex emergency, elective surgery, and medical emergencies will constitute the patient population. The power of technological medicine will continue to expand and will be applicable to an ever increasing spectrum of patients. That means that patients with less acute medical and surgical illnesses will be in secondary care hospitals. As a result, patients with chronic illness—indeed all long term care patients—will be cared for in facilities specifically designed to meet their particular needs. The acute intensive care hospital and the long term or chronic care facility will become functionally more widely separated than they are now.

Whether these two types of facilities will be under the same administration is an open question. Much will depend on how hospitals meet the challenges of a competitive ethos and fiscal survival. Many hospitals will be forced to redefine their roles. I am not certain whether it will be feasible economically to combine the administration of ambulatory care, long term care, and rehabilitation centers, for example. Competing needs and competing values will surely clash in the care of these different kinds of patients. It will be difficult for one institution to perform all these activities at the level of sophistication the year 2000 will demand.

Reprinted with permission from *Hospital Progress*, February 1983.

What will be the Church's role in those changes? How will the changes affect Catholic hospitals' and long term care facilities' identity?

Increasingly the Church will have to pick up the neglected areas of care: the chronically ill, the aged, the mentally retarded, the poor and the outcast, and those with illnesses not susceptible to tertiary care or not "profitable." All patients need humane and considerate treatment, but patients in these categories will be even more desperately in need of understanding and compassionate care than they are now.

The Church in its health ministry has Christ as its model. It must be concerned with those on the margins of society, or they will not receive care. Christian churches of all denominations must confront this reality. The Catholic Church is already an indispensable source of medical and health care throughout the world. In the future, it will be confronted in our own country with the casualties of our new competitive ethos.

Our government is defecting on its responsibilities to those who can't make their own way. Who will care for the poor? If that is not a unique responsibility of Christians, then it is difficult to comprehend what Christian charity means in practice. These problems will be accentuated if a procompetition bill is ever passed. Competition displaces the focus from care to profit and dominating the market. While such bills are seductive in a time of rising costs and overutilization, they are inconsistent with the care of all who are ill.

The new emphasis on reducing costs may force Christians to define consciously their responsibilities to those who are ill. The challenge to the Church is to manifest its Christian concern, to fill in the gaps, until we develop some realignment of responsibilities among the private, local, and federal sectors. A society that does not provide some adequate baseline of medical care can hardly call itself enlightened. To define that baseline is a matter of public policy, not the purview of each medical provider. Catholic hospitals will have to be more vigorously supported by Catholics if they are to provide care with a minimum of economic, social, or bureaucratic pressure. We all share this responsibility to reduce the mounting economic pressure to deprive patients of needed care—and this means sacrifices on our part as Christians.

Who is responsible for paying for health care? What is the physician's role in resolving the dilemma?

Payment, as I just pointed out, is a shared responsibility of all of us—neither a totally government-supported nor a free market program is adequate or ethically defensible. The physician's first responsibility is to be a vigorous advocate for proper care for all who are ill. The most important thing physicians can do in cost containment is to practice rational diagnostics and therapeutics. That means careful, critical workups—not a "saturation-bombing" with every diagnostic modality available. Physicians should be therapeutically parsimonious, using only those treatments known to change effectively the natural course of the disease or demonstrably ease pain and discomfort. Physicians should not become agents of fiscal or social policy deciding who is more deserving of care, or who should be given full treatment except on grounds of medical indication and patient choice. The physician's first responsibility must be to the patient.

Who should make decisions about who gets care?

I don't think we are really at the point where we have to deprive people of medical care for economic reasons. Look, for example, at our expenditures for such things as alcohol, gambling, illicit drugs, handguns, tobacco, sports, and recreation. If we are finally forced to "life raft" ethics, the decisions should be made in the realm of public policy. As a nation, we would have to decide not to make available certain kinds of technology, for example, renal dialysis, artificial hearts, or care for certain categories of patients. The physicians should not make such decisions on an individual basis. Otherwise, we face the danger of some people being classed as more valuable than others, and this leads us to making decisions about the "worth" of individual human beings. The dangers of leaving such decisions to any group, physicians included, are historically all too obvious. The physician's duty is to advocate effective medically indicated care of all patients who desire it. The physician must also take part in broader public policy decisions if they have to be made—on a category-by-category basis.

How should Catholics support health care?

Catholic hospitals are the responsibility of the Catholic community. As a community we must decide what our priorities as Christians will be. In comparison with some other denominations, we support our hospitals rather poorly as a whole. We must decide where care of the sick fits among our Christian obligations when compared with other needs like welfare, housing, and caring for the homeless or others in our society who need care, comfort, and compassion. Can a society be called Christian if it neglects those in need? Can we defend, as Christians, ignoring the call to sacrifice some of our pleasures for the sake of others? At the moment we seem to be drifting toward selfishness and indifference to a two-class society of haves and have-nots. How consistent is this with Christian teaching? . . .

What is your view of physicians' moving toward the entrepreneurial role? How does this affect hospitals and individual patients?

Physicians are being forced into an entrepreneurial role by the procompetition, price-is-the-bottom-line rules of the marketplace now being voiced as a national policy. A physician who becomes an entrepreneur is seeking self-interest, not the patient's interest. When a physician becomes the owner of a nursing home, or an investor in the health care industry, his judgment about what is "necessary," and who should do it, is bound to be clouded. How can the physician separate personal interest from the interest of the patient when fiscal advantage, not service, is the primary motive? Physicians shouldn't be putting their energies into marketing, pricing, and competing. They should be concentrating on the care of sick people. Our society is already overmedicalized; too many procedures are done and too many drugs given—"competition" will foster more overutilization for those who can pay and corner cutting for those who cannot.

Undoubtedly, utilization of hospitals, tests, and procedures is excessive. But I fear that a system that rewards physicians who treat large volumes of patients at a low "unit" cost per patient may encourage underutilization and cutting of corners. In the long run, if an illness goes undiagnosed or without effective treatment, it is more costly than proper diagnosis. Ironically, some of the more blatant examples of overutilization occur in localities where entrepreneurship is most evident.

Do you believe, then, that quality of care could suffer in a competitive environment?

Yes, if the rising prices and deteriorating quality of many goods and services in other so-called competitive markets are any indication. Shoddy workmanship, deceptive advertising, and creating markets for autos, clothes, and household goods are omnipresent. This is merely dishonest and costly. In medical care it is tragic. Fortunately, most of American medicine still holds to traditional ideals of service, and medical care has not deteriorated. Under competition, the consumer would choose between providers, presumably after "shopping around" for the best coverage at the lowest price. But how will consumers distinguish between a confusing variety of plans with different options? Who will advise them? Can they trust providers, whose interest must be profit? Trust between patient and care provider is an essential ingredient in healing.

What will be the consequences if consumers choose inadequate health plans?

Physicians and hospitals will face terrible moral dilemmas. If most hospitals become proprietary and physicians must make an annual profit, how do they help those who opted for the wrong plan, or no plan, or used up their "vouchers"? Those at the margins of society, who usually need more care and are the most likely to put off expenditures for a future illness, will bear the brunt of the questionable techniques of cost cutting. They are more vulnerable to the "bonus" of leaving the hospital soon or not going to the hospital at all.

Competition advocates insist that the poor will not suffer under a competitive model. Do you agree?

No. Most of the proposals specify legislation to prevent plans from selecting the profitable, low-risk, affluent patient, against the poor, aged, or chronically ill. Here we see the paradox, the "free" market must be "regulated," too, it seems, or the poor will suffer. Health care is simply not like other commodities, but this lesson has to be learned over and over again. I predict, as a consequence of the abuses competition will foster, that public reaction will in a few years call for much stricter governmental regulations than we've ever had. Then we will err on the other side of a totally bureaucratic medicine. Physicians, especially those in primary and family practice, are on the firing line. They are already seeing the victims of procompetition long before the rear-line planners have grasped the fact. They have an obligation to sound the warning signal. . . .

What area of the trustee's relationship to the hospital needs improvement? Is conflict of interest a problem?

Conflict of interest, especially as competition increases, is going to be a greater problem. Trustees have a responsibility not only for the fiscal and legal but also for the ethical practices in their institution because they, too, make a promise, enter a covenant, with society. They hold the hospital "in trust" for the community the hospital purports to serve. The law recognizes the responsibilities of trustees for a wide range of hospital functions. Certainly ethics, which should be more finely tuned to right and good human behavior than law, must recognize trustees' moral responsibility. This is a dimension of trusteeship that demands much greater attention than it has received.

The average age in many religious congregations is nearly 60. Do you envision lay sponsorship as an alternative to congregational sponsorship of Catholic hospitals?

The Church has a serious obligation to continue the Catholic hospital's unique mission in our pluralistic society: providing care based on a clear set of spiritual and moral values and ministering to the least fortunate as Christ did. Laypeople are no less bound by the apostolate of Christian service than religious. The laity are fully capable of operating Catholic hospitals, if necessity demands. Mechanisms and criteria will need to be established whereby authentically Catholic hospitals can be run under lay auspices. The presence of religious in Catholic hospitals offers invaluable comfort to patients and visible witness to the hospitals' Catholic identity. It would be a great loss if their presence were no longer a reality. Whether or not they sponsor hospitals, religious congregations should seek ways to maintain religious participation in hospital life at all levels, from administrative boards to pastoral care departments.

105.
Sanctity and Scarcity: The Makings of Tragedy

ALLEN VERHEY

Crisis is common to medicine. Coping with tragedy comes with the territory. But crises and tragedies come in different forms. The kind of crisis routinely handled by medicine is the medical emergency, but the crisis confronting medicine today is more financial than medical. The form of tragedy familiar to medicine is "the sad story," for people can tell very sad stories indeed of or with their bodies. But the form of tragedy facing medicine in its financial crisis was familiar to Sophocles as a story in which "goods collide and evils gather."

As Sophocles knew, the really important issues in such cases are the issues of identity, of character, and of virtue, and it is not too much to claim that the financial crisis of medicine is an identity crisis for medicine. Medicine needs to address questions of public policy, doubtless, but no public policy "solution" will substitute for professional integrity. Authentic tragedies, after all, do not admit of being remedied—by public policy or by anything else human. They can, however, be endured by strength of character, by virtue. Our children may yet have a legacy of medical care in which they may take human delight as well as technological pride.

Medicine has always been best equipped to respond to the medical crisis. A fascinating and terrifying collection of technologies is quickly and skillfully brought to bear in such a crisis. Pumps make strange soft sounds. Other machines command our attention with little bleeping noises, while the blinking lights of still others demand our concentration. Even those like me who are uninitiated in such mysteries and cannot decipher any meaning in the sounds and lights find it hard to turn from them or to look past them. When we do, of course, we encounter not just technology but tragedy, the sad stories people tell of their bodies. The machines both point us toward tragedy and hide it from us. But anyone with eyes to see will finally see tragedy beyond the blinking lights; anyone with ears to hear will finally hear its sighs above the bleeping sounds.

The appropriate human and Christian response to this sort of tragedy has always been sympathy and care. All human beings, after all, even (or especially) those in crisis, those whose stories are sad stories, are the objects of God's unbounded love. Thus, as Gandhi said, "in that which is most basic, . . . the value of each life, we are all equal." That is all—but all of that—that I mean by "sanctity."

Some human beings have made it their business—no, more than their business, their *profession,* their avowed and public identity—to respond to such sad stories, to the stories of massive heart attacks and tumors growing slowly but surely or to the medical emergencies in the narratives of disaster and catastrophe, with the sympathy and care appropriate to a person's "sanctity." For centuries such sympathy and care were almost helpless in the face of tragedy. Medicine's duty was to care when there was no cure, when patients were "overmastered by their diseases." Everyone acknowledged the tragedy, but they also acknowledged that nothing could be done in the crisis.

Since Francis Bacon, who first insisted that to call any disease incurable "gives a legal sanction as it were to neglect and inattention, and exempts ignorance from discredit," medical science and technology have gradually developed to the point that we are not quite so helpless and hopeless in the medical emergency. Medicine has learned to care, if not more intensely, then at least more effectually. Moved by compassion for those who suffer, prompted by a sense of the sanctity of the life in crisis, medicine has learned to intervene in some sad stories of human suffering and premature dying, so that—sometimes at least—the sad story has a happy ending after all.

The very success of medicine, however, has led to another form of crisis and reminded it of another form of tragedy. The new crisis is not medical but financial: we simply do not have the resources to do all we can do and all we want to do for all patients. That is what I mean by "scarcity." It is "scarcity" which makes allocation necessary; if we do not have the resources to do all we can do and want to do for all patients, then we must limit what we will do for at least some patients.

I need hardly pause to demonstrate "scarcity." The United States now spends more than 10 percent of its gross national product on health care. Perhaps we can and will spend still more, but there is a limit. We value other things as well as health—education, other human services for the indigent and the elderly, the environment. There is a limit, and establishing that limit and then enforcing it will require decisions about allocation, about rationing the goods and services that we can provide. Public policy will decide what public resources will be allocated to health care and

From *The Reformed Journal* 35 (February 1985): 10-14. Used by permission.

what to other social goods, and public policy will also decide what resources within health care funds will be allocated to medical research, to preventive medicine, to crisis medicine, etc. And these decisions will necessitate other decisions, decisions within medical care about who will receive the scarce vaccine, the scarce artificial heart, the scarce bed.

If it is "scarcity" which makes allocation decisions necessary, it is "sanctity" which makes them tragic. For when the goods or services to be allocated are goods or services on which life or health may depend and when the unbounded love of God for each one requires that we regard each life as of equal value, then the necessary allocation decision is necessarily tragic.

The notion of tragedy here is not just the "sad story," but the Sophoclean sort in which goods collide and evils gather. Because goods collide, to choose one good is to choose against another good, and, of course, we should never choose against the good. Because evils gather, they cannot all be avoided, but, of course, we should never choose the evil. The financial crisis of medicine requires tragic choices of this sort, and medicine must learn to live with and to cope with this sort of tragedy as well.

Medicine is not unacquainted with tragedy of the Sophoclean sort, however, and its own experience may provide valuable lessons for enduring its financial crisis. Not all the sad stories of medical crises, after all, have happy endings. Sometimes medicine's interventions preserve a patient's life, but it is a life either full of pain or empty of a capacity for human relationships. The tragic consequences of medical choices frequently require choosing one good over another, rejecting one evil while accepting another.

Two lessons emerge from such tragic choices that are relevant to allocation decisions. The first thing we learn is that tragic choices are always a consequence of our finitude, of the fact that we are not gods, that our mortality is indefeasible, and that our resources, while considerable, are still finite. The point of this is obvious: medicine and medical technology do not and cannot provide an escape either from our mortality or from the finitude of our resources. Medicine does not and cannot eliminate tragedy of the Sophoclean sort.

This is obvious, I say, but we have not been disposed to acknowledge the obvious. Perhaps our enthusiasm for medicine and medical technology as a response to the sad story has blinded us to its limits. Perhaps because medicine reminds us so vividly of tragedy, we have used it ironically and self-deceptively to hide and deny tragedy and the limits imposed by our mortality and the finitude of our resources. We have been disposed to fight against our own mortality—but some, and finally all, of us *are* "overmastered by our diseases," in spite of Bacon. We have been disposed to promise "everything for everyone" when it comes to allocation—but our limited resources forbid our fulfilling that promise. Doctors and nurses may not deny the tragic truth about our world or the tragic limits of medicine either to their patients or to themselves.

The truthfulness necessary to acknowledge tragedy and the humility necessary to cope with it can be sustained by piety, for piety knows it is God, not medicine, who brings a new age. For all its benefits, medicine has yet to deliver us, and will not deliver us, from our finitude and to our flourishing. The final victory over disease and death, pain and tears, is a divine victory, not a technological one. Such truthfulness and humility, nurtured by piety, might make it possible to lower the expectations and demands laid against medicine and to sustain a medical character identified less with the technological wizard than with the professional covenanted to care in the midst of tragedy, to care even when she cannot—or may not—cure.

If the first thing we learned from tragic choices in the care of dying patients is that we cannot successfully and may not truthfully deny our finitude, the second thing we learn is that the choice to use medical technology—or the refusal to use it even when we can—can be irremediably ambiguous. To claim to "solve" these problems, to arrive at some unambiguously "right" answer, makes one a comic character in the midst of tragedy, demonstrating either that one does not understand the limits of medicine (not to mention the limits of philosophy and theology) or that one lacks an appropriately awful sense of sanctity. When medical technology is being used to sustain a life, but a life either full of pain or empty of a capacity for human relationships, it may be morally appropriate to withdraw the medical technology—but it is not simply "good." A person should not choose either death or a lingering dying for someone else—but choose one must. The choice is not right or wrong, but right *and* wrong; not good or bad, but good *and* bad. The choice is tragic and irremediably ambiguous.

Goods, genuine goods, come into conflict, genuine conflict. Evils gather and cannot all be avoided. The ambiguity is hard, but it can be endured. It becomes destructive only when we refuse to recognize our choices for what they are, when, for example, we call death a "good," or when we refuse to acknowledge each other and ourselves for what we are: loved by God. In what is most basic, life itself, we are all equal, but finite and mortal, tragic figures in need finally of

God's grace and God's future. Piety can help sustain such truthfulness and nurture the confidence in God's final triumph and forgiveness necessary to endure it and to make the necessary even though ambiguous choices.

The financial crisis now confronts medicine with such tragic choices in its allocation decisions. Allocation decisions, of course, are not new in medicine. What nurse has not experienced the finitude of her own resources for helping? Who will receive care when a dying patient needs someone to talk to, when a patient with a heart condition needs constant monitoring, and too many others need more care than can be provided? What doctor has not put off one patient for the sake of another? What hospital administrator has not faced hard and tragic choices constrained because funds to purchase equipment and to operate medical units are finite? The financial crisis has only made such choices more public, more frequent, and more urgent. Medicine's response to its financial crisis, if what it has learned from the care of dying patients is true, will not be a response that denies or avoids moral ambiguity. Many proffered responses, however, attempt to do exactly that.

In allocation decisions there are two strategies for denying tragedy: one is to deny sanctity; the other is to deny scarcity. Both strategies are illustrated in the response to the crisis of kidney dialysis. In 1961 a committee at the Seattle Artificial Kidney Center was formed to select those patients who would receive treatment when not all could. It allocated the scarce medical treatment to those whom it considered the most deserving; it denied sanctity, denied the equal value of each of the lives of the medically acceptable candidates. Most of the criticism of this committee focused on the denial of what we called "sanctity." Paul Freund, for example, argued that "in a matter of choosing for life or death, not involving specific wrongdoing, no one should assume the responsibility of judging *comparative* worthiness to live on the basis of unfocused criteria of virtue and social worthiness." Such a strategy was and remains morally unacceptable.

The next strategy was to deny *scarcity,* to provide almost universal funding for kidney dialysis, in order to acknowledge and affirm sanctity. The strategy was, of course, self-deceptive, for a policy which promises kidney dialysis for everyone distinguishes those dying from renal failure from those dying from other diseases. There are limits, and the tragedy of the necessary allocation decisions cannot be hidden or denied for long.

In any context of scarce resources, of course, the notion of distributive justice is applicable, and decisions which violate that principle are not only tragic but wrong. To provide ordinary health care to the wealthy because they can pay or to the nice because we like them or to the promising because of their social utility while we withhold it from the poor, the outcast, and the handicapped is not only tragic but unjust. Just what justice requires in the distribution of health care is, of course, a much debated and very debatable topic. Without attempting to enter fully into that discussion, let me simply propose Charles Fried's conclusion that justice requires that all citizens be entitled to "a decent minimum of health care," without supplying his argument or spelling out what "a decent minimum" might be. This seems to be the position recommended for future public policy by the president's commission in its report "Securing Access to Health Care." The authors of the report retreated from the "equal access—equal care" goal of the last twenty years. They recognized scarcity, that there simply are not the resources to do all we can do and would like to do for all patients. They accepted—because in recognizing scarcity, they had to accept—the notion of "two-track care."

My point is not that this is wrong. Public policy must deal with scarcity and in dealing with scarcity the claims of justice are properly adamant. My point is that such a policy does not "solve" or remove tragedy. Physicians and nurses commit themselves to provide not a decent minimum of health care to their patients, but to offer their *best* efforts with their *best* tools. To provide the best care for all is impossible; there are limits to our resources. To provide "a decent minimum" for all patients may be possible, and it is required by justice. But not to provide the best care for any patient is not, therefore, "good." It remains tragic.

Some health planners have urged a policy of cost containment that decides whether to create a new technology or to keep an existing one available based on its cost-effectiveness. Preventive medicine is ordinarily favored above critical care on this basis because it is generally cheaper and results in better health for more people. There is some wisdom here—and some folly. But it does not solve the tragedy. Physicians and nurses are not committed to the health of some distant patient, some statistical patient, or society as a patient; they are committed to the life and the flourishing of the patient on the table or in the bed in front of them. And society signals its compassion by allocating resources to those in the midst of suffering, not those who are prospective sufferers. To provide the best care for all is impossible; there *are* limits to our resources. To be concerned about cost-effectiveness is a legitimate concern. But not to provide a costly but genuine therapy is not therefore "good." It remains tragic.

The constraints of justice and cost containment are just that for medicine: they are constraints, not virtues. Public policy based on such considerations will set the limits within which medicine can act with integrity. But medicine must act with integrity within those constraints. That is important to say, for the financial crisis in medicine has created an identity crisis. Rival and alien definitions are being used to understand medicine and to shape its response to the financial crisis. The rational and impartial perspectives of justice and utility are legitimate, but they threaten to alienate medicine from itself, from its own moral interests and loyalties, from the projects and passions which give it moral character. How medicine deals with its financial crisis will determine the character of our children's medicine. Medicine must reassert an identity of care in the midst of tragedy, of care even when it cannot—or may not—cure. The definition of medicine must continue to center on caring, intensive caring, for the patient in crisis, but it will have to acknowledge truthfully that its story is a tragic story. Medicine will have to make allocation decisions, and how it makes those decisions will express its sense of itself, its values, integrity, and character. The questions answered by allocation decisions are: "What is medicine?" and "What shall it become?"

In this crisis some are suggesting that medicine be defined by that quintessentially American story of the marketplace, where you get rich by supplying what the buyer wants. Then medicine is simply a commodity, that collection of skills to get what we want, a value-free enterprise which may be bought and sold to satisfy consumer desires, hired to do the autonomous bidding of the one who pays. But we are all uncomfortable with the marketplace definition of medicine, for such medicine cannot and will not sustain the dispositions of care and trust which have sometimes defined the characters of doctor and patient. Marketplace medicine will become a medicine in the service of the rich and powerful, while the poor and weak watch and pray.

If medicine is true to itself as a profession prompted by and practiced in care for those in tragedy, born and nurtured by its sense of the sanctity of the life in crisis, then it cannot and will not regard the marketplace definition as its definition. Piety provides a resource to support this fragile identity, for it acknowledges that we are enlisted on the side of life and health in a world where death and evil still apparently reign, and it owns a story, told elegantly by the physician Luke, of good news to the poor, to the sick, to the despised.

In response to the financial crisis and in rejecting a pure market allocation of medical resources, medicine may honor and applaud proposals for guaranteeing access to "a decent minimum" and for assessing cost-effectiveness. But medicine may not identify with the impartial perspective which prompts these proposals. Medicine should not allow itself to become an agent of public or economic policy, even good public or economic policy. It must preserve its own identity, its own integrity, even when that requires acknowledging the moral ambiguity of abiding by the constraints public policy and an impartial perspective may impose.

I suggest that it is not only medical integrity which is at stake but the success of the public policies as well. A lively sense of medicine's professional identity and its awful sense of the sanctity of all lives in crisis may keep a two-track medical delivery system from becoming a two-class system. At least such a medicine will constantly remind the rest of us not only of scarcity but also of sanctity, of the tragedy and the moral ambiguity of allocation decisions where life and health are at stake.

A lively sense of medicine's professional identity may also preserve us from a society where cost-effectiveness is the only relevant consideration, from the sort of society prepared to stand impassively by in the face of medical crises because it is disposed to let present victims die for the sake of future possibilities. At least such a medicine will force the rest of us to ask whether a society which can ignore a cry for help even as it "maximizes protection" is the sort of society we want to be or to become.

Medicine must be true to itself—for its own sake and for ours. The financial crisis may be an opportunity for medicine to reassert its identity, not as a Promethean character denying the limits of our resources and of our mortality, not as a way of overcoming tragedy, but as a way to signal care for one another in the midst of tragedy.

Such a medicine will nurture and sustain certain virtues. One virtue is sensitivity to economic factors. The physician and the nurse, with integrity to their loyalty to the patient, can make contributions to the careful use of resources. They can have—and should have—a "cost conscience." They can cultivate diagnostic and therapeutic "elegance," not accepting the technologic that "if we can, we must," avoiding the shotgun workups and roulette therapies. These produce excessive costs and are indefensible both economically and clinically. A physician and a nurse with a "cost-conscience" will not give in to the patient's every whim as little more than hired hands on the marketplace model. That is poor—and costly—medicine. These are not tragic choices. These are choices coherent with the definition of medicine as a profession committed to the care of the patient. But these are not final solutions to the problem of scarce resources either; they will not finally eliminate the necessity of tragic choices.

We cannot eliminate tragedy when scarcity and sanctity meet, but we must not deny it either. A second virtue is truthfulness; doctors and nurses and hospital administrators should not deny the truth about our world, about the limits imposed by our mortality or the finitude of our resources, either to their patients or to themselves.

Joined to truthfulness is humility, the acknowledgment that we are not gods, but the creatures of God, finite and mortal creatures, human beings loved and cherished by God, so that in what is most basic, we are all equal.

Truthfulness and humility can sustain another virtue—care. Without them, without acknowledging limits, without an appropriate sense of the tragic, the capacity and responsibility to care (and to care intensively) may not be sustainable. And intensive care in response to crisis, it will be recalled, is what inspired and prompted medicine in the first place.

Let me add, finally, piety to this catalogue of virtues. There is nothing alien about piety to medicine. After all, the oath was sworn by Apollo, Asclepius, Panaceia, Hygeia, and all the gods and goddesses. The story of medicine has its beginnings among the gods and it will end with the story of a new heaven and a new earth when death and disease and pain will be no more. While we wait and watch for that day, piety can nurture and sustain truthfulness about our finitude, gratitude for the opportunities within our limitations, respect and care for the sanctity of each human life, and a sense of God's forgiveness in the midst of moral ambiguity.

Such a medicine will allocate the resources provided and limited by public policy in a way determined by its character, its identity, its virtue. That way, I suggest, will not rely on the marketplace to make the allocation decision and will not deny sanctity by using the criteria of social worth or potential social benefit. It will rely instead first on medical criteria and medical judgment. Techniques and procedures will be used only on persons who may and probably will benefit from them. But medical criteria may only define the candidates for medical procedures or techniques. The final allocation decision should be based on *random* selection. When scarcity makes allocation necessary, sanctity requires random selection and forbids godlike judgments that one life is worth more than another. Random selection alone will nurture medicine's capacity to care even when it may not cure. Random selection alone will sustain a relationship of truthfulness and trust between physician and patient. Random selection alone will encourage us to find less costly ways of responding to those threats to human life which menace those about whom we care intensively but may not cure.

When goods collide and evils gather, we may not deny scarcity, we may not deny sanctity; the best we can do is to act with integrity. The financial crisis is an identity crisis, and the allocation decisions it forces are decisions about the character and virtues of medicine. May medicine be true to the integrity of its character, to care when it cannot or may not cure.